OXFORD MEDICAL PUBLICATIONS

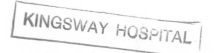

BRAIN'S
DISEASES OF THE
NERVOUS SYSTEM

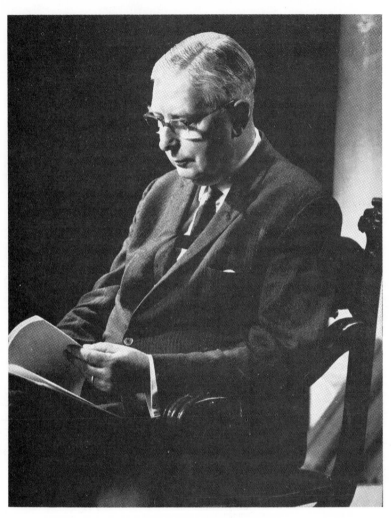

LORD BRAIN OF EYNSHAM
1895–1966

BRAIN'S
DISEASES OF THE
NERVOUS SYSTEM

EIGHTH EDITION

REVISED BY

JOHN N. WALTON

T.D., DR. DE L'UNIV. (Hon., Aix-Marseille)

M.D., D.SC., F.R.C.P.

Professor of Neurology and Dean of Medicine,
University of Newcastle upon Tyne
Consultant Neurologist,
Newcastle Area Hospitals

OXFORD
OXFORD UNIVERSITY PRESS
NEW YORK   TORONTO
1977

Oxford University Press, Walton Street, Oxford OX2 6DP

OXFORD LONDON GLASGOW NEW YORK
TORONTO MELBOURNE WELLINGTON CAPE TOWN
IBADAN NAIROBI DAR ES SALAAM LUSAKA ADDIS ABABA
KUALA LUMPUR SINGAPORE JAKARTA HONG KONG TOKYO
DELHI BOMBAY CALCUTTA MADRAS KARACHI

First edition 1933
Eighth edition 1977

British Library Cataloguing in Publication Data

Brain, Walter Russell, *Baron Brain*
  Brain's diseases of the nervous system—8th ed.—(Oxford medical publications)
  1. Nervous system—Diseases
  I. Walton, John Nicholas II. Diseases of the nervous system
  III. Series
  616.8   RC346
  ISBN 0 19 261309 X

Printed in Great Britain
at the University Press, Oxford
by Vivian Ridler
Printer to the University

CONTENTS

PREFACE TO THE EIGHTH EDITION

IN my preface to the Seventh Edition, I noted that before Lord Brain's untimely death in 1966, he had revised about one-third of *Diseases of the Nervous System* in preparation for that new edition. In accepting the honour which his executors and publishers did me by inviting me to complete the preparation of that edition and in assuming the authorship of subsequent versions, I remarked that that edition was inevitably something of a hybrid as I felt in duty bound to leave untouched those sections which Lord Brain had revised before his death. These included most of the previous Chapters 1, 2, and 4, much of Chapter 17, several sections of Chapters 3 and 23, and other isolated sections of the book. For that edition, however, I added an introductory commentary on general principles, based largely upon the opening chapter of my own *Essentials of Neurology* (Pitman Medical Publishing Company Ltd.) but including also some comments upon the structure, function, and pathology of the neurone and of the glia. The chapter on disorders of muscle was completely rewritten, drawing widely upon that written with Dr. D. Gardner-Medwin in the Second Edition of *Disorders of Voluntary Muscle* (Churchill Livingstone Ltd.) and many other chapters, notably numbers 3, 6, 10, 11, 13, 18, and 22, were extensively revised. Many new illustrations and references to the neurological literature were also added.

The previous editions of this book will stand as a permanent monument to Lord Brain's clinical expertise, to his thoughtful approach to neurological medicine, and to his outstanding literary skills. In preparing this Eighth Edition I have felt it right to maintain the traditional structure of the volume so carefully conceived by Lord Brain over many years. It was difficult to decide whether or not to remove, for instance, many of those disorders due to inborn errors of metabolism whose biochemical basis has been elucidated recently, from the chapter on congenital and degenerative disorders, or to transfer tetanus from the chapter on intoxications and metabolic disorders into a new section on bacterial infections, to quote but two examples. In the end I decided to leave the original arrangement unchanged, believing that with a comprehensive Table of Contents and Index, the reader will readily find the topics he is seeking, even if some seem illogically placed.

So much new knowledge has emerged in the field of neurology since the last edition was published in 1969 that this revision has been a massive task. Every chapter has been extensively modified, many have been totally rewritten, and there have been substantial additions to virtually every section of the volume, with many up-to-date references being provided. Although some outdated and redundant material has been deleted, the book is inevitably much longer than the last edition, a consequence which could not be avoided if it were to remain a comprehensive reference text. Virtually all of the illustrations of radiographs and the clinical photographs, and many of the histological sections, have been replaced, as many of the blocks of the illustrations used in previous editions were no longer serviceable. Some readers will miss the old familiar pictures, but I hope that those which have replaced them and the many new ones which have been included (illustrating, for example, new methods of radiological examination including computerized transaxial tomography, and electrophysiological methods of investigation) are as clear or even clearer than those which have been supplanted.

In the Seventh Edition, new illustrations were included by kind permission of Dr. D. Denny-Brown and the Liverpool University Press, Dr. C. S. Hallpike and the editors and publishers of *Proceedings of the Royal Society of Medicine*, Professor W. Blackwood and E. & S. Livingstone Ltd., publishers of *Atlas of Neuropathology*, Dr. J. R. Smythies and Blackwell Scientific Publications Ltd., publishers of *The Neurological Foundations of Psychiatry*, and Dr. P. Hudgson and the editors and publishers of *Neurology (Minneapolis)*. Others were kindly supplied by Dr. G. L. Gryspeerdt and Dr. G. W. Pearce, and I provided some of my own, prepared in the Photography and Teaching Aids Laboratory of the University of Newcastle upon Tyne. These photographs and diagrams have all been retained. However, I am also deeply indebted to Dr. Arnold Appleby who has supplied a large number of new radiographs, Dr. James Ambrose for the illustrations of the EMI scan, Professor B. E. Tomlinson for many new neuro-pathological illustrations both macroscopic and microscopic, Dr. R. Madrid for electron micrographs of peripheral nerve, Dr. J. D. Spillane who not only provided me with a series of new clinical photographs from his own extensive collection but also allowed me to reproduce several from his Second Edition of *An Atlas of Clinical Neurology* (Oxford University Press), Professor A. Brodal who agreed to the reproduction of one illustration from *Neurological Anatomy in Relation to Clinical Medicine* (Oxford University Press), Dr. D. D. Barwick and Dr. R. Weiser who provided reproductions of electro-encephalographic and electromyographic recordings (one previously published in *Essentials of Neurology*, Pitman Medical), Professor W. G. Bradley who allowed me to reproduce electrophysiological and histological illustrations previously published in his book *Disorders of Peripheral Nerves* (Blackwell Scientific Publications Ltd.), Dr. J. C. Brown who provided new illustrations and Dr. R. J. Johns and the Editor of the *Bulletin of the Johns Hopkins Hospital* who agreed to the reproduction of one diagram. I have also drawn extensively on material published elsewhere, as acknowledged in the reference lists, and especially upon *Child Neurology* by J. L. Menkes (Lea and Febiger, Inc.). To all of these authors and publishers I express my sincere thanks, as I do also to Dr. James Bull, Dr. D. Gardner-Medwin, Professor L. P. Garrod, Professor A. J. McComas, Professor F. W. O'Grady, and Dr. J. B. Selkon, all of whom gave help with the last or with this edition in many different ways.

The preparation of this volume would never have been possible but for the efficient and tireless help of my secretary Miss Rosemary Allan who typed many hundreds of pages of inserts and corrections and was a tower of strength in the arduous revision of the index. To Dr. J. C. Gregory, and the staff of the Oxford University Press, I must express my thanks for their patience, understanding, and tolerance during the gestation period. I can but hope that I have done justice to some at least of what Lord Brain's aims and intentions for this edition would have been.

JOHN N. WALTON

Newcastle upon Tyne
February 1977

PREFACE TO THE FIRST EDITION

THE last twenty years have witnessed a remarkable development in neurology. Investigation of the effects of war injuries of the spinal cord has greatly increased our knowledge of reflex action in man. The appearance of encephalitis lethargica and the multiplication of forms of acute disseminated encephalitis have added a new field to clinical neurology and brought it into relationship with the new branch of bacteriology which studies the filterable viruses. The discovery of important metabolic centres in the hypothalamus has enhanced the importance of neurology to general medicine. Advances in the technique of neurological surgery have aroused fresh interest in the symptoms and in the pathology of intracranial tumours. Other developments, scarcely less important, have occurred.

Much of this new knowledge is physiological, and in one respect I have departed from the traditional arrangement of a textbook of nervous diseases. Neurology is more dependent than many other branches of medicine upon anatomy and physiology. These subjects, the essential basis of neurological diagnosis, are usually dismissed in a few introductory pages, with the result that much clinical neurology is apt to be both unintelligible and uninteresting to the student. In the first part of this book, as an introduction to the subject, I have discussed—at greater length than usual—the application of anatomy and physiology to the interpretation of the physical signs of nervous disease. Elsewhere will be found sections dealing with anatomy and physiology as introductions to clinical sections. In planning the clinical sections I have used what seemed the most practical, if not always the most logical, arrangement, for there is no entirely satisfactory way of arranging subjects, many of which might be placed in more than one group.

Limitations of space restrict the number of references which it is possible to quote. I have, therefore, chosen only those of special interest and those which form the best introduction to a subject, or are themselves useful sources of references. To the many other writers upon whose work I have freely drawn I express my indebtedness. I am indebted also to a number of my colleagues for the loan of illustrations.

Finally, I welcome this opportunity of expressing my gratitude to my colleagues at the London Hospital for their teaching, encouragement, and help, especially to Dr. Charles Miller, Professor Arthur Ellis, and Dr. George Riddoch, under whom I had the privilege of working on the Medical Unit, and to Mr. Hugh Cairns, Dr. Dorothy Russell, and Dr. S. Phillips Bedson.

W. RUSSELL BRAIN

London
June 1933

1

DISORDERS OF FUNCTION IN THE LIGHT OF ANATOMY AND PHYSIOLOGY

SOME GENERAL CONSIDERATIONS

THOUGH there can be no absolute distinction between diseases of the nervous system and those which affect other organs or systems of the human body, by convention the clinical science of neurology embraces those many disorders which affect the functioning of the central and peripheral nervous systems and the voluntary muscles. In this first chapter it is proposed to review briefly current knowledge of the means by which disorders of nervous function may be brought about by a variety of pathological processes. For the purposes of convenience, this review has been organized on an anatomical and physio-logical basis so that descriptions of the anatomy and, where necessary, of the physiology of certain structures and pathways in the nervous system will be con-sidered, together with the disorders of function which result when they are diseased. First, however, it is important to recognize that the manifestations of disordered function of the central nervous system may be greatly modified by mental, as by pathological processes, and may also be altered by the influence of the individual's constitution and inherited characteristics. Furthermore, before considering the applied anatomy and physiology of some of the more important pathways in the nervous system which are commonly affected by disease, it will be necessary to consider the nature of some important units of structure of the nervous system, as well as to classify some of the pathological processes which commonly influence their behaviour.

It must be admitted that there are still many problems in neurology which are not clearly understood. We have, for instance, no definite evidence as to how the brain controls thought processes; while disordered activity of the mind is commonly present and is attributed to dysfunction of the brain even when modern techniques fail to demonstrate any abnormality of structure or any measurable disorder of function in physiological terms, conversely the influence of the mind upon the behaviour of the organs of the body can also be profound. Mental disorders frequently initiate or accentuate symptoms of physical disease, while some organic diseases are regularly accompanied by psychological mani-festations. The importance of these mechanisms must be recognized by the physician who deals with sick people, as disease is an abstraction; it is the patient who suffers from the disease who is real and who shows a personal and individual reaction to it. Thus although many physical disorders of the nervous system regularly produce a consistent series of symptoms and physical signs independent of the personality and constitution of the individual, the severity of the resultant symptoms and the rate of recovery or of deterioration, depending upon the pathological process involved, can be influenced by factors which are independent of the physical process present within nervous tissue. While a simple peripheral nerve lesion is likely to produce a consistent clinical syndrome, its effects upon the patient may depend upon the nature of the lesion responsible, in that in industrial injuries, for instance, the patient's disability may be excessive and his recovery unduly delayed, particularly if financial compensation is involved.

In disorders of the nervous system, more perhaps than in any other group of diseases, the physical signs discovered on examination often indicate the anatomical localization of the lesion or lesions responsible for the abnormalities of function which are present, while it is the history of the illness, revealing the detailed evolution of the patient's symptoms, which generally indicates the nature of the pathological process. Thus although the intelligent interpretation of the significance of physical signs demands an adequate knowledge, first, of neuroanatomy for localization of the lesion, and secondly of neurophysiology in order to assess the means by which function has been disordered, it is also necessary that the student should have some understanding of neuropathology in order to be able to analyse the nature of the pathological process which is present. Admittedly there are many neurological disorders, such as migraine and epilepsy, for instance, which give characteristic clinical pictures but in which physical examination may be negative and diagnosis must rest upon analysis of the history alone. Furthermore, as already indicated, the clinical effects of pathological processes are not immutable and the resultant disease can be greatly influenced by the personality and constitution of the individual and by his state of mind. Some patients are born physically and mentally less perfect than others and yet show no obvious defect, but constitutionally they are less capable of resistance to stress, both mental and physical, and are seriously disturbed by environmental influences which would leave others unaffected. Hence the possible effects of fatigue, of ageing processes, and of other contributory influences which cannot easily be measured by scientific parameters must be also stressed. In his analysis of the interplay of these many factors, the doctor may be required to bring into play all his reserves of experience and understanding. It is also important to consider at this stage the concept of 'functional' illness or 'functional' disorder. In the strictest anatomical and physiological terms, it would be reasonable to regard as 'functional' those diseases in which there is an important disorder of the function of some organ of the body but which do not depend upon any recognizable pathological change in the organ concerned. By convention, however, the term 'functional disorder' is more often applied in medicine to symptoms and signs which result from a disordered state of mind. Thus headaches due to anxiety or nervous tension are 'functional', and so, too, is hysterical aphonia, while other forms of anxiety or hysterical reaction are commonly included in this category. Functional disorders, therefore, are those conditions in which symptoms and signs result not from any primary physical disease but from conscious or subconscious mental processes; it must be appreciated that these processes may profoundly affect the physical functioning of the body, giving rise to such manifestations as increased cardiac output, tachycardia, perspiration, and insomnia. Hence the clinical use of the term 'functional', if not strictly correct in a semantic sense, is hallowed through common usage and can usefully be employed provided the doctor using it understands its meaning and does not regard this as a final diagnosis. It is important also to recognize at this stage that the distinction between organic and functional disease is often one of the most difficult to make in medicine since even when there is clear evidence of a primary physical abnormality, the symptoms may readily be accentuated or distorted by concurrent psychological factors.

Disordered function depends not only upon the localization of pathological change but upon its severity, its extent, and the effects it has upon contiguous nervous tissue and upon interconnected though anatomically remote structures in the nervous system. Thus an acute and extensive lesion may affect a greater area of the brain than its anatomical extent would lead one to expect, for around the edge of the lesion itself the activity of the surrounding nervous tissue is disturbed by oedema, vascular changes, and other ill-defined abnormalities. Furthermore, an acute lesion can produce a state of 'shock' or temporary dissolution of function in related areas of the brain or spinal cord. By contrast, lesions of equal extent which are slow to develop produce far fewer symptoms and physical signs as it is only the structures which are actively invaded or destroyed by the lesion whose function is disturbed; the surrounding tissues have more time to adapt themselves to the presence of the lesion. Adaptation of other forms may also occur, particularly in the cerebral cortex, for here, particularly in children rather than in adults, a function which has been lost through a cortical lesion may be 'adopted', though usually much less efficiently, by another area of the brain. The younger the patient the greater the flexibility of cerebral organization. This type of re-organization is much less likely to occur in the spinal cord for the pathways followed here are more stereotyped and probably less complex. No such adoption of functions can occur in peripheral nerves, but, on the other hand, peripheral nerves are able to regenerate effectively following injury, while effective regeneration does not occur within the spinal cord or brain.

CONSTITUTION AND HEREDITY

It is only too easy to overlook the important influences which may be derived from inherited characteristics. Some neurological disorders are clearly inherited in a strictly Mendelian manner. Diseases such as migraine, Huntington's chorea, and facioscapulohumeral muscular dystrophy are generally inherited by an autosomal dominant mechanism, meaning that they result from a dominant gene situated on one of the autosomes and are thus passed on by an affected individual to half his or her children of either sex if penetrance or expressivity of the gene is complete. An autosomal recessive gene, however, can only produce its phenotypic effect if it is paired with a similar gene lying on the other chromosome of the pair. Hence such a disease is only expressed when two unaffected heterozygous carriers marry; usually, therefore, there is no previous history of the disease in the family unless there has been intermarriage between relatives (consanguinity). In such families the likelihood is that the disease will affect 1 in 4 of a series of brothers and sisters; Friedreich's ataxia, hepatolenticular degeneration (Wilson's disease), and spinal muscular atrophy of infancy are usually inherited in this way. A recessive gene can produce an effect, however, if it is situated on the unpaired portion of the X-chromosome, so that this type of condition occurs in males and is carried by apparently unaffected females. This is the typical pattern of sex-linked recessive (or X-linked) inheritance when the disease may have been found in maternal uncles and now occurs in half the male children of an apparently normal female carrier. Red-green colour blindness, haemophilia, and muscular dystrophy of the Duchenne type are inherited in this way. Any inherited disease can, of course, appear anew in a family if a previously normal gene has undergone a process of spontaneous change or mutation. It must also be remembered that apart from those diseases which are clearly inherited by recognizable genetic mechanisms, there are many other disorders of the nervous system in which genetic influences are of importance, though these factors are difficult to define.

Before going on to discuss individual anatomical pathways in the nervous system and the clinical effects of their dysfunction, it will now be important to consider certain units of nervous structure and some of the ways in which they may be affected by pathological processes. This commentary will perforce be superficial and introductory in nature and for fuller information the reader is referred to textbooks on neuroanatomy, neurophysiology, and neuropathology.

THE NEURONE

The nerve cell is one of the few types of cell in the human body which cannot be replaced if it is destroyed; it does not undergo division nor is it capable of regeneration after the first few weeks of extra-uterine life. The neurone theory was first proposed by Cajal and his colleagues in 1889–91; this stated that each neurone is a separate cellular entity which consists first of a cell body, secondly of dendrites or short processes which extend for a short distance from the cell, and thirdly of a long (or sometimes short) axon which makes contact by means of nerve endings of various types with the dendrites or cell bodies of other neurones or with muscle or other effector cells. This theory was opposed by many earlier workers who thought that nerve processes merged or became continuous with one another but it has now been shown conclusively that each neuroblast in the embryo forms a single adult nerve cell and that in the mature human and animal synaptic junctions are invariably present when axons and dendrites meet so that neurofibrils never pass from one cell to another. Furthermore, studies of degeneration have shown that neither chromatolysis nor any other form of degeneration in a cell necessarily spreads to involve other neurones. It has also been concluded from tissue culture studies that nerve processes always arise by direct growth from parent cells and not by differentiation from intercellular material. Many millions of neurones are present within the central nervous system; they are linked together to form functional conducting pathways and are supported or held together by a framework of specialized but non-conducting cells which constitute the neuroglia.

Neurones vary greatly in size, shape, and functional characteristics. Those with long processes are frequently called Golgi Type I, and those with short processes Golgi Type II. The cytoplasm of a neurone contains granules of Nissl substance which stain with basic dyes such as cresyl violet or toluidine blue, while within its cytoplasm there are minute neurofibrils which extend into its processes and can be demonstrated by special silver stains. Typically the nucleus of a neurone looks pale but it has a single dense central nucleolus [FIG. 1 (a)].

It is now evident that most of the dendrites of a neurone are afferent, while the longer axons are generally efferent. Most dendrites contain small quantities of Nissl substance and have many branches, while axons do not contain Nissl granules and their main branches come off terminally; the point of origin of the axon from the nerve cell is called the axon hillock [FIG. 1 (b)].

In the central nervous system many large axons, such as those of the pyramidal cells of the cerebral cortex and of the cerebellar Purkinje cells, give off

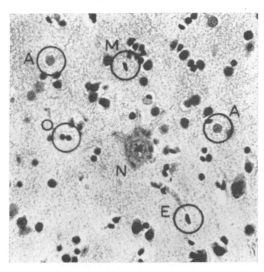

FIG. 1 *a*. Cells of normal precentral cortex stained by
Nissl's method. N = nerve cell; A = astrocyte; O = two
oligodendrocytes; M = microglial nucleus; E = capillary
endothelial cell nucleus. Thionin, × 350

(FIG. 1 (*a–g*) is reproduced from Blackwood, W., Dodds, T. C., and Sommerville, J. C.
(1964) *Atlas of Neuropathology*, 2nd ed., by kind permission of the authors and E. and
S. Livingstone Ltd.)

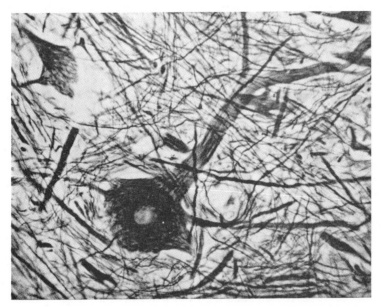

FIG. 1 *b*. Anterior horn cell, spinal cord, showing neurofibrils and the axon.
Hortega's silver, × 350

collateral fibres close to their origin, and many large axons of sensory neurones in the posterior root ganglia branch shortly after entering the spinal cord. Close to their termination axons usually divide into a number of fine terminal twigs or telodendria which either enter a peripheral end-organ or else make synaptic contact with the cell bodies or dendrites of other neurones; the resultant ring-like endings are called *boutons terminaux*.

The large axons of the lower motor neurones (alpha-neurones) which arise from large anterior horn cells in the spinal cord usually divide after entering voluntary muscle (the effector organ) and each main branch then divides further to innervate a group of extrafusal muscle fibres. The lower motor neurone and the muscle fibres which it supplies form a functional unit called the motor unit; some groups of fibres supplied by single large branches have been called sub-units. The intrafusal muscle fibres within the muscle spindles are innervated by axons arising from smaller anterior horn cells (the so-called gamma-neurones).

THE MYELIN SHEATH

In the vertebrate central and peripheral nervous systems it appears that all axons with a diameter greater than 1 μm are surrounded by a myelin sheath; this can be seen best in sections stained with osmic acid which demonstrate the myelin but not the axon. The myelin sheath is a complex of lipids and contains cerebroside, sphingomyelin, and cholesterol. In the peripheral, but not in the central nervous system, the myelin sheath is enclosed by the processes of Schwann or neurilemmal cells and this sheath is interrupted at regular intervals at the nodes of Ranvier. At this point, though the myelin is interrupted, the Schwann cells nevertheless appear to be continuous. It is the integrity and continuity of the sheath of Schwann around peripheral nerves which allows effective regeneration of axons to occur after injury or degeneration. Whereas in the central nervous system sprouting of damaged axons may also take place when a disease process resolves, these axons cannot be properly directed by a surviving neurilemmal sheath so that such regeneration usually proves to be abortive.

GROUND SUBSTANCE

Apart from the nerve and neuroglial cells and their processes which constitute the grey matter of the central nervous system, it seems that there is also a background substance which probably contains mucopolysaccharides. Though electron microscopy seems to indicate that the cortex is almost wholly made up of the branching processes of neurones and of neuroglial and oligodendroglial cells, there also appears to be a small amount of intercellular fluid (which is increased in cerebral oedema) or ground substance but its function is still unknown.

SYNAPSES OR NEURONAL JUNCTIONS

While peripherally axons may end in effector organs such as muscle, in the central nervous system each small terminal branch or telodendron makes contact with a dendrite (axodendritic contact) or with a cell body (axosomatic contact). In these junctional regions, which are called synapses, cell membranes are in close contact but do not fuse. As already mentioned, a synaptic contact between a telodendron and a dendrite or a cell body may take the form of a small swelling or ring-like structure (a *bouton terminal*). But a telodendron may make one synaptic contact, in passing, by a *bouton de passage* but then continues to its termination on another part of the same cell or on another cell, so that one axon may have synaptic junctions with many cells. Similarly, a single cell may have many hundreds of surface synaptic contacts derived from many axons. The arrangement and variety of these synapses determine the means by which a nerve cell can be activated, and also, of equal importance in nervous activity, by which it may be inhibited. Physiologically, learning, memory, and the acquisition of skills probably depend upon the progressive facilitation of synapses in certain specific pathways in the brain. Transmission of nervous activity across synapses is mediated by chemical substances released from axon terminals. At the synapse most extensively studied, namely the neuro-muscular junction, there is convincing evidence that the arrival of a nerve impulse causes a release of acetylcholine, probably from synaptic vesicles in the subneural apparatus, and that this in turn depolarizes the muscle fibre membrane. There is good evidence to suggest that acetylcholine is also responsible for synaptic transmission at many sites within the central nervous system, but many other neurotransmitter substances have been identified recently; thus dopamine acts in this way in some parts of the basal ganglia.

NEUROGLIA

The supporting cells of the brain and spinal cord are known as the neuroglia. Special silver stains are usually necessary in order to demonstrate fully these glial cells which differ in size and shape and have processes which not only inter-mingle with the axons and dendrites but which are frequently attached to the wall of blood vessels. Larger stellate neuroglial cells are called astrocytes; they can be divided into protoplasmic and fibrous forms, the fibrous being dis-tinguished from the protoplasmic form chiefly by the presence in the cell body and its processes of fine fibres [FIG. 1 (*c*)]. The processes of fibrous astrocytes are longer and finer and branch less frequently than do those of the proto-plasmic variety, in which the rather thicker and shorter branches which come off at a wider angle give a rather 'mossy' appearance to the cell [FIG. 1 (*d*)]. Under the light microscope neuroglial fibres seem fine and relatively straight, being seen only with high magnification, but under the electron microscope they are seen to be beaded. Undoubtedly astrocytes have a metabolic function, but their exact role in the metabolism of nervous structure is as yet undetermined. The oligodendroglia are smaller neuroglial cells with fewer and shorter processes [FIG. 1 (*a*)]; they may be seen close to axons and around cell bodies but are much more common in the white matter; almost certainly they play an important role in the formation and maintenance of myelin. Microglial cells are much smaller [FIG. 1 (*e*)] and unlike other glial cells which are of ectodermal origin, they are derived from the mesoderm which is carried into the nervous system by blood vessels. They frequently enlarge and become phagocytic [FIG. 1 (*f*)] and thus play an important role in removing damaged tissue in the course of pathological processes. The proliferation of neuroglial cells almost always occurs as a reaction to the degeneration of neurones or else as a secondary part of the disease process which causes the neurone to degenerate. The prolifera-tion of astrocytes is called astrocytosis or gliosis, while the proliferation of microglial cells is comparable to the scavenging activity of histiocytes in other organs of the human body.

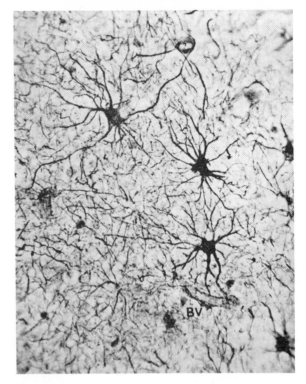

FIG. 1 *c*. Fibrillary astrocytes in the cortex. Cajal's gold sublimate, ×350

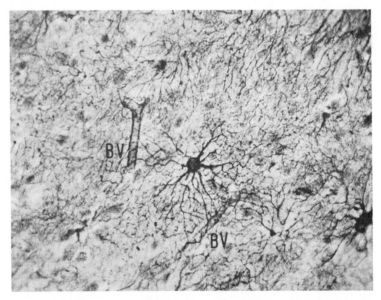

FIG. 1 *d*. Protoplasmic astrocytes in the cortex. Cajal's gold sublimate, ×350

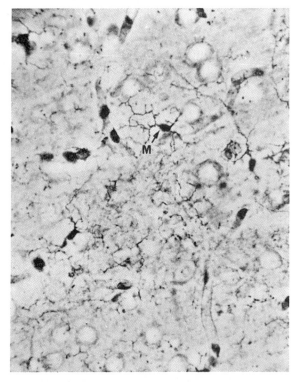

FIG. 1 e. Normal microglia in the cortex of a rabbit (human
cells are similar). Hortega's silver, × 450

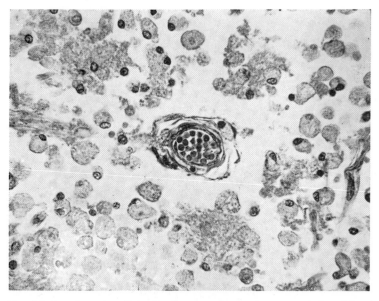

FIG. 1 f. Reactive microglial cells ('compound granular corpuscles' or 'gitter'
cells) which are distended with phagocytosed lipid

DEGENERATION AND REGENERATION IN THE NERVOUS SYSTEM

An adult nerve cell, once destroyed, can never be replaced. With increasing age there is undoubtedly a progressive fall-out of certain cortical and spinal neurones. In elderly individuals it is not uncommon to find within the cerebral cortex neurofibrillary tangles or so-called senile argyrophilic placques which develop in relation to degenerating neurones. Such lesions, if seen in profusion in the cerebral cortex at a relatively early age, are virtually diagnostic of pre-senile dementia and the changes in senile dementia are similar, but it is the age at which they are found and their profusion which is important as they are almost invariably seen to occur in some degree as a result of normal ageing processes in the eighth or ninth decades.

When certain processes of a nerve cell are destroyed, the cell body may survive, but if as a result, say, of peripheral nerve injury, the axon of an anterior horn cell is divided, the Nissl substance in the cell of origin at first aggregates and later disappears (chromatolysis) and the nucleus shifts towards the periphery [FIG. 1 (g)]. These changes are more easily seen in large cells which have

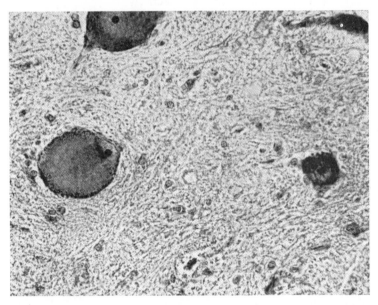

FIG. 1g. Chromatolysis of an anterior horn cell. The cell is swollen and rounded, the Nissl substance is accumulated at the periphery and the nucleus is eccentric.
H & E, ×350

abundant Nissl substance; their severity is related to the distance of the axonal lesion from the parent cell body and they are more severe when the break is close. It is rare for cells with bodies and processes confined to the central nervous system to survive axonal section and hence these cellular changes may sometimes be used to locate the cells of origin of degenerating axons in a peripheral nerve or in a specific fibre pathway. It is, however, important to recognize that appearances somewhat similar to those of chromatolysis may occasionally be seen in control material and can result from post-mortem autolysis. When degeneration of a cell body proceeds even further, due either to damage to its axon or to a primary degenerative process, it may be surrounded by microglial cells and later disappears leaving only a small glial cluster (neuronophagia).

An axon that has been severed from its cell body undergoes Wallerian degeneration. Within a few days the terminal part of the axis-cylinder begins to swell and subsequently it becomes beaded and then disintegrates. This process of swelling and progressive disintegration then moves slowly proximally (dying back of the neurone). If the axon is myelinated, the myelin sheath begins to break down within a few days and it seems that the neurilemmal cells then proliferate, subsequently appearing to ingest or enfold both the disintegrating axis-cylinder and the myelin within Schwann cell processes. Histiocytes have a phagocytic role and proliferating connective tissue cells also play a part in the degenerative process. Similar axonal changes occur in the central nervous system, except that gliosis results from astrocytic proliferation and the microglia act as phagocytes. The degeneration of myelin secondary to such axonal damage may be identified by certain specific stains which form the basis of the Marchi method which demonstrates degenerating myelinated fibres in such a way that these fibres can be traced in microscopic sections.

In peripheral nerves, soon after an axon has been divided, its tip begins to grow out distally into the surviving neurilemmal sheath which directs its growth. Collateral sprouting often occurs alongside the growing axon, though it is usual for one of these axons to grow distally more rapidly than its collateral sprouts; this distal growth only occurs when the cell body survives and the chromatolytic process is then reversed. Growth occurs at a rate of a millimetre or two a day at first, but after a few weeks it slows down; myelin gradually begins to re-form until eventually the axon re-establishes distal contact. Although profuse axonal sprouting may be seen in the brains or spinal cords of very young animals and infants after injury, it is doubtful as to whether it is ever effective as the axonal sprouts rarely, if ever, make contact with any effector organ.

It must also be recognized that in clinical neurology there are many disease processes which cause demyelination in peripheral nerves or in the central nervous system but which initially leave the axon intact, though incapable of conducting normally. In peripheral nerves such demyelination may begin at or close to the nodes of Ranvier (perinodal demyelination) and may then spread to involve one or many internodal distances. Subsequently if the disease process is reversed, remyelination may occur. In teased specimens of nerve fibres obtained by biopsy or at autopsy in such cases it is often found that the regenerated myelin sheath is thinner than normal and in such areas the internodal distances are often irregular and much shorter than normal. A demyelinating type of neuropathy frequently produces marked slowing of conduction in peripheral nerves, but as the disease process recovers this may eventually return to normal. Demyelination within the central nervous system also affects conduction in the parent axon. The process by means of which remyelination occurs in the central nervous system is unknown, but this process presumably accounts for the remissions which may occur in demyelinating disorders such as multiple sclerosis.

SOME PHYSIOLOGICAL CHARACTERISTICS OF NEURONES

Nerve cells are excitable; this means that they can respond or react to stimuli and these reactions alter the physiological state of the organism. Some cells react specifically; thus stimulation of the lower motor neurone causes muscular contraction while stimulation of neurosecretory neurones causes glandular secretion. In some cells, the change once initiated by the stimulus spreads throughout the cell and its processes and is then independent of the stimulus. This spread or conduction is particularly rapid in muscle and nerve. The conducted response which begins in a nerve cell and spreads along its axon is known as the nerve impulse, while the activity which spreads along a muscle fibre from the neuromuscular junction once depolarization has occurred is called the propagated action potential. These reactions are accompanied by the utilization of oxygen and of glucose, the formation of carbon dioxide and the production of heat and they are also accompanied by certain specific electrical changes.

Nerve and muscle fibres are each normally polarized in such a way that the interior of the fibre is negative to the exterior; the potential difference across the fibre membrane is called the resting membrane potential. This can be measured in a neurone by inserting a micro-electrode into a nerve cell body; in the giant axon of the squid, the axon itself may be impaled. A stimulus adequate to excite the neurone alters the permeability of its membrane to many ions; it develops a high specific permeability to sodium, so that sodium rapidly enters the fibre. In less than a millisecond the polarity of the resting potential is reversed, so that the external surface becomes negative to the interior and the membrane is said to be depolarized. The electrical accompaniment of this change can be recorded as a spike potential and typically the depolarization and this spike potential are propagated along the fibre, forming the so-called nerve action potential. The spread of excitation along a muscle fibre is very similar. As the peak of the action potential moves on, the entry of sodium stops, potassium permeability increases, and potassium leaves the fibre so that the original membrane potential is eventually restored. The so-called sodium pump helps slowly to restore the original differences in sodium concentration. A nerve action potential can be measured by means of electrodes inserted into a nerve trunk or, in certain situations, surface electrodes applied to the overlying skin are sufficient. Muscle action potentials can also be recorded with surface electrodes but for diagnostic electromyography needle electrodes are inserted into the muscle. The form of the nerve action potential depends upon recording methods. The conduction velocity in peripheral nerves can be measured either by recording the rate of propagation of the nerve action potential (which is the usual method of measuring conduction in sensory nerves) or by measuring the latencies of the evoked muscle action potential induced by stimulation of a motor nerve at two points a known distance apart. The conduction velocity in a nerve depends upon the fibre diameter. In general, heavily myelinated, thick nerve fibres conduct rapidly and finely myelinated or unmyelinated fibres conduct slowly. In myelinated fibres the nerve impulse passes rapidly from one node of Ranvier to the next. The maximum rate of conduction known is about 100–120 metres per second, but in human peripheral nerves 50–70 metres per second is more usual and the slowest myelinated fibres conduct at about 40 metres per second. Demyelination in peripheral nerves causes marked slowing of conduction. When a nerve impulse has passed, the nerve may show an absolute and a relative refractory period, while small negative and positive after-potentials may be recorded. These after-potentials and accompanying changes in excitability of the nerve are related to the recovery process which follows the passage of the impulse. Just as in muscle miniature end-plate potentials may be recorded close to the neuromuscular junction and are believed to be due to the spontaneous release of amounts of acetylcholine which are insufficient to evoke a propagated action potential, so in a nerve a subthreshold stimulus produces a local excitatory state in a fibre; another subthreshold stimulus may then raise this local excitation to a threshold value and thereby set off a nerve impulse.

It will now be important to consider, as an introduction to the more specific commentaries which follow, some simple principles concerning pathological processes in the nervous system.

SOME PATHOLOGICAL REACTIONS IN THE NERVOUS SYSTEM

Pathological changes in the nervous system can be classified into three broad groups, namely focal lesions, which cause a disturbance in the function of a strictly localized area; diffuse or generalized disorders, whether of metabolic, toxic, vascular, or other aetiology, which affect nervous and supporting elements throughout the nervous system; and systemic nervous diseases, in which the pathological process shows a predilection for a particular neuronal structure or group of structures such as, for instance, the anterior horn cells, the cerebellum and its connections, or the pyramidal tracts. Many focal lesions and diffuse disorders affect nervous tissue more or less by accident and many of these are not primarily neurological diseases. Thus cerebral vascular disease, which may produce infarction or haemorrhage, is usually a complication of atherosclerosis or hypertension, while the diffuse pathological changes which occur in the brain in syphilis, for instance, form only one part of the changes resulting from infection of the entire human organism. In the systemic nervous diseases, by contrast, as in motor neurone disease, there is clearly some biochemical or other factor which causes the pathological process to be confined to a particular group of nerve cells or fibre pathways. In this context one must note that the tissues of the nervous system vary considerably in their response to a variety of different noxious influences. Thus ischaemia affects nerve cells more severely than myelin and neuroglia, while plaques of demyelination, as in multiple sclerosis, have a more profound influence upon the nerve fibres of the white matter. There are also considerable differences in the effects of ischaemia, compression, and various toxins upon nerve fibres depending upon whether they conduct motor or sensory impulses.

There are a number of methods of classifying pathological processes on an aetiological basis. Thus one can recognize that certain lesions are congenital or due to developmental abnormality. Others may be traumatic, the lesion then being the result of physical or possibly chemical injury. A third large group is that of the inflammatory disorders which in turn may be subdivided according to whether the inflammation is of infective or allergic origin. In either category the infection may be acute, subacute, or chronic. Neoplastic disorders are next to be considered and these in turn may be benign or malignant, while malignant processes may involve the nervous system primarily, or secondarily as a result of metastasis from a tumour elsewhere. Within a further large group of conditions classified at present as being degenerative because their nature is not yet understood, one must include cerebral vascular disease, but there are also many other conditions of unknown aetiology which must still be so classified. Finally, a variety of metabolic and endocrine disorders may also affect the functioning of the nervous system.

To mention a number of congenital disorders, these are most often apparent as gross disorders of anatomical development and configuration and include such conditions as anencephaly, hydrocephalus, and meningomyelocele. Vascular malformations are almost certainly also of congenital origin. Trauma to the nervous system will produce the familiar effects of necrosis, haemorrhage, and subsequent scar formation, the scar consisting of proliferated neuroglial cells and fibrils (gliosis) and of mesenchymal fibrous tissue derived from fibroblasts and microglial cells in the supporting tissue of the blood vessels. In the group of acute inflammatory disorders, one must consider the meningitides producing the typical pathological changes of inflammation and exudation in the meninges. It must, however, be noted that meningitis may give rise to superficial degenerative changes in underlying nervous tissue or to ischaemic changes in the nervous parenchyma resulting from an obliterative endarteritis of blood vessels which traverse the subarachnoid space. Pyogenic infection in the brain, as elsewhere, begins with diffuse suppuration, but localization and abscess formation generally follow with the formation of a capsule through gliosis and fibrosis. Most neurotropic viruses, such as those of encephalitis and poliomyelitis, show an affinity for nerve cells and inflammatory changes with perivascular cellular infiltration and degeneration of nerve cells are therefore seen in the grey matter of the brain and/or spinal cord and inclusion bodies may be found within the nucleus or cytoplasm of infected cells. Syphilis, and to a lesser extent tuberculosis, are still two of the most important chronic infections of the central nervous system. The pathological changes they produce will be considered under the appropriate sections later in this volume as they do not differ significantly from the pathological changes produced by these diseases elsewhere, except in so far that in general paresis there are degeneration of nerve cells, gliosis, and minimal inflammatory changes in the cerebral cortex, while in tabes dorsalis the most prominent pathological change is gliosis and meningeal fibrosis of the entry zones of the posterior spinal nerve roots with secondary ascending degeneration of the posterior columns of the spinal cord. In allergic or postinfective encephalomyelitis, by contrast to the virus infections, inflammatory changes, consisting largely of perivascular collections of inflammatory cells with loss of myelin, are seen particularly in the white matter of the nervous system. These pathological changes show some resemblance to those observed in the demyelinating disorders of unknown aetiology such as multiple sclerosis and diffuse sclerosis. In these disorders there is patchy loss of myelin of variable extent and severity occurring generally throughout the white matter of the brain and spinal cord. This type of degenerative change in which the axis-cylinders of the nerve fibres are initially preserved is eventually replaced by a glial scar.

So far as neoplastic disorders are concerned, the pathology of these conditions will be considered in greater detail in the sections on intracranial and intraspinal tumours, but it should first be remarked that the commonest benign tumours which compress and distort nervous tissues are the meningioma, which probably arises from cells of the arachnoidal membrane, and the neurofibroma, which grows from the sheath of Schwann of the cranial nerves, spinal roots, or peripheral nerves. The commonest of the malignant tumours of the central nervous system is the glioma; these are infiltrating and invasive tumours whose relative malignancy depends upon whether the principal constituent cell of the tumour is a relatively mature astrocyte or one of its more rapidly multiplying primitive precursors. Metastatic malignant neoplasms are also very common in the nervous system.

Vascular disorders are a common cause of pathological change. Bleeding into the subarachnoid space produces an aseptic meningeal inflammation comparable to that of meningitis and sometimes chronic arachnoiditis may result, while chronic bleeding can give rise to a state of haemosiderosis of the meninges. Haemorrhage into the nervous parenchyma gives a central area of total necrosis which is eventually walled off by gliosis and fibrosis. Sometimes a scar results, but more often a cavity is left which is filled with a clear straw-coloured fluid containing bilirubin. An infarct shows an area of central ischaemic necrosis but within 24 hours activated microglial cells invade the necrotic area and soon become distended with the fatty remnants of the necrotic myelin which they have ingested. A minute infarct produced by embolic occlusion of a tiny cortical vessel may consist of nothing more histologically than a small cluster of activated microglial cells, whereas a large one will show an extensive central area of necrosis surrounded by distended phagocytes ('gitter' cells) and proliferating astrocytes. A large area of infarction may eventually be replaced by a contracted glial scar or cavity, while multifocal infarction sometimes leads to the formation of multiple small cavities (status lacunosus).

There remain a large group of degenerative disorders of the central nervous system whose aetiology is at present unknown, but in some of which specific neuropathological changes are seen. In motor neurone disease, for instance, the cells of the motor nuclei of the brain stem and the anterior horn cells of the spinal cord and the corticospinal or pyramidal tracts show a progressive degeneration. In Huntington's chorea there is a selective degeneration of the caudate nucleus and of the nerve cells of the frontal cortex. But in these and in many other disorders which will be considered in the appropriate sections of this volume, though the anatomical distribution of the pathological lesions has been well defined, their nature is little understood. Nor do we know why anoxia should affect particularly the cells of the deepest layer of the cerebral cortex, the Ammon's horn area of the hippocampus, or the Purkinje cells of the cerebellum, nor why hypoglycaemia should also involve the Purkinje cells, or even why deficiency of vitamin B_{12}, as in subacute combined degeneration of the spinal cord, should damage so selectively the sensory nerves, posterior columns, and pyramidal tracts.

Many metabolic disorders which seriously disturb nervous function produce relatively little pathological change, but in hepatic failure there is astrocytic proliferation, particularly in the basal ganglia but also in the brain stem. The pathological changes in many different forms of polyneuropathy are also non-specific since in some cases the damage is primarily axonal with swelling and fragmentation of axis-cylinders, but in many others it is essentially a demyelinating process.

The purpose of this section has been to comment briefly upon some of the basic pathological reactions which may occur in the diseased nervous system and not to give comprehensive descriptions of the detailed changes which occur in individual disease entities as these will be described in subsequent sections. It will now be convenient to consider in greater detail some of the important neuronal and fibre systems and pathways in the central nervous system and the disorders of function which may be produced by disease in these specific structures.

REFERENCES

BLACKWOOD, W., DODDS, T. C., and SOMMERVILLE, J. C. (1964) *Atlas of Neuropathology*, 2nd ed., Edinburgh.
BLACKWOOD, W., and CORSELLIS, J. A. N. (1976) *Greenfield's Neuropathology*, 4th ed., London.
EMERY, A. E. H. (1974) *Elements of Medical Genetics*, Edinburgh and London.
GARDNER, E. (1968) *Fundamentals of Neurology*, 5th ed., Philadelphia.
KREIG, W. J. S. (1966) *Functional Neuroanatomy*, 3rd ed., Evanston, Ill.
McKUSICK, W. A. (1964) *Human Genetics*, Englewood Cliffs, N.J.
MATTHEWS, W. B. (1976) *Practical Neurology*, 3rd ed., Oxford.
PRATT, R. T. C. (1967) *The Genetics of Neurological Disorders*, London.
WALSH, E. G. (1964) *Physiology of the Nervous System*, 2nd ed., London.
WALTON, J. N. (1975) *Essentials of Neurology*, 4th ed., London.
ZACKS, S. I. (1971) *Atlas of Neuropathology*, New York.

THE CORTICOSPINAL (PYRAMIDAL) TRACT

ANATOMY

THE PRECENTRAL GYRUS

THE corticospinal tracts are the pathways by which the nervous impulses which excite voluntary movements pass from the cerebral cortex to the lower motor neurones which arise in the brain stem and spinal cord. The corticospinal fibres or upper motor neurones are the axons of cells of the precentral gyrus. It is probable that their cells of origin include not only the Betz cells but also the simple giant cells and the large ordinary pyramidal cells of the fifth layer of the cortex lying anterior to the central sulcus, and extending over Brodmann's areas 4 and 6 (Walshe, 1942).

Since the electrical excitation of different parts of the precentral gyrus evokes movements of different parts of the opposite side of the body, we are justified in speaking of the representation of parts of the body in this part of the brain. The order in which the parts of the body are thus represented is shown in FIGURES 2 and 3.

Individual movements are represented widely and in overlapping areas in the motor cortex, the function of which is the organization of movements in space and time. The cortical centre or focus of a movement is merely the area in which that movement is predominantly represented. Denny-Brown's (1966) observations on stimulation and ablation of area 4 in the monkey and division of the pyramidal tract led him to the conclusion that 'the pyramidal system is concerned not so much with "discrete" movements of individual muscles, or individual joints as with those spatial adjustments that accurately adapt the movement to the spatial attributes of the stimulus'.

THE INTERNAL CAPSULE

The axons of the corticospinal tract after leaving the grey matter of the cortex pass through the corona radiata and converge upon the internal capsule, a band of

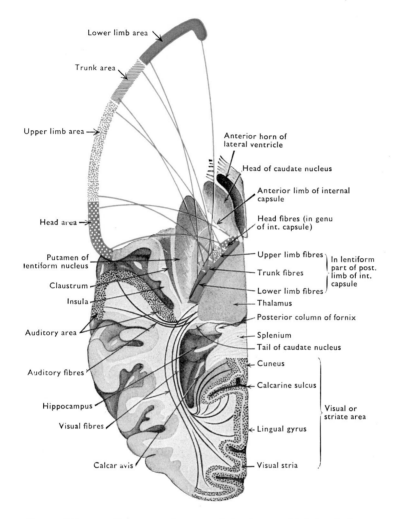

Lower limb area

Trunk area

Upper limb area →

Head area →

Putamen of
lentiform nucleus

Claustrum

Insula

Auditory area

Auditory fibres

Hippocampus

Visual fibres

Calcar avis

Anterior horn of
lateral ventricle

Head of caudate nucleus

Anterior limb of internal
capsule

Head fibres (in genu
of int. capsule)

Upper limb fibres ⎫ In lentiform
                   ⎪ part of post.
Trunk fibres   ⎬ limb of int.
                   ⎪ capsule
Lower limb fibres ⎭

Thalamus

Posterior column of fornix

Splenium

Tail of caudate nucleus

Cuneus

Calcarine sulcus

Lingual gyrus

Visual stria

Visual or
striate area

FIG. 2. Diagram of motor, auditory, and visual areas of left hemisphere
and their relations to the internal capsule

white matter lying deep in the substance of the cerebral hemisphere [FIG. 4]. Seen in horizontal section [FIG. 2], it has the head of the caudate nucleus and the optic thalamus on its medial side and the lentiform nucleus on its lateral side. Above, it expands into the corona radiata, and below it is continuous with the cerebral peduncle. The capsule is divided into a shorter, anterior, and a longer, posterior, limb separated by the genu.

The Corticospinal Tract. This occupies the posterior one-third of the anterior limb, the genu, and the anterior two-thirds of the posterior limb. The representation of different parts of the body in the capsule can be seen in FIGURE 2.

The Thalamocortical Tract. This is a sensory tract running from the optic thalamus, a great sensory relay-station, to the cerebral cortex. It is divided into an anterior and a posterior thalamic radiation, the former running in the

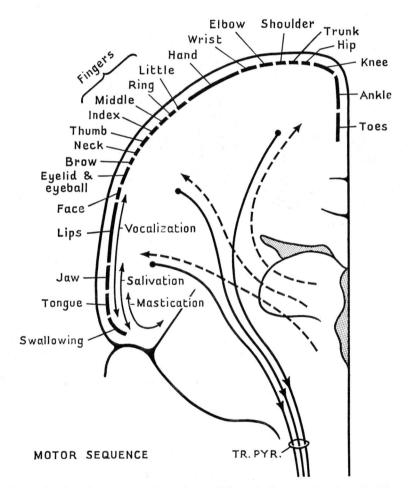

FIG. 3. Corticospinal motor pathway (pyramidal tract). Cross-section through right hemisphere along the plane of the precentral gyrus. The sequence of responses to electrical stimulation of the surface of the cortex (from above down, along the motor strip from toes through arm and face to swallowing) is unvaried from one individual to another

B

anterior limb of the capsule to the cortex of the frontal lobe, and the latter in the posterior limb to the postcentral and supramarginal gyri and to the temporal and occipital lobes.

The *optic* and *auditory radiations* are also shown in FIGURE 2.

The Frontopontine and the Temporopontine Tracts. These run from the frontal and temporal lobes to lower parts of the nervous system through the anterior and posterior limbs of the capsule respectively.

Fibres of the Corpus Striatum. Fibres linking the optic thalamus and caudate and lentiform nuclei also run in the internal capsule, and the main efferent path of the corpus striatum, the ansa lenticularis, passes in the posterior limb of the capsule from the globus pallidus to the red nucleus, substantia nigra, and subthalamic nucleus.

THE MIDBRAIN

In the midbrain the corticospinal fibres occupy the middle three-fifths of the crus cerebri, the medial fifth being occupied by the frontopontine fibres and

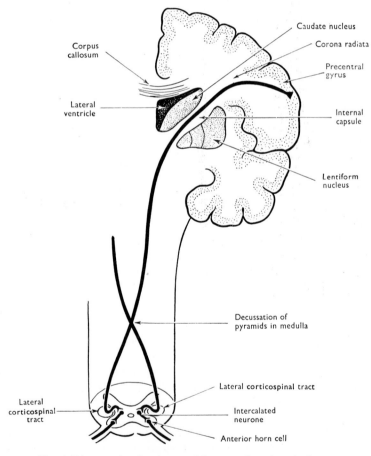

FIG. 4. Diagram showing course of the crossed corticospinal tracts

the lateral fifth by the temporopontine fibres. The crus cerebri is separated from the tegmen by the substantia nigra, which is thus a posterior relation of the corticospinal tract. Posteromedially to this is the red nucleus, through which pass the bundles of the oculomotor nerve, which emerges from the brain stem on the medial aspect of the crus [FIG. 5].

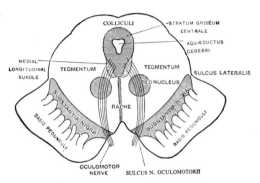

FIG. 5. Diagrammatic view of the cut surface of a transverse section through the superior part of the mesencephalon

THE PONS, MEDULLA, AND SPINAL CORD

On entering the pons the corticospinal tract ceases to be compact and becomes broken into scattered bundles by the transverse pontine fibres and the nuclei pontis. At the junction of the pons and the medulla these scattered bundles reunite, and each corticospinal tract constitutes a visible prominence on the anterior aspect of the medulla, the pyramid, which lies between the median fissure and the anterolateral sulcus from the bottom of which emerge the radicles of the hypoglossal nerve.

At the junction of the medulla and the spinal cord the corticospinal tract divides into three parts. (1) The larger medial part decussates with the corresponding fibres of the opposite tract and sinks back to take up a position in the lateral column of the spinal cord, the crossed corticospinal tract. (2) The smaller lateral portion remains in the anterior column of the spinal cord, moving to a medial position next to the median fissure. Although the medullary decussation is known as the decussation of the pyramids, corticospinal fibres cross the midline at all levels of the brain stem to reach the motor nuclei of the cranial nerves on the opposite side. The fibres of the direct corticospinal tract also gradually cross the midline in the anterior white commissure of the spinal cord, and this tract has usually disappeared in the mid-thoracic region. (3) Uncrossed fibres are also found in the lateral column (Fulton and Sheehan, 1935). The corticospinal fibres ultimately enter the grey matter of the spinal cord. Most of them end, not in relation with the anterior horn cells, but with internuncial fibres in the intermediate zone of the grey matter (Hoff and Hoff, 1934) which enables them to activate inhibitory as well as excitatory fibres; however, some do appear to end directly on anterior horn cells [see FIG. 6, p. 29].

UNILATERAL CORTICOSPINAL LESIONS

HEMIPLEGIA

The commonest cause of hemiplegia is a vascular lesion involving the motor cortex or internal capsule. We shall therefore consider this as typical of a unilateral corticospinal lesion, pointing out later the distinctive features of lesions in various situations. Let us suppose then that we are investigating a patient two months after such a lesion, when the effects of shock have passed off.

POSITIVE AND NEGATIVE ELEMENTS

We must first consider a concept which we owe to Hughlings Jackson which is important in the interpretation of nervous symptoms, namely, the distinction between the positive and negative elements in nervous symptomatology. In hemiplegia we find a loss or impairment of certain functions, e.g. voluntary movement. The functions lost, or the negative elements, were clearly dependent upon the integrity of the structures destroyed, i.e. the corticospinal tract. We also observe new phenomena which were not previously present, e.g. muscular hypertonia and an extensor plantar reflex. These, the positive elements, cannot be the direct result of a destructive lesion, but must be manifestations of the activity of other intact parts of the nervous system which have been released or have escaped from control as a result of damage to the fibres destroyed. If this distinction is borne in mind it will greatly clarify neurological symptomatology.

Negative Signs

Since the corticospinal fibres carry impulses which excite voluntary movements, the negative signs of a corticospinal lesion consist of impairment or loss of such movements.

Ocular Movements. The ocular movements are dealt with in detail in a later section [see p. 75]. Immediately after a lesion of the corticospinal fibres in one cerebral hemisphere there may be weakness of conjugate deviation of the eyes to the side opposite to the lesion. If the patient is unconscious the eyes are deviated to the side of the lesion. These ocular abnormalities usually pass off within a few hours or days of the onset; they are due to involvement of the so-called 'frontal eye field' (Brodmann's area 8) which lies immediately anterior to the face area of the motor cortex.

Movements of the Head. Lateral rotation of the head is a movement closely associated physiologically and anatomically with lateral deviation of the eyes. Hence we find that for a short time after the onset of hemiplegia there may be weakness of rotation of the head to the opposite side, and the unconscious patient usually lies with the head, like the eyes, rotated to the side of the lesion by the unantagonized action of the rotating muscles innervated from the normal hemisphere. This abnormal posture is also transitory, disappearing when consciousness returns.

Facial Movements. The facial movements are not all equally weakened by a unilateral corticospinal lesion. Movements of the upper part of the face, such as elevation of the eyebrows and closure of the eyes, are little affected, probably because, like other bilaterally synchronous movements, movements of each side of the upper part of the face are under the control of both cerebral hemispheres. In contrast there is marked weakness of voluntary movements of the lower part of the face, such as retraction of the angle of the mouth in showing the teeth and pursing the lips in whistling. Emotional movements of the lower face, such as smiling and crying, and associated movements, such as involuntary retraction of the angle of the mouth on voluntary closure of the eyes, are little affected by a cortical or capsular lesion because the nervous pathways controlling these movements originate at a lower level.

Movements of the Lower Jaw, Soft Palate, and Tongue. Movements of the lower jaw, soft palate, and tongue are for the most part bilaterally symmetrical and synchronous. We find therefore that they are less affected by a unilateral corticospinal lesion than are movements exclusively under the control of one hemisphere. After such a lesion, however, there is usually slight weakness of the mandibular, palatal, and lingual movements on the opposite side, indicated by deviation of the jaw on opening the mouth and of the tongue on protrusion, to the side opposite to the lesion, while on phonation the palate is less arched on the opposite side and the uvula tends to be drawn to the side of the lesion.

Movements of the Limbs. In the limbs the finer and more skilled movements suffer more than the grosser and less skilled. Hence movements of the fingers and toes are weaker than movements at the proximal joints. After a slight corticospinal lesion clumsiness in carrying out fine movements with the fingers, e.g. buttoning, sewing, or playing the piano, may be more evident than actual weakness. Hughlings Jackson's 'law of dissolution' states that the movements most recently acquired in the process of evolution are the first to be lost following a corticospinal tract lesion. Thus the 'precision grip' which depends upon opposition of the thumb and the individual fingers, a pattern of movement not seen in primates, is impaired when the 'power grip' which is produced by finger flexion, is relatively unaffected. It also becomes difficult to move the thumb in isolation from the other digits. This is the basis of *Wartenberg's sign*. If a normal individual is made to flex the terminal phalanges of his fingers against the resistance offered by the observer's fingers similarly flexed, his thumb remains abducted and extended. After a corticospinal lesion, however, the thumb becomes strongly adducted and flexed. After a corticospinal lesion also, movements are not confined to the appropriate parts, but the limbs tend to move as a whole. Finally, probably owing to the distribution of the muscular hypertonia, movements of flexion tend to be stronger than those of extension in the upper limb, while the reverse is the case in the lower limb.

Respiratory Movements. As Hughlings Jackson first demonstrated, during quiet breathing the amplitude of the thoracic expansion tends to be greater on the paralysed than on the normal side, but during vigorous voluntary breathing the opposite occurs.

Gait. The hemiplegic patient in walking circumducts his paralysed leg, swinging it outwards at the hip to obviate the difficulty arising from inability to flex it at the knee. The foot is plantar-flexed, hence the toe tends to drag and the sole of his shoe thus becomes worn at the toe.

Positive Signs

Muscular Hypertonia. Immediately after a vascular lesion the paralysed limbs are usually completely flaccid owing to the occurrence of neural shock. After a variable interval, usually two or three weeks, tone gradually returns to the affected muscles and they ultimately become hypertonic or 'spastic'. This is a state in which an attempt to stretch a muscle group by passive movement at a joint evokes resistance which increases in proportion to the velocity of stretch. As stretching continues the reflex is inhibited by impulses from Golgi tendon organs and secondary endings in the muscle spindles causing a sudden 'give' (the clasp-knife effect). The tendon reflexes are exaggerated. Not all muscle groups exhibit hypertonia in equal degree in hemiplegia. In the upper limb the adductors and internal rotators of the shoulder, flexors of the elbow, wrist, and fingers, and the pronators of the forearm are usually more spastic than their antagonists. Very rarely the increase of tone is more marked in the extensors of the elbow than in the flexors. In the lower limb the hypertonia predominates in the adductors of the hip, the extensors of the hip and knee, and in the plantar-flexors of the foot and toes. In time contractures tend to develop in the spastic muscles.

It was at one time assumed that hemiplegic spasticity is a release phenomenon due to corticospinal tract damage. Tower (1940), however, stated that a pure corticospinal lesion in the monkey causes a flaccid paralysis, and Fulton (1943) believed that a lesion of area 4 leads to flaccid paralysis while ablation of area 6 causes spasticity, amongst other symptoms. The subject was reviewed by Magoun and Rhines (1947) who regarded cerebral spasticity as an uncontrolled and augmented stretch reflex, produced by loss of descending inhibitory pathways running from area 4s, a suppressor zone between areas 4 and 6, to the bulbar reticular system and thence to the spinal cord, and receiving contributions from the striatum and the cerebellum. These pathways are not corticospinal. Certainly in man upper motor neurone paralysis and spasticity, though usually parallel in severity, sometimes behave as independent variables. Denny-Brown and Botterell (1948) concluded from their ablation studies in the monkey that spasticity does occur after removal of area 4 alone, but the additional removal of area 6 increases the spasticity in the flexors of the elbow and the extensors of the knee and ankle. Removal of area 6 alone causes a plastic type of rigidity in both flexors and extensors of the upper and lower limb on the affected side.

Denny-Brown (1966) subsequently concluded that hemiplegic spasticity is a mixed phenomenon. Its earliest manifestation is a soft, yielding resistance that appears only towards the end of passive stretch and is associated with increased amplitude of tendon reflex. At this stage clonus and its associated repetitive tendon reflex, and the clasp-knife phenomenon are absent. These together with the hemiplegic posture are 'epiphenomena'. Hemiplegic spasticity resulting from area 4 ablation is a postural automatism resulting from release of subcortical reactions; and its primary basis is direct facilitation of alpha neurones. But a substantial part is due to release of gamma innervation [see p. 28]. Lance (1970) agrees that in the early stages of spasticity there is hyperactivity of the gamma efferent system which can be reduced by injection of procaine or phenol into muscle or intrathecally, but points out that after some time, when contractures begin to develop, alpha mechanisms predominate. There is also evidence to indicate that in long-standing spasticity irreversible physico-chemical changes may occur in the muscles as a result of shortening, thus obscuring the effects of 'neurogenic tone'. In other words, increased resistance to stretch then results at least in part from loss of muscular elasticity.

Posture. The hemiplegic posture is the outcome of the selective distribution of hypertonia in the limb muscles, the more spastic muscles determining the position of the limb segments. Hence we find the upper limb usually adducted and internally rotated at the shoulder, flexed to a right angle at the elbow, somewhat pronated, and flexed at the wrist and fingers. In the exceptional cases in which hypertonia predominates in the extensors of the upper limb its attitude is one of extension at the elbow, and flexion of the wrist and fingers is less marked. The lower limb is extended, with plantar flexion and often slight inversion of the foot. The extensor attitude of the lower limb maintained by hypertonia of the extensor muscles may be regarded biologically as the posture of reflex standing, a condition akin to the extensor rigidity of the decerebrate animal.

Reflexes. The tendon reflexes on the paralysed side become exaggerated when shock has passed off, and clonus may be present in the flexors of the fingers, the quadriceps femoris, and the calf muscles. The superficial abdominal and cremasteric reflexes are diminished or lost and the plantar reflex becomes extensor. These reflex changes are more fully described on page 53. Wasting does not occur in the muscles as a result of a lesion of the corticospinal tract.

THE LOCALIZATION OF LESIONS OF THE CORTICOSPINAL TRACT

The following are the distinctive symptoms of lesions of the corticospinal tract at different points in its course.

CORTICAL LESIONS

The chief characteristic of cortical corticospinal lesions arises out of the wide surface distribution of the tract in this region. As a result a lesion of moderate size involves only a part of the motor cortex. In contrast to the conditions obtaining in the internal capsule, where the fibres are so crowded that even a small lesion usually produces a complete hemiplegia, cortical corticospinal lesions usually produce a monoplegia, that is, paralysis of the face or of one limb only, without, or with only slight, implication of parts of the body controlled by adjoining cortical areas.

Jacksonian Convulsions. Since the precentral cortex contains the bodies of the corticospinal cells, a lesion in this region may lead to excitation of the corticospinal fibres, which expresses itself as a focal convulsion. This is of the well-recognized type described by Hughlings Jackson and hence known as Jacksonian. Such a convulsion begins as a rule with clonic movements, rarely with tonic spasm, of a small part of the opposite side of the body, usually the thumb and index finger, the angle of the mouth, or the great toe, these movements being 'those that have the widest fields of low threshold excitability' (Walshe, 1943).

As the convulsion becomes more severe the initial movement becomes more violent and the movement spreads, in the case of a limb, centripetally, involving the flexor muscles predominantly. A convulsion beginning in a limb then involves the other limb on the same side centrifugally, and the face, and finally may become bilateral, when consciousness is usually lost. Up to a point it is true to say that the spread of the convulsion corresponds to the representation of movements in the motor cortex, but the cortical march must be interpreted in physiological and not in purely anatomical terms (see Walshe, 1943).

SUBCORTICAL LESIONS

In the corona radiata the corticospinal fibres are converging towards the internal capsule and are closer together than in the cortex. Subcortical lesions tend therefore to involve more fibres than cortical lesions of equal size, and it is usual to find that, though the weakness predominates in one limb, the whole of the opposite side of the body is to some extent affected. Adjacent thalamo-cortical sensory fibres may also be involved, causing impairment of postural sensibility and tactile discrimination and localization in the affected limbs. Damage to the optic radiation causes crossed homonymous hemianopia. A lesion in the internal capsule itself is likely to cause motor symptoms on the whole of the opposite side.

LESIONS IN THE MIDBRAIN

Here the proximity of the corticospinal fibres to the third nerve sometimes adds signs of localizing value. Thus we may encounter paralysis of the third nerve with hemiplegia on the opposite side (*Weber's syndrome*). Throughout the brain stem the two corticospinal tracts lie close together. Vascular lesions are often strictly unilateral, but space-occupying lesions, such as tumours, frequently involve both corticospinal tracts. The corticospinal fibres decussate at different levels, those destined for the opposite facial nucleus, for example, crossing at the junction of the midbrain and the pons, while those which are concerned in the movements of the limbs do not cross till they reach the corticospinal decussation in the medulla. A lesion in the midline situated anteriorly at the junction of the midbrain and pons may thus involve only the decussating fibres running to the facial nuclei, and so produce facial diplegia of the supranuclear type. This may be associated with bilateral paralysis of lateral conjugate ocular deviation, the supranuclear fibres for this movement crossing the midline at the same level.

LESIONS IN THE PONS

Owing to the higher level of decussation of the corticofacial fibres a unilateral corticospinal lesion in the pons does not cause weakness of the opposite side of the face, but only of the opposite bulbar muscles and limbs. But the lesion may also involve the facial nucleus or the intrapontine fibres of the facial nerve on the same side, thus causing one form of 'crossed hemiplegia'. Many forms of this have been described and named after their earliest observers.

Millard-Gubler syndrome consists of paralysis of the lateral rectus, with or without facial paralysis of the lower motor neurone type on one side and supranuclear paralysis of the bulbar muscles and limbs on the opposite side.

Foville's syndrome is similar to the Millard-Gubler syndrome, except that paralysis of conjugate ocular deviation to the side of the lesion takes the place of lateral rectus paralysis.

Ipsilateral paralysis of the jaw muscles due to involvement of the motor nucleus of the fifth nerve may be associated with either of these syndromes. When the lesion is situated deeply in the pons, near the midline, involvement of the medial lemniscus causes impairment of postural sensibility on the opposite side of the body. When the lesion is mainly in the lateral region of the pons the lemniscus escapes, but damage to the spinothalamic tract causes crossed analgesia and thermo-anaesthesia, with or without some impairment of sensibility in the trigeminal area on the side of the lesion, owing to involvement of the trigeminal fibres within the pons.

Horner's syndrome, paralysis of the ocular sympathetic, may also result from a lesion in the tegmentum of the pons.

LESIONS IN THE MEDULLA

Many varieties of crossed hemiplegia have been described as a result of unilateral medullary lesions. A lesion near the midline will involve the cortico-spinal fibres to the limbs above their decussation, together with the fibres of the hypoglossal nerve, causing unilateral paralysis of half of the tongue, with crossed hemiplegia of the limbs, to which loss of postural sensibility in the paralysed limbs may be added. When the lateral region of the medulla is affected as well there will also be paralysis of the soft palate and vocal cord, with Horner's syndrome and trigeminal analgesia and thermo-anaesthesia and some cerebellar deficiency, all on the side of the lesion, with loss of appreciation of pain, heat, and cold in the limbs and trunk on the opposite side. Vascular lesions in the midline of the medulla may involve both corticospinal tracts, leading to quadriplegia with unilateral paralysis of the tongue.

SPINAL HEMIPLEGIA

A unilateral lesion of the corticospinal tract in the spinal cord below the medulla and above the fifth cervical segment causes hemiplegia involving the limbs on the affected side but without paralysis of the muscles innervated by the cranial nerves.

DECEREBRATE MAN

Decerebrate rigidity in animals, according to Denny-Brown (1966), is due to overactivity of the gamma efferent fibres to the muscles resulting from release of a structure in the reticular formation of the lower pons from higher control. Its influence is mediated by the medial reticulospinal tract and it is seen when the brain stem is transected above the vestibular nuclei. There is increased tone in all the extensor muscles (see Brodal, 1969).

A condition which appears to be physiologically homologous with decerebration in the animal may occur in man, either in the form of a convulsion or as a prolonged state of muscular hypertonia without consciousness being invariably lost. The convulsions—'tonic' fits, or 'cerebellar' fits of Hughlings Jackson—are characterized by opisthotonos and rigid extension of all four limbs. The upper limbs are internally rotated at the shoulder, extended at the elbow and hyperpronated, and the fingers are extended at the metacarpophalangeal joints and flexed at the interphalangeal joints. The lower limbs are extended at the hip and knee, and the ankles and toes are plantar flexed. This human decerebrate attitude has been observed to result from lesions at the level of the upper part of the midbrain, such as tumours arising in the midbrain, and pineal tumours and tumours of the cerebellar vermis, which compress the midbrain from without. It may also be produced by diffuse cerebral disorders, such as anoxia, hydrocephalus, and diffuse sclerosis.

REFERENCES

BRAIN, W. R. (1927) On the significance of the flexor posture of the upper limb in hemi-plegia, with an account of a quadrupedal extensor reflex, *Brain*, **50**, 113.

BRODAL, A. (1969) *Neurological Anatomy in Relation to Clinical Medicine*, 2nd ed., New York.

CLARK, G. (1948) The mode of representation in the motor cortex, *Brain*, **71**, 320.

CURTIS, B. A., JACOBSON, S., and MARCUS, E. M. (1972) *An Introduction to the Neuro-sciences*, Philadelphia.

DENNY-BROWN, D. (1966) *The Cerebral Control of Movement*, Liverpool University Press, Liverpool.

DENNY-BROWN, D., and BOTTERELL, E. H. (1948) The motor functions of the agranular frontal cortex, *Res. Publ. Ass. nerv. ment. Dis.*, **27**, 235.

FOERSTER, O. (1931) The cerebral cortex in man, *Lancet*, **ii**, 309.

FOERSTER, O. (1936) The motor cortex in man in the light of Hughlings Jackson's doctrines, *Brain*, **59**, 135.

FULTON, J. F. (1943) *Physiology of the Nervous System*, 2nd ed., New York.

FULTON, J. F., and SHEEHAN, D. (1935) The uncrossed lateral pyramidal tract in higher primates, *J. Anat. (Lond.)*, **69**, 181.

GRANIT, R. (1970) *The Basis of Motor Control*, New York and London.

HOFF, E. C., and HOFF, H. E. (1934) Spinal terminations of the projection fibres from the motor cortex of primates, *Brain*, **57**, 454.

KREIG, W. J. S. (1966) *Functional Neuroanatomy*, 3rd ed., Evanston, Ill.

LANCE, J. W. (1970) *A Physiological Approach to Clinical Neurology*, London.

MAGOUN, H. W., and RHINES, R. (1947) *Spasticity*, Springfield, Ill.

PENFIELD, W., and JASPER, H. (1954) *Epilepsy and the Functional Anatomy of the Human Brain*, p. 60, London.

TOWER, S. S. (1940) Pyramidal lesions in the monkey, *Brain*, **63**, 36.

WALSH, E. G. (1963) *Physiology of the Nervous System*, 2nd ed., London.

WALSHE, F. M. R. (1942) The giant cells of Betz, the motor cortex and the pyramidal tract: a critical review, *Brain*, **65**, 409.

WALSHE, F. M. R. (1943) On the mode of representation of movements in the motor cortex, with special reference to 'convulsions beginning unilaterally' (Jackson), *Brain*, **66**, 104.

WALSHE, F. M. R. (1965) *Further Critical Studies in Neurology*, Edinburgh.

WILSON, S. A. K. (1920) On decerebrate rigidity in man and the occurrence of tonic fits, *Brain*, **43**, 220.

THE LOWER MOTOR NEURONE

The cell bodies of the lower motor neurones are situated in the motor nuclei of the brain stem and the anterior horns of the grey matter of the spinal cord. The larger cell bodies of the anterior horns give rise to the alpha motor neurones which act as the final common path of motor activity and innervate the voluntary muscles. Smaller cell bodies give origin to the gamma neurones which supply the intrafusal fibres of the muscle spindles. Each motor neurone is influenced by impulses reaching it from many nerve fibres—from the corticospinal tracts by way of interneurones and also from those nerve fibres which act as con-ductors in the reflex arcs. Between each such nerve terminal and the body of the motor neurone lies a synapse. An excitatory nerve fibre alters the synapse so as to depolarize the cell membrane of the motor neurone; an inhibitory fibre acts by hyperpolarizing it (Eccles, 1957).

The axons of the motor neurones pass into the cranial and spinal nerves, reaching the latter by way of the ventral roots, the motor functions of which were first recognized by Bell in 1811. From the spinal nerves they are distributed to the peripheral nerves, those destined for the limbs passing *en route* through the cervical, lumbar, and sacral plexuses. An alpha motor neurone and the muscle fibres which it supplies together constitute a motor unit; the physiological and histochemical characteristics of the different types of muscle fibres (so-called Types I and II) appear to be determined by the innervating neurones so that it can be inferred that there are at least two types of alpha neurones [see p. 990]. In human limb muscles, motor units each contain between 500 and 2,000 muscle fibres (see Sissons, 1974). Injury to the lower motor neurone leads to characteristic symptoms.

SYMPTOMS OF LESIONS OF THE LOWER MOTOR NEURONE

MUSCULAR WEAKNESS AND WASTING

Weakness or complete paralysis occurs in the affected muscles, according to the severity of the lesion. This is an impairment of the function of the muscle itself, and therefore is manifest equally in all movements in which the affected muscle normally plays a part.

MUSCULAR WASTING

Muscular wasting occurs in the affected muscles. This is conspicuous within two or three weeks of an acute lesion, such as acute poliomyelitis or division of a motor nerve, but develops very gradually in chronic disorders such as motor neurone disease.

DISTRIBUTION

The distribution of the weakness and wasting is the outcome of the grouping of the lower motor neurones at the point at which the damage occurs [see p. 30].

HYPOTONIA

Since muscle tone is dependent upon the integrity of the lower motor neurones [see p. 28], a lesion of this pathway causes hypotonia, which is manifested in flaccidity and a diminished resistance to stretching of the affected muscles.

REFLEXES

The reflexes in which the affected muscles take part are usually diminished or lost. An apparent exception to the rule that hypotonia and loss of reflexes result from lower motor neurone lesions is found when the same patient has also a lesion of the upper motor neurone, as in motor neurone disease. In such cases the hypertonia and increased tendon reflexes produced by the upper motor neurone lesion may more than counterbalance the opposite effects of the lower motor neurone lesion, depending upon which lesion predominates. Such patients may show increased tendon reflexes in the wasted muscles.

MUSCULAR FASCICULATION

Fascicular twitching of muscles is seen in its most typical form as a result of chronic degeneration of the anterior horn cells in progressive muscular atrophy. In such cases each twitch involves a group of muscle fibres. It does not occur when these cells are rapidly injured or destroyed as in the acute stage of poliomyelitis; and it is rare when they suffer from compression as in syringomyelia or spinal tumour. It is occasionally seen in peripheral nerve or root lesions but is absent in muscular dystrophy; it occurs rarely in thyrotoxic myopathy and polymyositis. Benign fasciculation may occur in normal individuals, especially in the orbicularis oculi (myokymia of the lower eyelid) and less often in the first interosseous space or calf muscles; it is rarely diffuse, as in generalized myokymia [p. 1001].

MUSCULAR CONTRACTURES

Muscular contracture, leading to permanent shortening, may occur in muscles of which the lower motor neurones are damaged, for example in the facial muscles after Bell's paralysis. More often it develops in their antagonists, the action of which is no longer opposed by the paralysed muscles. An example of this is contracture of the calf muscles following paralysis of the anterior tibial group and the peronei in poliomyelitis. Appropriate splinting and passive movements are required to prevent such contractures.

TROPHIC CHANGES

Lesions of the lower motor neurones are often attended by so-called trophic changes. The affected extremity is cold and cyanosed, the finger- and toe-nails are brittle, and the bones are smaller and lighter than normal. These changes are probably due partly to disuse, with loss of the influence of muscular action upon the circulation and the development of the bones, and partly to vasomotor paralysis from destruction of the vasoconstrictor fibres of the sympathetic.

ELECTRODIAGNOSIS

Many methods of investigation are now available in order to detect evidence of lower motor neurone lesions. The traditional technique of seeking Erb's so-called reaction of degeneration (loss of the response to faradism with retention of a response to galvanism) has been supplanted by the charting of strength-duration curves, utilizing square-wave stimuli of known duration delivered by a constant-current or constant-voltage stimulator. Even this method which, when carefully applied, can often distinguish between partial and complete denervation of a muscle, is now used much less often in view of the much more precise information concerning neuromuscular function which can be obtained by means of measurements of motor nerve conduction velocity and of terminal latency [see pp. 886–8] and/or by electromyography, a technique which involves recording of the electrical activity occurring in voluntary muscle at rest and during activity, using a needle electrode inserted into the muscle [pp. 882–6].

MUSCLE TONE

Muscle tone, as Sherrington showed, is reflex in origin. The muscle spindles are the receptors in the muscles which respond to stretch by sending impulses which travel in the largest afferent fibres from the muscles to the spinal cord. The muscle spindles are themselves innervated by the smallest, gamma, efferent fibres in the ventral spinal roots [FIG. 6], and these have been shown to regulate the response of the muscle spindles, acting synergically with external stretch. So by means of the stretch or myotatic reflex and the lengthening and shortening reactions, also described by Sherrington, muscle tone is reflexly maintained and adjusted to the needs of posture and movement. Hence interruption of the reflex arc on its afferent or efferent side leads to hypotonia.

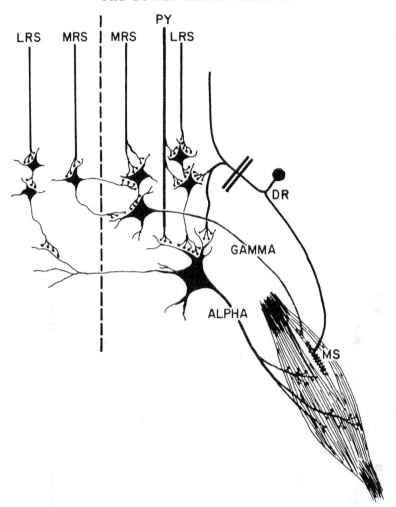

FIG. 6. Diagram to show how the gamma neurone providing motor innervation to the muscle spindle (MS) can, by increasing its sensitivity, facilitate afferent impulses from the annulospiral ending to provide excitation for alpha motor neurones of the same muscle. The medial reticulospinal tracts (MRS) drive the gamma neurone. The lateral reticulospinal tract (LRS) and pyramidal tract (PY) end on the alpha system. The broken line represents the midline. Decussating pathways from the opposite side of spinal cord have access to both types of activation of the alpha motor neurones. Section of the dorsal roots (DR) at the point shown by the bars blocks activation via the gamma neurone. (From Denny-Brown, D. (1966) *The Cerebral Control of Movement*, by kind permission of the author and Liverpool University Press)

This spinal reflex mechanism is profoundly influenced by higher levels of the nervous system. It is depressed by spinal shock. As the cerebellum is facilitatory to the stretch reflex cerebellar deficiency causes hypotonia. The reticular formation is also facilitatory, as is seen when removal of higher inhibitory control over it causes decerebrate rigidity [see p. 25]. Loss of corticospinal influence also causes spasticity [see p. 22]. The influence of the striatum is complex, but damage to the substantia nigra causes hypertonia (Magoun and Rhines, 1947; Kuffler and Hunt, 1952).

SEGMENTATION IN THE SPINAL CORD

It will be remembered that early in fetal development the body shows a division into a series of segments or metameres. This primitive segmentation to a large extent determines the subsequent plan of the lower motor and first sensory neurones at their emergence from, and entrance into, the spinal cord. Corresponding to each spinal segment is one pair of spinal nerves composed of the ventral and dorsal roots of that segment. The cell bodies of the first sensory neurone, which lie in the dorsal root ganglia, are completely separated in each segment from those of the segments above and below. The cell bodies of the alpha motor neurones, however, lie in longitudinal columns in the anterior horns, hence their segmental grouping is less distinct. Nevertheless, the emergence of their axons by a series of separate ventral roots is the basis of a motor segmental arrangement, for we may regard as a segment of the cord, from the aspect of motility, that group of anterior horn cells of which the axons emerge by one pair of ventral roots and join one pair of spinal nerves.

THE SEGMENTAL REPRESENTATION OF MUSCLES

As we have seen, the cells of the anterior horns lie in longitudinal columns and those which innervate a single muscle commonly extend over more than one segment longitudinally. Further, a number of such longitudinal columns may be recognized cut transversely in a transverse section of the cord. Hence several muscles may be represented in the same segment. It follows that complete destruction of the anterior horn cells in one segment, or of their axons in one ventral root or spinal nerve, causes weakness of all those muscles which are innervated from that segment, but completely paralyses only such as have no nerve supply from adjacent segments. Sharrard (1955) showed that groups of anterior horn cell bodies which innervate specific muscles occupy a constant position in certain spinal segments, and Tomlinson et al. (1973) have shown that the numbers of limb motor neurones in different segments of the human spinal cord are also remarkably constant.

Through the cervical and lumbosacral plexuses the axons of the lower motor neurones are redistributed and enter into new groupings in the peripheral nerves. Consequently, the fibres from a single spinal segment may reach several peripheral nerves, and conversely, a single peripheral nerve may receive fibres from several spinal segments. Thus we can distinguish between a lesion of a spinal segment, ventral root, or spinal nerve, on the one hand, and a lesion of a peripheral nerve on the other, because the resulting muscular weakness has a distinctive anatomical distribution. For example, the fifth cervical spinal segment innervates the supraspinatus and infraspinatus, deltoid, biceps, brachialis, and brachioradialis, muscles which receive their peripheral nerve supply from the suprascapular, axillary, musculocutaneous, and radial nerves respectively. These muscles cannot be paralysed by a lesion involving any single peripheral nerve, nor could a peripheral nerve lesion affect them without affecting others. Such a distribution of muscular weakness indicates a segmental lesion.

On the other hand, if the brachioradialis muscle is paralysed in association with the triceps and the extensors of the wrist and fingers, this grouping points to a lesion of the radial nerve which supplies all these muscles.

MUSCULAR SUPPLY OF PERIPHERAL NERVES

[Modified from Bing, R. (1927).]

A. PLEXUS CERVICALIS (C_1–C_4)

Nn. cervicales	Mm. longus colli	Flexion, extension, and rotation of the neck
	Mm. scaleni	Elevation of ribs (inspiration)
N. phrenicus	Diaphragma	Inspiration

B. PLEXUS BRACHIALIS (C_5–T_2)

N. thoracic. ant.	M. pect. maj. et min.	Adduction and forward depression of the arm
N. thoracic. long.	M. serrat. ant.	Fixation of the scapula during elevation of the arm
N. dorsalis scap.	M. levator scapul.	Elevation of the scapula
	Mm. rhomboidei	Elevation and drawing inwards of the scapula
N. suprascap.	M. supraspinatus	Elevation and external rotation of the arm
	M. infraspinatus	External rotation of the arm
N. subscapul.	M. latissimus dors. }	Internal rotation and dorsal adduction of the arm
	M. teres major }	
	M. subscapularis	Internal rotation of the arm
N. axillaris	M. deltoideus	Elevation of the arm to the horizontal
	M. teres minor	External rotation of the arm
N. musculocut.	M. biceps brach.	Flexion and supination of the forearm
	M. coracobrachialis	Flexion and adduction of the forearm
	M. brachialis	Flexion of the forearm
N. medianus	M. pronator teres	Pronation
	M. flexor carpi rad.	Flexion and radial flexion of the hand
	M. palm. long.	Flexion of the hand
	M. flex. digit. superficialis	Flexion of the middle phalanges of the fingers
	M. flex. poll. long.	Flexion of the terminal phalanx of the thumb
	M. flex. digit. (radial portion)	Flexion of the terminal phalanges of the index and middle fingers
	M. abduct. poll. brev.	Abduction of the first metacarpal
	M. flex. poll. brev.	Flexion of the first phalanx of the thumb
	M. opponens poll.	Opposition of the first metacarpal
N. ulnaris	M. flexor carpi uln.	Flexion and ulnar flexion of the hand
	M. flex. digit. prof. (ulnar portion)	Flexion of the terminal phalanges of the ring and little fingers
	M. adductor poll.	Adduction of the first metacarpal
	Mm. hypothenares	Abduction, opposition, and flexion of the little finger
	Mm. lumbricales	Flexion of the first phalanges, extension of the others
	Mm. interossei	The same; in addition, abduction and adduction of the fingers
N. radialis	M. triceps brach.	Extension of the forearm
	M. brachioradialis	Flexion of the forearm
	M. extensor carpi rad.	Extension and radial flexion of the hand
	M. extensor digit.	Extension of the first phalanges of the fingers
	M. extensor digit. minimi	Extension of the first phalanx of the little finger

N. radialis	M. extensor carpi uln.	Extension and ulnar flexion of the hand
	M. supinator brevis	Supination of the forearm
	M. abduct. poll. longus	Abduction of the first metacarpal
	M. extensor poll. brevis	Extension of the first phalanx of the thumb
	M. extensor poll. longus	Abduction of the first metacarpal and extension of the terminal phalanx of the thumb
	M. extensor indic. prop.	Extension of the first phalanx of the index finger

C. Nn. Thoracales (T_1–T_{12})

| | Mm. thoracici et ab-dominales | Elevation of the ribs, expiration, compression of abdominal viscera, etc. |

D. Plexus Lumbalis (T_{12}–L_4)

N. femoralis	M. iliopsoas	Flexion of the hip
	M. sartorius	Internal rotation of the leg
	M. quadriceps	Extension of the leg
N. obturatorius	M. pectineus	⎫
	M. adductor longus	
	M. adductor brevis	⎬ Adduction of the thigh
	M. adductor magnus	
	M. gracilis	⎭
	M. obturator extern.	Adduction and external rotation of the thigh

E. Plexus Sacralis (L_5–S_5)

N. gluteus sup.	M. gluteus med.	⎫ Abduction and internal rotation of the thigh
	M. gluteus min.	⎭
	M. tens. fasciae latae	Flexion of the thigh
	M. piriformis	External rotation of the thigh
N. gluteus inf.	M. gluteus max.	Extension of the thigh
N. ischiadicus (sciatic nerve)	M. obturator int.	⎫ External rotation of the thigh
	Mm. gemelli	⎬
	M. quadratus fem.	⎭
	M. biceps femoris	⎫
	M. semitendinosus	⎬ Flexion of the leg
	M. semimembranosus	⎭
N. peroneus:		
(a) Prof.	M. tibialis ant.	Dorsal flexion and inversion of the foot
	M. extens. digit. long.	Extension of the toes
	M. extens. hall. long.	Extension of the great toe
	M. extens. digit. brev.	Extension of the toes
	M. extens. hall. brev.	Extension of the great toe
(b) Superf.	Mm. peronei	Dorsal flexion and eversion of the foot
N. tibialis	M. gastrocnemius	⎱ Plantar flexion of the foot
	M. soleus	⎰
	M. tibialis post.	Plantar flexion and inversion of the foot
	M. flex. digit. long.	Flexion of the terminal phalanges, II–V
	M. flex. halluc. long.	Flexion of the terminal phalanx of the great toe
	M. flex. digit. brev.	Flexion of the middle phalanges, II–V
	M. flex. halluc. brev.	Flexion of the first phalanx of the great toe
	Mm. interossei plant.	Movements of the toes
N. pudendus	Mm. perinei et sphinct.	Closure of sphincters, co-operation in sexual act

SEGMENTAL INNERVATION OF MUSCLES OF UPPER EXTREMITY
(Modified from Bing, R. (1927))

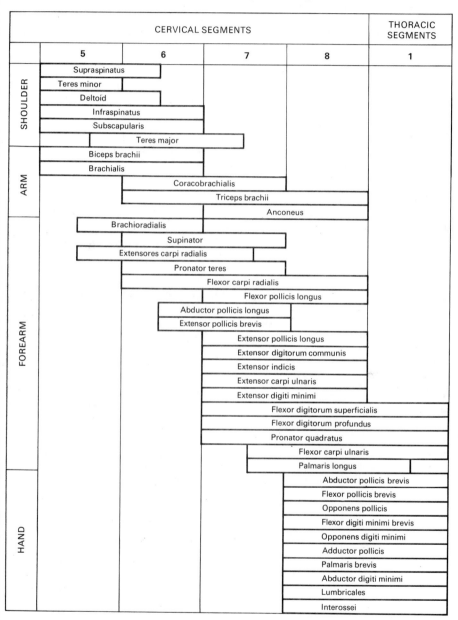

SEGMENTAL INNERVATION OF TRUNK MUSCLES
(Modified from Bing, R. (1927))

SEGMENTAL INNERVATION OF MUSCLES OF LOWER EXTREMITY
(Modified from Bing, R. (1927))

Region	Muscle	T12	L1	L2	L3	L4	L5	S1	S2
HIP	Iliopsoas		●	●	●				
HIP	Tensor fasciae latae					●	●		
HIP	Gluteus medius					●	●	●	
HIP	Gluteus minimus					●	●	●	
HIP	Quadratus femoris					●	●	●	
HIP	Gemellus inferior					●	●	●	
HIP	Gemellus superior					●	●	●	
HIP	Gluteus maximus						●	●	●
HIP	Obturator internus						●	●	●
HIP	Piriformis							●	●
THIGH	Sartorius			●	●				
THIGH	Pectineus			●	●				
THIGH	Adductor longus			●	●				
THIGH	Quadriceps femoris			●	●	●			
THIGH	Gracilis			●	●				
THIGH	Adductor brevis			●	●				
THIGH	Obturator externus				●	●			
THIGH	Adductor magnus			●	●				
THIGH	Adductor minimus			●	●				
THIGH	Articularis genus				●	●			
LEG	Semitendinosus					●	●	●	
LEG	Semimembranosus					●	●		
LEG	Biceps femoris						●	●	●
LEG	Tibialis anterior					●	●		
LEG	Extensor hallucis longus						●	●	
LEG	Popliteus					●	●		
LEG	Plantaris					●	●		
LEG	Extensor digitorum longus					●	●	●	
LEG	Soleus						●	●	●
LEG	Gastrocnemius						●	●	●
LEG	Peroneus longus						●	●	
LEG	Peroneus brevis						●	●	
LEG	Tibialis posterior					●	●		
FOOT	Flexor digitorum longus						●	●	
FOOT	Flexor hallucis longus						●	●	
FOOT	Extensor hallucis brevis					●	●	●	
FOOT	Extensor digitorum brevis					●	●	●	
FOOT	Flexor digitorum brevis					●	●	●	
FOOT	Abductor hallucis					●	●	●	
FOOT	Flexor hallucis brevis						●	●	
FOOT	Lumbricales						●	●	
FOOT	Abductor hallucis							●	●
FOOT	Abductor digiti minimi							●	●
FOOT	Flexor digiti minimi brevis							●	●
FOOT	Opponens digiti minimi							●	●
FOOT	Quadratus plantae							●	●
FOOT	Interossei							●	●

REFERENCES

BING, R. (1927) *Compendium of Regional Diagnosis*, pp. 39–49, London.

DENNY-BROWN, D., and PENNYBACKER, J. B. (1938) Fibrillation and fasciculation in voluntary muscle, *Brain*, **61,** 311.

ECCLES, J. C. (1957) *The Physiology of Nerve Cells*, Baltimore.

KUFFLER, S. W., and HUNT, C. C. (1952) The mammalian small-nerve fibers, a system for efferent nervous regulation of muscle spindle discharge, *Res. Publ. Ass. nerv. ment. Dis.*, **30,** 24.

MAGOUN, H. W., and RHINES, R. (1947) *Spasticity*, Springfield, Ill.

MEDICAL RESEARCH COUNCIL (1976) *Aids to the Examination of the Peripheral Nervous System* (M.R.C. Memorandum No. 45), London.

SHARRARD, W. J. W. (1955) The distribution of the permanent paralysis in the lower limb in poliomyelitis, *J. Bone Jt Surg.*, **37B,** 540.

SISSONS, H. A. (1974) The anatomy of the motor unit, in *Disorders of Voluntary Muscle*, ed. Walton, J. N., 3rd ed., Edinburgh and London.

TOMLINSON, B. E., IRVING, D., and REBEIZ, J. J. (1973) Total numbers of limb motor neurones in the human lumbosacral cord and an analysis of the accuracy of various sampling procedures, *J. neurol. Sci.*, **20,** 313.

SENSATION

THE EXAMINATION OF SENSATION

The neurologist is concerned with sensibility primarily for the purpose of localizing lesions in the nervous system and determining their nature. His methods of investigation are therefore more 'rough and ready' than those of the experimental psychologist, and have been adopted on account of their practical value for his immediate purpose.

SPONTANEOUS SENSATIONS

The investigation should begin with a careful inquiry whether the patient has experienced any abnormal spontaneous sensations or paraesthesiae. The commonest such sensation is pain, but in addition parts of the body may be described as feeling hot, cold, numb, dead, or heavy, and such abnormal feelings as constriction, itching, tingling, 'pins and needles', and 'electric shocks' may be experienced or else the affected part may feel swollen or as if surrounded by a tight band or plaster cast. When a patient complains of an abnormal sensation it is necessary to ascertain its situation and duration, whether it irradiates and if so in what direction, whether it is excited by movement or by any external stimulus, and whether it is attended by hypersensitivity of the skin to painful or other stimuli.

'Root-pains' are pains due to a lesion of one or more spinal dorsal roots and are experienced in the segmental areas innervated by the affected roots. They may be excited or intensified by coughing or sneezing or changes of posture.

A patient with a lesion of the posterior columns of the spinal cord in the cervical region may complain of a feeling like an electric shock radiating through the body on flexing or extending the cervical spine (Lhermitte's sign).

A strange sensory abnormality is the 'phantom limb'. A patient who has lost a limb by amputation may continue to feel as if the limb were still there, and may even experience pain in the phantom limb. Similarly a patient who has lost postural sensation in a limb or limbs as a result of a lesion of the spinal cord or brain may imagine that he feels his anaesthetic limb and that it occupies a posture different from its real position.

OBJECTIVE SENSORY TESTS

Light Touch. The appreciation of light touch is most conveniently investigated by means of a very small wisp of cotton wool applied to the shaved skin, care being taken that no pressure is exerted upon the skin. The patient with his eyes closed is asked to reply each time he feels a touch.

Pressure Touch. Pressure touch is similarly investigated by pressing with a blunt object such as the unsharpened end of a pencil.

Localization of Touch. The part of the body under investigation is screened from the patient's eyes and after he has been touched he is asked to name the spot or to point to it. For greater accuracy he may indicate it upon a diagram.

Superficial Pain. Superficial pain is investigated by pricking the skin with a pin or needle. It should be noted that this stimulus evokes a tactile sensation of sharpness as well as a feeling of pain. The patient's attention must therefore be directed to the painful element in the feeling. Two sensory effects of pinprick have now been distinguished—an immediate and a slightly delayed sensation of pain, differing somewhat in quality and known as 'first' and 'second' pain. In mapping out cutaneous areas of analgesia or hyperalgesia the point of a pin may be dragged along the skin, the patient being asked to say when the change to normal or exaggerated painful sensibility occurs.

Pressure Pain. Deep pressure, if sufficiently vigorous, normally excites pain. This is most simply tested by compressing a muscle between the fingers and thumb or by squeezing a tendon such as the Achilles tendon.

Temperature. For testing appreciation of temperature, metal tubes, made of copper or silver, should be used, since glass is a relatively poor conductor of heat. For ordinary purposes one tube should be filled with ice and the other with water at a temperature of 45 °C. The tubes are applied to the skin and the patient is asked to describe his sensations. If the water is too hot confusion may arise, since a sensation of pain may be excited.

Perceptual Rivalry. Sometimes loss of cutaneous sensibility may be demonstrable only if corresponding points on both sides of the body are stimulated simultaneously, the stimulus on the abnormal side being ignored (tactile inattention) [see p. 119].

Postural Sensibility. Postural sensibility, or sense of position, is tested by placing a segment of a limb in a certain position and asking the patient with his eyes closed to describe its posture or to imitate it with the opposite limb.

Passive Movement. Power of appreciating passive movement is tested by passively moving a segment of a limb at a joint and finding the angle through which it has to be moved in order that the patient can appreciate the movement. The part to be moved should always be grasped in such a way that the observer's fingers are applied to surfaces parallel to the plane of movement to eliminate the perception of variations in their pressure. Minimal degrees of movement of less than a millimetre are appreciated at the joints of the fingers and toes more easily than at the more proximal joints of the limbs. Normally a movement of a few degrees is recognized at the interphalangeal and metacarpo- and metatarsophalangeal joints.

Vibration. To test the appreciation of vibration, a tuning-fork beating 128 times a second is struck and applied to the part to be investigated. Normally the characteristic tingling sensation is readily felt. Normally also the patient is asked to say when he ceases to feel the vibration and the fork is then transferred to another part of the body where the vibration again becomes perceptible. In this way the extent of the loss or impairment of vibration sense can be assessed.

Tactile Discrimination. Tactile discrimination is measured by ascertaining the distance which two compass-points require to be separated in order that the patient may appreciate them as two and not one. Special compasses with blunt points are used, and these are furnished with a scale which indicates the distance the points are separated. The part to be tested is successively touched with two points and with one in a random order, and the number of correct answers and errors noted. The corresponding part on the opposite side, when normal, is used as a control, and to determine the normal threshold, that is, the distance of separation necessary for accurate discrimination. The normal threshold for two-point discrimination is 1–2 mm on the lips, 2–3 mm on the tips of the fingers, and 2–3 cm on the soles of the feet.

Appreciation of Form. Stereognosis, or the appreciation of form in three dimensions, is tested by asking the patient with his eyes closed to recognize common objects placed in his hand. Astereognosis, an inability to recognize objects when all other sensory modalities are intact, a form of tactile agnosia, should be distinguished from stereoanaesthesia, a similar difficulty in recognizing shape due to impairment of tactile discrimination or other obvious sensory abnormalities. Defects in the appreciation of form in two dimensions can be recognized by asking the patient to identify numbers drawn with a blunt object on the affected part.

THE FIRST SENSORY NEURONE

ANATOMY AND PHYSIOLOGY

The first sensory neurone is the path by which sensory impulses from the periphery reach the central nervous system. The cell bodies of the first sensory neurones are situated in the spinal dorsal root ganglia and in the corresponding sensory ganglia of the cranial nerves. They are bipolar cells, one process being distributed to the periphery and the other entering the spinal cord or brain stem. The peripheral process in some instances enters into relation with sensory end-organs, which are the specific receptors for certain forms of sensibility though there is evidence that some receptors are sensitive to more than one kind of stimulus. The nerve fibres concerned in the appreciation of pain appear to be devoid of end-organs and to terminate as free nerve endings. The receptors for heat and cold are not evenly distributed throughout the skin, but are situated in localized heat and cold spots. Krause's end-bulbs are believed to be the specific endings for cold and Ruffini's corpuscles for heat, though some believe that the Golgi–Mazzoni endings are also responsive to heat. Merkel's discs and Meissner's corpuscles are end-organs which are probably concerned in the appreciation of light touch. The hairs are also tactile organs and the hair follicles are richly supplied with nerve endings. Tickle is a form of tactile sensation, and itching is conducted by pain fibres. The Pacinian corpuscles are distributed to the deeper parts of the dermis and to the tendons, periosteum, and the neighbourhood of the joints. These are responsive to pressure and other mechanical stimuli. In addition muscles and tendons possess specialized sensory end-organs—the muscle spindles and Golgi tendon organs. Each dorsal root fibre breaks up to supply many nerve endings, sometimes hundreds, disposed in three dimensions, i.e. surface area and depth.

Sensibility may be divided into somatic and visceral (interoceptive) forms of sensation. Somatic sensibility again may be divided into exteroceptive and proprioceptive forms. Exteroceptive sensibility is concerned with the appreciation of stimuli coming from outside the body and includes cutaneous sensibility and the special senses. Proprioceptive sensibility is the appreciation of the posture and movements of the body itself. Proprioceptive impulses are derived from the labyrinths and the muscles, tendons, and joints. Not all proprioceptive afferent impulses reach consciousness. Many are concerned in reflex activities at the spinal level or influence the cerebellum in its control of movement and posture.

Sensory fibres in the peripheral nerves vary in size and in the rate at which they conduct impulses. Group A fibres in peripheral nerves are heavily myelinated somatic efferent and afferent fibres, 1-22 μm in diameter, which conduct at 5-120 m/s. Group B fibres are finely myelinated fibres, 1-3 μm in diameter, conducting at 3-15 m/s, and are mainly preganglionic fibres of the autonomic system. Group C fibres are unmyelinated, 0·3-1·3 μm in diameter, which conduct at 0·5-2·0 m/s; some of these are postganglionic autonomic fibres but others carry somatic afferent impulses. Touch, pressure, and proprioception are believed to be carried by A fibres, while some painful and thermal impulses also travel in A fibres but most are believed to be subserved by C fibres. Two varieties of painful response to a single stimulus have been distinguished— first, pain which is 'bright' or pricking in quality, and second, pain which is burning and is experienced only after a brief delay.

There are two principal opposing theories relating to pain sensation; one, the specificity theory, suggests that pain is a specific sensory modality with its own specific central and peripheral apparatus for recording and perception; the other, the pattern theory, suggests that the nerve impulse pattern subserving pain is caused by excessive stimulation of non-specific receptors. As Melzack and Wall (1965) pointed out, neither theory satisfactorily explains the observed facts. In their so-called 'gate theory' they propose that interneurones in the substantia gelatinosa of the spinal cord exercise a modulating effect upon sensory input, before this activates the first central transmission (T) cells in the dorsal horn of the cord which stimulate central mechanisms responsible for response and perception. They suggest that tonic activity in small C fibres keeps open the gate and allows the onward transmission of painful sensations. Activity in large A fibres is, by contrast, essentially inhibitory and tends to close the gate. Hence the final discharge from the T cells and thus the perception of pain is dependent upon the relative activity in large and small fibres. Counter-irritation, as by scratching or rubbing, increases large fibre discharge and so reduces pain. Not all of the recent physiological evidence supports the gate theory in its entirety (Iggo, 1972) but it is a useful working hypothesis.

Hyperalgesia is a term which has been used to identify an increased sensitivity to painful stimuli when pain is apparently evoked from skin or deeper structures, apparently at a lower threshold than normally. In fact, however, in most such cases, attempts to measure the pain threshold quantitatively indicate that it is raised and the abnormal and unpleasant quality of the painful sensation evoked is better referred to as *hyperpathia*. This phenomenon can generally be explained by an excessive continuing stimulation of C fibres, thus keeping the 'gate' open, or by a selective loss of A fibres, thus reducing inhibition, such as may be seen in cases of post-herpetic neuralgia (Noordenbos, 1968). Hyperpathia may also occur as a result of lesions in the spinothalamic tract or thalamus. The phenomenon of *referred pain*, an irradiation of pain into a specific skin area when a viscus or a muscle is the site of the lesion (e.g. pain in the centre of the chest, left arm, and jaw in cardiac infarction) can be explained by central summation mechanisms in relation to the gate theory as there is a widespread, diffuse monosynaptic input to the T cells of the spinal cord, often from relatively distant afferents (Mendell and Wall, 1965).

CUTANEOUS SENSORY SEGMENTATION

Primitive organisms frequently exhibit metameric segmentation of the body, and this arrangement is evident in the human fetus during the early stages of its development. Each somatic segment or metamere is linked to the corresponding segment of the neuraxis by a pair of spinal nerves. In the course of evolution the specialization of the anterior end of the organism to form the head, and the growth of the complicated motor and sensory functions of the limbs have interfered with the primitive metameric segmentation of the nervous system, which in man is now found in its simplest form only in the thoracic region.

Each spinal nerve is formed by a fusion of one ventral and one dorsal spinal root, the ventral root conveying efferent and the dorsal mainly afferent fibres. The sensory character of the dorsal roots was first recognized by Magendie in 1822. After this fusion the spinal nerve divides peripherally into its ventral and dorsal primary divisions, both containing motor and sensory fibres. The dorsal primary division conveys motor fibres to the muscles of the spine and sensory fibres to the overlying cutaneous area. The ventral primary division in its simplest form, for example in the mid-thoracic region, supplies motor fibres to the intercostal muscles and sensory fibres to a narrow zone extending horizontally round the thorax on one side as far as the middle line. At the cervical and lumbosacral enlargements of the cord the arrangement is complicated by the formation of the limb plexuses, in which several of the ventral primary divisions unite and subsequently subdivide to form the peripheral nerves to the limbs. Through the intervention of the plexuses a single spinal nerve may send both motor and sensory contributions to several peripheral nerves, and, conversely, a single peripheral nerve may receive contributions from several spinal nerves. It follows that the sensory loss resulting from interruption of a peripheral nerve differs in its distribution from that produced by interruption of a posterior root or spinal nerve. A segmental or radicular cutaneous area—dermatome—is an area of skin which receives its sensory supply from a single dorsal root and spinal nerve. In the trunk these segmental areas still exhibit a metameric arrangement. In the limbs this has been modified, but as a rule the segmental areas occupy elongated zones in the long axis of the limb [FIG. 7]. Owing to the specialization of the ventral primary divisions of the lower cervical and first thoracic spinal nerves in the innervation of the upper limb, these have lost their cutaneous supply to the trunk anteriorly, and at the level of the second

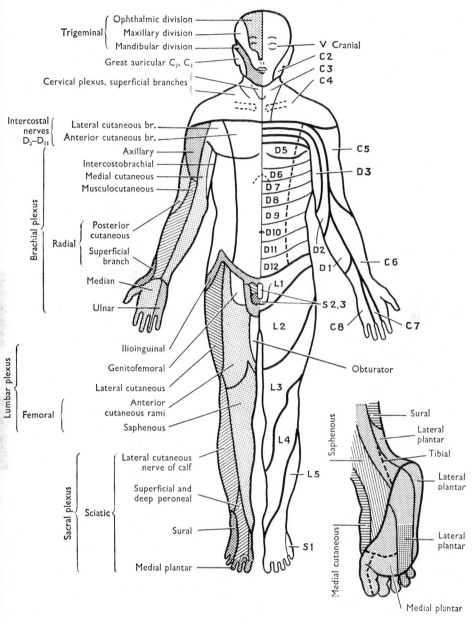

ANTERIOR ASPECT

FIG. 7 a. Cutaneous areas of distribution of spinal segments and the peripheral nerves

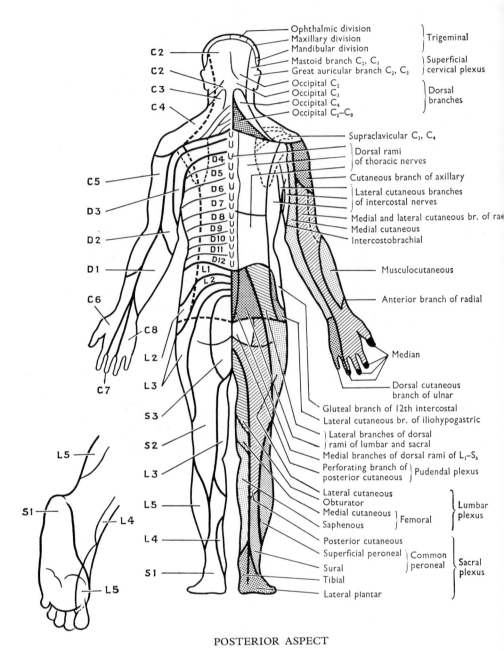

Ophthalmic division
Maxillary division — Trigeminal
Mandibular division
Mastoid branch C₂, C₃ — Superficial
Great auricular branch C₂, C₃ — cervical plexus
Occipital C₂
Occipital C₃ — Dorsal
Occipital C₄ — branches
Occipital C₅–C₈

Supraclavicular C₃, C₄

Dorsal rami
of thoracic nerves

Cutaneous branch of axillary

Lateral cutaneous branches
of intercostal nerves

Medial and lateral cutaneous br. of ra

Medial cutaneous

Intercostobrachial

Musculocutaneous

Anterior branch of radial

Median

Dorsal cutaneous
branch of ulnar

Gluteal branch of 12th intercostal

Lateral cutaneous br. of iliohypogastric

Lateral branches of dorsal
rami of lumbar and sacral

Medial branches of dorsal rami of L₁–S₆

Perforating branch of
posterior cutaneous — Pudendal plexus

Lateral cutaneous
Obturator
Medial cutaneous — Femoral — Lumbar plexus
Saphenous

Posterior cutaneous

Superficial peroneal — Common
Sural — peroneal — Sacral plexus
Tibial

Lateral plantar

POSTERIOR ASPECT

FIG. 7 b. Cutaneous areas of distribution of spinal segments and the peripheral nerves rib the fourth cervical segmental cutaneous area is contiguous with the second thoracic. The lower six thoracic spinal nerves supply the abdominal wall as low as the inguinal ligament. Probably owing to the fact that the dorsal primary divisions of the spinal nerves take no part in the formation of the limb plexuses, all spinal segments appear to be represented in the cutaneous supply of the back.

There is considerable overlapping of contiguous segmental cutaneous areas, hence the division of a single dorsal root does not cause any sensory loss detectable by ordinary clinical methods (Foerster). There is evidence that each root supplies fibres for pain, heat, and cold to a larger area than that to which it supplies fibres for light touch.

In the sensory innervation of the head the trigeminal nerve represents a fusion of the sensory supply of several segments, though the seventh, ninth, and tenth cranial nerves still possess rudimentary sensory branches distributed to the neighbourhood of the auricle. The posterior and inferior boundary of the trigeminal cutaneous area is contiguous with those of the first and second cervical segments respectively.

SENSORY PATHS IN THE SPINAL CORD

As we have seen, all sensory fibres from the limbs and trunk enter the spinal cord by the dorsal roots. After entering the cord these incoming fibres lie on the medial side of the apex of the posterior horn of grey matter, in the outer part of the fasciculus cuneatus, where they divide into ascending and descending branches. The unmyelinated descending branches, which form Lissauer's tract, terminate in the grey matter after passing downwards through a few segments. The myelinated descending fibres, which are relatively fewer, also synapse in the posterior horn after traversing a few segments. The ascending fibres, both myelinated and unmyelinated, pass upwards in the lateral part of the posterior column. They may be divided into three groups in accordance with their respective distributions [FIG. 8].

1. Some of the myelinated ascending fibres continue to pass upwards in the posterior column of the same side and terminate in the medulla in the nuclei

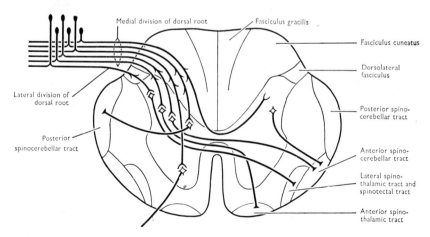

FIG. 8. Spinal cord and dorsal root, showing the divisions of the dorsal root, the collaterals of the dorsal root fibres, and some of the connections which are established by them

gracilis and cuneatus. In their upward course the fibres of lowest origin pass gradually towards the midline as they are joined on their outer side by fibres from higher roots. Thus the fibres from the sacral roots come to lie nearest the midline, with those from the lumbar roots to their lateral side, and fibres from the cervical roots are the most laterally placed. Hence those fibres derived from the lower limb pass upwards in the fasciculus gracilis, while those from the upper limb are found in the fasciculus cuneatus. The fibres of the posterior column convey impulses concerned with the appreciation of posture and passive movements of the joints and of the vibration of a tuning-fork. It is probable that some fibres concerned with the sensation of light touch also pass up in the posterior column as far as the medulla.

The fact that tactile discrimination, i.e. the ability to recognize as two the points of a compass simultaneously applied and that tactile localization may be impaired after lesions of the posterior columns, does not mean that these are distinct modalities of sensation mediated by the posterior columns but that they are judgements depending upon the integrity of the pathways subserving light touch.

2. The second group of entering fibres, again largely myelinated, pass up in the posterior column of the same side for a considerable distance, but ultimately enter the posterior horn of grey matter, round the cells in which they terminate. From these cells further fibres take origin and cross the midline in the grey and anterior white commissures to reach the opposite anterior column. There they turn upwards and constitute the anterior spinothalamic tract. These are the remaining fibres concerned in the relatively crude appreciation of touch.

3. The remaining fibres of the dorsal roots are those which ascend in the posterior column for the shortest distance, usually through only about three segments and never through more than five or six; many are unmyelinated. They also end among the cells of the posterior horn; it is at this point that dendrites from the cells of the substantia gelatinosa exercise their modulating influence, according to the gate theory. Fibres of the second relay take origin from these cells and, crossing the midline, like those of the previous group, enter the anterolateral column more posteriorly, and turning upwards constitute the lateral spinothalamic tract. These fibres conduct impulses concerned with the appreciation of pain, heat, and cold, those for pain lying dorsal to those for temperature. There is some evidence that there exists a lamination of the fibres of the spinothalamic tracts similar to that of the posterior columns, and that the fibres which convey sensation from the most caudal areas lie nearest to the surface of the cord in each tract and most posteriorly, while those entering at higher levels come to occupy successively deeper and more anterior layers. (For a full discussion see White (1954) and White and Sweet (1955).)

To complete our account of the destinations of the fibres entering the spinal cord by the dorsal roots we must mention two groups of fibres which are not concerned with sensation since they do not conduct impulses to consciousness, namely, those which are relayed upwards in the posterior and anterior spinocerebellar tracts. The end-organs of these fibres are probably mainly, if not exclusively, the proprioceptors of the muscles and tendons, and it is possible that the spinocerebellar tracts are supplied from collaterals of the fibres of the posterior columns. These impulses do not reach consciousness, but provide much of the 'raw material' of proprioceptor information which guides the activities of the cerebellum. Their existence explains why lesions of the dorsal roots and spinal cord may cause ataxia without gross loss of postural sensibility.

BROWN-SÉQUARD SYNDROME

Hemisection of the cord is a rare occurrence, but a lesion mainly involving one half is not uncommon. Destruction of the posterior column causes loss of appreciation of posture and passive movement of the joints, of the vibration of a tuning-fork, and of tactile discrimination below the level of the lesion. Destruction of the lateral spinothalamic tract causes analgesia and thermo-anaesthesia on the opposite side of the body. (Bilateral lesions seriously impair sexual sensibility.) Since fibres entering this tract do not cross the cord for several segments, the upper level of this sensory loss is likely to be a few segments below the level of the lesion. Conversely the fibres entering the cord just below the lesion may be caught before they cross, causing a narrow zone of similar analgesia and thermo-anaesthesia immediately below the lesion on the same side. Owing to the double route of fibres for light touch and tactile localization, partly crossed and partly uncrossed, there is rarely any loss of these forms of sensibility after a unilateral lesion of the cord. Any ataxia which might result from interruption of the spinocerebellar tracts is likely to be masked by that resulting from loss of posterior column sensibility. Hemisection of the cord, of course, interrupts descending as well as ascending tracts, and the clinical picture therefore includes the signs of corticospinal defect below the lesion; and destruction of the anterior horn causes a lower motor neurone lesion with a segmental distribution corresponding to the level of the lesion. The signs of this are likely to be conspicuous only when the lesion occurs at the cervical or lumbar enlargements.

SENSORY PATHS IN THE BRAIN STEM

The two principal modifications in the arrangements of the sensory fibres which distinguish the brain stem from the spinal cord are the entrance of the trigeminal nerve and the decussation of the lemniscus. The central connections of the trigeminal nerve are described elsewhere [see p. 172]. In summary it may be said that fibres concerned in the appreciation of pain, heat, and cold in one trigeminal area, after entering the spinal tract and nucleus of the fifth nerve, cross to the opposite side of the medulla as the quintothalamic or trigemino-thalamic tract and ascend in close relationship with the medial lemniscus joining the spinothalamic tract in the pons [FIG. 9].

The fibres of the posterior columns of the spinal cord have already been traced to their termination in the nuclei gracilis and cuneatus in the posterior part of the medulla. From these nuclei the second fibres of this sensory path take origin and cross to the opposite side as the internal arcuate fibres or the sensory decussation. After decussating they occupy a position on either side of the midline as the medial lemniscus and so pass upwards through the brain stem, to reach the optic thalamus. The medial lemniscus is joined in the pons by fibres from the principal sensory nucleus of the trigeminal nerve which are concerned in the appreciation of light touch, pressure, and postural sensibility over the trigeminal area.

Throughout the brain stem the spinothalamic tract, with which, above the medulla, the trigeminothalamic tract is associated, lies in the tegmentum, external to the medial lemniscus. As a result of this arrangement lesions involving the lateral part of the tegmentum of the brain stem are likely to cause hemi-analgesia and thermo-anaesthesia on the opposite side of the body, leaving postural sensibility and appreciation of passive movement and tactile discrimination intact. When the lesion is situated in the upper medulla or lower pons, below the point at which the spinothalamic tract has been joined by the trigemino-thalamic tract, analgesia and thermo-anaesthesia involve the opposite side of the body below the face only, while similar sensory loss is likely to occur on the face on the side of the lesion, owing to damage to the spinal tract and nucleus of the trigeminal nerve. Appreciation of pain, heat, and cold are frequently affected to a different extent by lesions of the brain stem. Deeply seated lesions may

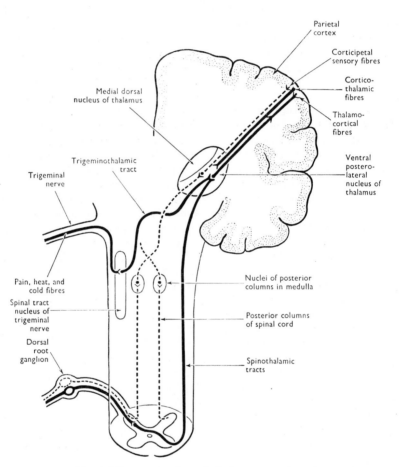

FIG. 9. Diagram showing principal sensory pathways

involve the medial lemniscus without the spinothalamic tract, thus producing loss of postural sensibility, of appreciation of passive movement and of tactile discrimination on one or both sides of the body, but leaving appreciation of pain, heat, and cold unimpaired. Massive lesions, such as tumours, are likely to involve all forms of sensibility, though often to a varying extent. In the midbrain the third nerve and red nucleus may be simultaneously involved, leading to *Benedikt's syndrome*—paralysis of the third nerve on one side with hemi-anaesthesia and tremor on the opposite side.

THE THALAMUS

Walker (1966) and Weddell and Verrillo (1972) have recently reviewed the internal structure and connections of the thalamus. Fessard and Fessard (1963) suggest that there are two systems of integrative structures at the thalamic level, the associative nuclei on the one hand, thus termed because they project to the association areas of the cortex after receiving afferents from the other nuclei of the thalamus, and on the other hand nuclei of the diffuse projection or non-specific system, comprising the intralaminar nuclei and certain mid-line nuclei. All sensory fibres pass upwards from the brain stem to the optic thalamus, whence many are redistributed in a further relay to the cerebral cortex [see p. 46]. Weddell and Verrillo (1972) suggest that two groups of thalamic nuclei are primarily involved in the mediation of pain. These are: (1) the ventrobasal complex (the ventral posterolateral nuclei or VPL); and (2) the intralaminar nuclei of the dorsal thalamus. The ventrobasal complex receives projections from the lateral spinothalamic tract and shows good somatotopic representation (Hassler, 1960). The posterior part of the complex receives fibres from both the lateral spinothalamic tract and from the dorsal column-lemniscal system and may be concerned more with the relay of touch and discriminatory sensation; here somatotopic representation is much less evident. The intralaminar and parafascicular nuclei receive fibres from the anterior spinothalamic tract. Projections from both VPL and from the intralaminar nuclei pass to the corpus striatum and to the sensory cortex, in the 'diffuse thalamic projection system' [Fig. 10] which is often regarded as the highest level of the reticular activating system. The dorsomedial nucleus is not concerned with direct sensory awareness, but is probably related to the affective response, especially to pain (see Henson, 1949). It projects to the prefrontal cortex. Since certain forms of sensibility are often unimpaired after lesions of the cerebral cortex, it has been argued that for these the optic thalamus must constitute the end-station: an alternative view is that they are bilaterally represented. These forms of sensation include the qualitative element in the appreciation of pain, heat, and cold, and the affective element, that is the pleasant or unpleasant character, of other forms of stimuli. Nevertheless, electrophysiology has shown that an intimate two-way relationship exists between the thalamus and the cerebral cortex (Jasper and Bertrand, 1966; Tasker and Organ, 1972). Lesions in and near the thalamus are likely to cause loss of various forms of sensibility owing to interruption of the fibres upon which they depend. In addition, peculiarities of sensory response, the interpretation of which has given rise to much discussion, occasionally occur. For the blood supply of the thalamus see page 313.

SENSORY LOSS

A severe and extensive lesion of the thalamus may cause gross impairment of all forms of sensibility on the opposite side of the body, as a result of damage to the ventral nuclei. Less severe lesions may cause less serious sensory disturbance and indeed in patients with thalamic tumours it is remarkable that sensory impairment is often slight. Appreciation of posture, passive movement, light touch, and tactile discrimination may all be impaired but, perhaps surprisingly, pain and thermal sensibility are often less affected (see Brodal, 1969), as in patients with 'pure sensory stroke' (Fisher, 1965); in one such case there was a small lacune in VPL at post-mortem. When the perception of pain is impaired, as a result of an extensive lesion, the pain threshold may be normal, but is frequently raised, even when painful stimuli cause an exaggerated response.

THALAMIC 'OVER-REACTION' OR 'THALAMIC SYNDROME'

This sensory abnormality which may follow lesions of the thalamus is rare, at least in a fully developed form. It is generally agreed that damage to the lateral nucleus is necessary for it to occur. Pain of central origin may be referred to the opposite side of the body. It may be extremely severe and fail to respond to analgesic drugs, including morphine. Although the threshold to sensory stimuli is usually raised on the affected half of the body, yet such stimuli, when they are effective, excite sensations of a peculiarly unpleasant character. This combination of a raised threshold with over-reaction is known as 'hyperpathia'. The painful stimulation of superficial and deep tissues and of the viscera excites more severe pain on the affected than on the normal side. Extremes of heat and cold similarly excite a feeling of great discomfort on the affected side, and the same is true of such stimuli as scraping, tickling, and a vibrating tuning-fork. Exceptionally, pleasurable stimuli, such as pleasant warmth, have been found to cause increased pleasure on the affected side, and this half of the body has been said to react to emotional states in a manner different from the normal half.

Thalamic over-reaction is most often seen after vascular lesions, and is rare with other types of lesion. Its nature has been much discussed and it has been attributed by some workers to irritation of the thalamus, by others to its escape from cortical control. The phenomenon of over-reaction to painful stimuli associated with a raised threshold to such stimuli is not a symptom of thalamic lesions only. It may, in fact, be observed as a result of a lesion involving pain fibres at any point between their endings in the skin and deeper tissues and the thalamus. Thus it occurs during regeneration of a peripheral sensory nerve and as a result of lesions of the spinothalamic tract within the spinal cord and brain stem. An imbalance between inhibitory and excitatory mechanisms as postulated in the gate theory may constitute a partial explanation.

SENSATION AT THE SUBCORTICAL LEVEL

A lesion involving the sensory fibres between the thalamus and the cerebral cortex usually causes severe and extensive sensory loss, since the fibres are here more closely crowded together than at the cortex. The appreciation of the qualitative element in pain, heat, and cold is unimpaired if the thalamus is undamaged. Other forms of sensibility are usually severely affected, there being as a rule marked loss of appreciation of posture, passive movement, tactile localization and discrimination, and of the appreciation of size, shape, and form. There may be an impairment of appreciation of temperatures in the middle of the thermal scale. A patient with a subcortical lesion does not exhibit the variability of response and threshold which characterizes patients with cortical lesions.

SENSATION AT THE CORTICAL LEVEL

As Head and his collaborators have shown, the cerebral cortex is concerned chiefly with the spatial and discriminative elements of sensibility, but it is now increasingly recognized that it plays a part in the perception of pain (Henson, 1949). The extent of the cerebral cortex concerned in sensation and the localization therein of different forms of sensory appreciation is somewhat uncertain.

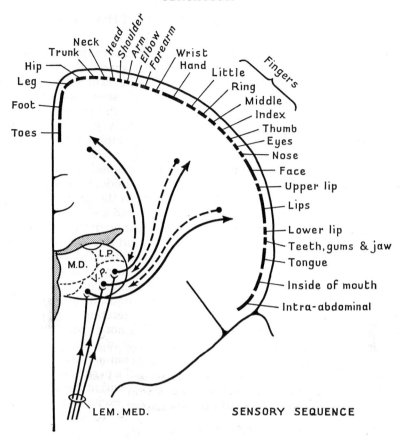

FIG. 10. Somatic sensation. Cross-section of the left hemisphere along the plane of the postcentral gyrus. The afferent pathway for tactile and kinaesthetic sensation is indicated by the unbroken lines coming up, through the medial lemniscus, and the posterolateral ventral nucleus of the thalamus, to the postcentral gyrus

There is no doubt that the postcentral gyrus is concerned in the appreciation of the posture and passive movements of the opposite half of the body, parts of which are represented there in a manner similar to their representation for purposes of motility in the precentral gyrus [see FIG. 10]. It is probable that the greater part of the parietal lobe behind the postcentral gyrus is also concerned in sensibility, and Penfield and Rasmussen's (1950) observations on cortical stimulation in the conscious patient have shown that the sensory cortex extends in front of the central sulcus also.

One striking feature of a lesion of the sensory cortex is the extreme variability of the patient's response to sensory stimuli and the difficulty or impossibility of obtaining a threshold. The appreciation of posture and of passive movement is frequently seriously impaired, together with the appreciation of light touch and its accurate localization and the discrimination of the duality of two compass-points. The appreciation of size, shape, form, roughness, and texture often suffers. The qualitative element in pain, heat, and cold is still recognized, but

C

in dealing with thermal stimuli in the middle of the scale the patient may find it difficult to say which of two is the hotter. (For recent reviews of sensory anatomy and physiology see Rose and Mountcastle, 1960; Weddell and Verrillo, 1972; and Schadé and Ford, 1973.)

PERCEPTUAL RIVALRY

This phenomenon, also known as sensory inattention, extinction, or suppression, is characteristic of a lesion of the parietal lobe, when a patient experiences a sensation if a stimulus is applied to the opposite side alone, but fails to experience it when a similar stimulus is simultaneously applied to a spot on the unaffected side of the body, which is the mirror-image of that first stimulated. It has been pointed out by Critchley (1953) and by Denny-Brown et al. (1952) that extinction does not occur if the interval between the two contacts is more than three seconds. (See also Bender (1945) and Henson (1949), who describe a similar suppression of thalamic over-reaction.)

REFERENCES

BENDER, M. B. (1945) Extinction and precipitation of cutaneous sensations, *Arch. Neurol. Psychiat. (Chic.)*, **54**, 1.
BISHOP, G. H. (1946) Neural mechanisms of cutaneous sense, *Physiol. Rev.*, **26**, 77.
BRODAL, A. (1969) *Neurological Anatomy in Relation to Clinical Medicine*, 2nd ed., New York.
CRITCHLEY, M. (1953) *The Parietal Lobes*, London.
DENNY-BROWN, D. (1966) *The Cerebral Control of Movement*, Liverpool University Press, Liverpool.
DENNY-BROWN, D., MEYER, J. S., and HORENSTEIN, S. (1952) The significance of perceptual rivalry resulting from parietal lesion, *Brain*, **75**, 433.
DYCK, P. J., SCHULTZ, P. W., and O'BRIEN, P. C. (1972) Quantitation of touch-pressure sensation, *Arch. Neurol. (Chic.)*, **26**, 465.
FESSARD, D. A., and FESSARD, A. (1963) in *Progress in Brain Research*, vol. i, ed. Moruzzi, G., Fessard, A., and Jasper, H. H., p. 115, Amsterdam.
FISHER, C. M. (1965) Pure sensory stroke involving face, arm and leg, *Neurology (Minneap.)*, **15**, 76.
FOERSTER, O. (1929) Spezielle Anatomie und Physiologie der peripheren Nerven, Lewandowsky's *Handbuch der Neurologie*, Ergänzungsband, 2, Berlin.
FOERSTER, O. (1933) The dermatomes in man, *Brain*, **56**, 1.
HASSLER, R. (1960) Die zentralen Systeme des Schmerzes, *Acta Neurochir (Wien)*, **8**, 353.
HEAD, H. (1920) *Studies in Neurology*, vols. i and ii, London.
HENSON, R. A. (1949) On thalamic dysaesthesiae and their suppression by bilateral stimulation, *Brain*, **72**, 576.
IGGO, A. (1972) The case for pain receptors, and critical remarks on the gate control theory, in *Pain*, ed. Janzen, R., Keidel, W. D., Herz, A., Steichele, C., Payne, J. P., and Burt, R. A. P., Stuttgart and London, pp. 60 and 127.
JASPER, H. H., and BERTRAND, G. (1966) Thalamic units involved in somatic sensation and voluntary and involuntary movements in man, in *The Thalamus*, ed. Purpura, D. P., and Yahr, M. D., New York.
MELZACK, R. (1973) *The Puzzle of Pain*, London.
MELZACK, R., and WALL, P. D. (1965) Pain mechanisms: a new theory, *Science*, **150**, 971.
MENDELL, L. M., and WALL, P. D. (1965) Responses of single dorsal cord cells to peripheral cutaneous unmyelinated fibres, *Nature*, **206**, 97.
NOORDENBOS, W. (1968) Physiological correlates of pain syndromes, in *Pain*, ed. Soulairac, A., Cahn, J., and Charpentier, J., London and New York.

PENFIELD, W., and RASMUSSEN, T. (1950) *The Cerebral Cortex of Man*, New York.

RIDDOCH, G. (1938) The clinical features of central pain, *Lancet*, **i**, 1093, 1150, 1205.

ROSE, J. E., and MOUNTCASTLE, V. B. (1960) in *Handbook of Physiology*, ed. Field, J., Neurophysiology, vol. i, 387, Washington, D.C.

SCHADÉ, J. J., and FORD, D. H. (1973) *Basic Neurology*, 2nd ed., Amsterdam.

SINCLAIR, D. C. (1955) Cutaneous sensation and the doctrine of perceptual rivalry, *Brain*, **78**, 584.

SINCLAIR, D. C., WEDDELL, G., and FEINDEL, W. H. (1948) Referred pain and associated phenomena, *Brain*, **71**, 184.

TASKER, R. R., and ORGAN, L. W. (1972) Mapping of the somato-sensory and auditory pathways in the upper midbrain and thalamus of man, in *Neurophysiology Studied in Man*, ed. Somjen, G. G., Amsterdam, p. 169.

WALKER, A. E. (1966) Internal structure and afferent-efferent relations of the thalamus, in *The Thalamus*, ed. Purpura, D. P., and Yahr, M. D., p. 1, New York.

WALSHE, F. M. R. (1942) The anatomy and physiology of cutaneous sensibility: a critical review, *Brain*, **65**, 48.

WEDDELL, G., SINCLAIR, D. C., and FEINDEL, W. H. (1948) An anatomical basis for alterations in quality of pain sensibility, *J. Neurophysiol.*, **2**, 99.

WEDDELL, G., and VERRILLO, R. T. (1972) Common sensibility, in *Scientific Foundations of Neurology*, ed. Critchley, M., O'Leary, J. L., and Jennett, B., London, p. 117.

WHITE, J. C., and SWEET, W. H. (1955) *Pain, its Mechanisms and Neurosurgical Control*, Springfield, Ill.

THE REFLEXES

General Considerations

A reflex is the simplest form of involuntary response to a stimulus. The anatomical basis of a reflex is the reflex arc, which consists of (1) a receptor organ, (2) an afferent path running from the periphery to the brain stem or spinal cord, (3) one or more intercalated neurones in the central nervous system linking the afferent path to (4) the efferent path which leaves the neuraxis by the lower motor neurones to reach (5) the effector organ. The reflex is elicited by a stimulus which may be a touch, a prick, the sudden stretching of a muscle, or some other event which excites an appropriate afferent impulse. The response is a muscular contraction, a modification in muscle tone, glandular secretion, etc., depending upon the nature of the reflex. Important though visceral reflexes are, the neurologist investigating the state of the nervous system is mainly concerned with reflexes which excite responses in the somatic musculature. Reflex action, conceived by Descartes, was first observed by Stephen Hales in a pithed frog about 1730. The concept was elaborated by Robert Whytt in 1755, and later by Marshall Hall in 1833.

A reflex is dependent upon the integrity of its arc. Lesions which interrupt this at any point abolish it. Loss of a reflex may thus be due to interruption of the afferent path by a lesion involving the first sensory neurone in the peripheral nerves, plexuses, spinal nerves, or dorsal roots, by damage to the central paths of the arc in the brain stem or spinal cord, or by lesions of the lower motor neurone at any point between the anterior horn cells and the muscles, or of the muscles themselves, or by the depression produced by neural shock. The activity of many bulbar and spinal reflexes is also profoundly influenced by the state of the muscle spindles and of the gamma efferent system of motor nerve fibres. In conditions causing hypotonia (e.g. cerebellar lesions) the tendon reflexes are depressed, but hypertonia associated with increased gamma efferent discharge gives exaggeration of these reflexes; this enhancement is greater in spasticity than in extrapyramidal rigidity. Anxiety, tension, and painful conditions may also give rise to some increase in the deep tendon reflexes. Paradoxically in severe long-standing spinal cord lesions, spasticity is sometimes so severe that the tendon reflexes in the lower limbs may be difficult to elicit, perhaps due to irreversible muscular shortening due to chronic spasticity, or else the flexor withdrawal reflex may be so dominant as to inhibit the tendon reflexes.

REFLEXES INVOLVING THE CRANIAL NERVES

The Pupillary Reflexes. These are described on page 92.

The Corneal Reflex. The stimulus which evokes the corneal reflex is a light touch upon the cornea, e.g. with a wisp of cotton wool, and the response is bilateral blinking. The afferent path is through the first division of the fifth cranial nerve; the central path consists of fibres uniting the spinal nucleus of the fifth nerve with both facial nuclei, and the efferent path passes through the facial nerves to both orbiculares oculi muscles. A lesion involving the fifth nerve or its spinal nucleus, since it interrupts the afferent path, causes bilateral loss of blinking in response to stimulation of the cornea on the side of the lesion. A lesion involving the nucleus or fibres of the seventh nerve interrupts the efferent path and hence causes loss of the reflex on the side of the lesion only, and blinking occurs on the opposite side. Loss of the corneal reflex is often an early sign of a lesion of the fifth nerve and may occur before any cutaneous anaesthesia can be detected. Apart from lesions involving the reflex arc, the corneal reflex is lost in states of deep coma.

Facial Reflexes. A brisk tap on the glabella above the bridge of the nose causes bilateral blinking. In the normal individual, on repeated tapping the blinking ceases after two or three taps, but in patients with Parkinsonism it may continue in time with the taps (the 'glabellar tap' sign). Electrophysiological recordings from the orbicularis oculi have shown that there is an initial monosynaptic reflex response of low amplitude, followed by a larger response of longer latency which is clearly polysynaptic (Kugelberg, 1952; Gandiglio and Fra, 1967) and which habituates in normal individuals but not in Parkinsonism.

The Oculocephalic Reflex (the Doll's Head Phenomenon). When the eyelids are held open and the head is rotated sharply from side to side, the eyes show conjugate deviation away from the side to which the head is moved and on flexion of the neck they move upwards; after each such movement they return rapidly to the mid position even if the head remains rotated or flexed. The exact physiological basis of this reflex is unknown but it persists in blind individuals, in coma, and after occipital lobectomy (Plum and Posner, 1972); it is, however, impaired when there are lesions of the oculomotor nerves.

The Oculovestibular (Caloric) Reflex. Irrigation of an external auditory meatus with warm or cold water causes nystagmus in normal individuals [see p. 192]. As this reflex depends upon the integrity of the vestibular nuclei, loss of this reflex may be a valuable sign of pontine damage if there is no reason to suspect a labyrinthine or eighth nerve lesion.

The Jaw Reflex. In response to a tap upon the chin, depressing the lower jaw, there is a bilateral contraction of the elevators of the jaw. Both afferent and efferent paths pass through the trigeminal nerve. This reflex is a stretch reflex, and, like these, becomes exaggerated as a result of bilateral corticospinal lesions.

The Sucking Reflex. In the infant the contact of an object with the lips evokes the movements of the lips, tongue, and jaw concerned in sucking. This sucking reflex is lost after infancy but may reappear in states of severe cerebral degeneration, for example, the presenile and senile dementias (Paulson and Gottlieb, 1968). It may be unilateral, and associated with a grasp reflex on the same side. When the lips follow the stimulating object this is sometimes called the 'rooting reflex'.

The 'Snout' Reflex. A tap on the centre of the closed lips will, in normal infants, provoke a pouting movement of the lips like the formation of a 'snout'. This reflex normally disappears with maturation but may reappear in the presence of bilateral corticospinal tract lesions in or above the upper brain stem and in cerebral degenerative disorders such as those in which the sucking reflex is re-established.

The Palatal Reflex. The palatal ('gag') reflex consists of elevation of the soft palate in response to a touch. The afferent path is by the second division of the fifth nerve; the efferent by the vagus. The palatal reflex is variable in intensity in normal individuals. It is abolished by lesions causing anaesthesia of the palate and by lesions of the vagus nuclei, and in lesions of one vagus nerve the response is unilateral and the uvula is displaced towards the normal side.

The Pharyngeal Reflex. The pharyngeal reflex consists of constriction of the pharynx in response to a touch upon the posterior pharyngeal wall. Its afferent path runs in the glossopharyngeal nerve, its efferent path in the vagus. Like the palatal reflex, it is abolished by lesions causing pharyngeal anaesthesia and by lesions of the vagus nuclei. In cases of unilateral paralysis of the vagus the response is confined to the opposite half of the pharynx.

REFLEXES OF THE LIMBS AND TRUNK

THE TENDON REFLEXES

Physiology

The basis of the tendon reflex is the myotatic reflex which is the reflex contraction of a muscle or part of a muscle in response to stretch. It is monosynaptic, i.e. it is mediated by a reflex arc consisting of two neurones with one synapse between them (Lloyd, 1952).

A so-called 'tendon reflex' or jerk is a sharp muscular contraction evoked by suddenly stretching the muscle. The sudden stretch may be brought about by tapping the tendon, or by suddenly displacing the segment of a limb into which the muscle is inserted. The response, a muscular contraction, is most evident in the muscle stretched, but may not be confined to this muscle. A tendon reflex is diminished or abolished by a lesion interrupting either the afferent, central, or efferent paths of the reflex arc or a disorder which makes the muscle incapable of responding to the nervous impulse. Reinforcement of the tendon jerks may be achieved by clenching the fists or by pulling the flexed fingers of the two hands against each other (Jendrassik's manœuvre), movements which cause increased activity of the gamma efferent system. Reflex activity in the legs may be studied electrically by recording the 'H' reflex, a contraction in the calf muscles which may be elicited by stimulating electrically the medial popliteal nerve. The H response, which is a monosynaptic reflex evoked by stimulation of Group I afferent fibres in the nerve, follows the so-called M response evoked in the muscle by the direct effect of the nerve stimulus upon alpha efferent fibres. In early polyneuropathy the tendon reflexes may be lost before sensory loss is detectable clinically, but in such cases abnormalities of conduction may be detectable electrically. Rarely the tendon reflexes are congenitally absent. The table which follows gives the principal tendon reflexes, their mode of elicitation, and their innervation.

Reflex	Mode of elicitation	Response	Spinal segment	Peripheral nerve
Biceps-jerk	A blow upon the biceps tendon	Flexion of the elbow	Cervical 5–6	Musculo-cutaneous
Triceps-jerk	A blow upon the triceps tendon	Extension of the elbow	Cervical 6–7	Radial
Supinator-jerk or radial reflex	A blow upon the tendon of brachio-radialis at the distal end of the radius	Flexion of the elbow	Cervical 5–6	Radial
Flexor finger-jerk	A blow upon the palmar surface of the semiflexed fingers	Flexion of the fingers and thumb	Cervical 7–8	Median and ulnar
Knee-jerk	A blow upon the quadriceps tendon	Extension of the knee	Lumbar 2–4	Femoral
Ankle-jerk	A blow upon the tendo calcaneus	Plantar flexion of the ankle	Sacral 1–2	Sciatic

Clonus. Clonus, a rhythmical series of contractions in response to the maintenance of tension in a muscle, associated with increased gamma efferent discharge, is often elicitable when the tendon reflexes are exaggerated after a corticospinal lesion. Clonus of the quadriceps, patellar clonus, is best elicited by a sudden sharp downward displacement of the patella. Ankle clonus is obtained by sharply dorsiflexing the ankle. Clonus of the flexors of the fingers can sometimes be elicited by suddenly extending the fingers.

Hoffmann's Reflex. The patient's hand is pronated and the observer grasps the terminal phalanx of the middle finger between his forefinger and thumb. With a sharp flick the phalanx is passively flexed and suddenly released. A positive response consists of a sharp twitch of adduction and flexion of the thumb and flexion of the fingers. This reflex is physiologically identical with the *flexor finger-jerk*, which is elicited by tapping the palmar surface of the slightly flexed fingers. It is an index of muscular hypertonia rather than of a corticospinal lesion as such. It is not always positive in the presence of such a lesion, and may be elicitable in a nervous individual with no organic disease; if present unilaterally, however, it is likely to be significant.

In states of muscular hypertonia a reflex response may spread beyond the muscles stretched, as when a tap on the styloid process of the radius elicits a contraction not only of the brachioradialis, but also of the long flexors of the fingers.

In the upper limbs, so-called 'inverted reflexes' may be a useful sign of lesions of the cervical cord. If there is a lesion at C5-6 which interrupts the arc for reflexes innervated by that segment, but which is also compressing the cortico-spinal tracts to give exaggeration of reflexes subserved by lower segments, tapping the tendon of the biceps may fail to elicit the biceps jerk but causes contraction of the triceps (the inverted biceps jerk); similarly, the radial jerk may be absent but the appropriate stimulus causes finger flexion (the inverted radial jerk).

CUTANEOUS REFLEXES

The Nociceptive Abdominal Reflexes. These are cutaneous reflexes con-sisting of a brisk unilateral contraction of a part of the abdominal wall in response to a cutaneous stimulus, such as a touch or a light scratch with a pin. It is convenient to elicit them at three levels on each side—just below the costal margin, at the level of the umbilicus, and at the level of the iliac fossa. Kugelberg and Hagbarth (1958) have shown that the abdominal and erector spinae reflexes are polysynaptic, and are reactions of the trunk to potential injury. They are plurisegmental, and lead to a local withdrawal from the stimulus. They are normally dependent, for a reason which is not fully understood, upon the integrity of the corticospinal tract. Hence a corticospinal lesion is usually associated with diminution or loss of the superficial abdominal reflexes upon the same side. If the corticospinal defect is slight the reflexes may be reduced but not completely abolished, the reflexes of the lowest segments being most impaired. Loss of the abdominal reflexes is not always proportional to the severity of the corticospinal lesion. In multiple sclerosis, for example, they may be lost early, at a stage of the disease when other signs of corticospinal lesions are slight. In congenital diplegia and motor neurone disease, on the other hand, they are often retained.

The reflex arcs of the superficial abdominal reflexes are localized in the spinal cord from the seventh to the twelfth dorsal segments. Lesions involving the arcs themselves may produce diminution or loss of the reflexes. The commonest such lesion is damage to the lower motor neurone by poliomyelitis. These reflexes may, however, be absent in some normal people, especially women, and especially in the aged, and obesity, abdominal scars, and repeated preg-nancies are not always responsible (Madonick, 1957).

The Cremasteric Reflex. The cremasteric reflex is a cutaneous reflex closely related to the abdominal reflexes. The appropriate stimulus is a light scratch along the inner aspect of the upper part of the thigh, and the response is a contraction of the cremaster muscle, with elevation of the testicle. This reflex, the arc of which runs through the first lumbar spinal segment, is diminished or abolished by a lesion of the corticospinal tract. It is usually extremely brisk in children, in whom it may sometimes be elicited by a stimulus applied to any part of the lower limb. It is usually diminished or absent on the affected side in a patient with varicocele.

The Gluteal Reflex. The gluteal reflex is physiologically akin to the abdominal reflexes. A scratch on the buttock evokes contraction of the glutei. The spinal segments concerned are lumbar 4 and 5.

The Plantar Reflex. The plantar reflex is one of the most important of all reflexes to the neurologist, because its meaning is unequivocal.

1. *The Flexor Plantar Reflex.* The flexor plantar reflex is normal after the first year of life. The stimulus which evokes it is a longitudinal scratch upon the lateral aspect of the sole of the foot from the heel towards the toes, and the response is plantar flexion of the toes sometimes associated with dorsiflexion of the foot at the ankle, contraction of the tensor fasciae latae muscle, and other variable muscular contractions. It is a spinal segmental reflex mediated by the first sacral segment of the cord and akin to the abdominal reflexes.

2. *The Extensor Plantar Reflex.* Babinski in 1896 first pointed out that in the presence of a corticospinal lesion the normal flexor plantar reflex did not occur, but its place was taken by an upward, extensor movement of the great toe. Riddoch, Walshe, and others showed that the extensor plantar reflex is not an isolated phenomenon, but is part of a general reflex flexion of the whole lower limb, homologous with the flexion reflex of the spinal animal in response to a nocuous or potentially painful stimulus. Clinical and physiological studies (Brain and Wilkinson, 1959; Landau and Clare, 1959; and Kugelberg *et al.*, 1960) have shown that the distinction between the flexor and extensor plantar reflexes is not absolute. Both are nociceptive reflexes, but 'the unique feature of the pathological extensor response is the recruitment of extensor hallucis longus into contraction with tibialis anterior and extensor digitorum longus' (Kugelberg and Hagbarth, 1958). The afferent focus, i.e. the region of easiest elicitation of this reflex, is the outer border of the sole and the transverse arch of the foot (Dohrmann and Nowack, 1973). The motor focus, or minimal response, is a contraction of the inner hamstring muscles. In its fully developed form the reflex consists of flexion at all joints of the lower limb with dorsiflexion of the great toe and abduction or fanning of the other toes.

Confusion has arisen from the application of the term extensor plantar reflex to a movement which forms part of a flexor reflex of the lower limb. The explanation of this misnomer is that the extensor hallucis longus muscle, though named extensor by the anatomists, is in fact a flexor muscle, since its action is to shorten the limb, and it contracts reflexly in association with other flexor muscles. The term extensor plantar reflex, however, appears to be too firmly established to be altered. 'Positive Babinski reflex' and 'upgoing toe' are alternative terms which are sometimes employed.

Physiological understanding illuminates several points of practical importance in the elicitation of the plantar reflex. The stimulus should always be applied first along the outer border of the sole; an extensor response may sometimes be obtained from this region when the inner border of the sole yields a flexor response. Dohrmann and Nowack (1973) have shown that the response is more consistently obtained if the stimulus is then continued medially across the anterior arch of the foot. Oppenheim's reflex, dorsiflexion of the great toe, evoked by firm moving pressure on the skin over the tibia, is physiologically the same as Babinski's reflex, differing only in the site of the stimulus. The same is true of Chaddock's and Gordon's reflexes. The extensor plantar reflex is not an all-or-none reaction: minor degrees of corticospinal tract damage lead to an incomplete flexor response or a failure of the great toe to move up or down (an 'equivocal' response).

Bilateral extensor plantar reflexes are often observed during sleep and deep coma from any cause, for a short time after an epileptic convulsion, and usually

in the first year of life, that is, when the corticospinal fibres are either functionally depressed or incompletely developed. Although this response has sometimes
been noted in cases in which no anatomical lesion of the corticospinal tract was
subsequently discovered, and is occasionally absent in the presence of such
a lesion (Nathan and Smith, 1955) and although it may occur transiently as
a result of physical fatigue, it can with confidence be accepted as indicating an
organic lesion or dysfunction of this tract in clinical practice. In the presence of
such a lesion, however, it may be lost if an associated lower motor neurone
lesion paralyses the extensor hallucis.

The Bulbocavernosus Reflex. The bulbocavernosus reflex consists of contraction of the bulbocavernosus muscle, which can be detected by palpation, in
response to squeezing the glans penis. The spinal segments concerned are sacral
2, 3, and 4. This reflex is frequently abolished in tabes and in lesions of the
cauda equina.

The Anal Reflex. The anal reflex consists of contraction of the external
sphincter ani in response to a scratch upon the skin in the perianal region. The
spinal segments concerned are sacral 4 and 5.

POSTURAL REFLEXES

'Postural reflexes' is a convenient term to apply to reflexes in which the
response consists not of a brief muscular contraction but of a sustained modification in the posture of one or more segments of the body.

Tonic Neck Reflexes. In the decerebrate animal it was found by Magnus and
de Kleijn that changes in the position of the head relative to the body caused
reflex modifications of the tonus and posture of the limbs. These reflexes, which
are excited from the proprioceptors of the cervical spine, are known as *tonic neck
reflexes* and may sometimes be observed in severe cerebral diplegia. Passive
turning of the head to one side may then evoke extension of the arm and leg on
the side to which the head is turned with flexion of the contralateral limbs.

Associated Reactions. Associated reactions, or associated movements, are
automatic modifications of the posture of parts of the body when vigorous
voluntary or reflex movement of some other part occurs. They are best observed
in the paralysed upper limb in hemiplegia, following a vigorous grasping movement with the sound hand. Other patterns of associated movement occur. Such
semi-voluntary activities as yawning, stretching, and coughing often evoke
associated movements in the paralysed limbs in hemiplegia, and may arouse in
the patient or his friends false hopes of recovery.

FORCED GRASPING AND GROPING

The Grasp Reflex of the Hand. In certain patients the contact of an object
with the palmar surface of the fingers, especially the region between the thumb
and the index finger, causes reflex flexion of the fingers and thumb so that the
hand involuntarily grasps the object. The patient is unable voluntarily to relax
his grasp, and efforts to pull the object away only cause it to be more firmly held.
The patient may notice that when he is holding an object he is unable to relinquish his hold of it in order to put it down. This phenomenon is known as the
grasp reflex. In some cases, when the patient's eyes are closed, if the palmar
surface of the hand or fingers is lightly touched, the fingers close upon the object

and the hand and arm move towards the stimulus and in this way may be drawn in any direction—*forced groping* or the *instinctive grasp reaction*. Even an object presented to vision may be groped for (Massion-Verniory, 1948; Seyffarth and Denny-Brown, 1948).

Forced grasping and groping, which have been considered a regression to the infantile stage of the function of grasping, usually indicate a lesion involving the upper part of the opposite frontal lobe, particularly areas 8s and 24s (Denny-Brown, 1951). A unilateral grasp reflex in a fully conscious patient is of localizing value. When the reflex is bilateral or the patient semi-conscious its value is much less. When the causative lesion produces a progressive hemiplegia the grasp reflex disappears when paralysis becomes complete, which appears to indicate that it utilizes the corticospinal tract as part of its motor path.

The Grasp Reflex of the Foot. An allied grasp reflex may sometimes be observed in the foot, light pressure or a stroking movement applied to the distal half of the sole and plantar surface of the toes evoking tonic flexion and adduction of the toes without other associated movements. Like the fingers, the toes may grasp and hold an object. This reflex is present in the normal infant up to the end of the first year, and in 50 per cent of children with Down's syndrome (mongolism). It may occur either with or without the hand-grasp reflex, and is caused by similar lesions.

REFERENCES

ADIE, W. J., and CRITCHLEY, M. (1927) Forced grasping and groping, *Brain*, **50,** 142.

BABINSKI, J. (1922) Reflexes de defense, *Brain*, **45,** 149.

BICKERSTAFF, E. R. (1973) *Neurological Examination in Clinical Practice*, 3rd ed., Oxford.

BRAIN, W. R., and CURRAN, R. D. (1932) The grasp reflex of the foot, *Brain*, **55,** 347.

BRAIN, W. R., and WILKINSON, M. (1959) Observations on the extensor plantar reflex and its relationship to the functions of the pyramidal tract, *Brain*, **82,** 297.

DENNY-BROWN, D. (1951) in *Modern Trends in Neurology*, ed. Feiling, A., London.

DOHRMANN, G. J., and NOWACK, W. J. (1973) The upgoing great toe: optimal method of elicitation, *Lancet*, **i,** 339.

GANDIGLIO, G., and FRA, L. (1967) Further observations on facial reflexes, *J. neurol. Sci.*, **5,** 273.

GRANIT, R. (1970) *The Basis of Motor Control*, New York.

HEAD, H., and RIDDOCH, G. (1917) The automatic bladder, excessive sweating and some other reflex conditions in gross injuries of the spinal cord, *Brain*, **40,** 188.

DE JONG, R. N. (1967) *The Neurologic Examination*, 3rd ed., New York.

KUGELBERG, E. (1952) Facial reflexes, *Brain*, **75,** 385.

KUGELBERG, E., EKLUND, K., and GRIMBY, L. (1960) An electromyographic study of the nociceptive reflexes of the lower limb, *Brain*, **83,** 394.

KUGELBERG, E., and HAGBARTH, K. E. (1958) Spinal mechanism of the abdominal and erector spinae skin reflexes, *Brain*, **81,** 290.

LANCE, J. W. (1970) *A Physiological Approach to Clinical Neurology*, London.

LANDAU, W. M., and CLARE, M. H. (1959) The plantar reflex in man, *Brain*, **82,** 321.

LANGWORTHY, O. R. (1930) The mechanism of the abdominal and cremasteric reflexes, *Arch. Neurol. Psychiat. (Chic.)*, **24,** 1023.

LLOYD, D. P. C. (1952) On reflex action of muscular origin, *Res. Publ. Ass. nerv. ment. Dis.*, **30,** 48.

MADONICK, M. J. (1957) Statistical control studies in neurology: 8. The cutaneous abdominal reflex, *Neurology (Minneap.)*, **7,** 459.

Massion-Verniory, L. (1948) Les réflexes de préhension, Suppl. ad *Mschr. Psychiat. Neurol.*, Fasc. 1 xxxviii.

Monrad-Krohn, G. H. (1918) *Om Abdominalreflexerne*, Christiania.

Monrad-Krohn, G. H. (1925) Reflexes of different order elicitable from the abdominal region, *Arch. Neurol. Psychiat. (Chic.)*, **13**, 750.

Nathan, P. W., and Smith, M. C. (1955) The Babinski response: a review and new observations, *J. Neurol. Neurosurg. Psychiat.*, **18**, 250.

Paine, K. S., and Oppé, T. E. (1966) *Neurological Examination of Children*, London.

Paulson, G., and Gottlieb, G. (1968) Developmental reflexes; the reappearance of foetal and neonatal reflexes in aged patients, *Brain*, **91**, 37.

Plum, F., and Posner, J. B. (1972) *The Diagnosis of Stupor and Coma*, 2nd ed., Oxford and Philadelphia.

Riddoch, G., and Buzzard, E. F. (1921) Reflex movements and postural reactions in quadriplegia and hemiplegia, with especial reference to those of the upper limb, *Brain*, **44**, 397.

Seyffarth, H., and Denny-Brown, D. (1948) The grasp reflex and the instinctive grasp reaction, *Brain*, **71**, 109.

Sittig, O. (1932) Über die Greifreflexe im Kindesalter, *Med. Klin.*, **28**, 934.

Walshe, F. M. R. (1914–15) The physiological significance of the reflex phenomena in spastic paralysis of the lower limbs, *Brain*, **37**, 269.

Walshe, F. M. R. (1919) On the genesis and physiological significance of spasticity and other disorders of motor innervation, with a consideration of the functional relationships of the pyramidal system, *Brain*, **42**, 1.

Walshe, F. M. R. (1965) *Further Critical Studies in Neurology*, Edinburgh.

Wartenberg, R. (1945) *The Examination of Reflexes*, Chicago.

THE CEREBELLUM

ANATOMY AND MORPHOLOGY

The cerebellum is situated in the posterior fossa of the skull and is joined to the brain stem by three peduncles, the superior, middle, and inferior. The tentorium cerebelli (see Bull, 1969) lies above, and below it is separated from the posterior aspect of the medulla and the dura mater covering the posterior atlanto-occipital membrane by a dilatation of the subarachnoid space, the cerebellomedullary cistern. To the naked eye it is composed of three main divisions, two lateral lobes and a median lobe, the vermis, but this is not a morphological division.

Phylogeny and experimental physiology provide a sounder basis for morphology. According to Larsell (1937) and Fulton and Dow (1937–8) the cerebellum has two primary divisions: (1) the flocculonodular lobe or archicerebellum, the most primitive part, with connections which are entirely vestibular, and (2) the corpus cerebelli, itself divided into (*a*) a palaeocerebellar division, receiving vestibular and spinocerebellar fibres, and composed anteriorly of lingula, lobus centralis, and culmen, and posteriorly of pyramis, uvula, and paraflocculi, and (*b*) a neocerebellar division, constituting the greater part of the corpus cerebelli, with connections mainly corticopontine. (For reviews see Jansen and Brodal, 1954; Kreindler and Steriade, 1958; Brookhart, 1960; Brodal, 1969; Granit, 1970; Schadé and Ford, 1973.)

The cerebellum consists mainly of white matter which is covered with a thin layer of grey matter, the cerebellar cortex, and contains several grey masses, the nuclei. These are divided into lateral nuclei, the nuclei dentatus and emboliformis, and middle and roof nuclei, the nuclei globosus and fastigius.

Microscopically the cortex consists of three principal layers of cells, the molecular layer, which lies most superficially, the granular layer, which is the deepest, and the layer of Purkinje cells, which lies between the two. In the three cortical layers are numerous fibres, impulses from which probably ultimately impinge upon the dendrites of the Purkinje cells. The so-called mossy and climbing fibres are the main cerebellar afferents which make synaptic contacts not only with dendrites of the Purkinje cells but also with those of the Golgi cells in the granular layer and with the small granular cells themselves. The axons of the Purkinje cells pass through the white matter of the cerebellar hemispheres, giving off collaterals to the Golgi cells, and are chiefly distributed to the dentate nuclei.

CEREBELLAR CONNECTIONS

AFFERENT FIBRES

The cerebellum receives numerous afferent fibres which are principally derived from the proprioceptor organs of the body, namely:

Vestibular Fibres. These, which are largely mossy fibres, come from the labyrinth and enter the cerebellum by the inferior peduncles, some being interrupted at the vestibular nuclei. They go mostly to the cortex of the vermis.

Spinal Fibres. These come from the skin and proprioceptors of the muscles and possibly also from the joints and tendons; they, too, are mainly mossy fibres. They reach the cerebellum by the posterior spinocerebellar tract, which ascends in the posterior part of the lateral column of the spinal cord and enters the cerebellum by the inferior peduncle, and by the anterior spinocerebellar tract, which passes up the cord in the anterolateral column, ascends as high as the midbrain, and turns backwards to the cerebellum through the superior peduncle. The posterior spinocerebellar tract probably receives a contribution from the trigeminal nerve. Fibres from the spinocerebellar tracts end throughout the cerebellar cortex.

Cortical Fibres. Impulses reach the cerebellum from the cerebral cortex by way of the corticospinal tracts with a relay station in the nuclei of the pons, whence fibres pass to the cerebellum by the middle peduncle. They are distributed mainly to the middle lobes.

Olivary Fibres. The olive, which receives spinal and thalamic connections, is intimately related to the opposite cerebellar hemisphere, to which it sends fibres through the opposite inferior peduncle; the olivary afferents are the so-called climbing fibres. Atrophy of one cerebellar hemisphere is usually associated with atrophy of the opposite olive.

EFFERENT FIBRES

Efferent fibres start from the cerebellar nuclei and leave the cerebellum by all three peduncles. The most important outgoing path from the cerebellum passes from the dentate nucleus and from the nuclei emboliformis and globosus through the superior peduncle and after decussation is distributed to the opposite red nucleus. From the red nucleus arises the rubrospinal tract, which decussates in the ventral tegmental decussation and passes down through the brain stem to the lateral column of the spinal cord. This is probably the principal route by which the cerebellum influences the lower motor neurone. Each cerebellar hemisphere is thus linked principally with the same side of the body by means of a double decussation in the midbrain. Other fibres from the red nucleus through the ansa lenticularis reach the thalamus and may thus bring the cerebellum into relationship with the basal ganglia and the cerebral cortex.

Other cerebellar efferent fibres reach the reticular formation of the midbrain, the pons, and the medulla by all three peduncles.

THE FUNCTIONS OF THE CEREBELLUM

Our earliest knowledge of the functions of the cerebellum was based upon Rolando's observations of the effects of removal of this organ in 1809. His observations were extended by Flourens in 1824. Luciani, in 1879, summarized the symptoms of cerebellar deficiency as asthenia, atonia, and astasia, that is, weakness and fatigability, diminution of tone, and tremor and a staggering gait. Recent experiments have yielded more precise information concerning cerebellar functions. Rademaker described extensor hypertonia in the limbs after removal of the whole cerebellum and Sherrington found that cerebellar stimulation could inhibit decerebrate rigidity. Denny-Brown et al. (1929) by stimulating the cerebellar cortex imposed modifications upon pre-existing spinal reflexes and observed inhibition and excitation of both extensor and flexor muscles, and Miller and Banting (1922) made similar observations in stimulating the cerebellar nuclei. These physiological observations, together with clinical investigation of the effects of cerebellar lesions by Holmes and others, have established the view that the neocerebellum is essentially a reinforcing and co-ordinating organ which plays an important part in graduating and harmonizing muscular contraction, both in voluntary movement and in the maintenance of posture. There is still much to be learned about the details of the physiology of the cerebellum. It is clearly involved in the regulation of the stretch reflex and in the control of motor activity, exercising a modulating effect upon the activity of the muscle spindles. It plays an important role in integrating a variety of afferent signals, many related to the length of skeletal muscle fibres, and thus acts as a kind of position servomechanism (Granit, 1970; Schadé and Ford, 1973).

The anterior lobe and the roof nuclei are largely concerned with the regulation of stretch reflexes and the anti-gravity posture. The flocculonodular lobe is an important equilibratory centre and lesions of this region cause swaying, staggering, and titubation. The neocerebellum is more concerned with the regulation of voluntary movement (Eccles, 1969; Snider, 1972).

SYMPTOMS OF CEREBELLAR DEFICIENCY IN MAN

The following are the principal effects of neocerebellar (cerebellar hemisphere) lesions in man:

MUSCULAR HYPOTONIA

Hypotonia is evident in the visible, palpable flaccidity of the muscles, in a diminished resistance to passive joint movements, and in the wide excursions occurring at the terminal joints when the limb is vigorously shaken. If the outstretched upper limb receives a sudden tap, it shows a greater displacement than a normal limb. When the lesion is confined to one cerebellar hemisphere the hypotonia is present only on the same side of the body. The hypotonia is probably due to loss of the facilitatory influence of the cerebellum upon the stretch reflex.

DISTURBANCES OF POSTURE

Abnormal Attitudes. With a unilateral cerebellar lesion the shoulder on the affected side is often held at a lower level than the normal shoulder and there may be scoliosis with the concavity towards the side of the lesion. In standing, the weight is thrown on the sound leg and the body is somewhat rotated, with the affected shoulder in advance of the sound one. In severe cases the patient is unable to stand or even sit without support and tends to fall towards the side of the lesion. When a lesion involves one cerebellar hemisphere the head is often rotated and flexed, so that the occiput is directed towards the shoulder on the side of the lesion. This rotated posture may be due either to cerebellar deficiency or to a coincident lesion of the vestibular tracts.

Static Tremor. Tremor develops if the patient attempts to maintain a limb in a fixed posture, probably owing to hypotonia of the agonists producing an irregular contraction of the muscles maintaining the attitude.

DISORDERS OF MOVEMENT (ATAXIA)

Several factors combine to produce disturbances of voluntary movement after a lesion of the cerebellum. Muscular contractions are weak and more easily fatigued than normally. Moreover, they are of an irregular, intermittent character, and there is delay both in initiating and in relaxing contractions.

Dysmetria. In dysmetria the range of the movement is inappropriate to its objective. Sometimes the harmonious synthesis of movements at different joints is lost, leading to the phenomenon known as 'decomposition of movement'. When a movement involves the whole arm, instead of its occurring to an appropriate extent at all joints simultaneously, one joint is moved before another.

Tremor. Tremor occurs on voluntary movement, owing partly to faulty fixation and partly to the factors responsible for static tremor. Fine movements, for example movements of the fingers, suffer especially from incoordination due to cerebellar deficiency, and the patient may find it impossible to button his clothes. Intention tremor, in which tremor increases markedly when, for instance, a pointing finger approaches a target, is a prominent feature of lesions involving cerebellar connections in the brain stem but is less often seen in lesions of one cerebellar hemisphere.

Adiadochokinesis. This is the term applied to an inability to carry out alternating movements with rapidity and regularity. For example, the patient is asked alternately to pronate and supinate his forearms or to flex and extend his fingers. After a unilateral cerebellar lesion alternating movements are accomplished slowly and in a jerky, incoordinated fashion on the affected side.

The Rebound Phenomenon. This is a disturbance of movement probably due to muscular hypotonia. If a normal individual is asked to flex his elbow against resistance offered by the observer and his forearm is suddenly released, its excursion in the direction of flexion is quickly arrested by contraction of the triceps. Cerebellar deficiency delays this contraction, with the result that flexion of the elbow is unchecked and the patient may strike himself in the face.

Associated Movements. After a lesion of the cerebellum the normal associated movements which occur on strong voluntary effort may be exaggerated. Vigorous grimaces may accompany speech after a lesion of the cerebellar vermis.

OCULAR DISTURBANCES

In the early stages of a unilateral cerebellar lesion there may be weakness of conjugate ocular deviation to the affected side, but this soon passes off. In cases of severe bilateral lesions, or if the vermis is affected, there may be a temporary impairment of conjugate movement in the vertical plane also.

Skew deviation of the eyes is occasionally observed for a few days after an acute cerebellar lesion. The eye on the affected side is deviated downwards and inwards, while the opposite eye is deviated outwards and upwards. This may be due either to cerebellar deficiency or to interference with the vestibular connections elsewhere.

Nystagmus is usually present in cerebellar disease. It is most evident when the eyes are deviated horizontally. The quick phase consists of a sharp jerk of the eyes towards the direction of gaze and is followed by a slow recoil towards the midline. In the case of unilateral cerebellar lesions the amplitude of the nystagmus is greater and its rate slower when the eyes are deviated towards the side of the lesion than when they are displaced to the opposite side. Nystagmus usually occurs in the horizontal plane, but there is occasionally a rotatory element also. Nystagmus on vertical deviation is inconspicuous except in lesions of the cerebellar tonsils at or near the foramen magnum. For a further discussion of nystagmus see page 85.

DISORDERS OF ARTICULATION AND PHONATION

Disturbances of articulation and phonation are more likely to occur when a lesion involves the vermis than when it is confined to one lateral lobe. Articulation is jerky and explosive. The voice is often too loud, and the syllables tend to be separated from each other. At the same time individual syllables are slurred owing to defective formation of consonants. Considerable recovery of speech usually occurs in the case of unilateral lesions.

DISORDERS OF GAIT

The patient with a unilateral lesion tends to stagger towards the affected side and to deviate to this side in walking. This may be well demonstrated by asking him to walk round a chair. When he is turning towards the affected side he tends to fall into the chair, when to the normal side, to move away from the chair in a spiral. The affected lower limb is markedly ataxic in the heel–knee test.

ABNORMALITIES OF THE REFLEXES

The cutaneous reflexes are unaffected by lesions of the cerebellum. The tendon reflexes, however, often exhibit a characteristic change, which is best seen in the 'pendular' knee-jerk. The knee-jerk is followed by a series of oscillations of the leg, which are normally prevented by the after-shortening of the quadriceps.

BÁRÁNY'S POINTING TEST

The patient, with his eyes closed and one arm outstretched, is asked to move the limb in a given plane and bring his finger back to its original position. Deviation of the limb occurs after a unilateral cerebellar lesion and is most conspicuous when the movement takes place in the vertical plane, the arm deviating outwards on the side of the lesion.

SYMPTOMS OF LESIONS OF THE FLOCCULONODULAR LOBE

Experimental lesions of this region in animals cause swaying, staggering, and titubation, symptoms identical with those of lesions of the vermis in man, especially the medulloblastoma of childhood. This so-called 'truncal ataxia' with difficulty in walking 'heel-to-toe', in stopping, and in turning, may be unaccompanied by any of the typical signs of cerebellar hemisphere lesions and is not evident if the patient is examined only in bed. The uninitiated may misconstrue this gait disturbance as hysterical.

CEREBELLAR VERTIGO

That cerebellar lesions may cause vertigo is not surprising in view of the postural and equilibratory functions of the cerebellum. It is stated that objects seem to move away from the side of the lesion and the sense of rotation of the body is in the same direction with intracerebellar tumours but in the opposite direction with extracerebellar tumours.

ACUTE AND CHRONIC LESIONS

The symptoms of a cerebellar lesion differ markedly in severity according to whether it develops rapidly or slowly. Most of our knowledge of the symptoms of cerebellar deficiency is based upon studies of acute lesions. When the lesion is slowly progressive, such as a tumour, symptoms of cerebellar deficiency are much less severe than when it is acute, and considerable recovery from the effects of an acute lesion can always be expected. These facts seem to imply that other parts of the nervous system can to a considerable extent compensate for loss of cerebellar function.

REFERENCES

BRODAL, A. (1969) *Neurological Anatomy in Relation to Clinical Medicine*, 2nd ed., New York.

BROOKHART, J. M. (1960) The cerebellum, in *Handbook of Physiology*, ed. Field, J., sect. 1, Neurophysiology, vol. ii, 1245, Washington, D.C.

BULL, J. W. D. (1969) The tentorium cerebelli, *Proc. roy. Soc. Med.*, **62**, 1301.

CLARKE, R. H. (1926) Experimental stimulation of the cerebellum, *Brain*, **49**, 557.

DENNY-BROWN, D. (1966) *The Cerebral Control of Movement*, Liverpool.

DENNY-BROWN, D., ECCLES, J. C., and LIDDELL, E. G. T. (1929) Observations on electrical stimulation of the cerebellar cortex, *Proc. roy. Soc. Med.*, **104**, 518.

DOW, R. S. (1942) Cerebellar action potentials in response to stimulation of the cerebral cortex in monkeys and cats, *J. Neurophysiol.*, **5**, 121.

DOW, R. S., and ANDERSON, R. (1942) Stimulation of proprioceptors and exteroceptors in the rat, *J. Neurophysiol.*, **5**, 363.

ECCLES, J. C. (1969) The dynamic loop hypothesis of movement control, in *Information Processing in the Nervous System*, ed. Leibovic, K. N., New York, p. 245.

FULTON, J. F., and DOW, R. S. (1937-8) The cerebellum. A summary of functional localization, *Yale J. Biol. Med.*, **10**, 89.

GRANIT, R. (1970) *The Basis of Motor Control*, London and New York.

HOLMES, G. (1917) The symptoms of acute cerebellar injuries due to gun-shot injuries, *Brain*, **40**, 461.

HOLMES, G. (1922) Croonian Lectures. The clinical symptoms of cerebellar disease and their interpretation, *Lancet*, **i**, 1177, 1231; and **ii**, 59, 111.

HOLMES, G. (1939) The cerebellum of man, *Brain*, **62**, 1.

INGVAR, S. (1923) On cerebellar localization, *Brain*, **46**, 301.

JANSEN, J., and BRODAL, A. (1954) *Aspects of Cerebellar Anatomy*, Oslo.

KREINDLER, A., and STERIADE, M. (1958) *La physiologie et la physiopathologie du cervelet*, Paris.

LARSELL, O. (1937) The cerebellum, *Arch. Neurol. Psychiat. (Chic.)*, **38**, 580.

MILLER, F. R., and BANTING, F. G. (1922) Observations in cerebellar stimulations, *Brain*, **45**, 104.

SCHADÉ, J. P., and FORD, D. H. (1973) *Basic Neurology*, 2nd ed., Amsterdam.

SNIDER, R. S. (1972) The cerebellum, in *Scientific Foundations of Neurology*, ed. Critchley, M., O'Leary, J. L., and Jennett, W. B., London.

THE VISUAL FIBRES AND THE VISUAL FIELDS

VISUAL ACUITY

The visual acuity is normally tested for both distant and near vision and if a refractive error is present it is reasonable in the neurological examination to allow the patient to wear his spectacles so that the 'corrected' acuity is assessed. For the testing of distant vision, Snellen's test types are used at a distance of 6 metres and the patient is asked to read the letters with each eye covered. The lines of type are each numbered; the patient with normal vision can read the line of letters numbered 6 at a distance of 6 metres so that his acuity is recorded as 6/6. When the acuity is grossly impaired, it may be recorded as 6/60; if a patient cannot read the largest type, then his acuity may be recorded as 'hand movements', 'light perception' only, or total blindness (amblyopia). For testing near vision, which depends upon the integrity of the macular area of the retina and the fibres derived from it, many reading types, including Jaeger's, are available. With the reading test types approved by the Faculty of Ophthalmologists, London, the smallest type is classified as N5, the largest N48. When testing the visual fields it should be noted that the results of perimetry may be prejudiced if visual acuity is grossly impaired in one or other eye due to refractive errors or other ocular abnormalities, so that the results may be unreliable if the acuity is 6/60 or worse.

THE VISUAL FIELDS

Investigation of the extent of the fields of vision and of the degree of visual acuity within them plays an important part in the routine examination of patients suffering from nervous diseases. 'Perimetry' is a term applied to the mapping of the visual fields. This may be carried out in the following ways:

CONFRONTATION PERIMETRY

This method is extremely rough and only gross defects of the visual fields are likely to be detected by it. The observer stands or sits opposite to the patient and

about a metre away from him. The patient is instructed to cover one eye with his hand and to fix the gaze of his other eye upon the opposite eye of the observer. The observer then brings a test object, such as a finger or preferably a hat-pin with a small white head, inwards from beyond the periphery of his own visual field, midway between himself and the patient, who is asked to say when he first sees it. This procedure is carried out above, below, and to either side, and the observer is able to determine the extent of the patient's visual field relative to his own. Besides ascertaining the outer boundaries of the visual field by the method described, the test object should be made to traverse the field in various directions and the patient should be asked to state if it disappears from view and when it reappears. In this way a *scotoma* (an area of defective vision within the field) may be detected. The 'blind spot' is a scotoma which results from the fact that the optic disc does not contain any visual receptors.

In young children and unco-operative patients a field defect may sometimes be detected by observing whether the patient notices an object brought in from the periphery in various directions, or whether he blinks in response to a feint with the hand towards the eye—the *menace reflex*.

MECHANICAL PERIMETRY

There are a large number of perimeters in use by which the visual fields can be tested and recorded. The patient is made to gaze at a fixation point and the test object is then moved in the arc of a circle towards the fixation point. The object is at a distance of from 250 to 330 mm from the eye and is usually between 3 and 10 mm in diameter. The visual acuity differs in different parts of the visual field. Although a moving object is readily perceived in the peripheral part, central vision for a stationary object is more acute than peripheral vision. Hence the smaller the test object the smaller the visual field in which it is perceptible. The conditions of the test are indicated by the fraction

$$\frac{\text{diameter of object}}{\text{distance}}.$$

If a 3-mm test object is used at a distance of 330 mm, this fraction is 3/330. Boundaries of the normal visual field for 3/330 are situated at about 60 degrees up, 60 degrees in, 75 degrees down, and 100 degrees, or a little more, out. The field for colours is smaller than that for white, that for blue and yellow being somewhat larger than that for red and green.

PERIMETRY BY BJERRUM'S SCREEN

A mechanical perimeter is a useful method for determining the boundaries of the visual fields. More refined methods, however, are often necessary for investigating the central fields. Bjerrum's screen enables test objects of 1 and 2 mm to be used at a distance of 2 metres—1/2000 and 2/2000. In this way very slight defects of central vision may be detected and, since they are projected upon a large area, accurately mapped. A depression of visual acuity in the centre of the field may not always be demonstrable with reading types. It is for the detection of such defects that Bjerrum's screen is of special value. The normal field for a 1/2000 test object by this method extends to nearly 26 degrees in all directions. If a defect exists to 1/2000 or 2/2000 objects, larger objects should be used until one is seen in the area of impaired vision.

ABNORMALITIES OF THE VISUAL FIELDS

The term 'hemianopia' indicates a loss of vision in half of the visual field. When this is present in the same half of both fields, for example both right halves, we speak of 'homonymous hemianopia'. When the field defect on one side is a mirror image of that on the other, the hemianopia is said to be bitemporal or binasal, according to the halves affected. A field defect limited to one quadrant is described as 'quadrantic hemianopia' or 'quadrantanopia'. When homonymous field defects are capable of being accurately superimposed one upon another, they are said to be congruous; when their corresponding boundaries differ, they are said to be incongruous.

Closely related disturbances of visual function are—visual inattention, indicated by a failure to notice movement of an object such as the observer's finger in one half-field, when there is a competing stimulus in the opposite half-field, and visual disorientation, which is inability to localize objects seen, especially to estimate relative distance [see p. 119].

Many more precise methods of assessing visual function are now available. Tachistoscopy is a complex method of assessing responses to and perception of visual stimuli presented independently or simultaneously in many parts of the visual field. The electroretinogram (ERG) is an electrical response of visual receptors in the retina which can be recorded with corneal electrodes, and the visual evoked response (VER) is an electrical potential arriving at the occipital cortex after stimulation of the retina by a flash of light or patterned stimuli; it can be recorded through the intact skull. Measurement of these electrical events and of the latency of the VER may be of considerable value in the differential diagnosis of disorders of visual function (Walsh and Hoyt, 1969; Harden and Pampiglione, 1970; Halliday et al., 1972).

THE PATH OF THE VISUAL FIBRES (FROM THE RETINA TO THE PRIMARY VISUAL CENTRES)

THE OPTIC NERVES

The fibres of the optic nerve are the axons of the ganglion cells of the retina. The macula is the region of most acute vision, and ocular fixation is so regulated as to bring on to the macula the image of any object at which we look. The macular fibres are thus the most important part of the visual afferent system.

In the retina these fibres run from the macula to the temporal side of the optic disc or papilla. Fibres from the upper and lower temporal quadrants of the retina are displaced by the macular fibres to the upper and lower parts of the disc, and fibres from the nasal quadrants occupy the nasal side. The optic nerves pass backwards and inwards through the optic foramina and terminate posteriorly at the optic chiasm.

THE OPTIC CHIASM

At the optic chiasm the two optic nerves unite and the decussation of the fibres derived from the nasal halves of the retinae occurs [FIG. 11]. The position of the chiasm is a variable one and assumes importance in relationship to the field defects produced by its compression by tumours in this region. It is usually situated a little behind the tuberculum sellae. It is rarely as far forward as the sulcus chiasmatis and is sometimes much further back behind the dorsum sellae and is then related to the posterior part of the pituitary. The relationship of the

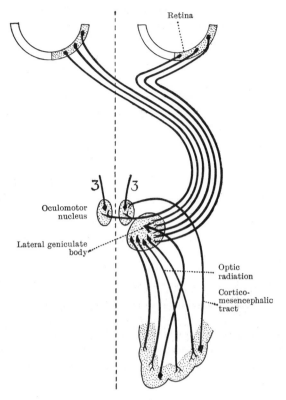

Fig. 11. Diagram of central connections of the optic nerve
and optic tract

chiasm to the sella turcica, pituitary body, and infundibulum is thus variable.
The most important of its other relations are, above, the floor of the third
ventricle and, laterally, the internal carotid arteries.

The decussating fibres from the nasal half of each retina expand within the
chiasm, those from the anterior part of the optic nerve passing inwards and
forwards to form a loop, entering the base of the opposite optic nerve before
passing backwards to the opposite optic tract, where they are joined by the nasal
fibres from the posterior part of the nerve which cross the chiasm more
posteriorly. The fibres from the temporal halves of the retinae do not decussate,
but are continued backwards on the same side in the optic tract. The blood
supply of the chiasm is derived from prechiasmal branches of the ophthalmic
artery, a few superior chiasmal branches from the anterior cerebrals, and inferior
chiasmal arteries which are branches of the internal carotids (Dawson, 1958).

THE OPTIC TRACT

Each optic tract is composed of fibres from the temporal half of the retina of
the same side and from the nasal half of the retina of the opposite side. Within
the tract the uncrossed fibres lie dorsolaterally and the crossed fibres ventro-
mesially. Each optic tract sweeps outwards and backwards between the cerebral
peduncle and the gyrus parahippocampalis, and finally inwards to terminate

in the superior colliculus, the lateral geniculate body, and the pulvinar of the optic thalamus, but experimental evidence throws doubt upon whether the last structure plays any part either in vision or in the optical reflexes. The lateral geniculate body appears to receive the fibres concerned in visual perception, and the superior colliculus those destined to excite reflex activity. Besides the localization in a lateral plane already described, there is in the optic nerves, chiasm, and tracts a considerable degree of localization of the fibres in the vertical plane also, fibres from the lower halves of the retinae lying below, and those from the upper halves above.

VISUAL FIELD DEFECTS DUE TO LESIONS OF THE OPTIC NERVES, CHIASM, AND TRACTS

We are now in a position to apply the anatomical facts just described to the interpretation of the visual field defects produced by lesions of the optic nerves, chiasm, and tracts.

LESIONS OF THE OPTIC NERVE

A lesion of one optic nerve produces a field defect limited to the same eye, since it lies anterior to the chiasmal decussation. The type of field defect produced varies according to the pathological nature of the lesion and is more fully discussed on pages 155–65. In general, inflammatory and compressive lesions of the optic nerve are likely to lead to a central scotoma [FIG. 12] or to a sector

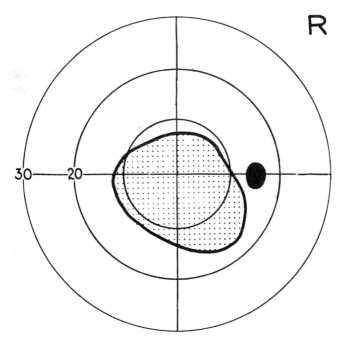

FIG. 12. A central scotoma due to retrobulbar neuritis

defect of irregular shape, but in papilloedema due to increased intracranial pressure the characteristic field defect is an enlargement of the blind spot, together with a peripheral concentric constriction.

LESIONS OF THE CHIASM

The commonest lesions of the optic chiasm are those due to pressure, either by tumours arising in the pituitary body or above the sella turcica, such as suprasellar cysts and meningiomas. In addition, the chiasm itself may be the site of a gliomatous tumour, or may be compressed by a tumour arising in the third ventricle, by distension of the third ventricle in hydrocephalus, or by an intracranial aneurysm. It may be involved in local chronic arachnoiditis, or in granulomatous meningitis due to syphilis, tuberculosis, or sarcoidosis, in demyelinating disorders such as multiple sclerosis and neuromyelitis optica, and, rarely, in vascular lesions and after head injury.

When the point of maximal pressure is in the midline the decussating fibres are first compressed, with the result that at some stage in the development of the growth there is bitemporal hemianopia, for, as we have seen, the decussating fibres are derived from the nasal halves of both retinae, and owing to the refractive effect of the optic lens these parts of the retinae receive images from the temporal halves of the visual fields. Binasal hemianopia may result from compression of the lateral aspects of the chiasm by atherosclerotic internal carotid or anterior cerebral arteries (O'Connell and du Boulay, 1973); O'Connell (1973) suggests that the medial fibres of the chiasm are most sensitive to the effects of tension, the lateral ones to pressure. When pressure is exerted upon the chiasm from below, the fibres from the lower nasal quadrants of the retinae are first affected. Hence the field defect begins in the upper temporal quadrants. When the pressure comes from above, the reverse is the case. This rather schematic explanation must now be qualified by the statement that pituitary and suprasellar tumours rarely exert a symmetrical pressure in the midline. Hence the decussating fibres are usually involved on one side before the other. Consequently, in the case of pituitary tumours, the field defect begins as a rule in the upper temporal quadrant on one side as an indentation which may be associated with a paracentral scotoma with which it subsequently fuses. It then spreads to the lower quadrant, while a similar change occurs a little later on the opposite sides [FIG. 13 (a) and (b)]. Further pressure leads to involvement of the nasal field of the eye first affected and at this stage there is blindness of one eye with temporal hemianopia of the other. Finally the remaining nasal field is lost.

Owing to the complicated paths of the fibres in the chiasm and the liability of pressure to involve also either the optic nerve or tract, many forms of visual field change are encountered.

The most characteristic feature of the visual field defects associated with lesions of the chiasm is their asymmetry compared with the more symmetrical character of the defects due to lesions of the optic tracts and radiation.

LESIONS OF THE OPTIC TRACT

Since the optic tracts are composed of fibres from the temporal half of the retina of the same side and the nasal half of the opposite retina, they carry impulses derived from visual images of objects in the opposite half of the visual field. Lesions of one optic tract, therefore, result in a crossed homonymous field defect which usually begins in one quadrant and rarely extends to a complete homonymous hemianopia. The defects in the two visual fields are not as a rule congruous, the visual field defect being usually slightly greater upon the side of the lesion than upon the opposite side. A homonymous field defect occurs in

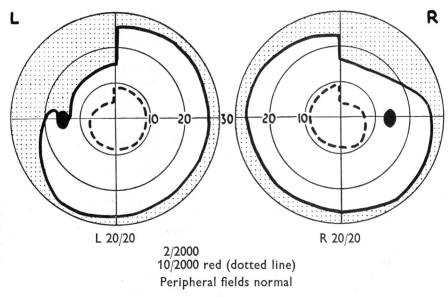

L 20/20   R 20/20

2/2000
10/2000 red (dotted line)
Peripheral fields normal

FIG. 13a. Visual fields of a patient with a chromophobe adenoma of the pituitary, showing early changes in the upper temporal quadrants

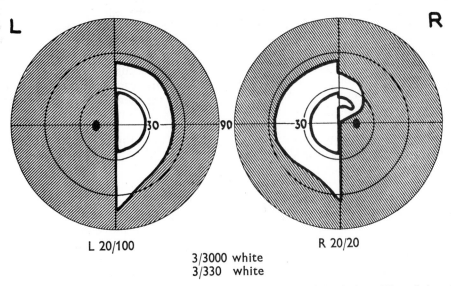

L 20/100   R 20/20

3/3000 white
3/330 white

FIG. 13b. Field changes in a patient with a chromophobe adenoma of the pituitary. The splitting of the macula which occurred in this case is unusual

cases of pituitary tumour about half as frequently as bitemporal hemianopia, and the optic tract may also be compressed by other tumours at the base of the brain, including the anterior part of the temporal lobe, and by aneurysm of the internal carotid and posterior communicating arteries; it may also be involved in inflammatory lesions, such as basal syphilitic meningitis.

THE GENICULOCALCARINE PATHWAY

The last stage of the path of the visual fibres to the cortex begins at the lateral geniculate body. From this they enter the posterior limb of the internal capsule, where they lie behind the somatic sensory fibres and internal to the fibres of the auditory radiation. They emerge from the capsule as the optic radiation, or geniculocalcarine pathway, which runs to the area striata of the occipital lobe. This path varies in directness for different fibres. The more dorsal fibres pass directly to the visual cortex, but those situated more ventrally in the optic radiation turn downwards and forwards into the uncinate region of the temporal lobe, and there spread out over the tip of the descending horn of the lateral ventricle before turning back along the inferior aspect of the ventricle to reach the inferior lip of the calcarine sulcus (Falconer and Wilson, 1958; van Buren and Baldwin, 1958). As we have seen, fibres derived from the lower half of the retina remain below those from the upper half throughout the optic chiasm and tracts, and this relationship persists in the geniculocalcarine pathway. Hence the more direct upper fibres of the optic radiation are derived from the upper halves of the retinae and are excited by images from the lower halves of the visual fields, and the reverse is true of the lower fibres, which pass by way of the tip of the temporal lobe. These facts explain the nature of the visual field defects produced by lesions involving the optic radiation in the temporal and parietal lobes respectively. A left temporosphenoidal abscess, for example, tends to damage the lower fibres rather than the upper, and the resulting field defect lies in the upper half of the visual fields. Since a unilateral lesion involves only the fibres concerned in vision in the opposite half-fields, the field defect is a crossed homonymous superior quadrantic one [FIG. 14]. Conversely a lesion involving the optic radiation in the parietal lobe may affect only the upper fibres and produce a crossed inferior quadrantic loss. Complete destruction of one optic radiation produces a crossed homonymous hemianopia. Homonymous field defects due to lesions of the optic radiation are congruous, sometimes with escape of a small area around the fixation point—'sparing of the macula' [FIG. 15] [and see below]. The commonest lesions involving the optic radiation are vascular lesions and tumours. The lower fibres may be involved in abscess of the temporal lobe. The radiations are early affected by degeneration in diffuse sclerosis (Schilder's disease).

THE VISUAL CORTEX

The cortical visual area or 'area striata' is situated above and below the calcarine sulcus and in adjacent portions of the cuneus and lingual gyrus, and sometimes extends slightly on to the lateral surface of the occipital pole. From what has been said previously concerning the representation of the retinae in the optic tracts, it will be realized that the visual cortex on one side receives impulses from the temporal half of the retina on the same side and the nasal

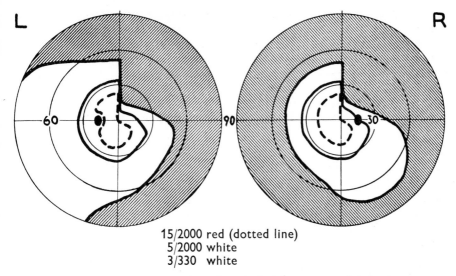

15/2000 red (dotted line)
5/2000 white
3/330 white

FIG. 14. Fields of a patient with a glioma in the left temporo-occipital region

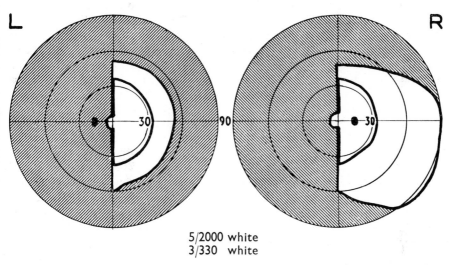

5/2000 white
3/330 white

FIG. 15. Fields of a patient with a metastasis from a breast carcinoma involving the right geniculo-calcarine pathway

half of the opposite retina, that is, those halves of the retinae which are excited by images derived from the opposite halves of the visual fields. Some workers believe that the macula is bilaterally represented at the cortex; others that each half is represented in the opposite visual cortex. This controversy remains unresolved (Walsh and Hoyt, 1969); Gassel and Williams (1962) believe that 'macular sparing' is an artefact due to a defect of gaze occurring during the charting of the visual fields, but Walsh and Hoyt (1969) disagree. The retinae may be regarded as projected upon the visual cortex as follows. The macular area occupies the depths of the calcarine fissure and a wedge-shaped area of the most posterior part of the visual cortex, extending slightly on to the lateral surface of the occipital lobe, the apex of the wedge being 2 or 3 cm anterior to the occipital pole. The periphery of the retina is represented in front of the macular area of the cortex, concentric zones of the retina from the macula to the periphery probably being represented from behind forwards in the visual area. The upper quadrants of the retina are represented in the upper part of the visual cortex, above the calcarine sulcus, and the lower quadrants below. From these facts the effects of lesions involving the visual cortex can readily be understood. Lesions of one visual cortex cause crossed homonymous field defects which are always congruous. Lesions involving the upper half, i.e. the area above the calcarine sulcus, produce inferior quadrantic field defects, and vice versa. Lesions confined to the calcarine sulcus and occipital pole produce central or paracentral scotomas. Lesions more anteriorly placed tend to produce scotomas involving the periphery of the visual fields, with escape of the central portions, provided the macular fibres of the optic radiation are not injured at the same time. Complete destruction of the visual cortex on one side produces a crossed homonymous hemianopia.

The main arterial supply of the visual cortex is the posterior cerebral artery. Thrombosis of the posterior cerebral artery therefore causes a crossed homonymous hemianopia, with, rarely, escape of the fixation point. Bilateral posterior cerebral artery occlusion usually gives total cerebral or cortical blindness (Symonds and Mackenzie, 1957); transient cortical blindness is also a common manifestation of cerebral anoxia, especially in children (Barnet *et al.*, 1970), and recovery is often incomplete. The commonest lesions of the visual cortex are vascular lesions and tumours. Many cases of gunshot wound of this part of the brain were observed during the First World War.

REFERENCES

BARNET, A. B., MANSON, J. I., and WILNER, E. (1970) Acute cerebral blindness in childhood, *Neurology (Minneap.)*, **20,** 1147.

BROUWER, B., and ZEEMAN, W. P. C. (1926) The projection of the retina in the primary optic neuron in monkeys, *Brain*, **49,** 1.

VAN BUREN, J. M., and BALDWIN, M. (1958) The architecture of the optic radiation in the temporal lobe of man, *Brain*, **81,** 15.

COGAN, D. G., and WILLIAMS, H. W. (1966) *Neurology of the Visual System*, Springfield, Ill.

CUSHING, H., and WALKER, C. B. (1914–15) Distortions of the visual fields in cases of brain tumor (4); chiasmal lesions with especial reference to bitemporal hemianopsia, *Brain*, **37,** 341.

DAWSON, B. H. (1958) The blood vessels of the human optic chiasma and their relation to those of the hypophysis and hypothalamus, *Brain*, **81,** 207.

FALCONER, M. A., and WILSON, J. L. (1958) Visual field changes following anterior temporal lobectomy; their significance in relation to 'Meyer's loop' of the optic radiation, *Brain*, **81,** 1.

GASSEL, M. M., and WILLIAMS, D. (1962) Visual function in patients with homonymous hemianopia. Part I, The visual fields, *Brain*, **85,** 175.

HALLIDAY, A. M., McDONALD, W. I., and MUSHIN, J. (1972) Delayed visual evoked response in optic neuritis, *Lancet*, **ii,** 982.

HARDEN, A., and PAMPIGLIONE, G. (1970) Neurophysiological approach to disorders of vision, *Lancet*, **ii,** 805.

HOLMES, G. (1918) Disturbances of vision by cerebral lesions, *Brit. J. Ophthal.*, **2,** 353.

HOLMES, G. (1931) A contribution to the cortical representation of vision, *Brain*, **54,** 470.

HOLMES, G., and LISTER, W. T. (1916) Disturbances of vision from cerebral lesions, with special reference to the cortical representation of the macula, *Brain*, **39**, 34.

HORRAX, G., and PUTNAM, T. J. (1932) Distortion of the visual fields in cases of brain tumour. The field defects and hallucinations produced by tumours of the occipital lobe, *Brain*, **55**, 499.

O'CONNELL, J. E. A. (1973) The anatomy of the optic chiasm and heteronymous hemianopia, *J. Neurol. Neurosurg. Psychiat.*, **36**, 710.

O'CONNELL, J. E. A., and DU BOULAY, E. P. G. H. (1973) Binasal hemianopia, *J. Neurol. Neurosurg. Psychiat.*, **36**, 697.

RIDDOCH, G. (1917) Dissociation of visual perception due to occipital injuries, with especial reference to appreciation of movement, *Brain*, **40**, 15.

SYMONDS, C. P., and MACKENZIE, I. (1957) Bilateral loss of vision from cerebral infarction, *Brain*, **80**, 415.

TRAQUAIR, H. M. (1938) *An Introduction to Clinical Perimetry*, 3rd ed., London.

TRAQUAIR, H. M., DOTT, N. M., and RUSSELL, W. R. (1935) Traumatic lesions of the optic chiasma, *Brain*, **58**, 398.

WALSH, F. B., and HOYT, W. F. (1969) The visual sensory system; anatomy, physiology and topographic diagnosis, in *Handbook of Clinical Neurology*, ed. Vinken, P. J., and Bruyn, G. W., Amsterdam.

THE OCULAR MOVEMENTS

The ocular movements are described as horizontal movement outwards, or abduction; horizontal movement inwards, or adduction; vertical movement upwards, or elevation; vertical movement downwards, or depression. The eye is, of course, capable of diagonal movements at any intermediate angle. The term 'rotation' should be reserved for wheel-like movements around an imaginary pivot passing from before backwards through the centre of the pupil. Such movements of rotation do not normally occur, but are observed only as a result of the unbalanced action of certain muscles. Inward rotation is a movement similar to that of a wheel rolling towards the nose, and outward rotation is the opposite rotatory movement. Normally the movements of the two eyes are harmoniously symmetrical and we then speak of conjugate ocular movements or deviation. Conjugate ocular deviation is described as horizontal or lateral, upward and downward. Conjugate adduction of the two eyes is known as convergence.

THE EXTRINSIC OCULAR MUSCLES

The extrinsic ocular muscles are the four recti, superior and inferior, lateral and medial, and the two obliques, superior and inferior. The action of each of these muscles is shown in the following table and in the diagram [FIG. 16], in which the relative power of the muscles in different directions is indicated by the length of the arrows.

Superior rectus	Medial rectus	Inferior rectus	Inferior oblique	Lateral rectus	Superior oblique
Adductor	Adductor	Adductor	Elevator	. .	Depressor
Internal rotator	. .	External rotator	External rotator	. .	Internal rotator
Elevator	. .	Depressor	Abductor	Abductor	Abductor

It will be seen that only the lateral and medial recti act in a single plane. The other muscles always act in concert with each other in such a way that their conflicting tendencies cancel and a harmonious resultant is produced. Thus when the two obliques aid the lateral rectus in abduction their vertical and rotatory forces cancel each other; and when the superior rectus and inferior oblique contract together in elevating the eye their horizontal and rotatory components also cancel.

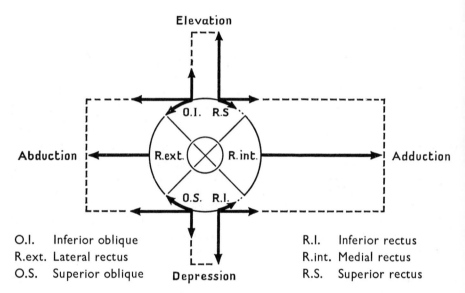

O.I.   Inferior oblique
R.ext. Lateral rectus
O.S.   Superior oblique

R.I.   Inferior rectus
R.int. Medial rectus
R.S.   Superior rectus

FIG. 16. Scheme to illustrate the action of the ocular muscles

But owing to the planes in which the superior and inferior recti and the obliques are placed their actions are influenced by the position of the eye in the orbit. When the eye is rotated outwards 23 degrees the superior rectus is a pure elevator and the inferior rectus a pure depressor. The more it is turned inwards the more they act as internal and external rotators. The converse is true of the obliques. In conjugate deviation there is a harmonious contraction of the appropriate muscles of the two eyes. In lateral conjugate deviation the lateral rectus of one eye and the medial rectus of the other are associated; in conjugate deviation upwards and downwards, the elevators and depressors of the two eyes respectively; and in convergence, the medial recti. Ocular movements must not be regarded as consisting merely of contractions of the prime movers, the muscles actively displacing the eye. There is evidence that graded contraction and relaxation of their antagonists play an important part in orderly movement.

PARALYSIS OF INDIVIDUAL OCULAR MUSCLES

The more important results of paralysis of an ocular muscle are (1) defective ocular movement, (2) squint, (3) erroneous projection of the visual field, and (4) diplopia.

DEFECTIVE OCULAR MOVEMENT

Defective ocular movement is demonstrated by asking the patient to fix his gaze on an object, such as the observer's finger, which is then moved upwards and downwards and to either side, convergence being tested by bringing it towards the patient. The movement is defective in the direction in which the eye is normally moved by the muscle which is paralysed. Slight weakness of a muscle, especially of one of the elevators or depressors, may not lead to any defect of ocular movement evident to the observer.

SQUINT

Squint, or strabismus, is the term applied to a failure of the normal co-ordination of the ocular axes. It is necessary to distinguish paralytic squint from concomitant or spasmodic squint. Paralytic squint may be present when the eyes are at rest, in which case it is due to the unbalanced action of the normal antagonist of the paralysed muscle, for example, the affected eye may be slightly adducted when the lateral rectus is paralysed. More often it is apparent only when the eyes are deviated in the direction in which the eye should be pulled by the paralysed muscle, or if squint is present at rest it is increased by such a movement. Concomitant squint, however, is present at rest and is equal for all positions of the eyes, and, if the fixing eye is covered, the movements of the squinting eye are found to be full. Concomitant squint is not usually associated with diplopia; paralytic squint, at least in the early stages, usually is. It should, however, be noted that when there is long-standing ocular muscle imbalance (latent concomitant squint or heterophoria) the patient may be able for many years to contract the ocular muscles so as to fuse the images from the two eyes; as he becomes older the effort may no longer be possible so that the latent squint breaks down and diplopia results. Similarly, in long-standing paralytic squint, one image may ultimately be suppressed so that diplopia disappears; suppression of this type often results in one eye becoming amblyopic as a result of untreated concomitant squint in early childhood.

When the lateral rectus is paralysed the ocular axes converge and the squint is said to be convergent. Paralysis of the medial rectus causes divergent squint. Divergent squint, however, may also occur in severe myopia, and is often present in an unconscious patient without indicating paralysis of an ocular muscle. The deviation of the axis of the affected eye from parallelism with that of the normal eye is called the 'primary deviation'. If the patient is made to fix an object in a direction requiring the action of the affected muscle and at the same time is prevented from seeing it with his normal eye, the latter is found to deviate too far in the required direction. This is called 'secondary deviation', and is due to the increased effort evoked by his attempt to move the affected eye.

ERRONEOUS PROJECTION OF THE VISUAL FIELD

If we look at a candle straight in front of us and then, turning the eyes but not the head, at a candle placed to one side, in each case the image of the candle falls upon the macula. Let us now consider what happens when the right lateral rectus is paralysed. On conjugate deviation to the right the left eye moves normally and the right eye remains directed forwards. The image of the object regarded falls in the left eye upon the macula, in the right eye upon the nasal half of the retina. The patient is accustomed to regard an object, the image of which falls upon the nasal half of the right retina, as situated to the right of one of which the image falls upon the macula. Consequently he sees two images and projects the false image perceived by his affected eye to the right of the true image perceived by his normal eye. If now his normal eye is covered and he is asked to touch the object, he will direct his finger to the right of its true position. The erroneous projection is always in the normal direction of action of the affected muscle. When it produces sufficient spatial disorientation vertigo may result. Hess's screen is an ingenious method of recording the position of the false image.

DIPLOPIA

Erroneous projection of the visual field of the affected eye is responsible for double vision. When both eyes are used, two images are seen, one correctly and one erroneously projected, the true and the false images. Let us apply our previous illustration to the interpretation of diplopia.

In paralysis of the right lateral rectus the right eye is not abducted. If the patient attempts to deviate his eyes horizontally to the right, the image of a small object falls in the left eye upon the macula. In the right eye, which is not displaced, it falls upon the nasal half of the retina, hence it is seen in (or projected into) the temporal field of the right eye. The false image is thus parallel with and to the right of the true image. The further the test object is moved to the right the further into the nasal half of the right retina its image moves, and the further the false image appears to move to the right. From these facts can be deduced two simple rules governing the appearance of diplopia:

1. The separation of the images increases the further the eyes are moved in the normal direction of pull of the paralysed muscle.
2. The false image is displaced in the direction of the plane or planes of action of the paralysed muscle.

It follows from the two rules that when the gaze is so directed that the separation of the images is greatest, the more peripherally situated image is the false one, derived from the affected eye, which can thus be ascertained. The simplest method is to cover one eye with a red, and the other with a green, glass. The patient is then made to look at a light, such as an ophthalmoscope lamp, or a small but well-illuminated piece of white paper. This is moved until the maximal separation of the images is obtained, and they are then distinguishable by their colour. If coloured glass is not available, an intelligent and cooperative patient is usually able to distinguish the images by noticing which disappears when each eye is covered separately.

When the affected eye has been discovered, the paralysed muscle can be determined. It is the muscle which normally displaces the eye in the direction of displacement of the false image. The positions of the false images resulting from paralysis of the various ocular muscles are described below for the right eye. The description will apply to the left eye if right be substituted for left and vice versa. The diplopia is said to be simple, or uncrossed, when the false image lies on the same side of the true image as the affected eye, and crossed when it lies on the opposite side.

POSITION OF FALSE IMAGE IN PARALYSIS OF THE OCULAR MUSCLES OF THE RIGHT EYE

Lateral Rectus. The diplopia is uncrossed and the maximal separation of the images occurs on abduction, when the false image is level with, and parallel with, the true.

Medial Rectus. The diplopia is crossed and the maximal separation of the images occurs on adduction, when the false image is level with, and parallel with, the true.

Superior Rectus. The false image is above and to the left of the true and tilted away from it. Vertical separation of the images is greatest on abduction, the tilting greatest on adduction. The diplopia is crossed.

Inferior Rectus. The false image is below and to the left of the true and tilted towards it. Vertical separation of the images is greatest on abduction, and tilting on adduction. The diplopia is crossed.

Inferior Oblique. The false image is above and to the right of the true and tilted away from it. The diplopia is uncrossed. Vertical separation of the images is greatest on adduction, and tilting on abduction.

Superior Oblique. The false image is below and to the right of the true and tilted towards it. The diplopia is uncrossed. Vertical separation of the images is greatest on adduction, and tilting on abduction. Since the diplopia occurs on looking downwards it is particularly troublesome to the patient when walking downstairs.

A patient suffering from diplopia usually rotates or tilts the head into the position in which the least demand is made upon the paralysed muscle.

THE NUCLEI OF THE OCULAR MUSCLES

The lower motor neurones which innervate the ocular muscles originate in the nuclei of the third, fourth, and sixth cranial nerves. The first two lie in the midbrain just anterior to the cerebral aqueduct at the level of the superior and inferior colliculi. The nuclei of the sixth nerve lie in the pons beneath the floor of the upper part of the fourth ventricle and partly encircled by the fibres of the seventh nerve.

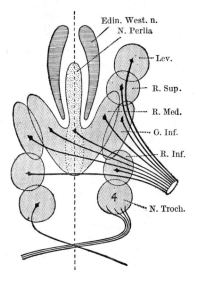

FIG. 17. Diagram of the oculomotor nucleus

The precise representation of muscles in the nucleus of the third nerve is still somewhat uncertain, but the diagram [FIG. 17] represents the probable arrangement. The median, unpaired, small-celled nucleus of Perlia is the centre for convergence and accommodation, while the lateral, paired, small-celled nucleus of Edinger-Westphal innervates the parasympathetic constrictor of the pupil. The remainder of the nucleus is the paired, large-celled, lateral nucleus in which the muscles are represented from above downwards as follows: levator palpebrae, superior rectus, inferior oblique, medial rectus, inferior rectus. Decussating fibres unite the lower parts of the nuclei. Immediately below the third nerve nucleus lies that of the fourth nerve which innervates the opposite superior oblique. This nucleus and the adjacent lowest part of the third nerve nucleus innervate the two muscles concerned in depression of the eye, and the two elevating muscles are innervated by mutually adjacent portions of the upper half of the third nerve nucleus.

THE SUPRANUCLEAR AND INTERNUCLEAR PATHS FOR OCULAR MOVEMENT

CONJUGATE LATERAL DEVIATION

Movements of the eyes can be evoked from two areas of the cerebral cortex by electrical stimulation (see Sachsenweger, 1969; Gay and Newman, 1972). One supranuclear path of the motor fibres concerned in conjugate lateral deviation begins in the posterior part of the middle frontal gyrus, anterior to the precentral gyrus. Electrical stimulation of this area produces deviation of the eyes to the opposite side. From the middle frontal gyrus the supranuclear path runs through the corona radiata to the internal capsule, where it is situated near the genu, and then to the cerebral peduncle. In the midbrain the fibres decussate and pass downwards into the upper part of the pons. Just above the sixth nucleus the path divides, some fibres running into that nucleus, while others cross the midline, turn upwards in the posterior longitudinal bundle, and terminate in that part of the third nerve nucleus which innervates the opposite medial rectus. Thus excitation of the supranuclear fibres causes a contraction of the opposite lateral rectus and the ipsilateral medial rectus, and so produces conjugate ocular deviation to the opposite side.

The other cortical area for eye movements is in or near the visual cortex in the occipital lobe (Bender *et al.*, 1957). From here fibres have been traced through the pulvinar to the midbrain. Recent neurophysiological evidence suggests that occipito-mesencephalic pathways are concerned especially with pursuit or following movements, fronto-mesencephalic pathways with rapid conjugate ocular movements including saccades (the movement when fixation is transferred from one object to another), and occipito-pretectal pathways subserve convergence (Gay and Newman, 1972).

CONJUGATE VERTICAL DEVIATION

Less is known about the supranuclear paths for conjugate vertical than about those for conjugate lateral deviation. Probably they also originate in the middle frontal gyrus, but it seems that bilateral activation is needed to evoke vertical movements and hence defective vertical conjugate gaze of cerebral origin only occurs in massive bifrontal lesions. The fibres probably run through the internal capsule and decussate in the upper part of the midbrain. Those concerned in conjugate elevation appear to cross at a higher level than those concerned in conjugate depression. After decussating they terminate in the appropriate regions of the third nerve nucleus and in the fourth nerve nucleus.

CONJUGATE CONVERGENCE

The supranuclear paths for conjugate convergence have been little studied. Since convergence is normally the response to the perception or imagination of a visual image, the path of excitation probably runs through the visual cortex, and then via occipito-pretectal fibres with the corticospinal fibres to the midbrain, to terminate after decussation in the nuclei of the medial recti.

REFLEX OCULAR FIXATION

In voluntary ocular deviation, the patient turns the eyes spontaneously or in response to a command. In addition, conjugate ocular deviation may be excited by various stimuli.

Retinal Stimulation. The retinal stimulus may be either (a) macular, or (b) peripheral.

(a) The patient's head is kept motionless and he is told to fix his gaze upon an object which is then moved in various directions. Appropriate conjugate ocular deviation occurs to keep the image of the object upon the macula. Continuous movement of a series of objects or lines in one direction evokes optokinetic nystagmus [p. 86].

(b) It is an everyday experience that a moving object in the periphery of the visual field excites deviation of the head and eyes so directed that its image is brought upon the macula.

Auditory Stimulation. In response to a sound the eyes are deviated in the direction from which the sound appears to come.

Labyrinthine Stimulation. Caloric, rotatory, and electrical excitation of the labyrinth evokes conjugate ocular deviation and nystagmus [p. 86].

Passive Movement of the Head. The patient is made to fix an object with his gaze and the head is then rotated, flexed, or extended at the neck. Afferent impulses from the cervical spine excite appropriate ocular deviation to keep the image of the object on the macula, whatever the position of the head. For example, if the head is passively rotated to the left, the eyes become deviated to the right. Movements of this nature are the basis of the so-called 'doll's head manœuvre' [p. 52].

The regions concerned in ocular fixation are the visual cortex and the descending path to the midbrain via the pulvinar and the posterior longitudinal bundle.

THE MEDIAL LONGITUDINAL FASCICULUS

The medial longitudinal fasciculus is an important path linking the oculomotor nuclei. It connects the lateral rectus with the opposite medial rectus in conjugate lateral deviation, and it carries impulses concerned in the reflex ocular movements described in the last section. It links together the cochlear and the vestibular parts of the eighth nerve with the oculomotor nuclei and the muscles which rotate the head.

SUPRANUCLEAR AND INTERNUCLEAR LESIONS

Dissociation of Voluntary Ocular Movement and Reflex Fixation. Bilateral lesions of the frontal centres or their descending paths interfere with voluntary movement of the eyes, which, however, can still follow a slowly moving object, or fix an object while the head is moved. In such cases reflex fixation is overactive and the eyes tend to remain fixed on an object until the gaze is obscured. The converse condition, a lesion interfering with reflex fixation, makes it impossible for the subject to fix, and hence to see clearly, a moving object or an object when he himself is moving (Holmes, 1938).

CONJUGATE LATERAL MOVEMENT

We may encounter either spasm, paralysis, or dissociation of conjugate lateral movement of the eyes.

Spasm of conjugate lateral movement may occur as an element in a focal epileptic attack, of which it may be the first symptom, when the exciting lesion is situated in the middle frontal gyrus, the eyes being deviated to the opposite

D

side. It may also occur in convulsions excited by an occipital lesion, in which case there is usually a visual aura. It is sometimes seen during a generalized epileptic convulsion. Spasmodic lateral deviation occasionally occurs in post-encephalitic Parkinsonism, though in this condition vertical deviation is more frequent. It may be excited reflexly by a lesion of the labyrinth, the eyes in this case being usually deviated towards the side of the lesion. In paralysis of conjugate lateral movement in an unconscious patient the eyes are often deviated to the non-paralysed side by the unbalanced action of the normal hemisphere.

Paralysis of conjugate lateral movement to one side may occur as a result of a lesion of the supranuclear fibres at any point in their course, but the effects of a unilateral lesion above the pons are always transitory. When the lesion is situated above the decussation of these fibres in the lower midbrain, lateral movement to the opposite side is paralysed. When the lesion is below the decussation, i.e. in the paramedian portion of the pons just above the sixth nucleus, the paralysis is to the same side as the lesion. A lesion involving the decussation leads to bilateral paralysis, and this may also occur as a result of one extending to both sides of the pons. Pathological evidence suggests that such lesions act by interrupting impulses descending to the contralateral abducens nucleus and to pontine reticular substance and then ascending in the medial longitudinal bundle (Halsey *et al.*, 1967; Goebel *et al.*, 1971). It must be remembered that the supranuclear fibres are concerned with voluntary movement of the eyes, and the true test of their conductivity is to tell the patient to look to one or the other side. To ask him to follow a moving finger with his gaze is to introduce a reflex element into the response. It is common to find in a patient, unconscious from a haemorrhage into the internal capsule, evidence of a paralysis of conjugate ocular deviation which apparently quickly disappears when he recovers consciousness. Such patients, however, often show slowness or weakness in deviating the eyes to the opposite side on command, though they are able to follow with their eyes a moving object.

A pontine lesion usually abolishes reflex conjugate lateral deviation as well as the voluntary movement—a point in favour of the existence in this region of a 'centre', from which starts a final common path shared by both voluntary and reflex movements.

In paralysis of conjugate lateral deviation the affected medial rectus contracts normally on convergence, unless the supranuclear path for convergence, which is separate from that for lateral deviation, is also involved. This is an example of the rule that supranuclear lesions cause paralysis of movements and not of muscles.

Dissociation of conjugate lateral movement occurs when either the lateral or the medial rectus contracts more strongly than its conjugate fellow, and the normal harmony of the two eyes is disturbed. Most commonly the lateral rectus contracts normally, but the opposite medial rectus is weak or paralysed for conjugate lateral movement but contracts normally on convergence. In its fully developed form, this so-called *anterior internuclear ophthalmoplegia* also causes nystagmus which is apparent only in the abducting eye and is associated with failure of medial movement of the adducting eye ('ataxic nystagmus' or Harris's sign). The lesion, usually due to multiple sclerosis, has been thought to involve the ascending fibres of the medial longitudinal fasciculus linking the two muscles together, while the supranuclear path for convergence which terminates at a higher level escapes; rarely it occurs as an early manifestation of brain stem tumour (Cogan and Wray, 1970). A lesion involving the nucleus of the medial rectus muscle in the third nerve nucleus, or the fibres running to this muscle in the third nerve, of course paralyses the muscle both for conjugate lateral movement and for convergence. A lesion of the sixth nerve or its nucleus causes paralysis of the lateral rectus, but the opposite medial rectus contracts normally on conjugate lateral deviation and on convergence. Rarely a similar sign (so-called *posterior internuclear ophthalmoplegia*) with paralysis of lateral movement in one eye with normal adduction of the other can result from a lesion immediately rostral to the abducens nucleus (Rothstein and Alvord, 1971).

Causes of Conjugate Lateral Paralysis

The commonest cause of conjugate lateral paralysis is tumour or infarction involving the pontine centre. It may also be produced by encephalitis, though less often than vertical paralysis, and by multiple sclerosis.

CONJUGATE VERTICAL MOVEMENTS

Spasm of conjugate vertical movement upwards may occur in an epileptic fit or in an attack of petit mal. It is also the commonest form of oculogyral spasm found in post-encephalitic Parkinsonism, though downward and lateral spasm occasionally occur. Upward deviation of the eyes also occurs normally during sleep, and on voluntary closure of the eyelids and blinking.

Paralysis of conjugate vertical movement rarely occurs as a result of lesions above the midbrain and then only with massive bifrontal lesions. At the level of the superior colliculus there exist supranuclear mechanisms for conjugate vertical movements and for convergence, since any of these movements may be abolished separately and without evidence of a nuclear lesion. Moreover, as in the case of conjugate lateral deviation, voluntary vertical deviation may be lost while the movement can still be excited reflexly, for example, by flexing or extending the head when the patient's gaze is fixed upon a motionless object. Such a loss of voluntary, with retention of reflex, movement indicates a lesion of the supranuclear path, while the final common path from the hypothetical midbrain 'centre' remains intact. The centre for vertical movement upwards is situated at a higher level in the midbrain than that for downward movement, since a tumour arising in the third ventricle and impinging upon the midbrain from above impairs the former before the latter. Upward deviation is much more frequently lost than downward deviation, and, as Collier pointed out, its loss is sometimes associated with retraction of the upper lids. In some cases the defect is congenital. The term 'Parinaud's syndrome' is often applied to isolated defects of upward conjugate gaze, but in the fully developed syndrome due to lesions of the midbrain tectum there is often loss of the pupillary reaction to light and paralysis of convergence in addition. It may result from encephalitis, neoplasm of the third ventricle, midbrain or pineal body, and vascular or other lesions of the upper midbrain.

PARALYSIS OF CONVERGENCE

Paralysis of convergence is rarely observed as a result of lesions of the cerebral hemispheres, probably because its supranuclear paths are bilateral. It is common, however, in extrapyramidal syndromes associated with rigidity, especially in post-encephalitic Parkinsonism. It is also met with as a result of lesions involving the convergence centre in the midbrain and may occur after head injury. In such cases there may be an isolated loss of convergence and accommodation. It may be one feature of Parinaud's syndrome (see above). Loss of convergence is occasionally, and spasm of convergence usually, hysterical; it may also occur with ageing and sometimes causes diplopia on near vision.

OCULAR MOTOR APRAXIA

Just as apraxia of limb movement identifies an inability to carry out skilled movements in the absence of paralysis [see p. 115], so ocular motor apraxia (Cogan and Adams, 1953) is an inability to move the eyes voluntarily in the desired direction when random and reflex eye movements are intact. The lesion which causes this rare manifestation appears to be in the prefrontal motor cortex.

PROGRESSIVE SUPRANUCLEAR DEGENERATION

In 1964, Steele, Richardson, and Olszewski described a rare degenerative disorder characterized by ophthalmoplegia affecting vertical and especially downward gaze and associated with variable Parkinsonian and dystonic features as well as dysarthria, pseudobulbar palsy, inconstant cerebellar and pyramidal signs, and variable dementia. Pathologically, such cases have shown neuro-fibrillary and granulovacuolar degeneration of neurones with gliosis and demyelination, especially in the brain stem, basal ganglia, and cerebellum, and the oculomotor nuclei are sometimes involved as well (Blumenthal and Miller, 1969). The disease is progressive and uninfluenced by levodopa or any other form of treatment.

NUCLEAR OPHTHALMOPLEGIA

By nuclear ophthalmoplegia is meant a paralysis of ocular muscles due to a lesion involving the nuclei of the oculomotor nerves. When the extrinsic ocular muscles are involved, the term external ophthalmoplegia is used: paralysis of the pupillary and ciliary muscles is known as internal ophthalmoplegia. When both are affected together we speak of total ophthalmoplegia. Internal ophthal-moplegia is dealt with in a later section. We are here concerned only with external ophthalmoplegia, including ptosis.

Nuclear ophthalmoplegia must be distinguished from supranuclear lesions and from lesions of the oculomotor nerve trunks. As we have seen, supranuclear lesions cause disturbances of conjugate ocular movement. Consequently the ocular axes remain parallel and diplopia is not produced. Nuclear lesions may be unilateral, but are more often bilateral. When bilateral they are not sym-metrical, and loss of parallelism of the ocular axes and diplopia occur. The varied degree of paralysis of the muscles of both eyes, with or without internal ophthal-moplegia, rarely simulates a lesion of the third nerve trunks, in which as a rule the muscles innervated by the nerve are all affected to an equal extent. Nuclear ophthalmoplegia confined to the fourth nerve has probably never been verified. Since the sixth nerve supplies only one muscle, an isolated lesion of the sixth nerve nucleus can only be distinguished from a lesion of the nerve trunk by the presence of associated symptoms of a lesion of the pons.

The following are the principal causes of nuclear ophthalmoplegia:

1. *Massive lesions involving the brain stem*, especially tumours of the third ventricle, midbrain, pineal body and pons, and vascular lesions.

2. *Avitaminosis.* The condition described by Wernicke as acute superior haemorrhagic polio-encephalitis is now ascribed to avitaminosis [see p. 846].

3. *Infections.* In this group fall syphilis, encephalitis lethargica, and disseminated encephalomyelitis. Syphilitic nuclear ophthalmoplegia may be vascular in origin, but a degenerative type sometimes occurs in tabes and in general paresis.

4. *Demyelination.* An isolated third or sixth nerve palsy is an occasional manifestation of multiple sclerosis, but internuclear ophthalmoplegia is more common. The syndrome of so-called acute idiopathic ophthalmoplegia with ataxia and areflexia (Fisher, 1956; Elizan *et al.*, 1971) is probably a form of polyneuropathy, involving the oculomotor nerve trunks and akin to the Guillain-Barré syndrome; hence the lesion is not nuclear.

5. *Progressive ophthalmoplegia* is the term which has been applied to a group of ophthalmoplegias of mixed aetiology, characterized by the insidious onset and slowly progressive course of ptosis and external ophthalmoplegia. The disorder may start at any age and is sometimes familial. Myopathy of the external ocular muscles accounts for some cases, but in others there is pigmentary retinal degeneration and cardiomyopathy with cerebellar and pyramidal tract signs, and the lesion may well be nuclear (Kearns and Sayre, 1958; Drachman, 1968) [see p. 1000]; mitochondrial abnormalities have been found in muscle and cerebellum in some such cases (Schneck *et al.*, 1973).

6. *Syringobulbia* rarely produces ophthalmoplegia.

7. *Head injury* is a rare cause of nuclear ophthalmoplegia, which may result from contusion of the brain stem.

8. *Congenital defects* of ocular movement occur. These may be hereditary and associated with other hereditary abnormalities. One of the commonest is *Duane's syndrome*, in which there is paralysis of abduction of the affected eye and on attempted adduction the globe retracts and the palpebral fissure narrows; the lateral rectus muscle is usually fibrotic. The condition may be bilateral.

NYSTAGMUS

Nystagmus is a disturbance of ocular posture characterized by a more or less rhythmical oscillation of the eyes. This movement may be of the same rate in both directions, or quicker in one direction than in the other. In the latter case the movements are distinguished as the quick and the slow phases (phasic nystagmus). The quick phase is taken to indicate the direction of the nystagmus, so that if the slow phase is to the left and the quick to the right, the patient is said to exhibit nystagmus to the right. Nystagmus may occur when the eyes are in the position of rest, or only on deviation in certain directions or on convergence, or only when the head is in a certain position—positional nystagmus. The movement may be confined to one plane, horizontal or vertical, or occur in more than one plane—rotary nystagmus. Nystagmus may rarely be associated with a rapid rotary tremor of the head, or with jerky vertical movements of the eyelids. The acquired forms may cause an apparent movement of objects seen by the patient. Nystagmus can be recorded by electronystagmography.

The nature of nystagmus can be best appreciated by recalling the statement made in a previous section [on p. 80] that the posture of the eyes is influenced reflexly by a number of factors of which the most important are impulses derived from the retinae, the labyrinths, and the cervical spine. Nystagmus is a disturbance of ocular posture which may be due to: (1) defective or abnormal retinal impulses; (2) disease or dysfunction of the labyrinths or of the vestibular nuclei or vestibular connections in the brain stem; (3) lesions of the cervical spinal cord; (4) lesions involving the central paths concerned in ocular posture. (5) It may also be a congenital abnormality of unknown aetiology; (6) it has been said to occur rarely in hysteria, but the irregular vertical ocular movements seen occasionally in hysterical subjects are not a true nystagmus; and (7) it may be toxic.

NYSTAGMUS OF RETINAL ORIGIN

1. *Amblyopia* coming on in early life may cause nystagmus if some vision is retained, and especially if macular vision is impaired. The visual impairment renders ocular fixation defective, and a pendular nystagmus results.

2. *Miners' nystagmus* has been attributed to the relative inefficiency of macular vision in a dim light as a result of the absence of rods in the macula. On this hypothesis the defectiveness of macular vision causes defective fixation. Patients with this disorder often showed in addition variable features of anxiety and even hysteria, especially in a compensation setting. The condition has virtually disappeared since underground lighting was improved.

3. *Optokinetic nystagmus.* Optokinetic nystagmus is the term applied to the nystagmus evoked by a succession of moving objects passing before the eyes. A familiar example is the nystagmus which occurs in an individual looking out of the window of a moving train. The slow phase is in the direction in which the landscape appears to move and the quick phase is in the direction in which the train moves. To test for optokinetic nystagmus a Bárány drum is used. This is a revolving, striped cylinder, the speed and direction of which can be altered easily. Horizontal and vertical nystagmus in each direction is produced by revolving the drum at the same speed. The amplitude and regularity of the nystagmus in each direction is noted.

Optokinetic nystagmus is a brain stem reflex, quite distinct from that for vestibular nystagmus and independent of the vestibular nuclei (Dix *et al.*, 1949). The cortical centre for optokinetic nystagmus is in the supramarginal and angular gyri (Carmichael *et al.*, 1956). Optokinetic nystagmus to the opposite side is suppressed in lesions of this area. Indeed, directional preponderance of optokinetic nystagmus towards the side of the lesion may occur not only as a result of parieto-occipital cortical or subcortical lesions but also with lesions of the upper brain stem. The test may be unreliable in the presence of a homonymous hemianopia, but absent, sluggish, or irregular optokinetic responses usually indicate a pontine lesion (e.g. tumour, infarct, or demyelination) (Cawthorne *et al.*, 1969).

LABYRINTHINE NYSTAGMUS

The clinical aspects of labyrinthine nystagmus are considered on page 191. Appropriate stimulation of the horizontal semicircular canals evokes horizontal nystagmus, and of the vertical canals, rotary nystagmus. Acute lesions of the internal ear, whether primary or secondary to disease of the middle ear, cause nystagmus, usually rotary, and with the quick phase as a rule towards the opposite side. The amplitude of the oscillation is increased when the eyes are deviated in the direction of the quick phase and diminished on fixation in the direction of the slow phase. Chronic labyrinthine lesions often lead to fine rotary nystagmus on lateral fixation to one or both sides, especially to the side of the lesion.

NYSTAGMUS DUE TO SPINAL CORD LESIONS

Nystagmus is very rarely seen after a lesion of the cervical region of the spinal cord, and has then been attributed to a defect of afferent impulses from the cervical spine (Biemond and de Jong, 1969). Many authorities have questioned whether an isolated lesion of the spinal cord alone can cause this sign, but vertical nystagmus commonly occurs as a result of lesions in the neighbourhood of the foramen magnum, especially in cases of the Chiari malformation, with or without syringomyelia (Barnett et al., 1973).

NYSTAGMUS DUE TO CENTRAL LESIONS

Nystagmus is a common symptom of lesions of the brain stem and cerebellum. With cerebellar lesions nystagmus may occur on fixation in any direction, the slow phase being towards the position of rest, and the quick phase towards the periphery. With a unilateral cerebellar lesion it is present in both eyes and is most marked on conjugate deviation to the side of the lesion. It may occur as a result of lesions involving the cerebellar connections within the brain stem, the vestibular nucleus, and the posterior longitudinal bundle. Multiple sclerosis is the commonest cause. Nystagmus of central origin also occurs in cases of Friedreich's ataxia and other hereditary ataxias, encephalitis, syringomyelia, tumours, and vascular lesions of the brain stem and cerebellum.

Positional nystagmus [see p. 193] has been used to distinguish central from labyrinthine lesions. A change in the direction of the nystagmus produced by a change in the position of the head favours a central lesion. Positional nystagmus elicited by rotation of the head to one side only is commonly seen in benign positional nystagmus (Nylén, 1950), due to a lesion of the utricle and saccule of one labyrinth. The positional nystagmus which may occur as a result of brain stem lesions (e.g. multiple sclerosis) but which more often results from posterior fossa tumours (especially ependymomas of the fourth ventricle or medulloblastomas in children and young adults or metastases in the elderly) is usually elicited by rotation to either side or by flexion or extension (Grand, 1971).

REBOUND NYSTAGMUS

Rebound nystagmus is an uncommon variety in which nystagmus of phasic type occurs on looking laterally but fatigues after about 20 seconds; when the eyes are then returned to the midline, phasic nystagmus to the opposite side develops and also quickly fatigues. The underlying pathology appears to be cerebellar degeneration (Hood et al., 1973).

SEE-SAW NYSTAGMUS

In this rare form of nystagmus one eye moves up while the other moves down; this disjunctive form of nystagmus has been described in patients with tumours of the third ventricular region but may also be a rare consequence of a pontine lesion (Mastaglia, 1974).

CONGENITAL AND FAMILIAL NYSTAGMUS

Nystagmus may be present from birth, and in several members of the same family, sometimes in successive generations. Congenital nystagmus is usually a fine pendular oscillation present at rest and increased on deviation in all directions, but more than one variety occurs. There may be an associated oscillation of the head. There is usually no subjective movement of objects. Its cause is unknown, but it may be associated with other ocular defects involving poor vision such as albinism, astigmatism, or amblyopia. It may be inherited as a Mendelian dominant or as a sex-linked recessive trait, and males are affected three times as often as females.

HYSTERICAL 'NYSTAGMUS'

Hysterical movements of the eyes superficially resembling nystagmus disappear when ocular fixation is unconscious and reappear on testing the eye movements. They may be associated with spasm of convergence or blepharospasm. *Pseudonystagmus*, often monocular, is also occasionally seen when there is weakness of external ocular muscles, as in myasthenia gravis.

TOXIC NYSTAGMUS

Phasic nystagmus occurring on lateral gaze to both sides is seen in alcoholic intoxication and as a result of many other drugs, including anticonvulsants and barbiturates.

OTHER SPONTANEOUS OCULAR MOVEMENTS

Opsoclonus is a term which has been given to rapid fluttering oscillations of the eyes, often interrupted by sudden, jerk-like myoclonic movements. It is seen most often in association with limb myoclonus in association with so-called acute myoclonic encephalopathy of infancy (Kinsbourne, 1962) but can also be a manifestation of encephalopathy or encephalitis in adults (Baringer et al., 1968; McLean, 1970).

Ocular bobbing is a syndrome of brisk, repetitive, downward conjugate deviation of the eyes, associated usually with pontine lesions in comatose patients (Fisher, 1964; Nelson and Johnston, 1970); recovery has been reported (Newman et al., 1971).

REFERENCES

BARINGER, J. R., SWEENEY, V. P., and WINKLER, G. F. (1968) An acute syndrome of ocular oscillations and truncal myoclonus, *Brain*, **91**, 473.

BARNETT, H. J. M., FOSTER, J. B., and HUDGSON, P. (1973) *Syringomyelia*, London.

BENDER, M. B. (1964) *The Oculomotor System*, New York.

BENDER, M. B., POSTEL, D. M., and KRIEGER, H. P. (1957) Disorders of oculomotor function in lesions of the occipital lobe, *J. Neurol. Neurosurg. Psychiat.*, **20**, 139.

BIEMOND, A., and DE JONG, J. M. B. V. (1969) On cervical nystagmus and related disorders, *Brain*, **92**, 437.

BLUMENTHAL, H., and MILLER, C. (1969) Motor nuclear involvement in progressive supranuclear palsy, *Arch. Neurol. (Chic.)*, **20**, 362.

CARMICHAEL, F. A., DIX, M. R., and HALLPIKE, C. S. (1956) Pathology, symptomatology, and diagnosis of organic affections of the eighth nerve system, *Brit. med. Bull.*, **12**, 146.

CAWTHORNE, T., DIX, M. R., HOOD, J. D., and HARRISON, M. S. (1969) Vestibular Syndromes and Vertigo, in *Handbook of Clinical Neurology*, vol. 2, ed. Vinken, P. J, and Bruyn, G. W., Amsterdam.

COGAN, D. G., and ADAMS, R. D. (1953) A type of paralysis of conjugate gaze (ocular motor apraxia), *Arch. Ophthalmol.*, **50**, 434.

COGAN, D. G., and WILLIAMS, H. W. (1966) *Neurology of the Visual System*, Springfield, Ill.

COGAN, D. G., and WRAY, S. H. (1970) Internuclear ophthalmoplegia as an early sign of brainstem tumors, *Neurology (Minneap.)*, **20**, 629.

DIX, M. R., HALLPIKE, C. S., and HARRISON, W. S. (1949) Some observations on the otological effects of streptomycin intoxication, *Brain*, **72**, 241.

DRACHMAN, D. A. (1968) Ophthalmoplegia plus. The neurodegenerative disorders associated with progressive external ophthalmoplegia, *Arch. Neurol.* (*Chic.*), **18**, 654.

ELIZAN, T. S., SPIRE, J. P., ANDIMAN, R. M., BAUGHMAN, F. A., and LLOYD-SMITH, D. L. (1971) Syndrome of acute idiopathic ophthalmoplegia with ataxia and areflexia, *Neurology* (*Minneap.*), **21**, 281.

FISHER, C. M. (1956) An unusual variant of acute idiopathic polyneuritis (syndrome of ophthalmoplegia, ataxia, and areflexia), *New Engl. J. Med.*, **255**, 57.

FISHER, C. M. (1964) Ocular bobbing, *Arch. Neurol.* (*Chic.*), **11**, 543.

GAY, A. J., and NEWMAN, N. M. (1972) Eye movements and their disorders, in *Scientific Foundations of Neurology*, ed. Critchley, M., O'Leary, J. L., and Jennett, W. B., London.

GOEBEL, H. H., KOMATSUZAKI, A., BENDER, M. B., and COHEN, B. (1971) Lesions of the pontine tegmentum and conjugate gaze paralysis, *Arch. Neurol.* (*Chic.*), **24**, 431.

GRAND, W. (1971) Positional nystagmus: an early sign in medulloblastoma, *Neurology* (*Minneap.*), **21**, 1157.

HALSEY, J. H., CEBALLOS, R., and CROSBY, E. C. (1967) The supranuclear control of voluntary lateral gaze. Clinical and anatomic correlation in a case of ventral pontine infarction, *Neurology* (*Minneap.*), **17**, 928.

HOLMES, G. (1938) The cerebral integration of the ocular movements, *Brit. med. J.*, **2**, 107.

HOOD, J. D., KAYAN, A., and LEECH, J. (1973) Rebound nystagmus, *Brain*, **96**, 507.

KEARNS, T. P., and SAYRE, G. P. (1958) Retinitis pigmentosa, external ophthalmoplegia, and complete heart block: unusual syndrome with histologic study in one of two cases, *Arch. Ophthal.*, **60**, 280.

KINSBOURNE, M. (1962) Myoclonic encephalopathy of infants, *J. Neurol. Neurosurg. Psychiat.*, **25**, 271.

LINDSAY, J. R. (1945) The significance of positional nystagmus in otoneurological diagnosis, *Laryngoscope* (*St. Louis*), **55**, 527.

LYLE, T. K., and JACKSON, S. (1949) *Practical Orthoptics in the Treatment of Squint*, 3rd ed., London.

MCLEAN, D. R. (1970) Polymyoclonia with opsoclonus, *Neurology* (*Minneap.*), **20**, 508.

MASTAGLIA, F. L. (1974) See-saw nystagmus: an unusual sign of brain-stem infarction, *J. neurol. Sci.*, **22**, 439.

NELSON, J. R., and JOHNSTON, C. H. (1970) Ocular bobbing, *Arch. Neurol.* (*Chic.*), **22**, 348.

NEWMAN, N., GAY, A. J., and HEILBRUN, M. P. (1971) Disjugate ocular bobbing: its relation to midbrain, pontine and medullary function in a surviving patient, *Neurology* (*Minneap.*), **21**, 633.

NYLÉN, C. O. (1950) Positional nystagmus: a review and future prospects, *J. Laryng.*, **64**, 295.

RADEMAKER, G. G. J., and TER BRAAK, J. W. G. (1948) On the central mechanism of some optic reactions, *Brain*, **71**, 48.

ROTHSTEIN, T. L., and ALVORD, E. C. (1971) Posterior internuclear ophthalmoplegia: a clinicopathological study, *Arch. Neurol.* (*Chic.*), **24**, 191.

SACHSENWEGER, R. (1969) Clinical localisation of oculomotor disturbances, in *Handbook of Clinical Neurology*, vol. 2, ed. Vinken, P. J., and Bruyn, G. W., Amsterdam.

SCHNECK, L., ADACHI, M., BRIET, P., WOLINTZ, A., and VOLK, B. W. (1973) Ophthalmoplegia plus with morphological and chemical studies of cerebellar and muscle tissue, *J. neurol. Sci.*, **19**, 37.

SMITH, J. LAWTON (1963) *Optokinetic Nystagmus*, Springfield, Ill.

STEELE, J. C., RICHARDSON, J. C., and OLSZEWSKI, J. (1964) Progressive supranuclear palsy: a heterogeneous degeneration involving the brain stem, basal ganglia and cerebellum with vertical gaze and pseudobulbar palsy, nuchal dystonia and dementia, *Arch. Neurol.* (*Chic.*), **10**, 333.

THE PUPILS AND THE EYELIDS

THE INNERVATION OF THE PUPILS

The size of the pupil is under the control of two mutually antagonistic muscles: the circular muscle of the iris, the sphincter pupillae, which causes contraction and is innervated by the third nerve, and the radial fibres of the iris which cause dilatation and receive their nerve supply from the cervical sympathetic.

THE IRIDODILATOR FIBRES

Little is known about the innervation of the pupil above the midbrain. The experimental work of Karplus and Kreidl, however, points to a path for pupillary dilatation from the frontal cortex to the hypothalamus and thence into the cerebral peduncle. Such a corticofugal path appears necessary to explain the occurrence of pupillary dilatation in states of emotion. The iridodilator fibres continue downwards in the tegmentum of the pons, medulla, and the cervical cord to the lateral horn of the grey matter of the eighth cervical and first and second thoracic segments. From the cells of these lateral horns the preganglionic fibres take origin, and leave the cord by the corresponding ventral roots. From the spinal nerves they pass by the white rami communicantes of the sympathetic to the cervical sympathetic nerve trunk to end in the superior cervical ganglion. The postganglionic fibres start from this ganglion and join the plexus in the coat of the internal carotid artery with which they enter the skull, and from which some pass to the ophthalmic division of the trigeminal nerve and reach the pupil by the nasociliary and long ciliary nerves, while others go from the carotid plexus through the ciliary ganglion without interruption, and into the short ciliary nerves.

THE IRIDOCONSTRICTOR AND CILIARY FIBRES

The iridoconstrictor fibres originate in the nuclei of Edinger-Westphal [see FIG. 17, p. 79]. Entering the third nerve, they terminate in the ciliary ganglion, from which postganglionic fibres arise which pass by the short ciliary nerves to the circular muscle of the iris. It is possible that this is true only of the fibres concerned in the reaction to light and that those involved in the reaction on accommodation by-pass the ciliary ganglion (see below). The ciliary fibres follow the same route except that they probably arise in the median nucleus of Perlia and terminate in the ciliary muscle, contraction of which allows the lens to become more convex and so accommodates the eye for near vision.

PARALYSIS OF THE SPHINCTER PUPILLAE

The constrictor muscle of the iris may be paralysed as a result of a lesion involving the iridoconstrictor fibres at any point between the nucleus of Edinger-Westphal and the eye. The pupil is widely dilated owing to the unantagonized action of the iridodilator muscle, and the reaction to both light and accommodation is lost. Paralysis of the sphincter pupillae occurring without paralysis of the extra-ocular muscles may be due to a lesion either of the nucleus of Edinger-Westphal or of the ciliary ganglion but can also be the first manifestation of compression of the trunk of the third nerve, for instance in herniation of one temporal lobe through the tentorial hiatus, as the pupillo-constrictor fibres lie superficially in the nerve trunk.

PARALYSIS OF THE DILATOR PUPILLAE: OCULAR-SYMPATHETIC PARALYSIS

Paralysis of pupillary dilatation is due to a lesion of the iridodilator fibres of the sympathetic. The pupil is constricted—myosis—by the unopposed iridoconstrictor muscle, and fails to exhibit the normal dilatation when the eye is shaded, in states of pain and emotional excitement, and reflexly when the skin of the same side of the neck is scratched with a pin—the ciliospinal reflex. The iridodilator fibres throughout their course are close to the other fibres of the ocular sympathetic, viz. those which produce tonic elevation of the upper lid and tonic protrusion of the eyeball by means of the unstriped muscle of the orbit. Paralysis of the dilator of the iris is therefore usually associated with paralysis of these muscles also, manifested in slight ptosis and enophthalmos (Horner's syndrome).

The myosis of the Argyll Robertson pupil has been attributed to a lesion of the iridodilator fibres in the midbrain. Myosis may also occur with lesions of the pons, as in the pin-point pupils of pontine haemorrhage, and of the lateral part of the medulla which interrupt descending fibres of the sympathetic, as in lateral medullary infarction due to thrombosis of the vertebral or posterior inferior cerebellar artery. In the spinal cord the lateral horns of the upper dorsal region may be involved in a variety of lesions. The sympathetic white rami may be destroyed by trauma, as in the Klumpke type of birth palsy of the brachial plexus; and the cervical sympathetic may be damaged in the neck by trauma or pressure, especially from enlarged cervical lymph nodes.

Within the cranium the postganglionic fibres may be damaged by the pressure of a tumour or aneurysm behind the orbit. In Raeder's paratrigeminal syndrome, division of the sympathetic fibres in or shortly after leaving the internal carotid artery gives the ocular manifestations of Horner's syndrome but without loss of sweating on the affected side of the face as the fibres responsible for the latter travel in the coat of the external carotid.

PARALYSIS OF ACCOMMODATION

Paralysis of accommodation may be produced by lesions involving the median nucleus of Perlia, the third nerve, or the ciliary ganglion. As an isolated ocular phenomenon it is found in diphtheria, in which condition the lesion is according to some authorities nuclear, according to others neuritic, and according to yet others in the ciliary muscle.

INEQUALITY OF THE PUPILS

Inequality of the pupils may occur when one is either pathologically small or pathologically large, or when one is of moderate size but fails to react to light; in this case the normal one will be the larger when it is dilated and the smaller when it is constricted. These various abnormalities can be interpreted in the light of the facts set out above. Irregularity of the pupils is frequently present in syphilis, and sometimes in encephalitis lethargica. In such cases it is probably due to lesions at or near the nucleus and must be distinguished from the irregularity produced by local lesions of the iris, especially iritis.

ACTION OF DRUGS ON THE PUPIL AND CILIARY MUSCLE

Certain drugs influence the pupil and accommodation when applied to the eye. Pilocarpine and physostigmine (eserine) cause constriction of the pupil and spasm of accommodation by stimulating the nerve endings of the third nerve in the pupil and ciliary muscle. Atropine causes dilatation of the pupil and paralysis of accommodation by paralysing the same nerve endings. Cocaine causes dilatation of the pupil by stimulating the nerve endings of the sympathetic fibres. The action of morphine in causing iridoconstriction is central, not peripheral.

THE PUPILLARY REACTIONS

THE LIGHT REFLEX

If one eye is exposed to light, a constriction of both pupils normally occurs. The response of the pupil of the eye upon which the light falls is called the direct reaction, that of the opposite pupil the consensual reaction. In eliciting the light reflex the patient should be asked to look at a distant object in order to eliminate the contraction of the pupil on accommodation, and the eye not being tested should be covered in order to eliminate the consensual reaction. The afferent impulses from the retina follow the path of the visual afferent fibres as far as the optic tracts, with a similar decussation of those from the nasal halves of the retina at the optic chiasma. It is unknown whether the reflex fibres are identical with those concerned in vision, or whether, as some have supposed, two separate sets of fibres exist for these functions. Fibres in the optic nerve vary in size and, correspondingly, in speed of conduction, and it has been shown in the cat that retinal impulses to the lateral geniculate body are conveyed by coarse fast-conducting fibres, while those passing to the midbrain centres are fine and slowly conducting (Clark, 1944). On leaving the optic tracts the reflex fibres separate from the visual and according to Magoun et al. (1936) in the monkey they pass through the brachium of the superior colliculus, but do not enter it, turning rostrally and medially into the pretectal region and then descending to the oculomotor nuclei. The decussating fibres cross, some in the posterior commissure and some ventral to the aqueduct near the nuclei. It is clear that both optic tracts must be connected with both oculomotor nuclei since a beam of light falling upon either half of either retina evokes a contraction of both pupils. The efferent path of the reflex runs from the nuclei of Edinger-Westphal by the iridoconstrictor fibres already described.

REACTION ON ACCOMMODATION/CONVERGENCE

When the gaze is directed from a distant to a near object, contraction of the medial recti brings about a convergence of the ocular axes and, in association with this, accommodation occurs by contraction of the ciliary muscle, and the pupil contracts. In these circumstances contraction of the pupil is in the nature of an associated movement, which is probably the outcome of impulses originating in the visual cortex and descending either directly or by way of the second frontal gyrus to the midbrain, there to terminate in the nuclei of Edinger-Westphal. In eliciting this reaction the patient is asked to look at a distant object and then at the examiner's finger, which is gradually brought to within 50 mm of the eyes.

There is evidence that constriction of the pupil may be associated with either convergence or accommodation, as it occurs on accommodation when convergence is paralysed and vice versa. Usually, however, the two actions cannot be dissociated; however, in post-encephalitic Parkinsonism, when convergence is lost, the accommodation reaction on focusing on a near object may be preserved, though it is often less brisk than normal. The reaction on accomodation/ convergence is impaired by any lesion which involves iridoconstrictor fibres; very rarely, in midbrain lesions this reaction is lost when that to light is impaired.

REFLEX IRIDOPLEGIA AND THE ARGYLL ROBERTSON PUPIL

The term 'reflex iridoplegia' indicates a failure of the pupil to react to light. The term 'Argyll Robertson pupil' should be reserved for a special form of reflex iridoplegia in which, as described by Argyll Robertson, the pupil 'is small . . . constant in size, and unaltered by light or shade; it contracts promptly and fully on convergence and dilates again promptly when the effort to converge is relaxed; it dilates slowly and imperfectly to mydriatics' (Adie). Most of the features had been described many years before Argyll Robertson by Romberg. Very rarely the Argyll Robertson pupil reacts paradoxically to light by a slight dilatation. In addition to loss of the light reaction, the typical Argyll Robertson pupils of syphilis are irregular and unequal, and there is atrophy and depigmentation of the iris and loss of the ciliospinal reflex. In congenital neurosyphilis the pupils are often dilated but unresponsive to light and so are not of the Argyll Robertson variety. Pupils showing most if not all of the typical Argyll Robertson features may also be seen rarely in diabetes, in alcoholic polyneuropathy, in chronic hypertrophic polyneuropathy, and in peroneal muscular atrophy.

Loss of the pupillary light reflex depends upon a lesion at some point on the reflex path, and the preservation of the reaction on accommodation implies that the lesion does not involve the fibres concerned in this reaction. Reflex iridoplegia may also occur as a result of lesions in the following situations.

Lesions of the Optic Nerve. Accommodation, convergence, and the associated iridoconstriction can occur in the absence of vision, for example, if an individual who has become blind tries to look at the end of his nose. Consequently a lesion of the optic nerve severe enough to impair the conduction of the afferent impulses concerned in the light reflex can cause loss of that reflex with retention of the reaction on accommodation.

Lesions of the Optic Tract. Destruction of one optic tract causes loss of the light reflex when the temporal half of the ipsilateral retina and the nasal half of the contralateral retina are illuminated, though the reflex remains elicitable from the other half of each retina. Homonymous hemianopia due to a lesion of the optic tract can sometimes thus be distinguished from a similar hemianopia due to a lesion of the optic radiation which does not interrupt the light reflex (Wernicke's hemianopic reaction).

Central Lesions. There is abundant evidence that reflex iridoplegia may be produced by lesions of the upper part of the midbrain. It has been observed in cases of tumour involving this region, as a result of vascular lesions, in encephalitis lethargica, as a rare manifestation of multiple sclerosis and syringomyelia, and as a result of a traumatic lesion of the upper midbrain. Syphilis is, of course, far the commonest cause of the Argyll Robertson pupil as above defined, which is usually present in general paresis and tabes and frequently in meningovascular syphilis. The site of the lesion responsible for this sign in syphilis of the nervous system is disputed. One hypothesis would place it in the upper half of the midbrain, near the cerebral aqueduct, where it may be supposed to interrupt the fibres approaching the iridoconstrictor nucleus (Lowenstein, 1956).

Lesions of the Motor Path. An alternative view is that the lesion lies in the ciliary ganglion, the fibres concerned in the reaction on accommodation reaching the ciliary body without passing through the ganglion and so escaping damage (Nathan and Turner, 1942; Naquin, 1954). It is stated that lesions of the third nerve may abolish the reaction of the pupil to light without that on accommodation. Such a dissociation can unquestionably occur as a result of lesions in or behind the eye, and it has been described in a number of cases of trauma involving the eye, and as a sequel of herpes zoster ophthalmicus. The explanation is probably the same as in the syphilitic Argyll Robertson pupil.

REFERENCES

CLARK, W. E. LE G. (1944) Discussion on the visual pathways, *Proc. roy. Soc. Med.*, **37**, 392.
COGAN, D. G., and WILLIAMS, H. W. (1966) *Neurology of the Visual System*, Springfield, Ill.
HARRIS, W. (1935) The fibres of the pupillary reflex and the Argyll Robertson pupil, *Arch. Neurol. Psychiat. (Chic.)*, **39**, 1195.
LOWENSTEIN, O. (1956) The Argyll Robertson pupillary syndrome; mechanism and localisation, *Amer. J. Ophthal.*, **42**, 105.
MAGOUN, H. W., ATLAS, D., HARE, W. K., and RANSON, S. W. (1936) The afferent path of the pupillary light reflex in the monkey, *Brain*, **59**, 234.
MERRITT, H. H., and MOORE, M. (1933) The Argyll Robertson pupil: an anatomic-physiologic explanation of the phenomenon, with a survey of its occurrence in neurosyphilis, *Arch. Neurol. Psychiat. (Chic.)*, **30**, 357.
NAQUIN, H. A. (1954) Argyll Robertson pupil following herpes zoster ophthalmicus with remarks on efferent pupillary pathways, *Amer. J. Ophthal.*, **38**, 23.
NATHAN, P. W., and TURNER, J. W. A. (1942) The efferent pathway for pupillary contraction, *Brain*, **65**, 343.
PATON, L., and MANN, I. C. (1925) The development of the third nerve nucleus and its bearing on the Argyll Robertson pupil, *Trans. ophthal. Soc. U.K.*, **45**, 610.
WILSON, S. A. K. (1928) Argyll Robertson pupil, *Modern Problems in Neurology*, p. 332, London.

TONIC PUPILS AND ABSENT TENDON REFLEXES

Definition. A syndrome of unknown aetiology characterized in its fully developed form by abnormalities in the reactions of one or both pupils to light and accommodation and absence of the tendon reflexes. The features of the tonic pupil were first described by Ware in 1813. They were rediscovered in 1902 by Strasburger and Saenger independently. An example of the complete syndrome was shown by Markus in 1905. Our present knowledge is based chiefly upon clinical observations of Moore (1924, 1931), Holmes (1931), Adie (1931 *a* and *b*, and 1932), and Russell (1956, 1958).

Synonym. The Holmes–Adie syndrome.

AETIOLOGY AND PATHOLOGY

The disorder occurs in females much more often than in males and the age of onset is usually during the third decade. Beyond this nothing is known as to its aetiology. Russell's (1956) work suggests that the lesion is in the efferent parasympathetic pathway to the eye, probably postganglionic. Harriman and Garland (1968) reported a case of tonic pupil which came to autopsy and Harriman (1970) added another. The pupils affected were the right ones and the right ciliary ganglia, in contrast to the left, showed degeneration of neurones, most of which were replaced by clumps of capsular cells. There was also a loss of large axons though many fine axons still traversed the ganglion. Some loss of neurones in dorsal root ganglia was also found.

SYMPTOMS

The onset is usually sudden, the patient or her friends noticing that one pupil has become larger than the other. Sometimes the first complaint is of mistiness of vision in one eye. The pupillary abnormality is unilateral in about 80 per cent of cases. The affected pupil is moderately dilated and is therefore usually larger than its fellow. When tested by ordinary methods the reaction of the affected pupil to light, both direct and consensual, is either completely or almost completely absent. Sometimes, however, a sluggish reaction to light can be elicited after the patient has remained in a dark room for about half an hour. The characteristic feature, however, is the response of the pupil to accommodation. Whereas a hasty examination may suggest that the pupil does not react at all on accommodation, nevertheless, if the patient be made to gaze fixedly at a near object, the pupil, sometimes after slight delay, contracts very slowly through a range which is often greater than normal, so that the affected pupil actually becomes smaller than the normal one. When accommodation is relaxed, dilatation of the pupil begins either at once or after a slight delay and proceeds even more slowly than contraction. This is the tonic pupillary reaction.

The tonic pupillary reaction, however, is not always present, but may be replaced by sluggishness or even absence of the reaction on accommodation. The pupil may thus be fixed to light and on accommodation. Russell (1956) distinguishes a 'paralytic' type of pupil attributed to parasympathetic paralysis and a 'tonic' type, due to supersensitization of the sphincter pupillae to acetylcholine liberated by intact parasympathetic fibres. The paralytic phase may thus be succeeded by the tonic phase. Accommodation may also be tonic, so that, after the gaze has been fixed on a near object, some seconds may elapse before this becomes clear. Russell (1958) explains the tonic ciliary muscle in the same way as the tonic pupil.

Some abnormality in the tendon reflexes is usually present, the ankle-jerks, knee-jerks, and arm-jerks being diminished or lost in this order of frequency. H-reflex studies suggest that there is depression of the monosynaptic spiral reflex arc (McComas and Payan, 1966). Occasionally the tonic pupil occurs with normal reflexes, or, less frequently, normal pupils with absent tendon reflexes. Usually no other abnormality is found in the nervous system or elsewhere.

DIAGNOSIS

It is important to distinguish the tonic pupil from the Argyll Robertson pupil, but this is not difficult as the Argyll Robertson pupil is smaller than normal, does not react to light, reacts promptly and fully on convergence, and dilates incompletely to mydriatics, differing in all these respects from the typical tonic pupil.

PROGNOSIS

The syndrome is permanent but has no ill effect beyond the inconvenience attaching to tonic accommodation. Patients have been observed in whom the condition of the pupil has remained unchanged for 30 or 40 years. Occasionally it spontaneously changes its size and, rarely, the other eye becomes affected some time after the first.

TREATMENT

No treatment is of any value, but eserine drops may be used if the dilated pupil leads to discomfort.

REFERENCES

ADIE, W. J. (1931 *a*) Pseudo-Argyll Robertson pupils with absent tendon reflexes, *Brit. med. J.*, **1**, 928.

ADIE, W. J. (1931 *b*) Argyll Robertson pupils true and false, *Brit. med. J.*, **2**, 136.

ADIE, W. J. (1932) Tonic pupils and absent tendon reflexes. A benign disorder *sui generis*; its complete and incomplete forms, *Brain*, **55**, 98.

ALAJOUANINE, T., and MORAX, P. V. (1938) La pupille tonique et ses rapports avec la syndrome d'Adie, *Ann. Oculist. (Paris)*, **175**, 205, 277.

HARRIMAN, D. G. F. (1970) Pathological aspects of Adie's syndrome, *Adv. Ophthal.*, **23**, 55.

HARRIMAN, D. G. F., and GARLAND, H. G. (1968) The pathology of Adie's syndrome, *Brain*, **91**, 401.

HOLMES, G. (1931) Partial iridoplegia associated with symptoms of other disease of the nervous system, *Trans. ophthal. Soc. U.K.*, **41**, 209.

McCOMAS, A. J., and PAYAN, J. (1966) Motoneurone excitability in the Holmes–Adie syndrome, in *Control and Innervation of Skeletal Muscle*, ed. Andrew, B. L., Edinburgh and London.

MOORE, R. F. (1924) Discussion on the pupil from the ophthalmological point of view, *Trans. ophthal. Soc. U.K.*, **44**, 38.

MOORE, R. F. (1931) The non-luetic Argyll Robertson pupil, *Trans. ophthal. Soc. U.K.*, **51**, 203.

RUSSELL, G. F. M. (1956) The pupillary changes in the Holmes–Adie syndrome, *J. Neurol. Neurosurg. Psychiat.*, **19**, 289.

RUSSELL, G. F. M. (1958) Accommodation in the Holmes–Adie syndrome, *J. Neurol. Neurosurg. Psychiat.*, **21**, 290.

THE INNERVATION OF THE EYELIDS

Two muscles act as elevators of the upper eyelid, the levator palpebrae superioris, which is innervated by the third nerve, and Müller's palpebral muscle, part of the smooth muscle of the orbit, which receives its nerve supply from the cervical sympathetic. Closure of the lids is brought about by the orbicularis oculi, the motor nerve of which is the facial.

RETRACTION OF THE UPPER LID

Retraction of the upper lid is attributable to a relative or absolute shortening of the elevating muscles, perhaps especially of the smooth muscle. When present it is exaggerated when the patient voluntarily elevates his eyes, and it is responsible for the lag of the upper lid in following the downward movement of the eye, which is known as von Graefe's sign. Lid retraction is most frequently encountered in ophthalmic Graves' disease, but, as Collier pointed out, it may be produced by a lesion in the upper part of the midbrain, especially one involving the posterior commissure. It may follow a vascular lesion in this situation and it is also sometimes met with in tabes, multiple sclerosis, post-encephalitic Parkinsonism, tumour of the midbrain, myasthenia gravis, and as a congenital abnormality.

Retraction of the upper lid may be unilateral or bilateral and may occur with or without exophthalmos. When it is due to a lesion in the upper part of the midbrain it may be associated with weakness of conjugate elevation of the eyes or with reflex iridoplegia.

PTOSIS OF THE UPPER LID

Ptosis of the upper lid may be the result of paralysis of either the levator palpebrae superioris or of the orbital smooth muscle. In the latter case the drooping of the lid is comparatively slight. Complete paralysis of the levator, however, causes closure of the eye. It is necessary to distinguish between ptosis due to a lesion of the sympathetic and that due to paresis of the levator. This may be done by observing the reaction of the lid when the patient voluntarily elevates the eyes. Normally, elevation of the upper lid occurs as an associated movement with elevation of the eyes. In ptosis of sympathetic origin the amplitude of this associated movement is normal. In ptosis due to paresis of the levator it is diminished. Over-action of the frontal belly of the occipitofrontalis muscle is commonly present in a patient with ptosis. This muscle normally contracts in association with the levator palpebrae, and when the latter muscle is paralysed the increased effort made by the patient to elevate the lid involves an increased contraction of the frontalis muscle, physiologically comparable to secondary deviation of a conjugate ocular muscle in paralytic strabismus. Paralysis of the levator may be due to a lesion involving the nucleus of the third nerve or the third nerve trunk or its superior division within the orbit, to disorder of function at the myoneural junction in myasthenia gravis, or to involvement of the muscle itself in ocular myopathy. It may be congenital and may occur intermittently on one side as a congenital synkinetic phenomenon with each movement of the jaw on chewing in the Marcus Gunn jaw-winking phenomenon (Gunn, 1883; Walsh, 1957). A lesion of the ocular sympathetic responsible for ptosis may occur within the brain stem, spinal cord, the eighth cervical and first and second thoracic ventral roots and spinal nerves, or the cervical sympathetic trunk. It is usually associated with other signs of ocular sympathetic paralysis, namely myosis and enophthalmos.

EXOPHTHALMOS AND ENOPHTHALMOS

The smooth muscle of the orbit is normally in a state of sufficient tonic contraction to produce some protrusion of the eyeball. Paralysis of this muscle causes slight enophthalmos: it is unlikely that exophthalmos is ever due to its over-activity. The commoner causes of exophthalmos are: (1) ophthalmic Graves' disease; (2) pseudotumour of the orbit; (3) primary tumours within the orbit, especially of the optic nerve and its sheath; (4) diseases of the nasal air sinuses, empyema, mucocele, and carcinoma; (5) retro-orbital intracranial tumours, especially meningiomas and aneurysms. Less common causes are carotid-cavernous sinus aneurysm, craniostenosis, xanthomatosis, Wegener's granulomatosis, chloroma, and metastatic tumour from the suprarenal (Hutchinson type) or breast (van Buren et al., 1975; Bedford and Daniel, 1960).

REFERENCES

BEDFORD, P. D., and DANIEL, P. M. (1960) Discrete carcinomatous metastases in the extrinsic ocular muscles, *Amer. J. Ophthal.*, **49,** 723.
BRAIN, W. R. (1955) Exophthalmic ophthalmoplegia, *Trans. ophthal. Soc. U.K.*, **55,** 351.
BUREN, J. VAN, POPPEN, J. L., and HORRAX, G. (1957) Unilateral exophthalmos, *Brain*, **80,** 139.

COLLIER, J. (1927) Nuclear ophthalmoplegia with especial reference to retraction of the lids and to lesions of the posterior commissure, *Brain*, **50**, 488.

GUNN, R. M. (1883) The jaw-winking phenomenon, *Trans. ophthal. Soc. U.K.*, **3**, 283.

POCHIN, E. E. (1939 *a*) Ocular effects of sympathetic stimulation in man, *Clin. Sci.*, **4**, 79.

POCHIN, E. E. (1939 *b*) The mechanism of lid retraction in Graves' disease, *Clin. Sci.*, **4**, 91.

WALSH, F. B. (1957) *Clinical Neuro-ophthalmology*, 2nd ed., p. 201, Baltimore.

SPEECH AND ITS DISORDERS

THE NATURE OF SPEECH

PSYCHOLOGICAL CONSIDERATIONS

Speech is an extremely complex activity. In order to understand its nature it is necessary to trace its development in the individual from infancy. Infant speech goes through a number of phases including babbling which is the spontaneous production of sounds, and echolalia, which is the imitation of sounds made by others. The foundation of speech is thus sensorimotor—the sounds produced by others causing the child to produce sounds which it hears itself and which are linked with proprioceptor impulses from its own muscles of articulation. The next stage is the long one of learning the meanings of words, which involves associating the sounds of the words with objects which are perceived in abstraction from their environment, and later increasing abstraction is involved in naming qualities, actions, and relationships. The meaning of words is also influenced by their arrangements in sentences, i.e. by their grammatical and syntactical modifications.

When the child learns to read it does so by associating visual signs, i.e. letters and words, with the sounds which it has already learned. Through reading aloud, written words become linked with heard words, and with the kinaesthetic sensations of speech. In writing, movements of the hand are employed to reproduce visual signs similar to those which form the basis of reading. Since in writing one reads as one writes there exists a close link between the perception of the visual signs which constitute letters and words, and the kinaesthetic sensations derived from the fingers.

Words therefore are symbols. A spoken word is to the hearer an auditory symbol of an object, action, or relationship; a written word in the first instance acquires its symbolic significance through its association with heard speech, that is, symbolic sounds. Words as symbols possess meanings, but these meanings are of an elementary nature. In fully developed speech individual words possess significance only in relationship with other words. The unit of meaning is then a sentence or even a series of sentences. Speech, therefore, is the communication of meanings by means of symbols, which usually take the form of spoken or written words. Meaning may, however, be communicated by gesture, and gesture meanings have been especially elaborated in the manual speech of the deaf and dumb. In reading Braille print the blind utilize tactile instead of visual sensations. Mathematics and music also involve the use of written symbols.

Hughlings Jackson first pointed out that speech is not always used for the communication of meanings—propositional speech, as he called it—but may also constitute the expression of feeling, in which case it may have no propositional value.

How far is thought dependent upon speech? It has been maintained that we think in words and that normal speech functions are therefore necessary for thought. The process of logical thought is probably subject to large individual variations depending upon whether the thinker chiefly utilizes visual or auditory images. It appears to be true, however, that internal verbal formulation is not necessary, at least for the simpler forms of logical thought. It is probably required for more abstract thinking, and is necessary for the communication of the products of thought to others.

PHYSIOLOGICAL AND ANATOMICAL CONSIDERATIONS

At the psychological level the meaning of a written or a spoken word is the outcome of the association of the given visual and auditory sensations with other forms of sensation in the past. A meaning is thus based upon a constellation of associations built up by experience. At the physiological and anatomical levels the basis of such meanings is presumably a linkage of neurones. Visual impulses reach the cerebral cortex in the region of the calcarine sulcus of the occipital lobes; auditory impulses in the posterior part of the superior temporal gyrus. Kinaesthetic impulses from the muscles of articulation and from the upper limb terminate in the lower half of the postcentral gyrus. It is to be expected therefore that the anatomical linkages of neurones upon which verbal meanings depend will join together these regions of the cerebral cortex, and these are found in the tracts of white matter known as association fibres, which underlie the grey matter of the cerebral cortex.

For reasons which are little understood, about 93 per cent of persons are right-handed, and in these the left cerebral hemisphere plays the predominant role in speech and is known as the dominant or major hemisphere: it is the site of the speech functions in about 40 per cent of left-handed people also. In the remainder of the left-handers the right hemisphere is the dominant one for speech, or speech functions may be bilaterally represented. There is evidence from cases of hemispherectomy in childhood that up to the age of four or five years, speech function can, after an extensive lesion of the dominant hemisphere, be transferred to the other, but little or no such adaptation can occur in older children or adults (Subirana, 1969). The important associational paths just described are therefore situated in the left hemisphere in right-handed persons, but sensory impulses concerned in the reception of speech also reach the auditory and visual regions of the right cerebral cortex, which are linked to the left hemisphere by paths passing through the corpus callosum. Their importance has recently been demonstrated by Gazzaniga et al. (1965), who found that, after division of the corpus callosum and the other commissural connections in man, speech could deal only with perceptual information reaching the left cerebral hemisphere. The right cerebral hemisphere still had capacities of its own but was isolated from verbal expression (see also Geschwind, 1965).

The posterior half of the left cerebral hemisphere is thus the site of those neuronal linkages which underlie the elaboration of meanings in response to auditory and visual stimuli, i.e. the comprehension of heard and written speech. Since articulated speech is the expression of meanings it must be the outcome of the activity of a part of the brain which at least overlaps that concerned in the reception of speech, for the anatomical basis of meanings is common to both. Articulation involves movements of the jaw, lips, tongue, palate, pharynx, and phonation involves the respiratory muscles, which are all represented in the lowest part of the precentral gyrus. If meanings are to gain articulate expression the posterior half of the left hemisphere must be linked to the lowest part of the precentral gyrus. An important part in this association is played by the arcuate fasciculus and the external capsule, which is a band of white matter running from the temporal lobe beneath the cortex of the inferior parietal lobe and insula to the lower part of the precentral gyrus and the posterior part of the middle and inferior frontal gyri. Speech requires co-ordinated bilateral movements of the muscles of articulation, and this co-ordination is effected by fibres passing from the lower part of the left frontal lobe to the corresponding region of the right hemisphere by the corpus callosum. From the lower part of the precentral gyri the motor fibres concerned in phonation and articulation pass downwards in the corticospinal tracts and after decussation end in the trigeminal and facial nuclei, the nuclei ambigui and the hypoglossal nuclei in the pons and medulla, whence the lower motor neurones run in the corresponding cranial nerves to the lips, soft palate, tongue, and larynx. Corticospinal fibres similarly innervate the diaphragm and intercostal muscles. As with other motor activities, the cerebellum and striatum exercise a regulating influence upon articulation.

DYSARTHRIA

We are now in a position to draw a distinction between speech, phonation, and articulation. Speech is the term employed for the whole process by which meanings are comprehended and expressed in words. Phonation is the process of driving a column of air across the vocal cords, with resonance in the larynx and pharynx, in order to produce a sound, and articulation is the process of moulding this sound into words. Aphonia means loss, and dysphonia impairment, of phonation. Dysarthria is a disorder of articulation. It does not therefore involve any disturbance in the proper construction and use of words. In the dysarthric patient symbolic verbal formulation is normal: only the mechanism of verbal sound production is faulty. When this is so severely affected that the patient is totally unable to articulate, he is said to be anarthric.

The following are the principal causes of dysarthria:

UPPER MOTOR NEURONE LESIONS

The articulatory muscles on each side appear to be innervated by both cerebral hemispheres. Hence a unilateral corticospinal lesion, for example in the internal capsule, may cause temporary but not permanent dysarthria; however, an extensive unilateral lesion involving the motor cortex may cause persistent dysarthria, especially when the dominant hemisphere is involved, when the dysarthria is often associated with some degree of Broca's aphasia (see below). Dysarthria is consistently produced, however, by bilateral corticospinal lesions, due, for example, to congenital diplegia, vascular lesions of both internal capsules, degeneration of both corticospinal tracts, as in motor neurone disease, and lesions such as tumours involving both corticospinal tracts together in the midbrain. With such lesions the articulatory muscles are weak and spastic and the tongue appears smaller and firmer than normal. The jaw-jerk and the palatal and pharyngeal reflexes are exaggerated. Speech is slurred, production of consonants, especially labials and dentals, being severely affected. Spastic dysarthria is usually associated with dysphagia and often with impairment of voluntary control over emotional expression, a syndrome which is often called 'pseudobulbar palsy'.

EXTRAPYRAMIDAL LESIONS

With lesions of the corpus striatum articulation is impaired, partly at least, as a result of muscular rigidity. Thus in hepatolenticular degeneration and in Parkinsonism articulation is slow and slurred owing to immobility of the lips and tongue and the pitch of the voice is monotonous, and in cases of athetosis, torsion dystonia, and Huntington's chorea, too, dysarthria is common; indeed in severe cases speech may be unintelligible. Irregular respiration may contribute to the dysarthria.

DISORDERS OF CO-ORDINATION

The co-ordination of articulation suffers severely when the vermis of the cerebellum is damaged and also when lesions involve the cerebellar connections in the brain stem. Speech in such cases is often explosive and associated with grimacing. Syllables may be slurred or unduly separated—scanning or syllabic speech. Ataxic dysarthria of this character is seen after acute cerebellar lesions and in multiple sclerosis and the hereditary ataxias.

LOWER MOTOR NEURONE LESIONS

Lower motor neurone lesions cause wasting and weakness, and often fasciculation, of the muscles of articulation (true bulbar palsy). In the early stages the pronunciation of labials suffers most. Later, progressive weakness of the tongue impairs the production of dentals and gutturals, and weakness of the soft palate gives the voice a nasal quality. To this may be added impairment of phonation, and finally there is total anarthria. Progressive bulbar palsy is the commonest cause, but paresis of the bulbar muscles may also be seen in syringobulbia, bulbar poliomyelitis, cranial polyneuritis, and brain stem tumours.

Combinations of these varieties of dysarthria are common; for example, in multiple sclerosis the articulatory muscles may be both spastic and ataxic and in motor neurone disease a combination of upper and lower motor neurone lesions may be present.

MYOPATHIES

Disease of the muscles, such as myasthenia gravis, polymyositis, and muscular dystrophy involving facial muscles, leads to dysarthria similar to that resulting from lesions of the lower motor neurones. In myasthenia fatigability may cause increasing slurring of speech if the patient is asked to count. In the myotonias impaired muscular relaxation may add a spastic quality to the speech.

TREATMENT

Little can be done when dysarthria is due to a progressive disorder, but in children suffering from congenital dysarthria or dysarthria due to diplegia, athetosis, and chorea much can be accomplished by speech therapy.

PALILALIA

Palilalia is a rare disorder of speech, the nature of which is obscure. As its name implies (from the Greek *palin*, again; *lalein*, to chatter), it is characterized by repetition of a phrase which the patient reiterates with increasing rapidity. Palilalia most frequently occurs in post-encephalitic Parkinsonism, in general paresis, and in pseudobulbar palsy due to vascular lesions. It is difficult to understand why a lesion involving the lower motor mechanisms of speech should cause a disorder of the formation of phrases.

MUTISM

Mutism is a term usually applied to a complete loss of speech in a conscious patient. It occurs in congenital deaf-mutes and also in akinetic mutism in which there is an abnormal state of consciousness [see p. 1159] but also in some cerebral lesions with preservation of consciousness, e.g. after severe head injury, after certain cerebrovascular lesions, in advanced Parkinsonism, after bilateral thalamotomy, and after anoxic states due to many causes, e.g. carbon monoxide poisoning. It also occurs in the psychoses, for example in cyclothymia, as a result of extreme depression or mental retardation, and in schizophrenia. It is also met with in hysteria. In the psychoses the severity of the mental disorder is always apparent and the mute patient is usually unable to write. In hysterical mutism other hysterical symptoms are usually present.

Hysterical mutism is usually transient; it often resolves following abreaction during intravenous anaesthesia or after speech re-education with the aid of a speech therapist.

APHONIA

In aphonia phonation is lost but articulation is preserved; hence the patient talks in a whisper. Aphonia may be the result of organic disease causing bilateral paralysis of the adductors of the vocal cords [see p. 212] or of disease of the larynx, for example, laryngitis. It is most commonly a symptom of hysteria, in which case the patient, though unable to phonate when speaking, can do so when coughing.

Like hysterical mutism, hysterical aphonia [see p. 1189] often resolves spontaneously once the precipitating stress is removed as in the singer or actress who loses her voice on the evening of an important performance; otherwise, it too may be helped by abreaction or speech therapy.

APHASIA

Whereas dysarthria is a disorder of the motor mechanism of articulation, aphasia is a disturbance of the higher and much more complex functions, described on pages 98–100, by which meanings are comprehended and expressed. It is thus a disorder of the use of symbols in speech. Since aphasia strictly interpreted means absence of speech, the term dysphasia, meaning disorder of speech, is sometimes employed. The terminology employed in the description of aphasia is still to some extent in bondage to old-fashioned views concerning the psychological nature of speech and outworn conceptions of cerebral localization. Confusion springs from a failure to distinguish between psychological, physiological, and anatomical accounts of speech and its disorders, and to recognize the complexity of the relations between them.

The Development of Thought about Aphasia

It is impossible to understand the terminology of aphasia without some knowledge of its historical development, which is described in more detail by Head (1920, 1926) and Weisenburg and McBride (1935).

The first attempt to localize functions in different parts of the brain was made by Gall (1758–1828), who distinguished six varieties of memory, including name-memory, verbal, and grammatical memory, all of which he localized in the frontal lobes. Dax in 1836 first drew attention to the special importance of the left cerebral hemisphere for speech. Broca (1824–80) in 1861 reported two cases which led him to take the view that the faculty of articulation was located in the inferior frontal gyrus (Broca's area). Damage to this area caused what he called 'aphemia'—a term altered by Trousseau to 'aphasia'. Broca distinguished two forms of speech disturbance—aphemia and verbal amnesia, the former being a defect of verbal expression and the latter a loss of memory for both spoken and written words.

Hughlings Jackson's (1835–1911) first paper on speech was published in 1864. It is difficult to summarize his views, which he elaborated in a series of communications. His great contribution was the introduction of a dynamic concept. Like Broca he recognized two main groups of aphasic patients. In one group speech is lost or gravely damaged; in the other the patient has numerous words but uses them wrongly. He pointed out that the higher and more voluntary aspects of speech tend to suffer more than the lower and automatic, and he distinguished what he called 'propositional' from emotional speech. Aphasia is essentially an inability to 'propositionize' in speech, and the same fundamental difficulty underlies spoken speech, reading, and writing. Internal speech is affected like external speech and the thinking of the aphasic patient is therefore also hampered, but in most cases of aphasia mental images are unimpaired.

Hughlings Jackson's work was little appreciated at the time and the main line of development of thought about aphasia was in the direction of increasing localization of function. Bastian (1837–1915) in 1869 maintained that we think in words and that words are revived in the cerebral hemispheres as remembered sounds. He localized auditory and visual word centres as well as other centres linked by association paths. He was thus the most notable of the 'diagram-makers' as Head called them. He prepared the way for the concept of word-deafness and word-blindness—terms introduced by Kussmaul—caused by lesions of these centres. Wernicke (1848–1905) in 1874 localized the centre for auditory images in the left superior temporal gyrus and described three varieties of aphasia—sensory, due to destruction of this centre, motor, due to a lesion of Broca's area, and a third due to interference with conduction between these two centres. When both centres were destroyed there was total aphasia.

In 1906 Pierre Marie (1853–1940) reopened the question by maintaining that lesions of Broca's area had nothing to do with speech disorders. He contended that there was only one form of aphasia—the sensory aphasia of Wernicke, which was not a specific loss of word memories but a defect of the special intelligence of language. He considered the motor speech disturbance to be an anarthria caused by a lesion of 'the lenticular zone'. Henschen and Kleist are among the modern workers who may be classed as localizationists.

Henry Head (1861–1940) returned to and developed the dynamic concepts of Jackson. He expressly avoided the question of localization, and developed a functional approach, seeking to discover by a specially devised series of tests how the function of speech broke down in aphasia, which he regarded as a disorder of 'symbolic formulation and expression'. In Head's (1926) view, 'disorders of language of this kind cannot be classified as isolated affections of speaking, reading, and writing, for these acts are more or less disturbed whatever the primary nature of the defect. Nor can they be attributed directly to destruction of auditory or visual images or to any other analogous processes, which belong to a relatively low order in the psychical hierarchy. Each clinical variety represents some partial affection of symbolic formulation and expression; the form it assumes depends upon the particular modes of behaviour which are disturbed or remain intact.' Head recognized four such forms of disturbance, which he termed verbal, nominal, syntactical, and semantic.

Some other points of view remain to be mentioned. Liepmann at one time regarded expressive aphasia as a form of apraxia, and word-deafness and word-blindness as forms of agnosia. Though he later abandoned this view it was subsequently adopted by Kinnier Wilson. Goldstein (1948) and others explain the various symptoms of aphasia in terms of the Gestalt theory as manifestations of a single functional disorder, loss of the ability to grasp the essential nature of a process, impairment of abstract attitude, etc.

Recent workers have applied to aphasic utterances phonetic analysis (Alajouanine and Mozziconacci, 1948; Alajouanine, 1956; and Bay, 1957), psychological testing (Bay, 1960), and the Gestalt theory (Conrad, 1954). For a review of the whole subject see Brain (1965); Lhermitte and Gautier (1969); Geschwind (1970); Critchley (1970); and Meyer (1974).

The Nature and Classification of Aphasia

Aphasia is a disorder of function and must therefore be interpreted in functional terms. The older concepts of aphasia were mostly inadequate because they treated of speech and its breakdown in terms of consciousness, i.e. of words and their auditory, visual, and kinaesthetic images. The neurophysiology of speech, however, embraces complex functions to which there is often no counterpart in consciousness, and which need new concepts for their interpretation (Goldstein, 1948; Alajouanine and Mozziconacci, 1948; Brain, 1965). A word is something more to the nervous system than any one of the innumerable ways in which it can be pronounced or written: its basis is a neurophysiological disposition, which Brain called a word-schema, and through which any specific instance of a word is able to evoke its appropriate meaning. Speech involves auditory phoneme-schemas, central word-schemas, sentence-schemas, meaning-schemas, and motor phoneme-schemas, and aphasia results from a breakdown of their receptive or expressive functions, or of both. It rarely happens, however, that a localized cerebral lesion disturbs only one physiological function, and the same psychological disorder may be the result of more than one kind of physiological disturbance. Hence the inadequacy of psychological classifications of aphasia and the failure of attempts to correlate anatomical lesions with clear-cut disorders of function. We have to fall back upon an empirical classification of aphasia. Experience shows that on the whole a lesion in one part of the brain disturbs speech in certain ways and a lesion in another situation in different ways. Hence there exists an anatomical classification of aphasia which roughly corresponds to a functional one. Thus, modified from Geschwind (1970), the principal forms of aphasia and related disorders can be classified as follows:

1. Broca's aphasia (expressive or motor aphasia, anterior aphasia)
2. Wernicke's aphasia (sensory or receptive aphasia):
    (a) pure word-deafness
3. Global or total aphasia
4. Conduction aphasia (central aphasia of Goldstein, syntactical aphasia)
5. The posterior (association) aphasias:
    (a) the syndrome of the isolated speech area;
    (b) nominal, anomic, or amnestic aphasia
6. Related disorders of language: agraphia, alexia, acalculia, amusia.

Broca's Aphasia

A lesion of Broca's area causes an inability to translate speech concepts into meaningful articulated sounds so that the content of speech is greatly reduced. Mutism rarely if ever occurs, however, and even in severe cases one or two words can usually be produced, though slowly and with considerable effort; there is commonly some degree of associated dysarthria. 'Propositional' speech suffers more than emotional so that expletives or other emotional expressions may be repeated spontaneously. Questions are often answered appropriately, but only in monosyllables, and spontaneous speech, when present, is telegraphic with lack of intonation, though word repetition is better than spontaneous formulation of thought concepts and the patient who is unable to think of a word readily recognizes it when offered to him. Comprehension of both written and spoken language is unimpaired, but reading aloud produces the same defective utterances as spontaneous speech.

As Broca's area lies close to the motor cortex, most patients have an associated hemiparesis so that if writing is to be tested this must be attempted with the unaffected hand (usually the left). The handwriting is usually markedly impaired and there is poverty and lack of precision of written language, though copying is relatively unimpaired.

The rare condition of so-called *pure word-dumbness* or subcortical motor aphasia, thought to be due to a lesion in the subcortical white matter which separates Broca's area from the motor cortex and the corpus callosum, is characterized by a similar impairment of spoken speech but comprehension and writing are unimpaired.

It has often been suggested that during recovery from Broca's aphasia in polyglots, ability to converse in the patient's mother tongue returns before the language subsequently acquired, but van Thal (1960) and others have shown that this is uncommon.

Wernicke's Aphasia

Lesions of Wernicke's area impair the comprehension of speech, as the meaning and significance of spoken words, received and recorded in the auditory cortex, are not understood. As Broca's area is unaffected, the production of speech is unimpaired so that the patient can produce fluent speech with normal rhythm and cadences, but its content is abnormal as he is also unaware of the meaning of many words which he himself produces. Paraphasias (incorrect word usage) are invariable in this form of aphasia and are either literal (the use of incorrect vowels or consonants within a word) or verbal (the use of incorrect words). In severe cases the patient produces meaningless jargon (*jargon aphasia*); it should, however, be noted that similar spontaneous speech occurs in conduction aphasia (see below). The repetition of words offered by the examiner is also impaired, as is the naming of objects; handwriting is usually normal but the content of written, as of spoken spontaneous language, is abnormal, though copying is relatively unaffected. The patient often shows striking lack of insight, being unaware that his speech is abnormal, and he is commonly frustrated by his inability to make himself understood.

Pure or *subcortical word-deafness* (auditory aphasia) is a very rare and fractional form of aphasia closely related to Wernicke's aphasia, but thought to be due to a lesion of the white matter deep to the posterior part of the left superior temporal gyrus (Hemphill and Stengel, 1940). The patient distinguishes words from other sounds but cannot understand them so that his own language sounds like a foreign tongue. He cannot repeat words or write to dictation but spontaneous speech, writing, and reading are unimpaired.

Global Aphasia

An extensive lesion of the dominant hemisphere involving both the frontal and temporal lobes often gives global aphasia (Mohr *et al.*, 1973) in which both the production of speech and the comprehension of spoken and written language are impaired.

Conduction Aphasia

A lesion in the arcuate fasciculus or external capsule which interrupts the main association pathway between Broca's and Wernicke's areas gives this form of aphasia in which speech is again fluent but with many paraphasic errors, usually of the literal type (see above). There may be slight impairment of articulation and object-naming is impaired, as is written spontaneous language, though the handwriting is usually normal. Hence as in Wernicke's aphasia the patient's fluent but inappropriate speech is usually that of jargon aphasia; and the ability to repeat words or to read aloud is markedly impaired. The only real distinction between this and Wernicke's aphasia is that in this variety the comprehension of spoken language is excellent as is that of written commands.

The Posterior (Association) Aphasias

Lesions in or near the angular gyrus of the dominant hemisphere may interrupt connections between Wernicke's area and most other areas of the brain but leave intact the association pathway to Broca's area via the arcuate fasciculus and external capsule.

A large lesion may produce '*the syndrome of the isolated speech area*' (Geschwind *et al.*, 1968) in which speech is fluent but paraphasic, while object-naming, spontaneous writing, and comprehension of both oral and written language are impaired. However, repetition of words spoken by the examiner is normal and the patient may show parrot-like repetition of a word or phrase ('echolalia').

If the lesion is less extensive, then speech may be fluent with only occasional paraphasia, and comprehension of written and spoken language as well as repetition are all normal, though written speech may be impaired. However, the most striking abnormality is often difficulty in naming objects and people (*anomia, nominal, or amnestic aphasia*). Typically the difficulty is most evident if the subject is asked to name unfamiliar rather than familiar objects and proper names, even of close friends, may be especially difficult to recall. It is also characteristic that the patient rejects a wrong name suggested by the examiner and insists that he knows the object and its purpose (which he may demonstrate by writing, say, with a pencil, or putting on spectacles), even though he is unable to name it.

Related Disorders of Language

Agraphia is an inability to produce written language, *alexia* an inability to understand written or printed speech.

Pure alexia without agraphia has also been called pure *subcortical word-blindness* or visual aphasia as the patient cannot recognize words, letters, or colours but can visualize colours. He cannot copy but can write and speak spontaneously and normally. The lesion responsible usually involves the visual cortex of the dominant hemisphere and the splenium of the corpus callosum, thus disconnecting the intact visual cortex of the opposite hemisphere from Wernicke's and Broca's areas. A contralateral homonymous hemianopia is invariably present.

Pure alexia with agraphia (also called *visual asymbolia* or *cortical word-blindness*) is usually due to lesions in the region of the dominant angular gyrus which divide the pathways between the visual association area and the speech areas. The patient can neither read, copy, nor write spontaneously. Benson *et al.* (1971) have shown that in pure alexia without agraphia the patient can read letters better than words, whereas patients with Broca's aphasia often have associated agraphia, and even in such anterior lesions, while the reading of words may be relatively unimpaired, the reading of letters may be abnormal. Geschwind has suggested that the outdated term *aphemia*, first introduced by Broca, may still reasonably be used to identify Broca's aphasia without agraphia.

Acalculia is a term applied to a defect in the ability to use mathematical symbols; a patient with Broca's aphasia may be unable to carry out mental arithmetic, but loss of the ability to understand and use mathematical symbols whether verbal or written is more commonly seen in lesions of the dominant parietal lobe, often in association with the other features of Gerstmann's syndrome [p. 119].

Amusia is the term given to a defect of musical expression or appreciation and, like aphasia, can be either expressive (in association with Broca's aphasia) or receptive (in association with Wernicke's aphasia).

Examination of a Patient with Aphasia

Examination of a patient with aphasia requires care and patience and should be carried out in a systematic manner. The following scheme of investigation fulfils all ordinary clinical requirements.

(1) Is the patient right- or left-handed, and, if the latter, did he write with the right hand? (2) What was his state of education as regards reading, writing, and foreign tongues? (3) Does he understand the nature and uses of objects, and can he understand pantomime and gesture, or express his wants thereby? (4) Is he deaf? If so, to what extent and on one or both sides? (5) Can he recognize ordinary sounds and noises? (6) Can he comprehend spoken language? If so, does he at once attempt to answer a question? (7) Is spontaneous speech good? If not, to what extent and in what manner is it impaired? Does he make use of paraphasias, either literal or verbal recurring utterances, or jargon? (8) Can he repeat words uttered in his hearing? (9) Is the sight good or bad; is there hemianopia, or impaired acuity? (10) Does he recognize written or printed speech and obey a written command? If not, does he recognize words, letters, or numerals? (11) Can he write spontaneously? What mistakes occur in writing? Is there paragraphia? Can he read his own writing some time after he has written it? (12) Can he copy written words, or from print into printing? Can he write numerals or perform simple mathematical calculations? (13) Can he read aloud? (14) Can he name at sight words, letters, numerals, and common objects? (15) Can he write from dictation? (16) Can he match an object with its name, spoken or written, when a series of objects and names are simultaneously presented?

Conclusions

In general, a fluent aphasic syndrome with paraphasia suggests that Broca's area is intact and suggests a posterior lesion, while speech which is slow, tele-

graphic, and dysarthric indicates one situated anteriorly. Impaired comprehension and repetition suggest Wernicke's aphasia, good comprehension and
poor repetition conduction aphasia; conversely, good repetition and poor
comprehension favour a lesion in the angular gyrus region isolating the speech
area. In global aphasia spontaneous speech, writing, reading, comprehension,
repetition, and object-naming are all impaired, while in nominal aphasia the
latter capacity is abnormal but comprehension is good and spontaneous speech
relatively unaffected. It must be remembered that comprehension should not
be tested simply by asking the patient to obey commands, as an individual with
apraxia [see p. 115] may understand the command but be unable to comply.

Associated neurological signs may also be helpful. A contralateral hemiparesis
is usually present in Broca's aphasia, less often in Wernicke's; a visual field
defect, on the contrary, is commonly present in association with the latter, rarely
with the former.

Kertesz and Poole (1974) have found that an aphasia quotient, based upon
numerical scores for fluency, comprehension, repetition, naming, and information can form a useful basis of clinical classification.

THE CAUSES OF APHASIA

Apart from developmental disturbances of speech described below, aphasia
is rare in childhood and increases in frequency with increasing age. It is most
frequently met with after middle life, since the commonest cause is a vascular
lesion, especially ischaemic. Cerebral haemorrhage causes aphasia less often
than thrombosis, because haemorrhage occurs deep in the white matter of the
hemisphere more often than in the cortex or subcortical regions. Transitory
attacks of aphasia may occur as a result of transient cerebral ischaemia whether
due to micro-embolism consequent upon arterial atheroma and stenosis or to
embolism from cardiac lesions. Aphasia may also occur as one feature of the
migrainous aura. The varieties of aphasia due to obstruction of the different
cerebral arteries are described elsewhere [see pp. 331–4].

Intracranial tumour is the commonest cause of aphasia during the first half of
adult life, when cerebral vascular lesions are rare. Abscess of the left temporal
lobe may also cause aphasia, and so may traumatic lesions involving the 'speech
areas' (Luria, 1970). Apart from abscess, infective lesions of the brain rarely
cause aphasia, though it occurs occasionally in acute necrotizing encephalitis,
and acute cerebral lesions causing hemiplegia and attributed to encephalitis or
vascular occlusion are almost the only causes of aphasia in childhood. Neurosyphilis may cause aphasia, either by leading to cerebral infarction or to general
paresis. In the latter, transitory aphasia may occur as an early symptom, while
a profound disintegration of speech may develop as a result of the widespread
deterioration of cortical function in the later stages, comparable to that which
occurs in the presenile and senile dementias.

PROGNOSIS

The prognosis of aphasia depends largely upon its cause. When it develops
as a result of a vascular lesion, neural shock is responsible for part of the
immediate disturbance of function. Consequently a considerable improvement
may be anticipated as this passes off. The prognosis seems rather better when
aphasia is due to haemorrhage than when an important artery has been obstructed
by thrombosis or embolism, and it is better also when the aphasia is of the
expressive, than when it is of the receptive, type and in the left-handed than in

the right-handed. The prognosis is good when aphasia is due to an extracerebral tumour, such as a meningioma, which has compressed but not invaded the brain. In the case of an intracerebral tumour, even if the tumour can be removed, the trauma of the operation is likely to cause an exacerbation of the speech disturbance and little ultimate improvement·can be expected. Recovery often occurs from aphasia due to acute inflammatory lesions, and from any lesion of the dominant hemisphere during the first four years of life.

TREATMENT

The treatment of aphasia requires unlimited patience and is likely to be more successful when the disturbance of speech affects the expressive than when it involves the receptive function. In the latter type of aphasia not only has the patient difficulty in understanding what is required of him, but he also fails to understand his own attempts at speech. The aphasic patient requires to be taught on lines similar to those used in teaching a backward child. The various vowel and consonant sounds must be taught separately, the patient being directed to watch the movements of his teacher's lips and tongue. He is then taught to pronounce the names of common objects when he sees them. The names have then to be associated with pictures and finally with simple written words. The scheme of instruction must be adapted to meet the requirements of each individual case and to utilize to the best effect those elements of speech which are least seriously impaired. Details are described by Weisenburg and McBride (1935), Goldstein (1942, 1948), and Alajouanine and Mozziconacci (1948).

REFERENCES

ALAJOUANINE, T. (1956) Verbal realization in aphasia, *Brain*, **79**, 1.
ALAJOUANINE, T., and MOZZICONACCI, P. (1948) *L'Aphasie et la désintégration fonctionelle du langage*, Paris.
BAY, E. (1957) Die corticale Dysarthrie und ihre Beziehungen zur sog. motorischen Aphasie, *Dtsch Z. Nervenheilk.*, **176**, 553.
BAY, E. (1960) Zur Methodik der Aphasie-Untersuchung, *Nervenarzt*, **31**, 145.
BENSON, D. F., BROWN, J., and TOMLINSON, E. B. (1971) Varieties of alexia—word and letter blindness, *Neurology (Minneap.)*, **21**, 951.
BRAIN, LORD (1965) *Speech Disorders*, 2nd ed., London.
BRAIN, W. R. (1945) Speech and handedness, *Lancet*, **ii**, 837.
CONRAD, K. (1954) Some problems of aphasia, *Brain*, **77**, 491.
CRITCHLEY, M. (1927–8) On palilalia, *J. Neurol. Psychopath.*, **8**, 23.
CRITCHLEY, M. (1970) *Aphasiology and Other Aspects of Language*, London.
CRITCHLEY, M. (1975), *Silent Language*, London.
CUMMING, W. J. K., HURWITZ, L. J., and PERL, N. T. (1970) A study of a patient who had alexia without agraphia, *J. Neurol. Neurosurg. Psychiat.*, **33**, 34.
GAZZANIGA, M. S., BOGEN, J. E., and SPERRY, R. W. (1965) Observations on visual perception after disconnexion of the cerebral hemispheres in man, *Brain*, **88**, 221.
GESCHWIND, N. (1965) Disconnexion syndromes in animals and man, *Brain*, **88**, 237, 585.
GESCHWIND, N. (1970) The organization of language and the brain, *Science*, **170**, 940.
GESCHWIND, N. (1974) *Selected Papers on Language and the Brain*, Boston Studies on the Philosophy of Science, vol. xvi, Dordrecht, Holland and Boston.
GESCHWIND, N., QUADFASEL, F. A., and SEGARRA, J. M. (1968) Isolation of the speech area, *Neuropsychologia*, **6**, 327.
GOLDSTEIN, K. (1942) *After-effects of Brain Injuries in War*, London.
GOLDSTEIN, K. (1948) *Language and Language Disturbances*, New York.

HEAD, H. (1926) *Aphasia and Kindred Disorders of Speech* (2 vols.), Cambridge.

HEMPHILL, R. E., and STENGEL, E. (1940) A study on pure word-deafness, *J. Neurol. Psychiat.*, **3**, 251.

HENSCHEN, S. E. (1926) On the function of the right hemisphere of the brain in relation to the left in speech, music and calculation, *Brain*, **49**, 110.

HENSCHEN, S. E. (1927) Aphasiesysteme, *Mschr. Psychiat. Neurol.*, **65**, 87.

HERMANN, G., and PÖTZL, O. (1926) Über die Agraphie, *Abhandlung aus der Neurol. Psychiat., Psychol. und ihr Grenzgetret*, Berlin.

JACKSON, J. H. (1932) *Selected Writings*, vol. ii, London.

KERTESZ, A., and POOLE, E. (1973) The aphasia quotient: the taxonomic approach to measurement of aphasic disability, *Canad. J. neurol. Sci.*, **1**, 7.

KLEIST, K. (1922) *Handbuch der ärztlichen Erfahrungen im Weltkriege*, iv, 491, Leipzig.

LHERMITTE, F., and GAUTIER, J. C. (1969) Aphasia, Chapter 5 in *Handbook of Clinical Neurology*, ed. Vinken, P. J., and Bruyn, G. W., vol. 4, Amsterdam.

LURIA, A. R. (1970) *Traumatic Aphasia*, The Hague and Paris.

MEYER, A. (1974) The frontal lobe syndrome, the aphasias and related conditions— a contribution to the history of cortical localization, *Brain*, **97**, 565.

MOHR, J. P., SIDMAN, M., STODDART, L. T., LEICESTER, J., and ROSENBERGER, P. B. (1973) Evolution of the deficit in total aphasia, *Neurology (Minneap.)*, **23**, 1302.

NIELSEN, J. M. (1946) *Agnosia, Apraxia, Aphasia. Their Value in Cerebral Localization*, 2nd ed., New York.

SUBIRANA, A. (1969) Handedness and cerebral dominance, Chapter 13 in *Handbook of Clinical Neurology*, ed. Vinken, P. J., and Bruyn, G. W., vol. 4, Amsterdam.

VAN THAL, J. H. (1960) Polyglot aphasics, *Folia phoniat.*, **12**, 123.

WEISENBURG, T. H., and McBRIDE, K. E. (1935) *Aphasia*, New York.

DEVELOPMENTAL SPEECH DISORDERS

Developmental speech disorders are of considerable importance, since, unless a correct diagnosis is made, the sufferer may be wrongly regarded as mentally retarded, and valuable opportunities of treatment may be missed. It is also essential to exclude congenital nerve deafness, which may cause severe delay in the acquisition of language, before concluding that a child with defective speech is suffering from a cerebral disorder of language or articulation. Lesser degrees of hearing loss may result in defective articulation; in particular, high-tone deafness causes difficulty in using the high-tone consonants such as 'f' and 's'.

Developmental expressive aphasia (Orton) is rare, developmental aphasia being usually of the receptive type. Two varieties of this, congenital word-deafness and developmental dyslexia, are distinguished, but combined forms occur.

DEVELOPMENTAL RECEPTIVE APHASIA

Congenital word-deafness, or congenital auditory imperception, as it has also been called, is a rare inborn defect of speech. It is frequently familial and may appear in different members of successive generations of a family. Males are affected more frequently than females in the proportion of 5 to 1. The essential disturbance of function appears to be an inability to appreciate the significance of sounds, although hearing is normal. It may be supposed that there is a lack of the anatomical or physiological mechanism whereby sounds become associated with other sensory impressions and with kinaesthetic sensations produced by speech and so acquire meanings. Since the disorder is more profound than merely a lack of appreciation of the significance of words, the term 'congenital auditory imperception' was proposed by Worster-Drought and Allen (1928-9).

The defect is present from birth but is not as a rule noticed until the age at which a normal child begins to understand speech and to learn to speak. It is then found that the patient takes no notice when spoken to and does not learn to repeat words. Hearing, however, is normal and the child responds to noises. Spoken language is not understood provided the patient has not learned to lip-read. The appreciation of musical sounds may or may not be defective. Worster-Drought and Allen pointed out that associated with the word-deafness there may be a defect in appreciating the meaning of written and printed symbols. This is not surprising in view of the large part which hearing plays in learning to read in normal individuals. Speech suffers seriously as a result of auditory imperception. For a number of years the child may not speak at all. Sooner or later, however, most patients acquire a vocabulary of their own, which is comprehensible only to those who have been closely associated with them. The words spoken bear little resemblance to normal words, though they possess meaning for the speaker. This defective form of speech has been identified by the now out-dated terms 'idioglossia' and 'lalling'.

Although sufferers from congenital word-deafness are frequently found in institutions for the mentally subnormal, they do not necessarily suffer from any defect in mental capacity but are severely handicapped by the inadequacy of the primary channel through which we learn the meaning of things around us. It is not surprising therefore that the victims of this disorder tend to develop abnormal psychological reactions to their surroundings, especially when they are treated as lazy or mentally subnormal.

The diagnosis is from general mental subnormality, and from high-tone deafness which can be excluded by audiometry.

The education of the congenitally word-deaf requires much care, and an intelligent appreciation of the nature of their disorder. As in the case of the deaf, they must be educated principally through the sense of sight and should be taught lip-reading, while their sense of touch may also be used to educate them in correct articulation. The nature of the disability must be taken into account in planning an occupation.

DEVELOPMENTAL DYSLEXIA

Developmental dyslexia seems the best term to apply to a mixed group of individuals who possess in common a defect in learning to read. This condition has been called congenital word-blindness (Drew, 1956), but a defect which can rightly be so described is the cause in only a small proportion of cases.

Developmental dyslexia is much commoner than congenital word-deafness, and Thomas (1905) estimated that it was present in 1 in every 2,000 London school-children. Like congenital word-deafness it is not uncommonly familial and may occur in more than one generation of the same family. In some cases it may be due to a congenital lack of the ability to appreciate the significance of visual symbols. In many patients, however, visual symbolization appears to be normal, and the defect appears to consist in an inability to differentiate the spoken word into its sounds and to break up a written word into its sounds and letters (Schilder, 1944). Consequently the printed word is wrongly pronounced, and conversely a dictated word is wrongly spelt. The writing of dyslexic children is very abnormal. The subject has been reviewed by Money (1962) and Critchley (1964).

Developmental dyslexia usually becomes apparent owing to the child's backwardness in learning to read. This may be wrongly attributed to a general defect of intelligence or to laziness. Yet by intelligence tests these children are frequently normal and their power of visual imagery is unimpaired. Such children are apt to develop psychoneurotic reactions to their environment owing to lack of understanding of their disability.

Children with congenital auditory imperception frequently have some difficulty in learning to read as well as to speak (Ingram, 1959), but in those with developmental dyslexia, spontaneous speech is usually normal in fluency and content.

MIRROR-WRITING

This is the term applied to script which runs from right to left, the letters being reversed and forming mirror-images of normal script. Normal individuals can frequently carry out mirror-writing with the left hand, either when writing with the left hand alone or with both hands simultaneously. Since this capacity is present without previous training we must assume that the education of the right hand in normal writing involves the unconscious education of the left hand to perform the same movements in the opposite direction. Such mirror-writing with the left hand may become evident in right-handed individuals who have developed right hemiplegia, and it has been known to follow an injury of the occipital region of the brain.

The situation is more complicated than this, however, in patients suffering from developmental dyslexia who exhibit mirror-writing, for in such individuals mirror-writing appears to be secondary to mirror-reading, as shown by Orton. These children tend to read words from right to left and pronounce them accordingly. For example, 'not' is pronounced 'ton', and if asked to copy words they frequently do so in the reversed order, with or without reversal of single letters. The frequent association of left-handedness with mirror-reading and writing suggests that these disorders may be secondary to a lesion of the left hemisphere which is normally dominant and to a substituted dominance of the right hemisphere. Many normal children pass through a temporary phase of mirror-writing, at least of certain letters, when first learning to write, especially when there is a family history of left-handedness or ambidexterity.

TREATMENT

Treatment of dyslexia must be based upon an understanding of the nature of the child's disability. Attention must be paid to educating the child in the association of syllables with the articulatory movements employed in their pronunciation. The phonetic method of teaching spelling, in which the child learns letters by their sounds and not by their names, should be employed. Special care must be taken in teaching the child to read from left to right. The teacher should point to the letters in this order and the child should be encouraged to do the same with the forefinger of the right hand (for details see Schonell, 1948 and Schiffman, 1962).

Stress should be laid upon reading for amusement, and in dictation the child should not depend solely upon ear, but should sit by a normal child and be allowed to see what he has written. Educational authorities throughout the child's career should be informed of his disability in order that allowances may be made, especially in examinations.

DEVELOPMENTAL DYSARTHRIA

Although dysarthria may be a striking feature of the various forms of cerebral palsy, and may even occur in some cases of 'minimal cerebral dysfunction' [p. 636], Morley *et al.* (1954) and Morley (1972) have pointed out that some children who show a relatively normal development of language and who have no evidence of spasticity, paresis, or dystonia of the articulatory muscles, demonstrate slow and clumsy articulation, associated with clumsiness of movement of the lips, tongue, and palate. They suggest that in some cases the defect is a form of articulatory dyspraxia. Some affected individuals also show associated clumsiness of limb movements or developmental apraxia [p. 118]. Ingram (1959) found that developmental dysarthria is often associated with variable defects in the acquisition of language and suggests that this syndrome rarely occurs in a 'pure' form.

DYSLALIA

This term was used by Morley (1957) to identify a syndrome in which speech is acquired at the normal age and soon becomes fluent but the child demonstrates many defects of consonant substitution and omission. The condition quickly responds to speech therapy and speech usually becomes normal in a few months. This is probably a syndrome of multiple aetiology (Ingram, 1959; Morley, 1972); in some cases the child imitates the defective articulation of other family members, in some there is mild mental retardation, and in yet others the condition may be a mild and rapidly reversible form of developmental receptive aphasia or developmental dysarthria.

STUTTERING (STAMMERING)

Definition. A dysrhythmia of speech leading to a disturbance of articulation characterized by abrupt interruptions of the flow of speech, or the repetition of sounds or syllables.

AETIOLOGY

There is still considerable controversy about the aetiology of stuttering. Orton (1937) suggested that this abnormality of speech is due to a defect in the establishment of dominance with respect to speech function in one or other cerebral hemisphere and found that it was commoner in left-handed persons and in shifted sinistrals. Others have suggested that the condition is of psychoneurotic origin. However, while recent studies have confirmed a clear association with partial or complete left-handedness or ambidexterity, Fransella (1970) has pointed out that stutterers do not have neurotic personalities or behaviour characteristics according to accepted psychological criteria. Transient stuttering may occur in adults as a result of dominant hemispheric lesions giving mild Broca's aphasia. The 'idiopathic' condition is much commoner in males, rarely develops after 7-8 years, and has been found in about 1 per cent of British schoolchildren (Andrews and Harris, 1964; Butler *et al.*, 1973). There is a strong familial incidence (Johnson *et al.*, 1948; Jameson, 1955) and the condition sometimes occurs in children with mild developmental dysarthria or apraxia or other evidence of minimal cerebral dysfunction. As Morley (1972) suggests, current opinion favours the view that the defect begins inadvertently in early life when neuromuscular control of speech is still unstable. The normal hesitations and repetitions of early childhood may be regarded as abnormal

E

by adults in the child's environment, and parental anxiety, communicated to the child, results in perpetuation of the defect. Anxiety, frustration, self-consciousness, and increasing attempts to correct the defect often have the effect of making it worse.

SYMPTOMS

The flow of speech may be broken by pauses, during which it is entirely arrested, or by the repetition of sounds or syllables. The pause may be filled with grunts or hisses, and stuttering is frequently associated with facial contractions or tics involving the limbs or even the whole body. The spastic element is usually called *tonus* and the repetitive *clonus*. Various stages in the development of stutter have been described. It is generally agreed that the first consists of reiteration of syllables. Stein (1942) describes six phases in the second stage. Dentals (t, d), labials (p, b), and gutturals (k and hard g) are the consonants which are usually the most troublesome to the stutterer, especially when they occur at the beginning of a word. Stutterers often go out of their way to avoid certain words by reconstructing sentences and may employ tricks to enable them to achieve correct pronunciation, for example, spelling a word before pronouncing it. They can usually sing, may be able to recite without hesitancy, and sometimes speak fluently when angry or when alone.

PROGNOSIS

Mild stuttering tends to disappear spontaneously. In some severe cases considerable improvement and even complete cure can be achieved by thorough treatment.

TREATMENT

When stuttering occurs in a left-handed child who has been made to use the right hand, a return to left-handedness may produce improvement. Re-education of speech by a trained teacher is essential. The role of muscular spasm in the production of stuttering must be explained to the patient, who should be taught to practise relaxation of the muscles concerned in speech. Relaxation should be followed by breathing exercises and by vocal gymnastics, exercises being prescribed in which the lips, tongue, jaw, and palate are moved without the production of sounds. Later the patient begins to practise words, and articulation may at first be facilitated by various devices such as singing, or speaking through a megaphone or in time with a metronome. The use of syllabic speech under the supervision of a trained speech therapist has proved to be remarkably successful in some cases.

In children psychological difficulties at home and at school should be dealt with if possible. In the pre-school child, treatment depends very much upon the mother, while in school, a teacher who understands the problem and is prepared to be patient can do a great deal. At all ages suggestion and the enthusiasm of the therapist play a vital role (Travis, 1959; Andrews and Harris, 1964; Morley, 1972).

REFERENCES

ANDREWS, G., and HARRIS, M. (1964) *The Syndrome of Stuttering*, London.
BRAIN, W. R. (1945) Speech and handedness, *Lancet*, **ii,** 837.
BUTLER, N. R., PECKHAM, C., and SHERIDAN, M. (1973) Speech defects in children aged 7 years: a national study, *Brit. med. J.*, **1,** 253.

CRITCHLEY, M. (1964) *Developmental Dyslexia*, London.

DREW, A. L. (1956) A neurological appraisal of familial congenital word-blindness, *Brain*, **79**, 440.

FRANSELLA, F. (1970) Stuttering—not a symptom but a way of life, *Brit. J. Dis. Commun.*, **5**, 22.

INGRAM, T. T. S. (1959) Specific developmental disorders of speech in childhood, *Brain*, **82**, 450.

JAMESON, A. M. (1955) Stammering in children. Some factors in the prognosis, *Speech*, **19**, No. 2, 60.

JOHNSON, W. (1959) in *Handbook of Speech Pathology*, ed. Travis, L. E., p. 897, London.

JOHNSON, W., BROWN, S. F., CURTIS, J. F., EDNEY, J. C., and KEASTER, J. (1948) *Speech Handicapped School Children*, New York.

MONEY, J. (1962) *Reading Disability. Progress and Research Needs in Dyslexia*, Baltimore.

MORLEY, M. E. (1957) *The Development and Disorders of Speech in Children*, London.

MORLEY, M. E. (1972) *The Development and Disorders of Speech in Childhood*, 3rd ed., London.

MORLEY, M. E., COURT, S. D. M., and MILLER, H. (1954) Developmental dysarthria, *Brit. med. J.*, **1**, 8.

ORTON, S. T. (1937) *Reading, Writing and Speech Problems in Children*, London.

SCHIFFMAN, G. (1962) in *Reading Disability. Progress and Research Needs in Dyslexia*, ed. Money, J., p. 45, Baltimore.

SCHILDER, P. (1944) Congenital alexia and its relation to optic perception, *J. genet. Psychol.*, **65**, 67.

SCHONELL, F. J. (1948) *Backwardness in the Basic Subjects*, 4th ed., Edinburgh.

STEIN, L. (1942) *Speech and Voice*, London.

THOMAS, C. J. (1905) Congenital word-blindness and its treatment, *Ophthalmoscope*, **3**, 380.

TRAVIS, L. E. (ed.) (1959) *Handbook of Speech Pathology*, London.

WEST, R. W., KENNEDY, L., and CARR, A. (1937) *The Rehabilitation of Speech*, New York.

WORSTER-DROUGHT, C., and ALLEN, I. M. (1928–9) Congenital auditory imperception, *J. Neurol. Psychopath.*, **60**, 193 and 289.

APRAXIA AND AGNOSIA

APRAXIA

Apraxia may be defined as an inability to carry out a purposive movement, the nature of which the patient understands, in the absence of severe motor paralysis, sensory loss, and ataxia. For example, a patient who is asked to protrude his tongue is unable to do so on request, though he may carry out inappropriate movements such as opening his mouth. A moment later he spontaneously protrudes his tongue to lick his lips. Apraxia may involve any movement normally voluntarily initiated—movements of the eyes, face, muscles of articulation, chewing and swallowing, manipulation of objects, gestures with the upper limb, walking, or sitting down.

Normal purposive movements depend upon the integrity not only of the corticobulbar and corticospinal tracts, but also of association tracts whereby these efferent paths are excited. The idea of the movement, whether formulated spontaneously or in response to an external command, thus passes into action. Apraxia is the result of interruption of the pathways thus acting as ideomotor links. In right-handed individuals purposive motor activity appears thus to be

controlled by the posterior part of the left hemisphere, especially by the supra-marginal gyrus. Thence fibres pass forwards in the left hemisphere to the precentral gyrus and cross to the same gyrus on the right side, through the corpus callosum. Lesions in the left parietal lobe are therefore likely to produce bilateral apraxia. Lesions between this region and the left precentral gyrus may lead to apraxia of the limbs on the right side, and lesions involving the anterior part of the corpus callosum or of the subcortical white matter on the right side may cause left-sided apraxia. The commonest form of apraxia is that involving the lips and tongue, which is frequently encountered in association with right hemiplegia due to a lesion of the left hemisphere. Dressing apraxia, in which the patient cannot dress because he is unable to relate the parts of his body to the parts of a garment, is essentially due to a disturbance of the body image (see below) and is usually the result of a lesion of the right parietal lobe.

Apraxia was classified by Liepmann (1905) into limb-kinetic apraxia, due to loss of kinetic memories of part of the body, ideokinetic apraxia, due to a dissociation between ideational and kinaesthetic processes, and ideational apraxia, in which the general conception of the movement is imperfect, its component parts being correctly carried out but wrongly combined.

Apraxia is usually associated with an impairment of the power to imitate movements. The disturbance of function which underlies apraxia is essentially the same as that responsible for motor aphasia, which may justly be regarded as an apraxia of the purposive movements concerned in speech. The nature of apraxia has recently been discussed by Geschwind (1965).

A special form of apraxia was named by Kleist (1922) *constructional or optical apraxia.* There is no apraxia of single movements but the spatial disposition of the action is disordered. The patient, for example, cannot copy a simple arrangement of matches, but recognizes his mistakes. Constructional apraxia may occur in association with lesions of either parietal lobe; when the dominant hemisphere is involved it is often associated with the other features of Gerstmann's syndrome [p. 119], but as an isolated defect it is commoner in lesions of the non-dominant hemisphere (Piercy *et al.*, 1960). *Apraxia of gait* is usually the result of bilateral frontal lesions (Meyer and Barron, 1960) and is sometimes seen in presenile dementia. Apraxia of ocular movements (Altrocchi and Menkes, 1960) has been described on page 84.

Apraxia is most frequently seen as a result of localized lesions of the brain, especially vascular lesions and tumours. It may also be a symptom of diffuse cerebral inflammatory or degenerative states, such as general paresis and the presenile cerebral degenerations.

AGNOSIA

The arrival of nerve impulses at the cortical areas concerned in vision, hearing, and cutaneous and postural sensibility excites crude sensations which have not yet attained the perceptual level involved in the recognition of objects. Recognition is brought about by the association of the sensations excited through one sensory channel with memories of sensations derived from other sensory channels during previous experiences of the object, which include our actions in regard to it. The perception of an object seen or felt is thus a constellation of sensory images and memories directed towards action, and the recognition of an object as having been seen before, and of its use, depends upon the capacity of the primary visual or tactile sensations which it evokes to excite the correct

motor or sensory associations. When, by reason of disease of the brain, this secondary process fails to occur, the patient fails to recognize the object. This defect is known as agnosia or mind-blindness. Its nature has been discussed by Geschwind (1965).

Visual agnosia is present when the patient, in whom the paths from the retina to the occipital cortex are intact and the latter is undamaged, nevertheless fails to recognize common objects which he clearly sees. This condition may result from lesions in the left parieto-occipital region in right-handed persons. Bender and Feldman (1972) point out that visual agnosias for form (Benson and Greenberg, 1969) and colour and object recognition (Rubens and Benson, 1971) rarely occur in 'pure' form but are usually associated with a contralateral hemianopia and with various other deficits of mental and cognitive function. *Prosopagnosia* is a restricted form of visual agnosia in which the patient is unable to recognize faces (Meadows, 1974). *Auditory agnosia* implies the failure to recognize sounds in a patient who is nevertheless not deaf. An individual suffering from this disability in a severe form will fail to appreciate not only the nature of words but also musical tunes. This results from a lesion of the left temporal lobe in right-handed persons. Word-deafness [p. 110] can be considered to be a form of auditory agnosia for spoken verbal symbols. *Tactile agnosia* is one form of the disorders comprised under the more general term *astereognosis*. The patient, though not suffering from gross sensory defect in the fingers or hand, is nevertheless unable to recognize an object placed in the hand. This may be produced by a lesion of the parietal lobe situated posteriorly to the post-central gyrus at the level of the hand area. One form of congenital indifference to pain (*pain asymbolia*) is thought to be an agnosia for painful sensations; it has been described in association with congenital auditory imperception (Osuntokun et al., 1968).

Agnosia usually affects only the recognition of objects through one sensory channel. Thus a patient suffering from visual agnosia, who cannot recognize a key when he sees it, can usually recognize it when it is placed in his hand. Conversely, a patient who cannot recognize objects placed in his hand recognizes them readily when he sees them. The various forms of agnosia, like apraxia, may result from focal vascular or neoplastic lesions and are sometimes seen in the presenile dementias. Visual agnosia is especially common as a consequence of cerebral anoxia, as in carbon monoxide poisoning.

REFERENCES

ALTROCCHI, P. H., and MENKES, J. H. (1960) Congenital ocular motor apraxia, *Brain*, **83,** 579.
BENDER, M. B., and FELDMAN, M. (1972) The so-called 'visual agnosias', *Brain*, **95,** 173.
BENSON, D. F., and GREENBERG, J. P. (1969) Visual form agnosia. A specific defect in visual discrimination, *Arch. Neurol. (Chic.)*, **20,** 82.
BRAIN, LORD (1965) *Speech Disorders*, 2nd ed., London.
BRAIN, W. R. (1941) Visual object-agnosia, with special reference to the Gestalt theory, *Brain*, **64,** 43.
GESCHWIND, N. (1965) Disconnexion syndromes in animals and man, *Brain*, **88,** 237, 585.
KLEIST, K. (1922) Die psychomotorischen Störungen und ihr Verhältnis zu den Motilitätsstörungen bei Erkrankungen der Stammganglien, *Mschr. Psychiat. Neurol.*, **52,** 253.
LIEPMANN, H. (1905) *Über Störungen des Handelns bei Gehirnkranken*, Berlin.
MEADOWS, J. C. (1974) The anatomical basis of prosopagnosia, *J. Neurol. Neurosurg. Psychiat.*, **37,** 489.

MEYER, J. S., and BARRON, D. W. (1960) Apraxia of gait: a clinico-physiological study, *Brain*, **83**, 261.

NATHAN, P. W. (1947) Facial apraxia and apraxic dysarthria, *Brain*, **70**, 449.

NIELSEN, J. M. (1938) Gerstmann syndrome: finger agnosia, agraphia, confusion of right and left and acalculia, *Arch. Neurol. Psychiat. (Chic.)*, **39**, 536.

NIELSEN, J. M. (1946) *Agnosia, Apraxia, Aphasia. Their Value in Cerebral Localization*, 2nd ed., New York.

OSUNTOKUN, B. O., ODEKU, E. L., and LUZZATO, L. (1968) Congenital pain asymbolia and auditory imperception, *J. Neurol. Neurosurg. Psychiat.*, **31**, 291.

PIERCY, M., HÉCAEN, H., and AJURIAGUERRA, J. DE (1960) Constructional apraxia associated with unilateral cerebral lesions—left and right sided cases compared, *Brain*, **83**, 225.

RUBENS, A. B., and BENSON, D. F. (1971) Associative visual agnosia, *Arch. Neurol. (Chic.)*, **24**, 305.

SITTIG, O. (1931) *Über Apraxie: eine klinische Studie*, Berlin.

DEVELOPMENTAL APRAXIA AND AGNOSIA

Gubbay *et al.* (1965) showed that some 'clumsy children' who presented with poor school performance due to delay in the development of motor skills could be shown to have defects of cognitive and executive performance which could be classified as various forms of apraxia and agnosia. Many such children also showed variable involuntary limb movements which superficially resembled chorea. In some children collateral clinical evidence suggested that perinatal brain damage may have been the cause, but in others the condition may have been due to a physiological disorder of the establishment of dominance in one or other hemisphere as there was evidence of crossed laterality. Most such children showed a discrepancy between a high verbal and low performance score on the Wechsler Intelligence Scale for Children. Improvement occurred with maturation but in several cases patient individual tuition was needed to overcome the disability. Minor degrees of this syndrome often go unrecognized and uncorrected in apparently normal schoolchildren (Walton *et al.*, 1962; Brenner *et al.*, 1967). A developmental form of Gerstmann's syndrome has been described (Benson and Geschwind, 1970).

REFERENCES

BENSON, D. F., and GESCHWIND, N. (1970) Developmental Gerstmann syndrome, *Neurology (Minneap.)*, **20**, 293.

BRENNER, M. W., GILLMAN, S., ZANGWILL, O. L., and FARRELL, M. (1967) Visuo-motor disability in schoolchildren, *Brit. med. J.*, **4**, 259.

GUBBAY, S. S. (1976) *Clumsy Children*, London.

GUBBAY, S. S., ELLIS, E., WALTON, J. N., and COURT, S. D. M. (1965) Clumsy children: a study of apraxic and agnosic defects in 21 children, *Brain*, **88**, 295.

WALTON, J. N., ELLIS, E., and COURT, S. D. M. (1962) Clumsy children: a study of developmental apraxia and agnosia, *Brain*, **85**, 603.

DISORDERS OF THE BODY-IMAGE

We are aware of the existence of our bodies, their position in space, and the relation of their parts to one another because we receive sense-data through numerous sensory channels, which include vision, cutaneous sensibility, and proprioceptor impulses from the muscles and joints and from the labyrinths. The paths carrying the somatic impulses pass by way of the ventral nucleus of

the optic thalamus to the supramarginal gyrus which is thus concerned with awareness of the opposite half of the body. This presentation of the body to consciousness is known as the body-image or body-schema.

Symptoms of disorder of the body-image may be positive or negative. The chief positive symptom is the phantom—an illusion of the persistence of a part of the body which has been lost by amputation, e.g. a phantom limb, or an illusory awareness of part of the body from which sensation has been lost owing to interruption of afferent pathways. Phantom limbs after amputation may be painless or painful (Riddoch, 1941). The painless phantom soon becomes less obtrusive, and gradually shortens, to disappear into the stump. A painful phantom is usually associated with abnormalities of the stump, especially large and tender terminal neuromas on the divided nerves. Painful phantoms may persist indefinitely and cause much distress. A phantom limb may be abolished by a lesion of the area of the opposite parietal cortex concerned with representation of the body-image.

Defects of the body-image are less easily demonstrated in patients with lesions of the dominant hemisphere as they are likely to be obscured by associated aphasia or other related phenomena. However, in Gerstmann's syndrome (Gerstmann, 1924, 1940, 1970) a lesion of the dominant angular gyrus gives finger agnosia, an inability to name or select individual fingers in the patient himself or in the examiner. In the syndrome as classically described, this abnormality is associated with agraphia, acalculia, and right–left disorientation; in some otherwise typical cases, alexia is also present.

Whereas visual agnosia for form and object recognition is also most often seen in lesions of the visual association areas of the dominant hemisphere, the most striking abnormalities of the body-image occur as a result of lesions of the non-dominant parieto-occipital region and can be regarded as various forms of visuo-spatial agnosia (Ettlinger et al., 1957). Thus the patient may be unaware of the opposite half of his body and of extrapersonal space on the same side—autotopagnosia, or contralateral visual neglect (Leicester et al., 1969). He ignores people and objects in that half of the visual field, may deny that his limbs on the affected side, even if hemiplegic, belong to him, and if he attempts to draw a clock face he will crowd all the figures into the opposite half of the circle. In severe cases, visual disorientation may be so severe that the patient is unable to find his way about, even in familiar surroundings. Denial of evidence of bodily disease, e.g. hemiplegia, is known as anosognosia, while denial of blindness has been identified as Anton's syndrome.

In parieto-occipital lesions of lesser severity the patient may be unable to localize visual stimuli in the opposite half-field or tactile stimuli on the opposite side of the body. When a stimulus, whether visual or tactile, is perceived when delivered independently on either side, but when one of two such stimuli presented simultaneously on the two sides is ignored, this is known as visual or tactile inattention [p. 50].

REFERENCES

CRITCHLEY, M. (1953) The Parietal Lobes, London.

ETTLINGER, G., WARRINGTON, E., and ZANGWILL, O. L. (1957) A further study of visual-spatial agnosia, Brain, **80**, 335.

FREDERICKS, J. A. M. (1969) Disorders of the Body Schema, chap. 11 in vol. 4 of Handbook of Clinical Neurology, ed. Vinken, P. J., and Bruyn, G. W., Amsterdam.

GERSTMANN, J. (1924) Fingeragnosie. Eine umschriebene Störung der Orientierung am eigenen Körper, *Wien. klin. Wschr.*, **37**, 1010.

GERSTMANN, J. (1940) Syndrome of finger agnosia, disorientation for right and left, agraphia and acalculia, *Arch. Neurol. Psychiat. (Chic.)*, **44**, 398.

GERSTMANN, J. (1970) Some posthumous notes on the Gerstmann syndrome, *Wien. Z. Nervenheilkunde*, **28**, 12.

LEICESTER, J., SIDMAN, M., STODDART, L. T., and MOHR, J. P. (1969) Some determinants of visual neglect, *J. Neurol. Neurosurg. Psychiat.*, **32**, 580.

LHERMITTE, J. (1939) *L'Image de notre corps*, Paris.

NIELSEN, J. M. (1938) Disturbances of the body scheme: their physiologic mechanism, *Bull. Los Angeles neurol. Soc.*, **3**, 127.

RANEY, A. A., and NIELSEN, J. M. (1942) Denial of blindness (Anton's syndrome), *Bull. Los Angeles neurol. Soc.*, **7**, 150.

REDLICH, F. C., and DORSEY, J. F. (1945) Denial of blindness by patients with cerebral disease, *Arch. Neurol. Psychiat. (Chic.)*, **53**, 407.

RIDDOCH, G. (1941) Phantom limbs and body shape, *Brain*, **64**, 197.

SCHILDER, P. (1935) *The Image and Appearance of the Human Body*, London.

THE SIGNS OF LOCAL LESIONS OF THE BRAIN

It is customary in textbooks on nervous diseases to describe in a separate section the signs of local lesions of the brain. Since these are dealt with in connection with anatomy and physiology, tumours, and vascular lesions, to avoid reduplication they will not be repeated, but for the convenience of the reader references are here given to the parts of the book in which are described the signs of local lesions in various situations.

The Prefrontal Lobe :

Tumours of the frontal lobe, pages 267–70.
Syndromes of the cerebral arteries—anterior cerebral artery, page 332.
Spasticity, page 22. The grasp reflex, page 57. Mental functions, page 1148.

The Precentral Gyrus :

The corticospinal tract, page 16.
Tumours of the precentral gyrus, pages 267–9.
Syndromes of the cerebral arteries—the middle cerebral artery, page 333.

The Temporal Lobe :

Tumours of the temporal lobe, page 270.
The geniculocalcarine pathway, page 72.

The Parietal Lobe :

Tumours of the parietal lobe, page 271.
Sensation at the cortical level, page 49.
The geniculocalcarine pathway, page 72.

The Occipital Lobe :

Tumours of the occipital lobe, page 272.
The visual cortex, page 72.
Syndromes of the cerebral arteries—the posterior cerebral artery, page 334.

The Corpus Callosum :

Tumours of the corpus callosum, page 273.

The Basal Ganglia:

The Internal Capsule:

The Third Ventricle and the Hypothalamus:

The Region of the Optic Chiasm:

The Midbrain:

The Pons and Medulla:

The Fourth Ventricle:

The Cerebellum:

THE CEREBROSPINAL FLUID

ANATOMY AND PHYSIOLOGY

FORMATION, CIRCULATION, AND ABSORPTION

Clinical and experimental observation has established that the cerebrospinal fluid is mainly formed by the choroid plexuses of the cerebral ventricles. That formed by the plexuses of the lateral ventricles passes through the interventricular foramina into the third ventricle. Thence the fluid flows through the cerebral aqueduct into the fourth ventricle, which it leaves by the median and two lateral foramina of the fourth ventricle to reach the subarachnoid space.

The subarachnoid space, which lies between the arachnoid membrane externally and the pia mater internally, constitutes a vessel which carries the fluid from the cerebral ventricles to its points of absorption. The inner surface of the arachnoid and the outer surface of the pia mater are covered with flattened mesothelial cells and these also cover the numerous trabeculae, which bridge the subarachnoid space, and the nerves and blood vessels which pass across it. The subarachnoid space is deepest at the base of the brain and between the inferior surface of the cerebellum and the medulla. In these regions its expansions constitute the various cisterns, the largest of which is the cerebellomedullary cistern beneath the cerebellum.

The subarachnoid space extends superficially over the whole surface of the brain and spinal cord. It is also prolonged into the substance of the nervous system by means of extensions which are known as the perivascular or Virchow-Robin spaces. Every blood vessel entering or leaving the nervous system must pass across the subarachnoid space. In so doing it carries with it into the nervous system a sleeve of arachnoid immediately surrounding the vessel and a sleeve of pia mater more externally. Between the two lies the extension of the subarachnoid space, which is known as the perivascular space and which subdivides on each division of the vessel to terminate where the pia mater and arachnoid become continuous. It is probable that products of metabolism and cell-containing inflammatory exudates pass from the perivascular spaces to mingle with the cerebrospinal fluid in the subarachnoid space, and it is in the perivascular spaces that cuffs of inflammatory cells are found in inflammatory disorders of the nervous system.

The cerebrospinal fluid of the subarachnoid space probably receives a contribution from the perivascular spaces, and possibly also from the lymphatics of the cranial and other peripheral nerves. After bathing the surface of the spinal cord and the base of the brain it passes upwards over the convexity of the hemispheres, to be absorbed into the intracranial venous sinuses. The bulk of the evidence shows that absorption takes place through the microscopic arachnoid villi, which are minute projections of the subarachnoid space into the lumen of the sinuses. The work of Welch and Friedman (1960) suggested that these operate as valves, opening in response to a rise of pressure of the cerebrospinal fluid, but electron-microscopic studies by Tripathi (1973) have demonstrated vacuoles within the cells of the villi which suggest that there is a dynamic system of transcellular channels or pores which allow the bulk outflow of cerebrospinal fluid across the mesothelial barrier.

CHEMICAL COMPOSITION OF THE CEREBROSPINAL FLUID

The following table, based upon the investigations of Fremont-Smith and Cohen, shows the principal differences in chemical composition between the cerebrospinal fluid and the blood plasma. It used to be thought that the cerebrospinal fluid was a dialysate of plasma, but Davson (1967) reviews the evidence that secretory activity is required to explain its chemical composition. Sweet et al. (1954) consider that it is both a secretion and an ultrafiltrate. Recent work (see Davson, 1967) has also defined comparative concentrations of amino acids in plasma and cerebrospinal fluid, and information upon the enzyme activity (LDH, GOT, CPK) in the fluid in health and disease is now being accumulated.

Comparison of Blood Plasma and Cerebrospinal Fluid

	Blood Plasma	Cerebrospinal Fluid
Group 1. (Substances normally present in greater quantity in the plasma than in the fluid.)	Protein, 6–7 g/100 ml	Ventricular, 5–15 mg/100 ml Cisternal, 15–25 mg/100 ml Lumbar, 15–45 mg/100 ml
	Inorganic phosphorus, 2–4 mg/100 ml	1·25–2 mg/100 ml
	Uric acid, 2–4 mg/100 ml	Trace
	Cholesterol, 150 mg/100 ml	Trace
	Calcium, 10 mg/100 ml	5–6 mg/100 ml
	Sulphates, 4 mg/100 ml	1 mg/100 ml
	Glucose, 100 mg/100 ml	50–80 mg/100 ml
Group 2. (Substances normally present in greater quantity in the fluid than in the plasma.)	Chloride (as NaCl), 560–620 mg/100 ml	725–750 mg/100 ml
	Folate, 5·20 μg/100 ml	20–25 μg/100 ml
Group 3. (Substances approximately equally distributed between plasma and fluid.)	Sodium, potassium, CO_2, urea, lactic acid, sulphonamides	
Group 4. (Substances which do not pass from the plasma to the fluid except in minute traces.)	Fibrinogen, iodides, salicylates, nitrates, lipids, bile pigments, organic arsenic, some enzymes, most antibodies, penicillin, streptomycin	

VOLUME AND RATE OF FORMATION

The volume of the cerebrospinal fluid in adults is normally about 130 ml. Its rate of formation can only be estimated by artificial methods, the accuracy of which is doubtful. It is probable that the total volume is completely replaced several times a day.

FUNCTIONS OF CEREBROSPINAL FLUID

Many functions have been attributed to the cerebrospinal fluid though most of them are somewhat speculative. There is no doubt, however, about its importance mechanically in protecting the nervous system from jars and shocks. Probably also it acts as a regulator of the intracranial pressure and as a support to the venous sinuses in postures in which the intracranial venous pressure is raised. Bowsher (1953, 1957) suggested that the resting pressure of the fluid is due to the pressure transmitted from the walls of blood vessels within the spinal and cranial subarachnoid space, and O'Connell (1970) pointed out that the pressure fluctuates rhythmically with changes in the calibre of intracranial vessels. Martins et al. (1972) have also shown that the spinal dural sac is a distensible reservoir, readily changing its capacity in response to pressure gradients developed within the subarachnoid space and in the spinal epidural venous plexus. It is also likely that the fluid plays a part in the nutrition and metabolism of the nervous system, though this aspect of its functions is little understood. However, the pH of the fluid, which is normally maintained at about 7·31 and is primarily determined by the $p\mathrm{CO_2}$, probably plays a part in the central regulation of respiration (Cameron, 1969; Johnson, 1972).

METHODS OF OBTAINING CEREBROSPINAL FLUID

To obtain cerebrospinal fluid for examination it is necessary to puncture either the cerebral ventricles or the subarachnoid space, which may be reached most easily either in the cerebellomedullary cistern or in the lumbar theca where it extends beyond the lower end of the spinal cord.

LUMBAR PUNCTURE

Lumbar puncture is the simplest method of obtaining access to the subarachnoid space and is so frequently used that every practitioner of medicine should be capable of carrying it out. The spinal cord terminates at the lower border of the first lumbar vertebra in the adult, and at a slightly lower level in the child. The arachnoid is continued downwards below the termination of the spinal cord as far as the second sacral vertebra, and forms a lumbar cul-de-sac of the subarachnoid space normally containing cerebrospinal fluid and crossed by the roots of the cauda equina. A needle can be introduced into this space without risk of injury to the spinal cord.

Indications and Contra-indications

Lumbar puncture is carried out for the following purposes: (1) to obtain cerebrospinal fluid for cytological, chemical, and other investigations and to estimate its pressure; (2) to introduce into the subarachnoid space therapeutic substances or local anaesthetics; (3) to introduce air into the subarachnoid space for encephalography or myelography; (4) to introduce opaque media for myelography.

There are several important contra-indications to lumbar puncture. In the presence of increased intracranial pressure, especially when there is reason to suspect a tumour in the posterior fossa of the skull, sudden withdrawal of fluid from the spinal canal may cause herniation of the medulla into the foramen magnum—the 'cerebellar pressure cone'—with fatal results. When a space-occupying lesion is present or suspected in one cerebral hemisphere a herniation of the medial part of the temporal lobe may occur through the tentorial hiatus and the resultant compression and distortion of the upper brain stem may be equally disastrous. Thus the investigation is better avoided if intracranial tumour, abscess, or haematoma are suspected and should be performed in such cases only if essential information can be obtained in no other way, and if immediate neurosurgical aid is at hand. In such cases, if a specimen of fluid *must* be obtained this can only be done safely by ventricular puncture through a burr hole. Skin sepsis in the lumbar region is a contra-indication to lumbar puncture, owing to the risk of infecting the spinal canal. Marked spinal deformity in the dorsal or lumbar regions may render lumbar puncture difficult or impossible.

Preparation for Lumbar Puncture

There are a number of patterns of lumbar puncture needle. Their gauge ranges from 17 to 19; a good length is 8 cm. Harris's needles for trigeminal injection made by Messrs. Weiss are excellent. A needle of larger diameter may be required in cases of meningitis when thick pus is to be withdrawn.

Method of Puncture

Lumbar puncture may be performed with the patient either sitting or lying on one side. As many patients cannot sit up, it is best to accustom oneself to performing the operation with the patient lying on his left side. In either position the most important point is to secure the greatest possible degree of flexion of the lumbar spine. If the patient is conscious and co-operative he should be asked to bend his legs until his knees approach his chin and then to clasp his hands beneath his knees, or an assistant can aid flexion of the spine by applying pressure with one hand behind the neck and the other beneath the knees. When the patient is in position the next step is to find the landmarks. A line joining the highest points of the iliac crests, which may be marked with a swab dipped in a suitable antiseptic, usually passes between the third and fourth lumbar spinous processes, and the puncture can be performed either at this point or between the fourth and fifth spines. The skin is now cleaned and anaesthetized with 1 per cent procaine solution. A general anaesthetic is necessary only in the case of delirious or excitable patients who cannot be maintained in position, or when there is a spasmodic extension of the spine which cannot otherwise be overcome, as may happen in meningitis.

The needle, with the stylet in position, is now introduced midway between the spinous processes in the selected interspace and either in the midline, or, as some prefer, 1 cm to one side. The cutting edges of the bevelled point should be directed upwards and downwards and not transversely, since the fibres of the ligamenta flava and of the dura run longitudinally and are less likely to be divided in the former case. After its point has entered the skin the needle is passed forwards and slightly upwards in the sagittal plane. If it has been introduced to one side of the midline slight medial deviation is also necessary. At an average depth of about 4·5 cm the point of the needle encounters the increased resistance of the ligamentum flavum, and after penetrating a further 0·5 cm it should enter the subarachnoid space. The stylet is now withdrawn and laid upon a sterile towel and if the puncture has been successful cerebrospinal fluid drips from the butt of the needle. After the pressure has been measured as described below the fluid is collected in two sterile test-tubes consecutively, about 3 ml being allowed to run into each. One sample is used for microbiological examination, the other for cytology and chemistry. The needle is then withdrawn. The patient sometimes complains of pain in one leg when the needle enters the subarachnoid space. This is due to the point having come into contact with one of the roots of the cauda equina, which, however, is not likely to be damaged. Care should be taken not to introduce the needle too far lest an intervertebral disc should be injured.

A Dry Tap

In many cases the failure to obtain fluid means that the puncture has been incorrectly carried out. The point of the needle may not have entered the subarachnoid space either because it has been introduced too obliquely in the longitudinal plane or because it has deviated to one side or because, on account of scoliosis or arthritis, the interspace is difficult to find. It may not have penetrated far enough, or it may have gone too far, the point having come into contact with the posterior wall of the body of the vertebra where puncture of a vein is the commonest cause of blood in the fluid. The stylet should be passed into the needle again to remove any possible obstruction and the depth of the point varied. If no fluid comes, the needle should be withdrawn and reinserted either in the same interspace or in the one above or below. A genuine dry tap, when the point of the needle is actually in the subarachnoid space, may occur when the spinal subarachnoid space is blocked at a higher level and hence the pressure of the fluid in the lumbar sac is low, or when the lumbar sac itself is filled by a neoplasm or by a developmental lesion, as in spina bifida.

Sequels of Lumbar Puncture

The only common sequel of lumbar puncture is headache, which comes on after a few hours, is throbbing in character, and may be associated with nausea, vomiting, giddiness, and pain in the neck and back. In severe cases it is literally prostrating, being much intensified by sitting up, and lasting for days or even exceptionally for weeks. It is due to lowered intracranial tension produced by a continued leakage of cerebrospinal fluid through the puncture wound in the theca. Certain precautions will do much to prevent the development of 'lumbar puncture headache'. The needle used should be small in calibre, and introduced with the cutting edges in the sagittal plane. A minimal amount of fluid should be withdrawn and it may be helpful if the patient lies down for one or two hours afterwards. Some workers feel that if the patient lies prone rather than supine, a positive rather than a negative pressure in the extradural space is produced and discourages leakage of fluid. If in spite of these precautions headache develops, analgesics may be needed and the drinking of large quantities of fluid may help to promote cerebrospinal fluid formation.

Lumbar puncture occasionally causes an intensification of symptoms of the disease from which the patient is suffering. Root pains, if present, may be intensified, and this is especially liable to occur in the presence of a lesion compressing the spinal cord, any of the symptoms of which may be exacerbated by the alterations of pressure induced by the withdrawal of fluid. In multiple sclerosis relapses have sometimes been attributed to lumbar puncture, but there is no convincing evidence to indicate that this is a significant risk. The risks attendant upon lumbar puncture when the intracranial pressure is greatly increased, especially when there is a tumour in the posterior fossa, have already been described. Meningitis following lumbar puncture is fortunately rare and is due to a failure to preserve asepsis during the procedure.

VENTRICLE PUNCTURE

The following are the principal indications for ventricle puncture: (1) the relief of increased intracranial pressure before operation for intracranial tumour; (2) the injection of air into the ventricles for ventriculography for the diagnosis of hydrocephalus or intracranial tumour; (3) the injection of an antibiotic; (4) for comparison of the pressure or chemical composition of the fluid in the two lateral ventricles or of the ventricular and spinal fluids; (5) in rare cases to obtain fluid for examination when there is a contra-indication to both cisternal and lumbar puncture. The first and second are the purposes for which ventricle puncture is most frequently carried out.

CISTERNAL PUNCTURE

The cerebellomedullary cistern which is penetrated in cisternal puncture is a dilatation of the subarachnoid space lying between the inferior surface of the cerebellum above, the posterior surface of the medulla in front, and the dura mater covering the posterior atlanto-occipital membrane below and behind.

Indications and Contra-indications for Cisternal Puncture

The principal indications for cisternal puncture are: (1) to obtain cerebrospinal fluid for examination when lumbar puncture is for some reason impossible, for example, on account of deformity of the spine; (2) for comparison of the composition or pressure of the cisternal and lumbar fluids; (3) for the injection of opaque media in the radiographic investigation of blockage of the spinal subarachnoid space and particularly when lumbar myelography is impossible, or when the upper as well as the lower limits of a spinal lesion must be defined; (4) for the introduction of therapeutic substances, such as an antibiotic; (5) very rarely, to introduce air for encephalography. Cisternal puncture should never be carried out when there is reason to suspect a tumour or abscess in the posterior fossa, when there is a marked rise of intracranial pressure, or when the cerebello-medullary cistern is likely to be obliterated by inflammatory adhesions, or to be the site of a congenital abnormality (e.g. a Chiari malformation).

Method of Cisternal Puncture

The patient is prepared by shaving the scalp up to a horizontal line at the level of the external occipital protuberance. The skin is then cleaned with a suitable antiseptic. The patient should be seated and his head is held by an assistant with both hands and well flexed. The operator places the tip of the forefinger of his left hand upon the spinous process of the second cervical vertebra, which is the highest palpable spinous process. A spot 1 cm above this point is anaesthetized with a 1 per cent solution of procaine. A lumbar puncture needle with the stylet in position is then inserted at this point and passed forwards in a plane which passes through the point of introduction, the middle of the external acoustic meatus, and the nasion. At a depth of about 3 cm the point of the needle will encounter the posterior atlanto-occipital membrane, which offers considerable resistance. On gently introducing it a further 0·5 cm it should penetrate the cerebellomedullary cistern, and on with-drawal of the stylet cerebrospinal fluid usually drips from the needle. Often, however, although the point of the needle is in the cistern, there is no flow of fluid. This may be promoted by exerting gentle suction with a syringe inserted into the butt of the needle. The medulla lies at a depth of about 3 cm in front of the posterior atlanto-occipital membrane. With care, therefore, there is no risk that the point of the needle will enter the medulla. It should not, however, be introduced more than 6 cm from the surface of the skin. If the operator is unaccustomed to cisternal puncture it is often rendered easier by directing the point of the needle slightly above the plane described, so that it comes into contact with the occipital bone. It is then slightly depressed to pass through the membrane. After withdrawal of the needle the point of puncture can be closed with antiseptic. Headache may follow cisternal puncture. Its prophylaxis and treatment are the same as those described above for lumbar puncture.

ROUTINE EXAMINATION OF THE CEREBROSPINAL FLUID PRESSURE

Method of Determination. The pressure of the cerebrospinal fluid is best determined by means of a simple manometer. A graduated glass tube is attached to the lumbar puncture needle and the observer reads the height to which the fluid ascends in the tube. The instrument designed by Greenfield consists of a lumbar puncture needle with a two-way stopcock which permits fluid to be withdrawn without removing the manometer. A glass tube 30 cm long is attached to the needle by a small piece of tubing. For routine purposes the pressure is determined with the patient lying on the left side, and it is important to see that the head is supported at the same level as the lumbar spine. Lumbar puncture having been performed in the usual way, the tap is turned so that the fluid rises in the manometer. At this point the patient should be allowed to straighten his spine and should be directed to relax his muscles and breathe quietly and regularly, as muscular tension and holding the breath raise the pressure. Pressure is measured in millimetres of cerebrospinal fluid and normally shows oscillations corresponding to respiration and finer variations synchronous with the arterial pulse. The normal pressure of the cerebrospinal fluid in adults in the horizontal position is 60–150 mm of fluid. According to Levinson it is lower in children, in whom it is normally from 45 to 90 mm of fluid. In adults in the sitting posture the normal pressure is from 200 to 250 mm of fluid, which, it should be noted, is usually less than the height of the vertex above the needle. Hence in the sitting posture the pressure in the ventricles and cerebello-medullary cistern may be negative.

Pathological Variations of Pressure. An abnormally high cerebrospinal fluid pressure is found in cases of intracranial tumour and haemorrhage, hypertensive encephalopathy, benign intracranial hypertension, hypervitaminosis A, hydrocephalus, intracranial sinus thrombosis, meningism, and in various forms of meningitis, encephalitis, and encephalopathy. The pressure may also be raised in uraemia and in some cases of emphysema. In a relaxed patient a pressure exceeding 300 ml of fluid is certainly abnormal and the needle should be withdrawn if the pressure exceeds this level and there will then be sufficient fluid in the manometer for examination.

A subnormal pressure is sometimes a sequel of head injury and may be found in cases of subdural haematoma. It is also encountered when the lumbar subarachnoid space is cut off from communication with the cerebral subarachnoid space. This is most commonly met with in cases of spinal subarachnoid block due to spinal tumour or localized spinal meningitis. It may also occur when a block exists at or near the foramen magnum as a result of a tumour in this situation or of meningeal adhesions following meningitis. The pressure may also be abnormally low if a second lumbar puncture is performed shortly after a previous one.

Queckenstedt's Test. Normally if one compresses the jugular veins of a patient during lumbar puncture there is an immediate and rapid rise in the pressure of the cerebrospinal fluid which quickly reaches 300 mm of fluid and almost as rapidly falls to normal when the veins are no longer compressed. The effect of compressing the veins is to cause raised pressure in the intracranial venous sinuses and hence in the cranium. The communication of this raised pressure or rather, displacement of fluid into, the manometer attached to the lumbar puncture needle (Bowsher, 1953) depends upon the patency of the subarachnoid space between the cranial cavity and the lumbar sac. In cases of obstruction of the subarachnoid space in the region of the foramen magnum or within the spinal canal, the rise of pressure normally produced by jugular compression is either absent or slight in extent and slow in appearing, according to whether the block is complete or incomplete. In cervical lesions the accuracy of the test may be improved by flexion or hyperextension of the neck as the block may vary in different positions of the head (Kaplan and Foster Kennedy, 1950). When there is a block, the normal variations in pressure due to respiration and the arterial pulse are also diminished or absent, but compression of the abdomen may cause an exaggerated rise of pressure as raised intra-abdominal pressure is transmitted to spinal veins.

Compression of either jugular vein separately may yield valuable evidence of thrombosis of the transverse sinus, for if the sinus is obstructed there will usually be no rise of pressure in the fluid when the jugular vein on the affected side is compressed.

Clinical experience has, however, shown that Queckenstedt's test is unreliable and with the increasing use of contrast methods of radiological investigation it is now used infrequently. The accuracy of the test can, however, be improved using electromanometrics with a minitransducer in the pressure recording system (Gilland and Nelson, 1970).

NAKED-EYE APPEARANCE

Turbidity. The normal cerebrospinal fluid is clear and colourless and resembles water. Turbidity, when present, is usually due to an excess of polymorphonuclear cells. In acute meningitis these are often present in such numbers that a deposit of pus forms at the bottom of the tube and the supernatant fluid may be yellow. It is rare for an excess of lymphocytes to cause turbidity, but malignant cells can do so in carcinomatous meningitis.

Fibrin Clot. The development of a clot of fibrin in a specimen of fluid implies the presence of fibrinogen. Such a clot may occur either in a fluid of which the protein content is only slightly raised or in the highly albuminous fluids characteristic of spinal subarachnoid block, and of certain forms of polyneuropathy. In the former case the clot forms a faint 'cobweb' which takes from 12 to 24 hours to appear. It is most frequently seen in tuberculous meningitis, but also occurs occasionally in other forms of meningitis and has been described in neurosyphilis and in poliomyelitis. The clot which forms in highly albuminous fluids may solidify the whole specimen.

Blood. Blood may be present in the cerebrospinal fluid, either as an accidental result of injury to an intrathecal vein by the lumbar puncture needle, or as the product of pre-existing haemorrhage into the subarachnoid space. This distinction is obviously of great importance. When a vein is injured at lumbar puncture the specimen of fluid collected in the first tube is often blood-stained, but the second usually shows no visible blood, whereas after subarachnoid haemorrhage both specimens are uniformly blood-stained. Further, in the former case if the red cells are given time to settle, the supernatant fluid is seen to be colourless, whereas within a few hours of subarachnoid haemorrhage the supernatant fluid shows a yellow coloration. In practice there is seldom any difficulty in distinguishing the accidental contamination of the specimen with blood from subarachnoid haemorrhage. *Subarachnoid haemorrhage* is usually due to head injury, or to the rupture of an intracranial aneurysm or angioma into the subarachnoid space, or to the bursting of an intracerebral haemorrhage into either the ventricular system or the subarachnoid space; other causes are uncommon [p. 357]. After subarachnoid haemorrhage the yellow coloration of the fluid appears in a few hours and reaches its greatest intensity at the end of about a week. It has usually disappeared in two to four weeks. The red cells generally disappear from the fluid in three to seven days. The presence of blood in contact with the leptomeninges excites a cellular reaction, and the fluid therefore usually contains a moderate excess of white cells. As a rule these are all mononuclear, but excess polymorphonuclear cells may be found in the early stages.

Xanthochromia. Xanthochromia, or yellow coloration of the cerebrospinal fluid, is found, as just described, after subarachnoid haemorrhage and also when pus is present in considerable amount in the fluid. In subarachnoid haemorrhage, faint xanthochromia due to oxyhaemoglobin appears within four to six hours, the deeper yellow coloration due to bilirubin in about two days; methaemoglobin is present in the fluid only if there is extensive brain destruction (Barrows *et al.*, 1955). Xanthochromic fluid is also often found after an intracerebral haemorrhage, or cerebral infarction, in some cases of intracranial tumour, especially when the tumour is near the ventricular system, and sometimes in the case of tumours of the eighth nerve. It is also characteristic of obstruction of the spinal subarachnoid space and may be seen in fluid from above a tumour of the cauda equina and sometimes in polyneuritis. A slight yellow coloration of the fluid may be present in cases of severe jaundice.

Kjellin and Söderstrom (1974) have shown that the spectrophotometric identification of pigments in the fluid may be of some value in the differential diagnosis of cerebral vascular disease.

CYTOLOGICAL AND CHEMICAL ABNORMALITIES

Since this is a textbook of clinical neurology, methods of carrying out cell counts and chemical investigations on the cerebrospinal fluid will not be described in more detail than is necessary for a discussion of their interpretation. Those who wish to acquaint themselves with the technique of these examinations are referred to the textbooks on the cerebrospinal fluid (see references).

Cells

The normal cerebrospinal fluid contains a small number of cells. These are normally lymphocytes and should not exceed three per cubic millimetre. In pathological states a variety of cells may be present and may occur in very large numbers. Those most frequently encountered are lymphocytes, large mononuclear cells, and polymorphonuclear cells. Less frequently eosinophils, plasma cells, macrophages, and compound granular corpuscles and fibroblasts are found. Tumour cells are rare but when present are of great diagnostic importance. Yeasts, actinomycotic granules, echinococci, and cysticerci may be found in cases of infection of the nervous system with these organisms.

Significance of Cell Content. Certain generalizations may be made with regard to the presence and numbers of different types of cell in the fluid. Most of the cells are probably derived from the meninges, though some may take origin within the nervous parenchyma and pass into the subarachnoid space from the perivascular spaces. In general a pleocytosis, or excess of cells in the spinal fluid, indicates meningeal irritation, though this does not necessarily imply the presence of meningeal infection. Whether the cellular increase is polymorphonuclear depends partly upon the acuteness of the pathological process and partly upon the nature of the infecting organism. A predominantly polymorphonuclear count is usually found in acute infections and in acute exacerbations of chronic infections, while a mononuclear count is characteristic of chronic infections. But while pyogenic organisms excite a mainly polymorphonuclear leucocytosis except in their most chronic stages, a mononuclear pleocytosis is characteristic of infection with neurotropic viruses, though polymorphonuclear cells are sometimes present when the infection is most acute. We thus encounter predominantly polymorphonuclear, predominantly mononuclear, and mixed cell counts.

A predominantly polymorphonuclear pleocytosis is found in meningitis due to pyogenic organisms, including the meningococcus, staphylococcus, streptococcus, pneumococcus, *Escherichia coli*, *Bacillus typhosus*, *Listeria monocytogenes*, and *Haemophilus influenzae*. In these conditions the polymorphonuclear cells are usually present in very large numbers. A very acute syphilitic meningitis may also excite a polymorphonuclear reaction in which the cells may number several thousands per cubic millimetre. Mononuclear pleocytosis rarely exceeds 200 cells per mm³ and more commonly lies between 10 and 50 cells per mm³. Counts of up to 1,000 per mm³, however, may occur in various forms of virus meningitis. A mononuclear reaction is characteristic of syphilis of the nervous system, encephalitis, multiple sclerosis, poliomyelitis (after the first few days of the infection), herpes zoster, acute lymphocytic choriomeningitis, and some cases of tuberculous meningitis. It may also be present in mumps, and has been described in infectious mononucleosis, whooping cough, malaria, trypanosomiasis, relapsing fever, and leptospirosis canicola or icterohaemorrhagica. Cerebral tumour may cause a slight mononuclear pleocytosis, especially when the tumour is in contact with the meninges. So also may cerebral abscess, intracranial sinus thrombosis, and subarachnoid haemorrhage. The mixed type of pleocytosis, in which polymorphonuclear and mononuclear cells are present in approximately equal numbers, is also found in cerebral abscess, in which case the number of cells is often small, and in cases of infection of the bones of the skull in the neighbourhood of the meninges. A mixed cell count is also present in many cases of tuberculous meningitis, in poliomyelitis during the first few days, and in the more acute forms of syphilitic meningitis.

Plasma cells, as well as the mononuclear forms mentioned above, are sometimes found in the fluid, usually in inflammatory disorders (Péter, 1967). Specialized cytological techniques (Sayk, 1960) are now employed increasingly and consistently detect malignant cells in the fluid in cases of carcinomatosis of the meninges. Even in cases of cerebral tumour, malignant cells may be found in the fluid, but positive findings are obtained in only about 10 per cent of cases of glioma and 20 per cent with intracranial metastases (Marks and Marrack, 1960; Jager, 1969). More recently it has been shown that immunofluorescent techniques of examining fresh or cultured cells obtained from the fluid may be helpful in the rapid diagnosis of viral encephalitis (Dayan and Stokes, 1973; Lindeman *et al.*, 1974).

Protein

The total protein content of the normal cerebrospinal fluid is from 0·015 to 0·045 g per 100 ml. This consists of albumin and globulin in a ratio of 8 to 1. Increase of the protein of the fluid is extremely common. A moderate increase, usually to below 0·2 g per 100 ml, is found in inflammatory diseases of the nervous tissue and meninges, such as the various forms of meningitis, encephalitis, poliomyelitis, multiple sclerosis, and syphilis of the nervous system. Intracranial tumour and cerebral haemorrhage and infarction may also cause a moderate rise of protein content. In cases of acoustic neuroma the protein often rises to more than 0·1 g per 100 ml, while in the Guillain–Barré syndrome increases to 1·0 g per 100 ml or more may occur.

Froin's syndrome is the name originally given to a condition in which the spinal fluid is xanthochromic, contains, as a rule, more than 500 mg of protein per 100 ml, and rapidly clots on standing. It is a phenomenon of multiple aetiology and may even be seen in cases of polyneuropathy, but more often results from a spinal block due to tumour, localized spinal meningitis, or epidural abscess. In such cases the block results in stagnation of the cerebrospinal fluid in the lumbar dural sac distal to the block with exudation or transudation of proteinaceous material from the tumour itself or of plasma from the blood vessels. Similar fluid is sometimes obtained when lumbar puncture is performed *above* a cauda equina tumour. In Froin's original cases there was also pleocytosis as his patients were suffering from localized spinal meningitis.

Fractionation of Cerebrospinal Fluid Proteins

A number of reactions have been used in the past to identify an excess of globulin in the cerebrospinal fluid. Various reagents (ammonium sulphate in the *Nonne–Apelt reaction*, butyric acid in the *Noguchi reaction*, carbolic acid in *Pandy's reaction*, and mercuric chloride in *Weichbrodt's reaction*) were used to precipitate the globulin, giving varying degrees of opalescence of the fluid. *Lange's colloidal gold reaction* was more precise and, until it was largely superseded by modern quantitative techniques of estimating the immunoglobulins in the fluid, it proved to be of great diagnostic value. In carrying out the test, increasing dilutions of cerebrospinal fluid were added to a series of 10 test tubes containing the reagent and the resultant colorimetric change from cherry-red to blue was graded on a six-point scale from 0 to 5 in each tube. Normal samples of fluid gave little or no precipitation and consequent colour change. The so-called 'paretic' curve (5555432100) was characteristic of general paresis and sometimes occurred in meningovascular syphilis and tabes; it was also found in up to 50 per cent of cases of multiple sclerosis and sometimes after subarachnoid haemorrhage. The *luetic or tabetic curve* (1233321000) was more characteristic of tabes dorsalis, while the *meningitic curve* (0012344310) was seen more typically in syphilitic and bacterial meningitis.

Kabat *et al.* (1942) examined cerebrospinal fluid using the Tiselius electrophoretic method and found increased concentrations of gamma-globulin in the fluid in cases of neurosyphilis and multiple sclerosis. They and other workers (Dencker and Swahn, 1961; Link, 1967) have shown that these changes are independent of those in the serum, suggesting that immunoglobulins are being produced in the central nervous system in some such diseases. Since that time paper and agar gel electrophoresis, immunoelectrophoresis, chemical precipitation, immunoprecipitation, and electroimmunophoresis have all been used, not only to estimate gamma-globulin as a fraction of the total protein, but also to estimate IgG, IgA, IgM, and IgD. An increase in gamma-globulin in relation to the total protein correlates well with the paretic Lange curve (Riddoch and Thompson, 1970). Using a simple zinc sulphate method for estimating gamma-globulin, Prineas *et al.* (1966) found that in 44 per cent of cases of multiple sclerosis this exceeded 29 per cent of total protein, but more sensitive electrophoretic methods give somewhat lower percentages (over 14 per cent is usually considered abnormal). Riddoch and Thompson (1970), using the single radial diffusion method for the estimation of immunoglobulins, found that the IgG was raised above the normal upper limit (more than 13 per cent of total protein) in 62 per cent of patients with multiple sclerosis and in only 14 per cent of patients with other neurological diseases, including neurosyphilis. However, Fischer-Williams and Roberts (1971) found that measurement of the total gamma-globulin electrophoretic fraction on concentrated fluid correlated better (over 14 per cent of total protein in 94 per cent of cases) with the diagnosis of multiple sclerosis than did the measurement of IgG by electroimmunodiffusion (over 14 per cent of total protein in 75 per cent of cases). IgD is not found in the cerebrospinal fluid and IgA and IgM are only present when the total protein is raised. In all forms of acute meningitis IgA and IgG levels are increased in the fluid (Smith *et al.*, 1973). The percentage of IgG in the fluid is lower in children (usually less than 8 per cent of total protein) (Nellhaus, 1971).

More recently still, isoelectric focusing of cerebrospinal fluid proteins (Latner, 1973; Kjellin and Vesterberg, 1974) has added even greater precision and this technique, with quantitative paper electrophoresis, has revealed minor abnormalities in the fluid in cases of hereditary ataxia (Kjellin and Stibler, 1975).

Phospholipids

The total phospholipid content of the fluid may be increased in a number of neurological diseases but a relative rise in the content of cephalin is seen in patients with demyelinating processes (Zilkha and McArdle, 1963).

Glucose

The normal glucose content of the cerebrospinal fluid is somewhat lower than that of the blood and lies between 50 and 85 mg per 100 ml. The glucose content of the fluid is diminished in meningitis as the glucose is consumed by the infecting organisms. In pyogenic meningitis, indeed, sugar is usually absent. A moderate decrease to 10–50 mg per 100 ml is characteristic of tuberculous meningitis, certain other chronic meningitides (e.g. torulosis), and carcinomatosis of the meninges. A rise in the glucose content of the fluid is found in diabetes parallel to that in the blood.

Chlorides

The chlorides are the only chemical constituent, apart from folate, to be maintained in the cerebrospinal fluid at a higher concentration than in the blood. The normal chloride content of the fluid is 720 to 750 mg per 100 ml estimated as sodium chloride. In purulent meningitis this figure is reduced to an average of from 650 to 680 mg per 100 ml. The reduction is much greater in tuberculous meningitis, in which condition Fremont-Smith and his collaborators obtained an average reading of 610 mg per 100 ml and a minimum of 520 mg. In the early stages the reduction is less marked. The chloride content of the fluid was in the past regarded as of diagnostic value in distinguishing tuberculous meningitis both from conditions such as poliomyelitis in which the chloride content of the fluid is normal and also from other conditions of meningeal inflammation in which the fall is less marked. However, it is now recognized that the fall of chloride content in the fluid is usually due to frequent vomiting and when the chloride content of the blood plasma varies from normal a corresponding change occurs in the fluid. Similarly we find the chloride content of the fluid to be above normal in many cases of uraemia.

Enzymes

Much work has been done in recent years upon the estimation of various enzymes in the cerebrospinal fluid. Among others, Green *et al.* (1957) and Katzman *et al.* (1957) found that *glutamic–oxalacetic transaminase* (aspartate aminotransferase) activity was raised in the fluid in some cases of cerebral infarction and multiple sclerosis, but Davies-Jones (1970), who studied that enzyme and *lactic dehydrogenase*, found normal activity in those conditions and in many other neurological disorders but the activity was raised in cases of carcinomatous neuropathy and of metastatic carcinoma in the nervous system. However, Wilcock et al. (1973) found that the Michaelis constants for these enzymes derived from brain tissue differed from those of the same enzymes when derived from blood and cerebrospinal fluid and concluded that these enzymes in the fluid are derived from those of the serum.

Cerebrospinal fluid *creatine kinase* activity is raised in cases of muscular dystrophy of the Duchenne type but does not parallel the level in the blood (Banerji et al., 1969). Sherwin et al. (1969) found the activity of this enzyme to be raised in the fluid in 70 of 185 patients with neurological disease, even after a generalized epileptic convulsion, and found that the enzyme did not cross-react immunologically with the enzyme from skeletal muscle; presumably, therefore, it was derived from brain. However, an elevated activity of this enzyme was of no diagnostic value.

Riekkinen and Rinne (1970) have also studied *non-specific esterases* and various *acid and alkaline proteinases* in the fluid. While increased activity of several of these enzymes was found in the acute phase of multiple sclerosis and in some cases of cerebral tumour, again little information of diagnostic value was obtained.

Sterols

The cholesterol and cholesterol ester content of the cerebrospinal fluid is raised in some neurological diseases, especially in multiple sclerosis (Cumings, 1953; Green et al., 1959) but this change is non-specific. However, Paoletti et al. (1969) showed that desmosterol (24-dehydrocholesterol) appears in the fluid of many patients with gliomas after the administration of triparanol. Weiss et al. (1972) found more cholesterol in the fluid of patients with gliomas than in controls and confirmed an increase in cerebrospinal fluid desmosterol in about 60 per cent of patients with glioma. The value of this test in diagnosis remains to be confirmed.

Amines

The cerebrospinal fluid contains 5-hydroxyindoleacetic acid (5-HIAA), a metabolite of 5-hydroxytryptophan (serotonin or 5-HT), and also homovanillic acid (HVA), a metabolite of dopamine. Patients with Parkinsonism in whom HVA is high in the fluid do not respond as well to treatment with levodopa as do those in whom it is low (Gumpert et al., 1973). While blood levels of 5-HT are low in patients with Down's syndrome (mongolism), the 5-HIAA in the fluid is normal (Dubowitz and Rogers, 1969). Studies of these metabolites in the fluid are throwing new light upon the biochemical basis of nervous disorders associated with abnormalities of the cerebral amines, perhaps even including endogenous depression (Moir et al., 1970).

Keratin

The presence of keratin in the cerebrospinal fluid may indicate the presence of an intracranial epidermoid cyst (Tomlinson and Walton, 1967).

Vitamin B$_{12}$ and Folate

In epileptic patients under treatment with anticonvulsant drugs the level of folate (which is normally three times as great as that in the blood) in the cerebrospinal fluid may fall, and it has been suggested that this may be associated with a fall in mental performance and even perhaps dementia (*see* Johnson, 1972). If folic acid is given, an increase in the number of fits may occur unless vitamin B_{12} is given as well, as the serum level of the latter may fall as the folate rises.

SEROLOGICAL REACTIONS

The Wassermann and V.D.R.L. reactions in the cerebrospinal fluid are discussed in the section on syphilis.

MICROBIOLOGICAL EXAMINATION

In most forms of pyogenic meningitis the direct staining of a smear of a centrifuged deposit of cells obtained from the fluid will reveal the infecting organism, but meningococci are often curiously difficult to find, whereas pneumococci, for instance, are usually found in profusion. For the detection of tubercle bacilli the Ziehl–Neilsen technique is required. Viruses in the fluid may be detected by direct immunofluorescent techniques. Culture of the fluid, using a variety of different techniques, or sometimes animal inoculation, may be required in order to confirm the nature of the infecting organism, whether this is a bacterium, a virus, or some other form of pathogen. For details the reader is referred to texts on microbiology.

CEREBROSPINAL FLUID FISTULAE

Following head injury, or as a consequence of raised intracranial pressure, or pituitary tumour, fistulous communications may develop between the subarachnoid space and the paranasal sinuses or middle ear, resulting in a leakage of cerebrospinal fluid. These fistulae may be detected and localized by means of a variety of biochemical and radiological techniques using such agents as radiosodium and radio-iodinated serum albumin (Crow *et al.*, 1956; Ommaya *et al.*, 1968; Brisman *et al.*, 1970).

REFERENCES

BANERJI, A. P., JAYAM, A. V., and DESAI, A. D. (1969) Creatine phosphokinase activity of cerebrospinal fluid in muscular dystrophy and other neurological disorders, *Neurology (Bombay)*, **17**, 123.

BARROWS, L. J., HUNTER, F. T., and BANKER, B. Q. (1955) The nature and significance of pigments in the cerebrospinal fluid, *Brain*, **78**, 59.

BOWSHER, D. (1953) The cerebrospinal fluid pressure, *Brit. med. J.*, **1**, 863.

BOWSHER, D. (1957) Further considerations on cerebrospinal fluid dynamics, *Brit. med. J.*, **2**, 917.

BRISMAN, R., HUGHES, J. E. O., and MOUNT, L. A. (1970) Cerebrospinal fluid rhinorrhea, *Arch. Neurol. (Chic.)*, **22**, 245.

CAMERON, I. R. (1969) Acid-base changes in cerebrospinal fluid, *Brit. J. Anaesth.*, **41**, 213.

CROW, H. J., KEOGH, C., and NORTHFIELD, D. W. C. (1956) The localisation of cerebrospinal-fluid fistulae, *Lancet*, **ii**, 325.

CUMINGS, J. N. (1953) The cerebral lipids in disseminated sclerosis and in amaurotic family idiocy, *Brain*, **76**, 551.

DAVIES-JONES, G. A. B. (1970) Lactate dehydrogenase and glutamic oxalacetic transaminase of the cerebrospinal fluid in neurological disease, *J. neurol. Sci.*, **11**, 583.

DAVSON, H. (1958) Some aspects of the relationship between the cerebrospinal fluid and the central nervous system, in *Ciba Foundation Symposium on the Cerebrospinal Fluid*, p. 189, London.

DAVSON, H. (1967) *The Physiology of the Cerebrospinal Fluid*, London.

DAYAN, A. D., and STOKES, M. I. (1973) Rapid diagnosis of encephalitis by immuno-fluorescent examination of cerebrospinal-fluid cells, *Lancet*, **i**, 177.

DENCKER, S. J., and SWAHN, B. (1961) *Clinical Value of Protein Analysis in Cerebrospinal Fluid*, London.

DUBOWITZ, V., and ROGERS, K. J. (1969) 5-hydroxyindoles in the cerebrospinal fluid of infants with Down's syndrome and muscle hypotonia, *Develop. Med. Child Neurol.*, **11**, 730.

FISCHER-WILLIAMS, M., and ROBERTS, R. C. (1971) Cerebrospinal fluid proteins and serum immunoglobulins: occurrence in multiple sclerosis and other neurological diseases, *Arch. Neurol. (Chic.)*, **25**, 526.

GILLAND, O., and NELSON, J. R. (1970) Lumbar cerebrospinal fluid electromanometrics with a minitransducer, *Neurology (Minneap.)*, **20**, 103.

GREEN, J. B., OLDEWURTEL, H., O'DOHERTY, D. S., FORSTER, F. M., and SANCHEZ-LONGO, L. P. (1957) Cerebrospinal fluid glutamic oxalacetic transaminase activity in neuro-logic disease, *Neurology (Minneap.)*, **7**, 313.

GREEN, J. B., PAPADOPOULOS, N., CEVALLOS, W., FORSTER, F. M., and HESS, W. C. (1959) The cholesterol and cholesterol ester content of cerebrospinal fluid in patients with multiple sclerosis and other neurological diseases, *J. Neurol. Neurosurg. Psychiat.*, **22**, 117.

GREENFIELD, J. G., and CARMICHAEL, E. A. (1925) *The Cerebrospinal Fluid in Clinical Diagnosis*, London.

GUMPERT, J., SHARPE, D., and CURZON, G. (1973) Amine metabolites in the cerebrospinal fluid in Parkinson's disease and the response to levodopa, *J. neurol. Sci.*, **19**, 1.

JAGER, W. A. D. H. (1969) Cytopathology of the cerebrospinal fluid examined with the sedimentation technique after Sayk, *J. neurol. Sci.*, **9**, 155.

JOHNSON, R. H. (1972) Cerebrospinal fluid, in *Scientific Foundations of Neurology*, ed. Critchley, M., O'Leary, J. L., and Jennett, B., London.

KABAT, E. A., MOORE, D. H., and LANDOW, H. (1942) An electrophoretic study of the protein components in cerebrospinal fluid and their relationship to the serum proteins, *J. clin. Invest.*, **21**, 571.

KAPLAN, L., and KENNEDY, F. (1950) The effect of head posture on the manometrics of the cerebrospinal fluid in cervical lesions: a new diagnostic test, *Brain*, **73**, 337.

KATZMAN, R., FISHMAN, R. A., and GOLDENSOHN, E. S. (1957) Glutamic-oxalacetic transaminase activity in spinal fluid, *Neurology (Minneap.)*, **7**, 853.

KJELLIN, K. G., and SÖDERSTRÖM, C. E. (1974) Diagnostic significance of CSF spectro-photometry in cerebrovascular diseases, *J. neurol. Sci.*, **23**, 359.

KJELLIN, K. G., and STIBLER, H. (1975) Protein patterns of cerebrospinal fluid in hereditary ataxias and hereditary spastic paraplegia, *J. neurol. Sci.*, **25**, 65.

KJELLIN, K. G., and VESTERBERG, O. (1974) Isoelectric focusing of CSF proteins in neurological diseases, *J. neurol. Sci.*, **23**, 199.

LATNER, A. L. (1973) Some clinical biochemical aspects of isoelectric focusing, *Ann. N.Y. Acad. Sci.*, **209**, 281.

LINDEMAN, J., MÜLLER, W. K., VERSTEEG, J., BOTS, G. T. A. M., and PETERS, A. C. B. (1974) Rapid diagnosis of meningoencephalitis, encephalitis. Immunofluorescent examination of fresh and in vitro cultured cerebrospinal fluid cells, *Neurology (Minneap.)*, **24**, 143.

LINK, H. (1967) Immunoglobulin G and low molecular weight proteins in human cerebro-spinal fluid, *Acta neurol. scand.*, **43**, suppl. 28.

MARKS, V., and MARRACK, D. (1960) Tumour cells in the cerebrospinal fluid, *J. Neurol. Neurosurg. Psychiat.*, **23**, 194.

MARTINS, A. N., WILEY, J. K., and MYERS, P. W. (1972) Dynamics of the cerebrospinal fluid and the spinal dura mater, *J. Neurol. Neurosurg. Psychiat.*, **35**, 468.

MERRITT, H. H., and FREMONT-SMITH, F. (1937) *The Cerebrospinal Fluid*, Philadelphia.

MILLEN, J. W., and WOOLLAM, D. H. M. (1962) *The Anatomy of the Cerebrospinal Fluid*, London.

MOIR, A. T. B., ASHCROFT, G. W., CRAWFORD, T. B. B., ECCLESTON, D., and GULDBERG, H. C. (1970) Cerebral metabolites in cerebrospinal fluid as a biochemical approach to the brain, *Brain*, **93**, 357.

NELLHAUS, G. (1971) Cerebrospinal fluid immunoglobulin G in childhood: measurement by electroimmunodiffusion, *Arch. Neurol. (Chic.)*, **24**, 441.

O'CONNELL, J. E. A. (1970) Cerebrospinal fluid mechanics, *Proc. roy. Soc. Med.*, **63**, 507.

OMMAYA, A. K., DI CHIRO, G., BALDWIN, M., and PENNYBACKER, J. B. (1968) Non-traumatic cerebrospinal fluid rhinorrhoea, *J. Neurol. Neurosurg. Psychiat.*, **31**, 214.

PAOLETTI, P., VANDENHEUVEL, F. A., and FUMAGALLI, R. (1969) The sterol test for the diagnosis of human brain tumors, *Neurology (Minneap.)*, **19**, 190.

PÉTER, A. (1967) The plasma cells of the cerebrospinal fluid, *J. neurol. Sci.*, **4**, 227.

PRINEAS, J., TEASDALE, G., LATNER, A. L., and MILLER, H. (1966) Spinal-fluid gamma-globulin and multiple sclerosis, *Brit. med. J.*, **2**, 922.

RIDDOCH, D., and THOMPSON, R. A. (1970) Immunoglobulin levels in the cerebrospinal fluid, *Brit. med. J.*, **1**, 396.

RIEKKINEN, P. J., and RINNE, U. K. (1970) Enzymes of human cerebrospinal fluid in normal conditions and neurological disorders, *Annales Universitatis Turkuensis*, suppl. 44.

SAYK, J. (1960) *Cytologie der Cerebrospinalflüssigkeit*, Jena.

SHERWIN, A. L., NORRIS, J. W., and BULCKE, J. A. (1969) Spinal fluid creatine kinase in neurologic disease, *Neurology (Minneap.)*, **19**, 993.

SMITH, H., BANNISTER, B., and O'SHEA, M. J. (1973) Cerebrospinal-fluid immunoglobulins in meningitis, *Lancet*, **ii**, 591.

SWEET, W. H., BROWNELL, G. L., SCHOLL, J. A., BOWSHER, D. R., BENDA, P., and STICKLEY, E. E. (1954) The formation, flow and absorption of cerebrospinal fluid, newer concepts based on studies with isotopes, *Res. Publ. Ass. nerv. ment. Dis.*, **34**, 101.

TRIPATHI, R. C. (1973) Ultrastructure of the arachnoid mater in relation to outflow of cerebrospinal fluid: a new concept, *Lancet*, **ii**, 8.

TOMLINSON, B. E., and WALTON, J. N. (1967) Granulomatous meningitis and diffuse parenchymatous degeneration of the nervous system due to an intracranial epidermoid cyst, *J. Neurol. Neurosurg. Psychiat.*, **30**, 341.

WEISS, J. F., RANSOHOFF, J., and KAYDEN, H. J. (1972) Cerebrospinal fluid sterols in patients undergoing treatment for gliomas, *Neurology (Minneap.)*, **22**, 187.

WELCH, K., and FRIEDMAN, V. (1960) The cerebrospinal fluid valves, *Brain*, **83**, 454.

WILCOCK, A. R., SHARPE, D. M., and GOLDBERG, D. M. (1973) Kinetic similarity of enzymes in human blood serum and cerebrospinal fluid: aspartate aminotransferase and lactate dehydrogenase, *J. neurol. Sci.*, **20**, 97.

WOLSTENHOLME, G. E. W., and O'CONNOR, C. M. (1958) *Ciba Foundation Symposium on the Cerebrospinal Fluid Production, Circulation and Absorption*, London.

ZILKHA, K. J., and MCARDLE, B. (1963) The phospholipid composition of cerebrospinal fluid in diseases associated with demyelination, *Quart. J. Med.*, **32**, 79.

HISTORY AND EXAMINATION

THE HISTORY OF THE ILLNESS

GENERAL CONSIDERATIONS

In the diagnosis of nervous disease, the history of the patient's illness is just as important and indeed often more so, than the elicitation of physical signs. Thus in disorders such as migraine and epilepsy the diagnosis will generally be made on the history alone, though examination should not be neglected lest the symptoms be symptomatic of an underlying structural abnormality such as an intracranial vascular malformation or neoplasm. On the other hand, a particular combination of abnormal physical signs (e.g. those of a hemiplegia) may indicate that the pathological process responsible lies in the opposite cerebral hemisphere, but the history of the development of the symptoms is then all-important in assessing the nature of the pathological change; thus a sudden onset may suggest that the lesion is vascular, a very gradual evolution that it is neoplastic.

The history obtained from the patient should always be supplemented, if possible, by an account of his illness given by a relative or by someone who knows him well. This is essential when the patient suffers from mental impairment and also when his complaint includes attacks in which he loses consciousness, but it is always desirable, since a relative or friend will often remember an important point which the patient himself has forgotten to mention.

First note the patient's name and address, age, and exact details of his occupation. The last named is often of importance as a source of exposure to injury or to toxic substances. Ascertain if he is right-handed.

It is well to begin by asking the patient of what he complains and when he was last in normal health, in this way fixing, at least provisionally, the date of onset of his symptoms. After this he should be allowed to relate the story of his illness as far as possible without interruption, questions being put to him afterwards to expand his statements and to elicit additional information. In the case of all symptoms it is important to ascertain not only the date but also the mode of onset, whether sudden, rapid, or gradual, whether the symptom since its first appearance has fluctuated in intensity and whether the patient's condition is improving, stationary, or deteriorating at the time of examination.

HISTORY OF PRESENT ILLNESS

Inquiry should always be made with regard to the following symptoms, whether or not the patient mentions them spontaneously:

Mental State. The patient's mental history should be ascertained, not only as far as possible from himself, but also from relatives or friends, on the lines laid down below for the examination of his mental condition. If mental abnormality is suspected it is necessary to ascertain the patient's normal level of intelligence and temperament.

Sleep. Has he suffered from disturbances of sleep, either from paroxysmal or persistent sleepiness or from insomnia?

Speech. Has he had difficulty in speaking? If so, of what nature? Has he been able to understand what is said to him and to read? Has his writing been affected? [see p. 107]. If his speech has been slurred, has there been associated dysphagia or difficulty in chewing?

Attacks of Loss of Consciousness. Has he suffered from attacks of loss or impairment of consciousness? If so, for further inquiries see pages 321 and 1097.

Headache. Has he suffered from headache? If so, further inquiries should be made as described on page 296. Has there been associated vomiting? If so, of what character?

Pain. Has he suffered pain in the face, trunk, or limbs? If so, what is its character, distribution, time of occurrence, constancy, or intermittency? Are there any precipitating or aggravating factors?

Special Senses. Has he had hallucinations of smell or taste or noticed an impairment of these senses? Has he had visual hallucinations? If so, what has been their character and distribution in the visual fields? Has there been any visual impairment: if so, of one or both eyes and of what nature? Has it been transitory or progressive? Has he had double vision? If so, has this been transitory or progressive and has he noticed this symptom when looking in any special direction? Is his hearing impaired? If so, is this unilateral or bilateral and is the deafness associated with tinnitus? Does he suffer from giddiness? If so, he should describe precisely its nature and state whether it is associated with a sense of rotation of himself or of his surroundings, and with deafness, tinnitus, or vomiting.

Movement and Sensibility. Does he complain of muscular weakness or wasting, of loss of control over the limbs or of involuntary movements, and if so, what is the distribution of these symptoms? Has his gait been abnormal, and if so, how? Has he tended to fall, and if so, in what direction? Has he had any spontaneous sensory disturbances, especially pain, numbness, or tingling? If so, further inquiries should be made, as described on page 36.

The Sphincters and Reproductive Functions. Has there been any disturbance of sphincter control? Has he experienced difficulty in holding or passing urine or faeces? Has he had polyuria? In the case of a man, is his sexual power normal for his age? In the case of a woman, has there been any abnormality in menstruation, especially amenorrhoea?

Disorders of Other Systems. Are there any symptoms of respiratory disease or insufficiency, of cardiac or arterial disease or any complaints to suggest renal, hepatic, gastrointestinal, or endocrine dysfunction?

Nutrition. Is the weight stationary, diminishing, or increasing?

HISTORY OF PREVIOUS ILLNESSES

Inquiry as to previous illnesses should always include a tactful inquiry as to venereal disease. A history of aural discharge or of tuberculosis may be important in relation to intracranial abscess or tuberculous meningitis. A history of convulsions or of meningitis in childhood or of encephalitis lethargica may be significant in relation to a later illness. A history of 'influenza' should be amplified by details of the illness thus described. Inquiry should always be made for a history of accidental injury, especially to the head and spine. A difficult birth may be significant in relation to epilepsy.

SOCIAL HISTORY

This should include inquiry as to the patient's educational and occupational career, adjustments to family life, military service career, residence abroad, and personal habits in respect of recreation, tobacco, alcohol, and other drugs. If alcoholic excess is admitted or if the patient has been taking drugs, the amount and duration should be ascertained.

FAMILY HISTORY

The family history is often of great importance, since many diseases of the nervous system are hereditary. The patient should always be asked whether cases of nervous or mental disease have occurred among his relatives and if so the precise nature of the illness should, if possible, be ascertained. Consanguinity in the parents should be inquired for. If the patient is married, inquiry should be made as to the state of health of the spouse. Death of a husband or wife from general paralysis or aneurysm may afford an important clue to a syphilitic disorder in a patient. For the same reason the number of children and the occurrence of miscarriages and stillbirths should be ascertained.

EXAMINATION OF THE PATIENT

The brief commentary given below will serve as a general guide to some important principles to be followed in examining the nervous system. Detailed descriptions of methods of testing the motor and sensory systems have already been given and methods of eliciting other signs of nervous dysfunction are given in other appropriate sections of this book. Techniques of neurological examination are described in greater detail by de Jong (1967) and Bickerstaff (1973). Useful guides to the neurological assessment of neonates, infants, and children are given by André-Thomas et al. (1955) and by Paine and Oppé (1966).

STATE OF CONSCIOUSNESS

Is the patient conscious or unconscious? If unconscious, how far does he respond to stimuli, such as pinching the skin? Can he be roused, and if so, when he is roused is his mental condition normal or abnormal? Detailed methods of assessment in stupor and coma are described on pages 1166–70. If he is conscious, how far can he think with normal clarity and speed, and perceive, respond to, and remember current stimuli? Can he swallow? The following psychological investigations are, of course, applicable only to conscious patients.

INTELLECTUAL FUNCTIONS

Is the patient orientated in space and time? Does he recognize his surroundings and does he know the date? Is his memory normal, and, if impaired, is it better for remote than for recent events? Does he fill gaps in his memory by confabulating, that is, by relating imaginary events or others taken out of their temporal context? Retentiveness may be tested by asking the patient to retain and repeat a series of digits—normally seven can be repeated—or retain a name, address, and the name of a flower for five minutes. Concentration and immediate recall can also be tested by asking the patient to repeat the Babcock sentence— 'One thing a nation must have to be rich and great is a large secure supply of wood'; normally this can be repeated accurately in not more than three attempts. It is also usual to ask for the names of well-known people (e.g. the last three Prime Ministers or U.S. Presidents) and to test simple calculation by requesting the patient to subtract serial sevens from 100.

What is his level of intelligence? Is he in touch with current events? Can he grasp the meaning of a passage which he reads from a newspaper, or of a picture depicting an incident?

Does he suffer from delusions or hallucinations? A delusion is an erroneous belief which cannot be corrected by an appeal to reason and is not shared by others of the patient's education and station. An hallucination is a sensory impression occurring in the absence of a corresponding external stimulus. A patient may conceal both delusions and hallucinations. The latter may sometimes be suspected on account of his behaviour. For example, a patient who is subject to visual hallucinations may behave as though manipulating invisible objects, while one who is experiencing auditory hallucinations, for example voices, may adopt a listening attitude.

EMOTIONAL STATE

Is the patient's emotional state normal? Is he excited or depressed? If excited, is his condition one of elation, that is, excitement associated with a sense of well-being, or of fear and anxiety? Apart from excitement, does he experience an abnormal sense of well-being—euphoria? Is he anxious and, if so, to what does he attribute his anxiety? Is he irritable? Is he emotionally indifferent and apathetic? Does he take normal care of his dress and appearance, or is he indifferent and dirty? Personal neglect may be due to a disorder of affect such as depression but is more often the result of disintegration of the personality and intellect (i.e. dementia).

SPEECH AND ARTICULATION

Are speech and articulation normal? If there is reason to suspect that the patient is suffering from aphasia, the appropriate tests must be carried out [see p. 107].

THE CRANIAL NERVES

Test the sense of smell for each nostril separately [see p. 154].

Test the visual acuity and visual fields [see pp. 65–7].

Examine the ocular fundi [see p. 155].

Are the pupils equal, central, and regular? Are they abnormally dilated or contracted? Test the reactions to light, both direct and consensual, of each eye separately, and the reaction on accommodation/convergence.

Test the ocular movements, upwards and downwards and to either side, and ocular convergence. Is squint, diplopia, or nystagmus present? Note the size of the palpebral fissures. Does the patient exhibit ptosis or retraction of the upper lids? Is exophthalmos present?

Is there wasting of the temporal muscles and masseters? Test the jaw movements and the jaw-jerk.

Examine sensibility to light touch, pin-prick, heat and cold over the trigeminal area, and test the corneal reflexes.

Is the facial expression normal? Is there wasting of the facial muscles? Is the face the site of involuntary movements? Test the following voluntary movements —closure of the eyes, elevation of the eyebrows, frowning, retraction of the lips, pursing the lips, whistling or the ability to retain air in the cheeks under pressure. Test emotional facial movements—smiling. In some cases of facial paralysis it is necessary to test the sense of taste [see p. 205].

Test the hearing, both air-conduction and bone-conduction. If hearing is defective, apply both Weber's and Rinne's tests [see p. 188]. In certain cases it may be necessary to test the vestibular reactions [see p. 191].

Is the soft palate elevated normally on phonation? Test the palatal and pharyngeal reflexes.

Examine the movements of the vocal cords, if necessary.

Test the movements of the sternomastoids and trapezii.

Examine the tongue. Is it wasted? Is fasciculation present? Is it tremulous? Is it protruded normally or does it deviate to one or other side?

Note the presence or absence of head retraction and test for cervical rigidity.

THE SKULL AND SKELETON

Inspect and then palpate the skull and spine, noting any evidence of abnormal configuration, local tenderness, or deformity. Note if there are any deformities of the limbs (e.g. contractures or pes cavus). Auscultate over the temporal fossae, over both orbits, and over the great vessels in the neck, noting the presence of bruits; on occasion it may be necessary to auscultate over the spinal column in an attempt to detect a spinal bruit.

THE LIMBS AND TRUNK

The following is a convenient routine for the examination of the limbs and trunk. Examine the upper limbs while the patient is lying down; then ask him to sit up, or, if he is unable to do so, to turn on to one side, and examine the scapular muscles and the back; then ask him to lie down again and examine the front of the thorax and the abdomen, and finally the lower limbs. Sensibility as well as motor functions should first be examined in this order, but in many cases, especially when there is reason to suspect a lesion of the spinal cord, it may be convenient to review the sensibility of the body as a whole.

Muscular Power and Co-ordination. In examining the limbs note first their *posture* and the presence or absence of *muscular wasting* and *fasciculation*. Next note the presence or absence of *involuntary movements*, of which the following are those most commonly encountered. A tic is a co-ordinated, repetitive movement involving as a rule a number of muscles in their normal synergic relationships. Choreic movements are quasi-purposive, jerky, irregular, and non-repetitive, and are characterized by dissociation of normal muscular synergy. Athetosis consists of slow, writhing movements, which are most marked in the peripheral segments of the limbs. Tremor is a rhythmical movement at a joint, brought about by alternating contractions of antagonistic groups of muscles. Myoclonus is a shock-like muscular contraction affecting part or the whole of the muscle independently of its antagonists. If involuntary movements are present, note their relationship to rest, posture, and voluntary movement.

Next examine *muscle tone* by passive movement at the various joints and note the presence or absence of *muscular contractures*. Next test voluntary power by asking the patient to carry out against resistance the movements possible at the various joints, comparing successively the same movement on the two sides of the body. If it is desired to record the degree of power present in a muscle the following scale may be used: no contraction, 0; flicker or trace of contraction, 1; active movement, with gravity eliminated, 2; active movement against gravity, 3; active movement against gravity and resistance, 4; normal power, 5. When attempting to identify weakness due to upper motor neurone lesions, it may be sufficient to examine the power of a few selected muscles only (e.g. deltoid, biceps, finger flexors, and extensors in the upper limbs, hip flexors, quadriceps, and tibialis anterior in the lower). In the assessment of suspected peripheral nerve lesions and in cases of neuromuscular disease, however, a more extensive examination of individual muscles is needed; full details may be found in the Medical Research Council Memorandum 'Aids to the Examination of the Peripheral Nervous System' (1976). In such an examination, grade 4 power as defined above may have to be divided into two subgroups (e.g. 4+, 4−). The detection of early corticospinal tract lesions may require the testing of manual dexterity and the ability to move the various fingers independently.

Muscular co-ordination is tested in the upper limbs by asking the patient to touch the tip of his nose with the tip of his forefinger, first with the eyes open and then with the eyes closed. He should also be asked to carry out alternating movements of flexion and extension of the fingers, or pronation and supination of the forearms simultaneously on both sides. When the patient is in bed, co-ordination of the lower limbs may be tested by asking him to place one heel on the opposite knee, or to raise the leg from the bed and touch the observer's finger with his toe.

Movements of the abdominal wall are tested by asking the patient to raise his head from the bed against resistance and noting by palpation the degree of contraction of the abdominal muscles and also whether displacement of the umbilicus occurs.

Sensibility. As a routine, the patient's appreciation of light touch, pin-prick, heat and cold, posture, passive movement, and vibration should be tested, attention being paid not only to defective sensibility but also to the presence of tenderness or sensitivity to pressure of the superficial and deep structures. In some cases additional tests may be needed [see p. 37]. Since the spinal segmental areas run longitudinally along the long axis of the upper limbs, sensibility on the ulnar border should be compared with that on the radial border, either by applying successive stimuli transversely to the limb, or by dragging the stimulus, for example a pin, along the skin. On the trunk the segmental areas are distributed almost horizontally. Changes of sensibility are therefore best detected by moving the stimulus from below upwards or vice versa. In the lower limbs the sacral segmental areas, which are represented on the sole and the posterior aspect of the limb and in the perianal area, should always be tested.

The Reflexes. The following reflexes should be examined as a routine: in the upper limbs, the supinator-, biceps-, and triceps-jerks; on the trunk, the abdominal reflexes; in the lower limbs, the knee- and ankle-jerks and the plantar reflexes; at the same time tests for patellar and ankle clonus should be carried out.

The Sphincters. Note the state of the sphincters and examine the abdomen for evidence of distension of the bladder.

Trophic Disturbances. Note the state of the patient's nutrition, especially the presence of wasting or excessive obesity and the condition of the external genitalia. Note the distribution of hair on the body, anomalies of sweating, and the presence or absence of cutaneous pigmentation and trophic lesions of the skin, nails, and joints.

A complete general physical examination should be made. Examination of the peripheral blood vessels, especially the carotids, is important. Inequality of carotid or radial pulsation should be noted, and if there is any difference the blood pressure should be recorded in both arms.

GAIT

If the patient is well enough to leave his bed, observe whether he is able to stand without support with the feet together, and whether the steadiness of his stance is affected when he closes his eyes. Ask him to walk, if necessary with support, and note the presence of spasticity or ataxia of the lower limbs in walking. Slight disturbances of stance and gait may be detected by asking the patient to stand first on one foot and then on the other, first with the eyes open and then with the eyes closed; and to walk along a line, placing one heel in front of the toes of the other foot. The 'scissors' gait of spastic diplegia, the hemiplegic gait, the stiff gait with dragging of both feet in spastic paraparesis, the high steppage gait of tabes dorsalis, the slow shuffle or festinant gait of Parkinsonism, the broad-based, staggering gait of central cerebellar lesions, the waddling gait of some neuromuscular disorders such as muscular dystrophy, and the foot-slapping gait of bilateral foot drop, to name but a few, are distinctive.

INVESTIGATION OF THE PATIENT WITH NEUROLOGICAL DISEASE

In considering the ancillary investigations which may be used as aids to diagnosis in a patient whose symptoms and signs suggest a disorder of the nervous system, it is of course important to appreciate that symptoms of neurological dysfunction may result from disease in some other part of the body. The patient must therefore be viewed as a whole if he is not to be subjected to a series of unpleasant tests designed to demonstrate an abnormality in the nervous system when the lesion responsible may be in some other organ apart from the brain and spinal cord. A second important principle is that investigations should always be planned to give the maximum required information about the patient's illness with the least possible discomfort and risk. In some patients with neurological symptoms, there may be no need for investigations either for diagnosis or to give guidance in management. Migraine, for instance, is a condition in which the diagnosis can usually be made on the clinical history alone and in which ancillary tests are rarely indicated. In other cases, investigation should be carefully designed in order to establish or exclude the diagnoses which are brought to mind by the patient's symptoms and signs. It is reasonable to begin by carrying out the simpler tests which the doctor is able to do himself before proceeding, if the diagnosis remains in doubt, to the more difficult investigations which require specialized apparatus and skilled technical help.

From this brief commentary it follows that in many patients it will be necessary to carry out examination of the urine and haematological and biochemical tests on blood samples, whereas electrocardiography, various microbiological studies, and in some situations biopsy of muscle, peripheral nerve, or of other tissues and organs may be required in order to clarify the nature of the patient's illness. A detailed commentary upon these tests would be out of place, but where necessary these studies are described in detail in subsequent chapters. Indications for, and methods of, examination of the cerebrospinal fluid have already been considered [pp. 124–35]. Certain specialized neurophysiological and radiological techniques are also considered in later chapters, as are some methods of investigation of particular relevance in the assessment of the special senses. In addition, methods of measurement of nerve conduction velocity, studies of neuromuscular transmission and electromyography are described in the sections on disorders of the peripheral nerve and muscle. It would, however, be appropriate here to consider some general principles underlying the use of electroencephalography, echo-encephalography, isotope studies, and radiological methods.

ELECTROENCEPHALOGRAPHY

Electroencephalography is a technique of recording the electrical activity of the brain through the intact skull. Electrodes are applied to the scalp and the potential changes so recorded are amplified and presented for interpretation as an ink-trace on moving paper. Machines in common use today have sixteen or more channels so that the activity from many different areas of the head can be recorded simultaneously. The technique is simple and harmless.

In the normal adult the dominant electrical activity in the EEG from the post-central areas is usually a sinusoidal wave form with a frequency of 8–13 Hz [FIG. 18 a]. This is the alpha rhythm; it commonly disappears on attention, as when the eyes open [FIG. 18 b]. Normally there is some faster so-called beta activity (14–22 Hz) in the frontal regions; this is greatly accentuated by the administration of barbiturates and sometimes by anxiety. In young infants the EEG is dominated by generalized slow activity of so-called delta frequency (up to 3·5 Hz); gradually during the processes of maturation this is replaced by theta activity (4–7 Hz) and subsequently by the alpha rhythm. Theta activity disappears last from the posterior temporal regions and the record is usually completely mature, showing no such activity, by the age of 12–14 years. During

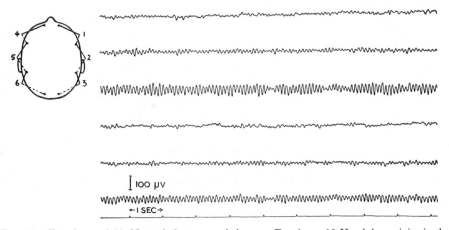

FIG. 18 a. Female, aged 23. Normal electroencephalogram. Dominant 10 Hz alpha activity in the posterocentral regions

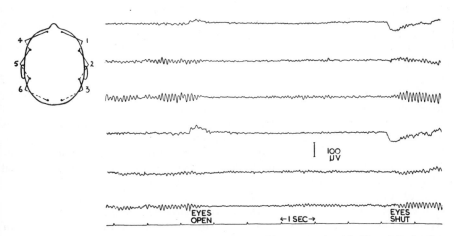

FIG. 18 b. Female, aged 23. Normal electroencephalogram. Almost complete blocking of the dominant alpha rhythm to eye opening

F

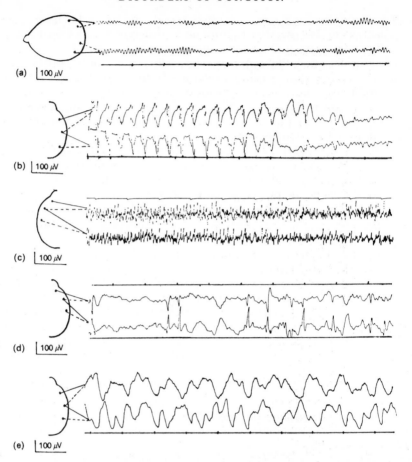

Fig. 19. Some common appearances in the electroencephalographic (EEG) recordings (from *Essentials of Neurology*, 4th ed., by J. N. Walton, Pitman Medical, 1975). A, a normal alpha rhythm recorded from both occipital regions and disappearing (in the centre of the recording) when the eyes are open. B, a 3 Hz spike and wave discharge of petit mal epilepsy, recorded in this illustration from the right temporal region. C, high frequency discharges (mainly muscle artefact) recorded from the left fronto-temporal region during a major epileptic seizure. D, a right anterior temporal focus of spike discharge in a patient suffering from temporal lobe epilepsy. E, a focus of high-amplitude delta activity seen in the right mid-temporal region in a patient suffering from a cerebral abscess in this situation.

drowsiness and sleep in the normal individual, theta activity and later delta activity reappear.

The EEG is of particular value in the diagnosis of epilepsy [FIG. 19]. In cases of petit mal it may show regular rhythmical generalized outbursts of repetitive complexes, each consisting of a spike and a delta wave (spike-and-wave), and recurring at a frequency of about 3 Hz. In idiopathic or centrencephalic major epilepsy, the interseizure record may sometimes show brief generalized out-bursts of spikes or sharp waves or of mixed spikes and slow activity. Similarly in patients suffering from focal epilepsy, including temporal lobe attacks, there may be spikes, sharp waves, or rhythmical outbursts of slow delta or theta activity arising in the epileptogenic area of the cortex. Unfortunately, a single record taken in an epileptic patient is often normal; positive findings are more common in children and less common the older the patient. Many other patients show non-specific abnormalities between attacks such as excessive temporal theta activity. Hence it is often necessary to take repeated recordings or alternatively to use various activation techniques in order to uncover epileptic discharges. Overbreathing for two to three minutes is particularly effective in evoking the discharges of petit mal, while photic stimulation (repetitive light flashes of variable frequency) can also bring out epileptic discharges. Since temporal spikes or sharp waves often appear in early sleep, it is usual to carry out recordings after oral or intravenous barbiturate sedation in cases of suspected temporal lobe epilepsy. In some such cases, recordings with a needle electrode inserted to lie in contact with the basi-sphenoid underneath the medial surface of the temporal lobe are helpful.

It can be concluded that a single routine EEG is of limited value but should generally be performed, using simple activating techniques if necessary, in most patients suspected to be suffering from epilepsy. If epileptic discharges are found, this will confirm the diagnosis and the nature of the discharge may help in deciding upon appropriate treatment. Negative findings, however, cannot be taken to exclude this diagnosis.

The EEG is also of value in the diagnosis of focal cerebral lesions. A relatively acute lesion of one cerebral hemisphere usually give a focus of delta activity in or around the area of the lesion [FIG. 19]. It is not the lesion itself which produces this abnormal discharge, but the changes which it has produced in the surrounding brain. A cerebral abscess usually produces a slow-wave focus of high amplitude, and similar though less striking abnormalities may result from tumour, haemorrhage, local injury, or infarction. Thus the EEG may help in localization but rarely if ever gives any indication of the pathological diagnosis, which must depend upon clinical or other information. An abnormality due to a tumour will usually become worse, while that due to an infarct often improves. In the case of lesions which are more chronic or more deeply situated in the cerebral hemisphere, focal theta activity of low amplitude or even an absence of alpha or beta activity on one side may be the only abnormality. Indeed, in some patients with intracranial tumours the record may be consistently normal. Whereas some localized abnormality may be found in up to 70 per cent of patients with intracranial neoplasms, the EEG is never sufficiently accurate in localization to be a safe guide to subsequent surgery and the neurosurgeon will invariably require information derived from other diagnostic methods.

A subdural haematoma may sometimes produce a unilateral suppression of the alpha rhythm and irregular slow activity on the affected side. Certain rare conditions such as subacute sclerosing panencephalitis give characteristic findings, but in many chronic neurological disorders such as Parkinsonism and multiple sclerosis the EEG is often normal. In subacute encephalitis isolated bizarre slow-wave complexes occur simultaneously in all channels against a background of comparative electrical silence, while in some children with cerebral lipidosis or in adults with Creutzfeldt-Jakob disease generalized and almost continuous irregular spike and wave discharge may be seen. A similar severe abnormality, often called hypsarrhythmia, may be found in records from infants suffering from so-called infantile spasms. Tumours in the posterior fossa or deeply situated lesions near the midline often give paroxysmal outbursts of theta or delta activity at the surface, but these changes are not specific as they occur in patients with many diffuse disorders including meningitis, subarachnoid haemorrhage, and encephalitis or conditions giving a generalized disorder of cerebral metabolism such as anoxia, uraemia, hyperglycaemia, hepatic coma, or pernicious anaemia.

The EEG is of comparatively little value in psychiatric diagnosis, though anxious and obsessional patients may show excessive frontal fast activity, while psychopaths and children with behaviour disorders have immature records with excessive temporal slow activity. Patients with organic dementia often show a dominant rhythm of theta rather than alpha frequency; in a sense this represents a reversion to the childhood pattern and may even occur naturally as a result of ageing.

It will thus be seen that the EEG is of some value in the diagnosis of epilepsy and of certain uncommon brain diseases in which relatively specific changes may sometimes be found. It is also of limited value in the investigation of patients with cerebral vascular disease and intracranial space-occupying lesions. It must not, however, be expected to give information which it is incapable of providing, and a single negative recording is of little value.

ECHO-ENCEPHALOGRAPHY

A number of simple and relatively inexpensive machines using ultrasonics for neurological diagnosis are now available commercially. An ultrasonic beam is passed horizontally through the intact skull and an 'echo' can be recorded from midline structures. A 'shift' of the midline can readily be demonstrated and this method, which is without risk, and may be helpful in confirming rapidly the presence of a space-occupying lesion in or overlying one cerebral hemisphere. The method is particularly useful for the rapid screening of patients in whom a subdural or extradural haematoma or a tumour in one cerebral hemisphere is suspected. More complicated and refined techniques have been introduced in order to define echoes arising from intracranial structures other than those in the midline.

GAMMA-ENCEPHALOGRAPHY

Scanning of the radioactivity recorded over the surface of the skull following the intravenous injection of a suitable isotope (^{99}Technetium is now most commonly used) is increasingly employed in many neurological and neuro-surgical units as an aid to the diagnosis of intracranial lesions. The blood vessels, and probably the cells of certain tumours, show a selective affinity for such isotopes so that the tumour is shown as an area of increased radioactivity. When lateral and antero-posterior scans are recorded, localization may be very accurate. Increased uptake is also seen in cerebral abscesses and in areas of infarction. Thus a single scan may not give a firm pathological diagnosis, but the technique is of particular value in demonstrating multiple intracranial lesions (e.g. metastases).

ISOTOPE VENTRICULOGRAPHY

If a small amount of radio-iodinated serum albumin (RISA) is injected by lumbar puncture in a normal individual and the skull is then scanned a few hours later, radioactivity is demonstrated in the subarachnoid space over the surface of the brain and not, as a rule, in the cerebral ventricles. If, however, the lateral ventricles soon show evidence of radioactivity and little or no isotope flows over the brain surface towards the superior longitudinal sinus, some degree of communicating hydrocephalus is probably present. This method is thus of particular value in detecting cases of so-called low-pressure hydrocephalus, and it is also helpful in detecting fistulous communications between the subarachnoid space and the middle ear or paranasal sinus such as may occur after head injury, otitis media, or sinusitis. Measurement of the rate of clearance of the isotope into the systemic circulation may also be used as a means of detecting the rate of cerebrospinal fluid absorption in a case of suspected hydrocephalus.

RADIOLOGY

Radiological methods are among the most helpful and widely used of all the ancillary techniques used in neurological diagnosis. While final diagnosis often depends upon the use of specialized methods involving the injection of air or other contrast media, each of these techniques is time-consuming, expensive, and often disturbing to the patient. It is therefore important to remember that valuable and sometimes even conclusive information may be obtained from plain radiographs of the skull and/or spine and of other parts of the body. Thus in patients with a clinical picture suggestive of intracranial neoplasm or in others with a subacute meningitic illness, X-rays of the chest are all-important, revealing perhaps a bronchogenic carcinoma or evidence of pulmonary tuberculosis. In other cases changes in the skeleton will throw light upon the significance of neurological symptoms and signs, as for instance in cases of prostatic carcinoma or multiple myelomatosis.

Straight Radiography of the Skull. It is usual to take routine anteroposterior and lateral views of the skull, while in most centres an antero-posterior view is also taken with the brow depressed some 35 degrees so that the petrous temporal bones become visible (Towne's view) and another of the skull base. Stenver's view is also utilized to examine the petrous temporal bone. Usually the skull vault is first examined to see if there is reasonable uniformity of bony thickness or whether there is any erosion or bony overgrowth such as may result from a meningioma, or abnormal vascular markings due to dilatation of the middle meningeal artery supplying a meningeal tumour or vascular malformation. Sometimes, as in carcinomatosis or myelomatosis, there may be multiple areas of bony rarefaction in the skull vault or a general thickening or 'woolliness' of the bone as in Paget's disease. In young children, hydrocephalus due to any cause may give separation of the cranial sutures and a characteristic 'beaten copper' mottling of the bone; however, the latter appearance is so often seen in normal individuals even in adult life that in itself it is not diagnostic. Fractures of the vault are noted if present, and it is also wise to examine the frontal, maxillary, and sphenoidal paranasal sinuses for opacities which may suggest infection or neoplasia. Hyperostosis of the inner table of the frontal bone is not uncommon but is of no pathological significance.

The base of the skull is next examined, first in the lateral projection. Here the relationship of the upper cervical spine to the foramen magnum is observed and it is noted whether there is any protrusion of the odontoid process of the axis above a line joining the posterior margin of the hard palate to the posterior lip of the foramen magnum (Chamberlain's line). If the odontoid does not show above this line, or if there is an abnormal tilt of the body of the atlas implying invagination of the basi-occiput, then basilar impression is present. The most important structure at the base of the skull visible on the lateral projection is the sella turcica. The size and shape of the sella and the integrity and density of the anterior and posterior clinoid processes which form its lips are noted. In patients with primary pituitary neoplasms the sella is expanded or ballooned and partially decalcified, while in those with suprasellar lesions it is also expanded but is shallower and flattened and there is often erosion of the clinoid processes. A moderate degree of flattening and expansion of the sella with decalcification of the posterior clinoid processes may occur in any patient with increased intracranial pressure.

Also to be noted on the lateral projection is the presence or absence of intra-cranial calcification. If present, such calcification can then be more accurately localized by means of antero-posterior views or by stereoscopic lateral pro-jections. In about 50 per cent of adults and even in some normal children, the pineal gland is calcified and may measure up to 0·5 cm in diameter. If the gland is calcified, it is important to measure its distance from the inner table of the skull on antero-posterior radiographs, as displacement to one or other side may indicate the presence of a space-occupying lesion in one cerebral hemisphere. Other intracranial structures which occasionally calcify in the normal individual are the choroid plexuses, the falx cerebri, and the petro-clinoid ligaments. Pathological intracranial calcification, if mottled in type and suprasellar in situation, usually indicates a craniopharyngioma, but many other intracranial tumours including meningiomas, gliomas, and oligodendrogliomas occasionally show a fine spidery pattern of calcification. Fine curvilinear lines of calcification may be seen in the wall of a large aneurysm, while calcific stippling can occur in a haematoma or arteriovenous angioma. Rare additional causes of intracranial calcification include cysticercosis, toxoplasmosis, and hypoparathyroidism. A form of widespread calcification outlining the gyri of one occipital and/or parietal lobe is seen in diffuse cortical angiomatosis associated with a port-wine naevus of the face (the Sturge–Weber syndrome).

In antero-posterior, Towne's, Stenver's, and the basal views, the most important feature to look for is enlargement or erosion of cranial exit foramina. Sclerosis and overgrowth of bone may also occur, particularly in the wings of the sphenoid in patients who have a meningioma in this region. Otherwise it is usual to examine the optic foramina, superior orbital fissures, and internal auditory meati in particular. A funnel-shaped erosion of the internal auditory meati, revealed by Towne's and Stenver's views, is characteristic of an acoustic neuroma. The basal view may also reveal bony erosion due to malignant infiltration of the base of the skull or enlargement of one foramen spinosum in a patient with a meningioma producing dilatation of one middle meningeal artery.

Radiology of the Spinal Column. In examining radiographs of the spine, we are concerned first with changes in the vertebrae themselves, secondly with the intervertebral discs, and thirdly with the intervertebral foramina. It is usual to carry out antero-posterior and lateral views to study the vertebrae and discs, but for examination of the intervertebral foramina, oblique views are necessary. In the vertebrae themselves one may first observe congenital abnormalities such as fusion of several vertebral bodies (if in the cervical region this may be called the Klippel–Feil syndrome) or spina bifida, either of which may be responsible for or associated with neurological signs. Fracture, fracture-dislocation, Paget's disease, osteomyelitis, neoplasia, either benign or malignant, of vertebral bodies, any one of which might give vertebral collapse and spinal cord compression, will generally be revealed by routine X-rays. Bony erosion and in particular enlargement of the relevant intervertebral foramen is typically seen, often with the extraspinal soft tissue shadow of a dumb-bell tumour, in cases of spinal neurofibroma. Less striking but of equal diagnostic importance is a variation in interpedicular distance. The distance between the vertebral pedicles is large in the cervical region, gradually diminishes to a minimum in the mid-dorsal region, and then expands again in the lumbar region, corresponding to the cervical and lumbar enlargements of the spinal cord. If successive interpedicular distances are measured and one or more measurements falls outside the expected arithmetical progression, this indicates the presence of an expanding lesion within the spinal cord or spinal canal in this region. Dorsal meningiomas may produce no more radiological change than this, whereas neurofibromas commonly give bony erosion as well. Measurement of the anteroposterior diameter of the spinal canal is also of value, particularly in the cervical region; an unduly wide canal is seen, for instance, in some cases of syringomyelia.

In a patient with an acute prolapse of an intervertebral disc, radiographs of the spine are often normal or reveal simply a narrowing of the disc space concerned. The prolapsed disc is not itself radio-opaque. If one or more disc protrusions have been present for some months or years, the margins of the prolapsed tissue gradually become calcified, giving posterior (and often anterior) osteophyte formation at the upper and lower borders of the contiguous vertebrae. As the prolapsed tissue often projects laterally as well, osteophytes also tend to encroach upon the intervertebral foramina and this change is shown on oblique views. A combination of changes of this type, which are most commonly observed in the cervical and lumbar regions, is referred to as spondylosis.

Computerized Transaxial Tomography. This new and exciting technique of radiological diagnosis (the so-called EMI scan) seems likely to transform the practice of neuroradiology and to supplant some of the more traditional contrast methods. Without the use of any contrast medium, this technique allows one to carry out rapid serial tomographic cuts in multiple planes and it has been found possible with the complex equipment which is needed to obtain remarkably accurate outlines of the cerebral ventricles and subarachnoid space and to identify and localize space-occupying lesions; differentiation between infarction and neoplasia is often possible. Without question, refinements of this method are likely to make it necessary in the future to carry out fewer studies involving the use of air or other contrast media. Some representative scans are given in FIGURE 20.

Contrast Methods. The contrast methods most often used in neurological diagnosis are air encephalography, ventriculography with air or myodil (pantopaque), carotid, vertebral, and aortic arch angiography, and myelography. Each of these methods carries certain possible hazards to the patient and all involve some degree of pain or discomfort; hence they must not be regarded as routine methods of investigation but should only be utilized when an accurate diagnosis can be reached in no other way. When this is the case, it must be decided which method is likely to give the most helpful information and whether the one chosen is likely to be safe or whether there are contra-indications. Sometimes it is necessary to carry out a number of these studies successively, but

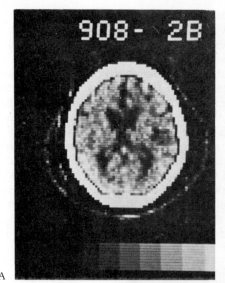
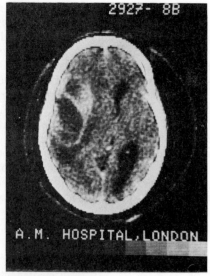

A   B

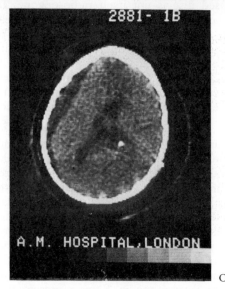

C

FIG. 20. A number of representative EMI scans. A, dilatation of the lateral ventricles and an increased size of the subarachnoid space, particularly in the Sylvian regions, is seen in a patient with cortical atrophy due to presenile dementia. B, a left-sided partially cystic glioma in the left fronto-temporal region, displacing the lateral ventricles to the right. C, a subdural haematoma in the left fronto-parietal region. (Scans kindly supplied by Dr. J. Ambrose.)

they should always be kept to the minimum necessary to give adequate information concerning the patient's disease.

The place of these investigations in the diagnosis of cerebral vascular disease, of intracranial space-occupying lesions, and other disease processes, and the place of myelography in the diagnosis of spinal lesions will be considered in appropriate chapters.

REFERENCES

ANDRÉ-THOMAS, CHESNI, Y., and ST-ANNE DARGASSIES (1955) *Examen Neurologique du Nourrisson*, Paris.

BICKERSTAFF, E. R. (1973) *Neurological Examination in Clinical Practice*, 3rd ed., Oxford.

BULL, J. W. D. (1951) Diagnostic neuroradiology, in *Modern Trends in Neurology*, ed. Feiling, A., chap. 20, 1st series, London.

DAVIS, C. H., and MARTIN, J. F. (1969) Ordering X-rays and performing contrast studies, in *Special Techniques for Neurologic Diagnosis*, ed. Toole, J. F., Contemporary Neurology Series, vol. 3, Philadelphia.

HILL, D., and DRIVER, M. V. (1962) in *Recent Advances in Neurology and Neuropsychiatry*, 7th ed., ed. Brain, W. R., p. 169, London.

HILL, D., and PARR, G. (1963) *Electro-encephalography*, 2nd ed., London.

DE JONG, R. N. (1967) *The Neurological Examination*, 3rd ed., New York.

KILOH, L. G., McCOMAS, A. J., and OSSELTON, J. W. (1972) *Clinical Electroencephalography*, 3rd ed., London.

MAYNARD, C. D., and JANEWAY, R. (1969) Radioisotope studies in diagnosis, in *Special Techniques for Neurologic Diagnosis*, ed. Toole, J. F., Contemporary Neurology Series, vol. 3, Philadelphia.

McKINNEY, W. M. (1969) Echoencephalography, in *Special Techniques for Neurologic Diagnosis*, ed. Toole, J. F., Contemporary Neurology Series, vol. 3, Philadelphia.

PAINE, R. S., and OPPÉ, T. E. (1966) *Neurological Examination of Children*, Clinics in Developmental Medicine, vol. 20/21, London.

SUTTON, D. (1969) Recent advances in neuroradiology, in *Recent Advances in Neurology and Neuropsychiatry*, 8th ed., ed. the late Lord Brain and Wilkinson, M., chap. 10, London.

2

THE CRANIAL NERVES

THE FIRST OR OLFACTORY NERVE

THE OLFACTORY FIBRES

THE olfactory portion of the nasal mucous membrane contains bipolar sensory cells which constitute the olfactory neurones of the first order. Their central processes, which are unmyelinated, form small bundles, the filaments of the olfactory nerve, which pass through the cribriform plates of the ethmoid bone and enter the olfactory bulb. From the olfactory bulb further fibres reach the brain through the olfactory tract (for details see Le Gros Clark, 1947). As this approaches the cerebral hemisphere it divides into a median and a lateral root on either side of the anterior perforated space. The lateral root is the more important in man and carries fibres to the olfactory area of the cerebral cortex, which consists of the peri-amygdaloid and pre-piriform areas of the so-called piriform lobe and, in spite of traditional views, does not include the hippocampus (Brodal, 1947). The anterior commissure unites the olfactory cortical regions of the two hemispheres and probably also carries fibres from each olfactory tract to the opposite hemisphere.

DISTURBANCES OF THE SENSE OF SMELL

By the sense of smell we perceive not only scents but also flavours, the sense of taste being concerned only with the recognition of the four primary tastes—sweet, bitter, salt, and acid. It is a commonplace observation that a cold in the head, or any lesion which abolishes the sense of smell, abolishes also flavours but not the primary tastes.

In testing the sense of smell small bottles containing coffee, oil of peppermint, oil of cloves, camphorated oil, and other scents are applied in turn to each nostril, and the patient is asked if he recognizes them. It must be remembered that many normal individuals with an acute sense of smell find difficulty in naming scents. After head injury, especially in a compensation setting, anosmia may be feigned in the hope of material gain; it may therefore be useful to ask the patient to smell concentrated ammonia which stimulates the trigeminal sensory terminals in the nose as well as the olfactory; if a patient claims not to be affected by ammonia it is likely that the anosmia is spurious.

Anosmia, or loss of the olfactory sense, is occasionally congenital, and sometimes hereditary. It may occur either temporarily or permanently as a result of infections of the nose. Total anosmia is a rare complication of anoxia; it most often results from division or compression of olfactory nerve fibres as they pass through the cribriform plate of the ethmoid. Complete or partial loss may occur on one or both sides as a result of head injury either with or without fracture of the base of the skull in the anterior fossa. Sumner (1964) found an incidence of 7·5 per cent, the liability increasing with increasing severity of the head injury. Anosmia may be temporary, lasting for only a few days, weeks, or months, but if it persists for more than a year it is unlikely to recover. Even trivial injuries occasionally produce this sign; recovery is much more likely to occur, however, after minor injury than after injuries giving 24 hours or more of post-traumatic amnesia (Sumner, 1972). The olfactory tract may be compressed by tumours, especially by meningiomas growing from the olfactory groove, or less frequently by tumours of the frontal lobe or in the region of the optic chiasm, or by the distended cerebral hemispheres in obstructive hydrocephalus. Thus unilateral anosmia may be a useful sign of an anteriorly situated space-occupying lesion. The tract may also be involved in meningitis, both purulent and syphilitic and, like the optic nerves, degenerate in tabes. It is doubtful whether complete anosmia is ever produced by lesions of the olfactory cortex on one side, probably because fibres from each olfactory tract reach both cerebral hemispheres. A lesion of one uncus, however, may cause a reduction in olfactory acuity in the nostril of the same side. Irritative lesions in the neighbourhood of the uncus are liable to cause olfactory hallucinations, which are usually associated with disturbance of consciousness and involuntary convulsive movements of the lips, jaw, tongue, and pharynx—uncinate fits [see p. 270].

Parosmia may occur especially after head injury. Strong scents then smell abnormal, usually unpleasant, and a persistent unpleasant olfactory hallucination may be experienced. A similar symptom sometimes occurs in depressive illness.

REFERENCES

Brodal, A. (1947) The hippocampus and the sense of smell, *Brain*, **70**, 179.
Clark, W. E. Le G. (1947) *Anatomical Pattern as the Essential Basis of Sensory Discrimination*, Oxford.
Dana, C. L. (1889) The olfactory nerve, *N.Y. med. J.*, **50**, 253.
Elsberg, C. A., and Stewart, J. (1938) Quantitative olfactory tests: value in localization and diagnosis of tumors of the brain with analysis of results in three hundred patients. *Arch. Neurol. Psychiat. (Chic.)*, **40**, 471.
Leigh, A. D. (1943) Defects of smell after head injury, *Lancet*, **i**, 38.
McCartney, W. (1972) Olfaction, sect. V, chap. 4, in *Scientific Foundations of Neurology*, ed. Critchley, M., O'Leary, J. L., and Jennett, W. B., London.
Sumner, D. (1964) Post-traumatic anosmia, *Brain*, **87**, 107.
Sumner, D. (1972) Clinical aspects of anosmia, sect. V, chap. 5, in *Scientific Foundations of Neurology*, ed. Critchley, M., O'Leary, J. L., and Jennett, W. B., London.

THE SECOND OR OPTIC NERVE

The course of the optic nerve and the situation of the retinal fibres within it are described on page 67 and methods of testing the visual acuity and visual fields are described on pages 65–7.

Ophthalmoscopy

Examination of the fundus oculi is of such importance in the investigation of cases of nervous disease that it should form part of the routine examination of every patient. Except when the pupil is greatly contracted, it is usually possible to examine the optic disc; but to make a complete examination of the macular region and of the periphery of the retina, the pupil should previously be dilated with homatropine. The normal optic disc is circular and rosy pink in colour, though slightly paler than the surrounding retina. It possesses a well-defined edge and a depression—the physiological cup—from which the arteries and veins emerge. The normal appearance of the disc and its vessels can be learned only from experience. The following are the most important abnormalities. The disc may be pinker than normal, from hyperaemia, or abnormally pale from optic atrophy. Its edge may be indistinct. The physiological cup may be filled or the disc may be actually swollen above the level of the surrounding retina, the swelling being measured in dioptres. Abnormal 'cupping' of the entire disc is characteristic of glaucoma. Streaks of white medullated nerve fibres extending on to the retina from one part of the disc are occasionally seen but have no pathological significance. A white crescentic area at one side of the disc (a myopic crescent) is commonly present in myopic individuals. The veins of the disc may be congested, the arteries may be thickened and tortuous, or both arteries and veins may be abnormally fine and narrow. Pulsation of the arteries is abnormal, but pulsation of the veins is sometimes seen in normal individuals. Finally, the disc and surrounding area of the retina may be the site of exudate or haemorrhages.

The macular region is situated about two disc-breadths horizontally outwards from the outer edge of the disc. It is somewhat darker than the rest of the fundus and is almost devoid of blood vessels. The principal abnormalities to be found in the macula are an extension of oedema from the optic disc—the macular 'fan'—and a stippled, star-shaped, or haemorrhagic exudate in cases of hypertensive retinopathy. A cherry-red spot is seen at the macula in cases of obstruction of the central artery of the retina and in the infantile form of cerebromacular degeneration, and pigmentation is seen in the late infantile and juvenile forms of this disease. Since the macula is the most sensitive part of the retina and is concerned in central vision, macular lesions cause great impairment of visual acuity.

Finally the whole of the periphery of the retina should be inspected. The condition of the arteries and the veins should be noted. Retinal arteriosclerosis first manifests itself in displacement of the veins at the point where they are crossed by the arteries, with congestion of the portion distal to the crossing. Greater degrees of arterial thickening lead to tortuosity and irregularity of the arteries, with an increased light refraction from their surface—silver-wire arteries. In retinal arteriosclerosis and hypertensive retinopathy haemorrhages and exudate may be seen in the peripheral parts of the retina and in diabetic retinopathy similar patches of white exudate may be seen, sometimes associated with microaneurysms, though for the accurate demonstration of the latter, fluorescein retinal angiography may be needed. In cases of recurrent micro-embolism of the retina (say as a consequence of carotid stenosis) it is sometimes possible to visualize micro-emboli of platelets or cholesterol in the smaller retinal arteries. Occlusion of individual arterial branches may occasionally occur in migraine; marked narrowing of all of the retinal arteries with pallor of the fundus can result from central retinal artery occlusion in cranial arteritis. Patchy black pigmentation of the retina may be seen in choroidoretinitis, but longitudinal streaks of pigment lying between the vessels, when accompanied by optic atrophy and attenuation of arteries is typical of retinitis pigmentosa, while similar pigmentary degeneration without changes in the disc and vessels is sometimes observed in various hereditary ataxias. A retinal angioblastoma may sometimes be seen in cases of Lindau's disease and a phakoma in tuberous sclerosis or neurofibromatosis, and in cases of general miliary tuberculosis and tuberculous meningitis tubercles may be seen in the retina as roundish, yellow bodies about half the size of the disc.

LESIONS OF THE OPTIC NERVE

PAPILLOEDEMA (CHOKED DISC)

By papilloedema is meant simply an oedema of the optic papilla or disc, without reference to its underlying cause. Like oedema in other parts of the body, papilloedema may be due to different pathological states, of which the following are the most important:

1. Increased intracranial pressure.
2. Inflammatory conditions of the optic nerve, optic neuritis, and retrobulbar neuritis.
3. Oedema associated with disease of the retinal arteries and retinal exudation, as in malignant hypertension and giant-cell arteritis.
4. Venous obstruction, due to space-occupying lesions in the orbit, thrombosis of the central vein of the retina, some cases of cavernous sinus thrombosis, traumatic arteriovenous aneurysm of the internal carotid artery and the cavernous sinus, intrathoracic venous obstruction, as by neoplasms, aneurysm of the aorta.
5. In conditions associated with a massive increase in the protein content of the cerebrospinal fluid (e.g. some cases of the Guillain-Barré syndrome).
6. Changes in the composition of the blood, as in severe anaemia, erythraemia, and severe emphysema.
7. Obscure causes. Disseminated lupus erythematosus, carcinomatous neuropathy, the reticuloses, infective endocarditis, low intraocular pressure as in uveitis or perforation of the globe, and Graves' disease with severe exophthalmos.

For the study of nervous diseases the papilloedema due to increased intracranial pressure and that associated with optic and retrobulbar neuritis are the forms of greatest importance. The single most useful distinguishing feature is that in papilloedema due to raised pressure, visual failure occurs late if at all, while in oedema due to optic neuritis severe loss of visual acuity is usually the first manifestation.

Papilloedema due to Increased Intracranial Pressure

The optic nerve, which developmentally and histologically is part of the brain, is surrounded like the brain by the three meninges. Immediately covering the nerve is the pia mater and superficially to that the arachnoid, both of which are prolonged forwards to fuse with the sclerotic. Outside both is the dura mater, which is continuous anteriorly with the periosteum of the orbit. The optic nerve, therefore, is surrounded by a subarachnoid space which is continuous with the cerebral subarachnoid space. A rise in the pressure in the cerebrospinal subarachnoid space is freely conducted to the optic subarachnoid space, where it has a double effect, causing compression of the central vein of the retina where it crosses the space, and impeding lymphatic drainage from the retina and optic nerve. The result of this combined venous and lymphatic obstruction is congestion and oedema of the optic disc and retina. Behrman (1966) has also drawn attention to the production of papilloedema by general brain swelling conducted to the optic nerves. The following are the principal causes of increased intracranial pressure leading to papilloedema:

Intracranial Tumour. Not all intracranial tumours cause papilloedema. The presence or absence of this symptom and its severity when present may, therefore, be an aid to the localization of a tumour. Generally speaking, the occurrence of papilloedema depends upon whether the tumour is so placed as to cause a rise in the tension of the cerebrospinal fluid, and also upon its rate of growth. It is almost constantly present at some stage in the case of tumours occupying the temporal lobe, the cerebellum, and the fourth ventricle, but is absent in many cases of subcortical and pontine tumours. It is frequently late in developing when the tumour is in the prefrontal region or arises near the vertex. Posterior fossa tumours give rise to papilloedema of the greatest severity. The more rapidly a tumour grows the more likely is it to cause papilloedema. Inequality of the degree of oedema in the two eyes is not uncommon, but if the difference is not great it is of no localizing value. A tumour arising near one optic foramen tends to prevent the development of papilloedema in that eye by cutting off the optic sheath from communication with the cerebral subarachnoid space. In such cases primary optic atrophy may develop on the side of the tumour and may be associated with papilloedema on the opposite side (syndrome of Gowers, Paton, and Foster Kennedy).

Cerebral Abscess. Papilloedema is inconstant in cerebral abscess and may be late in developing.

Hydrocephalus. Hydrocephalus from any cause may lead to papilloedema, but in some cases the pressure of the distended floor of the third ventricle upon the optic chiasm and nerves causes primary optic atrophy.

Meningitis. Meningitis causes papilloedema less frequently than might be expected, in view of the rise in pressure of the cerebrospinal fluid which occurs in this condition, possibly because meningeal adhesions tend to wall off the optic sheaths. Papilloedema is commonest in tuberculous and other forms of granulomatous meningitis.

Intracranial Sinus Thrombosis. This leads to an increase in the pressure of the cerebrospinal fluid by diminishing its paths of absorption into the intracranial venous system.

Cerebral Oedema. Generalized brain swelling (as after head injury) or focal oedema (as after massive infarction or cerebral haemorrhage) sometimes causes papilloedema. This sign is almost invariable in benign intracranial hypertension, a syndrome of diffuse cerebral oedema of multiple (often unknown) aetiology [p. 227].

Subarachnoid Haemorrhage. Haemorrhage into the subarachnoid space may cause papilloedema, the blood being driven into, and distending, the subarachnoid space of the optic sheaths. The commonest cause is leakage from an intracranial aneurysm.

Some Unusual Causes. Rarely emphysema leads to papilloedema by raising the pressure of the cerebrospinal fluid, as may hypervitaminosis A, and encephalopathy due to hypoparathyroidism.

Ophthalmoscopic Appearances of Papilloedema

In the earliest stage of papilloedema the retinal veins appear congested and the optic disc is pinker than normal. The disc edge appears blurred at its upper and lower margins, and this blurring extends to the nasal side before the temporal.

An increase in the oedema causes filling of the physiological cup, and later the nerve head becomes elevated above the general retinal level, sometimes by as much as 8 or even 10 dioptres. The oedema in severe cases spreads into the retina causing a macular 'fan'. Distension of the retinal veins is extreme, and haemorrhages may be found on the retina and on the disc itself. In severe papilloedema, transient amblyopic episodes or other obscurations of vision may occur, especially on stooping or on coughing, and the patient may see 'haloes' around lights. These symptoms demand urgent measures to reduce the intracranial pressure as they indicate retinal ischaemia due to pressure upon the central retinal artery; if they continue unchecked the artery may be permanently occluded, resulting in irreversible blindness. If chronic papilloedema persists, alternatively the condition progresses to so-called secondary optic atrophy. The swelling of the disc diminishes, and it becomes paler. The arteries become constricted and the perivascular lymph spaces thickened. Finally, in a typical case, the disc is pale and flat, the physiological cup remaining filled, and the edges of the disc being less distinct than formerly. The arteries are constricted, but the veins often remain congested for a considerable time.

The Visual Fields in Papilloedema

In the earlier stages of papilloedema the only change in the visual fields may be enlargement of the blind spots. Later there is concentric constriction of the fields. It should be noted that papilloedema may be associated with other changes in the visual fields due to lesions involving other parts of the visual system.

Pseudopapilloedema: Diagnosis from true Papilloedema. Slight elevation of the optic disc due to increased myelin anterior to the lamina cribrosa is sometimes seen in hypermetropic individuals and is one cause of pseudo-papilloedema. More difficult to distinguish are hyaline bodies or drusen, congenital lesions of no pathological significance which may be buried in the disc and may cause it to be elevated with blurred margins. The absence of venous congestion is a valuable sign in distinguishing this change from true papilloedema but when doubt persists fluorescein retinal angiography (Dollery et al., 1962; Hoyt, 1963; Haining, 1966) is helpful as in true papilloedema this shows swollen and proliferated capillaries around the disc margin and fluorescence in the swollen disc itself.

OPTIC NEURITIS AND RETROBULBAR NEURITIS

The term 'optic neuritis' used to be employed for all conditions associated with oedema of the optic disc, so that 'optic neuritis' was described as a symptom of intracranial tumour. Since neuritis implies inflammation this was a misnomer, and the name is now confined to infective, demyelinating, or toxi-infective conditions of the optic nerve giving acute unilateral or bilateral visual loss. The distinction between optic neuritis and retrobulbar neuritis is based upon an ophthalmoscopic rather than a pathological difference, and is apt to be misleading. If a neuritis of the optic nerve is sufficiently anterior to cause oedema of the disc it is described as optic neuritis or papillitis; if it is more posteriorly situated so that the direct effects of the inflammation are not visible ophthalmoscopically it is called retrobulbar neuritis. This accident of localization is of no pathological import.

Causes of Optic and Retrobulbar Neuritis

Bradley (1968) listed over twenty causes of optic neuritis, including local inflammatory causes (syphilis, orbital cellulitis, sinusitis, and meningitis), demyelination (as in multiple sclerosis and encephalomyelitis), toxic causes (alcohol, tobacco, drugs), metabolic causes (diabetes, vitamin deficiency, anoxia), vascular causes (ischaemia, arteritis), and familial disorders (e.g. Leber's optic atrophy). He suggested that the condition should be subdivided into symptomatic and idiopathic varieties. Bradley and Whitty (1968) pointed out that multiple sclerosis accounts for at least a third of all cases, but many remain completely unexplained, even after prolonged follow-up.

In fact, many of the causes listed are not inflammatory; some of the toxic, metabolic, and familial disorders if untreated go on to give optic atrophy so that the visual failure is irreversible, whereas an episode of this type in multiple sclerosis is usually followed by complete or at least partial recovery of visual acuity. Nevertheless the term optic or retrobulbar neuritis or neuropathy can reasonably be used to identify a syndrome of acute unilateral or bilateral visual loss provided it is recognized that it is one of multiple aetiology, but that multiple sclerosis remains the commonest cause.

Multiple Sclerosis. The optic nerve lesion, which is usually but not always unilateral, may be the first symptom and may precede other manifestations by many years. In other cases other symptoms or signs may have preceded it and may be found on routine examination of the nervous system. Examination of the cerebrospinal fluid may show abnormalities suggestive of multiple sclerosis, especially an abnormal gamma-globulin or colloidal gold curve. The changes in the optic nerve are the same as those of multiple sclerosis elsewhere in the nervous system, namely, demyelination and, later, gliosis. Recovery of vision in such cases is usually complete, but a permanent central scotoma may remain and the size of the scotoma may increase and reading acuity correspondingly diminish in some such cases on exercise or exposure to heat or vasodilator drugs (Uhthoff's symptom). Commonly after recovery, even if complete, there is pallor of the temporal half of the affected disc; measurement of the latency of the visual evoked responses recorded over the occipital region of the intact skull (Halliday et al., 1972; Heron et al., 1974) is a useful means of detecting evidence of a previous attack of retrobulbar neuritis [p. 67].

Disseminated Myelitis with Optic Neuritis (Devic's Disease or Neuro-myelitis Optica). This is a rare disease, closely allied to multiple sclerosis, both clinically and pathologically. Bilateral optic or retrobulbar neuritis is associated with transverse myelitis. Acute bilateral retrobulbar neuritis occurring without other lesions of the nervous system is probably a closely related disorder, but may be a self-limiting disorder akin to encephalomyelitis (Hierons and Lyle, 1959); it sometimes occurs also in multiple sclerosis.

Syphilis. A syphilitic lesion of the optic nerve, with the characteristic endarteritis of the secondary or tertiary stage (Graveson, 1950), is a rare cause of retrobulbar neuritis. Diagnosis with the aid of serological tests and cerebrospinal fluid examination is usually easy.

Zoster. Optic neuritis, going on to atrophy, with complete loss of vision, has been described in ophthalmic herpes zoster.

Orbital Infections. The optic nerve may be involved in inflammation spr
ing directly from the orbit, where it may be secondary to orbital cellu
infection of the nasal air sinuses or dental abscess.

Meningitis and Encephalitis. Infection may spread into the nerve from the
meninges in any form of meningitis, and optic neuritis sometimes occurs in
acute disseminated encephalomyelitis and in Schilder's disease.

Toxic and Metabolic Causes. Tobacco amblyopia, a form of sudden bilateral
visual failure, giving rise as a rule to bilateral centrocaecal scotomas, occurs
usually in middle-aged males who smoke strong pipe tobacco; there is often
evidence of excessive alcohol consumption as well. The syndrome has been
attributed to cyanide in pipe tobacco causing a disorder of vitamin B_{12} metabolism
(Heaton *et al.*, 1958). Freeman and Heaton (1961) suggested that tobacco
smoking might similarly lead to visual failure and optic atrophy in patients
with pernicious anaemia, but a primary dietary deficiency of vitamin B_{12} may
lead to optic atrophy in non-smoking vegans (who eat no meat products),
and in India Wadia *et al.* (1972) found no convincing evidence that vegetarianism,
smoking, or B_{12} deficiency contributed to the aetiology of optic neuritis in
20 cases. Increased dietary consumption of cassava root which contains cyanide
is the probable cause of optic neuritis in tropical ataxic neuropathy in Nigeria
(Williams and Osuntokun, 1969) and a disorder of thiocyanate metabolism
has been postulated as a cause of the acute bilateral optic neuritis which occurs
in Leber's optic atrophy (see below). Hydroxocobalamin has been recommended for the treatment of tobacco amblyopia but seems to be without effect
in Leber's disease. Most of the other toxic causes of acute 'optic neuritis'
(e.g. methyl alcohol) lead to optic atrophy.

Vascular Causes. Sudden unilateral visual loss may result from occlusion of
the central retinal artery (as in cranial arteritis) and as the optic disc may be
swollen this event may be thought to be due to optic neuritis. Acute optic
neuropathy in older patients was found often to be associated with diabetes,
hypertension, and atherosclerosis by Ellenberger, Keltner, and Burde (1973)
and was attributed to ischaemia. Chronic atherosclerotic ischaemia of the optic
nerve and/or anoxia due to severe blood loss or anaemia have also been noted
to give bilateral or unilateral visual loss and low tension glaucoma (Drance
et al., 1973).

Clinical Features of Optic and Retrobulbar Neuritis

Acute optic neuritis leads to pain in and behind the eye on ocular movement
and on pressure. If the inflammation extends to the optic disc it causes papillitis,
with the appearances of papilloedema, though the swelling of the disc is usually
slight, and haemorrhages are uncommon. When the inflammation is confined
to the retrobulbar portion of the nerve the disc appears normal until and if signs
of atrophy appear. This is indicated by pallor of the disc, involving in mild
cases the temporal fibres, in severe cases the whole disc. The physiological cup
is usually restored and the disc edge and vessels appear normal except that in
temporal pallor the temporal margin seems unusually clearly defined.

In inflammation of the optic nerve the macular fibres suffer most, either
because the central part of the nerve is most involved or because, being the most
highly evolved part of the visual afferent system, they are the most susceptible to
damage. In consequence the characteristic visual field defect is a central scotoma,

the loss for red and green objects being greater than that for white. In most cases improvement occurs in a few weeks, but the functional manifestation of the residual atrophy is often a central scotoma, much smaller than that of the acute phase. Helpful points of distinction between optic neuritis with papillitis, and papilloedema due to increased intracranial pressure, are that in the former the swelling of the disc is slight in comparison with the loss of vision, in the latter the reverse is usually the case; and in optic neuritis the usual field defect is a central scotoma, in papilloedema a peripheral concentric constriction.

The so-called retrobulbar pupil reaction may also be helpful; direct light stimulation of the affected eye gives a sluggish reaction while stimulation of the unaffected eye by contrast gives a brisk response in both eyes. Alternatively, in less severe cases, a reasonably brisk direct reaction in the affected eye may be followed by slow pupillary dilatation.

AMAUROSIS FUGAX

Transient monocular blindness, lasting for seconds, minutes, or occasionally for hours, sometimes occurs in migraine or as a consequence of atherosclerosis but is most often due to micro-embolism of the central retinal artery resulting from occlusion or stenosis of the ipsilateral internal carotid artery (Fisher, 1959; Marshall and Meadows, 1968). However, in many patients no cause is ever discovered and in young patients particularly the prognosis may be excellent though the aetiology remains obscure (Eadie et al., 1968).

OPTIC ATROPHY

'Primary' and 'Secondary' Optic Atrophy

As the foregoing sections of this chapter show, optic atrophy may follow a variety of pathological states, and other causes have yet to be mentioned. When the pathology of optic atrophy was less understood a confusing distinction was drawn between 'primary' and 'secondary' optic atrophy. This is purely an ophthalmoscopic distinction, 'secondary' optic atrophy being the term used when atrophy follows some observable change in the optic disc which influences the appearance of the atrophied nerve, and 'primary' atrophy when no such cause is ophthalmoscopically obvious. We now recognize that even the 'primary' atrophies are secondary to some pathological state such as pressure upon, demyelination of, or toxic damage to the optic nerve. The term 'consecutive' optic atrophy is sometimes used when the atrophy is consequent upon retinal lesions.

Causes of Optic Atrophy

Familial Disorders. In these obscure diseases the optic atrophy is probably due to a primary degeneration which affects various parts of the nervous system including the retinae and optic nerves.

1. *Cerebromacular Degeneration.* The infantile form, amaurotic family idiocy or Tay-Sachs disease [see p. 640], is characterized by a lipid degeneration of the ganglion cells of the retina, atrophy of which at the macula is responsible for the cherry-red spot.

In the late infantile and juvenile forms (Batten-Mayou type) the cherry-red spot is absent, but the macula may be pigmented. Macular degeneration may occur also at puberty or early in adult life as an inherited disorder (Behr).

2. *The Hereditary Ataxias* [see p. 669]. In this group of closely related

disorders there is degeneration of various parts of the nervous system, especially of the cerebellum and its tracts. Any form of hereditary ataxia may be associated with optic atrophy. Hereditary spastic paraplegia of early onset with optic atrophy is known as Behr's syndrome.

3. *Retinitis Pigmentosa*. This is an hereditary disease which is inherited in some sibships as a Mendelian dominant, less often as a recessive. It is often associated with nerve deafness and with a family history of epilepsy. There is a characteristic spidery black pigmentation of the periphery of the retina, and the optic disc exhibits a yellowish waxy pallor and much reduction in the calibre of the vessels. The victims of this disease suffer from night-blindness and progressive concentric constriction of the visual fields.

Retinitis pigmentosa is also a feature of the Laurence-Moon-Biedl syndrome.

4. *Leber's Hereditary Optic Atrophy*. This is a rare X-linked recessive disease which affects young males (François, 1961). There is a sudden onset of bilateral visual impairment, usually between the ages of 15 and 30. The fields of vision show central scotomata. Papillitis may be present in the acute stage: later the discs are atrophic. In about one-third of cases vision improves after the initial episode of acute unilateral or bilateral visual loss, only to deteriorate progressively later; occasionally involvement of one eye is followed by a similar episode in the other after days, weeks, or months. In the remaining two-thirds large bilateral central scotomata persist indefinitely with severe impairment of visual acuity. In some patients clinical and pathological evidence suggests involvement not only of the optic nerves but also of other parts of the central nervous system (cerebellum, posterior and lateral columns of the spinal cord) and there is some evidence of an inability to detoxicate cyanide to thiocyanate in such cases (Adams *et al.*, 1966). Wallace (1970) has suggested that viral infection may play a role in some cases.

Consecutive Optic Atrophy. In this group the cause of the optic atrophy is obvious on retinoscopy. It includes the various forms of retinitis and choroidoretinitis, glaucoma, and vascular lesions of the retina, especially obstruction of the central artery.

Secondary Optic Atrophy following Papilloedema. Optic atrophy following papilloedema has already been described [see p. 157].

Optic Atrophy following Acute Optic and Retrobulbar Neuritis. The causes of this are discussed on page 159.

Syphilitic Optic Atrophy. Syphilis once accounted for 40 per cent of cases of optic atrophy but is now a rare cause. This sign, leading to progressive visual loss and sometimes to total blindness, used to be seen in 10 to 15 per cent of cases of tabes dorsalis, was rare in acquired general paresis but occurred in up to 50 per cent of cases of congenital taboparesis. The lesion begins in the superficial fibres of the optic nerve, giving peripheral constriction of the visual fields, but is not due to optochiasmatic arachnoiditis (Bruetsch, 1948). Optic atrophy due to vasculitis or local inflammation occurs rarely in meningovascular syphilis. For details of prognosis and treatment see pages 460 and 463.

Toxic Optic Atrophy. The optic nerve fibres are susceptible to a number of poisons, though their mode and site of action are little understood. Among these are cyanide, lead, arsenic (especially tryparsamide), methyl mercuric iodide, methyl alcohol, carbon bisulphide, thallium, certain insecticides [see p. 960], quinine, and aspidium filix mas. It is uncertain whether methyl alcohol and carbon bisulphide cause degeneration of the retinal ganglion cells or act on the nerve fibres. Tobacco amblyopia [p. 161] seems to be due to cyanide which may produce conditioned vitamin B_{12} deficiency. The optic atrophy which rarely results from isoniazid administration is probably due to vitamin B_6 deficiency, while the retinopathy resulting from sensitivity to chloroquine may be accompanied by pallor of the optic discs. Quinine and aspidium filix mas are said to produce spasm of the retinal arteries and hence retinal atrophy. Ischaemia and anoxia are discussed on pages 162 and 301.

Pressure. Pressure is a common and important cause. In the eye itself it is produced by glaucoma. It may occur in the optic canal, if this is narrowed by bony overgrowth, as in Paget's osteitis, or if a tumour arises from the optic nerve or its sheath, or even as the result of a sclerotic ophthalmic artery. Behind the foramen the commonest cause of pressure is a tumour, either of the hypophysis, or of the craniopharyngeal pouch, or a meningioma arising above the sella turcica or in the olfactory groove, or a glioma of the optic chiasm, of the frontal lobe, or of the tip of the temporal lobe. Pressure may also arise from localized arachnoiditis of the optic chiasm, the distended floor of the third ventricle in obstructive hydrocephalus, from an intracranial aneurysm, or from arteriosclerotic internal carotid arteries. In the diagnosis of pressure upon the optic nerve radiography of the optic foramina is often of value.

Trauma. Primary optic atrophy may occur after head injury, usually in only one eye. The lesion is the immediate result of the blow, and there is often no radiographic evidence of fracture. The eye is usually completely blind, but rarely an incomplete lesion gives a localized visual field defect.

Visual Fields in Optic Atrophy

No generalization can be made about the visual fields in optic atrophy, since they depend entirely upon the cause. After papilloedema there are usually enlargement of the blind spot and peripheral concentric constriction. Retrobulbar neuritis and the toxic amblyopias are usually associated with central scotomas. In tobacco amblyopia the scotoma is centrocaecal. Pressure lesions may produce central scotomata or other partial field defects. It must be remembered, too, that optic atrophy following both papilloedema and pressure upon the optic nerve may indirectly be due to an intracranial lesion which also involves the visual fibres more posteriorly, and itself causes visual field defects.

Prognosis of Optic Nerve Lesions

The prognosis of lesions of the optic nerve depends chiefly upon the extent to which the cause can be removed. When papilloedema is due to increased intracranial pressure, relief of this is usually followed by marked improvement in vision, provided optic atrophy has not already developed. Similarly, improvement in vision often follows rapidly upon the removal of direct pressure upon the optic nerve. A considerable degree of recovery can usually be expected in optic neuritis and retrobulbar neuritis due to multiple sclerosis, and also in sporadic cases of acute bilateral optic and retrobulbar neuritis, though occasionally vision is permanently lost. The outlook is less satisfactory in toxic optic atrophy, though some improvement may occur if exposure to the toxin can be terminated; recovery from tobacco amblyopia is usually satisfactory. Tabetic optic atrophy, when severe enough to cause visual impairment, often progresses in spite of treatment.

Treatment of Optic Nerve Lesions

The treatment of lesions of the optic nerve is primarily that of the causal disorder. Controlled trials of treatment suggest that full doses of prednisone or ACTH given early in cases of acute optic or retrobulbar neuritis may shorten the course of the illness and reduce sequelae.

REFERENCES

ADAMS, J. H., BLACKWOOD, W., and WILSON, J. (1966) Further clinical and pathological observations on Leber's optic atrophy, *Brain*, **89**, 15.

ASHWORTH, B. (1973) *Clinical Neuro-Ophthalmology*, London.

BEHRMAN, S. (1966) Pathology of papilloedema, *Brain*, **89**, 1.

BELL, J. (1931) Hereditary optic atrophy (Leber's disease), *Treasury of Human Inheritance*, vol. ii, part iv, Cambridge.

BRADLEY, W. G. (1968) Symptomatic optic neuritis (aetiological factors in acute optic neuritis), *Diseases of the Nervous System*, **29**, 668.

BRADLEY, W. G., and WHITTY, C. W. M. (1968) Acute optic neuritis: prognosis for development of multiple sclerosis, *J. Neurol. Neurosurg. Psychiat.*, **31**, 10.

BRUETSCH, W. L. (1948) Surgical treatment of syphilitic primary atrophy of the optic nerves (syphilitic optochiasmatic arachnoiditis), *Arch. Ophthal. (Chic.)*, **38**, 735.

DOLLERY, C. T., HODGE, J. V., and ENGEL, M. (1962) Studies of the retinal circulation with fluorescein, *Brit. med. J.*, **2**, 1210.

DRANCE, S. M., MORGAN, R. W., and SWEENEY, V. P. (1973) Shock-induced optic neuropathy: cause of nonprogressive glaucoma, *New Engl. J. Med.*, **288**, 392.

EADIE, M. J., SUTHERLAND, J. M., and TYRER, J. H. (1968) Recurrent monocular blindness of uncertain cause, *Lancet*, **i**, 319.

ELLENBERGER, C., Jun., KELTNER, J. L., and BURDE, R. M. (1973) Acute optic neuropathy in older patients, *Arch. Neurol. (Chic.)*, **28**, 182.

FERGUSON, F. R., and CRITCHLEY, M. (1928–9) Leber's optic atrophy and its relationship with the heredo-familial ataxias, *J. Neurol. Psychopath.*, **9**, 120.

FISHER, C. M. (1959) Observations of the fundus oculi in transient monocular blindness, *Neurology (Minneap.)*, **9**, 333.

FRANÇOIS, J. (1961) *Heredity in Ophthalmology*, p. 500, St. Louis.

FREEMAN, A. G., and HEATON, J. M. (1961) The aetiology of retrobulbar neuritis in Addisonian pernicious anaemia, *Lancet*, **i**, 908.

GRAVESON, G. S. (1950) Syphilitic optic neuritis, *J. Neurol. Neurosurg. Psychiat.*, **13**, 216.

HAINING, W. M. (1966) Diagnostic value of intravenous fluorescein studies, *Brit. J. Ophthal.*, **50**, 587.

HALLIDAY, A. M., McDONALD, W. I., and MUSHIN, J. (1972) Delayed visual evoked response in optic neuritis, *Lancet*, **i**, 982.

HEATON, J. M., McCORMICK, A. J. A., and FREEMAN, A. G. (1958) Tobacco amblyopia: a clinical manifestation of vitamin-B_{12} deficiency, *Lancet*, **ii**, 286.

HERON, J. R., REGAN, D., and MILNER, B. A. (1974) Delay in visual perception in unilateral optic atrophy after retrobulbar neuritis, *Brain*, **97**, 69.

HIERONS, R., and LYLE, T. K. (1959) Bilateral retrobulbar optic neuritis, *Brain*, **82**, 56.

HOYT, W. F. (1963) Neuro-ophthalmology, *Arch. Ophthal.*, **70**, 679.

MARSHALL, J., and MEADOWS, S. (1968) The natural history of amaurosis fugax, *Brain*, **91**, 419.

WADIA, N. H., DESAI, M. M., QUADROS, E. V., and DASTUR, D. K. (1972) Role of vegetarianism, smoking and hydroxocobalamin in optic neuritis, *Brit. med. J.*, **3**, 264.

WALLACE, D. C. (1970) A new manifestation of Leber's disease and a new explanation for the agency responsible for its unusual pattern of inheritance, *Brain*, **93**, 121.

WILLIAMS, A. O., and OSUNTOKUN, B. O. (1969) Peripheral neuropathy in tropical (nutritional) ataxia in Nigeria: light and electron microscopic study, *Arch. Neurol. (Chic.)*, **21**, 475.

THE THIRD, FOURTH, AND SIXTH NERVES

The control of ocular movements, movement of the eyelids, the pupillary reactions, and nystagmus have been considered on pages 75–98.

THIRD-NERVE PARALYSIS

After leaving the nucleus [see p. 79] the fibres of the third nerve sweep outwards and forwards through the medial longitudinal fasciculus, the red nucleus, and the medial margin of the substantia nigra to emerge from the brain stem along the bottom of the sulcus oculomotorius on the medial aspect of the crus cerebri [FIG. 5, p. 19]. The nerve passes forwards between the posterior cerebral and superior cerebellar arteries, close to the posterior communicating artery, and pierces the dura mater beside the posterior clinoid process in a small triangular space between the free and attached borders of the tentorium cerebelli. It then passes through the lateral part of the cavernous sinus, where it lies close to the fourth and sixth nerves and the first division of the fifth, and enters the orbit through the superior orbital fissure between the two heads of the lateral rectus muscle. Here it divides into two branches, the upper supplying the levator palpebrae and the superior rectus, and the lower the medial and inferior recti and the inferior oblique, the nerve to which supplies the short root to the ciliary ganglion.

Paralysis of the third nerve causes ptosis, complete internal ophthalmoplegia, and paralysis of the superior, medial, and inferior recti, and inferior oblique. The pupil is widely dilated owing to paralysis of the sphincter pupillae and the unantagonized action of the dilator, and fails to react. Accommodation is paralysed. The unantagonized lateral rectus causes outward deviation of the eye, and the only possible ocular movements are abduction, carried out by the lateral rectus, and a movement of depression, internal rotation, and abduction by the superior oblique. Paralysis of the levator palpebrae superioris causes ptosis of the upper lid, and the resulting closure of the eye masks the diplopia, which becomes evident to the patient when the lid is passively raised [FIG. 21].

Although lesions of the third nerve usually cause both external and internal ophthalmoplegia, it may happen that in a partial lesion the iridoconstrictor fibres escape, or that in recovery from a complete lesion the intrinsic fibres may recover before the extrinsic. When both the third nerve and the ocular sympathetic are injured, as may happen with a lesion just behind the orbit, the pupil is not dilated but is fixed in the mid-position and unreacting. As the pupillo-constrictor fibres and those innervating the levator palpebrae lie superficially in the trunk of the nerve, a fixed dilated pupil is often the first sign of third nerve compression and ptosis the second, before external ophthalmoplegia develops (Sunderland and Hughes, 1946).

FOURTH-NERVE PARALYSIS

The fibres of the fourth nerve after leaving the nucleus turn backwards through the peri-aqueductal grey matter on the medial aspect of the mesencephalic root of the trigeminal nerve, and then downwards and medially to decussate in the anterior medullary velum, whence the nerve emerges just behind the colliculi. It then passes round the cerebral peduncle, lying between the peduncle and the temporal lobe, and pierces the free border of the tentorium cerebelli lateral to the third nerve to enter the lateral wall of the cavernous sinus. It enters the orbit through the superior orbital fissure above the ocular muscles and terminates in the superior oblique. A lesion of the fourth nerve causes paralysis of this muscle with weakness of downward and outward movement of

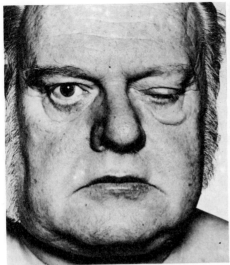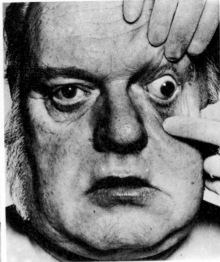

FIG. 21. A left third nerve palsy in a diabetic subject who also had a carcinoma of the left ethmoid sinus (figure kindly supplied by Dr. J. D. Spillane). Note the ptosis and the abduction of the eye due to the unopposed action of the lateral rectus

the eye. For the character of the resulting diplopia, see page 78. When the lesion involves the nucleus or the fibres of the nerve within the midbrain before their decussation, the paralysis of the superior oblique is on the opposite side to the lesion. When the nerve is damaged in its extracerebral course the paralysis is ipsilateral.

SIXTH-NERVE PARALYSIS

The fibres of the sixth nerve, after leaving the nucleus just below the floor of the fourth ventricle, pass forwards through the pons to emerge at its inferior border above the lateral side of the pyramid of the medulla. It has a long extracerebral course along the base of the brain and over the apex of the petrous temporal bone before it pierces the dura mater of the posterior fossa, just below the dorsum sellae. Like the third and fourth nerves, it lies in the lateral wall of the cavernous sinus, whence it passes through the superior orbital fissure to terminate in the lateral rectus muscle. A lesion of the sixth nerve causes paralysis of this muscle with loss of abduction of the eye, which is deviated inwards by the unantagonized medial rectus [FIG. 22]. For the character of the resulting diplopia, see page 78.

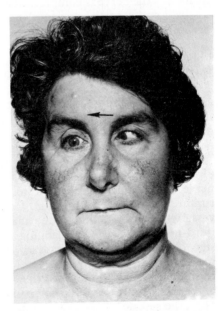

FIG. 22. A right sixth nerve palsy, evident on right lateral gaze (from *An Atlas of Clinical Neurology*, 2nd ed., 1975, by J. D. Spillane, reproduced by kind permission of the author)

CAUSES OF PARALYSIS OF THE THIRD, FOURTH, AND SIXTH NERVES

The third, fourth, and sixth nerves may be damaged singly or together, and on one or both sides.

Within the brain stem their nuclei or intracerebral fibres may be damaged by trauma, neoplasms, vascular lesions, encephalitis, poliomyelitis, or multiple sclerosis, and in the case of the sixth nerve, syringobulbia. Congenital aplasia of the nuclei may cause bilateral ptosis, absence of elevation of the eyes, or lateral rectus paralysis with or without facial paralysis (Moebius syndrome).

Duane's syndrome is a name which has been given to a benign congenital abnormality of ocular movement, commoner in females and often familial, in which there is impaired abduction of the eye; on attempted adduction there is retraction of the globe and narrowing of the palpebral fissure. The condition seems to be due to fibrous replacement of the lateral rectus muscle; though the condition resembles a sixth nerve palsy, there is probably no abnormality of the sixth nerve or its nucleus.

Intracranial tumour may cause direct compression of the nerves at any point in their course, but, in addition, *increased intracranial pressure* due to intracranial tumour or abscess remote from the nerves, or to hydrocephalus, may indirectly impair their conductivity. The sixth nerve most often suffers in this way, and sixth-nerve paralysis may occur as a false localizing sign of a tumour in any situation. Supratentorial tumours probably cause this by displacing the brain stem downwards and so stretching the nerve across the petrous apex. The third nerve may also suffer, especially with tumours of the temporal lobe. In such cases the nerve is compressed as it traverses the free edge of the tentorium cerebelli and a partial or complete third-nerve palsy is an important warning sign of herniation of the temporal lobe through the tentorial hiatus; a fixed dilated pupil may be an important early sign. The fourth nerve escapes. An isolated third-nerve palsy is an occasional sign of a rapidly expanding *chromophobe adenoma of the pituitary* [see p. 277].

Neoplastic infiltration of the meninges may compress the nerves in their passage across the base of the skull and through the dura mater. Such meningeal metastases may be due to extension of a primary growth in the nasopharynx, or there may be diffuse carcinomatosis of the meninges due to metastasis from a tumour elsewhere, e.g. in the lung, breast, stomach, or prostate.

Intracranial aneurysm, especially when arising near the circle of Willis, may directly compress one or more of the oculomotor nerves, especially the third nerve, or they may be subjected to pressure by extravasated blood or clot after rupture of the aneurysmal sac. Compression may also arise from a normal vessel which is congenitally abnormal in position (Sunderland, 1948). A unilateral third-nerve palsy, often developing rapidly with pain behind the eye, is a common sign of a supraclinoid aneurysm of the internal carotid or posterior communicating arteries. An infraclinoid aneurysm of the internal carotid, by contrast, lying within the walls of the cavernous sinus, more often causes paralysis of the third, fourth, and sixth nerves, and involvement of the first division of the fifth; the second division of the fifth nerve, which passes through the inferior part of the sinus, sometimes, but not invariably, escapes.

Ophthalmoplegic migraine is the term applied to cases of recurrent third- or sixth-nerve palsies, the onset of which is associated with severe headache, and which tend to recover in the course of days or weeks, only to relapse subsequently, sometimes becoming permanent. The relationship of this condition to true migraine is doubtful [see p. 304].

Inflammatory disorders of the meninges may involve any or all of the oculo-motor nerves, most often the third and the sixth. Sixth-nerve palsies are common in some severe cases of *pyogenic meningitis*, whereas unilateral or bilateral third- or sixth-nerve palsies may also develop in *meningovascular syphilis*, in *tuberculous or cryptococcal meningitis*, or in *sarcoidosis*.

Osteitis of the base of the skull and particularly of the apex of the petrous temporal bone due to otitis media may give a unilateral sixth-nerve palsy; there is often thrombosis of the inferior petrosal sinus. In this condition (Gradenigo's syndrome) there may also be facial pain and paraesthesiae due to involvement of the Gasserian ganglion.

A transient third- or sixth-nerve palsy may be due to a misplaced alcohol injection intended for the Gasserian ganglion and is an occasional complication of *spinal anaesthesia*.

Polyneuritis cranialis is a term which has been used to identify a syndrome of multiple unilateral or bilateral cranial-nerve palsies, often involving the third, fourth, and sixth nerves as well as others. Certainly any form of polyneuropathy, and particularly that of diphtheria or the Guillain–Barré syndrome, may involve the cranial nerves as well as the limbs and occasionally cranial nerves only are involved, as may also be the case in cephalic tetanus. Usually the cerebrospinal fluid protein content is raised. It is, however, important to exclude in such cases other causes of multiple cranial-nerve palsies (e.g. nasopharyngeal carcinoma). Rarely multiple recurrent cranial-nerve palsies occur and are unexplained (Symonds, 1958).

Vascular lesions of the oculomotor nerves are not uncommon, especially in diabetes and in other individuals with hypertension and atherosclerosis. An isolated painless third- or sixth-nerve palsy is the most usual presentation, often followed by complete recovery in three to six months; in some patients attacks of ophthalmoplegia recur and facial pain has also been described (Currie, 1970). Pathological evidence indicates that these attacks are usually due to ischaemic infarction of the trunk of the nerve (Dreyfus et al., 1957; Weber et al., 1970; Asbury et al., 1970). *Thrombosis of the cavernous sinus* may also damage the third, fourth, and sixth nerves, and these nerves can also be contused or divided in their intracranial course by *head injury*.

Finally, *orbital lesions* must be considered. A syndrome of the superior orbital fissure, or so-called painful ophthalmoplegia, has been attributed to orbital periostitis or to granulomatous vasculitis in the cavernous sinus (the Tolosa–Hunt syndrome). It is characterized by pain in the eye and by the development of a unilateral third-, fourth-, and sixth-nerve palsy, often with involvement of the first division of the fifth. The erythrocyte sedimentation rate is usually raised and there is a rapid response to prednisone. Orbital tumours or pseudo-tumour due to orbital granuloma of multiple aetiology (Jellinek, 1969) may also give ophthalmoplegia, as may ophthalmic Graves's disease and *paranasal sinusitis* (Dimsdale and Phillips, 1950). A mucocele of the ethmoid sinus may give asymmetrical painless proptosis and ophthalmoplegia; carcinoma of the paranasal sinuses will give a similar picture but with considerable local pain.

TREATMENT OF LESIONS OF THE OCULOMOTOR NERVES

Treatment is primarily that of the causal condition. When diplopia is present the patient may be helped by wearing a shade or a frosted glass in front of the eye. Orthoptic exercises are helpful during the recovery phase and it is sometimes possible to diminish diplopia by the use of a prism.

REFERENCES

ASBURY, A. K., ALDREDGE, H., HERSHBERG, R., and FISHER, C. M. (1970) Oculomotor palsy in diabetes mellitus: a clinico-pathological study, *Brain*, **93,** 555.

COGAN, D. G. (1966) *Neurology of the Visual System*, Springfield, Ill.

CURRIE, S. (1970) Familial oculomotor palsy with Bell's palsy, *Brain*, **93,** 193.

DIMSDALE, H., and PHILLIPS, D. G. (1950) Ocular palsies with nasal sinusitis, *J. Neurol. Neurosurg. Psychiat.*, **13,** 225.

DREYFUS, P. M., HAKIM, S., and ADAMS, R. D. (1957) Diabetic ophthalmoplegia, *Arch. Neurol. Psychiat.*, **77,** 337.

JELLINEK, E. H. (1969) The orbital pseudotumour syndrome and its differentiation from endocrine exophthalmos, *Brain*, **92,** 35.

LYLE, T. K., and JACKSON, S. (1949) *Practical Orthoptics in the Treatment of Squint*, 3rd ed., London.

SPILLANE, J. D. (1975) *An Atlas of Clinical Neurology*, 2nd ed., London.

SUNDERLAND, S. (1948) Neurovascular relations and anomalies at the base of the brain, *J. Neurol. Neurosurg. Psychiat.*, **11,** 243.

SUNDERLAND, S., and HUGHES, E. S. R. (1946) The pupillo-constrictor pathway and the nerves to the ocular muscles in man, *Brain*, **69,** 301.

SYMONDS, C. (1958) Recurrent multiple cranial nerve palsies, *J. Neurol. Neurosurg. Psychiat.*, **21,** 95.

WALSH, F. B., and HOYT, W. F. (1969) *Clinical Neuroophthalmology*, 3rd ed., Baltimore.

WEBER, R. B., DAROFF, R. B., and MACKEY, E. A. (1970) Pathology of oculomotor nerve palsy in diabetics, *Neurology (Minneap.)*, **20,** 835.

THE FIFTH OR TRIGEMINAL NERVE

PERIPHERAL DISTRIBUTION

The fifth nerve contains both motor and sensory fibres. It is the principal sensory cranial nerve and represents a fusion of the sensory nerves of a number of metameric segments. It arises from the inferior surface of the pons on its lateral aspect by two roots, a large sensory root and a small motor root. The two roots pass forwards in the posterior fossa and, piercing the dura mater beneath the attachment of the tentorium to the tip of the petrous part of the temporal bone, enter a cavity in the dura mater overlying the apex of the petrous bone. Here the sensory root expands to form the trigeminal or Gasserian ganglion, which contains the ganglion cells of the sensory fibres and is homologous with the dorsal root ganglia of the spinal nerves. The ganglion gives rise to three large nerve trunks, which constitute the three divisions of the trigeminal nerve, namely the ophthalmic or first division, the maxillary or second, and the

FIG. 23. The cutaneous distribution of the trigeminal nerve and its branches (from *Neurological Anatomy in Relationship to Clinical Medicine* by A. Brodal, 2nd ed., 1969, reproduced by kind permission of the author). ST = supratrochlear nerve, IT = intratrochlear nerve, NC = nasociliary nerve

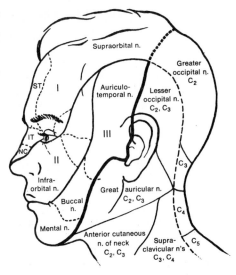

mandibular or third [FIG. 23]. The motor root of the nerve passes forwards beneath the ganglion and becomes fused with the third division.

THE OPHTHALMIC NERVE

The ophthalmic nerve, after lying in the lateral wall of the cavernous sinus together with the third, fourth, and sixth nerves, enters the orbit through the superior orbital fissure. It supplies the skin of the face and scalp, as follows: a narrow zone adjacent to the midline throughout the length of the nose; the upper eyelid and the scalp from the base of the nose and the eyelid as far back as the lambdoidal suture in the midline and for about 8 cm laterally to this. The first division also supplies sensory fibres to the eye, including the conjunctiva and the cornea, to the iris, and to the mucous membrane of the frontal sinuses and the upper part of the nose.

THE MAXILLARY NERVE

The maxillary nerve, after leaving the trigeminal ganglion, passes through the inferior part of the cavernous sinus and then via the foramen rotundum into the sphenopalatine fossa. Here it is joined by postganglionic parasympathetic fibres from the sphenopalatine ganglion which are secretory to the lacrimal gland. It enters the orbit as the infra-orbital nerve through the inferior orbital fissure, and then passing through the infra-orbital canal reaches the face through the infra-orbital foramen. It supplies the skin of the upper lip as far as the midline and the skin of the cheek between the area on the nose supplied by the ophthalmic nerve and a line passing upwards and slightly outwards from the angle of the mouth, crossing the zygoma about midway between the outer canthus of the eye and the ear, and continuing upwards to join the lateral boundary of the area of supply of the first division on the scalp, about the middle of the temporal ridge. The maxillary division also supplies the mucous membrane of the maxillary sinus and of the lower part of the nose, together with the mucous membrane of the upper lip, the hard palate, and the soft palate, except its posterior aspect, together with the teeth of the upper jaw.

THE MANDIBULAR NERVE

The mandibular nerve is formed by a fusion of the third division of the trigeminal ganglion with the motor root. These two roots pass out of the skull by the foramen ovale and unite to form a single trunk in the infratemporal fossa. The mandibular nerve supplies the skin of the lower lip and chin, together with a zone of the cheek about 2·5 cm wide laterally to the lateral boundary of the cutaneous supply of the maxillary nerve and bounded below by the border of the area supplied by the cervical plexus. Above this its distribution includes the tympanic membrane, the external auditory meatus, and the skin of the temple, where its distribution is bounded anteriorly by the lateral border of the second division, above by the lateral border of the first division, and behind by a line drawn upwards from the external meatus to the vertex in the region of the lambdoid suture. Anatomical and embryological evidence indicates supply of the tragus and upper part of the pinna by the auriculotemporal branch of the mandibular division. Clinical evidence suggests that there is some variation in precise distribution and the possibility of overlap cannot be excluded. In addition to this cutaneous area the mandibular nerve supplies the mucous membrane of the cheek, lower jaw, floor of the mouth, and anterior two-thirds of the tongue, and the teeth of the lower jaw. From the chorda tympani taste fibres pass to the anterior two-thirds of the tongue by the lingual nerve, which is a branch of the mandibular nerve; postganglionic parasympathetic fibres destined via the submaxillary ganglion for the submaxillary and sublingual glands also travel in this nerve. Meningeal branches from the trigeminal nerve supply the dura mater of the greater part of the skull above the tentorium and of the tentorium itself.

The cervical plexus supplies a zone of the cheek about 2·5 cm wide overlying the angle of the jaw.

THE MOTOR ROOT

The motor root of the trigeminal nerve innervates the following muscles: the temporal, the masseter, the medial and lateral pterygoids, the anterior belly of the digastric and the mylohyoid muscle, the tensor tympani, and the tensor veli palatini.

CENTRAL CONNECTIONS

The motor nucleus of the trigeminal nerve lies in the lateral part of the tegmental portion of the pons. The mesencephalic root is probably also motor. Incoming sensory fibres of the trigeminal divide, some passing into the principal sensory nucleus, which is situated in the substantia gelatinosa in the lateral part of the pontine tegmentum, while others turn downwards to form the spinal tract which descends on the lateral side of the substantia gelatinosa. As the spinal tract passes downwards its fibres gradually terminate in the substantia gelatinosa which constitutes its terminal nucleus, the nucleus of the spinal tract. In a sense, therefore, the trigeminal sensory nucleus consists of two parts, the nucleus spongiosus or principal nucleus which is like an upward extension of the stratum spongiosum of the cord, receiving impulses from the posterior columns, and the nucleus gelatinosus corresponding to an upward extension of the substantia gelatinosa of the dorsal horn of grey matter of the cord. Both the spinal tract and its nucleus end in the upper part of the spinal cord at about the level of the second spinal nerve. The sensory fibres entering the principal sensory nucleus are concerned with tactile and postural sensibility. From this nucleus relay fibres cross the midline and form the quintothalamic tract or trigeminal lemniscus at the inner end of the medial lemniscus. The descending fibres of the spinal tract are concerned with the appreciation of pain and thermal sensibility and with the convergence and co-ordination of stimuli arising in areas of overlapping innervation on the surface of the head supplied by the fifth, seventh, and tenth cranial nerves and the second and third cervical sensory roots (Denny-Brown and Yanagisawa, 1973). Fibres from the ophthalmic division end in the lowest part of the spinal nucleus, fibres from the mandibular division in the highest part, and those from the maxillary division intermediately so that 'representation' of cutaneous sensation on the face is inverted. Relay fibres from this nucleus cross the midline and pass upwards in close relationship with the medial lemniscus to join the spinothalamic tract in the pons [see p. 45].

LESIONS OF THE TRIGEMINAL NERVE

PERIPHERAL LESIONS

The nerve may be involved between the pons and the trigeminal ganglion in inflammatory lesions such as subacute or chronic meningitis, or it may be compressed by a tumour or an aneurysm. This part of the nerve commonly undergoes degeneration in tabes. In the trigeminal ganglion it may be compressed by a tumour of the ganglion itself, or by a meningioma or acoustic neuroma arising in its neighbourhood, or damaged by fracture of the base of the skull involving the middle fossa. With the sixth nerve it may be involved in inflammation spreading from the petrous bone in mastoiditis to the inferior petrosal sinus— Gradenigo's syndrome. Inflammation of the ganglion occurs in trigeminal herpes zoster. Like the third, fourth, and sixth nerves [p. 168], its upper two divisions may be damaged after leaving the ganglion by lesions in the cavernous sinus or its first division in the superior orbital fissure, and more peripherally still its divisions and their major branches may be injured as a result of fracture of the bones of the face; this is particularly true of the supraorbital and infra-orbital nerves. Lesions of the nerve often cause pain, which is referred to the cutaneous area of its distribution, and may be associated with cutaneous anaesthesia and analgesia. When the nerve is involved between the pons and the ganglion, all three divisions are likely to be affected, but lesions involving the ganglion itself may lead to symptoms which are confined to one division, most frequently the first. Lesions of the motor root cause weakness and wasting of the muscles of mastication on the affected side. Wasting of the temporal muscle and of the masseter leads to hollowing above and below the zygoma, and, when the patient is made to clench his teeth, palpation reveals that contraction of these muscles is less vigorous than on the normal side. When the mouth is opened, the jaw deviates to the paralysed side as a result of the unantagonized action of the lateral pterygoid on the opposite side.

CENTRAL LESIONS

The central connections of the trigeminal nerve may be involved in lesions, especially tumours, syringobulbia, and vascular lesions, affecting the pons, medulla, and uppermost cervical segments of the spinal cord. A plaque of demyelination may occur at the point of entry of the sensory root into the brain stem in multiple sclerosis so that trigeminal neuralgia or unilateral facial sensory loss involving all modalities of sensation, subsequently remitting, are among the less common manifestations of this disease. The motor nucleus may be affected by a lesion in the lateral part of the tegmentum of the pons, in which case weakness of the muscles of mastication is usually associated with paresis of the lateral rectus and facial paresis on the affected side. Owing to the divergence of the sensory fibres of the trigeminal nerve within the brain stem, dissociation of sensibility over the face commonly results from central lesions. A lesion of the pons which involves the principal sensory nucleus will cause anaesthesia to light touch over the trigeminal distribution, with preservation of appreciation of pain, heat, and cold. On the other hand, lesions involving the medulla and the upper cervical segments of the spinal cord, by injuring the spinal tract and its nucleus, will cause analgesia and thermo-anaesthesia, with preservation of sensibility to light touch and sometimes severe and persistent spontaneous pain referred to the trigeminal area. This latter dissociation is characteristic of syringobulbia and of the lateral medullary syndrome due to thrombosis of one vertebral or posterior inferior cerebellar artery. Since the first division of the nerve is represented lowest and the third division highest in the nucleus of the spinal tract a lesion of the lowest part of the medulla will cause analgesia limited to the first and second divisions only. Syringobulbia, however, leads to a characteristic progressive advance of the border of the analgesia, which begins posteriorly and gradually converges upon the tip of the nose and the upper lip, these being usually the last places to lose painful sensibility.

A lesion of the pons may also cause analgesia and thermo-anaesthesia on the opposite side of the face through damage to the crossed trigeminothalamic tract.

NEUROPATHIC KERATITIS

Neuropathic keratitis is a degenerative lesion of the cornea which may follow a lesion of the fifth nerve in any part of its course, including the pons, provided corneal analgesia results. It may occur as a complication of any lesion of the nerve, but was often seen in the past after alcohol injection of the trigeminal ganglion. It is probably due to trauma to the insensitive cornea and can usually be avoided by the use of protective drops or, if necessary, tarsorrhaphy. The corneal surface becomes hazy; if unchecked loss of the surface epithelium, ulceration, and secondary infection may develop.

TRIGEMINAL NEURALGIA

Synonym. Tic douloureux.

Definition. A disorder characterized by paroxysmal brief attacks of severe pain within the distribution of one or more divisions of the trigeminal nerve usually without evidence of organic disease of the nerve.

AETIOLOGY, INCIDENCE, AND PATHOLOGY

The aetiology of the condition is unknown (Penman, 1968). While the typical syndrome is rarely a presenting symptom of multiple sclerosis (Harris, 1926) or develops during the course of this disease, which is therefore the commonest cause of the condition in young patients, and while it may rarely develop in patients with ipsilateral or contralateral tumours in the posterior fossa (Hamby, 1947), in which case traction on the sensory root is postulated as a possible cause, most cases are 'idiopathic'. The condition is slightly commoner in females than males and usually develops after the age of 50 years, not uncommonly in those over 70. There is a slightly greater familial incidence (2 per cent) than could be accounted for by chance, and rarely the condition may be bilateral. Traction upon the sensory root of the nerve, non-specific inflammation of the ganglion, dental malocclusion (Carney, 1967), and ischaemia have all been postulated as the cause, but this is a disease without a known pathology. Kugelberg and Lindblom (1959) suggest that the pain is due to central dysfunction in the brain stem in structures related to the spinal nucleus of the fifth nerve; this could be comparable to a disorder of the spinal cord 'gating' mechanism [p. 39].

SYMPTOMS

The characteristic feature of trigeminal neuralgia is the occurrence of brief, lancinating paroxysms of pain, which are usually for a long time confined to the distribution of one division of the nerve. The second and third divisions are the site of the pain with approximately equal frequency. The first division is rarely affected and then usually only after the second division has been involved. Whether the pain first involves the second or third division, it usually in the course of time spreads to the other of the two lower divisions. In a small proportion of cases it is bilateral, though rarely from the onset. By definition, there is freedom from pain between paroxysms, though a slight background ache is occasionally present, the pain is confined to the cutaneous distribution of the trigeminal nerve, does not cross the midline, and may be precipitated by more than one 'trigger' (see below).

In an attack the pain is usually most intense in, and may be confined to, part of the region supplied by the affected division. Thus it may be most marked in the cheek, the upper jaw, the lower jaw, or the tongue. It tends to spread, however, through the rest of the divisional area. It is usually described as burning or stabbing. One of the most striking features of the attacks is that they tend to be precipitated by chill, by touching the face, as in washing or shaving, by talking, mastication, and swallowing. Many patients describe 'trigger zones', touching of which will invariably excite an attack. The attacks are always brief and do not last longer than one or two minutes. The pain is very severe and during the attack the patient may be in agony. The pain often reflexly evokes spasm of the muscles of the face on the affected side, hence the term 'tic douloureux'. Flushing of the skin, lacrimation, and salivation may also occur.

In trigeminal neuralgia there is no reduction of sensibility over the distribution of the nerve. So-called trophic changes in the skin have been described, but probably these are the result of the patient rubbing the face during the attack or of remedies applied in his attempts to relieve the pain. The attacks may interfere with the taking of food, and the recurrence of severe pain over a long period tends to cause loss of weight and depression. Fortunately the attacks usually cease at night, though they sometimes awaken the patient from sleep. Long remissions of pain, lasting weeks or months, are the rule in the early stages.

DIAGNOSIS

There is usually little difficulty in diagnosis if attention is paid to the cardinal symptoms, especially the paroxysmal character of the attacks with freedom from pain in the intervals, the factors which precipitate them, and the absence of signs of an organic lesion of the nerve. In the rare cases in which this syndrome is associated with organic disease, for example, multiple sclerosis or tumour of the eighth nerve, other signs of these disorders are usually present. It is important to distinguish trigeminal neuralgia from the pain due to a gross lesion of the nerve, especially compression by a tumour. In such cases the pain is more persistent and is usually associated with impairment of sensibility in the distribution of the nerve, and weakness of the muscles supplied by the motor root is often present. Trigeminal pain may follow lesions of the central connections of the nerve within the brain stem, for example, lateral medullary infarction or syringobulbia. In such cases, however, other signs of a brain stem lesion are present. Post-herpetic pain of trigeminal distribution is distinguished by the history of the zoster eruption, which leaves characteristic residual cutaneous scars, by the persistence of the pain, and by the impairment of sensibility. Tabes dorsalis is an occasional cause of paroxysmal attacks of pain within the trigeminal area. The characteristic signs of tabes, however, render the diagnosis of the cause of the pain easy. Attacks of similar neuralgic pain confined to the distribution of the supraorbital and infraorbital nerves sometimes occur and may be similar in aetiology to the more fully developed syndrome, or else they may be due to local irritative lesions of the respective nerves in or near their foramina of exit from the skull, in which case there may be local tenderness over the upper margin of the orbit or maxilla. Costen's syndrome (pain radiating into the lower jaw and temple on chewing) may resemble trigeminal neuralgia but is provoked only by chewing and no other trigger; this often results from temporomandibular arthrosis and dental malocclusion and may be relieved by building up the bite.

Referred pain is extremely common within the trigeminal distribution, and possible causes of this must always be excluded. Frontal sinusitis and infection of the maxillary sinus tend to cause pain which is referred to the areas of the first and second divisions respectively. In such cases there may be oedema of the tissues overlying the infected air sinus and in addition to tenderness of the supraorbital and infra-orbital nerves the bone also is tender. Radiography of the sinuses, and examination of the nose may be necessary to establish the diagnosis. Similar facial pain may result from malignant disease of the head and neck. Diseases of the eye may cause severe referred pain, especially glaucoma, in which the pain is referred to the temple. Examination of the eye immediately reveals the cause of the trouble. The teeth are a common source of referred pain. In addition to dental caries, which is easily detected, pain may be due to a peri-apical abscess or to an unerupted wisdom tooth. In case of doubt, radiograms of the teeth should be taken. Pain provoked by hot or cold fluids or food is usually of dental origin. Severe pain in the lower jaw developing on exertion is sometimes experienced in angina of effort.

Psychogenic pain in the face may lead to diagnostic difficulties. In this syndrome of so-called atypical facial neuralgia, which most often occurs in young and middle-aged women, the pain is dull and constant, often occurring unilaterally in the upper jaw (though it may spread to other parts of the head and neck) and there are usually associated manifestations of chronic anxiety and depression. It fails to conform to the characteristics either of trigeminal neuralgia or of any form of pain due to an organic disease, signs of which are absent, nor does it respond to analgesic drugs. Some improvement is often achieved with antidepressive and tranquillizing remedies.

Migrainous neuralgia ('cluster headache') causes severe paroxysmal pain within the trigeminal distribution [p. 309], but is distinguished from trigeminal neuralgia by its periodicity, the absence of precipitating factors, and the much longer duration of each paroxysm.

PROGNOSIS

Spontaneous recovery from trigeminal neuralgia is rare. The interval between the bouts of pain may be long, remissions lasting months or even years. As a rule, however, once the disorder is established attacks follow each other fairly frequently and the intervals between them become shorter. Trigeminal neuralgia caused by multiple sclerosis may cease spontaneously.

TREATMENT

The most effective drug is carbamazepine (*Tegretol*) in doses of 200 mg three or four times daily depending upon tolerance (Blom, 1962; Campbell *et al.*, 1966; Killian and Fromm, 1968). This drug, an anticonvulsant chemically related to the phenytoins, is remarkably effective in the great majority of cases, but it causes dizziness and nausea in some patients and in others skin rashes and leucopenia develop and occasionally necessitate withdrawal. Usually after a few weeks or months of treatment the drug can be withdrawn but may have to be reintroduced if the pain recurs.

For patients who do not respond or who are intolerant of carbamazepine, injection or surgical treatment may be required. When pain is limited to the distribution of the supraorbital or infraorbital nerves, alcohol or phenol injection or surgical division of these nerves sometimes gives relief for months or years. Pain in the distribution of the third division, too, is occasionally relieved by the provision of improved dentures or by injection of the inferior dental nerve. If these relatively minor measures fail, then it is necessary to consider alcohol injection of the Gasserian ganglion (Harris, 1926, 1937, 1938) or surgical division of the sensory root intracranially. Surgical treatment is usually to be preferred in younger patients, first because pain may return after alcohol injection in 1–3 years and secondly because with injection in the hands of the inexperienced it may be difficult to spare the cornea. Hence many workers reserve alcohol or phenol injection of the ganglion for use in the elderly, though the method using radiological control devised by Penman (1949, 1950), though time-consuming, is very effective and gives long-lasting relief in experienced hands. The surgical operation usually employed is partial extradural division of the sensory root, approached via the middle fossa; care is taken, when appropriate, to spare the corneal fibres. Some surgeons prefer an approach via the posterior fossa but this operation is more hazardous. Division of the spinal tract of the nerve in the medulla (Sjöqvist, 1937) and decompression of the sensory root and ganglion (Woolsey, 1955) are now outmoded. An occasional troublesome sequel of the operation is dull aching pain in the anaesthetic area (anaesthesia dolorosa) but in most cases the operation is successful and relief permanent. It is, however, important to warn the patient in advance that the affected side of the face will be permanently numb, and before operation is performed it is important to be sure that the pain is severe enough to justify this inevitable consequence.

TRIGEMINAL NEUROPATHY

This term has been used by Spillane and Wells (1959) to describe a disorder characterized by 'persistent sensory disturbance of the face, usually numbness

G

in the territory of one or more divisions of the trigeminus'. Pain may occur, and in one case there was trophic ulceration of the nose. Hughes (1958) found at operation on similar cases evidence of a chronic inflammatory process causing atrophy of the sensory root and Ashworth and Tait (1971) described persistent unilateral facial sensory loss in cases of progressive systemic sclerosis and systemic lupus erythematosus. A similar picture in Sjögren's syndrome (keratoconjunctivitis sicca) has been described (Kaltreider and Talal, 1969), but Blau *et al.* (1969) have shown that many such cases remain unexplained and run a benign course. As already mentioned, a transient trigeminal neuropathy is sometimes seen in multiple sclerosis.

REFERENCES

ASHWORTH, B., and TAIT, G. B. W. (1971) Trigeminal neuropathy in connective tissue disease, *Neurology (Minneap.)*, **21**, 609.

BLAU, J. N., HARRIS, M., and KENNETT, S. (1969) Trigeminal sensory neuropathy, *New Engl. J. Med.*, **281**, 873.

BLOM, S. (1962) Trigeminal neuralgia; its treatment with a new anticonvulsant drug (G32883), *Lancet*, **ii,** 839.

BRODAL, A. (1969) *Neurological Anatomy in Relation to Clinical Medicine*, 2nd ed., Oxford.

CAMPBELL, F. G., GRAHAM, T. G., and ZILKHA, K. J. (1966) Clinical trial of carbamazepine (Tegretol) in trigeminal neuralgia, *J. Neurol. Neurosurg. Psychiat.*, **29**, 265.

CARNEY, L. R. (1967) Considerations on the cause and treatment of trigeminal neuralgia, *Neurology (Minneap.)*, **17**, 1143.

DANDY, W. E. (1929) An operation for the cure of tic douloureux, *Arch. Surg.*, **18**, 687.

DENNY-BROWN, D., and YANAGISAWA, N. (1973) The function of the descending root of the fifth nerve, *Brain*, **96**, 783.

FRAZIER, C. H. (1925) Subtotal resection of sensory root for relief of major trigeminal neuralgia, *Arch. Neurol. Psychiat. (Chic.)*, **13**, 378.

GOLDSTEIN, N. P., GIBILISCO, J. A., and RUSHTON, J. G. (1963) Trigeminal neuropathy and neuritis, *J. Amer. med. Ass.*, **184**, 458.

HAMBY, W. B. (1947) Trigeminal neuralgia due to contralateral tumors of the posterior fossa. Report of 2 cases, *J. Neurosurg.*, **4**, 179.

HARRIS, W. (1926) *Neuritis and Neuralgia*, London.

HARRIS, W. (1937) *The Facial Neuralgias*, London.

HARRIS, W. (1938) Alcohol injection in inoperable malignant growths of the jaws and tongue, *Brit. med. J.*, **2**, 831.

HUGHES, B. (1958) Chronic benign trigeminal paresis, *Proc. roy. Soc. Med.*, **51**, 529.

JEFFERSON, G. (1931) Surgical treatment of trigeminal neuralgia, *Brit. med. J.*, **2**, 309.

KALTREIDER, H. B., and TALAL, N. (1969) The neuropathy of Sjögren's syndrome: trigeminal nerve involvement, *Ann. intern. Med.*, **70**, 751.

KILLIAN, J. M., and FROMM, G. H. (1968) Carbamazepine in the treatment of neuralgia: use and side effects, *Arch. Neurol. (Chic.)*, **19**, 129.

KUGELBERG, E., and LINDBLOM, U. (1959) The mechanism of the pain in trigeminal neuralgia, *J. Neurol. Neurosurg. Psychiat.*, **22**, 36.

PATON, L. (1926) The trigeminal and its ocular lesions, *Brit. J. Ophthal.*, **10**, 305.

PENMAN, J. (1949) A simple radiological aid to Gasserian injection, *Lancet*, **ii,** 268.

PENMAN, J. (1950) The differential diagnosis and treatment of tic douloureux, *Postgrad. med. J.*, **26, 627.**

PENMAN, J. (1968) Trigeminal neuralgia, in *Handbook of Clinical Neurology*, ed. Vinken, P. J., and Bruyn, G. W., vol. 5, chap. 28, Amsterdam.

PENMAN, J., and SMITH, M. C. (1950) Degeneration of the primary and secondary sensory nerves after trigeminal injection, *J. Neurol. Neurosurg. Psychiat.*, **13**, 36.

SJÖQVIST, O. (1937) Eine neue Operationsmethode bei Trigeminusneuralgie: Durchschneidung des Tractus spinalis trigemini, *Zbl. Neurochir.*, **i–ii,** 274.

SMYTH, G. E. (1939) The systematization and central connections of the spinal tract and nucleus of the trigeminal nerve, *Brain*, **62,** 41.

SPILLANE, J. D., and WELLS, C. E. C. (1959) Isolated trigeminal neuropathy, *Brain*, **82,** 391.

WOOLSEY, R. D. (1955) Trigeminal neuralgia: treatment by decompression of the posterior root, *J. Amer. med. Ass.*, **159,** 1733.

THE SEVENTH OR FACIAL NERVE

ORIGIN, COURSE, AND DISTRIBUTION

The seventh cranial nerve contains motor fibres only, though it is associated in part of its course with a small number of sensory fibres going to the external acoustic meatus, with fibres which excite salivary secretion, and with others which convey taste impulses from the anterior two-thirds of the tongue. These secretory and gustatory fibres travel in the nervus intermedius. The motor nucleus is situated in the ventral part of the tegmentum of the pons. The fibres which take origin from this nucleus pass backwards in the pons almost as far as the floor of the fourth ventricle, where they form a loop around the nucleus of the sixth nerve before turning forwards to emerge from the lateral aspect of the lower border of the pons, on the medial side of the eighth nerve, from which the seventh is separated by the nervus intermedius [FIG. 24]. The three nerves then pass together from the pons to the internal acoustic meatus. Within the petrous portion of the temporal bone the facial nerve occupies the aqueductus Fallopii or facial canal. After passing outwards it turns sharply backwards on the medial side of the middle ear and then downwards behind it to emerge from the skull at the stylomastoid foramen. At the backward turn of the nerve it expands to form the geniculate ganglion which receives the nervus intermedius and which contains the ganglion cells of the taste fibres of the chorda tympani. It sends branches to the pterygopalatine and otic ganglia, carrying fibres for the secretion of saliva. Within the facial canal the facial nerve gives off a nerve to the stapedius muscle, and the chorda tympani nerve which carries gustatory fibres to the anterior two-thirds of the tongue. The chorda tympani after crossing the tympanic cavity emerges from the skull by the anterior canaliculus for the chorda tympani and unites with the lingual nerve, a branch of the mandibular nerve, beneath the lateral pterygoid muscle. The facial nerve after emerging from the stylomastoid foramen gives branches to the stylohyoid muscle, to the posterior belly of the digastric and the occipital belly of the occipitofrontalis, and then turns forwards to divide within the parotid gland into a number of branches which innervate the muscles of expression, including the buccinator and the platysma.

FACIAL PARALYSIS

Facial paralysis may be due to:

1. A supranuclear lesion involving the corticospinal fibres concerned in voluntary facial movement.
2. A supranuclear lesion involving the fibres concerned in emotional movement of the face—mimic paralysis.
3. Nuclear and infranuclear lesions involving the lower motor neurones.
4. Primary degeneration or disorder of function of the facial muscles.

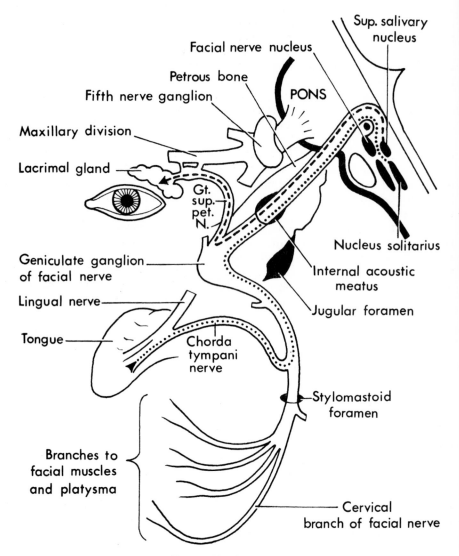

FIG. 24. The facial nerve

Lesions involving the facial nerve trunk above the geniculate ganglion will cause loss of lacrimation (greater petrosal nerve), and loss of taste in the anterior two-thirds of the tongue (chorda tympani nerve), as well as paralysis of both upper and lower facial muscles.

Lesions between the geniculate ganglion and the point where the chorda tympani nerve leaves the facial nerve (6 mm above the stylomastoid foramen), will cause loss of taste sensation in the anterior two-thirds of the tongue, as well as paralysis of the facial muscles, but lacrimation will still be present.

Lesions below the point where the chorda tympani nerve leaves the facial nerve will cause paralysis of the facial muscles, but both taste and lacrimation will be present.

(Redrawn from an original drawing by Mr. Charles Keogh)

1. *Facial paralysis due to a supranuclear corticospinal lesion* is distinguished by the fact that movements of the lower part of the face are affected more severely than those of the upper part, and that although voluntary retraction of the angle of the mouth is weak, emotional and associated movements of the face are little, if at all, affected. There are no electrophysiological signs of denervation in the facial muscles.

2. The occasional occurrence of *weakness or abolition of emotional movements of the face* with retention of voluntary movements and the escape of the former after corticospinal lesions indicates that the nervous impulses concerned in emotional movement of the face employ a different supranuclear path from the corticospinal tract. This path appears to originate in the frontal lobe, anterior to the precentral gyrus, and most cases of mimic facial palsy are due to lesions of the anterior part of the frontal lobe. This dissociated form of facial weakness has also been described as a result of lesions in the neighbourhood of the thalamus.

3. *Lesions involving the lower motor neurones* supplying the facial muscles, since they destroy the final common path, affect to an equal extent all forms of facial movement, and as a rule the upper and lower facial muscles are equally weakened. The symptoms of facial paralysis due to lower motor neurone lesions are described in detail in the section dealing with Bell's paralysis. The facial lower motor neurones may be involved by a lesion:

(*a*) within the pons;
(*b*) within the posterior fossa, between the pons and the internal acoustic meatus;
(*c*) within the temporal bone;
(*d*) after emergence from the skull.

(*a*) *Pontine lesions.* Massive lesions involving the facial nucleus or the fibres of the facial nerve inevitably affect neighbouring structures as well. Facial paralysis due to such lesions is, therefore, usually associated with paralysis of the lateral rectus, or of conjugate ocular deviation to the same side, and often with paralysis of the ipsilateral jaw muscles. There may also be sensory loss due to involvement of the spinal tract and nucleus of the trigeminal nerve and of the spinothalamic tract, or a corticospinal lesion of the upper and lower limbs on the opposite side. Acute and chronic degenerative lesions of the facial nuclei are likely to involve other bulbar motor nuclei. Pontine lesions causing facial paralysis include tumours, syringobulbia, vascular lesions, poliomyelitis, multiple sclerosis, and encephalomyelitis. Bilateral facial paralysis occasionally occurs as a congenital abnormality, probably due to a failure of development of the facial nuclei, and is then usually associated with congenital ocular palsies (Moebius' syndrome).

(*b*) *Within the posterior fossa* the proximity of the facial nerve to the nervus intermedius and the eighth nerve is responsible for the fact that these nerves usually suffer together. Lesions in this situation, therefore, may cause deafness and loss of taste in the anterior two-thirds of the tongue, in association with facial paralysis. The commonest of such lesions are acoustic neuroma and other tumours in the region of the cerebellopontine angle such as meningioma, cholesteatoma, chordoma, and tumours of the glomus jugulare. In its extracerebral course, the facial, like the other cranial nerves, may be damaged by polyneuritis cranialis [p. 986], granulomatous meningitis, and sarcoidosis, but is less often affected by these processes than the oculomotor nerves.

(c) *Within the temporal bone* the facial nerve may be involved in fractures of the skull, and is exposed to infections of the middle ear and mastoid, and facial paralysis may be the direct result of spread of infection from the middle ear to the facial canal, or may follow surgical operations on the ear, in which case the nerve may be merely contused or actually divided or exposed to invasion by the infecting organism. Slow progressive facial palsy may be caused by an epidermoid within the temporal bone, and is then associated with deafness (Jefferson and Smalley, 1938). Herpes zoster infecting the geniculate ganglion [p. 520] usually causes facial paralysis through secondary involvement of the motor fibres of the nerve (syndrome of Ramsay Hunt). Facial paralysis caused by a lesion within the middle ear is usually associated with loss of taste in the anterior two-thirds of the tongue, as a result of interruption of the fibres of the chorda tympani within the facial nerve, or in its passage through the middle ear. Inflammation of the facial nerve within the stylomastoid foramen is probably the cause of facial paralysis occurring spontaneously or following exposure to cold and known as Bell's palsy.

(d) *After leaving the skull* the fibres of the facial nerve may be involved in inflammation from suppurating glands behind the angle of the jaw or in compression by tumours or other lesions of the parotid gland. Various inflammatory and malignant processes are known sometimes to cause unilateral or bilateral facial palsy, probably due to involvement of the nerve within the parotid. This may occur in uveoparotid fever (Heerfordt's syndrome), which is probably a form of sarcoidosis, in infective mononucleosis and in acute leukaemia.

Melkersson's syndrome is a name which has been given to a condition of benign course and unknown aetiology in which recurrent episodes of facial oedema and unilateral or bilateral facial palsy occur in patients with deeply furrowed tongues.

The fibres of the facial nerve may also be compressed or divided, due to trauma to the face, as by obstetric forceps during delivery.

4. *Primary dysfunction of the facial muscles* is seen in myasthenia gravis, in which the retractors of the angle of the mouth suffer earlier and more severely than the elevators and depressors of the lips, in the facioscapulohumeral type of muscular dystrophy, and in dystrophia myotonica. Facial muscle weakness rarely occurs in polymyositis, motor neurone disease, and other forms of spinal muscular atrophy, and involvement of the orbicularis oculi is usual in cases of ocular myopathy.

BELL'S PALSY (FACIAL PARALYSIS)

Definition. Facial paralysis of acute onset due to non-suppurative inflammation of the facial nerve within the stylomastoid foramen.

AETIOLOGY AND PATHOLOGY

The most plausible explanation of Bell's paralysis (named after Sir Charles Bell, 1774–1842) is that it is due to acute inflammation or oedema involving the nerve within the stylomastoid foramen. This leads to compression of the nerve fibres, with resulting paralysis. At first the nerve is swollen, later it is reduced to a fibrous cord (Morris, 1938, 1939).

Bell's paralysis may occur at any age from infancy to old age. It appears to be most common in young adults, and males are affected more frequently than females. A careful epidemiological survey carried out by Leibowitz (1969) has suggested that small epidemics occur, suggesting an infective aetiology.

In some cases no predisposing cause can be found, but not uncommonly there is a history of exposure to chill, for example, riding in a vehicle or sleeping next to an open window. In other cases the paralysis follows an acute infection of the nasopharynx. While facial paralysis (often with ipsilateral deafness, facial numbness, and vesicles in the external meatus or on the soft palate) may occur in herpes zoster (the Ramsay Hunt syndrome) this is a comparatively rare cause. McCormick (1972) suggests that herpes simplex virus may be a commoner cause, while in older patients with diabetes Korczyn (1971) has suggested that it is more likely to be due to ischaemia; Abramsky et al. (1975) have advanced immunological evidence to suggest that the condition may be due to a lymphocyte-mediated hypersensitivity phenomenon like that which probably accounts for the Guillain–Barré syndrome.

SYMPTOMS

Bell's palsy is almost always unilateral, very rarely bilateral. The onset is sudden and frequently the patient awakens in the morning to find the face paralysed. He or his friends observe that his mouth is drawn to one side. There is frequently pain at the onset within the ear, in the mastoid region, or around the angle of the jaw.

There is paralysis of the muscles of expression [FIG. 25]. The upper and lower facial muscles are usually equally affected and the muscles are paralysed to an equal extent for voluntary, emotional, and associated movements. The eyebrow droops, and the wrinkles of the brow are smoothed out. Frowning and raising the eyebrow are impossible. Owing to paralysis of the orbicularis oculi the palpebral fissure is wider on the affected than on the normal side and closure of the eye is impossible. When the patient attempts to close the eye, the globe rolls upwards and slightly inwards (Bell's phenomenon). Eversion of the lower lid, and lack of approximation of the punctum to the conjunctiva impair the absorption of tears, which tend to overflow the lower lid. The nasolabial furrow is smoothed out, and the mouth is drawn over to the sound side. The patient is unable to retract the angle of the mouth, and to purse the lips, as in whistling. Owing to paralysis of the buccinator the cheek is puffed out in respiration, and food tends to accumulate between the teeth and the cheek. The displacement of the mouth causes deviation of the tongue to the sound side when it is protruded, and

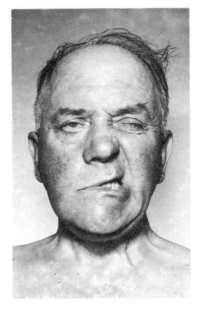

FIG. 25. An acute right-sided facial paralysis. The patient is trying to close his eyes and show his teeth (from *An Atlas of Clinical Neurology*, 2nd ed., 1975, by J. D. Spillane, reproduced by kind permission of the author)

may thus cause paralysis of the tongue to be suspected in error.

When the inflammatory process extends upwards to involve the nerve above the point at which the chorda tympani leaves it, there is loss of taste on the anterior two-thirds of the tongue, and when the branch to the stapedius is also involved the patient may complain of hyperacusis, an intensification of loud noises in the affected ear.

DIAGNOSIS

Bell's palsy of the facial nerve is distinguished from facial paralysis due to a lesion of the pons by the presence in the latter case of symptoms of involvement of other pontine nuclei, especially the fifth and sixth, and sometimes of the long tracts. Lesions in the posterior fossa often involve the eighth nerve as well. A history of aural discharge and examination of the tympanic membrane makes it easy to recognize facial paralysis secondary to otitis media. Unilateral facial palsy is sometimes an early symptom of multiple sclerosis, especially in young adults. A recurrent form associated with headache has been termed 'facioplegic migraine'.

PROGNOSIS

In many cases of Bell's palsy complete recovery occurs, though this may take months. In Taverner's (1955) series about half the patients made a complete recovery. If at the end of three weeks from the onset there is some return of voluntary power in the face, recovery is likely to be rapid and will probably be complete in a few weeks. Electromyography is a useful guide to prognosis. If within a few days after the onset there are motor units under voluntary control in the facial muscles and if facial nerve conduction remains normal or only slightly slowed, then in all probability the lesion is mainly neurapraxial and recovery is likely to be rapid and complete. If, on the other hand, paralysis is complete, if no motor units can be detected by needle electrode exploration of the facial musculature and if within a few days the facial nerve is totally unresponsive to stimulation, then the prognosis is much less good and the appearance of spontaneous fibrillation potentials in the muscle within two or three weeks indicates that at least some of the fibres have undergone Wallerian degeneration.

In those cases in which recovery is never complete, contracture usually develops in the paralysed muscles, and this does much to improve the appearance of the face at rest, although the paralysis is evident when the patient smiles. When marked contracture develops, the nasolabial furrow may become actually deeper on the paralysed side than on the normal side and the affected eyebrow may be drawn downwards. Clonic facial spasm is an occasional sequel of incomplete recovery, but usually is not very severe. The syndrome of 'crocodile tears'—unilateral lacrimation on eating—occurs in a small proportion of cases. It is due to regenerating facial nerve fibres running from the geniculate ganglion through the greater petrosal nerve and the pterygopalatine ganglion to the lacrimal gland. Recurrent 'idiopathic' facial palsy is rare. It may occur first on one side and a year or two later on the other, while very occasionally it may develop simultaneously on the two sides.

TREATMENT

When the patient is seen during the acute stage, treatment should be directed to relieving the inflammation. Robison and Moss (1954) advocate the use of cortisone but Taverner et al. (1966) suggested, after a controlled trial, that ACTH was more effective if given early enough. More recently, however, Taverner et al. (1971) found that prednisone, 40 mg four times a day for 5 days followed by diminishing doses thereafter was superior to ACTH. It is sound treatment to try to prevent stretching of the paralysed muscles, which occurs when the mouth is drawn over to the sound side. The usual wire splint is unphysiological. It is better to apply two strips of adhesive strapping or transparent tape ('Sellotape' or 'Scotch Tape') above and below the mouth to counteract the pull of the muscles on the normal side (Pickerill and Pickerill, 1945).

Since Ballance and Duel (1932) first advocated decompression of the facial nerve in its canal for the treatment of Bell's palsy, there have been many advocates of early operative treatment (Morris, 1938, 1939) and in recent years the operation has been revived for the treatment of cases presumed, on electrophysiological grounds, to carry a poor prognosis. A recent controlled trial, however (Mechelse et al., 1971), showed that the natural history of the condition was not favourably influenced by decompression in the second or third week after the onset.

After the acute stage, direct electrical stimulation of the facial muscles has its advocates but others believe that such treatment may predispose to the development of contracture and it is not now widely used. Once voluntary power returns, exercises are, however, helpful. When there is little or no recovery, facio-hypoglossal anastomosis, autografting of the facial nerve itself, and various plastic and cosmetic surgical procedures have been advocated but none is uniformly successful and most patients adjust to the residual deformity and weakness. Even after total resection of the parotid gland for malignant tumour, some facial movement may return after months or years due to misdirection into the facial nerve of regenerating axons from branches of the motor division of the trigeminus (Trojaborg and Siemssen, 1972).

CLONIC FACIAL SPASM (HEMIFACIAL SPASM)

Definition. A disorder which chiefly affects middle-aged or elderly women. There are frequent shock-like contractions of the facial muscles, usually limited to one side. Its cause is unknown.

AETIOLOGY AND PATHOLOGY

The causation of clonic facial spasm is uncertain. It is probably the result of an irritative lesion at some point in the course of the nerve and has been ascribed to a lesion of the geniculate ganglion. Others suggest that it is due to a compressive lesion of the nerve (usually fibrosis of unknown aetiology) within its canal. Similar spasms may certainly develop after incomplete recovery from Bell's palsy.

SYMPTOMS

Clonic facial spasm is much more common in women than in men and is rare before middle life. It usually begins in the orbicularis oculi as a fine intermittent twitching resembling the benign myokymia of the lower eyelid which occurs in normal individuals in states of debility and fatigue and which is known as 'live flesh'. The spread of the spasm is extremely slow, but gradually the muscles of the lower part of the face are involved, especially the retractors of the angle of the mouth. Finally strong spasms involve all the facial muscles on one side almost continuously. At this stage there is always slight weakness and wasting of the facial musculature. Taste may be lost over the anterior two-thirds of the tongue. Bilateral clonic facial spasm is less common: in such cases one side is usually affected after the other. The involuntary closure of both eyes in such cases causes much inconvenience. Clonic facial spasm may be associated with trigeminal neuralgia on the same or the opposite side.

DIAGNOSIS

Clonic facial spasm must be distinguished from other involuntary movements involving the face. The commonest of these is habit spasm, a brief compulsive movement usually seen in children and young adults. When the face is the site of habit spasm the movements are usually bilateral. Blepharospasm, prolonged spasm of the orbicularis oculi, is usually seen in elderly patients, and in this case also the movements are bilateral and there is no clonic twitching of the lower facial muscles. However, it may sometimes be associated with choreic movements of the lips in cases of senile chorea while intermittent blepharospasm is a common 'hysterical' phenomenon and may sometimes be severe and disabling in patients of either sex suffering from severe depression or anxiety. The involuntary movements of chorea and athetosis are also bilateral, and are usually associated with similar movements in the limbs.

PROGNOSIS

In the absence of treatment clonic facial spasm is a slowly progressive disorder and spontaneous recovery does not occur. It may terminate after many years in complete facial paralysis on the affected side, and the twitching then ceases.

TREATMENT

Drugs are of no lasting value although the condition is accentuated by tension and embarrassment so that chlordiazepoxide (*Librium*) in doses of 5–10 mg three times a day, or diazepam (*Valium*) 2–5 mg three times a day, are sometimes helpful. Relief can sometimes be obtained by means of a temporary interruption of conduction in the facial nerve by alcoholic injection. The method of injection of the nerve trunk in the region of the stylomastoid foramen was described by Harris (1926). A selective paresis can be produced by the simple procedure of injecting with alcohol the appropriate branches of the nerve as they lie behind the mandible or by partial surgical division of several branches.

Alcoholic injection of the branches of the facial nerve gives relief from the involuntary movements for a period of from six to twelve months while after partial division the effects last longer; both procedures produce some degree of facial paralysis and the movements are liable to recur as the muscles recover their power. Many patients are better left without any form of definitive treatment as the movements have no more than a minor nuisance value in the majority. Decompression of the nerve in the facial canal is more logical and is sometimes successful.

REFERENCES

ABRAMSKY, O., WEBB, C., TEITELBAUM, D., and ARNON, R. (1975) Cellular immune response to peripheral nerve basic protein in idiopathic facial paralysis (Bell's palsy), *J. neurol. Sci.*, **26**, 13.

BALLANCE, C., and DUEL, A. B. (1932) Operative treatment of facial palsy by introduction of nerve grafts into fallopian canal and by other intratemporal methods, *Arch. Otolaryng.*, **15**, 1.

HARRIS, W. (1926) *Neuritis and Neuralgia*, p. 371, London.

JEFFERSON, G., and SMALLEY, A. A. (1938) Progressive facial palsy produced by intra-temporal epidermoids, *J. Laryng.*, **53**, 417.

KORCZYN, A. D. (1971) Bell's palsy and diabetes mellitus, *Lancet*, **i**, 108.

LEIBOWITZ, U. (1969) Epidemic incidence of Bell's palsy, *Brain*, **92**, 109.

McCORMICK, D. P. (1972) Herpes-simplex virus as cause of Bell's palsy, *Lancet*, **i**, 937.

MECHELSE, K., GOOR, G., HUIZING, E. H., HAMMELBURG, E., VAN BOLHUIS, A. H., STAAL, A., and VERJAAL, A. (1971) Bell's palsy: prognostic criteria and evaluation of surgical decompression, *Lancet*, **ii**, 57.

MILLER, H. (1967) Facial paralysis, *Brit. med. J.*, **3**, 815.

MORRIS, W. M. (1938) Surgical treatment of Bell's palsy, *Lancet*, **i**, 429.

MORRIS, W. M. (1939) Surgical treatment of facial paralysis, *Lancet*, **ii**, 558.

PICKERILL, H. S., and PICKERILL, C. M. (1945) Early treatment of Bell's palsy, *Brit. med. J.*, **2**, 457.

ROBISON, W. P., and MOSS, B. F. (1954) Treatment of Bell's palsy with cortisone, *J. Amer. med. Ass.*, **154**, 142.

SPILLANE, J. D. (1975) *An Atlas of Clinical Neurology*, 2nd ed., London.

TAVERNER, D. (1955) Bell's palsy. A clinical and electromyographic study, *Brain*, **78**, 209.

TAVERNER, D., COHEN, S. B., and HUTCHINSON, B. C. (1971) Comparison of cortico-trophin and prednisolone in treatment of idiopathic facial paralysis (Bell's palsy), *Brit. med. J.*, **4**, 20.

TAVERNER, D., FEARNLEY, M. E., KEMBLE, F., MILES, D. W., and PEIRIS, O. A. (1966) Prevention of denervation in Bell's palsy, *Brit. med. J.*, **1**, 391.

TROJABORG, W., and SIEMSSEN, S. O. (1972) Reinnervation after resection of the facial nerve, *Arch. Neurol. (Chic.)*, **26**, 17.

THE EIGHTH OR VESTIBULOCOCHLEAR NERVE

The eighth nerve contains two groups of fibres, those which supply the cochlea and are concerned in hearing, and those which supply the semicircular canals, the utricle and the saccule, and are concerned in postural and equilibratory functions. These two parts of the eighth nerve are described as the cochlear and vestibular nerves. They run together in the eighth nerve from the internal acoustic meatus to its entry into the brain stem in the lateral aspect of the lower border of the pons, but they differ in their peripheral distribution and their central connections. The eighth nerve in its passage across the posterior fossa lies on the lateral side of the seventh nerve, from which it is separated by the nervus intermedius.

THE COCHLEAR FIBRES

The ganglion cells of the cochlear nerve are situated in the spiral ganglion of the cochlea. These are bipolar cells of which the peripheral processes terminate in relationship with the cells of the spiral organ. Their central processes pass through the eighth nerve into the pons, where they terminate in the cochlear nucleus. Relay neurones originate in the cochlear nucleus and cross to the opposite side by two alternative paths. Fibres from the more dorsal portion of the nucleus cross just beneath the floor of the fourth ventricle, where they form the striae acousticae; those from the ventral portion enter the olive of the same side, whence arise further neurones which cross in the ventral region of the pons and are known as the fibres of the trapezium. Both dorsal and ventral fibres meet in the lateral lemniscus in which they pass upwards through the brain stem to the inferior colliculus and the medial geniculate body, whence further fibres are distributed to the cortical auditory centre in the transverse temporal gyrus and adjacent portion of the superior temporal gyrus.

TESTS OF AUDITORY FUNCTION

Interruption of the cochlear fibres causes impairment of hearing—nerve deafness. Since loss of hearing is also a symptom of lesions involving the auditory conducting mechanism in the middle ear, it is necessary to distinguish nerve deafness from conductive or middle-ear deafness. For this purpose the following tests are employed.

Weber's Test. A vibrating tuning-fork (C = 256) is applied to the forehead or vertex in the midline and the patient is asked whether the sound is heard in the midline or is localized in one ear. In normal individuals the sound appears to be in the midline. In conductive deafness it is usually localized in the affected ear, in nerve deafness in the normal ear. This is due to the fact that in nerve deafness bone-conduction of sound is reduced as well as air-conduction, whereas in conductive deafness air-conduction is reduced but bone-conduction is relatively enhanced.

Rinne's Test. This is based upon the same fact. A vibrating tuning-fork is applied to the patient's mastoid process, the ear being closed by the observer's finger. The patient is asked to say when he ceases to hear the sound, and the fork is then held at the acoustic meatus. In conductive deafness the sound cannot be heard by air-conduction after bone-conduction has ceased to transmit it. In nerve deafness, as in normal individuals, the reverse is the case. It is usual also to occlude the opposite ear during the performance of the test; even so, the results of Rinne's test may be misleading in unilateral nerve deafness when the sound of the tuning fork applied to the mastoid process of the deaf ear is heard in the opposite normal ear.

A further distinction between nerve deafness and conductive deafness is that in the former loss of hearing is most marked for high-pitched tones; in the latter for low-pitched tones.

Audiometry and Other Quantitative Methods. Pure tone audiometry, a quantitative method of testing hearing, should now be a routine procedure in all patients suspected of hearing loss. The threshold in decibels for the perception of pure tones of different frequencies is measured in each ear using both air- and bone-conduction, with the other ear masked. Characteristic patterns are then obtained for nerve deafness (of high and low frequencies or both), for conductive deafness and for mixed types of deafness. A 'peep-show' technique has been devised for the examination of young children (Dix and Hallpike, 1952).

Loudness recruitment is a technique of particular value in detecting unilateral sensorineural deafness (due to cochlear end-organ disease, as in Ménière's syndrome). A pure tone of constant frequency is applied with increasing intensity (in decibels) to each ear alternately. In conductive deafness and in nerve deafness due to disease of the cochlear nerve central to the sensory end-organs in the cochlea, the ratio between the intensities required to produce sounds of equal loudness in the two ears remains constant; in sensorineural deafness, however, with increasing loudness the sound eventually seems equally loud in the two ears (Dix *et al.*, 1948).

More refined tests have been introduced more recently including the tone decay test (Rosenberg, 1958; Green, 1963), Békèsy audiometry (Jerger, 1960), measurement of the short increment sensitivity index (Jerger *et al.*, 1959), and speech audiometry (Johnson and House, 1964). Hood and Poole (1971) point out that the greatest social disability of the deaf is inability to hear and understand the spoken word; they point out that free-field speech audiometry is useful in the distinction between conductive, cochlear, and retrocochlear hearing loss and in helping to correct cochlear deafness with hearing aids. Cortical evoked response audiometry may prove to be especially useful in detecting deafness in children but is still being developed (Doig, 1972).

LESIONS RESPONSIBLE FOR NERVE DEAFNESS

Nerve deafness may result from involvement of the terminals of the cochlear part of the eighth nerve in lesions of the internal ear. The commonest causes are sensorineural deafness due to Ménière's disease, trauma, damage by drugs, spread of acute or chronic infection from the middle ear, virus infection causing so-called acute labyrinthitis, ageing (presbyacusis), and occlusion of the internal auditory artery due to atherosclerosis. Streptomycin and its analogues probably cause deafness by damaging the cochlear end-organ (Cawthorne and Ranger, 1957). The internal ear may also be involved in congenital syphilis, in congenital deaf-mutism, one form of which is associated with adenoma of the thyroid, and in otosclerosis. The many causes of hereditary deafness in man have been reviewed by Konigsmark (1969). The vestibulocochlear nerve may be damaged within the petrous bone by fractures of the skull or by an intratemporal epidermoid, in both of which cases deafness may be associated with facial palsy, and is sometimes compressed by bony hyperplasia of the internal acoustic meatus in osteitis deformans. In its passage across the posterior fossa the eighth nerve may be the site of a tumour, an acoustic neuroma, or may be involved in an inflammatory lesion, e.g. meningovascular syphilis or other forms of granulomatous meningitis. Rare causes are avitaminosis, mumps, and polyneuritis cranialis, the deafness in both being bilateral. Deafness is a rare symptom of lesions within the central nervous system, though unilateral deafness may be caused by a vascular lesion of the pons, and by multiple sclerosis, and total bilateral deafness and loss of vestibular function may be associated with other signs of brain-stem damage in a case of head injury. Compression of the midbrain in the region of the inferior colliculi by tumours of the midbrain or pineal body may cause impairment of hearing. Clinical deafness does not occur as a result of lesions of the temporal lobe unless the lesion is bilateral. Central deafness in childhood may be due to birth injury, perinatal anoxia, maternal rubella, or kernicterus. Cooper *et al.* (1974) have shown that in elderly deaf patients there is an increased incidence of paranoid psychosis and to a lesser extent of affective illness.

TINNITUS

Tinnitus is a sensation of noise caused by abnormal excitation of the acoustic apparatus or of its afferent paths or cortical areas. Tinnitus may be continuous or intermittent, unilateral or bilateral. The noise heard may be high- or low-pitched and is variously described as hissing, whistling, or, in severe cases, as resembling the noise made by a steam-engine or by machinery. It may possess a rhythm corresponding to that of the pulse. Apart from associated deafness, tinnitus when severe may interfere with hearing, and is most evident to the patient at night, when objective noises are diminished. Persistent tinnitus often leads to much distress and depression in elderly people, and there is evidence to suggest that it may be a manifestation of endogenous depression in such cases and can be relieved by appropriate treatment of the depression. Tinnitus is often associated with deafness and sometimes with vertigo.

The causes of tinnitus are various. Wax in the external acoustic meatus, catarrh of the Eustachian tube, and acute otitis media probably act by causing obstruction of the conducting apparatus of the ear. The tinnitus produced by hemifacial spasm is attributed to an associated spasm of the stapedius. In a large group of cases tinnitus is probably due to ischaemia of the internal ear, and it may be produced by drugs, for example, quinine, salicylates, and amyl nitrite, by acute labyrinthitis, generalized arteriosclerosis, severe anaemia, aortic incompetence, and otosclerosis. Tinnitus precedes the deafness sometimes caused by streptomycin [see p. 189]. Abnormal sounds arising within the cranium may be conducted to the ear and so cause tinnitus. Thus a rhythmical bruit is sometimes heard by the patient in cases of carotico-cavernous fistula, congenital intracranial aneurysm, and arterial angioma. Irritation of the acoustic afferent paths may lead to tinnitus when the eighth nerve is the site of a tumour or is involved in inflammation due, for example, to meningitis. Tinnitus is rarely the result of a lesion of the central nervous system, but may occur in association with deafness after vascular or other lesions of the lateral part of the tegmentum of the pons. Noises heard as a result of irritative lesions of the auditory cortex in the temporal lobe are usually more complex than those caused by irritation of the acoustic apparatus and its lower pathways. In this group fall auditory hallucinations comprising the aura of an epileptic fit and those which sometimes occur as symptoms of a neoplasm or other lesion involving the temporal lobe. But Frazier and Rowe (1932) reported that tinnitus occurred in 25 per cent of their fifty-one verified cases of temporal lobe tumour.

The treatment of tinnitus is disappointing. Local lesions of the ear should receive appropriate treatment. Sedatives, tranquillizers, and nocturnal hypnotics have some palliative action and vasodilator drugs have been tried, usually with little benefit; when depression is severe, antidepressive drugs are sometimes dramatically successful. In severe cases, in which the tinnitus is intolerable, it may be justifiable to destroy the cochlea by ultrasound, but the patient must be informed that complete deafness in the ear thus treated will result and that tinnitus may persist in spite of the operation.

THE VESTIBULAR FIBRES AND THE FUNCTIONS OF THE LABYRINTH

The membranous labyrinth is concerned with hearing and balance. The end-organs for balance are the semicircular canals, utricle and saccule. This membranous structure is a closed system surrounded by perilymph, lying within the bony labyrinth of the temporal bone. It is filled with endolymph, which has a high potassium and low sodium content closely resembling intracellular fluid (Citron et al., 1956). On the wall of the canal of the cochlea is a gland-like structure, the stria vascularis, which is thought to be concerned with the production of endolymph. Perilymph has a composition similar to extracellular fluid and it communicates with the subarachnoid space through the saccus endolymphaticus.

The semicircular canals, three in number, are arranged approximately in the three planes of space at right angles to one another, and are so placed that, when the head is inclined 30 degrees forwards from the erect position, the lateral canal is horizontal. The anterior canal lies in a plane midway between the frontal and sagittal planes with the outermost portion anteriorly and runs inwards and backwards. The posterior canal lies in a vertical plane at right angles to the anterior canal with its outermost part posteriorly and runs inwards and forwards. Each canal exhibits a dilatation, the ampulla, which contains epithelium, and the crista, bearing hair cells, which are the vestibular receptors. Somewhat similar receptors, the maculae, exist in the utricle and saccule, but in these the hair cells are in contact with small crystals, the otoliths. The semicircular canals are excited by movements, especially angular acceleration. Movement of the endolymph bends the hairs causing their parent cells to fire off impulses. The utricle conveys information concerning the position of the head in space. The position of the otoliths with reference to the hair cells varies under the influence of gravity. The saccule may be concerned with vibration.

The vestibular nerve arises from cells in the vestibular ganglion and is joined in the internal meatus by the cochlear nerve which arises from cells in the spiral ganglion of the cochlea. These two nerves form the eighth cranial nerve. On reaching the cranial cavity this nerve crosses the cerebellopontine angle and enters the pons. The vestibular division passes medial to the cochlear division which soon becomes separated from it by the inferior cerebellar peduncle. The vestibular fibres terminate in a group of nuclei in the brain stem.

Recent research and clinical observation have led to the concept that each vestibular system is divided into two functional parts, the canal and tonus elements. The right and left lateral canals act together as a pair, while each superior canal acts with the opposite posterior canal; phasic impulses, evoked by endolymph movements in the canals, travel to the brain-stem vestibular nuclei and thence to the various oculomotor nuclei. This is the pathway taken when nystagmus is evoked during the caloric test. The right and left tonus elements, from the utricles, are believed to have their own brain-stem nuclei and cortical centres in the posterior parts of the temporal lobes. Each tonus system is functionally opposed and balanced by the other. The brain-stem nuclei of the canal, and the tonus elements, are interconnected. A knowledge of this working hypothesis is necessary for the interpretation of the caloric test for vestibular function.

EXAMINATION FOR VESTIBULAR DYSFUNCTION

Examination for vestibular dysfunction must include observations for spontaneous manifestations—nystagmus, disorders of gait and of muscular control—as well as induced manifestations. Investigation of cochlear function should accompany this examination.

Spontaneous Vestibular Nystagmus

Spontaneous nystagmus [p. 85] consists of a slow and a rapid component. It is described by the direction of the rapid component. It may be first, second, or third degree.

First-degree nystagmus to the left is seen only on looking to the left.

Second-degree nystagmus to the left is present on looking straight ahead and is increased on looking to the left.

Third-degree nystagmus to the left is present on looking straight ahead, is increased to the left, and is present, though decreased, on looking to the right.

Observation for spontaneous nystagmus should always be made with the patient's head in the erect position. The lateral gaze must not be extended beyond the limits of binocular vision.

In dysfunction of the semicircular canals or their peripheral neurones, the nystagmus is always accompanied by vertigo and is limited in duration because central compensation occurs. If nystagmus persists for more than a few weeks it is usually due to changes in the central vestibular pathways. With central lesions the subjective symptoms are frequently less severe. Dix (1969) points out that nystagmus of peripheral origin is unidirectional, always conjugate, and is enhanced by removing ocular fixation, while central nystagmus may be multidirectional, dissociated in the two eyes, and unchanged or inhibited on cessation of fixation.

Induced Manifestations of Vestibular Dysfunction

Induced manifestations are shown by various clinical tests for vestibular function. The caloric test and tests for positional and optokinetic nystagmus are necessary for diagnosis. Electronystagmography makes it possible to record details of the nystagmus.

Caloric Test. The caloric test of Fitzgerald and Hallpike is a means of demonstrating dysfunction of the canal and tonus elements of the vestibular system. The results remain remarkably constant regardless of repetition.

A moderate but effective thermal stimulus is applied to each labyrinth separately. The stimulus used is water at 7 °C below and 7 °C above body temperature. This produces equal and opposite horizontal nystagmus lasting approximately two minutes in the normal individual.

During the test the patient lies on a couch with his head raised 30 degrees from the horizontal. In this position the lateral semicircular canals are vertical, the position of maximal thermal sensitivity. The patient is asked to look at a suitable spot so that a fixed gaze is maintained. Water at 30 °C is run into one ear continuously for 40 seconds, not less than 250 ml being used. In the normal subject second-degree nystagmus away from the stimulated labyrinth occurs. The time is recorded in seconds from the beginning of irrigation to the point when second-degree nystagmus can no longer be seen with a good light at a distance of 25 cm. Irrigation at 30 °C is repeated in the other ear. Water at 44 °C is then used in each ear in turn, when the induced nystagmus is towards the irrigated side. Accuracy of temperature and duration of irrigation are essential. Experience in observation of the end point and in interpretation of the caloric patterns is necessary for reaching a correct diagnosis.

The caloric test is of great value in the diagnosis of organic lesions at all levels of the vestibular system. It may show suppression of activity on one side, canal paresis, or a directional preponderance of nystagmus, which means that nystagmus in one direction, from whichever canal it is obtained, is stronger and lasts longer than in the other direction, according to whether the canal or tonus elements of the vestibular system are affected. Combined responses showing directional preponderance and canal paresis frequently occur [FIGS. 26–30].

In cerebral lesions involving the posterior temporal lobe, the cortical centre for the tonus pathway, marked directional preponderance of caloric nystagmus towards the side of the lesion is found (Carmichael *et al.*, 1956).

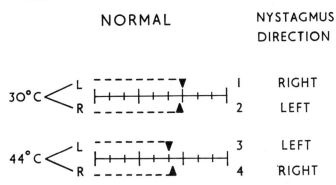

FIG. 26. Caloric responses: normal. (From Fitzgerald, G., and Hallpike, C. S. (1942), *Brain*, **65**, 115. By kind permission of the Authors and Editor.)

In brain-stem lesions directional preponderance away from the lesion is found more frequently than canal paresis, which occurs when the lesion is at or above the level of the entry of the eighth nerve. Combined responses sometimes occur (Carmichael *et al.*, 1965). Simple stimulation of one ear with a small quantity of ice-cold water in an attempt to induce nystagmus is a useful rapid test of the responsiveness of pontine vestibular nuclei in comatose patients; absence of any response implies a severe disturbance of brain-stem function [p. 1168].

In peripheral lesions the commonest abnormality found is canal paresis, due to a lesion of the lateral semicircular canal or its peripheral neurones. Canal paresis is found in a high proportion of patients with Ménière's disease, vestibular neuronitis, and acoustic neuroma. Combined lesions indicating a change in the utricle or its peripheral neurones as well as the lateral canal occur in 21 per cent in cases of Ménière's disease (Hallpike, 1950). Directional preponderance of caloric nystagmus alone is found less commonly in peripheral disease.

Positional Tests. Dix and Hallpike (1952) showed that nystagmus on sudden movement of the head in certain directions is produced by changes in the otolith organ of the utricle. The cause of this syndrome of so-called benign positional vertigo or nystagmus (Barány's syndrome) [p. 199] is unknown.

Tests for otolith function cannot be confined to one ear, but there is a useful and easily performed test to elicit positional nystagmus (Barány 1921; Nylén, 1939). The patient is seated on a couch. His head is held and he is briskly laid back so that his head becomes 30 degrees below the horizontal and rotated 30 to 40 degrees towards the observer [FIG. 31]. In the normal subject no nystagmus or vertigo occur. In benign paroxysmal positional nystagmus, after a short, characteristic latent period, severe vertigo and rotary nystagmus towards the lowermost ear (the affected one) occur and last for several seconds. If the critical position is maintained, the nystagmus and vertigo gradually stop. On returning to a sitting position a similar, though usually less severe, episode occurs. If the test is then repeated the phenomenon may not be observed, as adaptation occurs rapidly.

Positional nystagmus is sometimes seen in posterior fossa lesions and especially in patients with ependymomas or metastases (Cawthorne and Hinchcliffe, 1961) in the fourth ventricle or in others with brain-stem lesions of multiple sclerosis. In contrast to those with the benign syndrome, in these individuals nystagmus

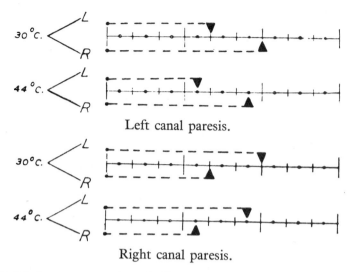

Left canal paresis.

Right canal paresis.

FIG. 27. Caloric responses: canal paresis. (From Fitzgerald, G., and Hallpike, C. S. (1942) *Brain*, **65,** 115. By kind permission of the Authors and Editor.)

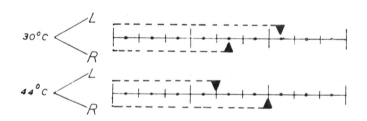

DIRECTIONAL PREPONDERANCE TO RIGHT.

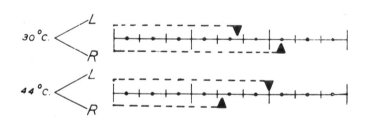

DIRECTIONAL PREPONDERANCE TO LEFT.

FIG. 28. Caloric responses: directional preponderance. (From Fitzgerald, G., and Hallpike, C. S. (1942) *Brain*, **65,** 115. By kind permission of the Authors and Editor.)

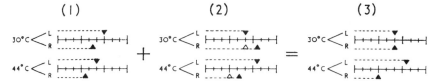

FIG. 29. Caloric responses: from a case of Ménière's disease of the right labyrinth. Combination of right canal paresis (1) and directional preponderance to the left (2). (From Hallpike, C. S. (1965) *Proc. roy. Soc. Med.*, **58**, 185. By kind permission of the Author and Editor.)

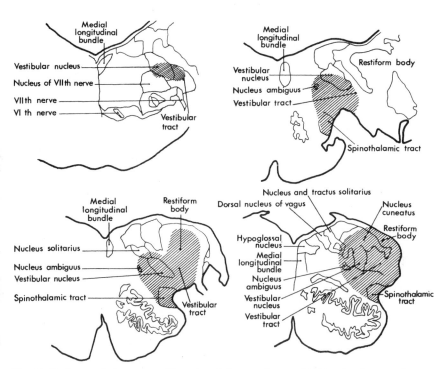

FIG. 30. Brain-stem lesion; a case of lateral medullary syndrome with directional preponderance of the caloric responses to the left. (From Carmichael, E. A., Dix, M. R., and Hallpike, C. S. (1965) *Brain*, **88**, 51. By kind permission of the Authors and Editor.)

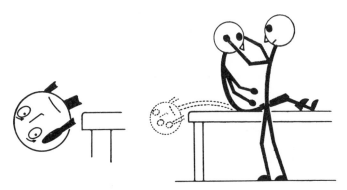

FIG. 31. The method of eliciting positional nystagmus. (From Hallpike, C. S. (1955) *Postgrad. med. J.*, **31**, 330. By kind permission of the Author and Editor.)

develops without a latent period, neither adapts nor fatigues and is variable in direction depending upon how the head is moved and there is less severe subjective vertigo or even none at all (Dix, 1969).

REFERENCES

BARÁNY, R. (1921) Diagnose von Krankheitserscheinungen im Bereiche des Otolithen-apparates, *Acta Oto-lar.*, **2**, 434.

CARMICHAEL, E. A., DIX, M. R., and HALLPIKE, C. S. (1956) Pathology, symptomatology and diagnosis of organic affections of the eighth nerve system, *Brit. med. Bull.*, **12**, 146.

CARMICHAEL, E. A., DIX, M. R., and HALLPIKE, C. S. (1965) Observations upon the neuro-logical mechanism of directional preponderance of caloric nystagmus resulting from vascular lesions of the brain-stem, *Brain*, **88**, 51.

CAWTHORNE, T. E., and HINCHCLIFFE, R. (1961) Positional nystagmus of the central type as evidence of subtentorial metastases, *Brain*, **84**, 415.

CAWTHORNE, T. E., and RANGER, D. (1957) Toxic effect of streptomycin upon balance and hearing, *Brit. med. J.*, **1**, 1444.

CITRON, L., EXLEY, D., and HALLPIKE, C. S. (1956) Formation, circulation and properties of the labyrinthine fluids, *Brit. med. Bull.*, **12**, 101.

COOPER, A. F., KAY, D. W. K., CURRY, A. R., GARSIDE, R. F., and ROTH, M. (1974) Hearing loss in paranoid and affective psychoses of the elderly, *Lancet*, **ii**, 851.

DIX, M. R. (1956) Loudness recruitment, *Brit. med. Bull.*, **12**, 119.

DIX, M. R. (1969) Modern tests of vestibular function, with special reference to their value in clinical practice, *Brit. med. J.*, **3**, 317.

DIX, M. R., and HALLPIKE, C. S. (1952) Further observations upon the diagnosis of deaf-ness in young children, *Brit. med. J.*, **1**, 235.

DIX, M. R., HALLPIKE, C. S., and HARRISON, M. S. (1949) Some observations upon the otological effects of streptomycin intoxication, *Brain*, **72**, 241.

DIX, M. R., HALLPIKE, C. S., and HOOD, J. D. (1948) Observations upon the loudness recruitment phenomenon, with especial reference to the differential diagnosis of disorders of the internal ear and VIII nerve, *Proc. roy. Soc. Med.*, **41**, 516.

DOIG, J. A. (1972) Auditory and vestibular function and dysfunction, sect. V, chap. 3 in *Scientific Foundations of Neurology*, ed. Critchley, M., O'Leary, J. L., and Jennett, W. B., London.

FRAZIER, C. S., and ROWE, S. N. (1932) Certain observations upon the localization in 51 verified tumours of the temporal lobe, *Res. Publ. Ass. nerv. ment. Dis.*, **13**, 251.

GREEN, D. S. (1963) Modified tone decay test (MTDT) as screening procedure for eighth nerve lesions, *Speech Hearing Dis.*, **28**, 31.

HALLPIKE, C. S. (1950) in Discussion on the medical treatment of Ménière's disease, *Proc. roy. Soc. Med.*, **43**, 288.

HALLPIKE, C. S. (1955) Ménière's disease, *Postgrad. med. J.*, **31**, 330.

HALLPIKE, C. S. (1965) Clinical otoneurology and its contributions to theory and practice, *Proc. roy. Soc. Med.*, **58**, 185.

HALLPIKE, C. S. (1967) Some types of ocular nystagmus and their neurological mechanisms, *Proc. roy. Soc. Med.*, **60**, 1043.

HOOD, J. D., and POOLE, J. P. (1971) Speech audiometry in conductive and sensorineural hearing loss, *Sound*, **5**, 30.

HOUSE, W. F. (1965) Subarachnoid shunt for drainage of hydrops, *Laryngoscope (St. Louis)*, **75**, 1547.

JERGER, J. F. (1960) Békèsy audiometry in analysis of auditory disorders, *J. Speech Res.*, **3**, 275.

JERGER, J. F., SHEDD, J. L., and HARFORD, E. (1959) On the detection of extremely small changes in sound intensity, *Arch. Otolaryng.*, **69**, 200.

JOHNSON, E. W., and HOUSE, W. F. (1964) Auditory findings in 53 cases of acoustic neuroma, *Arch. Otolaryng.*, **80**, 667.

KONIGSMARK, B. W. (1969) Hereditary deafness in man, *New Engl. J. Med.*, **281**, 713, 774, 827.

NYLÉN, C. O. (1939) The otoneurological diagnosis of tumours of the brain, *Acta oto-lar.*, Suppl. 33.

ROSENBERG, P. E. (1958) Clinical Measurement of Tone Decay: read before the American Speech and Hearing Association Convention, 1958.

VERTIGO

THE NATURE OF VERTIGO

Vertigo may be defined as the consciousness of disordered orientation of the body in space. The derivation of the term implies a sense of rotation of the patient or of his surroundings, but this, though frequently present, is not the only form of vertigo as just defined. There are three ways in which the spatial orientation of the body may be felt to be disordered.

1. The external world may appear to move, often in a rotatory fashion, but other forms of movement, such as oscillation, may be experienced.

2. The body itself may be felt to be moving, either in rotation or as a sensation of falling, or the movement may be referred to within the body, e.g. within the head.

3. The postures and movements of the limbs, especially the lower limbs, are felt to be ill-adjusted and unsteady.

The motor accompaniments of vertigo consist of forced movements of the body, such as falling, and disordered orientation of parts of the body, manifested in the eyes as nystagmus and sometimes diplopia, and in the limbs as pass-pointing, while visceral disturbances, such as pallor, sweating, alterations in the pulse rate and blood pressure, nausea, vomiting, and diarrhoea may be present.

Since vertigo is due to a disturbance of spatial orientation, a brief review of the organization of this function is desirable. The maintenance of an appropriate position of the body in space depends in man upon several groups of afferent impulses, of which the following are the most important.

1. From the retinae are derived visual impulses which, in contributing to our perception of visual space, are intimately concerned in spatial orientation.

2. The labyrinth is a highly specialized spatial proprioceptor. The otoliths are mainly concerned in the orientation of the organism with reference to gravity, while the semicircular canals respond to movement and to angular momentum.

3. The proprioceptors of the joints and muscles of the neck are of importance in relating labyrinthine impulses, which convey information solely concerning the position of the head, to the attitude of the rest of the body.

4. The proprioceptors of the lower limbs and trunk are concerned with the position of the body in relation to the acts of sitting, standing, and walking.

The afferent impulses derived from these various sense organs are mutually related by central mechanisms, of which the cerebellum, the vestibular nuclei, the medial longitudinal fasciculus, and the red nuclei are probably the most important, and which constitute reflex paths by which the position of the body is normally appropriately orientated. From these lower centres impulses reach the cerebral cortex mainly in the temporal and parietal lobes and so influence voluntary movement. Vertigo may result from the disordered function either of the sensory end-organs or of the afferent paths or of the central mechanisms concerned.

THE CAUSES OF VERTIGO

It is clear from the anatomical and physiological considerations outlined above that vertigo may be the result of a disturbance of function at many different levels. We may therefore recognize (1) psychogenic dizziness, (2) vertigo due to cortical disturbances, (3) vertigo of ocular origin, (4) vertigo of cerebellar origin, (5) vertigo due to brain-stem lesions, (6) vertigo due to lesions of the eighth nerve, and (7) aural vertigo. In diffuse conditions, such as head injury and circulatory disease, it may be difficult to say what is the site of origin of the symptoms.

Psychogenic Dizziness

In lay terminology, 'giddiness' is the term most often to be equated with genuine vertigo, while dizziness is used more often to identify a variety of less well-defined symptoms including vague feelings of instability, swimming in the head, feelings of faintness, and many more. Confusion results from the fact that some patients and doctors use these two terms as if they were interchangeable; as Matthews (1970) suggests, analysis of these symptoms and differential diagnosis may be very difficult, and Drachman and Hart (1972) in an article on '. . . the dizzy patient' were clearly referring to vertigo.

While subjective sensations which, in their description, cannot be distinguished from true vertigo, may be one manifestation of hysteria, vague feelings of dizziness and instability, often with features of depersonalization, are common in patients with anxiety states or depressive illness and are prominent in those with panic attacks and hyperventilation.

Vertigo due to Cortical Disturbances

The aura of an epileptic attack may be a feeling of giddiness, as is not uncommon in minor epilepsy of temporal lobe origin. Vertigo may also occur uncommonly in association with other localized temporal lobe lesions.

Vertigo of Ocular Origin

Vertigo may occur in normal individuals in consequence of unusual visual perceptions. Giddiness at heights and on looking from the platform at a swiftly moving train are examples of this. Paralysis of one or more external ocular muscles is sometimes associated with vertigo. This is due to the spatial disorientation which is produced by false projection of the visual fields [see p. 77].

Vertigo of Cerebellar Origin

Vertigo may be slight or absent in spite of a massive lesion of the cerebellum, especially if this is limited to the lateral lobe. A cerebellar lesion is most likely to cause vertigo when it involves the flocculonodular lobe which is closely linked anatomically with the vestibular system. Thus severe vertigo may occur as a symptom of cerebellar infarction and it is an invariable symptom in those patients with primary intracerebellar haemorrhage who remain conscious.

Vertigo due to Brain-Stem Lesions

Vascular or neoplastic lesions of the brain stem may cause vertigo if they involve the vestibular connections. Neoplasms in the fourth ventricle (ependymoma in young patients or metastases in the elderly) commonly produce vertigo induced by change in posture or sudden head movement. Streptomycin may damage the vestibular nuclei and cerebellum (Winston *et al.*, 1948; Burns and

Westlake, 1949) but its principal toxic effect is probably upon the labyrinth itself (Cawthorne and Ranger, 1957). Other drugs such as barbiturates and anticonvulsants (e.g. phenytoin) probably produce giddiness, drowsiness, and ataxia by an action on central vestibular and cerebellar connections and a similar mechanism probably accounts for vertigo in metabolic disorders such as hypoglycaemia. A plaque of multiple sclerosis in the pons may cause severe vertigo with conspicuous nystagmus, vomiting, and prostration: so too may syringobulbia. Acute vertigo is a prominent presenting symptom of lateral medullary infarction due to vertebral or posterior inferior cerebellar artery occlusion; transient attacks due to brain-stem ischaemia are common in basilar artery migraine, in patients with basilar aneurysm or brain-stem angioma and especially in vertebro-basilar insufficiency. Transitory ischaemia of the brain stem is the probable cause of the vertigo evoked by head movement in patients with atheroma of the vertebral arteries, especially in the presence of cervical spondylosis.

Vestibular Neuronitis and Epidemic Vertigo

Dix and Hallpike (1952) applied the term vestibular neuronitis to a disorder causing acute vertigo unassociated with deafness or tinnitus. Tests of cochlear function showed no abnormality: the caloric vestibular responses, however, were abnormal, often grossly so, on one or both sides. The onset was often associated with an infective illness and the prognosis was good. *Epidemic vertigo* produces a very similar clinical picture occurring in epidemics sometimes with symptoms of gastro-intestinal or respiratory infection. There is evidence that it may be due to a mild viral encephalitis affecting the brain stem (Leishman, 1955; Pedersen, 1959). The onset is acute and prostrating; vertigo is precipitated by any movement of the head; the condition may last for days or even weeks and relapses have been described. Most cases of so-called acute labyrinthitis are probably of this type.

Vertigo due to Lesions of the Eighth Nerve

Since the eighth nerve carries the vestibular fibres, lesions of this nerve may cause giddiness associated with deafness and tinnitus but severe vertigo is uncommon. The commonest such lesion is an acoustic neuroma, but the nerve may also be compressed by abnormal vessels or involved in meningeal inflammation.

Other Causes of Aural Vertigo

Mild vertigo can result from wax in the external auditory meatus and from blockage of the Eustachian tube. When inflammation due to acute or chronic otitis media invades the labyrinth, more severe vertigo results and a fistula sign (vertigo induced by sudden pressure upon the external meatus) will be present. Sudden acute vertigo can result from occlusion of the internal auditory artery and is then associated with sudden unilateral deafness, and a similar syndrome of less abrupt onset may result from herpes zoster of the geniculate ganglion.

Other important causes include head injury, benign positional vertigo, the instability of motion sickness, and recurrent aural vertigo (benign, in childhood; and Ménière's syndrome in adults).

Benign Positional Vertigo

Benign positional vertigo usually comes on relatively acutely between the ages of 30 and 60. It is attributed to irritation of the otolith apparatus, and is occasionally associated with middle-ear disease but is more often 'idiopathic'. Giddiness occurs on head movement and may be evoked by the test described on page 193. The condition is characterized by vertigo evoked by one specific movement of the head; it is often self-limiting and clears up spontaneously in a few months but occasionally persists for much longer. A similar syndrome in which any movement of the head (turning, or looking upwards or downwards) causes transient vertigo, presumed to be due to damage to the utricle, is a relatively frequent sequel of closed head injury (Harrison, 1956) and may take many months or even one or two years to resolve.

MÉNIÈRE'S DISEASE

Definition. The characteristic feature is the recurrence of attacks of severe giddiness leading to vomiting and prostration, and usually associated with tinnitus and increasing deafness. The disorder runs a protracted course with a tendency to disappearance of the vertigo as the deafness increases. All these characteristics were described by Ménière (1860–1).

AETIOLOGY AND PATHOLOGY

Men suffer from Ménière's syndrome more often than women in a proportion of about 3 to 2. It is a disorder of middle age, especially late middle age, the average age of onset being 50, and more than one-third of all patients are first affected after the age of 60. Little is known about the aetiology. An affinity between recurrent aural vertigo and migraine was first pointed out by Ménière himself. Allergy may possibly be a factor in some cases (Atkinson, 1941, 1943). Pathological investigations by Hallpike and Cairns (1938) demonstrated a gross dilatation of the endolymph system of the internal ear, the cause of which is unknown.

SYMPTOMS

The usual history is that the patient has suffered from slowly progressive deafness and tinnitus in one or both ears for months or even years, and then suddenly has an attack of giddiness. In some cases the giddiness develops so rapidly that the patient may fall; more often it takes a few minutes to become severe. In a severe attack the patient is literally prostrated, and there is an intense sensation of rotation of the surroundings, less often of the patient himself. Vomiting soon develops with severe nausea, and lasts as long as the patient remains giddy. Rarely there is also diarrhoea. The pulse may be rapid or slow, and the blood pressure raised or lowered, and there may be profuse sweating. Double vision occurs rarely, and in very severe cases consciousness may be lost. Deafness and tinnitus are sometimes intensified during the attack. The vertigo may last from half an hour to many hours, and then gradually subsides. On attempting to stand and walk the patient is unsteady and staggers.

During the attack the patient usually lies on the sound side and exhibits a rotary nystagmus which is most evident on looking towards the affected ear. In the intervals between the attacks giddiness is occasionally brought on by sudden movements of the head and there may be a fine rotary nystagmus on extreme lateral fixation to either side. There may be some persistent unsteadiness, indicated by an inability to stand steadily with the eyes closed or to walk heel-to-toe. Deafness is usually unilateral, rarely bilateral. Both air- and bone-conduction are usually impaired and there is a selective loss of the higher tones.

Loudness recruitment is always present. The caloric test usually shows a canal paresis in the affected ear. Directional preponderance is less frequent. Less often still, both are present.

DIAGNOSIS

Aural vertigo may sometimes be confused with minor epilepsy, but when giddiness is a symptom of the latter condition the attacks last only a few seconds, consciousness is always impaired or lost, and the giddiness disappears as rapidly as it develops. In Ménière's disease tinnitus and some impairment of hearing are almost always present, and a lesion which involves both the cochlear and the vestibular functions must be situated either in the internal ear or in the eighth nerve. A lesion of the latter rarely gives severe vertigo and the corneal reflex is usually reduced or lost on the affected side. When vertigo is due to lesions of the brain stem or cerebellum hearing is usually unimpaired and other symptoms and signs of lesions in these situations are usually present.

PROGNOSIS

The attacks tend to recur at irregular intervals and with varying severity. Usually the intervals of freedom last only a few weeks; in rare cases the patient is free from attacks for years. There is a tendency for the attacks to diminish in severity spontaneously, and finally to cease *pari passu* with an increase of the deafness. Exceptionally, in the absence of radical treatment, the attacks continue for many years.

TREATMENT

During an attack the patient must rest lying perfectly still. An intramuscular injection of 50 mg of chlorpromazine will relieve the discomfort in severe cases. Dimenhydrinate 50 mg, promethazine 25 mg, thiethylperazine maleate 10 mg, or prochlorperazine 5 mg may be used regularly as vestibular sedatives. The patient should be warned about the risk of a sudden attack. If, after six months, there is no response to medical measures, and especially if the vertigo incapacitates him from following his occupation, surgical treatment should be considered. Section of the vestibular nerve abolishes the vertigo while preserving the hearing and the tinnitus, but is a major neurosurgical operation. Ultrasonic irradiation destroys vestibular function. Some reduction of hearing occurs in one-third of cases. Endolymphatic subarachnoid shunt is a method of correcting the causal endolymphatic hydrops with occasional good results (House, 1962). Labyrinthectomy may abolish the vertigo but also causes total deafness and may be followed by troublesome ataxia in the elderly; hence the ultrasonic method is probably now to be preferred.

BENIGN PAROXYSMAL VERTIGO OF CHILDHOOD

This benign and self-limiting disorder gives recurrent severe but brief attacks of vertigo in children, usually below the age of three years. The episodes are distressing but generally resolve spontaneously within months or at the most a few years (Basser, 1964; Koenigsberger *et al.*, 1970). The disorder is of labyrinthine origin but of unknown aetiology and is usually relieved substantially by treatment with dimenhydrinate.

REFERENCES

ATKINSON, M. (1941) Observations on the aetiology and treatment of Ménière's syndrome, *J. Amer. med. Ass.*, **116**, 1753.

ATKINSON, M. (1943) Ménière and migraine. Observations on a common causal relationship, *Ann. intern. Med.*, **18**, 797.

BASSER, L. S. (1964) Benign paroxysmal vertigo of childhood, *Brain*, **87**, 141.

BRAIN, W. R. (1938) Vertigo. Its neurological, otological, circulatory, and surgical aspects, *Brit. med. J.*, **2**, 605.

BURNS, P. A., and WESTLAKE, R. E. (1949) in *Streptomycin*, ed. Waksman, S. A., p. 524, Baltimore.

CAIRNS, H., and BRAIN, W. R. (1933) Aural vertigo. Treatment by division of eighth nerve, *Lancet*, **i**, 946.

CAWTHORNE, T. E., FITZGERALD, G., and HALLPIKE, C. S. (1942) Studies in human vestibular function: III. Observations on the clinical features of 'Ménière's' disease: with especial reference to the results of the caloric tests, *Brain*, **65**, 161.

CAWTHORNE, T. E., and RANGER, D. (1957) Toxic effect of streptomycin upon balance and hearing, *Brit. med. J.*, **1**, 1444.

DANDY, W. E. (1933) Treatment of Ménière's disease by section of only the vestibular portion of the acoustic nerve, *Bull. Johns Hopk. Hosp.*, **53**, 52.

DANDY, W. E. (1934) Ménière's disease, *Arch. Otolaryng.*, **20**, 1.

DANDY, W. E. (1937) Pathologic changes in Ménière's disease, *J. Amer. med. Ass.*, **108**, 931.

DIX, M. R., and HALLPIKE, C. S. (1952) The pathology, symptomatology and diagnosis of certain disorders of the vestibular system, *Proc. roy. Soc. Med.*, **45**, 341.

DRACHMAN, D. A., and HART, C. W. (1972) An approach to the dizzy patient, *Neurology (Minneap.)*, **22**, 323.

FITZGERALD, G., and HALLPIKE, C. S. (1942) Studies in human vestibular function: II. Observations on the directional preponderance ('Nystagmusbereitschaft') of caloric nystagmus resulting from cerebral lesions, *Brain*, **65**, 115.

HALLPIKE, C. S. (1965) Clinical otoneurology and its contributions to theory and practice, *Proc. roy. Soc. Med.*, **58**, 185.

HALLPIKE, C. S., and CAIRNS, H. (1937–8) Observations on the pathology of Ménière's syndrome, *Proc. roy. Soc. Med.*, **31**, 1317, also (1938) *J. Laryng.*, **53**, 625.

HARRISON, M. S. (1956) Notes on the clinical features and pathology of post-concussional vertigo, with especial reference to positional nystagmus, *Brain*, **79**, 474.

HOUSE, W. F. (1962) Subarachnoid shunt for drainage of endolymphatic hydrops, a preliminary report, *Laryngoscope*, **72**, 713.

KOENIGSBERGER, M. R., CHUTORIAN, A. M., GOLD, A. P., and SCHVEY, M. S. (1970) Benign paroxysmal vertigo of childhood, *Neurology (Minneap.)*, **20**, 1108.

LEISHMAN, A. W. D. (1955) 'Epidemic vertigo' with oculomotor complication, *Lancet*, **i**, 228.

MATTHEWS, W. B. (1970) *Practical Neurology*, 2nd ed., London.

PEDERSEN, E. (1959) Epidemic vertigo, *Brain*, **82**, 566.

WINSTON, J., LEWEY, F. H., PARENTEAU, A., MARDEN, P. A., and CRAMER, F. B. (1948) An experimental study of the toxic effects of streptomycin on the vestibular apparatus of the cat, *Ann. Otol. (St. Louis)*, **57**, 738.

THE NINTH OR GLOSSOPHARYNGEAL NERVE

The glossopharyngeal nerve contains both sensory and motor fibres. The ganglion cells of the former are situated in the inferior ganglion of the nerve. Their central processes mostly pass into the tractus solitarius and terminate in the nucleus of this tract. A few also enter the dorsal nucleus of the vagus. The motor fibres originate partly in the inferior salivary nucleus and partly in the

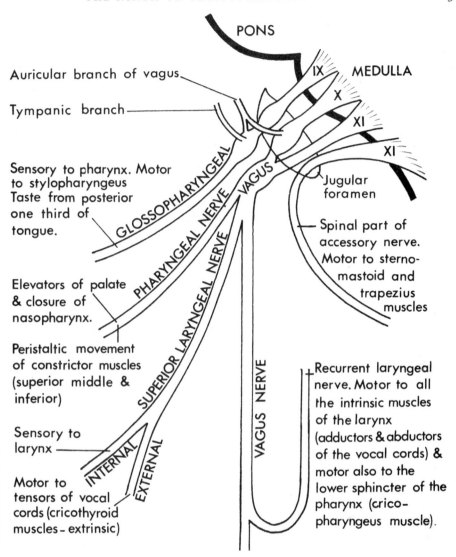

FIG. 32. The motor and sensory nerves supplying the pharynx and larynx, explaining the various patterns of paralysis commonly met with. (Redrawn from an original drawing by Mr. Charles Keogh.)

nucleus ambiguus. The glossopharyngeal nerve arises by a series of radicles from the posterior lateral sulcus of the medulla between the fibres of origin of the vagus and accessory nerves [FIG. 32]. After crossing the posterior fossa of the skull it emerges through the anterior compartment of the jugular foramen. In the neck it arches downwards and forwards between the internal carotid artery and the internal jugular vein, and then between the internal and external carotid arteries to the side of the pharynx. Within the skull it gives off the tympanic nerve which enters the tympanic cavity, to which it supplies sensation, and joins the tympanic plexus, from which the lesser petrosal nerve carries to the otic ganglion fibres which excite salivary secretion. In the neck the glosso-pharyngeal nerve gives a branch to the stylopharyngeus muscle, its sole motor supply, and branches to the mucous membrane of the pharynx. The terminal branches of the nerve supply the tonsil, the lower border and posterior surface of the soft palate, and the posterior third of the tongue. The glossopharyngeal nerve is thus the motor nerve of the stylopharyngeus and carries fibres concerned in the secretion of saliva, especially by the parotid gland. It supplies common sensibility to the posterior third of the tongue, the tonsils, and the pharynx, and taste-fibres to the same region.

Isolated lesions of the glossopharyngeal nerve are almost unknown. It is most frequently damaged in association with the vagus and accessory nerves at the jugular foramen (see below).

GLOSSOPHARYNGEAL NEURALGIA

Glossopharyngeal neuralgia in its general characteristics resembles the much commoner paroxysmal trigeminal neuralgia. As in the latter, the pain occurs in brief attacks, which may be of great severity. It usually begins in the side of the throat and radiates down the side of the neck in front of the ear and to the back of the lower jaw. Exceptionally, the pain may begin deep in the ear. Attacks tend to be precipitated by swallowing or by protruding the tongue, and the ear may be extremely sensitive to touch.

Glossopharyngeal neuralgia is distinguished from trigeminal neuralgia by the situation of the pain and the precipitation of the attacks by swallowing. Pain of a similar distribution but of more continuous character may occur as a result of new growths involving the tonsil and pharynx, and this cause must therefore be excluded.

Carbamazepine (*Tegretol*) in doses of 200 mg three or four times daily may completely control the pain. If it fails, treatment consists in interruption of the afferent fibres of the nerve. Harris successfully injected the nerve with alcohol after its emergence from the skull, but this is a difficult procedure. To obtain permanent relief it is better to carry out surgical avulsion of the nerve, which may be performed in the neck when the pain is predominantly pharyngeal, but should be carried out intracranially in the posterior fossa when the deep part of the ear is also the site of pain (Jefferson, 1931). Chawla and Falconer (1967) give reasons for suggesting that the condition is more aptly named glosso-pharyngeal and vagal neuralgia as the areas of supply of the auricular and pharyngeal branches of the vagus nerve are also involved. They recommend intracranial section of the glossopharyngeal nerve and of the upper two rootlets of the vagus as the operation of choice.

REFERENCES

ADSON, A. W. (1924) The surgical treatment of glossopharyngeal neuralgia, *Arch. Neurol. Psychiat.* (*Chic.*), **12**, 487.

CHAWLA, J. C., and FALCONER, M. A. (1967) Glossopharyngeal and vagal neuralgia, *Brit. med. J.*, **3**, 529.

DANA, C. L. (1926) The story of the glossopharyngeal nerve and four centuries of research concerning the cranial nerves of man, *Arch. Neurol. Psychiat.* (*Chic.*), **15**, 675.

DANDY, W. E. (1927) Glossopharyngeal neuralgia (tic douloureux), *Arch. Surg.*, **15**, 198.

FAY, T. (1927–8) Observations and results from intracranial section of the glossopharyn-geus and vagus nerves in man, *J. Neurol. Psychopath.*, **8**, 110.

Harris, W. (1926) *Neuritis and Neuralgia*, London.
Jefferson, G. (1931) Glossopharyngeal neuralgia, *Lancet*, **ii,** 397.
Stookey, B. (1928) Glossopharyngeal neuralgia, *Arch. Neurol. Psychiat. (Chic.)*, **20,** 702.

THE SENSE OF TASTE

There are only four tastes: sweet, salt, bitter, and acid. All other flavours are olfactory sensations. The acuity of taste, especially on the anterior two-thirds of the tongue, varies considerably in normal individuals and tends to decline with increasing age (Brodal, 1969).

The sense of taste is tested by means of weak solutions of sugar, common salt, quinine, and acetic acid or vinegar. The patient must keep his tongue protruded and must reply to questions by nodding or shaking his head. It is convenient to have the names of the four tastes written on cards, to which he can point. The protruded tongue is dried and a drop of the testing solution applied to the lateral border on one side. The patient is then asked to indicate what he tastes. The anterior two-thirds and the posterior one-third of the tongue must be tested separately but testing on the posterior third is very difficult. The tongue is dried between successive tests. Stimulation of the tongue with a galvanic current applied by a naked copper electrode has also been used to examine taste (de Jong, 1967) and Krarup (1958) has designed a quantitative technique of electro-gustometry.

THE TASTE FIBRES

PERIPHERAL PATH

The fibres carrying taste impulses from the anterior two-thirds of the tongue pass at first through the lingual nerve to the chorda tympani, through which they reach the facial nerve, and the geniculate ganglion which contains their ganglion cells. From the geniculate ganglion they pass to the pons by the nervus intermedius. Lesions of the third division of the trigeminal nerve have been said to be followed by loss of taste on the anterior two-thirds of the tongue, though this loss is often only temporary. It is possible that the loss of taste in such circumstances is not due to an interruption of the taste fibres but to loss of the background of somatic sensation (Rowbotham, 1939). It is possible that in certain individuals some of these taste fibres travel via the otic ganglion and then centrally in the greater superficial petrosal nerve and in the trigeminal, but this seems to be uncommon (Brodal, 1969).

Taste fibres from the posterior one-third of the tongue, from the pharynx, and from the lower border of the soft palate are carried by the glossopharyngeal nerve.

CENTRAL CONNECTIONS

The taste fibres after entering the pons pass into the tractus solitarius, the upper part of which, sometimes called the gustatory nucleus of the trigeminal, may receive taste fibres from the trigeminal nerve, while the middle part receives fibres from the nervus intermedius, and the lower part fibres from the glosso-pharyngeal. The fibres of the tractus solitarius terminate in a column of grey matter known as the nucleus of this tract, from which relay-neurones arise, which cross the midline and turn upwards in the tegmentum of the pons and medulla to form the gustatory lemniscus, which lies near the midline to the outer side of the medial longitudinal fasciculus. The gustatory lemniscus ascends to the VPM nucleus of the thalamus, from which taste fibres are further relayed to the cortical centre for taste at the foot of the postcentral gyrus.

LOSS OF TASTE

Loss of taste (ageusia) on the anterior two-thirds of the tongue may occur as a result of lesions of the chorda tympani or of the geniculate ganglion and perhaps of the mandibular nerve. There is no clear evidence as to whether or not it results from lesions of the nervus intermedius. Lesions of the glosso-pharyngeal nerve cause loss of taste on the posterior one-third of the tongue. Lesions of the tractus solitarius and its nucleus cause unilateral ageusia, and lesions near the midline of the pons may cause bilateral loss of taste from destruction of both gustatory lemnisci (Harris).

Little is known with regard to loss of taste resulting from cerebral lesions, though taste is occasionally lost, together with the sense of smell, as a result of head injury. Sumner (1967) described 10 cases of post-traumatic ageusia, 9 of which also had anosmia. Rarely ageusia follows bilateral thalamotomy for Parkinsonism.

Hallucinations of taste may occur in association with those of smell as a result of an irritative lesion involving the neighbourhood of the uncus. Lesions in this region may also cause parageusia, a perversion of taste in which many substances possess the same unpleasant flavour; this symptom occasionally develops without apparent cause in elderly subjects, causing anorexia and showing little if any response to treatment.

REFERENCES

BRODAL, A. (1969) *Neurological Anatomy in Relation to Clinical Medicine*, 2nd ed., London.
HARRIS, W. (1926) *Neuritis and Neuralgia*, London.
DE JONG, R. N. (1967) *The Neurological Examination*, 3rd ed., New York.
KRARUP, B. (1958) Electro-gustometry; a method for clinical taste examination, *Acta oto-laryng.*, **49,** 294.
ROWBOTHAM, G. F. (1939) Observations on the effect of trigeminal denervation, *Brain*, **62,** 364.
SCHWARTZ, H. G., and WEDDELL, G. (1938) Observations on the pathways transmitting the sensation of taste, *Brain*, **61,** 99.
SUMNER, D. (1967) Post-traumatic ageusia, *Brain*, **90,** 187.

THE TENTH OR VAGUS NERVE

CENTRAL CONNECTIONS

The vagus nerve contains both sensory and motor fibres. The ganglion cells of the former are situated in the superior ganglion and in the inferior ganglion of the nerve. The cells of the superior ganglion are concerned in the supply of common sensibility to part of the external ear and terminate in relation to the spinal tract of the trigeminal nerve and its nucleus. The cells of the inferior ganglion are concerned in the carriage of afferent impulses from the pharynx, larynx, trachea, oesophagus, and thoracic and abdominal viscera. Their central processes terminate in relation to the tractus solitarius, and the dorsal nucleus of the vagus. The motor fibres of the vagus are derived from two nuclei in the medulla. The dorsal nucleus of the vagus is situated near the midline, a little beneath the floor of the fourth ventricle. It sends fibres to the parasympathetic ganglia of the vagal plexuses for the innervation of the thoracic and abdominal viscera. The nucleus ambiguus is an elongated column of grey matter situated deep in the medulla between the dorsal accessory olive and the spinal nucleus of the trigeminal nerve. Its fibres are distributed through the glossopharyngeal, vagus, and accessory nerves to the striated muscles of the palate, pharynx, and larynx.

PERIPHERAL DISTRIBUTION

THE VAGUS TRUNK

The vagus leaves the medulla by a series of radicles at the anterior margin of the inferior cerebellar peduncle and in series with the roots of the glossopharyngeal nerve above and the accessory below [FIG. 32]. The roots form a single trunk, which leaves the skull through the jugular foramen, in which it occupies the same compartment as the accessory nerve. Within the neck it occupies the carotid sheath, lying behind the carotid arteries and the internal jugular vein. It enters the thorax behind the large veins, on the right side crossing over the subclavian artery, on the left side occupying the interval between the left common carotid and subclavian arteries. In the thorax the relations of the two nerves differ. The right nerve passes downwards beside the brachiocephalic trunk and the trachea and behind the right brachiocephalic vein and superior vena cava to the posterior surface of the root of the lung. The left nerve passes downwards between the left common carotid and subclavian arteries and behind the left brachiocephalic vein and the phrenic nerve. It passes over the aortic arch to the posterior surface of the root of the left lung. In the posterior mediastinum both nerves contribute to the pulmonary and oesophageal plexuses, and at the oesophageal opening of the diaphragm they enter the abdomen, the left nerve in front of the oesophagus and the right behind it, and terminate by supplying the stomach and other abdominal organs.

Branches. The superior ganglion of the vagus gives off a meningeal branch, which supplies the dura mater of the posterior fossa, and an auricular branch which supplies common sensibility to the back of the auricle and external acoustic meatus. The inferior ganglion supplies a pharyngeal branch which combines with the pharyngeal branches of the glossopharyngeal and superior cervical ganglion of the sympathetic to form the pharyngeal plexus, to which it contributes motor fibres destined for the muscles of the pharynx and soft palate, except the stylopharyngeus and the tensor veli palatini. The superior laryngeal nerve is derived from the inferior ganglion, and divides into internal and external branches. The internal laryngeal branch is the principal sensory nerve of the larynx. The external laryngeal branch, after supplying fibres to the inferior constrictor of the pharynx, innervates the cricothyroid muscle.

Within the neck the vagus gives off cardiac branches, and the recurrent laryngeal nerves, which pursue a different course on the two sides. The right recurrent laryngeal nerve arises at the root of the neck, where the vagus crosses the subclavian artery, around which it passes upwards and immediately behind the subclavian, the common carotid, and the thyroid gland. The left recurrent laryngeal nerve leaves the vagus as it crosses the aortic arch, and after passing beneath the arch turns upwards in the superior mediastinum, between the trachea and the oesophagus to the neck, where its course is the same as that of the right nerve. The terminal branches of the recurrent laryngeal nerves innervate all the muscles of the larynx (with the exception of the cricothyroid muscles, and possibly some fibres of the transverse arytenoid muscles), and also supply the cricopharyngeus muscles which form the lower sphincter of the pharynx.

SYMPTOMS OF LESIONS OF THE VAGUS

THE PHARYNX AND LARYNX

The function and neurology of the pharynx and larynx are so closely linked together that it is best to consider them together.

A unilateral lesion of the vagus will paralyse on one side the muscles of the soft palate, the three constrictors of the pharynx, the intrinsic and extrinsic laryngeal muscles, and the lower sphincter of the pharynx, giving the patient considerable difficulty in dealing with saliva and nasopharyngeal secretions and in coughing, clearing the voice, and swallowing.

The pharynx functions as a muscular peristaltic tube in the second (involuntary) stage of deglutition. In the anterior wall of the pharynx are (a) the opening into the mouth and the back of the tongue, and (b) the opening into the larynx, and the thyroid and cricoid cartilages. Above is the nasopharyngeal sphincter, separating the pharynx from the nasal passages, and below is the cricopharyngeal sphincter, separating the pharynx from the oesophagus. During respiration the nasopharyngeal sphincter and the larynx remain open and the cricopharyngeal sphincter is closed. In the act of swallowing the nasopharyngeal sphincter and the larynx are closed, and the cricopharyngeal sphincter opens.

PARALYSIS OF THE PALATE

The motor fibres to the soft palate originate in the upper part of the nucleus ambiguus and leave the vagus trunk at the inferior ganglion, just below the jugular foramen, in the pharyngeal nerve. Lesions of the vagus above the ganglion, or lesions involving the pharyngeal nerves, cause paralysis of the palate. It must be remembered that the tensors of the palate are supplied by the fifth nerve, and are unaffected by lesions of the vagus.

Unilateral palatal paralysis causes few apparent symptoms, because of the efficient compensation by the paired unparalysed muscles of the opposite side. Nevertheless the slight changes may cause the patient to have postnasal catarrh due to inefficient drainage of the nasopharynx, snoring, slight changes in phonation in singers, and ultimately slight changes in hearing because of inefficient function of the Eustachian tube on the same side.

Unilateral paralysis is detected on examination of the throat by the fact that when the patient phonates, for example in saying 'ah', elevation of the palate fails to occur on the affected side, and the uvula is drawn over to the normal side.

Bilateral palatal paralysis causes regurgitation of food into the nose on swallowing, because the nasopharyngeal sphincter fails to close off the nasal passages. The voice takes on a nasal quality for the same reason, and there is an alteration in the pronunciation of consonants which require the nasal passages to be occluded. This is most evident in the pronunciation of b and g, rub becoming rum, and egg, eng. There is a tendency to mouth-breathing and snoring at night, and there is difficulty in draining mucus from the nasal passages into the pharynx. There is no elevation of the paralysed palate, and the palatal reflex is lost.

The commonest causes of palatal paralysis are bulbar poliomyelitis, diphtheritic polyneuropathy, myasthenia gravis, polymyositis, and brain stem infarction. Palatal myoclonus is associated with lesions of the olivodentate system [p. 624].

PARALYSIS OF THE PHARYNX

The motor fibres to the three paired constrictors of the pharynx, which are the muscles mainly responsible for propelling food into the oesophagus, originate in the middle part of the nucleus ambiguus and leave the vagus trunk at the inferior ganglion. Lesions above the ganglion cause pharyngeal paralysis. The palatal muscles (superior sphincter of the pharynx), the laryngeal muscles (sphincter of the larynx), and the cricopharyngeal muscles (lower sphincter of the pharynx), are often involved at the same time. The pharyngeal wall droops on the affected side, and the pharyngeal reflex is present only on the other side.

There is a tendency to collect frothy mucus above the opening of the oesophagus indicating delay in pharyngeal emptying. This mucus overflows into the larynx causing troublesome efforts to clear the voice, and coughing. Compensation by the constrictor muscles on the unaffected side is often efficient, but the patient will find it easier to sleep on the affected side to prevent irritation to the larynx from mucus; there is always difficulty in clearing the throat, and swallowing has to be deliberate.

Bilateral pharyngeal paralysis causes marked dysphagia and bilateral loss of the pharyngeal reflex. Soft pulpy foods are sometimes more readily swallowed than the usual solids and liquids.

PARALYSIS OF THE LARYNX

The motor fibres to the larynx originate in the lowest part of the nucleus ambiguus and some at least probably leave the medulla by the accessory fibres of the accessory nerve, subsequently joining the vagus in the jugular foramen. The fibres destined for the cricothyroid muscle, which acts as a tensor of the vocal cords, leave the vagus by the superior laryngeal nerve and reach the muscle through its external branch. Fibres which innervate the abductors and adductors of the vocal cords leave the vagus by the recurrent laryngeal nerves.

Abduction of the vocal cords occurs during inspiration, and the cords are adducted in phonation and coughing. Reflex adduction occurs in response to irritation of the larynx.

Supranuclear Lesions

Little is known regarding the effects on the larynx of supranuclear lesions. Hemiplegia does not impair the movement of the vocal cords. Bilateral lesions involving the laryngeal centre in the cortex at the base of the precentral gyrus may do so. In such cases respiratory and reflex laryngeal movements are unaffected.

Nuclear and Infranuclear Lesions

The old terms adductor and abductor paralysis are misleading. The position of the vocal cords in varying forms of paralysis depends upon the site of the lesion, and the extent to which different peripheral nerves are involved, and whether wasting of paralysed muscles has taken place. The ability of the larynx

H

to overcome the handicap of varying forms of paralysis is a remarkable example of compensation by unparalysed muscle groups.

The following varieties of laryngeal paralysis may occur:

Unilateral Paralysis. (1) If the lesion affects the recurrent laryngeal nerve on one side only, there will be unilateral paralysis of all the muscles of the larynx with the exception of the tensors of the cords (cricothyroids) which are supplied by the external branch of the superior laryngeal nerve. The lower sphincter of the pharynx (cricopharyngeus) will also be paralysed on the same side. The appearance of the larynx when viewed through a laryngeal mirror shortly after the lesion [FIG. 33] shows a paralysed vocal cord lying near the midline, with the unparalysed cord coming across to meet it when the patient tries to say E. There will be pooling of frothy mucus round the opening of the oesophagus on the same side, showing delay in emptying the pharynx into the oesophagus. As compensation becomes established, this tendency to collect mucus may disappear. At first there is slight hoarseness of the voice and slight difficulty with swallowing fluids, but compensation by the unparalysed paired muscles is so efficient that the voice may appear normal, although it may tend to tire. For this reason unilateral paralysis of the larynx often remains undiagnosed. Slight movement can be seen on the affected side, because the tensors of the paralysed cord are still functioning, and the paralysed arytenoid will come to lie just in front of the arytenoid on the unparalysed side. This is a useful diagnostic aid. The presence of some motor fibres running in the internal branch of the superior laryngeal nerve to the transversus arytenoideus has been suggested, and this could account for some of the slight movements seen in the affected cord.

(2) If the lesion involves the superior laryngeal nerve as well as the recurrent laryngeal nerve (that is between the nucleus ambiguus and the inferior ganglion of the vagus) total paralysis of one half of the larynx will be present. Paralysis of the pharynx and palate on the same side will almost always be present, because the pharyngeal branch of the vagus is involved in the lesion. The vocal cord on the affected side will lie at rest slightly to one side of the midline, and the arytenoid cartilage on the same side will appear to lie in front of its fellow on the opposite side, and will often bend slightly inwards over the vocal process. There will be frothy mucus round the opening of the oesophagus. Cinematograph X-rays of patients swallowing opaque meals show that there is a tendency for the majority of the food to pass down one piriform recess into the oesophagus. The cricopharyngeus is seen to close firmly, shutting off the pharynx from the oesophagus, and oesophageal peristalsis continues to propel the food down the oesophagus. If the cricopharyngeus muscle is paralysed partly, or wholly, there is inefficient closure of this sphincter of the crico-pharyngeus, and some food regurgitates back into the pharynx. This accounts for the presence of frothy mucus in the lower pharynx in paralysis of the recurrent laryngeal nerves.

Bilateral Paralysis. This may be produced by bilateral lesions at any point between the nucleus ambiguus and the recurrent laryngeal nerves, but if the paralysis is really complete the lesions must be above the inferior ganglion of the vagus on both sides.

1. If the bilateral lesions are below the inferior ganglion, the motor fibres in the superior laryngeal nerve will escape, and the main tensors of both cords will then be intact and unopposed, because all the other muscles are paralysed. As described above, some motor fibres may run in the internal branch of the

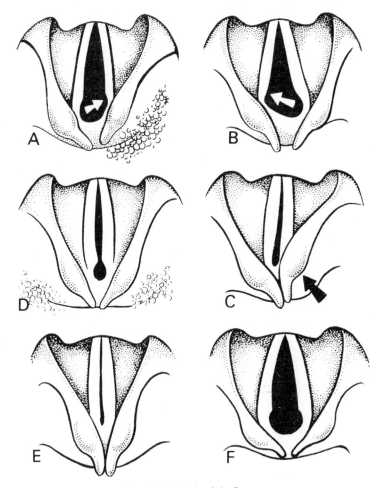

Fig. 33. Paralysis of the Larynx
(as seen through a laryngeal mirror)

(A) Paralysis of the left recurrent laryngeal nerve. (Neurofibroma)
The paralysed arytenoid always lies slightly in front of the non-paralysed right arytenoid. Froth tends to collect round the opening of the oesophagus, owing to paralysis of the left cricopharyngeus muscle (lower sphincter of the pharynx, supplied by the same recurrent laryngeal nerve). On adduction the non-paralysed right vocal cord moves across to meet the paralysed left cord.

(B) Paralysis of the right recurrent laryngeal nerve. (Thyroidectomy)
There is no collected froth at the opening of the oesophagus because compensation is so good by the intact left paired cricopharyngeus muscle that it has been able to overcome the delay due to the paralysis of the right cricopharyngeus muscle.

(C) The same case showing closure of the larynx on adduction.
The left non-paralysed cord now moves up to the paralysed cord, and the non-paralysed arytenoid now lies in front of the paralysed arytenoid.

(D) Paralysis of both vocal cords at the same time. (Thyroidectomy)
The cords are held in adduction because their muscles are all paralysed except for the chief tensors of the cords, the cricothyroid muscles (supplied by the external branch of the superior laryngeal nerve).

(E) Normal closure of the vocal cords as seen in a laryngeal mirror.

(F) Normal abduction of the vocal cords as seen in a laryngeal mirror.

(Redrawn from an original drawing by Mr. Charles Keogh.)

superior laryngeal nerve to the transversus arytenoideus. The cords are held close together, not more than 2 mm apart. Some apparent adduction can take place because the tensors are active, but abduction is impossible. There is pooling of mucus at the opening of the oesophagus indicating delay in emptying the pharynx into the oesophagus, because the lower sphincter of the pharynx (cricopharyngeus) is paralysed. The voice is weak but remarkably clear; there is dyspnoea on exertion, and inspiratory stridor on deep inspiration [Fig. 34]. Patients differ very greatly in their disabilities, some being unable to undertake ordinary duties without stridor and breathlessness and distress, whilst others manage very well except for breathlessness on exertion, and distress during upper respiratory infections.

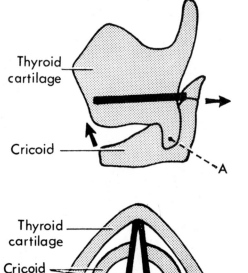

Thyroid cartilage

Cricoid

Thyroid cartilage

Cricoid cartilage

A — — A

Fig. 34. Diagram of the mechanism of the larynx to explain why there is severe respiratory stridor when both recurrent laryngeal nerves are paralysed. The unopposed contraction of the non-paralysed cricothyroid muscles tilt the posterior border of the cricoid cartilage backwards, tensing the vocal cords and drawing them together.

A–A shows the axis of tilt.

2. If bilateral paralysis of the larynx is complete, the lesions must involve both superior laryngeal nerves and both recurrent laryngeal nerves. The lesions are usually above the inferior ganglion of the vagus on both sides, or involve all four of the above peripheral nerves. Paralysis of the palate and pharynx often accompanies complete bilateral paralysis of the larynx. The cords are immobile and lie just to the side of the midline in the so-called cadaveric position. The voice is weak but clear. The airway is adequate for most normal duties. There is difficulty in clearing the cords of mucus, coughing is not efficient, and swallowing is difficult partly because there is overflow into the paralysed larynx, and partly because there is paralysis of the cricopharyngeus and the pharynx cannot empty itself properly.

Speech in Laryngeal Paralysis

It must be remembered that patients can develop astonishingly good voices after complete removal of the larynx for carcinoma with permanent tracheostomy. With practice, air is sucked into the open oesophagus on deep inspiration, and expelled through folds in the pharynx. It is not surprising therefore that patients retain remarkably clear voices in all forms of paralysis of the vocal cords, even though the voice may be weak and hoarse.

Recovery in Paralysis of the Recurrent Laryngeal Nerves

Paralysis of the recurrent laryngeal nerves most commonly follows thyroid operations or results from poliomyelitis, aortic aneurysm, or from involvement of the left nerve in the mediastinum by lymph node metastases from bronchial carcinoma or reticulosis. Occasionally paralysis of one nerve may take place without any apparent cause, even after exhaustive investigation; perhaps this rare event is comparable to Bell's palsy of the facial nerve. Recovery from a recurrent laryngeal nerve lesion, as after thyroid surgery, may occur either because the lesion was neurapraxial or it may result from regeneration even after division of axons if the epineurium remains in continuity. After prolonged paralysis of the larynx, wasting of the laryngeal muscles may occur with some subluxation of the cricoarytenoid joints. Indrawing of the arytenoid eminences and folds may then occur on forced inspiration.

Visceral Functions of the Vagus

Little is known concerning the effects of high lesions of the vagus upon its visceral functions. In animals section of both vagi is usually fatal. In man tachycardia may follow bilateral lesions of the vagus, for example, in the case of subtentorial tumours, and in various forms of polyneuropathy. The parasympathetic function of the nerve plays an important role in the regulation of cardiac and respiratory function and many abnormalities of cardiac rhythm and of respiration seen, for instance, in comatose patients [p. 1167] are presumably mediated via this nerve. The trigeminal is afferent, the vagus efferent in the oculocardiac reflex (slowing of the heart rate induced by pressure upon the globe of the eye); in the carotid sinus reflex [p. 323] the glossopharyngeal nerve is afferent and the vagus efferent.

LESIONS INVOLVING THE VAGUS

Nuclear Lesions

Lesions of the nucleus ambiguus may occur in lateral medullary infarction, syringobulbia, medullary tumour, motor neurone disease, encephalitis, poliomyelitis and rabies.

Nuclear lesions usually cause an associated paralysis of the soft palate, pharynx, and larynx, though when the upper part of the nucleus only is affected the larynx escapes (palatopharyngeal paralysis: syndrome of Avellis).

Bilateral paralysis of the larynx may be due to a nuclear lesion, of which one cause is tabes. It is more often due to progressive bulbar palsy or cranial polyneuritis but is a rare manifestation of lead poisoning.

Lesions in the Posterior Fossa

Lesions which involve the vagus between its emergence from the medulla and its exit from the skull in the jugular foramen almost invariably affect neighbouring cranial nerves, especially the ninth, eleventh, and twelfth. Such lesions include primary tumours (meningioma, glomus jugulare tumour) and metastases, and the extension of infection from the middle ear to the bone or dura mater of the posterior fossa. The commonest combinations of associated cranial nerve lesions in this region are glossopharyngeal, vagus, and accessory (the syndrome of the jugular foramen, and of Vernet); vagus and accessory (the syndrome of Schmidt); vagus, accessory, and hypoglossal (the syndrome of Hughlings Jackson).

Lesions of the Trunk

Lesions of the trunk of the vagus above the origin of the superior laryngeal nerve cause unilateral anaesthesia of the larynx, with total paralysis of the ipsilateral vocal cord.

Lesions of the Recurrent Laryngeal Nerve

Lesions of the recurrent laryngeal nerve do not affect the sensibility of the larynx. The left recurrent laryngeal nerve, owing to its longer course, is more exposed to damage than the right. Within the thorax it may be compressed by aneurysm of the aorta, and rarely by the enlarged left atrium in mitral stenosis, or by neoplasm of the mediastinum or enlargement of mediastinal glands due to neoplastic metastases, lymphosarcoma, or Hodgkin's disease. Within the neck both recurrent laryngeal nerves are exposed to surgical trauma, to the pressure of enlarged deep cervical glands, whether malignant or inflammatory, and of an enlarged thyroid, and may be involved in carcinoma of the oesophagus.

The Superior Laryngeal Nerve

Lesions of this nerve are of little clinical importance; impairment of its sensory function does not give rise to symptoms. In the past its internal laryngeal branch was sometimes injected with alcohol for the relief of laryngeal pain due to tuberculosis or neoplasm. Kaeser and Richter (1965), however, reported 4 cases of isolated palsy of the superior laryngeal nerve and pointed out that unilateral paralysis of the cricothyroid muscle may give rise to flabbiness of the corresponding vocal cord with impairment of the purity and strength of the voice. They found that stroboscopic examination of the vocal cords and electromyography of the cricothyroid muscle were helpful in diagnosis; in two of the cases the palsy was due to trauma, in one to hypothermia and in the other it followed thyroidectomy.

REFERENCES

FAY, T. (1927) Observations and results from intracranial section of the glossopharyngeus and vagus nerves in man, *J. Neurol. Psychopath.*, **8**, 110.

DE JONG, R. N. (1967) *The Neurologic Examination*, 3rd ed., New York.

KAESER, H. E., and RICHTER, H. S. (1965) La paralysie isolée du muscle cricothyroïdien, *Rev. neurol.*, **112**, 339.

SCHUGT, H. P. (1926) Tuberculosis of the larynx. Treatment by surgical intervention in the superior and inferior laryngeal (recurrent) nerve, *Arch. Otolaryng.*, **4**, 479.

TERRACOL, J., EUZIÈRE, J., and PAGÉS, P. (1930) Les Paralysies laryngées, *Rev. Oto-neuro-ophtal.*, **8**, 241.

THE ELEVENTH OR ACCESSORY NERVE

ORIGIN AND DISTRIBUTION

The accessory is a purely motor nerve, which arises partly from the medulla and partly from the spinal cord. The cranial portion, or internal branch, is derived from cells situated in the lower part of the nucleus ambiguus of the medulla. The spinal portion, or external branch, is derived from cells situated in the lateral part of the anterior horn of grey matter of the spinal cord, from the first cervical down to the fifth cervical segment. The cranial fibres emerge from the lateral aspect of the medulla below the roots of the vagus. The spinal fibres emerge from the lateral aspect of the spinal cord between the ventral and dorsal roots. The spinal rootlets unite to form a trunk, which ascends in the spinal subdural space, posterior to the ligamentum denticulatum, to the foramen magnum, where it joins the cranial portion to form a single trunk, which leaves the skull through the jugular foramen with the vagus. In the jugular foramen the cranial fibres join the vagus, and their subsequent course to the pharynx and larynx has already been described. The spinal portion, or external branch, enters the neck between the internal carotid artery and the internal jugular vein. Passing downwards and laterally across the latter it descends beneath the sternomastoid muscle, which it supplies as it pierces it on its deep aspect. After crossing the posterior triangle, the nerve ends by entering the trapezius on its deep surface. In its course it communicates with branches of the second, third, and fourth cervical nerves.

LESIONS OF THE ACCESSORY NERVE

NUCLEAR LESIONS

Lesions of the nucleus ambiguus, the nucleus of origin of the cranial fibres, have been described in the section dealing with the vagus nerve. The cells of origin of the spinal fibres may be attacked by poliomyelitis or degenerate in motor neurone disease, or may be compressed in syringomyelia or by tumours involving the spinal cord in the cervical region.

LESIONS OF THE NERVE TRUNK

Within the posterior fossa the nerve trunk may be damaged by tumours near the jugular foramen or involved in granulomatous meningitis or basal carcinoma, usually with the ninth, tenth, and twelfth nerves as described in the section on the vagus nerve. After emerging from the skull the nerve trunk may be compressed or involved in inflammation by the upper deep cervical glands, or may be severed by penetrating wounds or in operations in this region. When the lesion is deep to the sternomastoid, both sternomastoid and trapezius are paralysed; when it is in the posterior triangle of the neck the sternomastoid escapes.

LESIONS OF THE SPINAL BRANCH

UNILATERAL LESIONS

Paralysis of one sternomastoid causes no abnormality in the position of the head at rest. The muscle is wasted and less prominent than its fellow on the normal side. There is weakness of rotation of the head to the opposite side, and when the patient flexes the neck the chin is slightly turned to the paralysed side by the unopposed action of the normal opposite muscle. A lesion of the accessory nerve causes paralysis of only the upper fibres of the trapezius. This part of the muscle is wasted and the normal curve formed on the back of the neck by the lateral border of the trapezius becomes flattened. The shoulder is lowered on the affected side, and the scapula becomes rotated downwards, and outwards, the lower angle being nearer the midline than the upper. There is also slight winging of the scapula, which disappears when the serratus anterior is brought into action. There is weakness of elevation and retraction of the shoulder, and the patient is unable to raise the arm above the head after it has been abducted by the deltoid. It can still be raised above the head in front of the body, however, a movement in which the serratus anterior takes part.

BILATERAL LESIONS

Bilateral paralysis of the sternomastoids causes weakness of flexion of the neck, and the head tends to fall backwards when the patient is erect. Weakness of the sternomastoids is conspicuous in dystrophia myotonica. Paralysis of both trapezii causes weakness of extension of the neck, and the head tends to fall forwards. This is most frequently seen in motor neurone disease, polymyositis, and myasthenia gravis.

REFERENCES

SEDDON, H. (1976) *Surgical Disorders of the Peripheral Nerves*, 2nd ed., Edinburgh and London.
STRAUSS, W. L., and HOWELL, A. B. (1936) The spinal accessory nerve and its musculature, *Quart. Rev. Biol.*, **11**, 387.
SUNDERLAND, S. (1968) *Nerves and Nerve Injuries*, Edinburgh and London.

THE TWELFTH OR HYPOGLOSSAL NERVE

ORIGIN AND DISTRIBUTION

The hypoglossal nerve is the motor nerve of the tongue. Its fibres originate in the hypoglossal nucleus of the medulla, which represents an upward continuation of the anterior horn of spinal cord grey matter. It is an elongated column of grey matter, which in its upper part is subjacent to the floor of the fourth ventricle, near the midline, and below lies on the anterolateral aspect of the central canal. The nerve fibres pass forwards from the nucleus through the medulla to emerge from its ventral aspect between the olive and the pyramid. After a short course across the posterior fossa the rootlets of the nerve unite in the hypoglossal canal through which it leaves the skull. In the neck the nerve passes downwards and forwards towards the hyoid bone, and then turns medially towards the tongue, passing forwards and downwards over the two carotid arteries, lying beneath the digastric and stylohyoid muscles. It then passes between the mylohyoid and hypoglossus muscles to reach the tongue.

The chief branch of the hypoglossal nerve, its descending branch, passes downwards in the anterior triangle to join the descending cervical nerve and form the ansa hypoglossi, from which branches are distributed to the majority of the infrahyoid muscles. A further branch of the hypoglossal nerve supplies the thyrohyoid muscle but the fibres which leave the nerve by both the descending and the thyrohyoid branch are derived from a communication from the first and second cervical nerves.

LESIONS OF THE HYPOGLOSSAL NERVE

A unilateral lesion of the hypoglossal nerve causes weakness and wasting of the corresponding half of the tongue. The wasting of the tongue muscles throws the epithelium on the affected side into folds, and owing to the relative thickening of the epithelium fur tends to accumulate on the paralysed half of the tongue. The median raphe becomes concave towards the paralysed side, to which the tip is deviated. The tongue deviates to the paralysed side on protrusion [FIG. 35]. Unilateral paralysis of the tongue does not impair articulation.

Bilateral lower motor neurone lesions of the tongue cause marked wasting of both sides, associated, when the lesion is due to a progressive degeneration of the cells of the nuclei, with fasciculation. In severe cases of bilateral paralysis the tongue lies on the floor of the mouth and protrusion is impossible. Dysarthria and some degree of dysphagia are present. In dysarthria due to bilateral palsy of the tongue alone the patient finds it difficult to pronounce t and d, and the anteriorly produced lingual vowels, ĕ, ā, ĭ, and ē. But bilateral paralysis of the tongue is not usually an isolated phenomenon, and in such cases dysphagia and dysarthria are therefore due in part to paralysis of other muscles.

Unilateral lower motor neurone lesions of the tongue may occur as a result of lesions involving the hypoglossal nucleus or the fibres of the nerve in their course through the medulla, for example, acute poliomyelitis, syringobulbia, and thrombosis of median branches of the vertebral artery. In the last case one or both corticospinal tracts are usually also involved. Between the medulla and the hypoglossal canal the nerve roots may be compressed by a glomus tumour or meningioma or by an aneurysm of the vertebral artery, or may be involved in granulomatous or carcinomatous meningitis. In such cases the glossopharyngeal, vagus, and accessory nerves are likely to suffer in association with the hypoglossal (syndrome of Hughlings Jackson). Unilateral or, less often, bilateral atrophy and fasciculation of the tongue may also be due to congenital anomalies in the neighbourhood of the foramen magnum (the Arnold–Chiari malformation, basilar impression of the skull).

Unilateral hypoglossal paralysis has been ascribed to a periostitis of the hypoglossal canal analogous to the lesion of the stylomastoid foramen responsible for Bell's facial paralysis. It is a rare sequel of head injury. In the neck the nerve may be injured in operations in this region, accidentally or intentionally, as in the operation of facio-

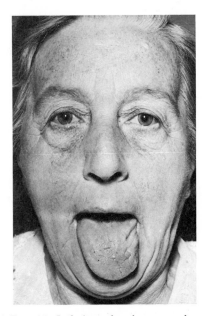

FIG. 35. Left hypoglossal nerve palsy showing wrinkling and furrowing of the left side of the tongue and deviation to the left on protrusion (from *Atlas of Clinical Neurology*, 2nd ed., 1975, by J. D. Spillane, reproduced by kind permission of the author)

hypoglossal anastomosis. Hemiatrophy of the tongue may occur as part of the syndrome of facial hemiatrophy.

The commonest cause of a bilateral lower motor neurone lesion of the tongue is involvement of the medullary nuclei in motor neurone disease—progressive bulbar palsy. In such cases fasciculation is conspicuous as long as active degeneration is occurring. It may also be caused by subluxation of the odontoid process or may follow retropharyngeal infection.

There should be no difficulty in distinguishing upper from lower motor neurone lesions involving the tongue. Bilateral upper motor neurone paralysis occurs as a result of lesions involving both corticospinal tracts above the medulla and forms part of the syndrome known as pseudobulbar palsy. The commonest causes are double hemiplegia of vascular origin, multiple sclerosis, motor neurone disease, and tumours of the brain stem. The tongue is somewhat smaller than normal owing to spastic contraction of the muscles, but true wasting does not occur. Neighbouring muscles are also the site of spastic paralysis and the jaw-jerk is exaggerated.

REFERENCES

GOLDENBERG, N. A., and SANDLER, J. G. (1931) Isolated paralysis of the hypoglossal nerve, *Rev. Oto-neuro-ophtal.*, **9,** 429.
DE JONG, R. N. (1967) *The Neurologic Examination*, 3rd ed., New York.

3

HYDROCEPHALUS, INTRACRANIAL TUMOUR, AND HEADACHE

HYDROCEPHALUS

Definition. An increase in the volume of the cerebrospinal fluid (CSF) within the skull.

AETIOLOGY

It is important at the outset to distinguish (1) increase in the volume of CSF without increase in its pressure, and (2) increase in the volume with increase in pressure. It should be noted that in cases initially due to obstruction to CSF flow with a consequent rise in pressure, the latter may subsequently become normal, as in cases of so-called 'low pressure hydrocephalus' (*vide infra*).

1. *Increase in the volume of CSF without increase of pressure* (*compensatory hydrocephalus*) is a situation in which more CSF than usual is present within the cranial cavity in order to compensate for cerebral atrophy and the hydrocephalus itself is of no clinical importance. This condition is observed in cases of congenital cerebral hypoplasia and of acquired cerebral atrophy due to diffuse sclerosis, general paresis, and senile or presenile degenerative changes, after severe head injury, and in some epileptics. There is an excess of fluid occupying the subarachnoid space over the shrunken gyri, and there is also usually some distension of the cerebral ventricles, which, however, is not due to increased intraventricular pressure but is a passive result of atrophy of the white matter of the hemispheres.

2. *Increased volume of the CSF with increased pressure* (at some stage) is due to a disturbance of the formation, circulation, or absorption of the fluid. In some cases one, in others more than one, of these factors operate.

As we have seen on pages 121-2, the CSF is formed by the choroid plexuses of the cerebral ventricles, flows through the ventricular system, reaches the subarachnoid space by the medial and lateral apertures of the fourth ventricle, bathes the surface of the brain and spinal cord, and is largely resorbed into the blood stream by the arachnoid villi of the intracranial venous sinuses.

Increased Formation

Papilloedema and increased intracranial pressure have been described in vitamin A deficient animals and Millen and Woollam (1958) suggested that deficient intake of this vitamin in infants, or in their mothers during pregnancy, might give rise to hydrocephalus. Whether this rare syndrome is due to over-production of CSF or to deficient absorption due to squamous metaplasia of the arachnoid villi (Davson, 1967) remains undecided. The only clinical disorder in which it seems likely that hydrocephalus results from increased production of fluid is that due to choroid plexus papilloma (Guthkelch, 1972); in such cases removal of the tumour is usually curative but occasionally, despite successful removal, hydrocephalus persists (McDonald, 1969).

Obstructed Circulation

Obstruction to the circulation of the CSF may occur at any point of its course. Within the ventricles the commonest cause is a neoplasm which may compress one or both interventricular foramina or fill the third ventricle. The cerebral aqueduct may be obstructed by a tumour arising in the third ventricle, in the midbrain, or in the pineal body, or may be congenitally narrowed or even absent. Owing to the small calibre of the cerebral aqueduct, slight swelling of its ependymal lining may lead to its obstruction, and cases have been reported in which hydrocephalus has been due to gliosis caused by ependymitis in this region. Aqueduct stenosis is one of the commonest causes of infantile hydrocephalus and may even give rise to symptoms of increased intracranial pressure for the first time in adult life (McHugh, 1964). The cause is unknown but the demonstration by Johnson et al. (1967) and by Johnson and Johnson (1968) that aqueduct stenosis and hydrocephalus can be induced in suckling hamsters by the inoculation of mumps virus may be relevant.

Subtentorial tumours may obstruct the fourth ventricle. The foramina of the fourth ventricle may be blocked by a congenital septum (the Dandy–Walker syndrome) or by adhesions following meningitis or by displacement of the medulla into the foramen magnum by the pressure of a tumour. The Dandy–Walker syndrome may be due to atresia of the foramina of Magendie and Luschka or to a dysplasia of the cerebellum developing early in fetal life, as the cerebellar vermis is often absent or vestigial in such cases (Benda, 1954; Brodal and Hauglie-Hanssen, 1959; Hart et al., 1972). The malformation may be accompanied by extra-axial leptomeningeal cysts in the posterior fossa (Haller et al., 1971), while such cysts alone may give a similar clinical and radiological picture. Within the subarachnoid space obstruction may again be due to tumour, to adhesions following trauma, inflammation, or haemorrhage, or to congenital abnormalities such as basilar impression or the Arnold–Chiari malformation.

The Arnold–Chiari malformation consists of a congenital displacement of the cerebellar tonsils and of an elongated medulla oblongata downwards into the cervical spinal canal [FIG. 36]. The malformation prevents the egress of CSF from the fourth ventricle into the subarachnoid space; it is sometimes associated with lumbosacral spina bifida and with meningocele or meningomyelocele, but the Chiari type I anomaly consists of a simple ectasia of the cerebellar tonsils unaccompanied by any other primary malformation of the neuraxis. MacFarlane and Maloney (1957) have observed congenital narrowing of the cerebral aqueduct sufficient to cause hydrocephalus in half of 20 cases of Arnold–Chiari malformation. Gardner (1965) has suggested that a Chiari malformation or, less often, the Dandy–Walker syndrome may result in dilatation of the central canal of the spinal cord early in life (hydromyelia) and that this, in turn, is the commonest mechanism by means of which syringomyelia is produced. The observations of Appleby et al. (1968) and Barnett et al. (1974) give some support to this view.

Impaired Absorption

Absorption of fluid from the arachnoid villi may be impaired by a rise in the intracranial venous pressure, due to compression of venous sinuses by an intracranial tumour, or impediment to the venous drainage from the head by raised intrathoracic pressure in cases of pulmonary or mediastinal neoplasm or pulmonary hypertension. Thrombosis of the superior sagittal sinus caused by

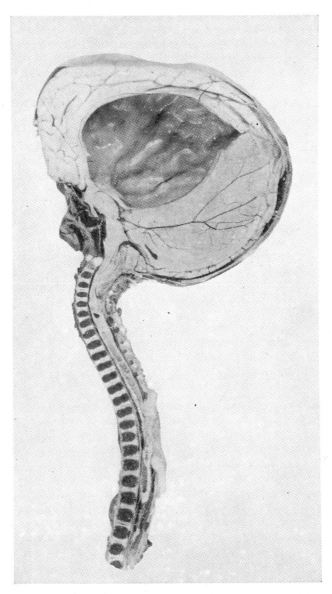

FIG. 36. Sagittal section of the nervous system in a case of hydro-cephalus due to the Arnold–Chiari malformation. Note the abnormal cerebellum and the spina bifida. (By courtesy of the Photographic Department of the Hospital for Sick Children, Great Ormond Street, London.)

extension of inflammation from the transverse sinus seems one probable cause of the condition described as 'otitic hydrocephalus' in which symptoms of hydrocephalus complicate otitis media or mastoiditis (Symonds, 1931, 1937) but Foley (1955) states that in such cases the ventricles are not enlarged and the condition should not therefore be called hydrocephalus. [See also p. 227.] Obliteration of the arachnoid villi by inflammatory material may occur in meningitis.

CLASSIFICATION

We can thus distinguish the following varieties of hydrocephalus:

1. Increased volume of CSF with normal pressure at all stages—*compensatory hydrocephalus* or *hydrocephalus ex vacuo*.

2. Increased volume of CSF with increased pressure at some stage—*hypertensive hydrocephalus*.

Hypertensive hydrocephalus can be further subdivided into:

(*a*) *Obstructive hydrocephalus*, in which there is an obstruction to the circulation of the CSF, either within the ventricles or aqueduct or at the outlet from the fourth ventricle, which prevents free communication between the ventricles and the subarachnoid space, and

(*b*) *Communicating hydrocephalus*, in which free communication between the ventricles and the subarachnoid space exists and hydrocephalus is due either to disturbance in the formation and absorption of CSF, or to an obstruction to its circulation in the subarachnoid space itself. Ḥakim and Adams (1965) distinguished a form of communicating hydrocephalus of unknown aetiology, usually occurring in late life, which they called *low-pressure hydrocephalus* since although the cerebral ventricles are dilated the pressure within them at the time of measurement is either normal or only slightly raised (see below).

The obsolete terms internal and external hydrocephalus should not be used, since the ventricles are usually dilated in all forms of hydrocephalus, both compensatory and hypertensive, and an increased volume of fluid in some parts of the subarachnoid space is common to both compensatory and hypertensive communicating hydrocephalus.

Laurence (1959) in 100 consecutive post-mortem examinations found that malformation alone was the cause in only 14 per cent of cases, but in association with infection or trauma it accounted for 46 per cent. Inflammatory reaction due to infection or haemorrhage without malformation accounted for another 50 per cent, the remaining 4 per cent being due to tumours. Thus malformation was present in 46 per cent and inflammation in 82 per cent. Cohen (1965) reviewing the radiological findings in Macnab's (1962) series of 200 found that 18 per cent were due to aqueduct block, 42 per cent to cistern block, and 40 per cent were associated with an Arnold–Chiari malformation [FIG. 36].

In the past, a distinction was often made between 'congenital' and 'acquired' hydrocephalus. What has just been said, however, shows that this distinction is an artificial one. A congenital abnormality alone is the most likely cause of hydrocephalus developing before birth but as the work of Laurence shows, both congenital and acquired factors frequently contribute to hydrocephalus in infancy. Nor do congenital factors cease to operate in later life since hydrocephalus developing in adult life may be the late result of a congenital abnormality of the aqueduct or an Arnold–Chiari malformation.

The commoner causes of hydrocephalus developing in the absence of congenital abnormalities are adhesions of the leptomeninges following meningitis, and arachnoiditis of obscure origin, thrombosis of the intracranial venous sinuses, and intracranial tumour. Syphilitic meningitis or arachnoiditis following subarachnoid bleeding are rare causes. Obstruction within the third or fourth ventricle or in the subarachnoid space, is occasionally due to parasitic cysts.

INCIDENCE

The incidence of all neural malformations, including hydrocephalus, has been shown to vary considerably between different countries, being much higher, for instance, in Scotland and Ireland than in Japan. In the United States, between 1959 and 1961 congenital malformations of the nervous system accounted for 94 deaths per 100,000 population in infants under one year of age, and 27 of these were due to hydrocephalus; the incidence was much higher in the east, and especially in the north-east of the country, than elsewhere (Kurtzke *et al.*, 1973).

PATHOLOGY

As we have seen, the causes of hydrocephalus are pathologically various. Distension of the cerebral ventricles is the most conspicuous feature. When obstruction occurs in the cerebral aqueduct only the lateral and third ventricles are distended. When the obstruction is more caudally situated the cerebral aqueduct and the fourth ventricle may also be enlarged. Ventricular distension causes thinning of the cerebral hemispheres, which in severe cases may be extreme and is associated with marked atrophy of the white matter and loss of cortical ganglion cells. The ependyma of the ventricles is normal, except in inflammatory cases, when a localized or more or less diffuse ependymitis may be present. Meningeal adhesions indicate a previous meningitis. Distension of the ventricles leads to pressure upon the bones of the skull, which become thin, especially where they overlie the cerebral gyri. Separation of the sutures occurs when hydrocephalus develops in early life, but is not as a rule seen after the age of 18. Compression of the base of the skull causes erosion of the clinoid processes and excavation of the sella turcica. The olfactory tracts and optic nerves are often atrophic.

SYMPTOMS AND SIGNS

Infantile Hydrocephalus

Enlargement of the head is the most conspicuous symptom in infantile hydrocephalus [FIG. 37]. It may occur before birth, but is usually noticed during the first few months of life owing to the large head, prominent scalp veins, and turning down of the eyes ('rising sun sign'). In most cases it is slowly progressive and the head may attain a huge size, with a circumference of 75 cm or even more. The cranial sutures are widely separated and the anterior fontanelle is much enlarged. There is marked congestion of the veins of the scalp. In extreme cases the head may be translucent and may yield a fluid thrill on percussion and an audible murmur on auscultation. Enlargement of the head occurs in all its diameters. The frontal region bulges forwards, and downward pressure upon the orbital plates causes the eyes to be protruded forwards and downwards. As the head becomes too heavy for the child to lift it, gravity, acting upon it in the supine position, in time causes it to become relatively larger in the coronal than in the sagittal plane.

Owing to the expansibility of the skull in infancy, the familiar symptoms of increased intracranial pressure are slight or absent. Hydrocephalic children seem little troubled by headache and rarely vomit. Convulsions are common. Bilateral anosmia may occur. Optic atrophy due to pressure upon the nerves is usually present, but in some cases there is papilloedema, and this may be superimposed upon optic atrophy. Papilloedema does not occur when the subarachnoid space is blocked. Visual acuity may be progressively reduced until in severe cases the child may become blind. Paralysis of other cranial nerves may occur, and squint

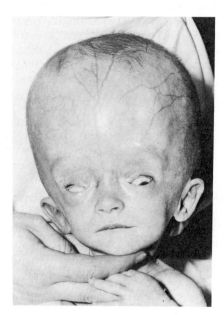 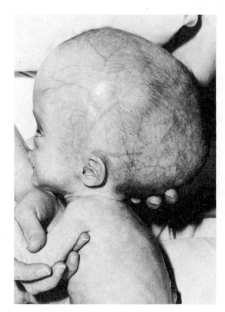

FIG. 37A and B. Gross enlargement of the head in an infant with obstructive hydrocephalus associated with a lumbar meningomyelocele and an Arnold–Chiari malformation (photographs kindly supplied by Mr. L. P. Lassman)

is not uncommon. Nystagmus may be present. In the limbs there are usually some weakness and inco-ordination, which are generally more marked in the lower than in the upper limbs. Spasticity with exaggeration of tendon reflexes is common in the lower limbs, though sometimes the tendon reflexes are lost. The plantar reflexes are usually extensor. There is little or no disturbance of sensibility. The mental state varies in different cases. In severe cases there is usually dementia, but in milder cases this may be slight or absent. Intelligence may be unimpaired even when the ventricular dilatation is such that only one centimetre thickness of cerebral substance remains between the ventricles and the inner table of the skull. In milder cases there may be obesity due to compression of the hypothalamus and pituitary. In more severe cases there is usually wasting. Cerebrospinal rhinorrhoea is a rare complication.

Hydrocephalus after Infancy

The clinical picture of hydrocephalus after infancy varies somewhat with its cause. In obstructive hydrocephalus symptoms of increased intracranial pressure are conspicuous. Headache and vomiting are the earliest symptoms and are followed after a short interval by the development of papilloedema. The headache is at first paroxysmal, but later becomes constant, and there are sometimes intense exacerbations characterized by severe headache radiating down the neck and associated with head retraction and even with opisthotonos, vomiting, and impairment of consciousness. Giddiness is a common symptom. Some mental deterioration usually occurs after a time, especially in later life, and hallucinations, delusions, and disturbances of emotional mood may occur. Convulsions are less common than in the infantile variety, and enlargement of the head is less conspicuous on account of the greater age of the patient, and does not occur after the age of 18. Before that age there is often slight separation of the cranial sutures, yielding a 'cracked-pot sound' on percussion and associated with venous congestion of the scalp. Cranial nerve palsies may occur, especially paralysis of the sixth and seventh nerves, and often fluctuate in severity from day to day. Slight exophthalmos is not uncommon. Gross weakness of the limbs is absent, though clumsiness and slight inco-ordination are common. The tendon reflexes may be exaggerated or diminished. The plantar reflexes are frequently extensor. There is as a rule no sensory loss. Symptoms of hypopituitarism, obesity, and genital atrophy, are common in children and adolescents.

The pressure of CSF is generally increased in communicating hydrocephalus, but is often normal or may even be diminished late in the course of obstructive hydrocephalus. In the syndrome of 'low-pressure hydrocephalus' (Hakim and Adams, 1965) fluctuating confusion, ataxia, and progressive dementia are the most prominent features; characteristically such patients often deteriorate strikingly following air encephalography which demonstrates marked dilatation of all the ventricles but no air diffuses over the cortex. The condition usually presents in middle or late life, sometimes with dementia alone (Crowell et al., 1973) or with the clinical picture of the Parkinsonism-dementia complex (Sypert et al., 1973) but as Messert and Wannamaker (1974) have pointed out, cases selected for surgical treatment should have: (1) dementia, apraxia of gait, and incontinence; (2) a progressive course; (3) diagnostic air encephalography; and (4) definite evidence of block on RISA cisternography (Spoerri and Rösler, 1966; Bannister et al., 1967; Harbert, 1973). McCullough et al. (1970) have shown that there is a good correlation between ventricular stasis demonstrated by such RISA cisternograms on the one hand and clinical improvement after a shunt operation (see below) on the other. Measurement of the rate of clearance of intrathecal RISA into the plasma is also a useful test (Abbott and Alksne, 1968). The cause of the communicating hydrocephalus in most such cases is unexplained though it may follow subarachnoid haemorrhage or many years after recovery from meningitis. In some such cases, although the CSF pressure is generally low or normal, there are episodes of raised pressure (Symon et al., 1972). Differential diagnosis from hydrocephalus *ex vacuo* consequent upon cerebral atrophy in presenile dementia is important as shunting operations are of no value in the latter condition; measurement of the size of the temporal horn demonstrated by air encephalography may be helpful (Sjaastad et al., 1969) but RISA cisternography is probably more reliable.

In most forms of obstructive and communicating hydrocephalus not resulting from tumour or meningeal inflammation the CSF is normal in composition, but Rogers and Dubowitz (1970) found that 5-HIAA (hydroxyindole acetic acid) was consistently raised in the ventricular CSF of 40 hydrocephalic children. Radiograms of the skull [FIG. 38] may show enlargement of the calvarium, with suture diastasis, thinning, and exaggeration of the convolutional markings, but the latter alone may be a normal finding and is an unreliable guide to raised intracranial pressure. Separation of the sutures may be present in children. The clinoid processes are often eroded and the sella turcica is deepened and expanded anteroposteriorly. Ventriculograms show enormous dilatation of the ventricular system [FIG. 38] and the concavity of the anterior cerebral

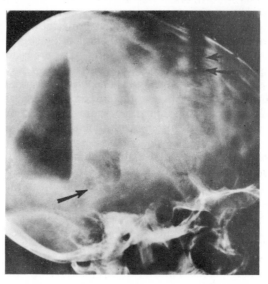

FIG. 38. A ventriculogram of a child with hydrocephalus due to aqueduct stenosis (single arrow) showing gross dilatation of the lateral ventricles. Note also the suture diastasis (double arrows)

arteries is increased in the angiograms. Ventriculography with a suitable contrast medium may be needed to show the site of an obstruction. Isotope ventriculography or cisternography is not only useful in the diagnosis of communicating hydrocephalus but may also identify the site of leakage of CSF into the nasal cavity (CSF rhinorrhoea) which is an occasional complication of all forms of hydrocephalus.

DIAGNOSIS

The diagnosis of infantile hydrocephalus is not usually difficult. Owing to the enlargement of the head it may be confused with rickets, but in rickets the enlargement of the head is due to localized thickening of the bone and other characteristic bony abnormalities are present elsewhere. The rare condition megalencephaly can be distinguished only by ventriculography.

After infancy hydrocephalus is often a complication of the many conditions which cause increased intracranial pressure. The recognition of the hydrocephalus is usually a simple matter. The discovery of its cause calls for the appropriate investigations. When the cause is a tumour focal signs may be lacking, and in hydrocephalus of long standing confusion may arise from the presence of signs produced by the hydrocephalus itself. Spina bifida should suggest the presence of the Arnold–Chiari malformation. Brock *et al.* (1974) and Wald *et al.* (1974) have shown that estimation of the maternal plasma alpha-fetoprotein may be a reliable guide to the presence of fetal anencephaly or spina bifida and may allow early antenatal diagnosis and therapeutic abortion.

Benign Intracranial Hypertension

This term was used by Foley (1955) to describe a persistent rise of pressure of the cerebrospinal fluid in the absence of a space-occupying lesion and with ventricles of normal or even reduced size, which makes the term hydrocephalus unsuitable. This syndrome, also called 'toxic hydrocephalus', occurs in two groups of patients. One consists predominantly of women, with a peak incidence in the fourth decade. The patient is often obese, and there is an association with pregnancy and miscarriage: in a smaller group, affecting the sexes equally, there is a previous history of infection or mild head injury. In these cases the condition appears to be due to a diffuse cerebral oedema of unknown cause. In a series of 34 cases reported by Boddie *et al.* (1974) only 44 per cent showed small lateral ventricles and in many others the ventricular volume was increased radiologically. In so-called 'otitic hydrocephalus', which is sometimes due to transverse or sagittal sinus thrombosis secondary to otitis, again the pressure of the fluid is raised but usually without ventricular enlargement. Papilloedema is constant, headache and vomiting are common though often not severe and diplopia may occur. The condition, whether 'idiopathic' or 'otitic', is benign and if appropriately treated (see below) the prognosis is excellent on follow-up (Boddie *et al.*, 1974) but in the acute stage papilloedema may constitute a serious threat to vision and blindness or permanent central scotomas have been recorded.

PROGNOSIS

In many cases untreated infantile hydrocephalus proves fatal during the first few years of life, but Macnab (1966) quotes figures showing that the average hydrocephalic alive at 3 months has a 26 per cent chance of reaching adult life without surgery, and if he survives to between 1 and 2 years he has a 50 per cent chance. Some who survive suffer from mental subnormality, epilepsy, or blindness. Laurence (1969) has confirmed that even in aqueduct stenosis, the hydrocephalic process often arrests spontaneously. In 41 per cent of 70 cases without spina bifida the IQ after 6 years was over 85, in 29 per cent below 50. There was a close relationship between IQ on the one hand and physical disability (e.g. spasticity and ataxia) and the severity of hydrocephalus on the other. In the past many children with the Arnold–Chiari malformation and myelomeningocele died either from infection of the sac or coning of the malformation in the foramen magnum. The introduction of the Spitz–Holter valve has reduced the mortality of hydrocephalus with myelomeningocele to 30 per cent at the end of 2 years and that of uncomplicated hydrocephalus to 20 per cent. The prognosis of hydrocephalus after infancy depends upon its cause and how far this is amenable to treatment.

TREATMENT

Infantile Hydrocephalus

In the past many operations, including excision of the choroid plexus, Torkildsen's ventriculo-cisternostomy, ventriculo-subdural, ventriculo-ureteric, and ventriculo-peritoneal drainage, were used with varying degrees of success, but there is now general agreement that the use of Spitz–Holter or Pudenz–Heyer or similar silastic valves inserted into one lateral ventricle with catheter drainage via a jugular vein into the cardiac atrium is the treatment of choice, even though there is a significant complication rate due to infection, thrombosis, and embolism (Nicholas *et al.*, 1970; Noble *et al.*, 1970) and Hammon (1971) still prefers ventriculo-peritoneal drainage. With increasing use of these methods, early closure of associated spina bifida sacs, with or without meningomyelocele, has become possible in the first few days and weeks of life, although the careful selection of cases, bearing in mind the prognosis of both the hydrocephalus and the spina bifida, is a matter for the expert and is still a controversial ethical problem. Neurological disability, including syringomyelia, resulting from the Arnold–Chiari malformation, may be alleviated in many cases by suboccipital decompression. In some neonatal cases with mild or moderate hydrocephalus and normal or slightly increased intracranial pressure, compressive head wrapping (Epstein *et al.*, 1973) appears to be helpful in promoting increased CSF absorption.

Hydrocephalus after Infancy

The appropriate treatment of hydrocephalus after infancy depends upon its cause. When it is due to an intracranial tumour this must receive appropriate surgical treatment whenever possible. When there is a tumour in the third ventricle or midbrain or in some other area which is causing obstruction but cannot be removed or treated effectively by radiotherapy, considerable temporary improvement may result from a shunting operation with insertion of a valve as in infancy, and a similar procedure may be dramatically successful in communicating 'low-pressure' hydrocephalus.

In benign intracranial hypertension and otitic hydrocephalus, treatment with high doses of steroids (dexamethasone or beta-methasone 5 mg four times a day) is obligatory and rapidly reduces cerebral oedema and the threat to vision. In occasional cases with severe papilloedema and rapidly failing vision, surgical subtemporal decompression may still be needed as an emergency measure. Repeated lumbar puncture and diuretics may also be of some value but are now recognized to be inferior to steroid treatment.

REFERENCES

ABBOTT, M., and ALKSNE, J. F. (1968) Transport of intrathecal I^{125} RISA to circulating plasma; a test for communicating hydrocephalus, *Neurology (Minneap.)*, **18,** 870.

APPLEBY, A., FOSTER, J. B., HANKINSON, J., and HUDGSON, P. (1968) The diagnosis and management of the Chiari anomalies in adult life, *Brain*, **91,** 131.

BANNISTER, R., GILFORD, E., and KOCEN, R. (1967) Isotope encephalography in the diagnosis of dementia due to communicating hydrocephalus, *Lancet*, **ii,** 1014.

BARNETT, H. J. M., FOSTER, J. B., and HUDGSON, P. (1974) *Syringomyelia*, vol. 1 in Major Problems in Neurology, London.

BENDA, C. E. (1954) The Dandy-Walker syndrome or the so-called atresia of the foramen Magendie, *J. Neuropath. exp. Neurol.*, **13**, 14.

BODDIE, H. G., BANNA, M., and BRADLEY, W. G. (1974) 'Benign' intracranial hypertension—a survey of the clinical and radiological features, and long-term prognosis, *Brain*, **97**, 313.

BROCK, D. J. H., BOLTON, A. E., and SCRIMGEOUR, J. B. (1974) Prenatal diagnosis of spina bifida and anencephaly through maternal plasma–alpha–fetoprotein measurement, *Lancet*, **i**, 767.

BRODAL, A., and HAUGLIE-HANSSEN, E. (1959) Congenital hydrocephalus with defective development of the cerebellar vermis (Dandy-Walker syndrome), *J. Neurol. Neurosurg. Psychiat.*, **22**, 99.

COHEN, S. J. (1965) *see* MACNAB, G. H. (1966).

CROWELL, R. M., TEW, J. M., and MARK, V. H. (1973) Aggressive dementia associated with normal pressure hydrocephalus. Report of two unusual cases, *Neurology (Minneap.)*, **23**, 461.

CUSHING, H. (1926) *Studies in Intracranial Physiology and Surgery*, London.

DANDY, W. E. (1918) Extirpation of the choroid plexus of the lateral ventricles in communicating hydrocephalus, *Ann. Surg.*, **68**, 569.

DAVSON, H. (1967) *The Physiology of the Cerebrospinal Fluid*, London.

EPSTEIN, F., HOCHWALD, G. M., and RANSOHOFF, J. (1973) Neonatal hydrocephalus treated by compressive head wrapping, *Lancet*, **i**, 634.

FOLEY, J. (1955) Benign forms of intracranial hypertension in 'toxic' and 'otitic' hydrocephalus, *Brain*, **78**, 1.

GARDNER, W. J. (1965) Hydrodynamic mechanism in syringomyelia: its relationship to myelocele, *J. Neurol. Psychiat.*, **28**, 247.

GLOBUS, J. H., and STRAUSS, I. (1928) Subacute diffuse ependymitis, *Arch. Neurol. Psychiat. (Chic.)*, **19**, 623.

GUTHKELCH, A. N. (1972) High pressure hydrocephalus, sect. VIII, chap. 3 in *Scientific Foundations of Neurology*, ed. Critchley, M., O'Leary, J. L., and Jennett, W. B., London.

HAKIM, S., and ADAMS, R. D. (1965) The special clinical problem of symptomatic hydrocephalus with normal cerebrospinal fluid pressure, *J. neurol. Sci.*, **2**, 307.

HALLER, J. S., WOLPERT, S. M., RABE, E. F., and HILLS, J. R. (1971) Cystic lesions of the posterior fossa in infants: a comparison of the clinical, radiological, and pathological findings in Dandy-Walker syndrome and extra-axial cysts, *Neurology (Minneap.)*, **21**, 494.

HAMMON, W. M. (1971) Evaluation and use of the ventriculo-peritoneal shunt in hydrocephalus, *J. Neurosurg.*, **34**, 792.

HARBERT, J. C. (1973) Radionuclide cisternography in adult hydrocephalus, *Proc. roy. Soc. Med.*, **66**, 827.

HART, M. N., MALAMUD, N., and ELLIS, W. G. (1972) The Dandy-Walker syndrome. A clinicopathological study based on 28 cases, *Neurology (Minneap.)*, **22**, 771.

JOHNSON, R. T., and JOHNSON, K. P. (1968) Hydrocephalus following viral infection: the pathology of aqueductal stenosis developing after experimental mumps virus infection, *J. Neuropath. exp. Neurol.*, **27**, 591.

JOHNSON, R. T., JOHNSON, K. P., and EDMONDS, C. J. (1967) Virus-induced hydrocephalus: development of aqueductal stenosis in hamsters after mumps infection, *Science*, **157**, 1066.

KURTZKE, J. F., GOLDBERG, I. D., and KURLAND, L. T. (1973) The distribution of deaths from congenital malformations of the nervous system, *Neurology (Minneap.)*, **23**, 483.

LAURENCE, K. M. (1959) The pathology of hydrocephalus, *Ann. roy. Coll. Surg. Engl.*, **24**, 388.

LAURENCE, K. M. (1969) Neurological and intellectual sequelae of hydrocephalus, *Arch. Neurol. (Chic.)*, **20**, 73.

McCULLOUGH, D. C., HARBERT, J. C., DI CHIRO, G., and OMMAYA, A. K. (1970) Prognostic criteria for cerebrospinal fluid shunting from isotope cisternography in communicating hydrocephalus, *Neurology (Minneap.)*, **20**, 594.

McDONALD, J. V. (1969) Persistent hydrocephalus following the removal of papillomas of the choroid plexus of the lateral ventricles, *J. Neurosurg.*, **30**, 736.

MACFARLANE, A., and MALONEY, A. F. J. (1957) The appearance of the aqueduct and its relationship to hydrocephalus in the Arnold–Chiari malformation, *Brain*, **80**, 479.

McHUGH, P. R. (1964) Occult hydrocephalus, *Quart. J. Med.*, **33**, 297.

MACNAB, G. H. (1962) *see* MACNAB, G. H. (1966).

MACNAB, G. H. (1966) The development of the knowledge and treatment of hydrocephalus, in *Hydrocephalus and Spina Bifida*, National Spastics Society, p. 1, London.

MESSERT, B., and WANNAMAKER, B. B. (1974) Reappraisal of the adult occult hydrocephalus syndrome, *Neurology (Minneap.)*, **24**, 224.

MILLEN, J. W., and WOOLLAM, D. H. M. (1958) Vitamins and the cerebrospinal fluid, *Ciba Foundation Symposium on the Cerebrospinal Fluid*, p. 168, London.

NICHOLAS, J. L., KAMAL, I. M., and ECKSTEIN, H. B. (1970) Immediate shunt replacement in the treatment of bacterial colonisation of Holter valves, in *Studies in Hydrocephalus and Spina Bifida, Develop. Med. Child Neurol.*, suppl. 22, p. 110.

NOBLE, T. C., LASSMAN, L. P., URQUHART, W., and AHERNE, W. A. (1970) Thrombotic and embolic complications of ventriculo-atrial shunts, in *Studies in Hydrocephalus and Spina Bifida, Develop. Med. Child Neurol.*, suppl. 22, p. 114.

ROGERS, K. J., and DUBOWITZ, V. (1970) 5-Hydroxyindoles in hydrocephalus. A comparative study of cerebrospinal fluid and blood levels, *Develop. Med. Child Neurol.*, **12,** 461.

RUSSELL, D. S. (1949) Observations on the pathology of hydrocephalus, *Spec. Rep. Ser. med. Res. Coun. (Lond.)*, No. 265.

SCARFF, J. E. (1963) Treatment of hydrocephalus; an historical and critical review of methods and results, *J. Neurol. Psychiat.*, **26**, 1.

SHELDON, W. D., PARKER, H. L., and KERNOHAN, J. W. (1930) Occlusion of the aqueduct of Sylvius, *Arch. Neurol. Psychiat. (Chic.)*, **23**, 1183.

SJAASTAD, O., SKALPE, I. O., and ENGESET, A. (1969) The width of the temporal horn in the differential diagnosis between pressure hydrocephalus and hydrocephalus ex vacuo, *Neurology (Minneap.)*, **19**, 1087.

SPOERRI, O., and RÖSLER, H. (1966) Isotope ventriculography with I^{131} and I^{125} in the evaluation of hydrocephalus, in *Hydrocephalus and Spina Bifida*, National Spastics Society, p. 88, London.

SYMON, L., DORSCH, N. W. C., and STEPHENS, R. J. (1972) Pressure waves in so-called low-pressure hydrocephalus, *Lancet*, **ii**, 1291.

SYMONDS, C. P. (1931) Otitic hydrocephalus, *Brain*, **54**, 55.

SYMONDS, C. P. (1937) Hydrocephalic and focal cerebral symptoms in relation to thrombophlebitis of the dural sinuses and cerebral veins, *Brain*, **60**, 531.

SYPERT, G. W., LEFFMAN, H., and OJEMANN, G. A. (1973) Occult normal pressure hydrocephalus manifested by Parkinsonism-dementia complex, *Neurology (Minneap.)*, **23**, 234.

TORKILDSEN, A. (1947) *Ventriculocisternostomy*, Oslo.

WALD, N. J., BROCK, D. J. H., and BONNAR, J. (1974) Prenatal diagnosis of spina bifida and anencephaly by maternal serum–alpha–fetoprotein measurement: a controlled study, *Lancet*, **i**, 765.

INTRACRANIAL TUMOUR

Definition. The term 'intracranial space-occupying lesion' is generally applied to identify any lesion, whether vascular, neoplastic, or inflammatory in origin, which increases the volume of the intracranial contents and thus leads to a rise in the intracranial pressure. In the strictest sense the term 'intracranial tumour' should be reserved for neoplasms, whether benign or malignant, primary or secondary, but conventionally this inclusive term is often used to embrace lesions such as vascular malformations and granulomas of inflammatory origin (e.g. gumma and tuberculoma) as well as parasitic cysts, which are not neoplastic in the strict pathological sense, and this convention will be followed here.

AETIOLOGY, INCIDENCE, AND PATHOGENESIS

Over 1 per cent of all deaths are due to intracranial tumours, which form about 10 per cent of all malignant neoplasms in man. Apart from those of inflammatory origin, the aetiology of intracranial tumours is little understood. In a minority of cases congenital abnormality appears to play an important part in causation, especially in the angiomatous malformations and the angioblastomas, the ganglioneuromas, the cholesteatomas, and the tumours of the craniopharyngeal pouch. Genetic factors are clearly important in the case of haemangioblastomas which are often familial, and in neurofibromatosis and tuberous sclerosis, both of which may be associated with intracranial growths; gliomas rarely occur in more than one member of a family (Zülch, 1956; Russell and Rubinstein, 1959). The causation of the gliomas is as obscure as that of neoplasms in general. It is uncertain whether the primitive character of the cells of which some gliomas are composed should be regarded as an indication that they are derived from embryonic cell rests, or should be considered as a cellular regression. While brain tumours have been induced in animals of various species by chemical means, using especially nitrosurea derivatives, or by virus infection (Bigner et al., 1972), there is no convincing evidence that chemical carcinogens, viruses, or other environmental factors play a significant role in the pathogenesis of intracranial neoplasia in man, although the description of intracranial neoplasms of mesenchymal origin (especially reticulum cell sarcoma) developing in patients after renal transplantation (Schneck and Penn, 1971) suggests that iatrogenic immunosuppression may rarely play a part. There is little evidence that trauma is a predisposing factor, except, rarely, in the case of meningiomas which have been known to arise beneath the site of a previous head injury.

An intracranial tumour may occur at any age, though, as will be seen later, certain types of glioma show a characteristic age incidence. The frequent occurrence of some forms of glioma in childhood accounts for the fact that the age incidence of intracranial tumours differs from that of most other malignant neoplasms, which are rare before middle life. Intracranial tumour affects the sexes with equal frequency and shows no significant variation in geographical incidence (Kurtzke, 1969) except that tuberculomas and some forms of parasitic cyst are much commoner in under-developed countries.

PATHOLOGY

The pathology of intracranial neoplasms has made great advances during the present century, following upon the early work of Cajal, Hortega, and Cushing and his pupils, and has assumed considerable clinical importance. The different types of tumour, even the different varieties of glioma, often exhibit a characteristic age incidence and rate of growth and a predilection for certain situations in the brain. It has become possible for the clinician to diagnose with increasing precision not only the presence and situation of an intracranial tumour, but also its precise pathological nature, and to form an accurate estimate of its prospects of removal, of the peculiar difficulties likely to be encountered in the task, and of its probable malignancy. Modern techniques of investigation, including angiography, isotope encephalography, and EMI scanning, will often not only localize the tumour but give some indication of its pathological nature, and histological examination of biopsy specimens, where appropriate, often gives information of considerable value in determining treatment and prognosis.

In Cushing's (1932 b) oft-quoted series of 2,023 intracranial tumours, about 43 per cent were gliomas, 18 per cent pituitary adenomas, 13 per cent meningiomas, 7 per cent sarcomas, and 4 per cent metastases, but since that time the proportion of metastases reported in all series has increased and that of sarcomas and pituitary adenomas has fallen. A representative recent series of 3,010 cases described by Courville (1967) gave the following percentage incidence:

Gliomas	41·5
Pituitary adenomas	3·4
Meningiomas	11·6
Acoustic neuromas	2·5
Congenital tumours	3·5
Metastases	23·7
Granulomatous tumours	2·5
Blood vessel tumours	7·8
Sarcomas	0·3
Parasitic cysts	0·7
Miscellaneous lesions	2·2

There is now general agreement that gliomas constitute 40–45 per cent of all intracranial neoplasms, metastases about 20 per cent, meningiomas about 10 per cent, and acoustic neuromas and pituitary tumours not more than 5 per cent each.

Gliomas

The gliomas are tumours derived from the cells which constitute the supporting tissue of the nervous system, but unlike connective-tissue tumours elsewhere they are of epiblastic origin. Their precise classification is still unsettled. Bailey and Cushing (1926) proposed a classification based upon the development of the glial cell, but this was criticized by Scherer (1940 a and b). He pointed out that too much stress had been laid upon specific staining methods, and that immature or anaplastic glioma cells cannot be identified with certainty. Systematic examination of complete tumours reveals different types of cell in a single tumour. Moreover, tumours which are histologically identical may behave quite differently, e.g. the cerebral and cerebellar astrocytomas and the more and less rapidly growing oligodendrogliomas. Sometimes a glioma seems to arise diffusely, as in so-called 'gliomatosis cerebri', or from multiple centres at the same time. Kernohan et al. (1949) recognized only five main groups of primary brain tumours, distinguishing within the group grades of malignancy. Though not universally accepted, their classification, based upon the characteristics of the predominant cell in the tumour in ascending grades of malignancy from 1 to 4, is widely used. Thus the astrocytoma of Bailey and Cushing (1926) is their astrocytoma grade 1, the astroblastoma grade 2, and the glioblastoma multiforme becomes an astrocytoma grade 3 or 4, depending upon the degree of malignancy. Similarly, the classical ependymoma becomes an ependymoma grade 1, the ependymoblastoma becomes the ependymoma grades 2–4, and the oligodendroglioma and oligodendroblastoma become oligodendrogliomas of grades 1–4. The classification of the medulloblastoma remains unchanged; the rare neurocytomas, ganglioneuromas, gangliocytomas, and gangliogliomas become the neuroastrocytoma grade 1, and the neuroblastoma, spongio-neuroblastoma, and glioneuroblastoma are included in the neuroastrocytomas, grades 2–4.

With the exception of the ependymoma the gliomas are all infiltrative tumours. This explains the great difficulty of complete surgical removal and the liability to recurrence after operation. Moreover, the fact that the glioma may leave nervous tissue which it infiltrates intact explains why a tumour may be much more extensive than would be supposed from the symptoms and physical signs. The gliomas most frequently encountered are the astrocytomas, about 36 per cent, glioblastomas, about 34 per cent, and medulloblastomas, about 11 per cent.

Medulloblastoma. These are rapidly growing tumours which are most frequently encountered in the cerebellum in children, where they arise in the region of the roof of the fourth ventricle, but they also occur rarely in adults. They are composed of masses of rounded undifferentiated cells [FIG. 39] and show a marked tendency to disseminate through the subarachnoid space both of the brain and of the spinal cord. Other gliomas may show a similar spread but much less commonly; the medulloblastoma is also unique in that it may metastasize outside the cranial cavity giving secondary deposits especially in

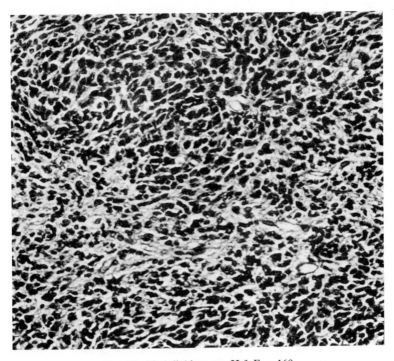

FIG. 39. Medulloblastoma, H & E, ×160

bone, particularly after partial operative removal or after a shunting operation carried out to relieve hydrocephalus. The medulloblastoma is one of the more malignant gliomas, and the average duration of illness is six months before and six months after operation though, especially in adults, survival for several years is not uncommon. Radiation appears to be of considerable value in retarding the growth of this tumour.

Glioblastoma Multiforme (Astrocytoma grades 3–4). This is an extremely malignant glioma arising in middle life and almost invariably found in the cerebral hemispheres. It tends to infiltrate the brain extensively and often attains an enormous size. It is a reddish, highly vascular tumour, and often exhibits haemorrhages and areas of necrosis [FIG. 40]. Microscopically it consists of relatively undifferentiated round or oval cells, together with spongioblastic and

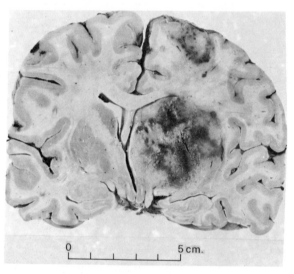

0   5 cm.

FIG. 40. Glioblastoma multiforme (astrocytoma grade IV) involving parietal cortex, centrum semiovale, and basal ganglia of the left cerebral hemisphere with oedema of the affected hemisphere and displacement of the ventricular system

astroblastic forms; cellular polymorphism with frequent mitoses indicates its anaplastic character [FIG. 41]. No form of treatment prolongs life for more than a few months, and the average survival period for those treated surgically is twelve months.

Astrocytoma (Astrocytoma grade 1). These tumours have been divided into protoplasmic, fibrillary, pilocytic, and gemistocytic types (Russell and Rubinstein, 1959) depending upon their predominant cellular constitution, but this subdivision has little clinical significance. They are white, infiltrating growths which may occur at any age, and in either the cerebral [FIG. 42] or the cerebellar hemispheres. They grow slowly, and are relatively benign, and the average survival period after the first symptom is 67 months in the case of the former and 89 months in the case of the latter. The cerebellar astrocytoma of

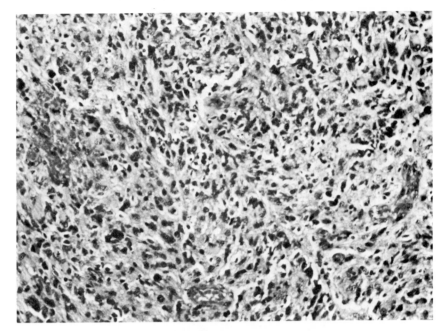

A, H & E, ×160

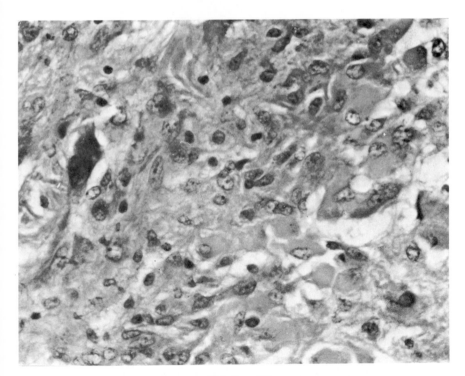

B, H & E, ×400

FIG. 41. Glioblastoma multiforme (astrocytoma grade IV)

childhood is a particularly benign tumour. Microscopically [FIG. 43] they exhibit abundant astrocytes and, in the case of the fibrillary astrocytomas, a dense fibril network, and the tumour cells exhibit attachments to the blood vessels characteristic of the astrocyte. Astrocytomas are particularly liable to undergo cystic transformation. Gliomatous cysts, therefore, have on the whole a favourable prognosis, though cystic change is also fairly common in the glioblastomas.

The *astroblastoma* is somewhat less benign though not as malignant as the glioblastoma multiforme and usually occurs in the white matter of one cerebral

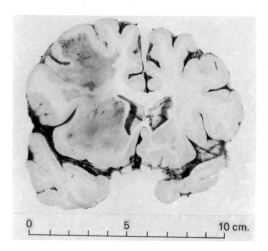

FIG. 42. An extensive astrocytoma grade II of the right cerebral hemisphere

hemisphere. Russell and Rubinstein (1959) still identify a so-called *polar spongioblastoma* as a relatively benign tumour of childhood or early adult life, occurring especially in the optic nerve and chiasm or brain stem, but others regard this neoplasm as merely an astrocytoma of pilocytic type.

Less common gliomas are:

Oligodendroglioma. This is a rare, slowly growing, usually relatively benign tumour occurring in the cerebral hemispheres in young adults. Oligodendrogliomas often calcify, giving a fine punctate or stippled pattern [FIG. 44] which, on a skull radiograph, may be virtually diagnostic; more malignant forms (oligodendroblastoma) are rare.

Ependymoma. This is a firm, whitish tumour, sometimes pedunculated, arising from the ependyma, frequently in the roof of the fourth ventricle and sometimes from the walls of the other ventricles or from the central canal of the spinal cord. Histologically it shows a characteristic 'rosette' formation [FIG. 45].

Neuroblastoma, Ganglioglioma, and Ganglioneuroma. These rare tumours all contain ganglion cells. The neuroblastoma is made up predominantly of neuroblasts (neuroastrocytoma grades 2–4), the ganglioglioma shows abnormal ganglion cells lying among proliferating astrocytes or astroblasts, and the ganglioneuroma contains not only ganglion cells and astrocytes but also nerve fibres, usually unmyelinated (neuroastrocytoma grade 1).

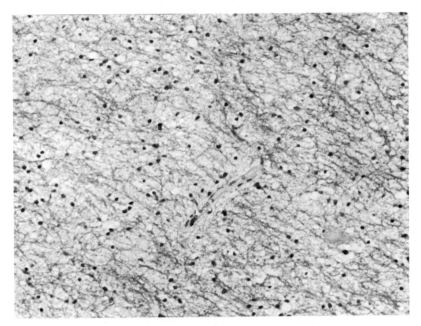

A, fibrillary type, H & E, ×160

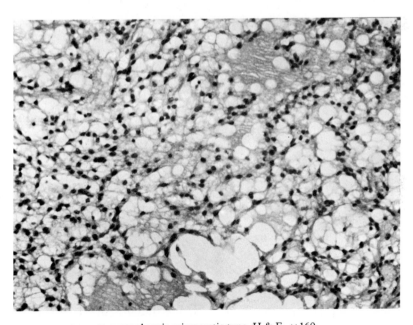

B, protoplasmic microcystic type, H & E, ×160

FIG. 43. Astrocytoma grade I

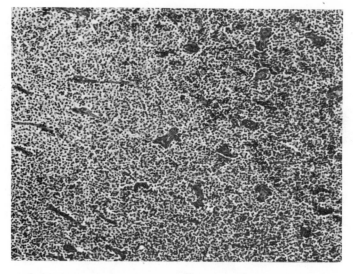

A, ×64

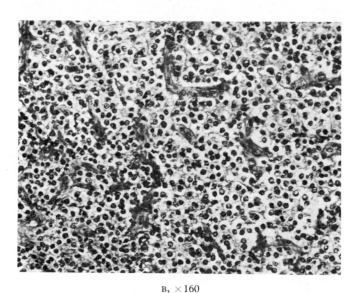

B, ×160

FIG. 44. Oligodendroglioma, H & E. Note the areas of calcification

Meningioma

These tumours [FIG. 46] were at one time thought to arise from the dura mater and hence were known as dural endotheliomas. It is now believed, however, that, although they are attached to the dura, most arise from the arachnoid cells which penetrate the dura to form the arachnoid villi, projecting into the dural venous sinuses. They are composed of specialized connective-tissue cells resembling the cells which constitute the arachnoid villus. These cells are

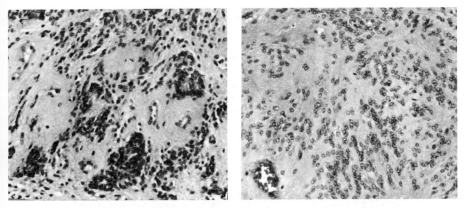

Fig. 45A and B. Two examples of 4th ventricle ependymomas showing variations in the histological appearance. H & E, × 160

present in columns or whorls [Fig. 47], and the tumour sometimes contains fibroglia together with collagen fibres and small calcified concretions known as psammoma bodies. Syncytial and angioblastic histological types have been described.

Commonly the meningioma is a single, large, more or less irregularly lobulated growth, but less frequently it may form a flat plaque spreading over the inner surface of the dura ('meningioma en plaque'). A distinctive feature of the meningiomas is their relationship to the bones of the skull. Though hyperostosis may occur as a reaction in the overlying bone without its having been invaded, these tumours tend to invade bone in about 20 per cent of cases, absorption of bone and new bone formation occurring simultaneously. In this process the outer table of the skull may be absorbed and rebuilt so as to constitute a bony boss. Microscopically, meningioma cells fill the Haversian canals and spaces.

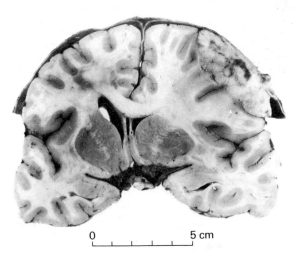

0   5 cm

Fig. 46. A left parietal meningioma

New bone is laid down in spicules perpendicularly to the surface of the skull, the osteogenetic cells being derived from the outer layers of the dura or from the bone itself. In rare cases a meningioma may perforate the skull and infiltrate the extracranial tissues. The meningioma, which is of mesodermal origin, does not usually invade the brain but compresses it, and the resulting disturbance of cerebral function is as a rule much less marked in proportion to the size of the tumour than is the case with the gliomas. A malignant invasive form (sarcomatous change) is described and seems particularly to occur in the rare instances when the tumour recurs after apparent total removal.

Since the meningiomas arise from the cells of the arachnoid villi they are commonly found along the course of the intracranial venous sinuses, and their

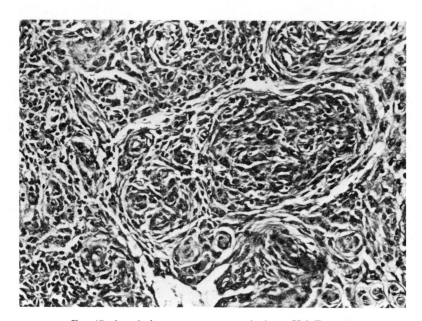

FIG. 47. A typical psammomatous meningioma, H & E, ×160

sites of greatest predilection are the superior sagittal sinus—parasagittal meningiomas; the sphenoparietal sinus and the middle meningeal vessels— meningiomas of the sphenoid ridge and the convexities; the olfactory groove of the ethmoid; and the circle of sinuses around the sella turcica—suprasellar meningiomas. Meningiomas are uncommon below the tentorium but may arise from the tentorium itself or at the torcula. Occasionally they are found within the lateral ventricles. All meningiomas are commoner in women than in men. Multiple meningiomas may occur in association with multiple neurofibromas [see p. 665].

Reticuloses

Deposits of lymphoma, lymphosarcoma, and of leukaemic cells may, on occasion, develop in the cranial and spinal meninges, giving symptoms of cerebral or spinal compression (John and Nabarro, 1955; Hutchinson *et al.*, 1958; Sohn *et al.*, 1967; Currie and Henson, 1971; West *et al.*, 1972). A solitary reticulum cell sarcoma arising in the cranial bones or spinal column may similarly compress or invade nervous tissue. In addition, a reticulum cell sarcoma sometimes arises within the brain itself giving symptoms and signs of a focal cerebral lesion; alternatively such a neoplasm may arise diffusely throughout the cerebral substance ('microgliomatosis cerebri') (Schaumburg *et al.*, 1972).

Acoustic Neuroma

Acoustic neuromas are usually unilateral [FIG. 48]. Rarely they are bilateral and are then usually, though not always, manifestations of generalized neurofibromatosis and may be associated with multiple meningiomas [see p. 665]. Familial examples of bilateral acoustic neuroma have been reported. Penfield believes that the solitary acoustic neuroma can be differentiated histologically from that associated with generalized neurofibromatosis. A solitary tumour consists of elongated cells like spindle fibroblasts with much collagen and reticulum, and exhibits marked palisading and parallelism of nuclei [FIG. 49]. Some workers believe that these tumours arise from the perineurial or endoneurial connective tissue and that the fibroblast is their type cell. They have therefore been termed 'perineurial fibroblastomas'. Russell and Rubinstein (1959), deriving them from the Schwann cells, call them schwannomas, but they are also called neurilemmomas or neurofibromas. Though the eighth cranial nerve is their commonest site, similar tumours may be found upon other cranial nerves, especially the optic and the trigeminal, upon spinal nerve roots, usually the dorsal, and upon peripheral nerves.

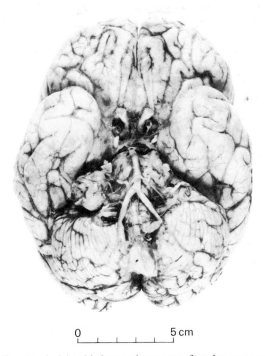

0   5 cm

FIG. 48. A right-sided acoustic neuroma found at autopsy

I

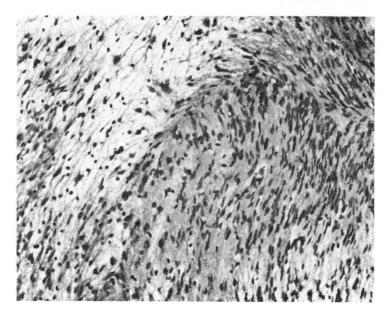

A, H & E, ×160, showing Antoni type A and B appearances, A to the right, B to the left

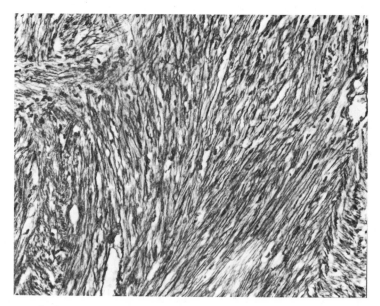

B, reticulin, ×160, showing the close reticulin net in an Antoni type A area

FIG. 49. An acoustic neuroma

Blood Vessel Tumours

The blood vessel tumours of the brain have been subjected to detailed study only comparatively recently and any classification is necessarily to some extent provisional. The following forms are encountered:

1. The angiomatous malformations.
2. The cavernous haemangiomas.
3. The haemangioblastomas.
4. The Sturge–Weber syndrome.

The first two groups are collectively known as blood vessel hamartomas. However, it should be noted that the term hamartoma has also been applied to areas of ectopic neuronal and glial tissue, often encapsulated, and clearly of developmental origin which have been found within the substance of the brain or in the meninges. Thus some, but not all, hamartomas have a blood vessel component.

1. *The Angiomatous Malformations.* These are probably to be regarded as congenital abnormalities of vascular development rather than as true neoplasms. They may be divided into (*a*) telangiectases, (*b*) arteriovenous malformations.

(*a*) *Telangiectases*, or capillary angiomas, consist of groups of greatly dilated capillaries. They may be associated with Osler's hereditary telangiectasia and are usually accidental post-mortem findings, though rupture has been known to cause death through haemorrhage.

(*b*) *Arteriovenous Malformations.* These consist of a mass of enlarged and tortuous cortical vessels, supplied by one or more large arteries usually derived from the blood supply of one, but sometimes of both, hemispheres, and sometimes fed also from below the tentorium, and drained by one or more large veins. Sometimes there is also a contribution from the middle meningeal artery. These malformations are most frequently encountered in the field of the middle cerebral artery, but may involve the brain stem (Logue and Monckton, 1954).

Angiography has revealed that the angiomatous malformations are commoner than used to be thought. Verified angiomas accounted in one series for 6·5 per cent of 200 cases of cerebral vascular disease. Increased vascularity of the scalp, with large and pulsating arteries, and hypertrophy of one or both carotids may be present, and even secondary cardiac hypertrophy may occur. A bruit is commonly heard over one or both carotid arteries in the neck and on the scalp overlying the angioma.

2. *The Cavernous Haemangiomas.* The cavernous haemangiomas appear to be congenital abnormalities rather than true neoplasms. They usually occur above the tentorium. They form a lobulated mass consisting of small and large spaces containing blood. Similar haemangiomas of vertebral bodies may cause vertebral collapse and spinal cord compression (McAllister *et al.*, 1975).

3. *The Haemangioblastomas.* The haemangioblastomas are tumours which, according to Cushing and Bailey (1928), are composed of angioblasts, the primitive cells which normally form the fetal blood vessels. They usually consist of vascular channels and spaces with sparse intercapillary tissue containing swollen fat-laden endothelial cells [FIG. 50]. They exhibit a marked tendency to form cysts in the surrounding nerve tissue, the cyst containing xanthochromic fluid which is probably an exudate from the tumour vessels. The cyst may be large and the tumour a small nodule in its wall, which must be excised if the cyst is not to refill. The haemangioblastomas are almost invariably subtentorial tumours, though they have been rarely observed above the tentorium. They are usually single, but there may be multiple growths in

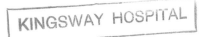

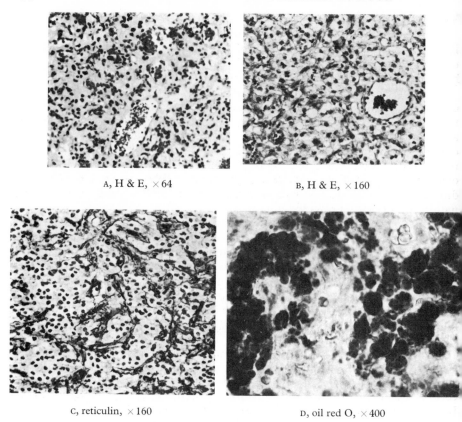

A, H & E, ×64

B, H & E, ×160

C, reticulin, ×160

D, oil red O, ×400

FIG. 50. Haemangioblastoma of cerebellum, showing fat-filled macrophages

the cerebellum or in addition to a cerebellar tumour a tumour in the medulla or spinal cord. An important feature is the association of haemangioblastomas with abnormalities in other parts of the body. The most important of these, because the most easily observed, is a haemangioblastoma of the retina (von Hippel's disease). This is a small tumour usually situated in the periphery of the retina and supplied by an enlarged artery and vein. Secondary proliferative changes in, and rarely even detachment of, the retina may render it difficult to recognize. Other abnormalities which may coexist are haemangioblastoma of the spinal cord, cysts of the pancreas and kidneys, hypernephromas of the kidneys or the suprarenal glands. The coincidence of these abnormalities is known as Lindau's disease and is familial in about 20 per cent of cases. Polycythaemia may occur.

4. *The Sturge–Weber Syndrome.* In the fully developed form of this disorder an extensive capillary-venous malformation affects one hemisphere, particularly in the parieto-occipital region and is associated with a characteristic 'wavy' pattern of subcortical calcification which outlines the gyri and is visible radiologically after the third to fifth year of life. There is a 'port-wine' stain on the face on the affected side, often with an associated buphthalmos (ox eye), while most patients have a contralateral hemiparesis and epilepsy.

Craniopharyngioma

These tumours are also described as tumours of the craniopharyngeal, or Rathke's, pouch, adamantinomas, and hypophysial epidermoids. In order to understand their origin it is necessary briefly to review the development of the hypophysis (pituitary gland) in the embryo.

The hypophysis develops as a result of fusion of an evagination of the ectoderm of the stomadaeum with a process which extends downwards from the floor of the forebrain. The former loses its opening into the mouth cavity and becomes a closed sac from which are derived the anterior lobe and the pars intermedia of the hypophysis. The process from the forebrain forms the posterior lobe and the infundibulum. The remnants of the craniopharyngeal pouch remain, and, owing to rotation of the developing gland, come to lie anterior to the infundibulum and at the upper angle of the anterior lobe. They may also be found within the sella turcica itself.

Tumours arising from these embryonic relics show characteristics resulting from their origin. They contain cells resembling those of the buccal epithelium of the embryo, including the ameloblasts of the embryonic enamel organ. These tumours are very liable to undergo cystic degeneration [FIG. 51] and calcification and may even develop bone. They usually arise above the sellar diaphragm, and extend upwards into the third ventricle and hypothalamic region, but occasionally are seen within the sella itself.

Tumours of the Hypophysis (Pituitary Gland)

The cells of the anterior lobe of the hypophysis are the alpha, eosinophil, or acidophil cells, which secrete growth hormone, luteinizing hormone, and prolactin; the beta or basophil cells, which secrete follicle-stimulating hormone, corticotrophin and thyrotrophin, and the poorly staining chromophobe cells. It is now thought that the small chromophobe cell may be a stem cell, the large chromophobe being an actively secreting cell (see Hubble, 1961).

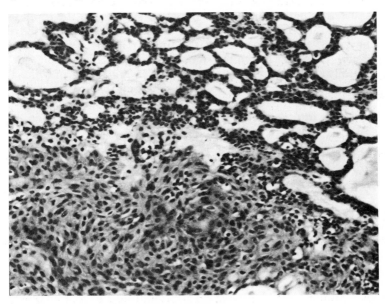

FIG. 51. Craniopharyngioma, H & E, ×160

The common hypophysial tumours are adenomas. The commonest of these is the chromophobe adenoma, composed of cells which sometimes show alveolar formation and resemble the chromophobe cells of the normal gland. The endocrine disturbances associated with chromophobe tumour are those of 'hypopituitarism'. The chromophil adenoma is composed of cells resembling the acidophil cells of the normal gland. It sometimes undergoes cystic degeneration. This tumour gives rise to symptoms of hyperpituitarism—gigantism if it develops before puberty and acromegaly in adults. The basophil adenoma is usually microscopic in size and only rarely causes pressure symptoms. It causes Cushing's syndrome; this condition is much more often due to hyperadrenalism.

The hypophysial adenomas arise within the sella turcica, which they expand, and later may pass through the sellar diaphragm and attain a considerable size, compressing the structures at the base of the brain.

Adenocarcinoma of the hypophysis is a rare, rapidly growing tumour which gives rise to metastases.

The occurrence within the sella turcica of metastases from extracranial tumours is rare and has been most frequently recorded in cases of carcinoma of the breast.

Osteoma and Osteochondroma

Ivory osteomas may develop in the frontal or ethmoidal sinuses and may occasionally be large enough to compress the frontal lobe. Osteochondroma of the base of the skull rarely gives neurological manifestations but has been known to produce subarachnoid haemorrhage.

Cholesteatoma

The cholesteatoma, or cerebrospinal epidermoid, is a rare tumour of adult life which affects males more frequently than females. It is regarded as a fetal epithelial inclusion and is most frequently found in the subarachnoid cisterns at the base of the brain. Those arising below the tentorium, a common site, may be situated either in the cerebellopontine angle or in the midline on the ventral aspect of the cerebellum, or within the fourth ventricle or in the temporal bone. The naked-eye appearance of the tumour in the fresh state is highly characteristic. It is pearly white, smooth, and glistening, firm but brittle. Microscopically a cholesteatoma is composed of several layers, of which the most characteristic—the stratum granulosum—consisting of several rows of large, finely granular cells, probably corresponds to the dermis. Rarely these tumours may leak keratin into the cerebrospinal fluid causing degeneration of cranial nerves and the spinal cord (Tomlinson and Walton, 1967).

Dermoid Cysts

Posterior fossa dermoid cysts have been described in children but are very uncommon.

Pinealoma

The commonest variety of tumour arising in the region of the pineal gland, and thus called a pinealoma, is in fact a teratoma (Russell, 1944; Russell and Rubinstein, 1959); growths arising from pineal cells are very rare.

Colloid Cysts of the Third Ventricle

These are rounded cystic tumours measuring from 1 to 3 cm in diameter and arising from the paraphysis, ependyma, or choroid plexus. They are lined with ciliated epithelium and contain thick glairy fluid or gelatinous material. Owing to their position they readily cause intermittent hydrocephalus.

Chordoma

These rare tumours, derived from primitive remnants of the notochord, arise either in the region of the clivus, causing cranial nerve palsies and backward displacement of the pons, or in the body of the sacrum and sacral canal, causing a cauda equina syndrome.

Papilloma of the Choroid Plexus

Up to half of these benign vascular tumours occur in the fourth ventricle, about one-third in the lateral ventricles (usually left) and one-sixth in the third ventricle. Recurrent or chronic subarachnoid bleeding and communicating hydrocephalus may result.

Glomus Tumours

These tumours arise from the glomus jugulare and may invade the middle ear or the posterior fossa giving rise to unilateral deafness and multiple palsies of lower cranial nerves; erosion of the base of the skull is often visible radiologically (Henson *et al.*, 1953; Siekert, 1956). Sometimes the tumour invades the internal and middle ear and may be seen with the auriscope. Glomus intravagale tumours also occur but, like the histologically similar carotid body tumours, are usually extracranial. Though they are similar pathologically to chromaffinomas in other sites these neoplasms rarely, if ever, secrete noradrenaline.

Metastatic Tumours

About 20 per cent of cerebral neoplasms are secondary to a primary growth elsewhere, usually in the lung, breast, stomach, prostate, kidney, or thyroid. The lung appears to be the commonest source of metastatic cerebral tumour and not infrequently the symptoms of the cerebral growth are more conspicuous than those of the primary. Secondary cerebral carcinomas are usually multiple and rapidly growing. Hence the history of symptoms is usually short. They are pinkish, rounded tumours, well defined from the oedematous and softened surrounding brain tissue. Metastases within the fourth ventricle may give in middle or late life the same triad of symptoms (morning headache, morning vomiting, and postural vertigo) as is seen in younger patients with ependymomas in the same site. An important variety of secondary carcinoma within the skull is constituted by a group of cases in which the tumour cells infiltrate the dura at the base of the skull and spread into the leptomeninges and the bones of the base. This condition is sometimes described as carcinomatosis of the meninges and may rarely lead to subdural haematoma. More often many of the cranial nerves are compressed or infiltrated and multiple cranial nerve palsies are accompanied by neck stiffness, headache, and confusion (Jacobs and Richland, 1951; Olson *et al.*, 1974). The hypophysis may be invaded and the tuber cinereum compressed, leading to metabolic and endocrine disorders. In such cases metastatic deposits may be present in the uppermost cervical lymph nodes. Secondary sarcoma of the brain is much rarer than secondary carcinoma. Melanotic sarcoma may metastasize with great rapidity to the brain and meninges and can produce subarachnoid haemorrhage.

Myeloma

Multiple myelomatosis frequently involves the cranial bones, giving multiple areas of osteolysis; it rarely involves the brain but extradural deposits from solitary or multiple myelomas may compress the spinal cord. Solitary myelomas have been described in the skull base or orbit (Gardner-Thorpe, 1970) and in the substance of the brain (French, 1947; Clarke, 1954).

Tumours of Infective Origin

Tuberculoma. Tuberculoma of the brain appears to be much less frequent in Britain than a generation ago, when it was regarded as one of the commonest of intracranial tumours. It is still one of the commonest intracranial tumours on the Indian sub-continent. Cerebral tuberculomas are more frequently subtentorial than supratentorial and vary in size from small nodules up to large masses which may occupy more than one lobe of the brain. They are usually at some point subjacent to the pia mater. There is a yellow caseous centre surrounded by a pinkish-grey outer zone. Microscopically, cerebral tuberculomas show the features characteristic of tuberculous lesions elsewhere. The caseous centre is surrounded by a zone containing giant cells and epithelioid cells and vessels showing endarteritis. Outside this area infiltration with compound granular corpuscles and fibrosis is conspicuous.

Gumma. Gumma of the brain is extremely rare. It is generally connected with the meninges, probably arising initially as a circumscribed patch of gummatous meningitis. Its pathology is described in the section on cerebral syphilis.

Parasitic Cysts. Intracranial hydatid cysts are rare even in countries in which hydatid infection is common, the brain being infected in only 5 per cent of cases. They may be single or multiple. They sometimes occur outside the dura, and in one of Brain's patients, an extradural collection of hydatids eroded the frontal bone, and some cysts were extruded through the scalp. More often the cysts, which frequently attain the size of a hen's egg, occupy the substance of the cerebral hemispheres or lie within the ventricles. Cysticercus cellulosae and coenurus cerebralis cysts may cause symptoms of increased intracranial pressure. Either may occur in the ventricles or cause an adhesive arachnoiditis in the posterior fossa. Cysticercus cellulosae may also behave as a space-occupying lesion in the cerebral hemisphere (Kuper *et al.*, 1958) [see also p. 451]. Rarely infection of the brain with the ova of *Schistosoma japonicum* may cause tumour-like masses.

PATHOLOGICAL PHYSIOLOGY

The functions of the brain depend upon the maintenance of the circulation of the blood and of the CSF at their appropriate pressures. The brain is unique among the viscera in being confined within a rigid box, the cranium. It follows that the total volume of the intracranial contents, the brain and its coverings, the blood vessels and the blood, and the CSF is constant, and that an increase in the volume of any one of them can only occur at the expense of the others. The intracranial contents, however, do not respond passively to changes in their volume or pressure, but react in complicated ways, so that any such alteration has far-reaching consequences. Four factors which influence the intracranial pressure require consideration—the mass of the brain, the circulatory system, the CSF, and the rigidity of the skull.

The Mass of the Brain

An intracranial tumour usually increases the mass of the brain, though in the case of certain slowly growing infiltrating tumours the increase in mass may be very slight, with the result that symptoms of increased intracranial pressure are slight or absent. The direct local effects of the increased mass of the brain produced by a tumour play a comparatively small part in raising intracranial pressure. Owing to the partial division of the cranial cavity into compartments by the falx and the tentorium, the local rise of pressure is to a considerable extent limited to the cranial compartment in which the tumour arises though it may cause local herniations, e.g. of the cingulate gyrus of the frontal lobe beneath the falx cerebri—subfalcial herniation, of the medial temporal lobe into the opening in the tentorium—tentorial herniation, or of the cerebellar tonsils into the foramen magnum—the cerebellar pressure cone.

The Cerebral Circulation

Compression of veins and venous sinuses increases venous pressure, thus contributing to the rise in intracranial pressure and is also one factor responsible for the induction of cerebral oedema, which is a common complication of intracranial tumour. Pressure upon arteries reduces blood flow either focally or generally (if the rise in pressure is severe), and rarely infarction may result. More often reflex arterial hypertension develops in an attempt to compensate for the increased cerebral arterial resistance.

The Cerebrospinal Fluid

Depending upon their size and situation, many tumours give rise to hydrocephalus, not only by increasing the volume of the intracranial contents but also by obstructing the circulation of the CSF; for example, a tumour in or near the midbrain which compresses or kinks the aqueduct is particularly likely to have this effect.

The Rigidity of the Skull

In the adult after union of the cranial sutures the skull is rigid and unyielding, and by preserving the volume of the intracranial contents constant is responsible for the far-reaching effects of a disturbance of the intracranial pressure. In the child the non-union of the sutures provides a partial safety-valve, and allows of some expansion. Hence a marked rise of intracranial pressure in childhood leads to separation of the sutures, and the skull yields a 'cracked-pot sound' on percussion. Some relief of the pressure results and other signs of raised intracranial pressure are often slighter in childhood than in later life.

MODE OF ONSET

The mode of onset of symptoms depends upon the nature and site of the tumour. It is slowest in the case of astrocytomas, oligodendrogliomas, meningiomas, acoustic neuromas, and pituitary adenomas which may be present for years before the patient consults a doctor, and most rapid in glioblastoma multiforme and secondary carcinoma. The commonest modes of onset are (1) progressive focal symptoms, e.g. focal epilepsy, monoplegia, hemiplegia, aphasia, cerebellar deficiency, associated with symptoms of increased intracranial pressure; (2) symptoms of increased intracranial pressure alone; (3) progressive focal symptoms alone, e.g. visual failure, unilateral deafness, dementia; (4) generalized epileptic attacks preceding other symptoms by many years; both slowly-growing gliomas and meningiomas may cause epilepsy for as long as 20 years, before causing other symptoms; (5) an apoplectiform onset with loss of consciousness, and perhaps hemiplegia.

SYMPTOMS OF INCREASED INTRACRANIAL PRESSURE

The symptoms of an intracranial tumour are conveniently divided into symptoms attributable to increased intracranial pressure, and focal symptoms which are due to the local effects of the growth. It might be expected that focal symptoms would arise before a tumour was large enough to disturb the intracranial pressure. More frequently, however, the reverse is the case, and the general symptoms often indicate the presence of a tumour which it is by no means easy to localize by physical examination alone. Headache, papilloedema, and vomiting may be described as the classical triad of symptoms of increased intracranial pressure, but they are not found with equal frequency. In one series headache was present in 88 per cent, papilloedema in 75 per cent, and vomiting in 65 per cent of cases of cerebral tumour. All three were found together in only 60 per cent. It is clearly unnecessary that all, or indeed any, of these symptoms should be present in order to diagnose an intracranial tumour.

Headache. The headache of intracranial tumour is probably mainly due to compression or distortion of the dura and of the intracranial blood vessels. It is often paroxysmal, at least in the earlier stages. It is usually described as a throbbing or a 'bursting' pain. It occurs chiefly during the night and in the early morning. Often the patient awakens with a headache which lasts from a few minutes to a few hours and then passes off, to recur the next day. With the gradual enlargement of the growth the headaches tend to become more prolonged and may ultimately be continuous. They always tend to be intensified by any activities which raise the intracranial pressure, such as exertion, excitement, coughing, sneezing, vomiting, stooping, and straining at stool. They may be influenced by posture, being worse when the patient is lying down, or lying upon one side, and may be relieved by adopting a sitting attitude.

Owing to the early occurrence of a diffuse rise of intracranial pressure in many cases of cerebral tumour, headache is of little localizing significance. The pain due to the local pressure of the growth may be predominantly unilateral, on the side of the tumour, and is occasionally associated with tenderness of the skull on percussion over a limited area overlying it. In the case of subtentorial tumours the headache in the early stages may be mainly suboccipital, with a tendency to radiate down the back of the neck. In such cases flexion of the neck may increase the pain and this sign may be a warning of a cerebellar pressure cone. As the intracranial pressure rises, the headache tends to be diffuse, and hydrocephalus may lead to paroxysms of severe diffuse pain radiating down the neck and sometimes associated with head retraction. Pressure upon the trigeminal nerve leads to unilateral pain, most commonly following the distribution of the first division and associated with hyperpathia or analgesia over the same area.

Papilloedema. The pathogenesis and appearances of papilloedema are described on pages 157-9. Its incidence varies according to the situation of the tumour. It is almost constant in tumours of the cerebellum, fourth ventricle, and temporal lobes, but is absent in half the cases of pontine and subcortical tumours. It is usually late in developing in the case of prefrontal tumours, and is often more severe with extracerebral than with intracerebral growths. Cerebellar tumours cause papilloedema of the greatest severity. A slight difference in the degree of swelling of the two optic discs is not uncommon, but is of little value as an indication of the situation of the tumour. A tumour arising sufficiently near the optic canal to cut off the subarachnoid space of the optic nerve from communication with the cerebral subarachnoid space causes primary optic atrophy on the affected side and occasionally contralateral papilloedema results from the general effect of the tumour (Foster Kennedy syndrome, often due to an olfactory groove meningioma).

The changes in the visual fields due to papilloedema consist of enlargement of the blind spot with concentric constriction at the periphery of the field. Visual acuity deteriorates, and, if the condition progresses, optic atrophy and complete blindness are likely to result. Patients with severe papilloedema are liable to brief transitory attacks of blindness which may give warning of impending irreversible visual failure due to arterial occlusion.

Vomiting. Vomiting, when due to intracranial tumour, usually occurs during the night or in the early morning when the headache is especially severe. Though sometimes, especially in children, it is preceded by little nausea, there is no ground for the belief that vomiting of cerebral origin is always of this precipitate character.

Epilepsy. While generalized epileptiform convulsions may occur in patients with hydrocephalus and increased intracranial pressure, in cases of intracranial tumour epileptic manifestations are usually due to the direct effect of the neoplasm upon the surrounding or underlying brain. Such attacks have been estimated to occur in about 30 per cent of cases (Hoefer et al., 1947; Nattrass, 1949); they are more likely when the tumour lies in or near the cerebral cortex and are infrequent when it lies deeply in the hemisphere, brain stem, or posterior fossa (Schmidt and Wilder, 1968). Such attacks are also more common with benign or slowly growing malignant neoplasms than with those of more rapid growth. In patients presenting with epilepsy the incidence of neoplasms rises steadily with increasing age and is greater in patients with focal rather than generalized seizures. Schmidt and Wilder (1968), reviewing a large number of published series, concluded that in patients with epilepsy beginning over the age of 20, about 10 per cent are eventually shown to have intracranial tumours. Penfield et al. (1940) found that about two-thirds of all patients with meningiomas or slowly growing astrocytomas and only about one-third of those with glioblastomas had fits at some stage.

Vertigo. While many patients with increased intracranial pressure due to intracranial tumour complain of unsteadiness or dizziness, true vertigo with an actual sense of rotation of the patient or his surroundings is uncommon, even in cases of acoustic neuroma. However, severe vertigo induced by change in posture is an important manifestation of ependymomas or metastases in or near the fourth ventricle and vertigo has also been reported as a very rare manifestation of temporal lobe tumour.

Disturbances of Pulse Rate and Blood Pressure. An acute or subacute rise of intracranial pressure, such as that due to intracranial haemorrhage or meningitis, often causes slowing of the pulse rate, usually to between 50 and 60 beats a minute. If the pressure continues to increase the pulse becomes extremely rapid. In either case it may be irregular. A gradual increase in the intracranial pressure, such as that due to an intracranial tumour, does not usually cause bradycardia, but moderate tachycardia is not uncommonly found in cases of subtentorial tumour.

A rapid rise of intracranial pressure usually causes a rise of blood pressure. Thus in intracranial haemorrhage a progressive rise of blood pressure probably indicates that the bleeding is continuing and in rapidly growing tumours or severe cerebral oedema there may be a similar sustained rise. Chronic rise of intracranial pressure does not have this effect, and in patients with more slowly growing tumours, especially when the lesion is below the tentorium, the blood pressure is often subnormal.

Respiratory Rate. A gradual rise of intracranial pressure does not at first affect the respiratory rate. A rise of sufficient rapidity and severity to produce loss of consciousness usually leads at first to slow and deep respirations. Later the respiratory rate may become irregular, e.g. of the Cheyne-Stokes type, in which periods of apnoea alternate with a series of respirations which wax and wane in amplitude. In the terminal stage of a fatal increase of intracranial pressure the respirations are rapid and shallow. These respiratory manifestations are in general due to compression or distortion of the brain stem, especially the medulla, where the respiratory centres lie. Central neurogenic hyperventilation [p. 1167] is not uncommon in such cases, but so-called apneustic or ataxic breathing (Plum and Posner, 1972) may each rarely occur. These abnormalities of respiratory rate and rhythm sometimes result from the median raphe haemorrhages or infarcts in the midbrain, extending down the brain stem, which may be a consequence of herniation of the medial temporal lobe through the tentorial notch; in such cases the patient usually lapses into irreversible coma. Hence these changes are not confined to posterior fossa neoplasms which directly compress or distort the brain stem but may also complicate supratentorial lesions.

'Hypopituitarism.' Any chronic state of increased intracranial pressure associated with internal hydrocephalus may lead to symptoms of 'hypopituitarism', namely, adiposity and genital atrophy in some cases, loss of body hair and hypoadrenalism with hypothyroidism in others. This is due to downward pressure of the floor of the distended third ventricle, which may erode the clinoid processes and diaphragma sellae and compress the hypophysis. These symptoms commonly arise in children and are most frequently seen in cases of cerebellar tumour. It is not easy to say whether they should be ascribed to compression of the hypothalamus or of the hypophysis itself. Possibly both are in part responsible. Radiography of the skull in such cases shows erosion of the clinoid processes and slight general enlargement of the sella turcica. This group of symptoms, if misinterpreted, may lead to the erroneous diagnosis of a hypophysial or suprasellar tumour.

Somnolence. Persistent somnolence is seen when hydrocephalus is pronounced and with tumours near the hypothalamus. Narcolepsy is uncommon.

Glycosuria. Glycosuria is occasionally encountered, sometimes with hyperglycaemia, more often with a normal blood-sugar and a lowered renal threshold.

Mental Symptoms. The most varied mental symptoms may be associated with increased intracranial pressure. If the pressure rises sufficiently high all mental activity is suspended in coma, and the more rapid the rise the more likely is this to occur. An acute or subacute rise of pressure insufficient to produce coma usually leads to confusion with disorientation in space and time. Chronic rise of intracranial pressure or frontal meningioma (Hunter *et al.*, 1968) may lead to progressive dementia, with a failure of intellectual capacity, emotional apathy, carelessness with regard to the person, and incontinence of urine and faeces. Less frequently, marked disturbances of mood are conspicuous, and the patient suffers from outbreaks of excitement or euphoria, or from depression in which he may be suicidal. In the mildest cases some impairment of memory and of power to concentrate, with irritability, may be the only mental symptoms.

In cases of intracranial tumour mental symptoms are most likely to occur when the tumour is situated in the frontal lobe or corpus callosum; but they may be produced by a tumour in any situation which causes a rise of intracranial pressure. Thus any of the mental disturbances described may be produced by a tumour of the cerebellum. Mental symptoms as a result of increased intracranial pressure are more likely to occur in the middle-aged and elderly than in younger patients.

False Localizing Signs

Collier first drew attention to the importance of symptoms, especially cranial nerve palsies, produced by intracranial tumours in other ways than by direct compression. Since these, unless properly interpreted, may lead to mistakes in localization, he termed them 'false localizing signs'. A sixth-nerve palsy on one or both sides, and, less frequently, a third-nerve palsy, may be thus produced and have been variously attributed to stretching of the nerves, to their compression by arteries, and to other modes of interference with their function resulting from displacement of the cranial contents, e.g. tentorial herniation compressing one third nerve at the edge of the tentorium. Other false localizing signs include bilateral extensor plantar responses or bilateral grasp reflexes resulting from interference with the function of the cerebral hemispheres by distension of the ventricles in hydrocephalus; 'hypopituitarism' resulting from hydrocephalus, as already described; an extensor plantar response occurring on the same side as a tumour of one cerebral hemisphere produced by compression of the opposite cerebral peduncle against the tentorium; cerebellar symptoms resulting from tumours of the frontal lobe, and midbrain signs, especially fixed dilated pupils, produced by a tumour of the cerebellar vermis.

EXAMINATION OF THE HEAD

Examination of the head may yield important information in cases of intracranial tumour and should never be neglected. There may be visible enlargement when hydrocephalus develops before the union of the cranial sutures. In such cases separation of the sutures may yield a 'cracked-pot sound' on percussion. Local tenderness of the skull may be present in the region overlying the tumour. A bony boss may overlie a meningioma. Venous congestion of the scalp is a not uncommon result of increased intracranial pressure in children with marked separation of the sutures. Dilatation and tortuosity of the arteries of the scalp are sometimes associated with a vascular intracranial tumour, especially a meningioma or an angioma. Such arterial congestion is usually confined to the side of the tumour and is often most evident in the superficial temporal artery. An audible bruit should be sought by auscultation. It is most frequently present over an arterial angioma, much less frequently over a highly vascularized meningioma, very rarely in the presence of an aneurysm. However, cranial bruits are not infrequently heard in normal children, while bruits heard in the neck in adults and resulting from stenosis of major vessels (carotid, vertebral, subclavian) may rarely be transmitted along temporal vessels so that ausculta-tion of the neck is also essential. A bruit over the orbit is usually present, along with pulsating exophthalmos, in cases of carotico-cavernous fistula.

Facial naevus may be associated with venous angioma, retinal haemangio-blastoma with haemangioblastoma of the cerebellum, and cutaneous pigmenta-tion with neurofibromatosis, while unilateral exophthalmos may be due to a retro-orbital meningioma.

Management of the Tumour Suspect

In any patient in whom symptoms and/or physical signs suggest the possi-bility of an intracranial tumour, it is reasonable to begin by employing succes-sively those investigations which are likely to give the maximum information with minimum risk to the patient and only subsequently to employ potentially hazardous investigations if the information necessary to localize and identify, or to exclude the presence of a neoplasm can be obtained in no other way. Thus radiography of the chest (to exclude, for instance, a bronchogenic carcinoma which may have metastasized to the brain) is invariably necessary, as are X-rays of the skull (see below). An echoencephalogram [p. 148] may confirm displace-ment of midline structures and may even be helpful in determining ventricular size and displacement, especially if the more sensitive B-scan is used (McKinney, 1969) though the simpler A-scan can give useful information (Garg and Taylor, 1968). An electroencephalogram [p. 144] may not only indicate a lesion in one cerebral hemisphere but may give some clue as to its situation; a negative recording, however, cannot exclude a tumour (Williams *et al.*, 1972). Gamma-encephalography [p. 148] should next be considered (van Eck, 1966) as in many cerebral hemisphere lesions it will show an area of increased uptake of radioactive isotope (Boller *et al.*, 1973; Penning *et al.*, 1973); it is less valuable in detecting posterior fossa lesions [FIG. 52] but may indicate the presence of more than one lesion when multiple metastases are present. Computerized transaxial tomography (the EMI scan) [p. 151] (Gawler *et al.*, 1974; Kistler *et al.*, 1975) is likely to be used increasingly in the future and will almost certainly supplant many of the more traditional radiological methods utilizing air or con-trast media as it is a safe and rapid technique of localizing intracranial tumours in many cases, but the role of this method is still being explored and developed and the expense of the equipment is such that it is not yet universally available.

Lumbar puncture is generally better avoided in the tumour suspect, certainly when symptoms and signs indicate raised intracranial pressure, because of the risk of tentorial or cerebellar herniation, even though a rise in the pressure of the fluid and in its protein content [pp. 131–3] may be of value, especially in cases of acoustic neuroma or meningioma; in such individuals a substantial rise in the CSF protein content is commonly observed, while lesser rises are also found in many patients with gliomas or intracranial metastases. Cytological examination of the fluid (Dyken, 1975) is sometimes of value in detecting malignant cells, occasionally in patients with gliomas but more especially in carcinomatosis of the meninges, while the lactate dehydrogenase and glutamic oxalacetic transaminase activity of the fluid is sometimes increased in patients with cerebral metastases (Davies-Jones, 1969). It has also been found that after triparanol treatment of human CSF, a concentration of desmosterol (a pre-cursor of cholesterol) of more than 0·1 μg/ml indicates the presence of an intra-cranial tumour (Paoletti *et al.*, 1969). Despite the value of these tests, the risks inherent in lumbar puncture mean that the technique is now used less often in the tumour suspect than in the past. Certainly the investigation should never be undertaken lightly and then only if evidence of raised pressure is lacking, if neurosurgical aid is immediately at hand, and if the information which the test is anticipated to give cannot be obtained by means of less hazardous methods.

For the same reasons, fractional pneumoencephalography (see below), which may be a valuable means of indicating ventricular distortion or displacement in the presence of a neoplasm, is now being employed less often, though it still has an important if limited role to play when there is no evidence of raised pressure

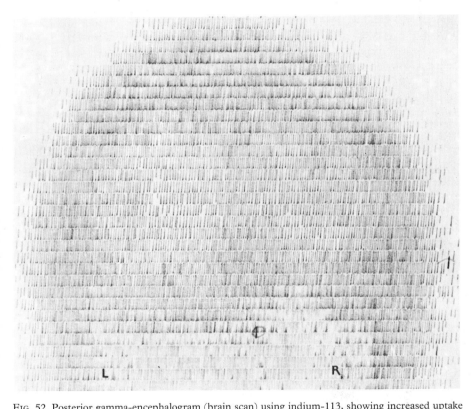

FIG. 52. Posterior gamma-encephalogram (brain scan) using indium-113, showing increased uptake on the right side of the posterior fossa due to a cerebellar haemangioblastoma

or of focal neurological signs, but when there is no other reasonable means of excluding a tumour and when facilities are immediately available for neuro-surgical exploration if a space-occupying lesion is demonstrated.

When no EMI scan is possible, when there is evidence of raised intracranial pressure, and certainly when signs of a focal lesion are present, cerebral angio-graphy is usually indicated, first because this may demonstrate the presence of hydrocephalus, or, in lesions of one cerebral hemisphere, it may indicate dis-placement of major vessels or a pathological tumour circulation. If no such localizing signs are found, or if the angiographic signs are those of hydro-cephalus, the next step will usually be ventriculography (see below), either with air, or, on occasion, using contrast medium, especially when a neoplasm in one of the cerebral ventricles or in the brain stem or posterior fossa is suspected.

Accessory Methods of Investigation

Radiography. Some principles have already been outlined [pp. 149–52]. In every suspected case of intracranial tumour lateral, anteroposterior, and postero-anterior views should be taken, and other positions, including basal views and Towne's view, are usually included in routine skull surveys (Bull, 1951). Radiographic examination of the skull may reveal abnormalities in the bones, calcification in the tumour [FIGS. 53, 54, and 55], or displacement of the pineal body.

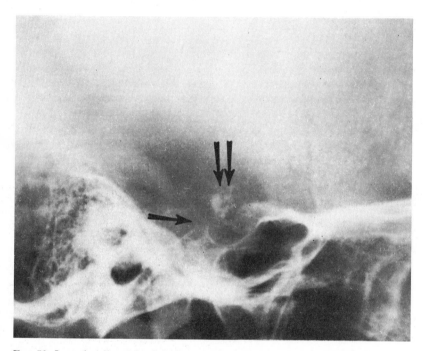

FIG. 53. Lateral radiograph of skull in a child with a suprasellar craniopharyngioma showing calcification (double arrows) and erosion of the tip of the dorsum sellae (single arrow)

Separation of the sutures may be seen when a rise of intracranial pressure occurs before the age at which these unite [FIG. 38, p. 226]. Erosion of the posterior clinoid processes and erosion or decalcification of the dorsum sellae is a safer guide to the presence of raised intracranial pressure (see below) but decalcification in this area is also a common result of normal ageing processes. Local erosion of bone is most frequently seen in the region of the skull superficial to a meningioma. Around the eroded area new bone formation occurs, often taking the form of spicules, perpendicular to the vault, and surrounding this there is frequently a network of deepened vascular channels in the bone. The petrous portion of the temporal bone may be eroded by an acoustic neuroma

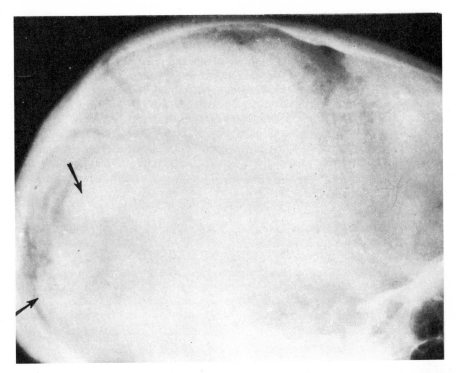

FIG. 54. Lateral radiograph of skull showing parallel lines of calcification in an occipital oligo-dendroglioma (arrows)

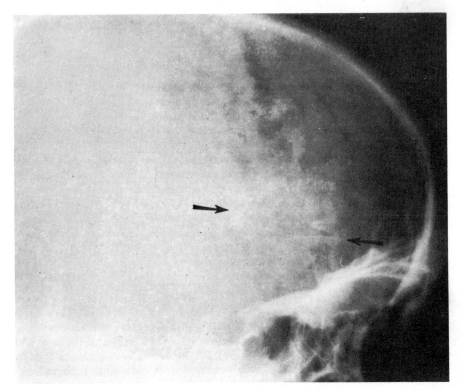

FIG. 55. Lateral radiograph of skull showing curvilinear calcification (arrows) in a frontal arteriovenous angioma

which may lead to unilateral enlargement of the internal acoustic meatus [FIG. 56].
Bony changes in the region of the sella turcica are produced not only by tumours
of the hypophysis itself and those arising in its neighbourhood, but also by a
general increase in the intracranial pressure [FIG. 57]. Hypophysial tumours
cause a uniform expansion of the sella turcica with thinning of its walls [FIG. 58].
The ballooned sella projects downwards and forwards into the sphenoidal
sinuses, and the upward pressure of the growth may erode the clinoid processes.
Tumours arising outside the sella, but immediately above it, cause erosion of the
clinoid processes and flattening of the sella, which is not, however, uniformly

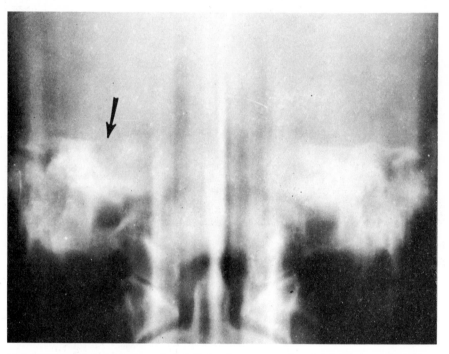

FIG. 56. Towne's view (tomogram) of skull showing gross erosion of the right internal auditory
canal produced by an acoustic neuroma

enlarged unless invaded by the tumour [FIG. 53]; while the downward pressure
of the floor of the distended third ventricle in internal hydrocephalus results in
a very similar radiographic appearance.

Calcification is most frequently observed in craniopharyngiomas [FIG. 53]
(in about 75 per cent of cases). These tumours may exhibit on the X-ray film
merely a few opaque flecks, or a mass the size of a hen's egg.

Calcification may occur also in the angiomas [FIG. 55], and may sometimes
present a characteristic convoluted appearance due to the deposit of calcium in
the walls of the vessels composing the tumour but more often the pattern is non-
specific. Meningiomas also sometimes show calcified areas, and these may be
encountered, though less frequently, in gliomas, especially oligodendrogliomas
[FIG. 54], teratomas, tumours of the choroid plexuses, and tuberculomas.
Chronic intracerebral haematomas, and, very rarely, subdural haematomas may

also calcify. A typical form of calcification is also seen in the very rare lipoma of the corpus callosum, while bilateral calcification in the basal ganglia may be familial or can occur in pseudohypoparathyroidism.

The pineal body is normally sufficiently calcified to be visible radiographically in 60 per cent of adults and is to be seen in the midline above and behind the

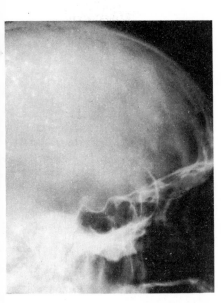 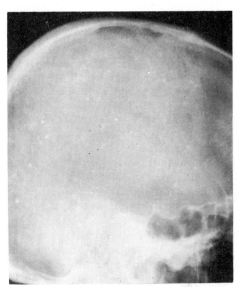

FIG. 57. On the left is a normal lateral radiograph of skull; on the right is a radiograph taken one year later of the same patient showing loss of the lamina dura of the dorsum sellae due to increased intracranial pressure

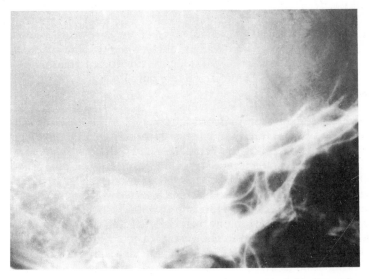

FIG. 58. Lateral radiograph of skull showing enlargement and thinning of the walls of the sella turcica due to a chromophobe adenoma of the pituitary

sella turcica. It may be displaced to the opposite side by a neoplasm of one cerebral hemisphere. Calcification may also be seen in the normal choroid plexuses, in the petroclinoid ligaments, tuberculum sellae and falx cerebri, and even in the dura mater of the vault of the skull.

Contrast Methods

As stated above, the contrast methods in common use for the localization and identification of intracranial tumours are carotid and vertebral angiography, pneumoencephalography and ventriculography with air or contrast media (*Myodil* or *Conray*).

Angiography. In carotid arteriography, the common carotid artery is injected with an iodine-containing contrast medium such as *Urografin* (60 per cent) or *Conray 80* (46 per cent). This technique is usually carried out by percutaneous injection under local or general anaesthesia; the internal carotid artery and its branches (the middle and anterior cerebral arteries and their radicals) are demonstrated and sometimes, but not often, one or both posterior communicating and posterior cerebral arteries may be filled. Vertebral angiography may also be performed by percutaneous puncture but the complications are fewer if a catheter inserted into a limb artery such as the femoral or radial is used to inject contrast medium into one of the vertebral vessels. Aortic arch angiography is particularly valuable in detecting lesions of the great vessels in the thorax and neck in patients with symptoms of cerebral vascular disease. This method is less valuable in detecting intracranial tumours when it is necessary to demonstrate the fine detail of intracranial vessels. However, selective filling of the external carotid artery and its branches may be necessary in order to demonstrate tumours in the neck (e.g. carotid body tumours) or others which are extracranial. Subtraction techniques (which subtract the bony shadows leaving a clearer demonstration of the vessels) as well as image intensification or magnification using television are being used increasingly, but for details of technique the reader is referred to textbooks of neuroradiology (Krayenbuhl and Yaşargil, 1968; Newton and Potts, 1974). Normally at least three lateral, anteroposterior, and oblique views are taken at one- or two-second intervals to give early and late arterial and venous filling, but in some cases the demonstration of vascular lesions or of pathological tumour circulations may require much more frequent films (rapid serial angiography).

In cases of intracranial space-occupying lesion, displacement of arteries and/ or veins may localize the lesion whether it be a tumour, an abscess, or a haemorrhage and an unusually wide 'sweep' of the anterior cerebral and pericallosal arteries around the corpus callosum may indicate ventricular dilatation due to hydrocephalus [FIG. 59]. Some tumours may show a characteristic pathological circulation. Astrocytomas tend to be relatively avascular [FIG. 60], glioblastomas and metastases commonly show tangles of small abnormal blood vessels [FIGS. 61 and 62], arteriovenous angiomas contain greatly enlarged and tortuous arteries and veins [FIG. 63], and meningiomas often give a typical 'blush' in the venous phase of the angiogram owing to retention of contrast medium in the vessels of the tumour [FIG. 64], to quote only a few examples. Vertebral angiography may similarly be successful in demonstrating lesions in the posterior fossa, especially haemangioblastomas of the cerebellum [FIG. 65], and displacement of the basilar artery is a valuable sign of tumours lying in or in relation to the brain stem.

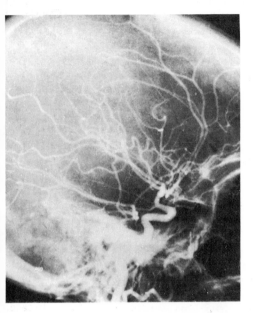 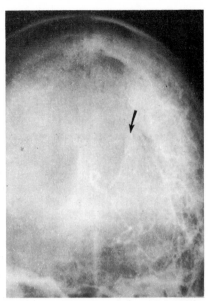

Fig. 59. Ventricular dilatation demonstrated by carotid angiography. On the left the anterior cerebral arteries are seen to take a wide sweep around the elevated corpus callosum. On the right, the thalamo-striate vein (arrow) indicates the width of the lateral ventricle

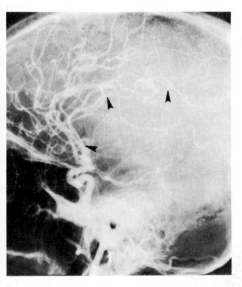 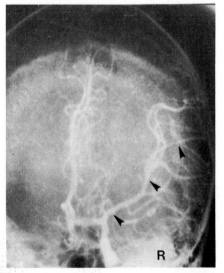

Fig. 60. Upward and inward displacement of the middle cerebral vessels produced by a temporal lobe glioma (there is no pathological circulation)

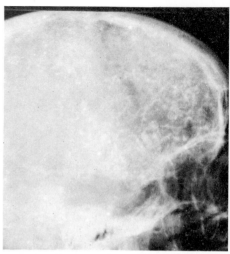
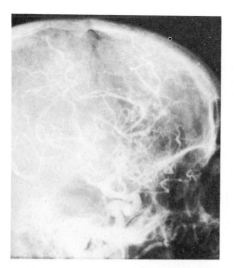

Fig. 61. A pathological circulation in a large frontal lobe glioma

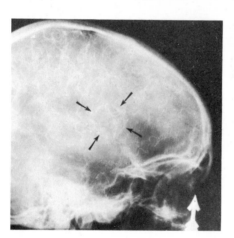
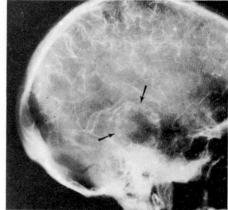

Fig. 62. Left carotid angiogram (left) showing a vascular metastasis in the fronto-parietal region (arrows). Right carotid arteriogram of the same patient (right) showing a similar lesion in the right temporal lobe

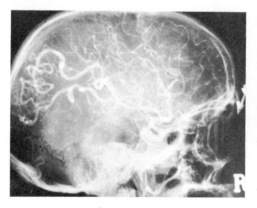
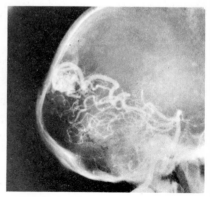

Fig. 63. An occipital arteriovenous angioma supplied by both the carotid (left) and vertebral (right) systems

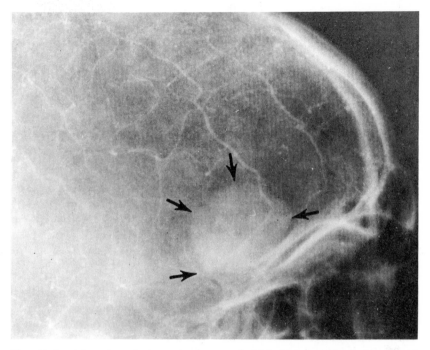

FIG. 64. A subfrontal meningioma showing a typical 'blush' (arrows) in the late arterial phase

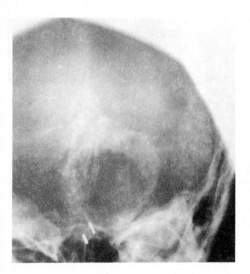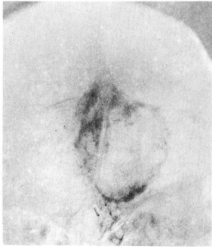

FIG. 65. A recurrent haemangioblastoma shown by vertebral angiography (left) to have a peripheral pathological circulation and an avascular centre; a subtraction print of the same angiogram is shown on the right

Pneumoencephalography. Some of the contra-indications to pneumo-encephalography have been mentioned above; this technique is better avoided when there is reason to suspect that the intracranial pressure is raised or when there are strong grounds for suspecting the presence of a tumour in one cerebral hemisphere or in the posterior fossa. Nevertheless, if other investigations (EEG, echoencephalogram, gamma scan, EMI scan, and angiography) have given negative or equivocal findings or when, for instance, it is necessary to define the upper limits of a tumour arising in the pituitary fossa, it may still be the appropriate examination in some tumour suspects but should only be carried out in a specialized unit with neurosurgical aid immediately available. This method is used more often nowadays to demonstrate cerebral atrophy in patients with presumed dementia or to confirm a diagnosis of communicating hydro-cephalus.

To perform a pneumoencephalogram (Robertson, 1967), a lumbar puncture is performed with the patient sitting upright. After a few drops of CSF have been allowed to flow, sufficient only to determine that the needle is in position, 5 ml of air or oxygen is injected slowly and radiographs are taken as the bubble passes through the basal cisterns and fourth ventricle. Then 5 ml of CSF is removed, 10 ml of air is injected, and subsequently another 10 ml of fluid is withdrawn. The procedure is continued until a total of 25–30 ml of air has been injected and adequate filling of the ventricular system has been obtained [FIG. 66]. The procedure consistently produces a severe headache and some-times prostration and vomiting; the severity of these symptoms is usually in direct proportion to the amount of air injected. It is usual to give pethidine or a similar analgesic both as a premedication and subsequently, and haloperidol or chlorpromazine may be required in order to prevent or relieve vomiting. General anaesthesia will usually be needed when the investigation is to be per-formed in children or restless or confused adults. As already mentioned, the technique is particularly valuable in defining the upper limits of a pituitary neoplasm [FIG. 67] and it is useful in demonstrating encroachment upon or distortion of the fourth ventricle produced by tumours in these areas such as brain stem gliomas, acoustic neuromas [FIG 68], or other lesions in the posterior fossa. Neoplasms of the cerebral hemispheres may be localized by signs of displacement of the lateral and/or third ventricles, but rarely is it possible to draw conclusions about the pathological character of the lesion except by inference according to its site.

Ventriculography. This technique requires shaving of the scalp and the insertion of bilateral posterior burr holes in the skull, after which air is injected into one lateral ventricle through a needle which is passed through a burr hole and then through brain tissue. The procedure is not without risk, first because the needle may pierce a vessel in its passage through the brain and secondly because a sudden release of pressure in one lateral ventricle may result in herniation of the opposite cerebral hemisphere beneath the falx cerebri. Immediate puncture of the opposite cerebral ventricle or operative decom-pression may then be required. Hence the investigation is only performed when it is possible to proceed at once with any necessary neurosurgical operation.

Once air has been injected, the radiologist will then manipulate the bubble throughout the cerebral ventricular system. As with pneumoencephalography, the technique localizes neoplasms displacing or encroaching upon the lateral,

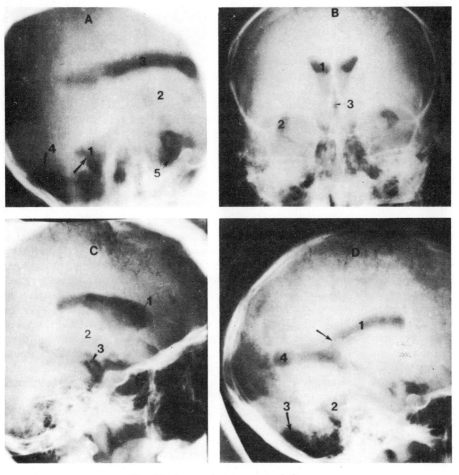

FIG. 66. A normal pneumoencephalogram.

A, erect mid-line tomogram.

1. 4th ventricle, the choroid plexus is arrowed
2. 3rd ventricle
3. Lateral ventricle
4. Cisterna magna
5. Pre-pontine cistern

C, lateral brow-up view.

1. Frontal horn of lateral ventricle
2. 3rd ventricle
3. Temporal horn

B, antero-posterior brow-up view.

1. Body of lateral ventricle
2. Temporal horn
3. 3rd ventricle

D, lateral brow-down view.

1. Lateral ventricle (choroid plexus arrowed)
2. 4th ventricle
3. Cisterna magna
4. Occipital horn

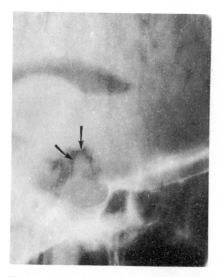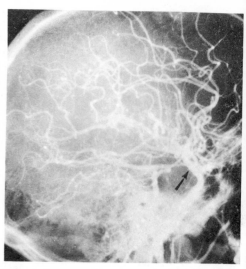

Fig. 67. Pneumoencephalogram (left) of the patient whose X-ray of skull is shown in Fig. 58. Air in the basal cisterns outlines a suprasellar extension of a chromophobe adenoma of the pituitary. Right carotid angiogram (right) shows deformity of the carotid siphon produced by the parasellar extension of the tumour

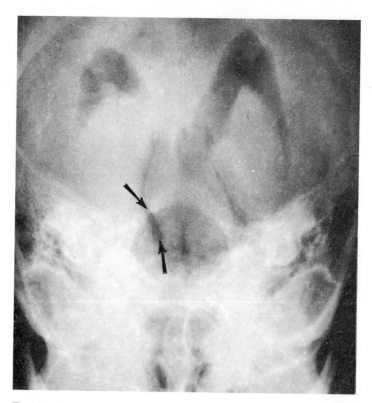

Fig. 68. Pneumoencephalogram of a case of acoustic neuroma showing displacement to the right of the cerebello-pontine angle cistern (arrows)

third, or fourth ventricles (provided that the air will pass down the aqueduct) with a considerable degree of success [FIGS. 69–72]. The method is also valuable in demonstrating the site of obstruction (e.g. the aqueduct) in cases of hydrocephalus [FIG. 38, p. 226]. Sometimes precise demonstration of the third or fourth ventricles requires injection of a contrast medium such as *Myodil* or *Conray* [FIG. 73]. The latter technique should be used only when absolutely necessary as the injected material may act as a cerebral irritant unless it can be made to pass downwards into the spinal theca at the conclusion of the examination and this is not always possible if the CSF pathways are obstructed.

FOCAL SYMPTOMS

Frontal Lobe

Prefrontal Tumours. By prefrontal tumours are meant tumours confined to that part of the frontal lobe lying anterior to the precentral gyrus. Headache as a rule occurs early, but papilloedema and vomiting usually develop late and may be absent. As we have seen, mental symptoms may occur with a tumour in any situation, even below the tentorium. There is evidence, however, that they are more likely to occur when the tumour is in the corpus callosum or frontal lobe than when it is elsewhere. Moreover, in the absence of other localizing signs the development of mental symptoms before signs of increased intracranial pressure favours a frontal localization. The mental disturbance is a progressive dementia, of which the characteristic feature is a defective grasp of situations as a whole, a failure of the synthetic function of thought. In more severe cases the patient's intellectual capacity suffers more seriously. He becomes stupid, fails to appreciate the gravity of his illness, is careless of his dress and appearance, and develops incontinence of urine and faeces without exhibiting any sense of impropriety. Such patients are sometimes jocular and facetious and repeatedly make simple jokes or puns (Witzelsucht). Irritability of temper and depression are not uncommon.

Generalized convulsions occur in up to 50 per cent of cases. When the tumour is situated near the base the patient may experience an aura associated with speech. He may feel as if he wishes to speak but cannot do so, and may actually stammer before losing consciousness. There may be a sensation of something gripping the throat. When the tumour is situated towards the superior aspect of the lobe the motor element in the convulsion is likely to consist of turning of the head and eyes to the opposite side (adversive attacks) with complex clonic and tonic movements of the contralateral limbs.

Catatonia is a very rare manifestation of organic brain disease, occurring much more often in schizophrenia, but it has been described as an uncommon manifestation of frontal lobe tumour. The patient tends to become immobilized for some time in one attitude; or may maintain indefinitely an attitude into which his limbs have been manipulated by the observer—waxy flexibility. Large frontal tumours sometimes cause considerable unsteadiness in walking or marked impairment of the gait, even in the absence of other evidence of paresis or reflex change. This ill-defined symptom has been thought of as being an apraxia of gait, but is sometimes called 'frontal lobe ataxia'.

Expressive aphasia (Broca's aphasia) may occur when the tumour involves the posterior part of the dominant inferior frontal gyrus.

The grasp reflex is an important sign, when present, as it is probably pathognomonic of a frontal lobe lesion. It is most frequently observed in the opposite hand, but may be found only in the foot when the tumour is situated in the superior part of the lobe.

A rare sign of a lesion of the frontal lobe which must not be confused with the grasp reflex is tonic innervation or perseveration, which consists of a persistence of muscular contraction voluntarily initiated, due to a failure of relaxation. Tonic perseveration is usually most evident after flexion of the fingers, but may occur after movements of other parts of the body on the side opposite to the lesion. Muscular relaxation is slow and may not be complete for several seconds.

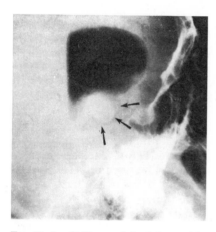

FIG. 69. A colloid cyst of the 3rd ventricle outlined by ventriculography

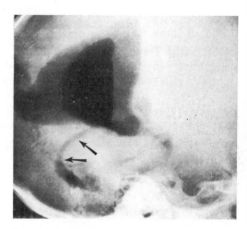

FIG. 70. A large ependymoma of the 4th ventricle demonstrated by ventriculography

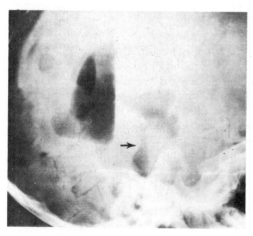

FIG. 71. A ventriculogram in a child with a medulloblastoma of the cerebellar vermis which is displacing the aqueduct and 4th ventricle forwards

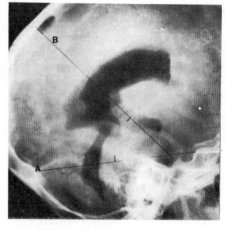

FIG. 72. A ventriculogram of a patient with a large glioma of the brain stem. A is Twining's line, the mid-point of which should normally lie in the 4th ventricle. B is the Swedish line; the aqueduct should be at the junction of the anterior one-third and posterior two-thirds of the line. Both structures are displaced backwards and upwards

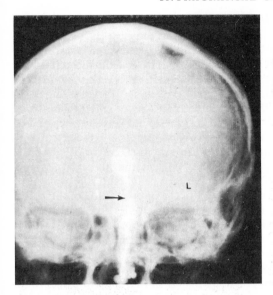 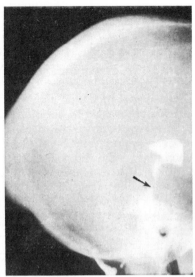

FIG. 73. Myodil ventriculogram of a patient with a cerebellar haemangioblastoma whose brain scan is shown in FIG. 52 [p. 255]. The aqueduct and 4th ventricle are displaced forwards and to the left. In the lateral view (right) contrast medium in the cisterna magna outlines the herniated cerebellar tonsils

Pressure upon neighbouring corticospinal fibres may lead to weakness upon the opposite side of the body, usually most marked in the face and tongue. Pressure upon the olfactory nerve, lying upon the floor of the anterior fossa, may lead to anosmia on the side of the lesion. This is most likely to occur in the case of meningiomas arising from the olfactory groove. Such tumours extending backwards may compress the optic nerve, causing primary optic atrophy on the side of the lesion, while the rise of intracranial pressure causes papilloedema on the opposite side (the Foster Kennedy syndrome).

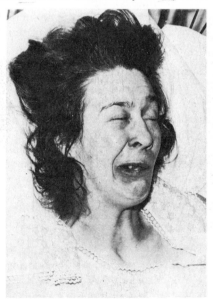

FIG. 74. Jacksonian epilepsy involving the right side of the face (photograph kindly provided by Dr. J. D. Spillane)

Precentral Tumours. Precentral tumours are perhaps the easiest to localize on account of the early development of symptoms of excitation and destruction of the corticospinal fibres.

Corticospinal excitation finds expression in a focal convulsion, of which several forms are encountered. In the typical Jacksonian fit [FIG. 74] the convulsion begins with clonic movements, rarely with tonic spasm, in a limited area of the opposite side of the body, e.g. the thumb, and slowly spreads, involving other parts in the order in which they are represented in the precentral gyrus [see p. 17]. When the whole of one side of the body is convulsed the opposite side may become involved, and at this stage consciousness is usually lost. Partial Jacksonian attacks may occur, in which the convulsion is limited to a small part of one side of the body, without loss of consciousness. Such a convulsion may be continuous—'epilepsia partialis continua'. Jacksonian attacks may occur at long intervals, or with great frequency, even up to several hundreds a day—serial Jacksonian epilepsy. When consciousness is not regained between successive attacks the condition is described as Jacksonian status epilepticus.

Motor weakness is the result of the destruction or compression of the cortico-spinal cells and fibres by the tumour, and exhibits a regional distribution corresponding to the representation of parts of the body in the precentral gyrus. Owing to the large surface extent of the cortical motor cells, even a large cortical tumour is likely to cause weakness of only a part of the opposite side of the body, that is, a monoplegia. With inferiorly placed tumours there is weakness, often accompanied by apraxia, of the face and tongue on the opposite side, and weakness of movements of the thumb, which is represented in the adjacent area. If the tumour is at a higher level the thumb may escape, though the fingers and arm are affected, while a tumour involving principally the medial aspect of the hemisphere is likely to cause a monoplegia involving only the foot or the whole lower limb. The usual reflex changes associated with a corticospinal lesion are found, and such reflex abnormalities may be limited to the paretic part.

A tumour of the falx in the region of the paracentral lobule (a parasagittal meningioma) is likely to produce weakness of both lower limbs, beginning in the feet, one being usually affected more than the other. Retention of urine may occur owing to compression of the cortical centres for initiating micturition. There may be an impairment of postural sensibility in the toes when the sensory area of the paracentral lobule is involved.

Jacksonian convulsions are usually associated with permanent weakness of the part of the body which is the focus of the fit, but after each convulsion there is often a temporary extension of this weakness to other parts (Todd's paralysis). Sensory loss is absent, unless the tumour extends to the postcentral gyrus.

Temporal Lobe

The focal symptoms of temporal lobe tumours are often slight, especially when the tumour is on the right side. When the lesion is anteriorly situated and involves the uncus there is often a very characteristic group of symptoms. This is the cortical centre for taste and smell, and the closely associated motor functions of licking, mastication, and swallowing are also represented nearby. Tumours of the uncus may cause so-called uncinate fits which are characterized by an olfactory or gustatory aura often with certain motor concomitants. The aura consists of an hallucination of taste or smell which is usually unpleasant but occasionally pleasant. It may be described as resembling paint, gas, acetylene, 'something burning', or even, as one patient put it, the monkey house at the Zoo. There may be abnormal sensations referred to the epigastrium. Involuntary licking, smacking the lips, or tasting movements frequently accompany the olfactory or gustatory aura and form the motor component of the uncinate fit.

Sometimes in association with such uncinate attacks other manifestations of temporal lobe epilepsy also occur as the epileptic discharge spreads more posteriorly. More often, and especially with small tumours situated in the medial temporal lobe (Cavanagh, 1958), other symptoms including automatism, disordered consciousness, and perversions of memory and of the emotions characterize temporal lobe attacks. The patient presents a dazed or dreamy appearance and usually stops what he is doing, but does not fall. He may have no recollection of the attack afterwards or he may describe peculiar disturbances of memory, for example, the *déjà vu* phenomenon, a feeling that everything that is happening has happened before, or experience a recurrent dream, or he may in a very short time relive in detail a large part of his past life. He may experience illusions relating to the external world or his own body. Objects may appear larger or smaller or more distant than normally, or unreal. There may be visual or auditory hallucinations. A sense of depersonalization or unreality (*jamais vu*) may occur. Emotional disturbances include fear (even 'panic attacks') and depression. Generalized convulsions sometimes occur, with or without a 'temporal lobe' aura.

Destruction in the region of the uncus leads to an impairment of taste and smell on the side of the lesion, though this does not as a rule proceed to complete loss.

Visual field defects may be produced by temporal lobe tumours. They are absent in at least half of all cases, but when present are of great localizing value. The lower fibres of the optic radiation are likely to be caught in their path around the tip of the inferior horn of the ventricle. The characteristic defect is therefore a crossed upper quadrantic hemianopia, the loss being usually more extensive in the ipsilateral field. Although the cortical centre for hearing is situated in the posterior part of the temporal lobe, temporal tumours do not cause complete deafness in either ear, though a unilateral lesion in this situation may lead to some bilateral impairment of hearing.

Tumours in or near the auditory cortex sometimes cause tinnitus, while if auditory association areas are involved other crude auditory hallucinations or even organized hallucinations (e.g. voices or music) rarely occur. Lesions of the dominant temporal lobe may cause either nominal, receptive (Wernicke's), or conduction aphasia [see pp. 102–9] depending upon which part of the speech pathway is involved. Most often the patient has difficulty in understanding spoken language and speaks in jargon with frequent paraphasia.

Commonly with larger lesions there is involvement of the lower cells and fibres of the corticospinal tract with contralateral weakness of the face of 'upper motor neurone' type, perhaps with weakness of the arm and hand. Herniation of the medial temporal lobe through the tentorial hiatus may give compression of the trunk of the third nerve causing a fixed dilated pupil on the same side and sometimes ptosis, while compression of the trigeminal ganglion rarely causes loss of the ipsilateral corneal reflex.

Parietal Lobe

The parietal lobe is the principal sensory area of the cerebral cortex. Sensory disturbances therefore constitute a prominent part of the symptoms of tumours of this region. The postcentral gyrus is the part of the parietal lobe most concerned with sensation. Parts of the body are here represented for purposes of sensation in a manner similar to their motor representation in the precentral gyrus. From below upwards we encounter in the following order the larynx and pharynx, the tongue, the buccal cavity, the face, neck, thumb, index, second, third, and fourth fingers, the hand, forearm, upper arm, shoulder, chest, abdomen, thigh, and leg. The foci of the foot and toes are situated at the superior border of the hemisphere, and on the medial aspect, in the paracentral lobule, lie the foci of the bladder, rectum, and genital organs [see p. 49].

Irritation of the postcentral gyrus causes sensory Jacksonian fits which consist usually of paraesthesiae, such as tingling or 'electric shocks', rarely of pain, and which begin in that part of the opposite side of the body corresponding to the focus of excitation. The paraesthesiae then spread to other parts in the order of their representation in the gyrus. Such sensory fits may occur alone, or may be followed by a similar spreading motor discharge due to the extension of the excitation to the precentral gyrus, in which case the clonic convulsion often lags behind the advance of the paraesthesiae.

A destructive lesion of the postcentral gyrus leads to sensory loss, the extent of which corresponds in distribution to the extent of the cortical lesion. The sensory loss is of the cortical type, that is, it involves the spatial and discriminative aspects of sensation, especially postural sensibility and tactile discrimination, while the crude appreciation of pain, heat, and cold is left intact. As a result of sensory loss the patient may be unable to recognize objects placed in his affected hand—'stereoanaesthesia'.

Postcentral lesions lead also to hypotonia and wasting of the affected parts and to both static and kinetic ataxia. When the patient is at rest there is often a conspicuous restlessness of the affected upper limb, sometimes amounting to 'pseudo-athetosis', and he may gesticulate exaggeratedly with the affected hand. There is likely to be considerable ataxia in the finger–nose test—'sensory ataxia'.

Parietal tumours reaching deep into the white matter may lead to 'thalamic over-reaction', an exaggerated response to unpleasant stimuli on the opposite side of the body, though this is usually present to only a slight extent. Involvement of the fibres of the optic radiation causes a crossed homonymous defect of the visual fields; and since the upper fibres are the more likely to be caught, the field defect may be confined to the lower quadrant.

The posterior part of the parietal lobe constitutes a 'watershed' between the three great cortical sensory areas, the optic, acoustic, and somatic. A left-sided lesion of this area may therefore be expected to cause considerable disturbance of speech on its receptive side. Lesions of the left angular gyrus usually cause alexia and agraphia with which may be associated finger-agnosia and acalculia. Lesions of the same area on the right side cause disturbances of awareness of the opposite side of the body and the opposite half of space. Such disturbances of the 'body image' in non-dominant parietal lobe lesions may be associated with dressing apraxia. Other forms of apraxia and agnosia [see pp. 115–17] more often result from dominant parietal lesions.

Lesions of either parietal lobe occasionally cause contralateral tactile inattention; there is no evident sensory impairment when each side is examined independently, but when bilateral simultaneous stimuli are applied, those on the opposite side of the body from the lesion may be ignored.

Occipital Lobe

Tumours of the occipital lobe are comparatively rare. Headache is an early symptom, and other signs of increased intracranial pressure are usually conspicuous. Epileptiform convulsions occur in a considerable proportion of cases —50 per cent in one series. They may be preceded by a visual aura, such as flashes of light moving from one side towards the middle line, but this is not constant. Such attacks may begin with turning of the eyes to the opposite side. Rarely, if the so-called visual association areas are involved, formed visual hallucinations may occur rather than crude unformed hallucinations such as flashes of light which result from irritation of the striate cortex. The characteristic focal sign of an occipital tumour is a visual field defect. This may consist of a crossed homonymous hemianopia extending up to the fixation point, or of a crossed homonymous quadrantic defect, or of a crescentic loss in the periphery of the opposite half-fields. Hemianopia may have been discovered by the patient owing to his collisions with people or objects on his blind side.

Lesions of the dominant occipital lobe may give visual object agnosia as well as a visual field defect and rarely agnosia for colours. Prosopagnosia (inability to recognize faces) is a rare manifestation. If the lesion spreads more anteriorly to involve the posterior temporal lobe, jargon aphasia and/or auditory hallucinations may occur, while extension to the posterior parietal region may cause apraxia, dyslexia, acalculia, or even contralateral sensory loss or inattention (see above). Just as lesions of the parietal lobe sometimes cause tactile inattention, those of the occipital lobe sometimes cause contralateral visual inattention; this phenomenon may be defined by tachistoscopy [p. 67].

Corpus Callosum

Tumours of the corpus callosum are more common than is generally realized. Bull (1967) has recently pointed out that one quarter of all hemisphere astrocytomas show macroscopic or microscopic evidence of invasion of the corpus callosum. Sometimes they yield a distinctive clinical picture but more often the clinical presentation is non-specific. Mental symptoms are prominent and are often the first to be noticed. It is said that mental changes are more frequently observed in cases of tumour of the corpus callosum than when the tumour is situated in any other part of the brain, including the frontal lobe. Apathy, drowsiness, and defect of memory are the commonest disturbances, but any of the mental symptoms already described as occurring in cases of cerebral tumour may be present. The defect of memory may be so severe that a patient who has suffered from an intense headache may in a few minutes have forgotten it completely. General convulsions are common. Indeed, a combination of progressive dementia with major (or focal) attacks of epilepsy must always raise the possibility of a tumour in this position. The situation of the tumour in the midline extending laterally into the central white matter on both sides soon leads to damage to the corticospinal tracts. This is usually asymmetrical at first, and it is then common to find hemiplegia on one side, while the other exhibits increased reflexes with little loss of power. Later, double hemiplegia may be found. Anteriorly placed tumours extending into the frontal lobes may cause a grasp reflex on one or both sides. Apraxia is present in a small proportion of cases. It may occur on the left side only, owing to interruption of fibres linking the left supramarginal gyrus with the right corticospinal tract. Tremor and choreiform movements sometimes occur and are probably due to involvement of the corpus striatum. Signs of increased intracranial pressure are often late in developing. The protein content of the CSF is likely to be high.

Centrum Semiovale and Basal Ganglia

The centrum semiovale consists mainly of corticospinal fibres converging on the internal capsule, and sensory fibres diverging from the latter to the various cortical sensory areas. Tumours in this region may cause little disturbance of the intracranial pressure, but they usually cause motor or sensory symptoms early. Owing to the concentration of fibres near the internal capsule the whole of the opposite side of the body is likely to be affected. Anteriorly placed tumours cause a progressive spastic hemiplegia. When the tumour is situated more posteriorly

K

or in the thalamus the presenting symptoms are sensory, and all forms of sensibility are usually impaired on the opposite side, and sensory ataxia is present. Hemianopia may be added if the optic radiation is involved. Somnolence is not uncommon when the tumour invades the thalamic or subthalamic regions; and signs of pressure upon the upper part of the midbrain may be found, especially weakness of conjugate deviation upwards and inequality of the pupil. The invasion of the third ventricle by the tumour is rapidly followed by the development of signs of increased intracranial pressure if these have not been present before (see McKissock and Paine, 1958).

Third Ventricle

The third ventricle may be the primary site of a tumour, e.g. a colloid cyst, or it may be invaded by a tumour arising below, in the interpeduncular space, above, in the falx or corpus callosum, or laterally, in the basal ganglia. Such extraventricular tumours usually yield ample evidence of their presence before they invade the ventricle. Tumours arising in the ventricle, however, are often difficult to localize. Astrocytomas arising in the wall of the ventricle are not uncommon in children (Stein et al., 1972). Hydrocephalus may be acute, subacute, intermittent, or chronic. Severe paroxysmal headaches are common, and may be influenced by changes ·in the position of the head. Headache and papilloedema may be the only symptoms. Progressive dementia may occur, or coma may suddenly develop. Impairment of memory, including a Korsakow-like syndrome, may occur. In cases of colloid cyst in the ventricle [FIG. 69, p. 268], attacks of loss of consciousness without convulsive features, occurring often at the height of an attack of headache, are common, as are 'drop' attacks with transient weakness of the lower limbs and falling but without loss of the senses; occasionally episodes of paraesthesiae in the limbs also occur (Kelly, 1951).

Somnolence, polyuria, hyperglycaemia and glycosuria, obesity, sexual regression, and irregular pyrexia may be produced by downward pressure by a tumour upon the tuber cinereum and pituitary body. Lateral extension of the growth in the region of the internal capsule causes signs of corticospinal defect on one or both sides.

Midbrain

Tumours arising in the midbrain usually cause internal hydrocephalus early owing to obstruction of the cerebral aqueduct. Headache, papilloedema, and vomiting are therefore conspicuous. Owing to the concentration in this region of the nuclei of the third and fourth cranial nerves and the supranuclear paths converging upon them, ocular abnormalities are prominent. Lesions of the upper part of the midbrain usually cause a paresis of conjugate ocular deviation upwards (Parinaud's syndrome, p. 83), and retraction of the upper lids may be associated with this. Lesions of the lower half cause paresis of conjugate ocular deviation downwards with which ptosis and paresis of convergence may be combined. Conjugate lateral movement of the eyes usually escapes, at least in the early stages, though a lesion just above the pons may involve the supranuclear fibres for lateral movement at their decussation and so cause a bilateral paralysis of lateral conjugate gaze.

The pupils are often unequal and tend to be dilated. The reactions both to light and on convergence-accommodation may be lost, or the latter may be preserved when the former is lost. Asymmetrical nuclear ophthalmoplegia may occur.

The corticospinal tracts are usually involved on both sides, though one is often more severely affected than the other. The characteristic reflex changes of corticospinal lesions are present. Weakness and spasticity, slight in the early stages, progress until in some cases a condition of virtual decerebrate rigidity supervenes. 'Tonic' fits characterized by opisthotonos with extension of all four limbs and loss of consciousness may occur; less severe episodes (which are also seen sometimes in brain stem multiple sclerosis) give rigid extension of one or more limbs or other sudden changes in posture of the limbs or trunk without loss of the senses. Tremor is common, and nystagmus and ataxia result from injury to the cerebellar connections.

Sensory changes are due to damage to the long ascending sensory paths. Extensive areas of analgesia and defects of postural sensibility may be encountered. Compression of the lateral lemniscus may lead to unilateral or bilateral deafness.

Pineal Body

The symptoms of tumours of the pineal body consist of: (1) signs of increased intracranial pressure; (2) signs of pressure upon neighbouring parts of the brain; and (3) in exceptional cases disturbances of growth and development. As previously mentioned, most tumours in this area are teratomas; growths arising in pineal cells are very rare. Since the pineal body is situated between the splenium of the corpus callosum above and the superior colliculi below, its enlargement speedily causes internal hydrocephalus, owing to obstruction to the drainage of the third ventricle, and symptoms of compression of the upper part of the midbrain. Signs of increased intracranial pressure therefore occur early, and are associated with the signs of a midbrain lesion as described in the previous section, namely, defect of conjugate ocular deviation upwards, less often downwards and laterally; paresis of convergence; retraction or ptosis of the upper lids; inequality of the pupils, which are usually dilated; reflex iridoplegia; bilateral signs of corticospinal lesion; nystagmus and ataxia; tremor and sensory loss, rarely including deafness.

The disturbances of growth are found only when the tumour develops in young boys, and not always then, occurring in less than 10 per cent of cases. They consist of precocity, abnormal growth of the skeleton, and premature development of the genitalia and secondary sexual characteristics, a syndrome which has received the name 'macrogenitosomia praecox'. The cause of these symptoms is unknown. There is some recent evidence to suggest that tumours in this area may rarely secrete aldosterone, or perhaps stimulate the output of aldosterone from the adrenals, giving the manifestations of aldosteronism. The internal hydrocephalus caused by a pineal tumour may lead to 'hypopituitarism', and obesity may then complicate the clinical picture.

The Region of the Optic Chiasm

The small region at the base of the brain lying between the optic chiasm and the cerebral peduncles is the site of tumours arising in four situations, namely: (1) tumours of the pituitary (hypophysis); (2) craniopharyngiomas; (3) suprasellar meningiomas; and (4) gliomas of the optic chiasm. Since these tumours are distinguished by differences in the general and focal symptoms to which they give rise it is convenient to consider them separately.

Tumours of the Pituitary Gland. As already described, three pathological types of pituitary tumour commonly occur, namely, (a) chromophil, (b) chromophobe, thus described in terms of the reaction of their cells to eosin staining, and (c) basophil adenomas. The symptoms of these tumours may be divided into: (1) endocrine disturbances which vary according to the pathological nature of the tumour; (2) pressure symptoms; and (3) alterations in radiographic appearance, which, though varying in severity, are common to the first two tumours by virtue of their situation within the sella turcica.

1. *Endocrine Disturbances*. (*a*) *Chromophil Adenoma*. In this tumour the eosinophil cells characteristic of the anterior lobe of the normal pituitary predominate, though chromophobe cells may also be present. The endocrine symptoms are due to an overproduction of growth hormone. When the tumour arises before growth has ceased, gigantism occurs; when, as more frequently happens, it begins during adult life, acromegaly is the result [FIG. 75]. This is

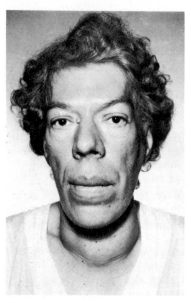

FIG. 75. The facial appearance of acromegaly from *An Atlas of Clinical Neurology*, 2nd ed., by J. D. Spillane, reproduced by kind permission of the author

characterized by slow changes in the skin and subcutaneous tissues, bones, viscera, general metabolism, and sexual activity. The skin and subcutaneous tissues, especially of the fingers, lips, ears, and tongue, exhibit a fibrous hyperplasia, and paraesthesiae may occur in the fingers due to compression of the median nerve in the carpal tunnel. Overgrowth of the bones is most evident in the skull, face, mandible, and at the periphery of the extremities. The calvarium is thickened and the bony ridges and points of attachment of muscles are increased in size. The zygomatic bones enlarge, and as a result of overgrowth of the mandible the lower jaw becomes prognathous, and separation of the teeth occurs. The hands become broad and spade-like and hyperostoses may develop on the terminal phalanges ('tufting'). Similar changes occur in the feet, and the patient frequently notices that he requires a larger size in gloves and shoes. Kyphosis in the upper dorsal spine is common and hypertrophy of many of the viscera has been described. Sugar metabolism is often disturbed, leading to hyperglycaemia and glycosuria, which frequently responds less to insulin than in diabetes mellitus. Thyrotoxicosis may occur, and hypertrichosis may be present. Impairment of sexual function occurs in both gigantism and acromegaly, impotence in the male and relative or complete amenorrhoea in the female being the rule. Enlargement of the breasts, and lactation persisting for months, and occurring even in nulliparous women, have been described in association with pituitary tumours, presumably due to an overproduction of prolactin.

(*b*) *Chromophobe Adenoma*. These tumours occur almost exclusively in adult life and according to Cushing are three times as common as the chromophil tumour which is associated with acromegaly. Since both their endocrine and their pressure symptoms are apt to be less obtrusive, the diagnosis is more likely to be missed. The endocrine symptoms of the chromophobe tumour are due to its destructive effect upon pituitary function giving hypopituitarism. The first symptom is usually a depression of sexual function, which in women takes the form of scanty menstruation, progressing to complete amenorrhoea, and in men to impotence. Women sometimes give a history of a late onset as well as an early cessation of menstruation. The skin becomes soft and pliable and there is often a loss of hair over the limbs and trunks (particularly in the axillae and pubic regions), and over the face in men. Moderate obesity often develops, associated with a lowered metabolic rate and increased sugar tolerance. The biochemical changes of hypothyroidism, hypo-adrenalism, and hypogonadism will be found. These symptoms may be present for many years before pressure symptoms occur. Rarely a chromophobe adenoma is associated with Cushing's syndrome.

(c) *Basophil Adenoma*. The basophil adenoma rarely attains a sufficient size to cause pressure symptoms. It has been found in association with Cushing's syndrome, but Crooke (1935) found that hyaline change in the basophil cells of the anterior lobe of the hypophysis was the only feature common to patients exhibiting this syndrome, whether it was associated with basophil adenoma of the pituitary, hyperplasia or neoplasm of the suprarenal cortex, tumour of the thymus, or bronchial carcinoma. Recently, however, true basophil adenomas have been discovered in patients who had previously undergone adrenalectomy for Cushing's syndrome (Montgomery et al., 1959). The individuals affected are usually young women, and their symptoms include painful, plethoric adiposity, 'moon-face' associated with purplish cutaneous striae, hirsutes, amenorrhoea, hyperglycaemia, hypertension, polycythaemia, osteoporosis, and myopathy. These symptoms are, of course, mimicked by the side-effects of corticosteroid drugs.

2. *Pressure Symptoms*. Pressure symptoms may be entirely absent particularly in the case of the basophil adenoma and less often with the chromophil (acidophil) adenoma which may for some time produce only endocrine effects. Headache is usually an early symptom of pituitary tumour, and is more marked as a rule when the tumour is of the chromophil, than when it is of the chromophobe, type. In the early stages it is due to expansion of the sella and pressure upon the diaphragma sellae and is usually described as a 'bursting' headache with a bitemporal distribution. If later the tumour extends beyond the diaphragma the headache is due to a general increase of intracranial pressure. Vomiting is usually absent, except in the later stages. Since the optic chiasm lies above the diaphragma sellae, visual field defects are an important and early symptom of tumours. Usually the tumour as it enlarges upwards first compresses the decussating fibres of the chiasm, hence bitemporal hemianopia is the field defect most frequently encountered [see p. 71]. This is as a rule asymmetrical, the defect beginning in the periphery of the upper temporal quadrant on one side, whence it extends towards the fixation point and downwards into the lower temporal quadrant. A similar change occurs either simultaneously or subsequently on the opposite side. In other cases the defect may begin as a scotoma on the temporal side of the fixation point. As the tumour grows, the nasal field of the eye first affected is encroached upon so that the patient often passes through a stage of complete blindness in one eye with a temporal hemianopia on the opposite side. Later, if the pressure is not relieved, the second eye also becomes blind. Less frequently one or other optic tract is compressed before the chiasm giving a homonymous hemianopia. Rarely the visual paths escape damage.

Compression of the optic chiasm causes optic atrophy, which is often more advanced in one eye than in the other. As the pressure at the same time obliterates the subarachnoid sheath of the optic nerves, papilloedema is rare. In the later stages of the development of the growth ocular palsies may be produced by compression of the third or sixth cranial nerves, and trigeminal pain, usually referred to the first division of the nerve and sometimes associated with analgesia. Rarely unilateral ocular palsies without a visual field defect may be the presenting symptom (Symonds, 1962). The title *'pituitary apoplexy'* has been given to the syndrome which may result from infarction in a chromophobe adenoma during a period of rapid growth. This may give rise to intense headache, prostration, and even loss of consciousness with subarachnoid haemorrhage (Walton, 1956); more often the tumour as it 'balloons' out of the sella causes compression of one third nerve and sometimes sudden blindness and optic atrophy (Jefferson and Rosenthal, 1959).

Cerebral symptoms do not occur until the tumour has expanded beyond the sella, when compression of the cerebral peduncles or invasion of one hemisphere from below may lead to unilateral or bilateral signs of corticospinal defect; uncinate fits may result from compression of the uncus, and pressure upon the frontal lobe may lead to marked mental deterioration, with or without abnormal emotional reactions. Somnolence, apathy, and confusion may be due to compression of the floor of the third ventricle and the hypothalamus; such mental symptoms usually indicate a large extension (White and Cobb, 1955).

3. *Radiographic Appearances.* Adenoma of the hypophysis, except the basophil variety, causes a uniform expansion of the sella, with thinning of its walls and an upward extension may be demonstrated by angiography or pneumoencephalography [FIG. 67, p. 266].

Craniopharyngioma. The pathology of these tumours has already been described. Since they depend upon abnormalities of development, symptoms often appear at an early age, and in more than one-third of the cases the patient comes for treatment before the age of 15. Less frequently, however, they cause no symptoms until middle life or even old age. In a series of 85 cases Bartlett (1971) found that the sexes were equally affected: 30 were under the age of 15 when first seeking medical advice but the others were evenly distributed through the decades, the oldest being 71 years of age. In those under 15 years of age, 76 per cent presented with visual failure, 43 per cent with papilloedema, 40 per cent with growth disturbance; over that age 74 per cent presented with visual symptoms, 32 per cent with dementia, and 32 per cent with pituitary failure, but only 5 per cent had papilloedema. These tumours usually arise above the sellar diaphragm, but exceptionally they develop within the sella itself.

1. *Endocrine Disturbances.* Since they are situated between the floor of the third ventricle and the pituitary and develop at an early age, they may produce many different disturbances of growth and metabolism, which may be due to their compression either of the pituitary or of the tuber cinereum, or of both of these structures. In Cushing's words, 'the patient may show extreme degrees of adiposity or emaciation, of polyuria or the reverse, of dwarfism, of sexual infantilism or of premature physical senility'. In the later stages the patient may be drowsy, and hyperpyrexia has not uncommonly followed operative interference with the growth. Diabetes insipidus is common and may develop for the first time after surgery (Northfield, 1957).

2. *Pressure Symptoms.* Symptoms of increased intracranial pressure are much more conspicuous than in the case of pituitary tumours. When the tumour arises in childhood the skull may be enlarged and the sutures separated. Headache and vomiting may be severe, and papilloedema is rather commoner than optic atrophy. The tumour may compress the optic nerves, chiasm, or tracts leading to corresponding field defects. The optic chiasm is compressed from above, hence

the resulting bitemporal hemianopia usually begins in the lower quadrants. The frontal lobes, temporal lobes and cerebral peduncles may also be compressed.

3. *Radiographic Appearances.* These consist of: (i) general signs of increased intracranial pressure; (ii) erosion of the clinoid processes and flattening of the sella turcica, the result of downward pressure by the tumour; (iii) radiographic evidence of calcification within the tumour [FIG. 53, p. 256], which is present in about 75 per cent of cases and varies from faint, opaque flecks to a mass the size of a hen's egg, lying above the sella turcica. Occasionally there are also areas of calcification within the sella.

Suprasellar Meningioma. Suprasellar meningiomas are tumours of adult life arising from the meninges which cover the circle of venous sinuses around the diaphragma sellae. Headache is not as a rule severe and endocrine symptoms are usually absent. The principal symptoms are visual and are due to compression of the optic nerve, chiasm, or tract, according to the position of the tumour. Primary optic atrophy is the rule and the visual field defects may consist either of hemianopia or a central or temporal paracentral scotoma. One eye is usually affected before the other and to a greater extent. Pressure of the tumour upon the base of the brain may lead to uncinate attacks, general convulsions, and hemiparesis. Radiograms may show no abnormality, or the optic canal or clinoid processes may be eroded and the sella flattened, and there may be opacities due to calcification within the growth. Occasionally the tumour surrounds and may occlude one internal carotid artery. Extension upwards of metastases in the sella may have a similar effect (Scatliff and Bull, 1965).

Glioma of the Optic Chiasm. This is a rare tumour which usually occurs in childhood, and may be associated with generalized neurofibromatosis. Owing to the situation of the tumour visual deterioration usually draws attention to its presence before a marked rise of intracranial pressure occurs. Primary optic atrophy is the rule and the visual field defects are often bizarre, and may not conform to the more familiar bitemporal or homonymous hemianopia. Exophthalmos may occur. Endocrine disturbances are absent. Radiograms usually show enlargement of one optic foramen [FIG. 76] and less often enlargement of

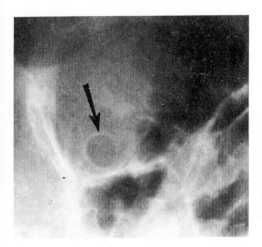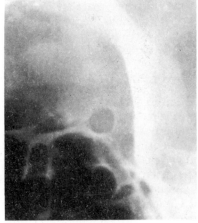

FIG. 76. Glioma of the right optic nerve. Radiographs show that the diameter of the right optic foramen (on the left) is 3 mm greater than the left (on the right)

the sella turcica forwards beneath the anterior clinoid processes. Gliomas in this situation in childhood tend to run a very slow course, often of many months or even years, before extending along the optic tracts into the midbrain. Rarely, if the diagnosis is made early it is possible to remove one eye and optic nerve before the chiasm is involved. Optic nerve gliomas in adult life, however, are often aggressively malignant and rapidly invasive, presenting with a picture like retrobulbar neuritis, giving total blindness within a few weeks and death in less than a year (Hoyt et al., 1973).

Cerebellum

The cerebellum is a common site of tumour, especially in childhood. Medulloblastomas are usually found in the cerebellum during the first decade of life. They arise in the midline in the region of the roof of the fourth ventricle. Astrocytomas, though they may occur either in the cerebrum or in the cerebellum, are common in the cerebellar hemispheres during childhood or early adult life, and are often cystic. Haemangioblastomas are almost exclusively cerebellar tumours, and are also usually cystic. The symptoms differ considerably according to whether the tumour is median or lateral.

Midline Cerebellar Tumours. In this group the history is usually short and the patient, generally a child, is likely to be brought for examination within a few weeks of the onset. Symptoms of increased intracranial pressure occur early, and often become severe. Headache, vomiting, and papilloedema are conspicuous, and in children hydrocephalus often leads to enlargement of the skull, with separation of the sutures. Symptoms of cerebellar deficiency are usually most marked on standing and walking (truncal ataxia), and there may be little or no ataxia of the limbs on examination. Giddiness is common, and there is usually unsteadiness on standing, especially with the eyes closed. The patient usually tends to fall backwards, sometimes forwards. The gait tends to be broad-based and unsteady, especially on turning. Nystagmus is often absent, but there is often muscular hypotonia which may be unequal on the two sides of the body. Compression of the midbrain may lead to 'tonic fits', characterized by extension of all four limbs and opisthotonos, with loss of consciousness, and the pupils are occasionally dilated and exhibit sluggish reactions, a misleading sign which may suggest a tumour of the third ventricle or pineal body. The remaining cranial nerves are often little affected, though weakness of one or both lateral recti and slight facial weakness may be encountered. There is as a rule little weakness of the limbs, though an extensor plantar response on one or both sides may be found. The tendon reflexes are sometimes sluggish. Sensory loss is exceptional.

Tumours of the Cerebellar Hemisphere. As in the case of midline cerebellar tumours, signs of increased intracranial pressure usually occur early, but a cystic haemangioblastoma may attain a large size without causing conspicuous symptoms. In addition to suboccipital headache early symptoms include clumsiness of the ipsilateral hand, a tendency to stagger to the side of the lesion, and giddiness on turning the head.

Nystagmus is usually marked and is most evident on conjugate lateral ocular deviation to the side of the lesion. The quick phase is directed towards the periphery and the slow phase towards the centre. Nystagmus is usually confined to the plane in which the eyes are deviated, but may occasionally be rotary. Other signs of a deficiency of cerebellar function are most marked in, and often confined to, the limbs on the side of the lesion. Hypotonia is usually conspicuous. The outstretched upper limb on the affected side tends to sway if unsupported. Ataxia is present on the affected side, being most evident in the upper limb on carrying out fine movements, for example in the finger–nose test, and in the lower limb in walking. The gait is unsteady. The patient tends to walk with a wide base and to deviate to the affected side, and is liable to fall to the affected side when standing up with the feet together and the eyes closed. Rapid alternating movements are carried out with the affected limb in an irregular, jerky manner or may even be impossible. The shoulder on the affected side is sometimes held lower than the normal shoulder, and there may be scoliosis with the concavity towards the side of the lesion.

There is occasionally an abnormal attitude of the head, which is flexed to one side and rotated so that the occiput is directed towards the shoulder, towards which the head is flexed. Speech is usually little affected in cerebellar tumours, whether of the midline or lateral lobes. [For other symptoms of cerebellar deficiency see p. 61.]

The symptoms of cerebellar deficiency associated with a tumour of the cerebellum often appear to be disproportionately slight with reference to the size of the tumour. It is known that after ablation of the cerebellum a considerable recovery of function may occur, and it is probable that the slow growth of the tumour permits a gradual compensation for cerebellar deficiency by other parts of the nervous system.

Neighbourhood symptoms are usually more conspicuous in the case of lateral cerebellar tumours than when the tumour is in the midline. Forward pressure by the tumour may cause a disturbance of function of any of the cranial nerves from the fifth to the twelfth on the same side, the fifth, sixth, and seventh being most frequently affected. Pressure upon the ipsilateral half of the pons and medulla not infrequently leads to slight signs of corticospinal defect on the opposite side of the body and occasionally to sensory loss, especially impairment of postural sensibility, though this is rarely marked. Sometimes ipsilateral signs of corticospinal tract dysfunction arise due to pressure of the contralateral crus cerebri against the free edge of the tentorium.

Eighth Nerve

Tumours of the eighth nerve (acoustic neuromas) may be either unilateral or bilateral. In the latter case they are usually manifestations of general neurofibromatosis. They rarely give rise to symptoms before the third decade of life and most commonly during the fifth decade. They are tumours of slow growth, and focal symptoms commonly exist for years before those of increased intracranial pressure develop. The first symptoms are due to a disturbance of the functions of the eighth nerve, and this feature is so constant that if a tumour situated in the cerebellopontine angle manifests itself through some other inaugural symptom it is unlikely to be an acoustic neuroma. Tinnitus is usually the first symptom, followed by progressive deafness, through sometimes labyrinthine symptoms, for example giddiness, precede disturbances of hearing. It is not uncommon to find that a patient, when he first comes under observation, is completely deaf in the affected ear as many patients fail to notice unilateral hearing loss. Headache at first is usually occipital, but sometimes frontal, and tends to radiate from back to front through the mastoid region. In the late stages it becomes general and there may be attacks of severe occipital pain radiating down the spine and associated with retraction of the head and neck, respiratory embarrassment, and, sometimes, loss of consciousness. Papilloedema and vomiting are comparatively late in developing. The patient may complain of paraesthesiae referred to the face on one or both sides, and attacks of unilateral facial spasm may occur. Diplopia is not uncommon. Dysphagia is a late symptom.

On examination there are signs of impaired conductivity in the affected eighth nerve. Hearing is much reduced and may be completely lost. Tests of vestibular function usually show loss of sensitivity—a canal paresis. This usually occurs alone but sometimes in combination with a directional preponderance to the unaffected side (Carmichael *et al.*, 1956). The head is sometimes rotated so that the occiput is directed towards the shoulder of the affected side.

Other signs result from pressure by the tumour upon neighbouring cranial nerves. There is usually some facial weakness on the affected side, though this may be slight. Sensory loss may occur in the trigeminal distribution, but reduction or loss of the corneal reflex may be the only sign of involvement of the fifth nerve. Nystagmus is almost invariable; if this sign is absent an acoustic neuroma is unlikely. Weakness of the lateral rectus may be present as a result of compression of the sixth nerve. The remaining cranial nerves are usually unaffected. Disturbance of function of the fifth, sixth, seventh, and eighth cranial nerves may occur on the opposite side as well as on the side of the tumour. Compression of the ipsilateral cerebellar hemisphere causes signs of cerebellar deficiency on the side of the tumour. Signs of compression of the brain stem are not as a rule conspicuous, but crossed hemiparesis and hemianaesthesia may occur as a result of compression of the long descending and ascending tracts, and weakness of conjugate ocular deviation to the side of the tumour, as a result of compression of the pons.

Atypical symptoms, occurring when the tumour arises more medially than usual, include acute or chronic hydrocephalus, causing rapid visual failure and slow mental deterioration, respectively, also paroxysmal disorders of consciousness, including epilepsy (Shephard and Wadia, 1956). Radiographic examination may show erosion of the petrous portion of the temporal bone [FIG. 56, p. 258] or of the internal acoustic meatus by the tumour. The size and situation of the tumour may be demonstrated by ventriculography [FIG. 68, p. 266] or by myodil cisternography.

Pons and Medulla

The commonest tumour of the brain stem is the pontine astrocytoma of childhood; less often these neoplasms occur in adults. Owing to the close association in the pons and medulla of important cranial nerve nuclei as well as of the descending and ascending fibre tracts, tumours in this region soon give rise to localizing signs and symptoms (Barnett and Hyland, 1952). Possibly for this reason signs of increased intracranial pressure are often slight when the patient first comes under observation. Vomiting is often absent, and papilloedema appears in under 50 per cent of cases. Headache, which in the early stages is mainly occipital, and vertigo are common, and both may be intensified by rotation of the head. Diplopia due to a unilateral sixth nerve palsy is usually the first focal symptom, a point of distinction from cerebellar medulloblastoma. At first the signs may point to a lesion confined to one-half of the brain stem but they eventually become bilateral. Weakness of the lateral rectus on one or both sides usually develops early, and may be followed by paresis of conjugate ocular deviation, or the latter may occur alone. Crossed paralysis is usually seen at an early stage, the distribution of the paresis on the two sides of the body depending upon the level of the tumour. Sometimes there is weakness of the jaw and facial muscles on one side and of the soft palate, tongue, and limbs on the other. Later bilateral paralysis of the bulbar muscles and limbs usually develops. Sensory loss in the region of the trigeminal distribution with reduction of the corneal reflex is usually present on one or both sides, and impairment of hearing may occur. Sensory loss on the limbs and trunk is variable. Analgesia and thermo-anaesthesia may occur without loss of postural sensibility or vice versa, or all forms of sensibility may be affected. Sensory changes may be predominantly unilateral or bilateral. Nystagmus and some degree of ataxia of the limbs are common, due to involvement of central cerebellar connections. Paralysis of the ocular sympathetic on one or both sides is frequent, and the visceral functions of the medulla may be disordered, leading to tachycardia or cardiac irregularity, alterations in the respiratory rate and rhythm, hiccup, and glycosuria. The course of the illness due to these tumours is sometimes protracted, lasting for several years, as many of them are very slow-growing (the condition which used to be called 'benign hypertrophy of the pons' is now known to be due to a slow-growing astrocytoma). Temporary remission of symptoms and signs is not infrequent (Sarkari and Bickerstaff, 1969).

A chordoma arising between the pons and the clivus may give a similar picture to that of an intrinsic brain stem tumour with cranial nerve palsies and long tract signs. These tumours sometimes calcify and an area of calcification posterior to the clivus may be diagnostic. Arteriovenous angiomas of the brain stem may give a similar picture. Vertebral angiography and/or pneumo-encephalography or ventriculography [FIG. 72] are the methods of radiological investigation which are most useful in localizing tumours in or near the brain stem.

Fourth Ventricle

Tumours arising in the fourth ventricle itself are usually ependymomas originating in the ependymal cells, though the fourth ventricle may be invaded by tumours arising in the vermis of the cerebellum or in the pons. The characteristic triad of symptoms are headache, morning vomiting and vertigo, with nystagmus increased or elicited by change in position of the head. In young patients ependymoma is the commonest cause but over the age of 50 the same syndrome may result from metastases in the fourth ventricle (usually from bronchial carcinoma). Headache is an early symptom and is liable to paroxysmal exacerbations, the pain radiating to the neck and even to the shoulders and arms. Vomiting and papilloedema and other evidences of hydrocephalus usually develop rapidly. But headache and papilloedema may be absent: one patient had no symptoms except vomiting, for which he had had a laparotomy, and an ataxic gait. There is often stiffness of the cervical muscles and disorders of equilibrium are prominent. Symptoms of cerebellar deficiency in the limbs may be slight or absent. 'Tonic fits' may occur. Disturbance of function of the cranial nerves is often slight, though there may be paresis of one or both lateral recti, and trismus has been noted. The tumour may lead to disturbances of the visceral centres of the medulla, causing attacks of tachycardia, dyspnoea and irregular respiration, hiccup, sweating, and vasomotor disturbances, polyuria, and glyco-suria. Sudden death may occur.

In rare cases the tumour grows out from the fourth ventricle and surrounds and compresses the spinal cord at the level of the foramen magnum, producing analgesia and thermo-anaesthesia of the face and upper limbs, with signs of corticospinal involvement, and leading to a clinical picture closely resembling syringobulbia.

Basal Meninges

Neoplastic infiltration of the basal meninges leads to a fairly distinctive clinical picture. This condition may be due to metastases from extracranial neoplasms, or to extension to within the cranial cavity of a primary carcinoma of the naso-pharynx or of a paranasal sinus. It leads to progressive cranial nerve palsies, which are usually unilateral but sometimes bilateral and asymmetrical. Often the neoplastic growth is wholly extradural, affecting particularly the third, fifth, and sixth cranial nerves as they emerge through their exit foramina, but sometimes the lower cranial nerves are selectively involved (tenth, eleventh, and twelfth). Radiographs of the skull base may demonstrate bony erosion [FIG. 77].

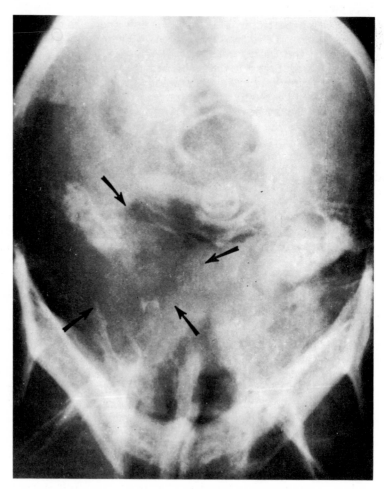

FIG. 77. Basal radiograph of skull demonstrating an ill-defined area of bony destruction (arrows) caused by a nasopharyngeal carcinoma. The foramina spinosum and ovale are completely destroyed on the left

In other instances, especially in the case of metastatic spread from extra-cranial visceral growths, the tumour is intradural and involves the arachnoid. Papilloedema may be present or absent. Invasion of the pituitary and tuber cinereum may cause polyuria, drowsiness, and other symptoms of hypothalamic disturbance. When the subarachnoid space is invaded cervical rigidity and pyrexia are present, the clinical picture then resembling that of tuberculous meningitis (carcinomatosis of the meninges). Neoplastic infiltration of the basal meninges may also be associated with focal symptoms due to other metastases within the brain, and signs of involvement of the cervical lymph nodes should be sought.

Gliomatosis Cerebri

In this rare condition [p. 232] dementia and personality change are the commonest presenting feature but headaches, papilloedema, fits, hemiparesis, ataxia, and brain stem signs may all occur (Couch and Weiss, 1974); often angiography and air pictures give non-specific findings and diagnosis may ultimately depend upon brain biopsy.

DIAGNOSIS

Other conditions may be confused with intracranial tumour, either because they give rise to increased intracranial pressure or because they lead to a progressive cerebral lesion, or for both of these reasons. The following are the conditions most likely to be mistaken for a growth.

Intracranial Abscess

In most cases intracranial abscess is readily distinguished from tumour, since its development is usually acute or subacute and a primary focus of infection is usually found either in the ears, sinuses, lungs, or elsewhere. Rarely, however, a chronic abscess may arise, its source of infection being latent or having disappeared. In such cases clinical diagnosis from tumour may be impossible. A sudden or apoplectiform onset, the occurrence of a leucocytosis in the blood and of a slight pleocytosis in the CSF, and the presence of slight pyrexia are points in favour of an abscess, but none of these is constantly present. The EEG is more often severely abnormal in the case of brain abscess than in intracranial tumour while gamma-encephalography and more particularly the EMI scan give distinctive appearances in cases of abscess.

Arachnoidal Cysts

Sometimes these cysts result from arachnoiditis following previous meningeal inflammation but most of those which mimic intracranial tumour are probably of developmental origin (Oliver, 1958). Localized cystic collections of CSF in the subarachnoid space may be indistinguishable from intracranial tumour before operation. Not uncommonly they occur in the cerebellopontine angle and at the base of the brain, where the optic chiasma may be involved. Pre-operative diagnosis from tumour may be impossible.

Benign Intracranial Hypertension

The raised pressure of the CSF in this condition due to venous sinus occlusion or cerebral oedema of cause unknown causes papilloedema, headache, and vomiting, but there are no progressive focal signs, the electroencephalogram may be normal (Foley, 1955) and the ventricles will be neither enlarged nor displaced; in fact they are usually small [see p. 227].

Cerebral Arterial Disease

Cerebral softening due to vascular occlusion usually causes symptoms apparently referable to a single lesion, though there is sometimes evidence that the lesions are multiple. The onset of symptoms with a slight 'stroke' is valuable evidence of their vascular origin, and confirmation is found in evidence of arteriosclerosis elsewhere. However, in some cases of cerebral infarction, particularly due to carotid occlusion, the evolution of symptoms is slow and diagnosis from tumour is difficult or impossible without contrast radiology. In malignant hypertension severe headache and papilloedema may coexist with a focal cerebral lesion, but the blood pressure is high and typical retinal changes are present. In some cases the diagnosis remains in doubt until investigation demonstrates the absence of a space-occupying lesion, but it must be remembered that in later life an intracranial tumour may coexist with arteriosclerosis and raised blood pressure.

Neurosyphilis

The meningovascular form of neurosyphilis may be mistaken for tumour on account of the presence of headache and papilloedema associated with an intracranial lesion, while the mental deterioration and convulsions of general paresis may suggest a tumour of the frontal lobe or corpus callosum. In both forms of neurosyphilis, however, reflex iridoplegia is likely to be present, and the V.D.R.L. reaction and other characteristic changes in the CSF reveal the true nature of the disorder. Gumma of the brain is now extremely rare, and the coexistence of symptoms of an intracranial tumour with a positive V.D.R.L. reaction must not be regarded as indicating that the patient is suffering from cerebral gumma. Syphilis and cerebral tumour sometimes occur in the same individual.

Epilepsy

Since epileptiform convulsions are a common symptom of intracranial tumour, the differential diagnosis of tumour from other causes of epilepsy frequently arises. Constitutional epilepsy usually begins before the age of 25, though even in later life no cause may be found for the fits even after prolonged observation. Convulsions beginning after this age should always suggest the possibility of tumour, though in late middle life and old age cerebral arteriosclerosis is probably the commonest cause. In idiopathic epilepsy headache is absent, except immediately after the fits, and there are no signs of a focal lesion of the nervous system. A focal onset of the fits or focal neurological signs in older patients always raise the possibility of tumour [p. 1110]. Full investigations should always be carried out in doubtful cases.

Migraine

Headache, vomiting, visual hallucinations, and visual field defects are common both to migraine and to tumours in the neighbourhood of the visual cortex of the occipital lobe, especially angioma. As a rule the field defects of migraine are transitory, lasting only for from one-half to one hour, but occasionally an exceptionally severe attack is followed by a permanent scotoma or hemianopia. Usually migraine begins at puberty, and there is often a family history of the disorder. Signs of increased intracranial pressure are absent and there is no evidence of a progressive intracranial lesion. Visual field defect associated with an occipital tumour is persistent. A bruit is sometimes to be heard over an angioma, and

X-rays may show calcification or abnormal vascular markings in the skull. Angiography usually settles the question.

Retrobulbar Neuritis

Acute bilateral retrobulbar neuritis may simulate intracranial tumour, because it causes disc swelling with impairment of vision. It is distinguished, however, by the acute onset and by the fact that the visual loss is disproportionately great compared with the papilloedema, which is usually slight. Headache is absent in retrobulbar neuritis, but pain in the eyes may be considerable, and they are usually tender on pressure.

Diffuse Sclerosis

Diffuse sclerosis may simulate tumour when papilloedema is present. However, the onset in early life, usually with visual failure of subcortical origin, and the bilateral distribution of the symptoms should enable the two conditions to be distinguished.

Chronic Subdural Haematoma

Since this is a slowly progressive space-occupying lesion it may be indistinguishable from tumour in the absence of a history of trauma. Electroencephalography may be helpful, and angiography usually settles the diagnosis.

Encephalitis

Herpes simplex encephalitis [p. 495] may give a picture suggesting an acute temporal lobe lesion but the apoplectiform onset is usually more suggestive of abscess than tumour. Other forms of encephalitis and especially subacute sclerosing panencephalitis sometimes give a 'pseudotumoural' picture of propressive hemiplegia in the early stages.

Aneurysm

Large intracranial aneurysms may present as space-occupying lesions, especially when suprasellar in situation, but are readily recognized on angiography.

Hydrocephalus and Dementia

Hydrocephalus of late onset, whether due to aqueduct stenosis first giving symptoms in adult life which may suggest a posterior fossa tumour, or to 'low-pressure communicating hydrocephalus' which usually presents with dementia and ataxia, must be distinguished by appropriate radiological studies. Similarly, pneumoencephalography may be needed to exclude the possibility of a corpus callosum glioma in some patients with presenile dementia.

DIAGNOSIS OF THE NATURE OF THE TUMOUR

Medulloblastoma

This is a rapidly growing, malignant tumour, most frequently found in the neighbourhood of the roof of the fourth ventricle in childhood. It should be suspected in children who present the symptoms of a midline cerebellar tumour with a history of a few weeks' or months' duration.

Glioblastoma Multiforme

This is a malignant and rapidly growing tumour arising in middle life and usually found in the cerebral hemispheres. It should be suspected in middle-aged persons presenting the symptoms of a tumour of one cerebral hemisphere with a history of a few weeks' or months' duration. Gamma-encephalography almost invariably shows an increased area of uptake of radioactivity and angiography a pathological circulation.

Astrocytoma

The astrocytoma is a slowly growing tumour which may arise either in the cerebral or cerebellar hemispheres. In most cases in which the history of an intracranial tumour in either of these situations extends over several years, the growth is an astrocytoma or an oligodendroglioma but the latter is more liable to show calcification on plain X-rays than the former. Owing to its situation, the cerebellar astrocytoma is likely to bring the patient under observation sooner than one situated in the cerebral hemisphere. The gamma-encephalogram is less often positive in these cases than in the more malignant growths and angiography usually shows displacement of vessels; as these growths are often avascular, a pathological circulation is relatively infrequent.

Meningioma

Meningiomas are almost exclusively supratentorial tumours and exhibit certain sites of election which have already been described. They are rare before middle life and are commoner in females. There may be a very long history, e.g. of epilepsy for many years. Owing to their extracerebral origin they compress but do not invade the brain. The focal symptoms to which they give rise are less severe in relation to the size of the tumour than is the case with the gliomas. Meningiomas, therefore, frequently cause a marked increase in intracranial pressure, with comparatively slight signs of a focal lesion. Symptoms and signs may increase during pregnancy and remit after delivery (Bickerstaff et al., 1958; Michelsen and New, 1969). Their proximity to the skull leads to erosion of bone in 20 per cent of cases, and this is often demonstrable on radiographic examination, which may also show calcification within the tumour. The meningiomas are usually associated with increased vascularity, which may be extracranial as well as intracranial, the latter being visible radiographically. Radiographs may also show enlargement of the foramen spinosum in the base of the skull and of the middle meningeal channels in the vault. Angiography often demonstrates filling of the tumour from the meningeal circulation and vascular displacement; the typical 'blush' in the venous phase or other types of tumour circulation are seen in only about 50 per cent of cases (Banna and Appleby, 1969).

Angioma

Since angiomas are of congenital origin two-thirds cause symptoms below the age of 30. Epilepsy, intracerebral or subarachnoid haemorrhage, and hemiparesis are the commonest presenting symptoms. The diagnosis is confirmed by angiography (Mackenzie, 1953).

Haemangioblastoma

These tumours are almost exclusively cerebellar and are sometimes associated with haemangioblastoma of the retina and spinal cord, and with cysts of the pancreas and kidneys, and hypernephromas of the kidneys or suprarenal glands. Only the first of these associated abnormalities, however, is likely to be discoverable clinically. As many of these tumours excrete erythropoietin, erythrocytosis is common (Jeffreys, 1975) with haemoglobin levels often exceeding

16 g/100 ml; this is a valuable confirmatory sign. These and other cerebral tumours occasionally cause paroxysmal hypertension mimicking the clinical picture of phaeochromocytoma (Cameron and Doig, 1970). Vertebral angiography, using a subtraction technique, commonly shows a typical tumour circulation.

Tumours in the neighbourhood of the Pituitary

Diagnosis of the nature of these tumours is described on pp. 275-8.

Acoustic Neuroma

The clinical picture of this tumour, which commonly arises in middle-aged persons, is distinctive, since the first symptoms are those of destruction of the eighth nerve on one side. A similar picture may result from a meningioma, cholesteatoma, or an arachnoid cyst in the cerebellopontine angle.

Metastatic Tumours

Metastatic tumours should be suspected in middle-aged or elderly individuals who present with the history of a rapidly developing intracranial growth. In all such cases a thorough clinical and radiographic search for a primary neoplasm should be made. A history of marked loss of weight is suggestive. Not infrequently an intracranial metastasis gives rise to symptoms before the primary lesion, especially when this is in the lung, and sometimes the primary lesion is not discovered until autopsy.

Tuberculoma

Tuberculoma may occur at any age, but is most frequent in childhood and early adult life. It is now rare in Europe and the U.S.A. but is still common in India (Dastur and Desai, 1965). These lesions are cortical or subcortical in the cerebral or cerebellar hemispheres and only rarely involve the brain stem. Remissions and relapses are somewhat characteristic, and increase in intracranial pressure is often disproportionately slight. A pleocytosis may be found in the CSF. The presence of a tuberculous lesion elsewhere will afford some confirmatory evidence, but this is so common that it may coexist with a glioma.

Gumma

Gumma is now a very rare tumour of the brain. Both glioma and syphilitic infection are comparatively common and both may occur in the same individual.

Parasitic Cysts

The possibility that the symptoms of an intracranial tumour may be due to parasitic cysts should always be considered in a patient who has been exposed to the infestation. The presence of such cysts elsewhere in the body affords strong confirmatory evidence, and the CSF often shows a mononuclear pleocytosis. The blood may exhibit an eosinophilia. Complement fixation and flocculation tests, and Casoni's intradermal sensitization test may be of diagnostic value in suspected cases of hydatid infection.

PROGNOSIS AND TREATMENT

The prognosis of intracranial tumour is influenced by the nature of the growth and its accessibility to the surgeon. In the absence of surgical interference almost all intracranial tumours increase in size, their rate of growth depending upon their nature. The resulting increase of intracranial pressure and destruction of brain tissue ultimately prove fatal. When papilloedema is severe, death may be preceded by blindness. The more malignant gliomas, such as the medullo-blastomas and the glioblastomas, grow rapidly and usually prove fatal within one or two years, though temporary remission of symptoms and signs resulting from a medulloblastoma may follow radiotherapy and even the skeletal meta-stases of such tumours which may develop following partial operative removal or 'shunt' operations [p. 228] may remit temporarily after treatment with vincristine sulphate (Lassman et al., 1969). The slowly growing astrocytomas may cause symptoms for many years before leading to a marked increase in intracranial pressure (see Penman and Smith, 1954).

Sudden death in cases of intracranial tumour is rare but occasionally results from rapidly developing cerebral oedema and/or tentorial or cerebellar hernia-tion. Increasingly severe headache, a unilateral dilated pupil, or increasing occipital pain and neck stiffness are important warning signs which may demand the urgent administration of high doses of steroids to reduce cerebral oedema, followed, where appropriate, by ventricular drainage or other appropriate neurosurgical measures.

Recent improvements in neurosurgical technique and anaesthesia, including the use of hypothermia whenever appropriate (Inglis and Turner, 1957) and a careful choice of anaesthetic agents (Jennett et al., 1969) have greatly improved the outcome of surgical procedures in patients with intracranial space-occupying lesions. Horrax (1954) pointed out that in almost half of all patients with intra-cranial tumours the course is relatively benign and in his series of 766 patients subjected to surgery the operative mortality was 13·2 per cent while almost 70 per cent engaged in useful activity for one to 20 years after operation. Even in cases of glioblastoma, partial removal of the tumour, creating an internal decompression, followed by the use of steroids may improve the outcome, although attempted removal is less appropriate in tumours lying in relation to the motor and/or sensory cortex, in relation to the speech areas of the dominant hemisphere or in those which are deeply situated. In slowly growing astro-cytomas and oligodendrogliomas of the cerebral hemispheres operative removal should not as a rule be attempted unless they lie in relatively silent areas, though exploration and biopsy may be necessary for diagnosis. By contrast, cerebellar astrocytomas can often be removed completely (see below), as is the case with many haemangioblastomas. Most convexity meningiomas and pituitary adenomas can be removed successfully but operation upon basal and parasellar meningiomas may be much more hazardous because of encroachment upon major vessels or cranial nerves. Recurrence of meningiomas after apparent total removal is not infrequent and sometimes the recurrent growth proves to be sarcomatous. Most colloid cysts of the third ventricle and other intra-ventricular tumours such as papillomas of the choroid plexus and ependymomas of the fourth ventricle can also be removed and partial removal of clivus chor-domas is also feasible, if hazardous. However, gliomas of the third ventricle and brain stem cannot be removed and the same is true of many pinealomas; in such cases if obstructive hydrocephalus develops a 'shunt' operation may give at least temporary relief of symptoms. In some patients with craniopharyn-giomas a similar palliative operation is all that can be done, but when the growth is relatively small partial or even total removal is feasible and may lead to preservation of residual vision and prolonged remission of symptoms; even the drainage of an associated cyst may be equally beneficial though a transient aseptic meningitis may result from the release of cholesterol into the sub-arachnoid space. Except in elderly patients with few focal signs and little evidence of raised pressure, all acoustic neuromas demand surgery but there is still some dispute among surgeons as to whether total or intracapsular removal is to be preferred; the outcome in such cases is clearly related to the experience of the surgeon in such procedures. There is also difference of opinion about the surgical treatment of arteriovenous angiomas; small malformations in relatively silent areas can be removed completely; few surgeons are prepared to operate upon large angiomas but some advocate ligation of major feeding vessels. The rare intracranial gumma responds little if at all to antisyphilitic treatment but may demand surgical removal; the same principle applies to tuberculomas which should be removed if possible after prior treatment with antituberculous drugs which should be continued for some months after removal in order to prevent meningitis. Surgery is of little or no value in the treatment of infiltrating basal neoplasms such as nasopharyngeal carcinoma and glomus tumours.

A major advance in the last few years has been the introduction of steroid drugs to reduce the intracranial pressure; the usual initial treatment is with dexamethasone 5 mg every six hours. This remedy has now supplanted other dehydrating agents such as intravenous sucrose, rectal magnesium sulphate, and urea (Javid, 1958). A dramatic reduction in cerebral oedema and in the intracranial pressure usually results and operation is facilitated (*British Medical Journal*, 1973). This treatment, followed by appropriate maintenance doses, may also produce prolonged remission of symptoms in many patients with intracranial metastases (Weinstein *et al.*, 1973), and similar maintenance treatment may prolong life and improve the quality of survival in some patients with other forms of intracranial tumour, including gliomas. The scope of radiotherapy in the treatment of intracranial tumour is still not clearly defined. Irradiation is indicated in most cases of pituitary adenoma and medulloblastoma, in association with surgical treatment, and also plays a valuable role in patients with pontine glioma and nasopharyngeal carcinoma. It is commonly used in patients in whom only partial removal of ependymomas of the fourth ventricle or of cerebellar astrocytomas or haemangioblastomas has been possible, as well as in cases of pinealoma, glomus tumour, and chordoma. It may also promote remission, along with steroids, in patients with cerebral metastases, particularly when the primary tumour (say in the lung) is known to be radiosensitive. The role of this treatment in gliomas of the cerebral hemisphere is less certain, though it is commonly employed in gliomas of moderate malignancy. No firm rules can at present be laid down; the aim must be not just to prolong life but to be sure that the quality of survival is improved; there is little point in prolonging life only to prolong suffering. The same dilemma relates to the use of antimitotic agents such as cyclophosphamide, azathioprine, and vincristine and other related remedies which have been utilized either systemically or, on occasion, by intracarotid injection, in patients with brain tumour; little objective evidence of their value is yet available, although it is clear that the combined use of radiotherapy and of such agents, including intrathecal methotrexate, is of considerable value in central nervous system leukaemia (*The Lancet*, 1972).

It is therefore possible to conclude that some benign intracranial tumours can be removed completely, and provided irreversible damage to nervous structures has not occurred, in these cases the prognosis is excellent. Even in the case of malignant or inaccessible neoplasms the judicious use of steroids, radiotherapy, antimitotic agents, and surgery in appropriate cases may greatly improve the prognosis, but in many cases, especially those with slowly growing astrocytomas, excessively radical or mutilating operations are contraindicated. Every individual case must be treated on its merits in the light of experience and new developments in therapy.

REFERENCES

ALEXANDER, G. L., and NORMAN, R. M. (1960) *The Sturge–Weber Syndrome*, Bristol.

BAILEY, P. (1932) Histologic diagnosis of tumors of the brain, *Arch. Neurol. Psychiat. (Chic.)*, **27**, 1290.

BAILEY, P. (1948) *Intracranial Tumors*, 2nd ed., Springfield, Ill.

BAILEY, P., and BUCY, P. C. (1931) The origin and nature of meningeal tumors, *Amer. J. Cancer*, **15**, 15.

BAILEY, P., and CUSHING, H. (1925) Medulloblastoma cerebelli, a common type of mid-cerebellar glioma of childhood, *Arch. Neurol. Psychiat. (Chic.)*, **14**, 192.

BAILEY, P., and CUSHING, H. (1926) *A Classification of the Tumours of the Glioma Group*, London.

BANNA, M., and APPLEBY, A. (1969) Some observations on the angiography of supra-tentorial meningiomas, *Clin. Radiol.*, **20**, 375.

BARNETT, H. J., and HYLAND, H. H. (1952) Tumours involving the brain-stem. A study of 90 cases arising in the brain-stem, fourth ventricle, and pineal tissue, *Quart. J. Med.*, **21**, 265.

BARTLETT, J. R. (1971) Craniopharyngiomas—a summary of 85 cases, *J. Neurol. Neurosurg. Psychiat.*, **34**, 37.

BICKERSTAFF, E. R., SMALL, J. M., and GUEST, I. A. (1958) The relapsing course of certain meningiomas in relation to pregnancy and menstruation, *J. Neurol. Neurosurg. Psychiat.*, **21**, 89.

BIGNER, D. D., KVEDAR, J. P., THOMAS, B. A., SHAFFER, C., VICK, N. A., ENGEL, W. K., and DAY, E. D. (1972) Factors influencing the cell type of brain tumors induced in dogs by Schmidt–Ruppin Rous sarcoma virus, *J. Neuropath. exp. Neurol.*, **31**, 583.

BOLLER, F., PATTEN, D. H., and HOWES, D. (1973) Correlation of brain-scan results with neuropathological findings, *Lancet*, **i**, 1143.

DU BOULAY, G. H. (1965) *Principles of X-ray Diagnosis of the Skull*, London.

BRADY, J. I., and RODRIGUEZ, F. (1961) Cerebellar hemangioblastoma and polycythemia, *Amer. J. med. Sci.*, **242**, 579.

BRITISH MEDICAL JOURNAL (1973) The swollen brain, *Brit. med. J.*, **3**, 463.

BULL, J. W. D. (1951) Diagnostic neuroradiology, in *Modern Trends in Neurology*, 1st Series, ed. Feiling, A., London.

BULL, J. W. D. (1967) The corpus callosum, *Clin. Radiol.*, **18**, 2.

BULL, J. W. D., and MARRYAT, J. (1965) Isotope encephalography: experience with 100 cases, *Brit. med. J.*, **1**, 473.

CAIRNS, H. (1935-6) The ultimate results of operations for intracranial tumors, *Yale J. Biol. Med.*, **8**, 421.

CAIRNS, H., and RUSSELL, D. S. (1931) Intracranial and spinal metastases in gliomas of the brain, *Brain*, **54**, 377.

CAMERON, S. J., and DOIG, A. (1970) Cerebellar tumours presenting with clinical features of phaeochromocytoma, *Lancet*, **i**, 492.

CARMICHAEL, E. A., DIX, M. R., and HALLPIKE, C. S. (1956) Pathology, symptomatology and diagnosis of organic affections of the eighth nerve system, *Brit. med. Bull.*, **12**, 146.

CAVANAGH, J. B. (1958) On certain small tumours encountered in the temporal lobe, *Brain*, **81**, 389.

CLARKE, E. (1954) Cranial and intracranial myelomas, *Brain*, **77**, 61.

COUCH, J. R., and WEISS, S. A. (1974) Gliomatosis cerebri. Report of four cases and review of the literature, *Neurology (Minneap.)*, **24**, 504.

COURVILLE, C. B. (1967) Intracranial tumors. Notes upon a series of three thousand verified cases with some current observations obtaining to their mortality, *Bull. Los Angeles neurol. Soc.*, **32**, suppl. no. 2.

CRITCHLEY, M., and FERGUSON, F. R. (1928) The cerebrospinal epidermoids (cholesteatomata), *Brain*, **51**, 334.

CROOKE, A. C. (1935) A change in the basophil cells of the pituitary gland common to conditions which exhibit the syndrome attributed to basophil adenoma, *J. Path. Bact.*, **41**, 339.

CURRIE, S., and HENSON, R. A. (1971) Neurological syndromes in the reticuloses, *Brain*, **94**, 307.

CUSHING, H. (1912) *The Pituitary Body and its Disorders*, Philadelphia.

CUSHING, H. (1917) *Tumors of the Nervus Acousticus and the Syndrome of the Cerebello-Pontine Angle*, Philadelphia.

CUSHING, H. (1927) Acromegaly from a surgical standpoint, *Brit. med. J.*, **2**, 1 and 48.

CUSHING, H. (1930) The chiasmal syndrome of primary optic atrophy and bitemporal defects in adults with a normal sella turcica, *Arch. Ophthal. (Chic.)*, **2**, 505 and 707.

CUSHING, H. (1932 *a*) The basophil adenomas of the pituitary body and their clinical manifestations (pituitary basophilism), *Bull. Johns Hopk. Hosp.*, **1**, 137.

CUSHING, H. (1932 *b*) *Intracranial Tumors. Notes upon a Series of Two Thousand Verified Cases with Surgical-mortality Percentages Pertaining Thereto*, Springfield, Ill.

CUSHING, H., and BAILEY, P. (1928) *Tumors Arising from the Blood-vessels of the Brain*, Springfield, Ill.

CUSHING, H., and EISENHARDT, L. (1938) *Meningiomas, their Classification, Regional Behavior, Life History, and Surgical End Results*, Springfield, Ill.

DANDY, W. E. (1928) Arteriovenous aneurysm of the brain and venous abnormalities and angiomas of the brain, *Arch. Surg.*, **17**, 190 and 715.

DANDY, W. E. (1933) *Benign Tumors in the Third Ventricle of the Brain*, London.

DASTUR, H. M., and DESAI, A. D. (1965) A comparative study of brain tuberculomas and gliomas based upon 107 case records of each, *Brain*, **88**, 375.

DAVIES-JONES, G. A. B. (1969) Lactate dehydrogenase and glutamic oxalacetic transaminase of the cerebrospinal fluid in tumours of the central nervous system, *J. Neurol. Neurosurg. Psychiat.*, **32**, 324.

DYKEN, P. R. (1975) Cerebrospinal fluid cytology: practical clinical usefulness, *Neurology (Minneap.)*, **25**, 210.

VAN ECK, J. H. M. (1966) Clinical value of isotope encephalography, *J. Neurol. Neurosurg. Psychiat.*, **29**, 145.

EDWARDS, C. H., and PATERSON, J. H. (1951) A review of the symptoms and signs of acoustic neurofibromata, *Brain*, **74**, 144.

FIELDS, W. S., and SHANKLY, P. C. (1962) *The Biology and Treatment of Intracranial Tumors*, Springfield, Ill.

FOERSTER, O., GAGEL, O., and MAHONEY, W. (1939) Die encephalen Tumoren des verlängerten Markes, der Brücke und des Mittelhirns, *Arch. Psychiat. Nervenkr.*, **110**, 1.

FOLEY, J. (1955) Benign forms of intracranial hypertension, *Brain*, **78**, 1.

FORD, R., and AMBROSE, J. (1963) Echoencephalography. The measurement of the position of midline structures in the skull with high-frequency pulsed ultrasound, *Brain*, **86**, 189.

FRENCH, J. D. (1947) Plasmacytoma of hypothalamus; clinical-pathological report of case, *J. Neuropath. exp. Neurol.*, **6**, 265.

GARDNER-THORPE, C. (1970) Presumed plasmacytoma of clivus producing isolated hypoglossal nerve palsy, *Brit. med. J.*, **2**, 405.

GARG, A. G., and TAYLOR, A. R. (1968) A-scan echoencephalography in measurement of the cerebral ventricles, *J. Neurol. Neurosurg. Psychiat.*, **31**, 245.

GAWLER, J., DU BOULAY, G. H., BULL, J. W. D., and MARSHALL, J. (1974) Computer-assisted tomography (EMI scanner): its place in investigation of suspected intracranial tumours, *Lancet*, **ii**, 419.

GLOBUS, J. H., and SILBERT, S. (1931) Pinealomas, *Arch. Neurol. Psychiat. (Chic.)*, **25**, 937.

HENSON, R. A., CRAWFORD, J. V., and CAVANAGH, J. B. (1953) Tumours of the glomus jugulare, *J. Neurol. Neurosurg. Psychiat.*, **16**, 127.

HOEFER, P. B., SCHLESINGER, E. B., and PENNES, H. H. (1947) Epilepsy, *Res. Publ. Ass. nerv. ment. Dis.*, **26**, 50.

HORRAX, G. (1924) Generalized cisternal arachnoiditis simulating cerebellar tumor, *Arch. Surg.*, **9**, 95.

HORRAX, G. (1939) Meningiomas of the brain, *Arch. Neurol. Psychiat. (Chic.)*, **41**, 140.

HORRAX, G. (1954) Benign (favorable) types of brain tumor. The end results (up to twenty years), with statistics of mortality and useful survival, *New Engl. J. Med.*, **250**, 981.

HORRAX, G., and BAILEY, P. (1925) Tumors of the pineal body, *Arch. Neurol. Psychiat. (Chic.)*, **13**, 423.

HOUDART, R., and LE BESNERAIS, Y. (1936) *Les Anévrismes artérioveineux des hémisphères cérébraux*, Paris.

HOYT, W. F., MESHEL, L. G., LESSELL, S., SCHATZ, N. J., and SUCKLING, R. D. (1973) Malignant optic glioma of adulthood, *Brain*, **96**, 121.

HUBBLE, D. (1961) The endocrine orchestra, *Brit. med. J.*, **1**, 523.

HUNTER, R., BLACKWOOD, W., and BULL, J. W. D. (1968) Three cases of frontal meningiomas presenting psychiatrically, *Brit. med. J.*, **3**, 9.

HUTCHINSON, E. C., LEONARD, B. J., MAUDSLEY, C., and YATES, P. O. (1958) Neurological complications of the reticuloses, *Brain*, **81**, 75.

INGLIS, J. M., and TURNER, E. (1957) Use of hypothermia in non-vascular intracranial tumours, *Brit. med. J.*, **1**, 1335.

IRONSIDE, R., and GUTTMACHER, M. (1929) The corpus callosum and its tumours, *Brain*, **52**, 442.

JACOBS, L. L., and RICHLAND, K. J. (1951) Carcinomatosis of the leptomeninges. Review of literature and report of four cases. *Bull. Los Angeles neurol. Soc.*, **16**, 335.

JAVID, M. (1958) Urea—new use of an old agent, *Surg. Clin. N. Amer.*, **38**, 907.

JEFFERSON, M., and ROSENTHAL, F. D. (1959) Spontaneous necrosis in pituitary tumours (pituitary apoplexy), *Lancet*, **i**, 342.

JEFFREYS, R. (1975) Pathological and haematological aspects of posterior fossa haemangioblastoma, *J. Neurol. Neurosurg. Psychiat.*, **38**, 112.

JENNETT, W. B., BARKER, J., FITCH, W., and McDOWALL, D. G. (1969) Effect of anaesthesia on intracranial pressure in patients with space-occupying lesions, *Lancet*, **i**, 61.

JOHN, H. T., and NABARRO, J. D. N. (1955) Intracranial manifestations of malignant lymphoma, *Brit. J. Cancer*, **9**, 386.

KELLY, R. (1951) Colloid cysts of the third ventricle, *Brain*, **74**, 23.

KERNOHAN, J. W., MABON, R. F., SVIEN, H. J., and ADSON, A. W. (1949) A simplified classification of the gliomas, *Proc. Mayo Clin.*, **24**, 71.

KILOH, L. G., and OSSELTON, J. W. (1973) *Clinical Electroencephalography*, 3rd ed., London.

KISTLER, J. P., HOCHBERG, F. H., BROOKS, B. R., RICHARDSON, E. P., NEW, P. F. J., and SCHNUR, J. (1975) Computerized axial tomography: clinicopathologic correlation, *Neurology (Minneap.)*, **25**, 201.

KRAYENBUHL, H., and YASARGIL, M. G. (1965) *Die zerebrale Angiographie*, Stuttgart.

KRAYENBUHL, H., and YASARGIL, M. G. (1968) *Cerebral Angiography*, 2nd ed., London.

KUPER, S., MENDELOW, H., and PROCTOR, N. S. F. (1958) Internal hydrocephalus caused by parasitic cysts, *Brain*, **81**, 235.

KURTZKE, J. F. (1969) Geographic pathology of brain tumors. 1. Distribution of deaths from primary tumors, *Acta Neurol. Scand.*, **45**, 540.

THE LANCET (1972) Treating the nervous system in acute leukaemia, *Lancet*, **i**, 297.

LASSMAN, L. P., PEARCE, G. W., BANNA, M., and JONES, R. D. (1969) Vincristine sulphate in the treatment of skeletal metastases from cerebellar medulloblastoma, *J. Neurosurg.*, **30**, 42.

LINDAU, A. (1921) Studien über Kleinhirncysten. Bau, Pathogenese und Beziehungen zur Angiomatosis Retinae, *Acta path. microbiol. scand.*, Supp. **i**, 1.

LOGUE, V., and MONCKTON, G. (1954) Posterior fossa angiomas, *Brain*, **77**, 252.

McALLISTER, V. L., KENDALL, B. E., and BULL, J. W. D. (1975) Symptomatic vertebral angiomas, *Brain*, **98**, 71.

MACKENZIE, I. (1953) The clinical presentation of the cerebral angiomas, *Brain*, **76**, 184.

McKINNEY, W. M. (1969) Echoencephalography, in *Special Techniques for Neurological Diagnosis*, Contemporary Neurology Series no. 3, ed. Toole, J. F., Philadelphia.

McKISSOCK, W., and PAINE, K. W. E. (1958) Primary tumours of the thalamus, *Brain*, **81**, 41.

MAYO CLINIC (1971) *Clinical Examinations in Neurology*, 3rd ed., Philadelphia, London, and Toronto.

MICHAUX, L., and FELD, M. (1963) *Les Phakomatoses cérébrales*, Paris.

MICHELSEN, J. J., and NEW, P. F. J. (1969) Brain tumour and pregnancy, *J. Neurol. Neurosurg. Psychiat.*, **32**, 305.

MONIZ, E. (1931) *Diagnostic des tumeurs cérébrales et épreuve de l'encéphalographie artérielle*, Paris.

MONTGOMERY, D. A. D., WELBOURN, R. B., McCAUGHEY, W. T. E., and GLEADHILL, C. A. (1959) Pituitary tumours manifested after adrenalectomy for Cushing's syndrome, *Lancet*, **ii**, 707.

MULLAN, S. (1962) Mortality of the surgical treatment of brain tumors, *J. Amer. med. Ass.*, **182**, 601.

NATTRASS, F. J. (1949) Clinical and social problems of epilepsy, *Brit. med. J.*, **1**, 1.

NEWTON, T. H., and POTTS, D. G. (1974) *Radiology of the Skull and Brain—Volume 2 (Angiography)*, St. Louis.

NORTHFIELD, D. W. C. (1957) Rathke-pouch tumours, *Brain*, **80**, 293.

OLIVER, L. C. (1958) Primary arachnoid cysts: report of two cases, *Brit. med. J.*, **1**, 1147.

OLSON, M. E., CHERNIK, N. L., and POSNER, J. B. (1974) Infiltration of the leptomeninges by systemic cancer. A clinical and pathologic study, *Arch. Neurol. (Chic.)*, **30**, 122.

PAOLETTI, P., VANDENHEUVEL, F. A., FUMAGALLI, R., and PAOLETTI, R. (1969) The sterol test for the diagnosis of human brain tumors, *Neurology (Minneap.)*, **19**, 190.

PENDERGRASS, E. P., SCHAEFFER, J. P., and HODES, J. P. (1956) *The Head and Neck in Roentgen Diagnosis*, 2nd ed., Oxford.

PENFIELD, W. (1931) A paper on classification of brain tumours and its practical application, *Brit. med. J.*, **1**, 337.

PENFIELD, W. (1932) Tumors of the sheaths of the nervous system, *Arch. Neurol. Psychiat. (Chic.)*, **27**, 1298.

PENFIELD, W., ERICKSON, T. C., and TARLOV, I. (1940) Relation of intracranial tumours and symptomatic epilepsy, *Arch. Neurol. Psychiat. (Chic.)*, **44**, 300.

PENMAN, J., and SMITH, M. C. (1954) Intracranial gliomata, *Spec. Rep. Ser. med. Res. Coun. (Lond.)*, No. 285.

PENNING, L., FRONT, D., BECHAR, M., GO, K. G., and RODERMOND, J. M. (1973) Factors governing the uptake of pertechnetate by human brain tumours—a scintigraphic study, *Brain*, **96**, 225.

PLUM, F., and POSNER, J. B. (1972) *Diagnosis of Stupor and Coma*, 2nd ed., Philadelphia.

RAIMONDI, A. J. (1966) Ultrastructure of brain tumours, in *Progress in Neurological Surgery*, ed. Krayenbuhl, H., Maspes, P. E., and Sweet, W. H., Basle.

ROBERTSON, E. G. (1967) *Pneumoencephalography*, 2nd ed., Springfield, Ill.

RUSSELL, D. S. (1944) The pinealoma: its relationship to teratoma, *J. Path. Bact.*, **56**, 145.

RUSSELL, D. S., and CAIRNS, H. (1930) Spinal metastases in a case of cerebral glioma of the type known as astrocytoma fibrillare, *J. Path. Bact.*, **33**, 383.

RUSSELL, D. S., and RUBINSTEIN, L. J. (1959) *Pathology of Tumours of the Nervous System*, London.

SARKARI, N. B. S., and BICKERSTAFF, E. R. (1969) Relapses and remissions in brain stem tumours, *Brit. med. J.*, **2**, 21.

SCATLIFF, J. H., and BULL, J. W. D. (1965) The radiological manifestations of suprasellar metastatic tissue, *Clin. Radiol.*, **41**, 66.

SCHAUMBURG, H. H., PLANK, C. R., and ADAMS, R. D. (1972) The reticulum cell sarcoma—microglioma group of brain tumours, *Brain*, **95**, 199.

SCHERER, H. J. (1940 a) The pathology of cerebral gliomas, *J. Neurol. Psychiat.*, **3**, 147.

SCHERER, H. J. (1940 b) The forms of growth in gliomas and their practical significance, *Brain*, **63**, 1.

SCHMIDT, R. P., and WILDER, B. J. (1968) *Epilepsy*, Contemporary Neurology Series, no. 2, Philadelphia.

SCHNECK, S. A., and PENN, I. (1971) De-novo brain tumours in renal-transplant recipients, *Lancet*, **i**, 983.

SHEPHARD, R. H., and WADIA, N. H. (1956) Some observations on atypical features in acoustic neuroma, *Brain*, **79**, 282.

SIEKERT, R. G. (1956) Neurologic manifestations of tumors of the glomus jugulare, *Arch. Neurol. Psychiat. (Chic.)*, **76**, 1.

SOHN, D., VALENSI, Q., and MILLER, S. P. (1967) Neurologic manifestations of Hodgkin's disease: intracerebral Hodgkin's granuloma, *Arch. Neurol. (Chic.)*, **17**, 429.

SPENCER, R. (1965) Scintiscanning in space-occupying lesions of the skull, *Brit. J. Radiol.*, **38**, 1.

STEIN, B. M., FRASER, R. A. R., and TENNER, M. S. (1972) Tumours of the third ventricle in children, *J. Neurol. Neurosurg. Psychiat.*, **35**, 776.

SYMONDS, C. (1962) Ocular palsy as the presenting symptom of pituitary adenoma, *Bull. Johns Hopkins Hosp.*, **111**, 72.

TAVERAS, J. M., and WOOD, E. H. (1964) *Diagnostic Neuroradiology*, Baltimore.

TOMLINSON, B. E., and WALTON, J. N. (1967) Granulomatous meningitis and diffuse parenchymatous degeneration of the nervous system due to an intracranial epidermoid cyst, *J. Neurol. Neurosurg. Psychiat.*, **30**, 341.

VAN WAGENEN, W. P. (1927) Tuberculoma of the brain, *Arch. Neurol. Psychiat. (Chic.)*, **17**, 57.

WALTON, J. N. (1956) *Subarachnoid Haemorrhage*, Edinburgh.

WEINSTEIN, J. D., TOY, F. J., JAFFE, M. E., and GOLDBERG, H. I. (1973) The effect of dexamethasone on brain edema in patients with metastatic brain tumours, *Neurology (Minneap.)*, **23**, 121.

WEST, R. J., GRAHAM-POLE, J., HARDISTY, R. M., and PIKE, M. C. (1972) Factors in pathogenesis of central-nervous-system leukaemia, *Brit. med. J.*, **3**, 311.

WHITE, J. C., and COBB, S. (1955) Psychological changes associated with giant pituitary neoplasms, *Arch. Neurol. Psychiat. (Chic.)*, **74**, 383.

WILLIAMS, J. O., HICKS, E. P., HERZBERG, L., WILLIAMS, N. E., and CROFT, D. N. (1972) Overall value of brain scans and electroencephalograms in detecting neurosurgical lesions, *Lancet*, **ii**, 642.

ZÜLCH, K. J. (1956) Biologie und Pathologie der Hirngeschwülste, in *Handbuch der Neurochirurgie*, ed. Aivecrana, H., and Tönnis, W., Berlin.

ZÜLCH, K. J. (1965) *Brain Tumors: Their Biology and Pathology*, New York.

HEADACHE

THE INVESTIGATION OF A CASE OF HEADACHE

Headache is one of the commonest symptoms. Though it is frequently a trivial disorder, it is also at times a symptom of the gravest significance. Every patient suffering from headache requires, therefore, careful consideration and sometimes thorough investigation. In taking the history, attention must be paid to the following points. How long has the patient suffered from headache? Is it increasing in severity? Is it constant or paroxysmal, and if paroxysmal what is the duration of the paroxysms, and do they occur at any special time of day? Are they precipitated by any circumstance or activity, and how, if at all, can they be relieved? What is the character of the headache, and what is its situation? Is it associated with tenderness of the scalp or skull, with visual disturbances, vomiting, or vertigo? Has there been an injury of the head? Are there symptoms of nasal obstruction or of a discharge, either from the nostrils or into the pharynx? Is the patient anxious, tense, or depressed?

The investigation of a case of headache involves a complete examination of all the systems of the body, special attention being paid to the ocular fundi, the nose and nasal air sinuses, the teeth, the blood pressure, and the urine. Radiography of the skull, including the nasal sinuses, of the cervical spine in cases of occipital headache, and other investigations (electroencephalography, gamma-encephalography, an EMI scan, or specialized neuroradiological studies) may be required in appropriate cases.

THE MODE OF PRODUCTION OF HEADACHE

All the tissues covering the cranium are sensitive to pain, especially the arteries but also the muscles and pericranium. The skull bone itself is insensitive. Within the cranium the venous sinuses and their tributaries, the dura mater and the cerebral arteries, the fifth, ninth, and tenth cranial nerves are the chief pain-sensitive structures.

The main factors in the causation of headache are: (1) inflammation of or about the pain-sensitive structures of the head; (2) referred pain; (3) meningeal irritation; (4) traction on or dilatation of the above-mentioned vessels; (5) direct pressure by tumours upon sensory nerves in the head; and (6) psychological causes, when the pain is often due to a state of tension in the muscles of the scalp and neck. The following is a convenient pathological classification.

THE CAUSES OF HEADACHE

Disease of the Bones of the Cranium

Osteitis of the cranial bones is an occasional cause of headache. Usually it is secondary to suppuration in the middle ear or paranasal sinuses; syphilitic osteitis is now rare but Paget's disease (which is not truly an osteitis despite its name, osteitis deformans) is quite common. Headache due to these causes is of a burning, boring character and is associated with tenderness of the skull, which often feels warmer than normal. Local or general thickening of the cranium is often present, and the characteristic changes in the bones are demonstrable by radiography. Metastases in the skull bones, whether osteolytic (e.g. in bronchial or breast carcinoma) or osteosclerotic (as in carcinoma of the prostate) may also give similar headache, as may multiple myelomatosis.

Neuralgia

Pain in the head occurs in many neuralgic syndromes. Thus paroxysms of pain may radiate along the distribution of the supraorbital or infraorbital nerves. Sometimes such neuralgic pain is due to local compression or irritation of the respective nerves produced, for instance, by local scarring after injury or arising without evident cause in their respective bony canals. In other cases paroxysmal pain which is localized in this way at first may be the initial manifestation of trigeminal neuralgia (tic douloureux), but the pain of the latter condition is commonest in the distribution of the second and third divisions of the trigeminus [p. 174]. Attacks of neuralgia of undetermined cause have also been described following the distribution of the auriculotemporal, posterior auricular, and occipital nerves, though auriculotemporal pain, like that in the distribution of the mandibular division of the fifth nerve, can be due to dental malocclusion with arthrosis of the temporomandibular joint (Costen's syndrome) and occipital pain can be a consequence of cervical spondylosis. Prolonged but paroxysmal attacks of severe boring pain in the eye ('ciliary neuralgia') or upper jaw (sphenopalatine or Sluder's neuralgia) are probably variants of periodic migrainous neuralgia [p. 309] while constant upper jaw pain in the absence of signs of organic disease (atypical facial neuralgia) is often of psychogenic origin [pp. 176 and 937]. Herpes zoster of the trigeminal ganglion is sometimes a cause of severe and persistent neuralgic pain. After the acute stage the scars of the eruption remain visible, and there is usually cutaneous anaesthesia. Pain in the distribution of the trigeminal nerve may also be due to pressure upon it in its intracranial course by intracranial neoplasm or aneurysm. Moreover, its central fibres may be involved in a lesion within the medulla. Thrombosis of the posterior inferior cerebellar artery, and syringobulbia, may in this way cause neuralgic pain over the face and scalp.

Referred Pain

Lesions of many viscera are attended by pain referred to the superficial tissues remote from the viscus involved, but innervated by the same segment of the nervous system. In this way visceral disease in many situations may be attended by pain in the head and localized hyperalgesia of the face or scalp. These symptoms may be produced by uncorrected visual refractive errors or latent squint, though this is not common (Waters, 1970), by iritis, glaucoma, lesions of the middle ear, nasal sinuses, teeth including unerupted teeth, pharynx, and tongue, and also by disease of the intrathoracic and intra-abdominal viscera [see p. 40]. The explanation of this reference of pain to the head from remote organs is that the trigeminal is the somatic sensory nerve corresponding to the vagus, by which so many viscera are innervated. Nasal obstruction, apart from infection of the nasal sinuses, is an occasional cause of persistent frontal headache. Occipital headache is often present in cases of cervical spondylosis.

Meningeal Irritation

Meningeal irritation is responsible for some of the most severe headaches. It may be due to the various forms of meningitis, or to the presence of non-infective irritant products such as extravasated blood in contact with the meninges. The pain is constant, severe, and throbbing or 'bursting', and is usually associated with other signs of meningeal irritation, such as cervical rigidity and Kernig's sign. Head movement increases discomfort and there is often photophobia and irritability.

Headaches of Vascular Origin

Paroxysmal throbbing or 'bursting' headaches may occur in patients with malignant hypertension, when the headache is not directly related to the height of the blood pressure but to the degree of stretch evoked at the time in the cranial arteries (Wolff and Wolf, 1948). Intracranial aneurysm is only rarely large enough to cause increased intracranial pressure before rupture. It may cause pain in the head, however, by compression of the trigeminal nerve. After rupture, subarachnoid haemorrhage leads to headache by causing both increased intracranial pressure and meningeal irritation.

Changes in the calibre and permeability of the cranial vessels are probably responsible for the headaches which accompany or follow numerous toxic states such as severe infections, alcoholic over-indulgence, general anaesthetics, uraemia, and diffuse cerebral inflammations—the various forms of encephalitis. In the 'hangover' headache dehydration and reduced intracranial pressure probably play a part. Sudden prostrating headache simulating that of sub-arachnoid haemorrhage has been described in patients who have eaten cheese or broad beans while taking mono-amine oxidase inhibitor drugs, mainly tranylcypromine, for the treatment of depression; similar headache has been described after ingestion of nitrite in frankfurter sausages (Henderson and Raskin, 1972) and all forms of vascular headache, including migraine, may be accentuated or precipitated by alcohol.

Migraine is probably also a vasomotor disorder, and on this hypothesis the headache is due to vascular dilatation following a preliminary constriction. The characteristics of migrainous headache are described on page 304.

Headache may also be caused by temporal or cranial arteritis; the scalp and the temporal arteries are usually tender [see p. 376].

Intracranial Space-occupying Lesions

The headache produced by intracranial neoplasm and abscess is considered elsewhere [see p. 250].

Trauma

In the more severe degrees of head injury headache is apt to be masked by impaired consciousness. It is a prominent symptom following concussion or cerebral contusion, and in this so-called post-concussional syndrome it may be paroxysmal, tends to be precipitated by noise, excitement, exertion, alcohol, and head movement, and is often associated with irritability, nervousness, and giddiness.

Lowered Intracranial Pressure

This may cause headache, as, for example, after lumbar puncture. Such headache is throbbing and may be literally prostrating, since it is intensified by sitting or standing and relieved by lying flat or with the feet raised above the level of the head. The pain may radiate from the head to the neck or dorsal spine.

Cough Headache

This is a very distinctive, brief, but often severe 'bursting' kind of pain experienced after coughing, usually by a middle-aged man, who may clasp his head when he coughs in an attempt to relieve it. Its cause is obscure, but rarely it is a symptom of an intracranial tumour. In most cases, however, it is benign and disappears spontaneously (Symonds, 1956).

Psychogenic Headache

Numerous abnormal cranial sensations are described by neurotic and psychotic patients. The commonest is a sense of pressure at the vertex, frequently encountered in anxiety states. One source of anxiety-headache is persistent con-traction of the frontal belly of the occipitofrontalis muscle. Such tension head-aches are typically dull and aching in character; they may be continuous but more often come on towards the end of the day, although in depressed patients the headache may be present on waking. Persistent 'neuralgic' pains associated with hyperaesthesia of the scalp and failing to respond to all analgesics may be encountered in hysteria as may bizarre headaches described in a florid manner ('like a nail being driven into the skull or an engine lifting off the top of the head'). Patients suffering from depressive states sometimes describe 'terrible pains in the head' of which they can give no more precise description [see also Chapter 23].

TREATMENT

Apart from palliative treatment with analgesics, which can safely be used in most cases, the treatment of headache is that of the causal disorder. Mild analgesics (aspirin, paracetamol) may be safely employed in all cases; opiates and other drugs of addiction must be avoided, especially in cases of recurrent headache but also because drugs which depress respiratory function should be avoided if the intracranial pressure is likely to be raised; nevertheless in severe headache due, for instance, to subarachnoid haemorrhage, pethidine or other similar powerful remedies may be needed. In a series of over 1,000 cases of chronic headache, Lance *et al.* (1965) found migraine (responding to ergot derivatives) and tension headache (responding to tranquillizers) to be the most common varieties.

REFERENCES

DALESSIO, D. J. (1972) *Wolff's Headache and Other Head Pain*, New York.
DRAKE, F. R. (1956) Tension headache; a review, *Amer. J. med. Soc.*, **232**, 105.
FRIEDMAN, A. P., and MERRITT, H. H. (1957) Treatment of headache, *J. Amer. med. Ass.*, **163**, 1111.
HENDERSON, W. R., and RASKIN, N. H. (1972) 'Hot-dog' headache: individual susceptibility to nitrite, *Lancet*, **ii**, 1162.
KUNKLE, E. C., and WOLFF, H. G. (1951) Headache, in *Modern Trends in Neurology*, 1st Series, ed. Feiling, A., London.
LANCE, J. W. (1969) *The Mechanism and Management of Headache*, London.
LANCE, J. W., CURRAN, D. A., and ANTHONY, M. (1965) Investigations into the mechanism and treatment of chronic headache, *Med. J. Aust.*, **2**, 909.
NORTHFIELD, D. W. C. (1938) Some observations on headache, *Brain*, **61**, 133.
SCHUMACHER, G. A., and WOLFF, H. G. (1941) Experimental studies in headache, *Arch. Neurol. Psychiat. (Chic.)*, **45**, 199.
SYMONDS, C. (1956) Cough headache, *Brain*, **79**, 557.
WATERS, W. E. (1970) Headache and the eye; a community study, *Lancet*, **ii**, 1.
WOLFF, H. G., and WOLF, S. (1948) *Pain*, p. 37, Springfield, Ill.

MIGRAINE

Synonyms. Hemicrania; bilious attack; sick headache.

Definition. A paroxysmal disorder characterized in its fully developed form by visual hallucinations, scotomas, and other disturbances of cerebral function, associated with unilateral headache and vomiting. While this definition is satisfactory for 'classical' migraine, there are many patients who never experience an aura and in whom the headache is always bilateral; the single most characteristic and constant feature is that migraine is a paroxysmal disorder, i.e. the headaches occur in attacks, separated by intervals of freedom.

AETIOLOGY, PATHOLOGY, AND INCIDENCE

Migraine has been known to medical science for nearly 2,000 years. In the first century of the Christian era Aretaeus of Cappadocia described it as heterocrania, and the term hemicrania, from which the word migraine was derived was introduced by Galen (A.D. 131–201). Among more modern studies Liveing's (1873) is a classic.

The aetiology of migraine is complex. It is not a fatal disease and pathological investigations are therefore scanty. Moreover, since it appears to be primarily a disorder of function little useful information is gained from morbid anatomy.

The Intracranial Disturbance of Function

It has long been held that the most plausible hypothetical explanation of migraine is that it is due to arterial spasm, followed by dilatation, occurring within the distribution of the common carotid artery. This view has now been confirmed. During the scotomatous phase of an attack focal electroencephalographic changes have been observed in the opposite cerebral cortex, consistent with cortical ischaemia (Engel et al., 1945), and during this phase it has also been observed that amyl nitrite will temporarily abolish the scotoma (Schumacher and Wolff, 1941). There is a generalized, rather than focal, reduction in cerebral blood flow during the aura (O'Brien, 1971). Occlusion of retinal arteries has been observed during an attack (Graveson, 1949), as has a persistent visual field defect due to ischaemic papillopathy (McDonald and Sanders, 1971). It appears, therefore, that arterial spasm in the retina and/or the visual cortex is responsible for the subjective visual disturbances and other cortical symptoms at the onset of the attack, while subsequent vasodilatation causes the headache and is manifest in flushing of the face, congestion of the superficial temporal artery and of the conjunctiva, and nasal mucosa on the side of the headache. Schumacher and Wolff have shown that the headache in migraine is due to dilatation mainly of the extracerebral arteries of the dura and scalp and branches of the external carotid. The specific effect of ergotamine tartrate on the headache is due to constriction of the branches of the artery. It is clear that the intracranial disturbance may be precipitated by more than one factor, and it is probable that in susceptible individuals more than one sort of stimulus may cause an attack, though in different patients different causal factors predominate.

Ocular Factors

Refractive errors and defective ocular muscle balance are often blamed for migraine, though probably usually with little justification. Attacks may certainly be precipitated, however, by unusual visual stimuli, such as bright light.

Allergy

The importance of allergy was stressed by Balyeat (1933). Sufferers from migraine may often be shown to be sensitive to one or more food proteins or other allergens, including pollen and tobacco, and may suffer from other disorders of an allergic nature.

Dietetic Factors

While allergy may explain the precipitation of attacks by protein to which the patient is sensitive, other dietary factors may play a part. Thus the excessive consumption of animal fat or of alcohol may be followed by an attack; so, too, may missing a meal (Hockaday et al., 1971).

Psychological Factors

Sufferers from migraine, though many are among the most intelligent and industrious members of the community, are not uncommonly of obsessional temperament, and attacks of migraine may be precipitated by mental fatigue or anxiety, or by other forms of stress. However, Waters (1971) found no evidence that individuals with migraine were more intelligent or of higher social class. Many women suffering frequent attacks at about the time of the menopause are found to be depressed and treatment of the depression is then beneficial.

Endocrine and Metabolic Factors

On the whole there is little evidence that endocrine abnormality is important. The occurrence of 'menstrual migraine' has been quoted in favour of an ovarian disturbance. Water-retention occurs in some cases (Goldzieher, 1941). Sicuteri *et al.* (1961) showed that the urinary excretion of 5-hydroxyindolacetic acid may be increased in severe attacks suggesting an intermittent release of 5-hydroxytryptamine (serotonin) into the circulation (Curzon *et al.*, 1966). Injection of reserpine, 2·5 mg intramuscularly, was found to precipitate attacks in 9 out of 16 female subjects (Curzon *et al.*, 1969), and similar observations were reported by Anthony *et al.* (1969) who also found evidence to suggest that the catabolism of serotonin and norepinephrine is increased in the first 12 hours of an attack and postulated that an endogenous serotonin-releasing factor is present in the plasma during migraine headache. Adams *et al.* (1968) biopsied temporal arteries during attacks in 6 subjects and found that the tunica adventitia of the arteries in such patients has a marked capacity to bind noradrenaline.

Heredity

Hereditary predisposition is important, but not perhaps as important as previously believed (Waters, 1971); nevertheless, migraine is often inherited as a Mendelian dominant trait. Here again appears a link with allergy, since asthma, hay fever, and other allergic disorders are common among the relatives of the migrainous.

Association with Epilepsy

Much stress has been laid by some writers on the association of migraine with epilepsy. Both are common disorders and many have thought that the relationship is coincidental, but Basser (1969), in a study of 1,800 cases, found the incidence of epilepsy in patients with migraine to be higher than in a control group. Occasionally a severe attack of migraine may terminate in an epileptic attack but loss of consciousness at the height of an attack is more often syncopal (Bickerstaff, 1961 *b*).

Age and Sex

The age of onset is usually at or shortly after puberty, much less frequently in middle life or later, though an onset at about the menopause is not uncommon in women. Migraine is rare before puberty, but cyclical vomiting and travel-sickness are common in childhood in those who subsequently develop it. Women are slightly more subject than men and usually suffer more severely.

SYMPTOMS

The Onset

Prodromal symptoms may be present or absent. The commonest of these are drowsiness and lassitude, hunger, and constipation or slight looseness of the bowels. Sometimes the subject feels exceptionally well before an attack. The onset may occur during the day, which is usually the case in migraine with a sensory aura. When headache is not preceded by such manifestations, the patient often awakens with it in the morning from a particularly heavy sleep.

Symptoms of Cortical Origin

Sensory symptoms, though not constant, are highly characteristic. Visual disturbances are the commonest. These usually have a homonymous distribution, involving the corresponding halves of both visual fields. They usually consist of a gradually developing hemianopia, which may be preceded by positive symptoms such as flashes of light. The hemianopia may begin in the periphery of the field and spread towards the centre, or vice versa. A common mode of onset is the appearance of a bright spot near the centre. This gradually expands towards the periphery, the advancing edge exhibiting scintillating figures which may be coloured and angular—*teichopsia*, or *fortification spectra*. The spreading scintillation leaves behind it an area of blindness, so that when it reaches the periphery of the half-fields the patient is left with homonymous hemianopia. The spread of these visual symptoms occupies from 15 to 20 minutes, and the hemianopia then gradually fades away in the order of its development, the whole disturbance lasting about half an hour, though objects in the affected fields may appear less bright than normally for several hours. Many varieties of migrainous visual disturbance occur. The symptoms may have a homonymous quadrantic distribution. Very rarely peripheral vision is lost in the whole of both fields, leaving only a 'telescopic' central field of vision. Exceptionally also the hemianopia is bilateral and leads to temporary complete blindness. In certain cases permanent visual field defects (hemianopia or a quadrantic defect) may persist after a severe attack.

Paraesthesiae and numbness of parts of the body occur next in frequency to visual disturbances. These symptoms possess a cortical distribution, involving the periphery of the limbs and the circumoral region. The upper limb is most often affected, a tingling sensation beginning in the periphery and gradually spreading up the limb, taking 15 or 20 minutes to do so. The lips, face, and tongue may be subsequently affected on one or both sides, or may be involved without the upper limb. The lower limb is rarely affected. Paraesthesiae usually develop shortly after the onset of the visual disturbances, but may occur without the latter as the first symptom. Less frequently they do not develop until after the headache has been present for several hours.

Gustatory and auditory hallucinations have been reported, but are rare.

Weakness of a limb, usually the upper, or of half of the body may develop and usually follows the paraesthesiae and in very occasional cases recurrent attacks are each accompanied by transient hemiparesis ('hemiplegic migraine').

Aphasia, usually of the expressive, less often of the receptive, type, may occur. In right-handed people it may be associated with visual disturbances in the right half-fields, and paraesthesiae on the right side of the body. There may be temporary disorientation in space.

Transitory diplopia may be complained of during an attack. Giddiness is not uncommon, and there may be slight mental confusion. Loss of consciousness or even an epileptiform attack rarely occurs. When the symptoms of the aura suggest ischaemia in the distribution of the hind-brain circulation the condition has been called 'basilar artery migraine' (Bickerstaff, 1961).

It is often assumed that in patients who show a permanent visual field defect, aphasia, ophthalmoplegia (see below), or motor weakness persisting after an attack of migraine it is likely that an intracranial vascular anomaly (e.g. aneurysm or angioma) will be present but an investigation of cases of 'complicated migraine' (Pearce and Foster, 1965) showed that investigations designed to demonstrate such lesions are usually negative.

Headache

Headache is the most characteristic symptom of migraine and the one from which it derives its name. It may be the only manifestation of the disorder, or may follow the sensory symptoms just described. It usually occurs as a boring pain in a localized area on one side, often in the temple, and gradually spreads till the whole of the affected side of the head is involved. Headache occurs on the side opposite to that to which the sensory symptoms are referred. Sometimes it extends to the whole head. It gradually increases in intensity and acquires a throbbing character, being intensified by stooping and by all forms of exertion. In milder cases it lasts for several hours but passes away if the patient can sleep, or after a night's rest. In more severe cases it persists for days.

Nausea is usually present during the stage of headache, and vomiting may or may not occur. In milder cases it seems to relieve the headache.

Vasomotor changes are often conspicuous (Appenzeller *et al.*, 1963). The face is often pale and the extremities are cold, until improvement begins, but congestion of the face, conjunctiva, and nasal mucous membrane may occur, and is often confined to the side of the headache. There may be subconjunctival haemorrhage or even bruising around the eyes. The superficial temporal artery on the affected side is congested and exhibits vigorous pulsation. There is often polyuria following the attack.

Electroencephalography

Dow and Whitty (1947) found a persistently abnormal EEG between the attacks in 30 of 51 patients examined and Slatter (1968) reported similar findings, with an unusual response to photic stimulation, but pointed out that some inter-ictal EEG abnormalities might well be the result of minor cerebral damage resulting from repeated attacks.

VARIETIES OF MIGRAINE

The commonest form of migraine is characterized by attacks of headache alone, or by headache and vomiting without other symptoms. Somewhat less frequently visual or sensory disturbances precede the headache. Less often still the visual or sensory symptoms, motor weakness, or aphasia are not followed by headache; in middle age, subjects who suffered from classical migraine in earlier life not infrequently experience an aura with associated malaise but without subsequent headache. Exceptionally vomiting may occur alone or in association with abdominal pain.

Ophthalmoplegic Migraine

This term has been applied to recurrent attacks of headache associated with paralysis of one or more oculomotor nerves, which persists for days or weeks after the attack and tends to become permanent. Although transitory diplopia is occasionally associated with true migraine the diagnosis of migraine should be accepted with reserve when it is used to account for ocular palsies lasting more than an hour or two. Probably many cases hitherto described as ophthalmoplegic migraine have been examples of intracranial aneurysm. However, in a review of the posterior limb of the internal capsule, part of the lateral nucleus of the thalamus, the anterior third of the crus cerebri, and part of the midbrain, including the subthalamic nucleus and Forel's field. The *anterior choroidal artery* passes backwards and outwards from the internal carotid to enter the anterior extremity of the descending horn of the lateral ventricle, where it supplies the choroid plexus. It is distributed also to the optic tract, to the uncus, to the posterior two-thirds of the posterior limb of the internal capsule, and the origin of the optic radiation, to part of the lentiform nucleus, and sometimes to the anterior third of the crus cerebri, which is usually supplied by the posterior communicating; sometimes it also supplies the posterior two-thirds of the crus cerebri which is more often supplied by the posterior cerebral.

The Anterior Cerebral Artery

The anterior cerebral artery passes forwards and medially from the internal carotid, turns round the genu of the corpus callosum, above which it runs backwards to terminate posteriorly, usually 2·5 cm anterior to the parieto-occipital sulcus. It gives off the following principal branches: (1) Basal branches, of which the most important has been called the recurrent branch (Heubner's artery). This branch enters the anterior perforated substance and supplies the anterior part of the caudate nucleus, the anterior one-third of the putamen, and the inferior half of the anterior limb of the internal capsule. (2) The anterior communicating artery, which is a short branch uniting the two anterior cerebrals and which gives off no branches. (3) Branches to the frontal and parietal lobes. These supply the medial aspect of the hemisphere and the upper part of its lateral aspect for from 2 to 2·5 cm from the median edge throughout the length of the artery and a corresponding area of the white matter of the frontal and parietal lobes, including the olfactory tract and lobe. The most important cortical branch of the anterior cerebral supplies the paracentral lobule, which contains the leg area of the motor cortex. Other branches of the anterior cerebral pass downwards to supply the genu, rostrum, and body of the corpus callosum.

The Middle Cerebral Artery

The middle cerebral artery passes laterally from the internal carotid in the stem of the lateral sulcus to the surface of the insula, where it divides into its terminal cortical branches. When crossing the base of the brain it gives off its striate branches. These branches supply part of the lentiform nucleus, the upper part of both anterior and posterior limbs of the internal capsule, and the horizontal part of the caudate nucleus behind the head. The cortical distribution of the middle cerebral artery is coterminous with that of the anterior cerebral as far back as the middle of the superior parietal lobule. It then extends to the edge of the median surface or is bounded by the territory of the posterior cerebral artery, passing downwards between the intraparietal sulcus and the occipital lobe to reach the middle of the inferior temporal or the lower border of the middle temporal gyrus. In about half of all cases the area of the middle cerebral artery extends to the occipital pole, or 1 cm anterior to it. It also supplies the tapetum of the corpus callosum and the white matter of the centrum semiovale corresponding to its cortical distribution. The cortical branches of the middle cerebral artery are the orbital, the frontal, which supply the inferior and middle frontal gyri, and are distributed to the precentral gyrus and the posterior part of the middle frontal gyrus; the parietal, which supply the postcentral gyrus and the adjacent superior parietal lobule; continuing in the direction of the main stem of

4

DISORDERS OF THE CEREBRAL CIRCULATION

THE CEREBRAL ARTERIAL CIRCULATION

THE intracranial blood supply is derived from the two internal carotid arteries and the two vertebral arteries which unite anteriorly to form the basilar artery. The circulus arteriosus cerebri (circle of Willis) which is situated at the base of the brain is formed by anastomoses between the internal carotid arteries, the basilar artery, and their branches, as follows.

The basilar artery divides into the two posterior cerebrals, which are joined to the two internal carotids by the posterior communicating arteries. The internal carotids give off the two anterior cerebral arteries, which are united by the single anterior communicating artery, which thus completes the circle.

In recent years it has become apparent that extracranial arterial disease, in the aorta and in the common and internal carotid and vertebral arteries in the neck, often accounts for symptoms of cerebrovascular insufficiency. Hence anomalies of origin and formation of the arteries themselves, and of the circle of Willis, and the efficacy of collateral channels must all be considered in the pathogenesis of cerebral vascular disease. Among the commoner developmental anomalies are: marked inequality in the size of the two vertebral arteries or of the posterior communicating arteries; hypoplasia or even absence of the anterior communicating artery and/or of the proximal portion of one anterior cerebral; an origin of one posterior cerebral artery from the carotid rather than the basilar; a persistent trigeminal artery joining the carotid to the basilar proximal to the cavernous sinus; an anomalous origin of one vertebral artery from the aorta or the carotid.

Many other rarer anomalies may occur but Hutchinson and Acheson (1975) in a recent review conclude that all such abnormalities are of theoretical interest only *unless* occlusive vascular disease develops, when the collateral circulation may be affected [see p. 315].

The principal intracranial arteries and their areas of distribution [see PLATES 1 and 2] are:

ARTERIES OF THE CEREBRAL HEMISPHERES
The Internal Carotid Artery

The internal carotid artery after entering the cranium gives off small branches to the wall of the cavernous sinus, and to the third, fourth, fifth, and sixth cranial nerves, including the trigeminal ganglion, the pituitary, and the dura mater of the middle fossa. The next branch is the *ophthalmic artery*, from which the central artery of the retina is derived. The internal carotid next gives off the *posterior communicating artery*, which unites it with the posterior cerebral artery. The posterior communicating artery supplies the optic chiasma, pituitary, tuber cinereum, and hypothalamic region, the lower part of the anterior third

REFERENCES

BALLA, J. I., and WALTON, J. N. (1964) Periodic migrainous neuralgia. *Brit. med. J.*, **i,** 219.

EKBOM, K. (1970) *Studies on Cluster Headache*, Stockholm.

EKBOM, K., and LINDAHL, J. (1971) Remission of angina pectoris during periods of cluster headache, *Headache*, **11,** 57.

HARRIS, W. (1926) *Neuritis and Neuralgia*, London.

HARRIS, W. (1940) Alcohol injection of the Gasserian ganglion for migrainous neuralgia, *Lancet*, **ii,** 481.

HORTON, B. T. (1941) Histamine cephalagia, *J. Amer. med. Ass.*, **116,** 377.

SYMONDS, C. (1956) A particular variety of headache, *Brain*, **79,** 217.

WOLFF, H. G. (1963) *Headache and Other Head Pain*, 2nd ed., New York.

SHAFAR, J., TALLETT, E. R., and KNOWLSON, P. A. (1972) Evaluation of clonidine in prophylaxis of migraine: double-blind trial and follow-up, *Lancet*, **i**, 403.

SICUTERI, F., TESTI, A., and ANSELMI, B. (1961) Biochemical investigations in headache; increase in the hydroxyindolacetic acid excretion during migraine attacks, *Int. Arch. Allergy*, **19**, 55.

SLATTER, K. H. (1968) Some clinical and EEG findings in patients with migraine, *Brain*, **91**, 85.

SUTHERLAND, J. M., HOOPER, W. D., EADIE, M. J., and TYRER, J. H. (1974) Buccal absorption of ergotamine, *J. Neurol. Neurosurg. Psychiat.*, **37**, 1116.

VON STORCH, T. J. C. (1938) Complications following the use of ergotamine tartrate, *J. Amer. med. Ass.*, **111**, 293.

WALTON, J. N. (1956) *Subarachnoid Haemorrhage*, Edinburgh.

WATERS, W. E. (1971) Migraine: intelligence, social class, and familial prevalence, *Brit. med. J.*, **2**, 77.

WIDERØE, T. E., and VIGANDER, T. (1974) Propranolol in the treatment of migraine, *Brit. med. J.*, **2**, 699.

ZAIMIS, E., and HANINGTON, E. (1969) A possible pharmacological approach to migraine, *Lancet*, **ii**, 298.

PERIODIC MIGRAINOUS NEURALGIA

This term was applied by Harris (1926) to a highly distinctive type of headache involving chiefly the eye and frontal region on one side and characterized by its periodicity. Attacks may occur once or several times in twenty-four hours and last from one to several hours. The pain is intense and continuous and 'boring' or 'burning' in character; typically the attacks may awaken the patient from sleep in the early morning. They may also be precipitated by alcohol or vasodilator drugs (Ekbom, 1970) and remission of the pain of angina pectoris has been described in the attacks (Ekbom and Lindahl, 1971). A bout tends to last for several weeks after which the patient is free from symptoms for months or even one or two years when the headache recurs in the same way. Lacrimation and nasal congestion on the affected side are apt to occur in the attacks. There are no abnormal physical signs, although a Horner's syndrome, either transient or permanent, sometimes develops on the affected side and has been attributed to damage to sympathetic fibres occurring in the wall of the carotid artery and resulting from recurrent dilatation of the vessel.

It now seems certain that the condition which has been variously referred to as 'histamine headache' (Horton, 1941) or 'cluster headache' (Wolff, 1963) is the same condition as periodic migrainous neuralgia and probably this syndrome also embraces the syndromes of ciliary neuralgia, vidian neuralgia, and sphenopalatine neuralgia described by the earlier neurologists. Harris (1940) recommended alcohol injection of the Gasserian ganglion but Symonds (1956) showed that ergotamine tartrate, 0·5 mg, given by subcutaneous injection once, twice, or even three times daily completely relieved the attacks. The injections are given for as long as may be necessary until the bout is over; this can only be determined by reducing or withdrawing treatment to see whether the attacks recur. Fortunately ergotism seems to be very rare in such cases. Balla and Walton (1964) found that in many cases ergotamine by mouth (*Migril*) was equally effective or, if this failed, dimethysergide, 1–2 mg three times daily. Dihydroergotamine (1–2 mg three times daily) is probably now the most favoured remedy. Probably oral medication should be tried first before going on to treatment with injections.

BARRIE, M. A., FOX, W. R., WEATHERALL, M., and WILKINSON, M. I. P. (1968) Analysis of symptoms of patients with headaches and their response to treatment with ergot derivatives, *Quart. J. Med.*, **37**, 319.

BASSER, L. (1969) The relation of migraine and epilepsy, *Brain*, **92**, 285.

BICKERSTAFF, E. R. (1961 *a*) Basilar artery migraine, *Lancet*, **i**, 15.

BICKERSTAFF, E. R. (1961 *b*) Impairment of consciousness in migraine, *Lancet*, **ii**, 1057.

BRADSHAW, P., and PARSONS, M. (1965) Hemiplegic migraine, *Quart. J. Med.*, **34**, 65.

CURRAN, D. A., and LANCE, J. W. (1964) Clinical trial of methysergide and other preparations in the management of migraine, *J. Neurol. Neurosurg. Psychiat.*, **27**, 463.

CURZON, G., BARRIE, M., and WILKINSON, M. I. P. (1969) Relationships between headache and amine changes after administration of reserpine to migrainous patients, *J. Neurol. Neurosurg. Psychiat.*, **32**, 555.

CURZON, G., THEAKER, P., and PHILLIPS, B. (1966) Excretion of 5-hydroxyindolyl acetic acid (5 HIAA) in migraine, *J. Neurol. Psychiat.*, **29**, 85.

DALESSIO, D. J. (1962) On migraine headache, serotonin and serotonin antagonism, *J. Amer. med. Ass.*, **181**, 318.

DALESSIO, D. J. (1972) *Wolff's Headache and Other Head Pain*, New York.

DOW, D. J., and WHITTY, C. W. M. (1947) Electroencephalographic changes in migraine, *Lancet*, **ii**, 52.

ENGEL, G. L., FERRIS, E. B., Jun., and ROMANO, J. (1945) Focal encephalographic changes during scotomas of migraine, *Amer. J. med. Sci.*, **209**, 650.

FRIEDMAN, A. P. (1963) The pathogenesis of migraine headache, *Bull. Los Angeles neurol. Soc.*, **28**, 191.

FRIEDMAN, A. P., and ELKIND, A. H. (1963) Methysergide in treatment of vascular headaches of migraine type, *J. Amer. med. Ass.*, **184**, 125.

GOLDZIEHER, M. A. (1941) Endocrine aspects of headaches, *J. Lab. clin. Med.*, **27**, 150.

GRAVESON, G. S. (1949) Retinal arterial occlusion in migraine, *Brit. med. J.*, **2**, 838.

HANINGTON, E. (1967) Preliminary report on tyramine headache, *Brit. med. J.*, **2**, 550.

HANINGTON, E. (1969) The effect of tyramine in inducing migrainous headache, in *Background to Migraine, Second Migraine Symposium, 1967*, pp. 113–19, ed. Cochrane, A. L., London.

HOCKADAY, J. M., WILLIAMSON, D. H., and WHITTY, C. W. M. (1971) Blood-glucose levels and fatty-acid metabolism in migraine related to fasting, *Lancet*, **i**, 1153.

JACOBS, H. (1972) A trial of opipramol in the treatment of migraine, *J. Neurol. Neurosurg. Psychiat.*, **35**, 500.

LANCE, J. W., ANTHONY, M., and SOMERVILLE, B. (1970) Comparative trial of serotonin antagonists in the management of migraine, *Brit. med. J.*, **2**, 327.

LEVITON, A., MALVEA, B., and GRAHAM, J. R. (1974) Vascular diseases, mortality, and migraine in the parents of migraine patients, *Neurology (Minneap.)*, **24**, 669.

LIVEING, E. (1873) *On Megrim, Sick-Headache, and Some Allied Disorders*, London.

McDONALD, W. I., and SANDERS, M. D. (1971) Migraine complicated by ischaemic papillopathy, *Lancet*, **ii**, 521.

MACKENZIE, I. (1953) The clinical presentation of the cerebral angiomas, *Brain*, **76**, 184.

MOFFETT, A., SWASH, M., and SCOTT, D. F. (1972) Effect of tyramine in migraine: a double-blind study, *J. Neurol. Neurosurg. Psychiat.*, **35**, 496.

O'BRIEN, M. D. (1971) The relationship between aura symptoms and cerebral blood flow changes in the prodrome of migraine, *Proceedings of the International Headache Symposium*, Elsinore, Denmark, 1971, pp. 141–3.

O'SULLIVAN, M. E. (1936) Termination of one thousand attacks of migraine with ergotamine tartrate, *J. Amer. med. Ass.*, **107**, 1208.

PEARCE, J. (1968) The ophthalmological complications of migraine, *J. neurol. Sci.*, **6**, 73.

PEARCE, J. M. S. (1969) *Migraine*, Springfield, Ill.

PEARCE, J. M. S., and FOSTER, J. B. (1965) An investigation of complicated migraine, *Neurology (Minneap.)*, **15**, 333.

SCHUMACHER, G. A., and WOLFF, H. G. (1941) Experimental studies in headache, *Arch. Neurol. Psychiat. (Chic.)*, **45**, 199.

et al., 1974) and suppositories containing ergotamine, which have had a vogue, are not demonstrably superior to oral medication. Often trial and error is necessary to find the most appropriate remedy for each individual patient. All such remedies must, however, be given early and preferably when the aura begins, if the attack is to be aborted. Vomiting is sometimes a troublesome side-effect. Some intelligent patients can be taught to inject themselves if oral medication fails.

In prophylaxis, antihistamine drugs such as prochlorperazine (*Stemetil*), 5 mg three times daily, are helpful in mild cases as are compound tablets containing ergotamine, atropine, and a barbiturate sedative (e.g. *Bellergal*, one tablet three times daily).

An effective prophylactic remedy is dimethysergide (Curran and Lance, 1964; Barrie *et al.*, 1968; Lance *et al.*, 1970) which is given in a dosage of 1–3 mg three times daily. There is, however, a risk that retroperitoneal fibrosis may result from prolonged ingestion of this drug which should not therefore be given in a dose of more than 3 mg daily for more than three months at a time. Other prophylactic remedies can be continued over much longer periods. More recent studies have shown that dihydroergotamine (1–2 mg three times daily) is as effective in prophylaxis as dimethysergide and has fewer side-effects; it can be continued for some months without significant risk of ergotism but must be used with caution in patients with coronary artery disease and is contra-indicated in pregnancy. Propanolol, 160 mg daily, has also been shown to be an effective prophylactic (Widerøe and Vigander, 1974) as has clonidine (Zaimis and Hanington, 1969) in a dose of 0·05 mg three times a day (Shafar *et al.*, 1972). Another remedy recently used with some success is opipramol 50 mg three times a day (Jacobs, 1972). In anxious and tense patients at any age, tranquillizing remedies such as trifluoperazine, 1 mg three times daily, or chlordiazepoxide, 5–10 mg three times daily, may be helpful, while in the many women in the paramenopausal age group in whom frequent attacks of migraine and depression coexist a similar tranquillizer along with phenelzine, 15 mg three times daily, or amitriptyline, 25–50 mg three times daily, may be dramatically successful in reducing the frequency and severity of attacks. Generally, because of potential side-effects, amine-oxidase inhibitors such as phenelzine are better avoided except in cases resistant to other remedies (Anthony and Lance, 1969).

REFERENCES

ADAMS, C. W. M., ORTON, C. C., and ZILKHA, K. J. (1968) Arterial catecholamine and enzyme histochemistry in migraine, *J. Neurol. Neurosurg. Psychiat.*, **31**, 50.

ADIE, W. J. (1930) Permanent hemianopia in migraine and subarachnoid haemorrhage, *Lancet*, **ii**, 237.

ANTHONY, M., and LANCE, J. W. (1969) Monoamine oxidase inhibition in the treatment of migraine, *Arch. Neurol. (Chic.)*, **21**, 263.

ANTHONY, M., HINTERBERGER, H., and LANCE, J. W. (1969) The possible relationship of serotonin to the migraine syndrome, *Res. clin. Stud. Headache*, **2**, 29.

APPENZELLER, O., DAVISON, K., and MARSHALL, J. (1963) Reflex vasomotor abnormalities in the hands of migrainous subjects, *J. Neurol. Neurosurg. Psychiat.*, **26**, 447.

BALYEAT, R. M. (1933) *Migraine, Diagnosis and Treatment*, Philadelphia.

BARRAQUER-BORDAS, L., PERES-SERRA, J., GRAU-VECIANA, J. M., and SAGIMON-RABASSA, E. (1970) Migraine prosoplégique familiale, *Acta neurol. belg.*, **70**, 301.

this should always suggest an organic lesion rather than migraine and angiography is usually indicated. Ultimately, on follow-up, there is a significantly higher incidence of hypertension and of cardiac infarction, but not of stroke, in sufferers from migraine (Leviton *et al.*, 1974).

DIAGNOSIS

It is important to distinguish migraine from similar symptoms resulting from organic disease of the brain. The early onset is an important point of distinction, since migraine usually begins at puberty whereas most organic conditions with which it may be confused are encountered in adult life. A tumour of the occipital lobe, especially an angioma, may lead to attacks of visual hallucinations associated with headache and vomiting. In these cases, however, careful perimetry usually shows a visual field defect, which persists between the attacks, and increases. Moreover, signs of increased intracranial pressure are likely to develop, and there may be evidence of pressure exerted by the tumour upon the neighbouring parts of the brain, and in the case of an arterial angioma a cranial bruit.

Migraine is occasionally confused with epilepsy, since visual hallucinations may constitute the prodromal symptoms of both. In migraine, however, the progress of the attack is slow, in epilepsy it is rapid; and the retention of consciousness in the former should put the diagnosis beyond doubt.

When transitory attacks of paraesthesiae, weakness, and aphasia occur in migraine without headache, the diagnosis may be difficult. Such disturbances may simulate cerebral ischaemia due to vascular lesions. In migraine, however, there is usually a history of previous attacks of headache, dating from an early age. The transitory ischaemic attacks of cerebral vascular disease occur chiefly in late middle and old age, and attacks of paraesthesiae in multiple sclerosis, which usually last for several days or weeks, thus differ from those of migraine, which usually last only half an hour or at the most a few hours. When headache occurs alone, it must be distinguished from pain in the head due to other causes: see pages 296–300.

TREATMENT

The sufferer from migraine should endeavour to regulate his life so as to avoid both mental and physical fatigue as far as possible. Refractive errors, if present, should be corrected. Diet is sometimes important, but individual idiosyncrasies are marked. Some patients benefit from a diet in which animal fats are restricted; and other articles of diet which seem occasionally to precipitate attacks include alcohol, eggs, chocolate, and raw fruit, especially apples and oranges. While tyramine-containing foods (e.g. cheese and red wine) have been thought to be particularly important (Hanington, 1967, 1969), Moffett *et al.* (1972), in a double-blind trial, did not find that capsules of tyramine consistently precipitated attacks.

Drug treatment can be divided into two categories, namely treatment of the attack and prophylaxis. While some attacks may be controlled by aspirin, paracetamol, or compound codeine tablets, the single most useful remedy is ergotamine tartrate which may be taken by mouth, sublingually, by suppository, by inhalation of a fine powder, or by intramuscular injection (0·5 mg). Useful commercial preparations in which ergotamine is combined with antihistamine or anti-emetic preparations include *Migril*, *Cafergot Q*, *Cafergot* suppositories, *Orgraine*, *Migraleve*, and *Medihaler ergotamine*. Buccal absorption of ergotamine seems to be no quicker than absorption from the stomach (Sutherland of the ophthalmological complications of migraine Pearce (1968) has found that ophthalmoplegia, either isolated or recurrent, occurring in attacks of migraine, may remain unexplained despite full investigation. A Horner's syndrome has been known to develop after repeated attacks.

Facioplegic Migraine

Recurrent facial palsy associated with migraine is very rare (Barraquer-Bordas *et al.*, 1970). It is probably to be explained by ischaemia of the nerve trunk or compression of it by a dilated artery as in ophthalmoplegic migraine.

Retinal Migraine

Retinal vascular lesions in migraine are fortunately rare. Thrombosis of the central artery of the retina, and of single branches may occur (Graveson, 1949), and recurrent attacks of retinal ischaemia may lead to bilateral optic atrophy due to ischaemic papillopathy (McDonald and Sanders, 1971). Retinal and vitreous haemorrhages may also occur.

Symptomatic Migraine

A history of migraine is common in patients with intracranial aneurysm, especially upon the internal carotid or posterior communicating arteries, but whether the relationship between the two disorders is real is dubious (Walton, 1956). However, recurrent but increasing retro-orbital pain and ophthalmoplegia due to a supraclinoid aneurysm may simulate ophthalmoplegic migraine. Many patients with intracranial arteriovenous angiomas suffer attacks of headache which may be indistinguishable from those of migraine; sometimes these occur consistently on the side of the head upon which the angioma lies (Mackenzie, 1953).

COURSE AND PROGNOSIS

The frequency of attacks of migraine varies considerably in different patients. Often the disorder seems to possess a rhythm which is little influenced by outside factors. The attacks may occur once a week, once a fortnight, or once a month, with great regularity. Attacks in which headache occurs alone are usually more frequent than those in which it is preceded by sensory symptoms. The latter usually recur at intervals of several months. Occasionally a patient has repeated frequent attacks, a condition which may be called status hemicranialis, by analogy with status epilepticus. Headache preceded by visual symptoms may occur more than once a day for a period of days. Apart from treatment, attacks tend to grow less frequent and less severe as the patient grows older and usually cease in late middle life. It is not uncommon for the character of the attack to change. For example, visual symptoms may cease to appear or occur without headache.

Migraine does not shorten life, but frequent severe and uncontrolled attacks may be exhausting and debilitating. Depression is a common accompaniment in middle life, especially in women, and vigorous treatment of the latter may improve the migraine dramatically. In some such cases it is difficult to be sure when migrainous headache ends and tension headache begins and in this circumstance the patient is rarely free from some form of pain in the head. In a small number of cases permanent hemianopia or other visual field defects have followed an exceptionally severe attack. In such cases teichopsia may persist for weeks. Very rarely permanent aphasia and hemiplegia occur, but

L

PLATE 1

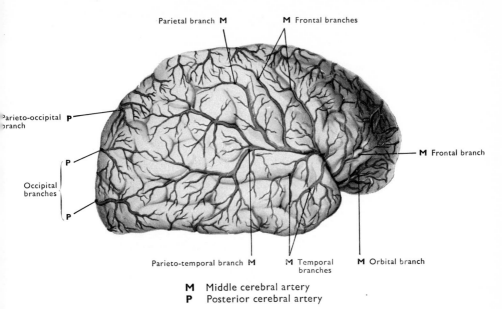

Parietal branch **M**   **M** Frontal branches

Parieto-occipital **P**
branch

P

Occipital
branches

P

M Frontal branch

Parieto-temporal branch **M**   **M** Temporal   **M** Orbital branch
branches

M Middle cerebral artery
P Posterior cerebral artery

Distribution of cerebral arteries on the supero-lateral surface of the right cerebral hemisphere

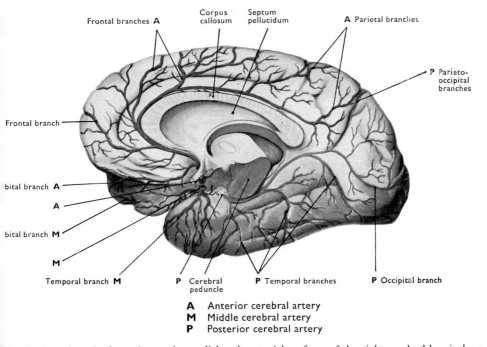

Frontal branches **A**   Corpus   Septum   **A** Parietal branches
callosum   pellucidum

P Parieto-
occipital
branches

Frontal branch

bital branch **A**

A

bital branch **M**

M

Temporal branch **M**   **P** Cerebral   **P** Temporal branches   **P** Occipital branch
peduncle

A Anterior cerebral artery
M Middle cerebral artery
P Posterior cerebral artery

Distribution of cerebral arteries on the medial and tentorial surfaces of the right cerebral hemisphere

PLATE 2

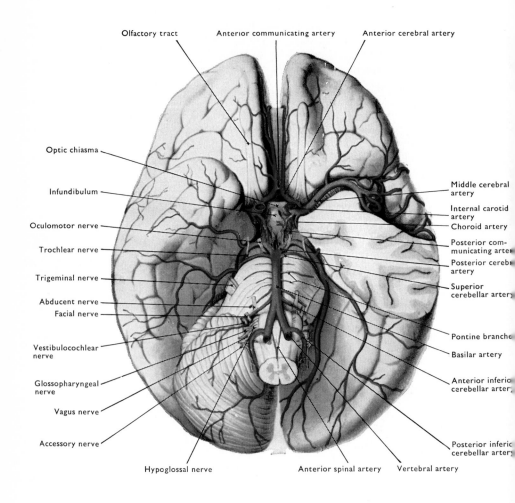

Olfactory tract   Anterior communicating artery   Anterior cerebral artery

Optic chiasma

Infundibulum

Oculomotor nerve

Trochlear nerve

Trigeminal nerve

Abducent nerve
Facial nerve

Vestibulocochlear
nerve

Glossopharyngeal
nerve

Vagus nerve

Accessory nerve

Middle cerebral
artery

Internal carotid
artery
Choroid artery

Posterior com-
municating arter

Posterior cereb
artery

Superior
cerebellar artery

Pontine branche

Basilar artery

Anterior inferio
cerebellar arter

Posterior inferic
cerebellar arter

Hypoglossal nerve   Anterior spinal artery   Vertebral artery

Arteries of the base of the brain

the artery these also supply the inferior parietal lobule, part of the lateral surface of the occipital lobe, and the posterior part of the temporal lobe; finally there are temporal branches, which supply the superior and middle temporal gyri.

The Posterior Cerebral Artery

The two posterior cerebral arteries are the terminal branches of the basilar. They run backwards and upwards around the cerebral peduncles and beneath the splenium of the corpus callosum to the calcarine sulcus of the occipital lobe. Close to its origin the posterior cerebral artery gives off basal branches which supply the posterior part of the thalamus, including the pulvinar, the posterior two-thirds of the crus cerebri, and the red nucleus. Other branches pass around the brain stem to supply the colliculi and the geniculate bodies. The *posterior choroidal arteries*, of which there are usually two, supply some branches to the thalamus, the brain stem, and the third ventricle, and terminate in the choroid plexus of the third and lateral ventricles. There are four *cortical branches* of the posterior cerebral: the anterior temporal and the posterior temporal, which supply especially the uncus; the calcarine branch, which passes along the calcarine sulcus and is distributed to the visual area of the cerebral cortex, and the parieto-occipital branch, which passes along the corresponding sulcus. The cortical area supplied by the posterior cerebral includes the medial surface of the temporal lobe, and of the occipital lobe as far forwards as the internal parieto-occipital sulcus, or to a point 2·5 cm anterior to this. The most anterior part of the temporal lobe, however, is supplied by the middle cerebral, and the anterior end of the uncus by the anterior choroidal artery. The cortical area of the posterior cerebral extends on to the outer surface for a distance of from 2 to 2·5 cm, being here bounded by the posterior limits of the anterior and middle cerebral arteries. Above, it usually extends anteriorly as far as the external parieto-occipital sulcus or in some cases to half-way along the superior parietal lobule; below, it supplies the medial aspect of the temporal lobe to within 2·5 cm of the tip.

Blood Supply of Internal Capsule, Basal Ganglia, and Optic Radiation

The superior half of the anterior limb of the *internal capsule* is supplied by the middle cerebral artery, the inferior half by the anterior cerebral; the posterior limb is supplied as follows: the superior half by the middle cerebral, the anterior one-third of the inferior half by the posterior communicating, the posterior two-thirds by the anterior choroidal. The *thalamus* is supplied by vessels derived from the posterior cerebral, the posterior communicating, the anterior and posterior choroidal arteries, and the middle cerebral. The posterior half of the lateral nucleus is supplied by the middle and posterior cerebral arteries, the anterior half by the middle cerebral and posterior communicating arteries. The posterior half of the lateral nucleus is supplied by the lenticulo-optic, retromammillary, and thalamo-geniculate (the artery of the thalamic syndrome), the anterior half by the lenticulo-optic and thalamo-tuberal vessels. The oral one-third of the *caudate nucleus* and *putamen* is supplied by perforating branches of the anterior cerebral, the rest by the striate branches of the middle cerebral. The greater part of the *globus pallidus* is supplied by the anterior choroidal. The *optic radiation* at its origin is supplied by the anterior choroidal artery: of the rest, the superior three-quarters is supplied by the middle cerebral and the inferior one-quarter by the posterior cerebral, unless the middle cerebral does not reach so far back, when the posterior cerebral supplies the whole.

ARTERIES OF THE BRAIN STEM

The arteries of the brain stem are mostly derived from the *basilar* and the two *vertebral arteries*, though the upper part of the midbrain receives in addition contributions from the posterior communicating artery, the anterior choroidal artery, and the posterior cerebral and its branches. The vertebral arteries enter a canal in the cervical spine at the level of the sixth cervical vertebra and then pass upwards to emerge at the level of the atlas and form a considerable loop before entering the foramen magnum. They fuse at the level of the junction between the pons and the medulla to form the *basilar artery*, which terminates at the upper border of the pons by dividing into the two posterior cerebrals. The arteries of the brain stem show considerable variations of distribution, but conform on the whole to the following general scheme:

Paramedian arteries enter the brain stem near the midline anteriorly and supply a narrow zone extending from before backwards close to the midline. Short circumferential arteries supply an area, often wedge-shaped, on the lateral aspect, and long circumferential arteries are distributed to the posterior part and to the cerebellum.

The superior cerebellar artery is the highest branch derived from the basilar before its bifurcation. It passes outwards and backwards around the brain stem, giving small branches to the cerebral peduncle and the colliculi, and terminates by dividing to supply the upper surface of the vermis and of the lateral lobe of the cerebellum.

The anterior inferior cerebellar artery arises from the middle of the basilar and passes backwards to supply part of the pons, including the lateral tegmental region and the anterior part of the lower surface of the lateral lobes of the cerebellum. The *internal auditory artery* leaves the anterior inferior cerebellar artery, or less often the basilar or the vertebral, to accompany the cochlear part of the eighth nerve and enters the internal acoustic meatus to supply the internal ear. Throughout its length the basilar gives off small vessels to the anterior part of the pons. Its lowest lateral branch supplies a wedge-shaped area of the lateral aspect of the upper part of the medulla corresponding to the area supplied by the posterior inferior cerebellar artery in the lower part of the medulla.

The posterior inferior cerebellar artery is the largest branch of the vertebral. Its site of origin is variable, but it usually arises from this artery a little distance below the lower border of the pons. It then passes outwards and backwards around the medulla, giving branches which supply a wedge-shaped area of the lateral aspect of the medulla, the base of which is on the surface, and the apex postero-internally, and the lower part of the inferior cerebellar peduncle. It also supplies the choroid plexus of the fourth ventricle. The main trunk divides into two terminal branches which supply the inferior vermis and the lower surface of the cerebellar hemisphere.

The vertebral artery, besides supplying the lateral aspect of the medulla through the posterior inferior cerebellar, gives off branches to the paramedian region, a narrow zone adjacent to the middle line, including the pyramids of the medulla and extending backwards as far as the floor of the fourth ventricle. This paramedian area at the lowest medullary level is supplied by the *anterior spinal artery*, which arises by the fusion of branches from each vertebral artery.

THE COLLATERAL CHANNELS

The experiments of McDonald and Potter (1951) showed that the internal carotid and vertebral arteries share the blood supply to their own half of the brain in such a way that there is normally no interchange of blood between them. Their respective streams meet in the posterior communicating artery at a 'dead point' at which the pressure of the two is equal, and do not mix there. If, however, both internal carotid or both vertebral arteries are occluded, blood passes backwards or forwards from the pair which are still patent. Similarly, if one internal carotid or one vertebral artery is occluded, blood crosses the middle line so that the area which would otherwise be deprived of blood is supplied by the contralateral fellow. Normally, the two streams from the vertebral arteries remain each on its own side of the basilar unmixed, like the Blue and White Nile for some miles below their union at Khartoum.

The circle of Willis is the principal collateral channel which helps to preserve circulation to the cerebral hemispheres if one of its principal feeding arteries is occluded (Sedzimir, 1959; Gryspeerdt, 1963). However, when there is occlusion of one internal carotid artery in the neck, important collateral channels may be established via the external carotid circulation with reverse flow through the ophthalmic artery. Less beneficial and indeed positively detrimental to the brain-stem circulation is the reverse flow down one vertebral artery into the distal subclavian artery (subclavian steal) which may follow proximal occlusion of one subclavian artery. An external carotid 'steal' has also been described (Barnett et al., 1970). In the cerebral cortex, areas of infarction due to occlusion of major arterial branches are limited by collateral flow through the profuse meningeal arterial anastomoses which exist at watershed areas between the anterior, middle, and posterior cerebral areas of supply (van der Eecken and Adams, 1953; Gillilan, 1959). However, perforating vessels which supply the internal capsule and basal ganglia are genuine end-arteries.

CEREBRAL BLOOD FLOW AND METABOLISM

While the extent and potency of the collateral channels is one factor of great importance in limiting the size of the area of infarction which results from arterial occlusion, another important factor is the 'ability of the cerebral blood vessels to compensate rapidly for sudden changes in blood supply' (Hutchinson and Acheson, 1975). These changes can be assessed by using the many methods now available to measure cerebral blood flow (CBF). Since Kety and Schmidt (1945) introduced the nitrous oxide method, many other techniques have been utilized. Cerebral 'transit time' can be measured by calculating the time taken for a radioactive bolus injected into the internal carotid artery to reappear in the jugular vein, but such measurements have been shown to be of little diagnostic value. Similarly, the recording of circulation time, by injecting radioactive hippuran intravenously and recording gamma radiation over the intact skull (Rowan et al., 1970) gives little useful information. An electromagnetic flow meter can be used to measure flow in the carotid artery (Hardesty et al., 1960; Meyer et al., 1967; Welch et al., 1974) but requires surgical exposure of the vessel. Gotoh et al. (1966) used hydrogen gas and measured hydrogen and other variables by means of electrodes inserted into the carotid artery and jugular vein, while Nylin et al. (1960) injected radioactive erythrocytes and studied the dilution curve in the jugular bulb. Techniques in common use nowadays, however, generally make use of an inert gas such as Xenon-133 or Krypton-85, either inhaled (Veall and Mallett, 1965) or injected, dissolved in 5 ml of sterile saline, into the internal carotid artery through a catheter (Ingvar and Lassen, 1962). With the latter technique it is possible, by using sixteen or more scintillation crystals placed laterally over the head, to measure regional blood flow in different areas of the cerebral hemisphere (Skinhøj et al., 1970); calculations may also be applied to compare flow in the cortex and in the white matter of the brain (Rees et al., 1971). Using these methods it is possible to measure CBF in ml of blood per 100 g of brain per minute, a ratio (mean arterial BP/CBF) indicative of cerebral vascular resistance (CVR) and another indicating cerebral oxygen utilization (arteriovenous O_2 difference/CBF) ($CMRO_2$).

Extensive studies using these techniques in recent years have shown first that the normal CBF is about 55 ml/100 g/min but diminishes with increasing age (Fazekas et al., 1955). The CBF is controlled by the perfusing pressure (which in normal subjects corresponds to the mean arterial blood pressure—MABP) and by the CVR; the ability of the brain to maintain CBF relatively constant despite variations in these parameters is known as autoregulation (Lassen, 1966), a facility which is highly developed under normal conditions but may be profoundly altered by cerebral vascular disease. Schmidt (1950) showed convincingly that cerebral vasomotor innervation plays little part in auto-regulation, but Fog (1939) had previously demonstrated that a rise in intra-vascular pressure caused constriction of pial arterioles and a fall caused dilatation. Recent work has, however, shown that the major factor which controls CVR in both man and animals is the CO_2 tension of the arterial blood (Kety and Schmidt, 1948; Gotoh et al., 1961; Harper and Bell, 1963; Reivich, 1964; Lassen, 1968); inhalation of gas containing more than 3·5 per cent CO_2 causes a significant increase in CBF. Changes in O_2 tension tend to have the reverse effect in that inhalation of O_2 causes vasoconstriction and hypoxia tends to cause dilatation (Heyman et al., 1952).

A vast literature has now accumulated upon the results of studies of CBF in various forms of cerebral vascular disease. In patients with hypertension and cerebral atherosclerosis earlier studies demonstrated consistent reductions in the over-all CBF and such reduction tended to be greater in patients with symptoms and signs of cerebral ischaemia (Scheinberg, 1950; Alman and Fazekas, 1957; Kempinsky et al., 1961). When angiography had demonstrated occlusion of a major vessel (internal carotid or middle cerebral) on one side, the total CBF was generally reduced more on the affected side of the head (McHenry, 1966; O'Brien and Veall, 1970) but in some cases, depending presumably upon the efficacy of the collateral circulation and the patency of small vessels, there was a general reduction of the CBF, even in the clinically uninvolved hemisphere. A similar unilateral reduction in CBF through the internal carotid circulation has been reported in the prodromal phase of a migraine attack (O'Brien, 1967; Skinhøj and Paulson, 1969).

Not surprisingly in the light of the experimental results described above, many workers suggested that cerebral ischaemia should be treated by the inhalation of CO_2, and Hegedus and Shackleford (1965) recommended the inhalation of 5 per cent CO_2 in cases of unilateral carotid obstruction, as this method in their hands produced a 40 per cent increase in total CBF. However, Fazekas and Alman (1964) found that in 9 of 22 patients with occlusion of major vessels, inhaled CO_2 did not increase CBF and actually reduced $CMRO_2$; they postulated that diseased small cerebral vessels were unresponsive.

Recent studies of regional blood flow (Høedt-Rasmussen et al., 1967; Paulson *et al.*, 1970; Skinhøj *et al.*, 1970; Rees *et al.*, 1970; Shah *et al.*, 1972) have clarified the position further. First, as Lassen (1966) showed, local hypoxia and tissue acidosis around an area of infarction may cause vasomotor vascular paralysis, vasodilatation, and loss of autoregulation which may in turn result in excessive blood flow around the periphery of such an area ('the luxury perfusion syndrome'). This phenomenon may give rise to venous engorgement (red venous blood) and sometimes even haemorrhage, and may extend the area of initial damage; inhaled CO_2 would be likely to increase flow into such areas and would thus be harmful. Høedt-Rasmussen *et al.* (1967) and McHenry *et al.* (1972) found evidence that this process not only caused local tissue damage but also tended to divert blood away from an ischaemic focus ('intracerebral steal syndrome'). Fortunately it seems that such hyperaemic foci with loss of autoregulation usually persist for only two or three days, though occasionally they last much longer, and Rees *et al.* (1970) found local areas of diminished CBF after transient cerebral ischaemic attacks for as long as 90 days. In occasional cases it appears that autoregulation may be temporarily impaired over the entire affected hemisphere.

The importance of luxury perfusion and the 'intracerebral steal' phenomenon in relation to treatment is indicated by the findings of Paulson *et al.* (1972) who found that hypocapnia induced by hyperventilation (Raichle *et al.*, 1970) was often effective in restoring autoregulation in patients in whom it was lost. Hence there is growing evidence to suggest that hyperventilation and hypocapnia do not cause cerebral ischaemic hypoxia in patients with cerebral ischaemia; on the contrary, they may increase local flow by producing vasoconstriction in the normal collateral channels, thus increasing the perfusing pressure to the ischaemic area (Hutchinson and Acheson, 1975). However, it is also important to note evidence that centres in the brain stem may exercise a neurogenic controlling effect upon CBF and metabolism (Meyer *et al.*, 1971).

The Blood-brain Barrier

All vessels within the central nervous system are surrounded by a thin covering formed by the processes of astrocytes. The plasma in the vessels is separated from the nervous tissue by the endothelium of the capillaries and their basement membrane, external to which is the extracellular space of the nervous system. The blood-brain barrier consists of the endothelial lining cells, the basement membrane, and the perivascular processes of astrocytes. The intravenous injection of trypan blue gives staining only of the astrocytic processes and the dye does not reach the nervous parenchyma except where the barrier is incomplete, as in the pineal, pituitary, area postrema of the brain stem, choroid plexus, and locus caeruleus (Dempsey and Wislocki, 1955; Brightman, 1965). Injected large molecules (ferritin, horseradish peroxidase) cannot pass the tight junctions of the capillary endothelial cells in either direction (Reese and Karnovsky, 1968). However, gases, water, glucose, electrolytes, and amino acids diffuse freely across the blood-brain barrier into the intracellular space (glial cells and neurons) and into the extracellular space of the brain. Acute cerebral lesions, whether due to trauma, inflammation, or infarction, increase the permeability of the barrier and thus alter the extra- and intracellular concentrations of protein, water, and electrolytes (Hess, 1955; Millen and Hess, 1958; Meyer, 1958; Lassen and Ingvar, 1963).

REFERENCES

ALEXANDER, L. (1942) The vascular supply of the strio-pallidum, *Res. Publ. Ass. nerv. ment. Dis.*, **21**, 77.

ALMAN, R. W., and FAZEKAS, J. F. (1957) Disparity between low cerebral blood flow and clinical signs of cerebral ischaemia, *Neurology (Minneap.)*, **7**, 555.

ATKINSON, W. J. (1949) The anterior inferior cerebellar artery, *J. Neurol. Neurosurg. Psychiat.*, **21**, 137.

BARNETT, H. J. M., WORTZMAN, G., GLADSTONE, R. M., and LOUGHEED, W. M. (1970) Diversion and reversal of cerebral blood flow: external carotid artery 'steal', *Neurology (Minneap.)*, **20**, 1.

BEEVOR, C. E. (1907) The cerebral arterial supply, *Brain*, **30**, 403.

BRIGHTMAN, M. W. (1965) The distribution within the brain of ferritin injected into the cerebrospinal fluid compartments, *Amer. J. Anat.*, **117**, 193.

CRITCHLEY, M. (1930) The anterior cerebral artery and its syndromes, *Brain*, **53**, 120.

DEMPSEY, E. W., and WISLOCKI, G. B. (1955) An electron microscopic study of the blood-brain barrier in the rat, *J. biophys. biochem. Cytol.*, **1**, 245.

VAN DER EECKEN, H. M. (1959) *The Anastomoses between the Leptomeningeal Arteries of the Brain*, Springfield, Ill.

VAN DER EECKEN, H. M., and ADAMS, R. D. (1953) The anatomy and functional significance of the meningeal arterial anastomosis of the human brain, *J. Neuropath. exp. Neurol.*, **12**, 132.

FAY, T. (1925) The cerebral vasculature, *J. Amer. med. Ass.*, **84**, 1727.

FAZEKAS, J. F., and ALMAN, W. R. (1964) Maximal dilatation of cerebral vessels, *Arch. Neurol. (Chic.)*, **11**, 303.

FAZEKAS, J. F., KLEIN, J., and FINNERTY, F. A. (1955) Influence of age and vascular disease on cerebral hemodynamics and metabolism, *Amer. J. Med.*, **18**, 477.

FOG, M. (1939) Reaction of pial arteries to increase in blood pressure, *Arch. Neurol. Psychiat. (Chic.)*, **4**, 260.

FOIX, C. (1925) Irrigation de la couche optique, *C.R. Soc. Biol. (Paris)*, **92**, 55.

FOIX, C., and HILLEMAND, P. (1925) Les artères de l'axe encéphalique jusqu'au diencéphale inclusivement, *Rev. Neurol. (Paris)*, **32**, 705.

GILLILAN, L. A. (1959) Significant superficial anastomosis in the arterial blood supply to the human brain, *J. Comp. Neurol.*, **112**, 55.

GOTOH, F., TAZAKI, Y., and MEYER, J. S. (1961) Transport of gases through brain and their extravascular vasomotor action, *Exp. Neurol.*, **4**, 48.

GOTOH, F., MEYER, J. S., and TOMITA, M. (1966) Hydrogen method for determining cerebral blood flow in man, *Arch. Neurol. (Chic.)*, **15**, 549.

GRYSPEERDT, G. L. (1963) Angiographic studies of the blood flow in the circle of Willis: the value of various arterial compression tests, *Acta Radiol.*, **1**, 298.

HARDESTY, W. H., BROOK, R., TOOLE, J. F., and ROYSTER, H. P. (1960) Studies of carotid artery blood flow in man, *New Engl. J. Med.*, **263**, 944.

HARPER, A. M., and BELL, R. A. (1963) The effect of metabolic acidosis and alkalosis on the blood flow through the cerebral cortex, *J. Neurol. Neurosurg. Psychiat.*, **26**, 341.

HEGEDUS, S. A., and SHACKLEFORD, R. T. (1965) Carbon dioxide and obstructed cerebral blood flow—correlation between cerebral blood flow crossfilling and neurological findings, *J. Amer. Med. Ass.*, **191**, 279.

HESS, A. (1955) Blood-brain barrier and ground substance of central nervous system, *Arch. Neurol. Psychiat. (Chic.)*, **74**, 149.

HEYMAN, A., PATTERSON, J. L., and WHATLEY DUKE, T. (1952) Cerebral circulation and metabolism in sickle cell and other chronic anaemias with observations on the effects of oxygen inhalation, *J. Clin. Invest.*, **31**, 824.

HØEDT-RASMUSSEN, K., SKINHØJ, E., PAULSON, O., EWALD, J., BJERRUM, J. K., FAHRENKRUG, A., and LASSEN, N. A. (1967) Regional cerebral blood flow in acute apoplexy. The 'luxury perfusion syndrome' of brain tissue, *Arch. Neurol. (Chic.)*, **17**, 271.

HUTCHINSON, E. C., and ACHESON, E. J. (1975) Strokes: Natural History, Pathology and Surgical Treatment, London.

INGVAR, D., and LASSEN, N. A. (1962) Regional blood flow of the cerebral cortex determined by Krypton[85], Acta Physiol. Scand., **54**, 325.

KEMPINSKY, W. H., BONIFACE, W. R., KEATING, J. B. A., and MORGAN, P. P. (1961) Serial hemodynamic study of cerebral infarction in man, Circulation Res., **9**, 1051.

KETY, S. S., and SCHMIDT, C. F. (1945) The determination of cerebral blood flow in man by use of nitrous oxide in low concentrations, Amer. J. Physiol., **143**, 53.

KETY, S. S., and SCHMIDT, C. F. (1948) Oxide method for the quantitative determination of cerebral blood flow in man. Theory, procedure and normal values, J. clin. Invest., **27**, 476.

LASSEN, N. A. (1966) The luxury perfusion syndrome, Lancet, **ii**, 1113.

LASSEN, N. A. (1968) Neurogenic control of cerebral blood flow, Scand. J. Clin. Lab. Invest., suppl. 102 VI:F.

LASSEN, N. A., and INGVAR, D. H. (1963) Regional cerebral blood flow measurements in man: a review, Arch. Neurol. (Chic.), **9**, 615.

McDONALD, D. A., and POTTER, J. M. (1951) The distribution of blood to the brain, J. Physiol. (Lond.), **114**, 356.

McHENRY, L. C., Jun. (1966) Cerebral blood flow studies in cerebrovascular disease, Arch. intern. Med., **117**, 546.

McHENRY, L. C., Jun., GOLDBERG, H. I., JAFFE, M. E., KENTON, E. J., WEST, J. W., and COOPER, E. S. (1972) Regional cerebral blood flow: response to carbon dioxide inhalation in cerebrovascular disease, Arch. Neurol. (Chic.), **27**, 403.

MEYER, A. (1958) in Neuropathology, ed. Greenfield, J. G., Blackwood, W., McMenemey, W. H., Meyer, A., and Norman, R. M., p. 230, London.

MEYER, J. S., YOSHIDA, K., and SAKAMOTO, K. (1967) Autonomic control of cerebral blood flow measured by electromagnetic flowmeters, Neurology (Minneap.), **17**, 638.

MEYER, J. S., TERAURA, T., SAKAMOTO, K., and KONDO, A. (1971) Central neurogenic control of cerebral blood flow, Neurology (Minneap.), **21**, 247.

MILLEN, J. W., and HESS, A. (1958) The blood-brain barrier: an experimental study with vital dyes, Brain, **81**, 248.

NYLIN, G., SILFVERSKIOLD, B. P., LOFSTEDT, S., REGNSTIONE, O., and HEDLUND, S. (1960) Studies of cerebral blood flow in man using radioactive-labelled erythrocytes, Brain, **83**, 293.

O'BRIEN, M. D. (1967) Cerebral-cortex-perfusion rates in migraine, Lancet, **i**, 1036.

O'BRIEN, M. D., and VEALL, N. (1970) The influence of carotid stenosis on cortex perfusion, Research in Cerebral Circulation, 3rd International Salzburg Conference, 165.

PAULSON, O. B., LASSEN, N. A., and SKINHØJ, E. (1970) Regional cerebral blood flow in apoplexy without arterial occlusion, Neurology (Minneap.), **20**, 125.

PAULSON, O. B., OLESEN, J., and CHRISTENSEN, M. S. (1972) Restoration of autoregulation of cerebral blood flow by hypocapnia, Neurology (Minneap.), **22**, 286.

RAICHLE, M., POSNER, J. B., and PLUM, F. (1970) Cerebral blood flow during and after hyperventilation, Arch. Neurol. (Chic.), **23**, 394.

REES, J. E., BULL, J. W. D., ROSS-RUSSELL, R. W., MARSHALL, J., and SYMON, L. (1970) Regional cerebral blood flow in transient ischaemic attacks, Lancet, **ii**, 1210.

REES, J. E., BULL, J. W. D., DU BOULAY, G. H., MARSHALL, J., ROSS-RUSSELL, R. W., and SYMON, L. (1971) The comparative analysis of isotope clearance curves in normal and ischaemic brain, Stroke, **2**, 444.

REESE, T. S., and KARNOVSKY, M. J. (1968) Fine structural localisation of a blood-brain barrier to exogenous peroxidase, J. Cell Biol., **34**, 207.

REIVICH, M. (1964) Arterial pCO_2 and cerebral hemodynamics, Amer. J. Physiol., **206**, 25.

ROWAN, J. O., CROSS, J. N., TEDESCHI, G. M., and JENNETT, W. B. (1970) Limitations of circulation time in the diagnosis of intracranial disease, J. Neurol. Neurosurg. Psychiat., **33**, 739.

SCHEINBERG, P. (1950) Cerebral blood flow in vascular disease of the brain with observations on the effects of stellate ganglion block, Amer. J. Med., **8**, 139.

SCHMIDT, C. F. (1950) *The Cerebral Circulation in Health and Disease*, Springfield, Ill.

SEDZIMIR, C. B. (1959) An angiographic test of collateral circulation through the anterior segment of the circle of Willis, *J. Neurol. Neurosurg. Psychiat.*, **22,** 64.

SHAH, S., BULL, J. W. D., DU BOULAY, G. H., MARSHALL, J., ROSS-RUSSELL, R. W., and SYMON, L. (1972) A comparison of rapid serial angiography and isotope clearance measurements in cerebrovascular disease, *Brit. J. Radiol.*, **45,** 294.

SKINHØJ, E., HØEDT-RASMUSSEN, K., PAULSON, O. B., and LASSEN, N. A. (1970) Regional cerebral blood flow and its autoregulation in patients with transient focal cerebral ischemic attacks, *Neurology (Minneap.)*, **20,** 485.

SKINHØJ, E., and PAULSON, O. B. (1969) Regional blood flow in internal carotid distribution during migraine attack, *Brit. med. J.*, **3,** 569.

STOPFORD, J. S. B. (1915–16 and 1916–17) The arteries of the pons and medulla oblongata, *J. Anat. Physiol.*, **50,** 131; and **51,** 250.

VEALL, N., and MALLETT, B. L. (1965) The partition of trace amounts of Xenon between human blood and brain tissues at 37°C, *Phys. Med. Biol.*, **10,** 375.

WELCH, K. M. A., SPIRA, P. J., KNOWLES, L., and LANCE, J. W. (1974) Effects of prostaglandins on the internal and external carotid blood flow in the monkey: possible relevance to cranial flow changes during migraine headache, *Neurology (Minneap.)*, **24,** 705.

CEREBRAL ISCHAEMIA

Cerebral ischaemia, or impairment of the blood supply to the brain, may be produced in a number of different ways. (1) Since, as we have seen, the cerebral blood flow is directly related to the blood pressure, a sudden fall of blood pressure from any cause may produce symptoms of cerebral ischaemia. The cause of this is discussed below. (2) The defective blood supply may be the result of disease of the cerebral arteries themselves due, for example, to atheroma or endarteritis. (3) A cerebral vessel may be obstructed by a substance carried into it from elsewhere by the circulation—cerebral embolism.

COMPLETE CIRCULATORY ARREST

The brain is very vulnerable to any interruption of its circulation. Irreversible dementia has been reported to follow severe blood loss in elderly subjects (Bedford, 1956) and permanent cortical blindness has been known to follow severe exsanguination resulting from haematemesis. It is generally agreed that loss of consciousness occurs within a few seconds after total interruption of the cerebral circulation as in cardiac arrest, and permanent damage is produced in about five to eight minutes (Plum, 1973), though Meyer (1958) reported a case in which irreversible brain damage followed after one minute of cardiac and respiratory arrest. Irreversible anoxic–ischaemic cell changes occur in experimental animals within 15 minutes. Bell and Hodgson (1974), in a study of 284 patients resuscitated from cardiac arrest, found that only 19 per cent of comatose patients lived to be discharged from hospital compared with 54 per cent of non-comatose individuals, and many of those surviving after initial coma showed persisting neurological deficits. The EEG is of some value in predicting the prognosis (Pampiglione and Harden, 1968). Brierley *et al.* (1971) found neuropathological evidence of almost total neocortical death in two patients who survived for 5 months in coma. The effects of anoxia due, for instance, to carbon monoxide poisoning [p. 810] are similar, if less profound than those of total circulatory arrest.

Neurological Complications of Open-Heart Surgery

Cerebral ischaemic episodes may develop as a consequence of open-heart surgery and vary in severity, sometimes simulating the effects of total cardiac arrest, sometimes those of diffuse cerebral anoxia (Gilman, 1965; Javid et al., 1969). Air or gas embolism due to the use of bubble oxygenators, which can be detected with Doppler ultrasonic flow detectors (Edmonds-Seal et al., 1970) is sometimes the cause, but more often these complications are due to micro-embolic encephalopathy, the emboli consisting of blood products, platelets, or denatured plasma proteins as well as gas bubbles (Williams, 1971; Brennan et al., 1971).

SYNCOPE

Definition. Syncope is a brief and transitory loss of consciousness, due to impairment of the cerebral circulation, and usually occurring in the absence of organic disease of the brain. If the fall in the cerebral circulation is sufficiently prolonged convulsions occur. Hence an isolated convulsion may sometimes be precipitated by circumstances which more usually cause syncope, but in pathogenesis, and electroencephalographically, syncope and epilepsy are quite distinct.

AETIOLOGY

The essential feature of syncope is a temporary fall in the cerebral circulation below the level necessary for the maintenance of consciousness. Apart from narrowing of the cerebral arteries, syncope is always the result of low cardiac output, which may be produced in a number of ways, some of them complex.

Postural Hypotension

This is a convenient term for the pathogenesis of fainting in a variety of circumstances which have this in common. Venous return to the heart is impaired because the blood accumulates in the veins in rapidly growing adolescents in hot rooms or in church, in young soldiers immobilized on parade, especially in hot weather, in patients getting up after long confinement to bed, in elderly men after emptying the bladder in the night (micturition syncope, The Lancet, 1962), in those too rapidly assuming the erect posture after sympathectomy, hypotensive drugs, spinal anaesthesia and high spinal cord injuries, and in certain diseases, e.g. tabes, polyneuritis, and porphyria. In all these conditions the reflex postural regulation of the blood pressure is inadequate. The reasons are often complex (Brigden et al., 1950). The pressor reflexes may be interrupted on their afferent side in tables and polyneuritis, or centrally depressed by alcohol or other drugs, including phenothiazines, levodopa, and amine-oxidase inhibitors.

Chronic Orthostatic Hypotension (the Shy-Drager Syndrome)

In this condition, which is often sporadic, but sometimes familial (Johnson et al., 1966), the blood pressure falls as soon as the patient assumes the upright posture but there is no compensatory vasoconstriction of peripheral vessels so that pallor, sweating, and tachycardia do not occur and there is abrupt loss of consciousness (Bradbury and Eggleston, 1925). Autopsy evidence (Shy and Drager, 1960; Chokroverty et al., 1969; Hughes et al., 1970; Roessmann et al., 1971; Thapedi et al., 1971; Bannister and Oppenheimer, 1972) has revealed degeneration of the cells of the intermediolateral column of the spinal cord, confirming evidence of autonomic denervation, and the condition has be[...] described in association with the Holmes–Adie syndrome (Johnson *et a[...]* 1971). While orthostatic hypotension may be symptomatic of many neurc[...] logical disorders (Martin *et al.*, 1968) and while the primary autonomic failur[...] is sometimes afferent and sometimes efferent (Love *et al.*, 1971), in many case[...] of the chronic syndrome Parkinsonian features, dysarthria, cerebellar ataxia, impotence and incontinence, and amyotrophy develop in varying combinations and with variable severity, so that the condition is often called progressive multi-system degeneration and widespread degenerative changes are found in the central nervous system. In the early stages attacks may be partially controlled by the use of drugs such as 9-α-fludrocortisone 0·1 mg twice daily with a high sodium intake to increase the blood volume; later the wearing of a G-suit may help but in most cases the disorder is progressive and ultimately fatal though the prognosis varies in individual cases.

Cough Syncope

Cough syncope is syncope produced by prolonged coughing, usually in middle-aged men with emphysema and chronic bronchitis. The changes in intrathoracic pressure produced by coughing interfere with the venous return of blood to the heart, and there may be atheromatous narrowing of the cerebral arteries as well. Treatment usually involves giving up smoking and other measures to prevent bouts of coughing. Another 'mechanical' mode of producing syncope by interfering with venous return is by stretching with the arms extended and raised and the spine hyperextended—'stretch syncope'—which may occur in young people.

Swallow Syncope

This rare disorder (Levin and Posner, 1972), in which swallowing induces fainting, can be the result of demyelination in the vagus nerve and may be controlled by anticholinergic drugs.

Psychological Causes

The occurrence of syncope as an immediate effect of sudden psychological shock is well known (Rook, 1947). Hysteria is a common cause of recurrent fainting in young girls. Here again there is a fall of blood pressure due to complex factors. Reflexly induced pooling in the peripheral circulation may be the most important, but McHenry *et al.* (1961) pointed out that hyperventilation, a common accompaniment of anxiety and hysteria, may lead to cerebral ischaemia by producing hypocapnia. Tachycardia, also due to anxiety, may lower the cardiac output. Fainting may be a conditioned reaction to particular circumstances.

Physical Shock

Many physical stimuli are capable of causing syncope, and in some cases it may be artificial to distinguish the physical from the psychological factor. Severe pain may cause loss of consciousness, but many stimuli which cause little or no pain may be equally effective, such as venepuncture, cisternal and lumbar puncture, and pleural puncture ('pleural epilepsy').

Anaemia of Sudden Onset

Anaemia due to severe haemorrhage may cause syncope, though an equally severe anaemia of gradual onset does not.

Polycythaemia Vera

In cases of polycythaemia vera the increased viscosity of the blood may pre-dispose to cerebral infarction but many patients also experience episodes of cerebral or brain-stem ischaemia similar to those of carotid or vertebro-basilar insufficiency (see below) (Silverstein et al., 1962). Others may present with symptoms suggesting an intracranial space-occupying lesion (Kremer et al., 1972).

Cardiac Disorder

Syncope may be caused by the impairment of the cerebral circulation resulting from low cardiac output caused by a disorder of the rate and rhythm of the heart in heart-block, auricular flutter, and paroxysmal tachycardia. Previously unrecognized episodes of cardiac dysrhythmia may be an important cause of episodes of transient cerebral ischaemia (McAllen and Marshall, 1973). Syncope due to heart-block (the Stokes–Adams syndrome) is well recognized. The loss of consciousness is most likely to occur during the cardiac asystole which may develop in the transition between partial heart-block and complete block, and the attacks may cease when the block is complete, but do not always do so. Many attacks may occur in a day. They usually occur when the patient is at rest and not during physical effort. Typically loss of consciousness and pallor occur during asystole and flushing with a few myoclonic jerks of the extremities occur when the pulse returns and consciousness is quickly restored. These attacks rarely occur in patients with bundle-branch block. In addition low cardiac output may be due to massive pulmonary embolism, mechanical obstruction of the mitral valve, and severe aortic stenosis.

Carotid Sinus Syncope

The important part played in the regulation of the circulation by the carotid sinus, the slight dilatation of the carotid in the region of the bifurcation, was first pointed out by Hering, though previously the vagus had been held respon-sible for the effects now known to originate in the sinus. A rise of pressure within the sinus causes a reflex fall in blood pressure with slowing of the heart rate, while a fall of pressure within the sinus has the opposite effect. These reflex changes are mediated by the nerve to the carotid sinus, a branch of the glosso-pharyngeal nerve, and the medullary vasomotor centres. Disease in the neigh-bourhood of the sinus, or even hypersensitivity of the reflex mechanism, may cause syncopal attacks which can be reproduced by digital pressure in this region. Precipitation of the attacks by spontaneous movements of the head is mentioned by Turner and Learmonth (1948).

Hutchinson and Stock (1960) reported 16 cases, all middle-aged or elderly males. Some had syncopal episodes alone, often with transient convulsive movements, but others experienced vertigo or focal symptoms suggesting transient brain stem or cerebral ischaemia in the attacks, presumably due to the effects of concomitant cerebral atheroma. Attacks were sometimes precipitated by head-turning. The diagnosis can readily be confirmed by recording the ECG during carotid sinus pressure when profound bradycardia and often transient asystole may occur (Reese et al., 1962).

The causes of carotid sinus attacks include lesions in the neighbourhood of the sinus, such as scarring from tuberculous adenitis, atheroma of the artery, and rarely carotid body tumour, but many cases are 'idiopathic'.

Cerebral Atheroma

Temporary cerebral ischaemia resulting from atheroma of the cerebral arteries is an unusual cause of syncope and is unlikely to occur unless the cerebral circulation as a whole is gravely impaired, or the ischaemia particularly involves the central reticular formation. Faintness may then be brought on particularly by turning the head or extending the neck, through impairment of the blood supply through one or other internal carotid or vertebral artery or both, independently of the carotid sinus reflex. Fainting attacks due to brain-stem ischaemia are particularly liable to occur when occlusion of the left subclavian artery close to its origin results in retrograde flow of blood down the homolateral vertebral artery in order to supply the upper limb (the 'subclavian steal syndrome').

SYMPTOMS

The onset of an attack of syncope may be sudden, but it often takes a few seconds to develop. There may be prodromal symptoms such as coldness of the extremities, sweating, 'swimming' in the head, or blurred vision. The patient becomes cold and limp, and sinks to the ground, though the premonitory symptoms often enable him to sit or lie down first. Respiration is usually sighing, the pulse is generally slow, and its tension low. The pupils may be dilated and react sluggishly to light, and the corneal reflexes are likely to be lost and the tendon reflexes diminished. Muscular twitching and urinary incontinence may occasionally occur, or, if the cerebral ischaemia is sufficiently prolonged, a general convulsion.

Electroencephalography

In syncope due to impairment of the cerebral blood flow slow waves of high voltage develop in the EEG concurrently with the loss of consciousness (Hill and Driver, 1962) and this is followed by complete flattening of the EEG record while clonic or tonic convulsions may occur (Gastaut and Fischer-Williams, 1957).

DIAGNOSIS

When syncope leads only to loss of consciousness it must be distinguished from epilepsy. Syncope, being secondary to a circulatory change, is usually more gradual in its onset and its cessation than an epileptic attack. Convulsive movements do not often occur, and the patient is limp rather than rigid, as in epilepsy. Syncopal convulsions, however, need to be distinguished from epilepsy. In many cases the cause of the syncopal attacks is obvious. Syncope of carotid sinus origin can be reproduced by pressure on the sinus, which, however, is no longer effective after procaine has been injected into this region. In the stage of partial heart-block the diagnosis may be impossible without an electrocardiogram: in complete block the heart rate is usually from 26 to 30. Paroxysmal or focal epileptic discharges in the EEG are absent: if syncope can be induced, e.g. by ocular compression, the EEG changes are those described above.

PROGNOSIS

A syncopal attack is rarely fatal and usually leaves no sequelae. However, prolonged and diffuse cerebral ischaemia which may, for example, occur during anaesthesia, particularly in the elderly, or severe recurrent faints, may lead to permanent anoxic brain damage. The prognosis is that of the causal condition.

TREATMENT

Little treatment is required for the ordinary attack of syncope, which is self-limiting. The patient should be placed in a horizontal posture. Any causal condition will require treatment. Syncope of carotid sinus origin is best treated with anticholinergic drugs of which atropine, 0·5 mg two or three times daily or propantheline bromide, 15 mg three times a day, are usually the most successful. In intractable cases it may be justifiable to denervate the sinus.

REFERENCES

BANNISTER, R., and OPPENHEIMER, D. R. (1972) Degenerative diseases of the nervous system associated with autonomic failure, *Brain*, **95**, 457.

BEDFORD, P. D. (1956) Adverse cerebral effects following acute haemorrhage in elderly people, *Lancet*, **ii**, 750.

BELL, J. A., and HODGSON, H. J. F. (1974) Coma after cardiac arrest, *Brain*, **97**, 361.

BRADBURY, S., and EGGLESTON, C. (1925) Postural hypotension: a report of three cases, *Amer. Heart J.*, **1**, 73.

BRENNAN, R. W., PATTERSON, R. H., and KESSLER, J. (1971) Cerebral blood flow and metabolism during cardiopulmonary bypass: evidence of microembolic encephalopathy, *Neurology (Minneap.)*, **21**, 665.

BRIERLEY, J. B., ADAMS, J. H., GRAHAM, D. I., and SIMPSON, J. A. (1971) Neocortical death after cardiac arrest: a clinical, neurophysiological, and neuropathological report of two cases, *Lancet*, **ii**, 560.

BRIGDEN, W., HOWARTH, S., and SHARPEY-SCHAFER, E. P. (1950) Postural changes in the peripheral blood-flow of normal subjects with observations on vaso-vagal fainting reactions as a result of tilting, the lordotic posture, pregnancy and spinal anaesthesia, *Clin. Sci.*, **60**, 79.

CHOKROVERTY, S., BARRON, K. D., KATZ, F. H., DEL GRECO, F., and SHARP, J. T. (1969) The syndrome of primary orthostatic hypotension, *Brain*, **92**, 743.

EDMONDS-SEAL, J., PRYS ROBERTS, C., and ADAMS, A. P. (1970) Transcutaneous Doppler ultrasonic flow detectors for diagnosis of air embolism, *Proc. roy. Soc. Med.*, **63**, 831.

FERRIS, E. B., Jun., CAPPS, R. B., and WEISS, S. (1935) Carotid sinus syncope and its bearing on the mechanism of the unconscious state and convulsions: a study of thirty-two additional cases, *Medicine (Baltimore)*, **14**, 377.

GASTAUT, H., and FISCHER-WILLIAMS, M. (1957) Electroencephalographic study of syncope, *Lancet*, **ii**, 1018.

GILMAN, S. (1965) Cerebral disorders after open-heart operations, *New Engl. J. Med.*, **272**, 489.

HILL, D., and DRIVER, M. V. (1962) in *Recent Advances in Neurology and Neuropsychiatry*, 7th ed., ed. Brain, W. R., p. 219, London.

HOHL, R. D., FRAME, B., and SCHATZ, I. J. (1965) The Shy–Drager variant of idiopathic orthostatic hypotension, *Amer. J. Med.*, **39**, 134.

HUGHES, R. C., CARTLIDGE, N. E. F., and MILLAC, P. (1970) Primary neurogenic orthostatic hypotension, *J. Neurol. Neurosurg. Psychiat.*, **33**, 363.

HUTCHINSON, E. C., and STOCK, J. P. P. (1960) The carotid-sinus syndrome, *Lancet*, **ii**, 445.

JAVID, H., TUFO, H. M., NAJAFI, H., DYE, W. S., HUNTER, J. A., and JULIAN, O. C. (1969) Neurological abnormalities following open heart surgery, *J. Thorac. Cardiovasc. Surg.*, **58**, 502.

JOHNSON, R. H., LEE, G. DE J., OPPENHEIMER, W. R., and SPALDING, J. M. K. (1966) Autonomic failure due to intermedio-lateral column degeneration, *Quart. J. Med.*, **35**, 276.

JOHNSON, R. H., McLELLAN, D. L., and LOVE, D. R. (1971) Orthostatic hypotension and the Holmes–Adie syndrome, *J. Neurol. Neurosurg. Psychiat.*, **34**, 562.

KERSCHMAN, J. (1949) Syncope and seizures, *J. Neurol. Neurosurg. Psychiat.*, **12**, 25.

KREMER, M., LAMBERT, C. D., and LAWTON, N. (1972) Progressive neurological deficits in primary polycythaemia, *Brit. med. J.*, **3**, 216.

THE LANCET (1962) Fainting on micturition, Leader, *Lancet*, **ii**, 286.

LEVIN, B., and POSNER, J. B. (1972) Swallow syncope. Report of a case and review of the literature, *Neurology (Minneap.)*, **22**, 1086.

LOVE, D. R., BROWN, J. J., CHINN, R. H., JOHNSON, R. H., LEVER, A. F., PARK, D. M., and ROBERTSON, J. I. S. (1971) Plasma renin in idiopathic orthostatic hypotension: differential response in subjects with probable afferent and efferent autonomic failure, *Clin. Sci.*, **41**, 289.

McALLEN, P. M., and MARSHALL, J. (1973) Cardiac dysrhythmia and transient cerebral ischaemic attacks, *Lancet*, **i**, 1212.

McHENRY, L. C., Jun., FAZEKAS, J. F., and SULLIVAN, J. F. (1961) Cerebral haemodynamics of syncope, *Amer. J. med. Sci.*, **241**, 173.

MARTIN, J. B., TRAVIS, R. H., and VAN DEN NOORT, S. (1968) Centrally mediated orthostatic hypotension: report of cases, *Arch. Neurol. (Chic.)*, **19**, 163.

MEYER, A. (1958) in *Neuropathology*, ed. Greenfield, J. G., Blackwood, W., McMenemey, W. H., Meyer, A., and Norman, R. M., p. 241, London.

PAMPIGLIONE, G., and HARDEN, A. (1968) Resuscitation after cardiocirculatory arrest. Prognostic evaluation of early electroencephalographic findings, *Lancet*, **i**, 1261.

PLUM, F. (1973) The clinical problem: how much anoxia-ischemia damages the brain?, *Arch. Neurol. (Chic.)*, **29**, 359.

REESE, C. L., GREEN, J. B., and ELLIOTT, F. A. (1962) The cerebral form of carotid sinus syncope, *Neurology (Minneap.)*, **12**, 492.

ROESSMANN, U., VAN DEN NOORT, S., and McFARLAND, D. E. (1971) Idiopathic orthostatic hypotension, *Arch. Neurol. (Chic.)*, **24**, 503.

ROOK, A. F. (1947) Fainting and flying, *Quart. J. Med.*, **40**, 181.

SHARPEY-SCHAFER, E. P. (1953) The mechanism of syncope after coughing, *Brit. med. J.*, **2**, 860.

SHY, G. M., and DRAGER, G. A. (1960) A neurological syndrome associated with orthostatic hypotension, *Arch. Neurol. (Chic.)*, **2**, 511.

SILVERSTEIN, A., GILBERT, H., and WASSERMAN, L. R. (1962) Hemiplegic complications of polycythaemia, *Ann. intern. Med.*, **57**, 909.

THAPEDI, I. M., ASHENHURST, E. M., and ROZDILSKY, B. (1971) Shy–Drager syndrome: report of an autopsied case, *Neurology (Minneap.)*, **21**, 26.

TURNER, R., and LEARMONTH, J. R. (1948) Carotid-sinus syndrome, *Lancet*, **ii**, 644.

WILLIAMS, I. M. (1971) Intravascular changes in the retina during open-heart surgery, *Lancet*, **ii**, 688.

CLASSIFICATION OF THE CEREBROVASCULAR DISEASES

In 1958 an *ad hoc* committee of the National Advisory Council of the National Institute of Neurological Diseases and Blindness published a 'classification and outline of the cerebrovascular diseases', which remains a useful basis of classification today. The principal types of cerebrovascular disease were classified as follows:

Cerebral infarction
Transient cerebral ischaemia without infarction
Intracranial haemorrhage
Vascular malformations and developmental abnormalities
Inflammatory diseases of arteries
Vascular diseases without changes in the brain
Hypertensive encephalopathy

Dural sinus and cerebral venous thrombosis
Strokes of undetermined origin

These broad diagnostic categories will in general be followed in the commentaries which follow.

THE INCIDENCE AND EPIDEMIOLOGY OF 'STROKES'

The accuracy of diagnostic information derived from epidemiological studies based upon death certificates must be treated with caution (Hutchinson and Acheson, 1975). Anderson and MacKay (1968) noted remarkable fluctuations in the incidence of recorded deaths due to cerebral thrombosis on the one hand and haemorrhage on the other between 1901 and 1961 but pointed out that in necropsy series the incidence had remained relatively constant. Statistics based upon hospital series are inaccurate as many elderly patients with strokes are not admitted to hospital. Whisnant et al. (1971) in a survey of strokes in the population of Rochester, Minnesota, found that the incidence of all forms of cerebral vascular disease was 194 per 100,000 of the population per year, and infarction accounted for 146 per 100,000; cerebral haemorrhage accounted for less than 10 per cent of all strokes, and it is generally agreed that subarachnoid haemorrhage is responsible for about 8 per cent. The incidence of cerebral haemorrhage has seemed at first sight to be much higher in Japan (Johnson et al., 1967) but Kurtzke (1969) in a detailed multinational survey concluded that the presumed high incidence of haemorrhage in Japan was an artefact as autopsy evidence has indicated that errors in diagnosis between haemorrhage and infarction may have varied from 10 per cent to as much as 40 per cent in different series. It is, however, clear that with an ageing population cerebrovascular disease imposes an increasingly heavy burden upon the hospital and community services (Acheson and Fairbairn, 1970). Though the prognosis of stroke may be somewhat better in females than in males (Marquardsen, 1969), paradoxically mortality may be slightly higher in females (Eisenberg et al., 1964); however, both morbidity and mortality are related in a linear manner to age (Hutchinson and Acheson, 1975). Cerebrovascular disease is ubiquitous in all races (Dalal et al., 1968; Williams et al., 1969); evidence suggesting a higher incidence of cerebral haemorrhage in the American negro (Kane and Aronson, 1969) is thought by some workers to be due to an artefact of reporting (Hutchinson and Acheson, 1975) but the incidence of cerebrovascular disease overall in that ethnic group appears to be higher than in Nigerians (Williams et al., 1969).

CEREBRAL INFARCTION

AETIOLOGY AND PATHOLOGY

The principal causes of cerebral infarction are atheroma, arterial hypertension, and cerebral embolism [p. 342] but rarer causes include direct trauma to the internal carotid artery in the neck (Hughes and Brownell, 1968) or to intracranial vessels in subarachnoid haemorrhage (Tomlinson, 1959), endarteritis due to meningovascular syphilis or other forms of meningitis [pp. 459 and 409], giant cell arteritis and granulomatous arteritis [pp. 376–7], collagen-vascular or connective-tissue disease [pp. 374–6], and fibromuscular hypoplasia of the internal carotid artery (Hartman *et al.*, 1971). Acute hemiplegia in child-hood (Solomon *et al.*, 1970) may be due to injury, infection, cardiac disease, or sickle cell anaemia but most often results from occlusive vascular disease, sometimes due to atheroma or perhaps to inflamed cervical lymph nodes involving the internal carotid artery (Bickerstaff, 1964). Disorders of the blood including anaemia, polycythaemia vera (Silverstein *et al.*, 1962), thrombotic microangiopathy [p. 378], and hypercoagulability due to oral contraceptive medication (Inman and Vessey, 1968; Schoenberg *et al.*, 1970; Bickerstaff, 1975) or pregnancy and the puerperium (Cross *et al.*, 1968) also play an important role. Occasionally, thrombosis in the carotid or vertebrobasilar system, even in young patients, occurs without demonstrable pathological cause (Graham and Adams, 1972).

Atheroma (often called arteriosclerosis) is a process which affects primarily the intima of the cerebral arteries. Intimal thickening is followed by the deposition of cholesterol and often by calcification and ulceration, often with consequent breaching of the internal elastic lamina, and ultimately there is some encroachment upon the media of the vessel. Atheromatous lesions often occur in the form of plaques, and thrombi may form on ulcerated areas so that emboli arising from such plaques are sometimes made up of platelet emboli, or sometimes so-called cholesterol emboli derived from breakdown of a dis-integrating plaque. The aetiology of atheroma is still uncertain but hyper-lipidaemia is certainly one factor and atheroma is often widespread in patients with diabetes and myxoedema. Atheroma is sometimes found in young children, and while its incidence certainly increases with age, some elderly individuals show very little. It is a process which principally affects large- and medium-sized arteries.

While many patients with widespread atheroma are also hypertensive, arterial hypertension *per se* tends to be associated with hypertrophy of the media of small arteries and arterioles and sometimes there is associated intimal thicken-ing (arteriolosclerosis). Miliary aneurysms are often found in such small vessels in the brain and retina in hypertensive subjects but may require special tech-niques of arterial injection at post-mortem or fluorescent retinal angiography during life for their demonstration.

By and large, therefore, it can be said that atheroma is primarily a disorder of large vessels, while hypertension is associated with thickening of small arteries and arterioles with diminution of their lumina, but the two often co-exist.

When nervous tissue is deprived of its blood supply for a few minutes due either to blockage of a vessel caused by thrombosis or embolism or when the flow through a narrowed but still patent artery falls below a critical level, nerve cells, nerve fibres, and glial cells degenerate to give an area of infarction or softening. The area is subsequently invaded by activated microglial cells ('gitter' cells) and eventually a cystic cavity or glial scar remains. Infarcts may be small (a few millimetres in diameter) or large, and can be single or multiple, cortical or subcortical. Some infarcts are pale (anaemic), some haemorrhagic, and some mixed. Adams (1954) showed that many haemorrhagic infarcts are embolic and suggested that as the embolus impacts in a major vessel the initial infarct is pale, but if the embolus then fragments and moves on, blood then extravasates freely in the necrotic area. Lacunes are small trabeculated cavities often found in the deeper parts of the brains of hypertensive subjects (Fisher, 1969) and while there is some dispute about their pathogenesis (Hughes, 1965) the view most widely accepted is that they are usually the result of small infarcts due to the occlusion of small perforating arteries.

If one excludes the rarer causes of cerebral infarction mentioned above, it is clear that atheroma, hypertension and/or embolism are usually responsible, but all authors are agreed that it is not invariably possible, even at post-mortem, to demonstrate a vessel occluded by a thrombus or embolus in such cases and infarction may result when various haemodynamic factors combine with the effects of arterial narrowing to cause a critical degree of ischaemia of one or more parts of the brain. Thus factors which may contribute include anaemia, sudden hypotension due to blood loss, cardiac infarction, poorly controlled anaesthesia, syncope, cardiac arrhythmias, and transient narrowing or kinking of a major artery (as of the vertebral artery on turning the neck when there is severe cervical spondylosis) (Bauer et al., 1961). The complexity of the situation is underlined by the fact that the cross-sectional area of a stenosed carotid artery may have to be reduced to 10-15 per cent of normal to cause a significant reduction in blood flow (Brice et al., 1964).

'Moyamoya Disease'

Takeuchi (1961) and Kudo (1968) were among the first to describe an unusual angiographic appearance in young Japanese patients in which the blood vessels supplying the cerebral hemispheres resembled the so-called 'rete mirabile' of lower animals; this appearance was entitled 'Moyamoya disease'. Patients demonstrating this appearance have sometimes presented with a choreiform syndrome, but more often with variable clinical features of cerebral ischaemia or of cerebral or subdural haemorrhage. In many of the Japanese reports a developmental anomaly of the circle of Willis was postulated, but it is now apparent that this angiographic appearance may be seen in adult non-Japanese patients as a result of atherosclerotic occlusion of both internal carotid arteries (Poór and Gács, 1974) and similar changes may be found in individuals with familial hypoplasia of these vessels (Austin and Stears, 1971). The exact nature of the pathological process which accounts for the frequency of this finding in Japanese children is uncertain but it is now apparent that this angiographic appearance results from the development of a collateral circulation following the occlusion of major arteries of the circle of Willis.

THE CLINICAL FEATURES OF 'STROKES'

The term 'stroke' is now used colloquially and medically to identify all forms of cerebrovascular accident; some such attacks are called 'seizures' by the layman, but seizure in medical terminology is more often used to identify an attack of epilepsy. The classical term apoplexy is still sometimes used for severe strokes (usually due to cerebral haemorrhage) which fell the patient, rendering him unconscious. A stroke or cerebrovascular accident can reasonably be defined (ad hoc Committee, 1958) as a focal neurological disorder of abrupt development due to a pathological process in blood vessels.

Although the clinical varieties of stroke are numerous, depending upon the nature of the primary pathological abnormality and the vessel or vessels involved, a few general principles may reasonably be stated here, provided it is recognized that there is no certain means of distinguishing clinically between haemorrhage and infarction. In general, the onset of cerebral embolism is abrupt, with the onset of hemiplegia, say, in a few seconds or minutes. Cerebral haemorrhage is often accompanied by headache at the onset, but loss of consciousness is usual with a neurological deficit which increases rapidly over 10–30 minutes, and the condition may develop during exertion or in other circumstances which raise the blood pressure. The onset in non-embolic cerebral infarction (cerebral 'thrombosis') may be equally abrupt and there may be headache if there is associated cerebral oedema; more often, however, the condition is noted on waking or soon after rising, or weakness, say of one arm and leg, develops over about 30 minutes; less often the neurological deficit slowly extends over hours or days (stroke-in-evolution), presumably due to spreading vascular occlusion and an expanding infarct, and the picture may then simulate that of an intracranial space-occupying lesion. In other cases the condition appears to increase in a step-wise manner (a so-called 'stuttering' stroke). Sometimes the established stroke is preceded by warning symptoms in the form of transient ischaemic attacks (see below) or a series of 'little strokes'. When there is neck stiffness suggesting blood in the subarachnoid space, this usually, but not invariably, indicates cerebral haemorrhage (a cerebellar infarct can cause neck stiffness at the onset). It must also be recognized that a massive infarct may cause loss of consciousness at the onset, while consciousness may be retained if a small, localized haemorrhage situated deeply does not reach the ventricles or subarachnoid space.

Before considering the specific clinical features associated with occlusion of the principal cerebral arteries and then going on to describe the clinical effects of embolism and intracranial haemorrhage, it will now be convenient to consider the general symptomatology of transient ischaemic attacks.

TRANSIENT CEREBRAL ISCHAEMIC ATTACKS

Transient cerebral ischaemic attacks are episodes indicating ischaemia of some part of one cerebral hemisphere or of the brain stem, lasting anything from a few minutes to a few hours in duration (some workers accept a duration of up to 24 hours) and followed by complete recovery. The episodes may be isolated and infrequent or may occur many times in a day and they tend to be consistent in their symptomatology in the affected individuals, suggesting that the recurrent episodes of ischaemia consistently involve the same area of the brain. The clinical features and natural history of these episodes have been reviewed in detail by Hutchinson and Acheson (1975). By definition these attacks are not accompanied by irreversible infarction of the affected brain substance, although in attacks which last as long as 24 hours it seems possible that minute areas of infarction may develop.

The importance of atheroma in the carotid and vertebral arteries in the neck and/or in other major branches of the aortic arch in the pathogenesis of such attacks was stressed by Fisher and Cameron (1953) and by Yates and Hutchinson (1961) and has been amply confirmed. Attacks indicating ischaemia in the distribution of one carotid artery are often referred to as episodes of carotid insufficiency, those involving the brain stem as vertebro-basilar insufficiency.

Denny-Brown (1951) suggested that the attacks often resulted from episodic hypotension, but Kendell and Marshall (1963) failed to reproduce attacks in affected individuals by lowering the blood pressure on a tilt table. Millikan et al. (1955), Fisher (1959), and Ross Russell (1961, 1963) suggested that the attacks are usually due to recurrent micro-embolism arising from mural thrombi developing upon atheromatous plaques in major vessels in the neck and observed such emboli in the retinal arteries in some cases. That this is the commonest cause of such episodes which are often due to carotid or vertebral stenosis is now well-recognized and the emboli may consist of platelets (McBrien *et al.*, 1963) or cholesterol (David *et al.*, 1963); the consistency of the symptomatology of the attacks seems to be due to the fact that blood flow in the major vessels is laminar so that emboli derived from the same thrombus or crumbling plaque ultimately reach the same peripheral intracranial vessel. Sometimes the attacks may result, alternatively, from 'steal' phenomena (Ross Russell and Green, 1971) [p. 315] or from episodes of cardiac arrhythmia (McAllen and Marshall, 1973). A bruit in the neck may be a useful indication of arterial stenosis but the absence of such a bruit does not exclude a surgically treatable stenosis and four-vessel angiography carried out by catheterization of the aortic arch is usually indicated and is relatively safe in such cases (Marshall, 1971).

The incidence of such episodes has been estimated at between 0.3 and 1.3 per 1,000 individuals in the population per year. Various publications (Baker *et al.*, 1968; Whisnant *et al.*, 1973 *a*; Toole *et al.*, 1975; Hutchinson and Acheson, 1975) have estimated the incidence of subsequent stroke in such cases at between 12 and 62 per cent, occurring from 12 to 30 months after the onset; occasionally the episodes develop for the first time after a stroke but this is uncommon. The attacks cease spontaneously in about 50 per cent of cases within 1–3 years; the prognosis is worse in patients under 65 than in those who are older, a fact which underlines the importance of investigation of younger patients who present in this way.

SYNDROMES OF THE CEREBRAL ARTERIES

Obstruction of a cerebral artery gives rise to a clinical picture which depends upon loss of function of the parts of the brain supplied by the vessel. This, of course, is influenced by the exact point at which the obstruction occurs, since blockage at the origin of a vessel may lead to loss of function of a larger region than is the case when the obstruction is situated more distally or involves only a single branch. However, as already mentioned, obstruction to a small perforating artery may have more profound and permanent effects (as these are end-arteries) than may proximal occlusion of a major trunk as the latter can be compensated for by meningeal arterial anastomoses. Variations in the clinical picture are also produced by the variability of the distribution of the arteries. As a result of the importance of the collateral circulation, obstruction of either the vertebral or the internal carotid artery may intensify symptoms due to obstruction of the other (Hutchinson and Yates, 1956).

The Internal Carotid Artery

Angiography [FIG. 78] has taught us much about the symptoms of occlusion of the internal carotid artery. There may be no symptoms. At the other extreme the hemiplegia may be complete almost at its onset—the 'completed stroke'. Progressive obliteration of the lumen by atheroma often causes recurrent transitory disturbances due to localized cerebral ischaemia, e.g. epilepsy, aphasia, confusion, or contralateral paraesthesiae or weakness, 'stuttering hemiplegia' terminating in a persistent hemiplegia. There may also be transitory amblyopia in the ipsilateral eye ('amaurosis fugax'). Transient ischaemic attacks may occur repeatedly within the territory of the internal carotid artery without a stroke resulting. Finally, a stroke may develop slowly over hours or a day or two—the 'stroke-in-evolution'. Unilateral frontal headache may occur with any of these. The symptoms of complete occlusion depend upon the adequacy of the collateral circulation through the circle of Willis and external carotid artery, and may include contralateral homonymous hemianopia, hemiplegia, and loss of spatial and discriminative sensibility on the opposite side of the body, and, when the lesion is on the left side, aphasia, both receptive and expressive.

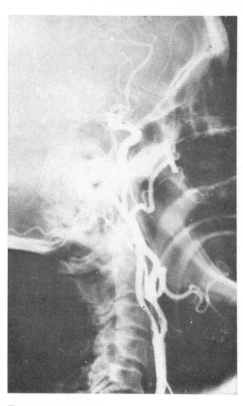

Symptoms of severe damage to the hemisphere suggest that thrombosis may have extended into the middle cerebral artery. The internal carotid pulse may be diminished or lost but the pulse in the neck may be difficult to distinguish from that of the external carotid artery and palpation with a finger in the lateral wall of the pharynx behind the tonsillar fossa is a safer guide. When the internal carotid artery is occluded, facial and orbital pulses may be accentuated (Fisher, 1970 a) and there may be a haemo-dynamic bruit over the contralateral internal carotid (Fisher, 1957). A bruit on the side of the lesion may be a useful guide to the presence of stenosis at or near the origin of the vessel, a lesion often associated with transient ischaemic attacks [FIG. 78] but Ziegler et al. (1971) found stenosis in the absence of a bruit in 73 per cent of cases and a bruit without stenosis in 10 per cent. Thermography of the supraorbital region indicating in-creased flow through supraorbital branches of the external carotid artery has been found by some workers to be a useful guide to the presence of internal carotid artery occlusion (Austin and Sajid, 1966; Mawdsley et al., 1968; Gross and Popham,

FIG. 78. Left carotid arteriogram demonstrating stenosis at the origin of the internal carotid artery. (From Walton, J. N. (1966) *Essentials of Neuro-logy*, 2nd ed. By kind permission of Pitman Medical Publishing Co. Ltd., London.)

1969). Ophthalmodynamometry (Heyman *et al.*, 1957) and electroencephalo-graphy may give useful information, and the angiogram is characteristic.

Occlusion of the ophthalmic branch of the internal carotid, if it extends into the central retinal artery, may give unilateral blindness; a perforating branch of the posterior communicating usually supplies the subthalamic nucleus (body of Luys) and an infarct here, seen usually in the elderly, usually gives contra-lateral hemiballismus. Thrombosis of the anterior choroidal artery is rare but may give contralateral hemiplegia and hemianalgesia; it is more often asympto-matic (Toole and Patel, 1974).

The Anterior Cerebral Artery

This long vessel may undergo occlusion at a number of different points with a corresponding variety of symptoms. The following are the most important of these:

Obstruction at its origin, proximal to Heubner's Artery. This causes hemiplegia on the opposite side together with sensory loss of the cortical type in the paralysed lower limb. When the lesion is on the left side there is in addition expressive aphasia, and apraxia on the left, non-paralysed side. This last symptom is due to interruption in the corpus callosum of fibres running from the left supramarginal gyrus to the right precentral gyrus.

Obstruction of Heubner's Artery. Since this artery supplies part of the frontal lobe, together with the anterior limb of the internal capsule, its obstruction leads to paralysis of the face, tongue, and upper limb on the opposite side, movements at the proximal joints of the limb being more affected than those at the distal joints. In addition, when the lesion is on the left side there is often expressive aphasia.

Obstruction distal to Heubner's Branch. This leads to hemiplegia on the opposite side, the weakness being most marked in the lower limb. In addition, there is often forced grasping and groping in the affected upper limb.

Obstruction of the Paracentral Artery. This is the branch of the anterior cerebral artery which supplies the paracentral lobule containing the cortical centres for movements of the lower limb. The result of this lesion is a crural spastic monoplegia on the opposite side, with or without sensory loss of the cortical type in the affected lower limb. Angiography may demonstrate obstruction of the anterior cerebral artery.

Obstruction of both Anterior Cerebral Arteries. This syndrome which not infrequently follows operation upon aneurysms of the anterior communicating artery, is characterized by profound dementia and apathy with variable long-tract signs and often incontinence. Bilateral grasp reflexes may be present and in the most severe cases the clinical picture resembles that of 'akinetic mutism' (Freemon, 1971).

The Middle Cerebral Artery

Obstruction of the middle cerebral artery at its origin [FIG. 79] causes hemiplegia with sensory loss on the opposite side. Lhermitte *et al.* (1968) suggest that the commonest cause is embolism and that thrombosis is relatively uncommon. The weakness is most marked in the face, tongue, and upper limb. When the lesion is on the left side there is also expressive aphasia and an impairment of the comprehension of spoken and written speech. Obstruction of the frontal branch which is distributed to the inferior frontal gyrus causes severe expressive aphasia with little or no weakness, except possibly of the face and tongue on the opposite side. Obstruction of the middle cerebral artery distal to this branch causes hemiplegia of the opposite side, the weakness being most marked in the upper limb, but speech disturbances are slight or absent. Obstruction of the parietal and temporal branches, when the lesion is on the left side, causes marked aphasia of the conduction type, with disturbance of comprehension of heard and written speech, and sometimes jargon aphasia. In addition, there may be a contralateral homonymous visual field defect (Lascelles and Burrows, 1965). Occlusion of small perforating branches has been thought by Fisher to cause small infarcts in the internal capsule giving rise to lacunes which

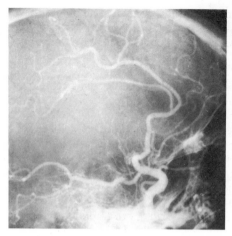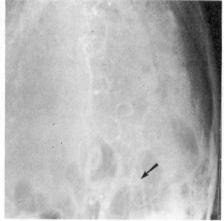

FIG. 79. Left carotid arteriogram (lateral view on right, anteroposterior view on left) showing total
occlusion of the trunk of the middle cerebral artery close to its origin

may be associated either with a 'pure sensory stroke' (contralateral hemianaesthesia) or a 'pure motor hemiplegia' (without sensory loss), though the
latter syndrome may also result from pontine infarction (Fisher *et al.*, 1974).

The Posterior Cerebral Artery

This artery supplies the visual cortex of the occipital lobe. Its occlusion, therefore, causes contralateral homonymous hemianopia, sometimes with 'macular
sparing' [p. 73]. If the obstruction is proximal to the supply to the thalamus
the thalamic syndrome may develop. Ischaemia of the left occipital lobe may
cause visual agnosia.

The Basilar and Vertebral Arteries

Complete obstruction of the main trunk of the basilar artery is usually rapidly
fatal. It leads to impairment of consciousness, small fixed pupils, pseudobulbar
palsy, and quadriplegia, but sensation may escape (Kubik and Adams, 1946;
Biemond, 1951). Incomplete obstruction of the vertebrobasilar arterial system,
however, is much commoner and may lead to a variety of transitory or permanent disorders of brain-stem function, including deafness, vertigo, drop-
attacks, ophthalmoplegia, ataxia, nystagmus, and bilateral dysaesthesiae over
the body and bilateral corticospinal tract signs (vertebrobasilar insufficiency).
Symonds and Mackenzie (1957) suggest that bilateral loss of vision from cerebral
infarction is due to embolism or thrombus in the basilar at or close to its bifurcation. Thrombi in this region may also cause occlusion of the posterior thalamo-
subthalamic paramedian artery, giving bilateral infarction of periventricular
grey matter around the posterior part of the third ventricle and of the upper
midbrain and part of the thalamus; clinically akinetic mutism is the usual
consequence (Segarra, 1970) ('*the syndrome of the mesencephalic artery*'). This
clinical state [see p. 1159] must be distinguished from the so-called '*locked-in
syndrome*' (Kemper and Romanul, 1967) which results from massive pontine
infarction, again often due to basilar artery occlusion; in this condition, the

patient, though tetraparetic and mute, may be alert and able to signal by means of voluntary eye movement. Small lacunar infarcts in the pons due to occlusion of single perforating branches of the basilar (Fisher and Caplan, 1971) have been noted to cause either a '*pure motor hemiplegia*' or the so-called '*dysarthria-clumsy hand syndrome*' (Fisher, 1967).

Many eponymous syndromes of brain-stem infarction due to occlusion of branches (especially perforating branches) of the vertebral and basilar arteries have been described and have been reviewed by Minderhoud (1971). Most are now included in the syndrome of vertebrobasilar insufficiency (Williams and Wilson, 1962). Some, however, occur with sufficient frequency to deserve separate identification. Hühn (1969) suggested that these include Weber's syndrome, Claude's syndrome, the Millard–Gubler syndrome, Foville's syndrome, and, most consistent of all, the lateral medullary syndrome of Wallenberg (see below).

Weber's syndrome (a unilateral third nerve palsy and contralateral hemiplegia) and *Claude's syndrome* (a unilateral third nerve palsy with ipsilateral tremor and contralateral hemiplegia) usually result from infarction of one cerebral peduncle and (in Claude's syndrome) one red nucleus, supplied by a branch of the posterior cerebral artery. The *Millard–Gubler syndrome* (unilateral sixth and seventh nerve palsy and contralateral hemiparesis) and the *Foville syndrome* (unilateral facial palsy with paralysis of conjugate gaze to the affected side with a contralateral hemiplegia) result from pontine infarction due to occlusion of perforating branches of the basilar. *Occlusion of the internal auditory artery* is another uncommon but identifiable syndrome giving acute severe vertigo, with unilateral deafness and tinnitus (Millikan *et al.*, 1959). Much less common are the syndromes of *Avellis* (ninth and tenth nerve palsy with contralateral hemiparesis and hemianaesthesia), *Babinski-Nageotte* (ataxia, Horner's syndrome, and contralateral hemiparesis), *Schmidt* (ninth, tenth, and eleventh nerve palsies with contralateral hemiparesis), and *Hughlings Jackson* (eleventh and twelfth nerve palsies and contralateral hemiplegia). Hühn (1969) and Minderhoud (1971) found that most patients with brain stem infarction did not present with manifestations of any of these so-called classical syndromes.

Occlusion of the *superior cerebellar artery* causes ipsilateral ataxia and sometimes choreiform movements and occasionally contralateral hemianalgesia. Massive cerebellar infarction sometimes gives rise to oedema sufficient to cause brain stem compression and a clinical picture simulating a posterior fossa tumour (Lehrich *et al.*, 1970).

Within recent years it has been noted that occlusion of the first part of one subclavian artery may result in a syndrome in which exercise of the affected arm induces retrograde flow of blood down the ipsilateral vertebral artery in order to supply the arm, thus effectively 'stealing' blood from the brain stem. In this '*subclavian steal syndrome*' (Mannock *et al.*, 1961; North *et al.*, 1962; Patel and Toole, 1965) there is often a bruit over the affected subclavian artery and the pulse and blood pressure in the affected arm are reduced when compared with the normal side. Symptoms of vertebrobasilar insufficiency (vertigo, transient bilateral blindness, syncope, and even olfactory hallucinations (Cameron and Wright, 1964)) may occur spontaneously or on exercising the affected arm. Similar symptoms may occur when one vertebral artery is occluded in the neck (Fisher, 1970 *b*).

The *lateral medullary syndrome of Wallenberg* has usually been attributed to obstruction of the posterior inferior cerebellar artery. It is probably more often due to thrombosis of one vertebral artery. In either case there is a characteristic clinical picture which results from infarction of a wedge-shaped area of the lateral aspect of the medulla and the inferior surface of the cerebellum. The onset of thrombosis is associated with severe vertigo, and hiccup and vomiting may occur. There is often dysphagia and, in some cases, pain or paraesthesiae, such as a sensation of hot water running over the face, may be referred to the trigeminal area on the affected side. There is some degree of cerebellar deficiency, with nystagmus, hypotonia, and inco-ordination on the side of the lesion. Ipsilateral paralysis of the soft palate, pharynx, and vocal cord results from involvement of the nucleus ambiguus. Horner's syndrome—myosis, enophthalmos, and ptosis—is present on the affected side. Dissociated sensory loss occurs, though its distribution is somewhat variable. Usually analgesia and thermo-anaesthesia are present on the face on the same side as the lesion and on the trunk and limbs on the opposite side. This is due to involvement of the spinal tract and nucleus of the trigeminal nerve and of the spinothalamic tract respectively. The sensory loss on the face may be confined to the first, or to the first and second, divisions of the nerve, since these regions are represented in the lowest part of the spinal nucleus, which may alone be supplied by the posterior inferior cerebellar artery. Persistent neuralgic pain in the face, on the side of the lesion, and sometimes in the limbs and trunk on the opposite side, and dysphagia are not uncommonly troublesome sequelae of this vascular lesion.

Diffuse Cerebral Atherosclerosis

Many cases of progressive dementia attributed in the past to cerebral atherosclerosis have undoubtedly been due to other forms of diffuse degenerative brain disease such as presenile dementia. Nevertheless, repeated episodes of cerebral infarction giving areas of softening of greater or lesser extent, sometimes unilateral but more often bilateral, may undoubtedly give rise to progressive impairment of memory and intellectual function, often accompanied by epileptic attacks, variable signs of focal brain damage, and ultimately an irreversible dementia with incontinence. When this syndrome results primarily from atheroma (large vessel disease) deterioration usually occurs in a step-like manner, in that each stroke tends to leave more evidence of mental and physical deterioration. Depending upon the areas of brain involved, dysarthria, aphasia, apraxia, hemiparesis, and other focal symptoms and signs may occur. Bilateral frontal lobe infarction may cause severe apraxia of gait, bilateral grasp reflexes, dementia, and incontinence. In such cases, deterioration often follows general anaesthesia.

The syndrome of pseudobulbar palsy (spastic dysarthria, brisk jaw and snout reflexes, and pathological overemotionalism with inappropriate laughter and crying) may occur as a late consequence of multiple bilateral infarcts as described above, but is more often seen in the slowly progressive syndrome of cerebral atherosclerosis, often without clinical evidence of actual minor strokes, which results from multiple small areas of softening occurring deep within the hemispheres and resulting from small vessel disease associated with severe hypertension. This syndrome has sometimes been called 'atherosclerotic Parkinsonism' as the patients show a slow, shuffling gait (marche à petits pas), usually with bilateral spasticity and rigidity of the limbs with extensor plantar responses; some degree of dementia is usual but facial masking and other stigmata of Parkinsonism are absent.

Accessory Investigations

The cerebrospinal fluid is usually normal except after an acute infarct, when the protein may be raised up to 100–200 mg per 100 ml for two or three weeks, and the fluid may be xanthochromic at first. There may also be a pleocytosis including a moderate excess of polymorphonuclear cells. Polymorphonuclear leucocytes are found more often in cases of intracranial haemorrhage and in haemorrhagic infarction than in patients with ischaemic infarcts (Sörnäs et al., 1972). The ECG is often abnormal but the abnormality is more often due to concomitant myocardial damage and hypertension than to any central effect caused by the cerebral infarct (Tomkin et al., 1968). The serum uric acid and serum triglycerides are often raised in patients with strokes (Pearce and Aziz, 1969, 1970). Moderate increases in serum and CSF creatine phosphokinase, aldolase, and lactic dehydrogenase occur but are less striking than those found in patients with intracranial haemorrhage (Wolintz et al., 1969). Norepinephrine and other catecholamines are also raised in the serum and CSF of patients with strokes, but again the rise is substantially greater in haemorrhage than infarction (Meyer et al., 1973). Electroencephalography may yield evidence of focal or diffuse lesions. Williams and Wilson (1962) and Phillips (1964) have drawn attention to the frequency of temporal lobe abnormalities in the EEG in basilar insufficiency.

Gamma-encephalography is of some value in diagnosis, in that a focal abnormality due to an infarct is likely to improve with the passage of time, while that due to a tumour will usually become worse. The EMI scan is also likely to prove of increasing value in the diagnosis and localization of infarcts. By far the greatest information, however, is likely to be derived from cerebral angiography which often reveals evidence of arterial occlusion or stenosis not previously diagnosed accurately on clinical grounds (Bull et al., 1960; Acheson et al., 1969; Weibel and Fields, 1969). Aortic arch catheterization is necessary in order to demonstrate the major vessels in the neck, while direct injection of the common carotid arteries is still the best method of revealing the detail of the intracranial vessels, especially if magnification and subtraction techniques are used. While the risks of the investigation are low in skilled hands, the examination should never be undertaken lightly, and much will depend upon the age and condition of the patient and the information which is likely to be derived from the examination. Angiography is usually indicated in young patients with strokes but should be employed more sparingly in the elderly. Its purpose is first to exclude a tumour, aneurysm, or angioma whose effects may be mimicking those of an infarct, secondly to exclude an intracranial haematoma, thirdly to demonstrate an arterial stenosis or occlusion which may be amenable to surgical or to some other form of treatment, and fourthly to give evidence relating to the collateral circulation if a vessel is occluded.

DIAGNOSIS

Cerebral atheroma commonly presents in one of four ways: (1) as a focal cerebral lesion of sudden onset; (2) as a focal cerebral lesion of insidious onset; (3) with remittent and recurrent symptoms; and (4) with diffuse and progressive symptoms.

1. *A focal cerebral lesion of sudden onset*, leading, for example, to hemiplegia, may be due to atheromatous occlusion of a large artery. This may be simulated by cerebral haemorrhage due to hypertension, or from a ruptured aneurysm or

M

angioma invading the substance of a cerebral hemisphere. Coma is more likely to be present, and, if present, deeper in cerebral haemorrhage than in cerebral infarction, unless the internal carotid artery is occluded. Severe hypertension favours haemorrhage. The cerebrospinal fluid is a valuable guide since it is likely to contain some red cells, as well as a raised protein, immediately after a cerebral haemorrhage, while if the haemorrhage has also reached the subarachnoid space the blood will be visible to the naked eye. Clinical evidence of a cardiac lesion may suggest that the infarct is embolic. When there is doubt whether a focal cerebral lesion is ischaemic or haemorrhagic the question can usually be settled by an EMI scan and/or angiography.

An intracranial tumour rarely causes sudden focal symptoms; when this does occur it is generally due to oedema and papilloedema is often present. Transient hemiplegia of sudden onset may occur in migraine, when the diagnosis rests upon its association with the familiar symptoms of migraine and the rapid recovery without residual symptoms or signs. General paresis is a rare cause of sudden hemiplegia. Very rarely a single lesion will develop in multiple sclerosis sufficiently suddenly to suggest a vascular lesion. Dissecting aneurysm of the aorta is a cause of sudden cerebral ischaemia. The lesions may be diffuse and will be accompanied by chest pain, and, usually, hypotension.

When it has been established that a lesion is ischaemic, and is associated with local vascular disease, it is usually easy to establish the cause. The diagnosis of atheroma will rest upon the age of the patient, the presence of atheroma elsewhere, particularly the retinal arteries, a bruit, if present, the absence of any other cause of vascular disease, and in some cases the presence of another predisposing disorder, e.g. diabetes or myxoedema. A syphilitic endarteritis will be associated with the characteristic changes in the cerebrospinal fluid and blood. Tuberculous endarteritis is the sequel of tuberculous meningitis. The rarer causes of arterial disease, such as polyarteritis nodosa and giant cell (temporal) arteritis can be diagnosed only through their systemic manifestations.

2. *Focal cerebral lesions of insidious onset.* Ischaemic brain disease, especially atheroma of one internal carotid artery, may cause a progressive focal lesion of gradual onset which it may be difficult to distinguish from a neoplasm. Conversely a glioma in an elderly atheromatous subject sometimes progresses so rapidly, and with so little evidence of increased intracranial pressure, that it closely simulates a cerebral vascular lesion. A third condition which may enter into the diagnosis is a chronic subdural haematoma. In such cases the diagnosis can often be made only with the help of accessory methods of investigation, such as an EMI scan or angiogram.

3. *Lesions producing remittent and recurrent symptoms.* Cerebral atheroma may lead to recurrent episodes of disturbance of cerebral function within the territory of a single artery (transient ischaemic attacks), or successive lesions involving different parts of the brain. These syndromes are unlikely to be confused with any other condition, but occasionally sensory Jacksonian epilepsy due to a glioma may simulate the former, while multiple metastatic neoplasms may produce symptoms resembling those of multiple vascular lesions. Recurrent epileptic attacks may be the sole manifestation of previous asymptomatic infarction, and other causes of epilepsy of late onset then have to be excluded. The rare 'pulseless disease' (Takayashu's disease) may cause intermittent cerebral ischaemia. This is an inflammatory arteritis of the aortic arch, occurring usually in young women and giving rise to progressive occlusion of those arteries which arise from the aortic arch.

4. *Lesions producing diffuse and progressive symptoms.* The failure of the intellectual powers and impairment of memory, characteristic of diffuse atheromatosis of the smaller cerebral vessels (multi-infarct dementia), may simulate dementia due to any other cause [see p. 1181]. General paresis is distinguished by the appropriate serological and other tests. In the absence of symptoms of increased intracranial pressure it may be difficult to exclude an intracranial tumour as the cause of dementia of insidious onset. Pneumo-encephalography is often helpful and in establishing the diagnosis of presensile dementia. 'Atherosclerotic Parkinsonism' needs to be distinguished from paralysis agitans [see p. 587] and some of the rarer degenerative cerebral diseases of the second half of life may also simulate cerebral atherosclerosis.

PROGNOSIS

The prognosis of cerebral ischaemia due to atheroma depends upon a number of factors, the chief among which are the age of the patient, the adequacy of the collateral circulation, the extent and degree of the atheromatous degeneration within the brain, the condition of the circulation as a whole, and the presence or absence of other metabolic disturbances, such as diabetes, renal disease, etc.

It may be difficult to assess the prognosis of a focal ischaemic lesion during the first two or three days after the onset. When the lesion is within the territory of the internal carotid artery, the greater the extent of the area of cerebral damage the worse the outlook. Unconsciousness, and the association of sensory loss and hemiplegia are bad prognostic signs. A small focal lesion in any part of the brain, however, is a less serious affair than evidence of a large infarct. An elderly patient may live for years after a small focal lesion, even hemiplegia, with no recurrence. Adams and Merrett (1961) reviewed the literature on the prognosis of cerebrovascular disease and themselves studied a series of 736 hemiplegics. Their figures showed that the expectation of life after a stroke is greatly shortened, being less than half the normal for people of the same age. They divided their patients into those who recovered in the sense of either becoming fully independent or were able to walk but handicapped by a useless arm, and those who failed to improve appreciably after three months of intensive treatment. They found that in the latter group a patient's chance of being able to get about and look after himself was little better than that of becoming a relatively helpless invalid. Age, however, did not in itself preclude a good recovery nor did a lesion of the dominant hemisphere. Adams and Hurwitz (1963) made a useful analysis of the associated defects of cerebral function which were held to be responsible for the failure to respond to treatment. These include defects of comprehension and various forms of apraxia and agnosia.

In an even more detailed survey based upon their personal experience and a thorough review of the literature, Hutchinson and Acheson (1975) found an immediate mortality of 30 per cent in cases of stroke in the first month. Long-term mortality at five years was 35–45 per cent; between 25 and 50 per cent of patients suffered recurrent strokes. Mortality and long-term prognosis were adversely influenced by the presence of hypertension which was the single most important adverse factor which emerged from a careful analysis, although an abnormal ECG was also significantly associated with the tendency to have a second or subsequent stroke. However, they found only minimal evidence that the arterial site of ischaemia influenced the prognosis; those with episodes involving the vertebro-basilar system did marginally better than those in whom the first stroke occurred in the territory of the internal carotid artery.

The clinical picture of diffuse cerebral ischaemia is insidiously progressive with or without focal exacerbations over a period of several years. In the terminal stage the patient is bedridden, with a variable degree of dementia, with or without hemiplegia, pseudobulbar palsy, 'arteriosclerotic Parkinsonism', or similar physical concomitants. Death occurs either in coma from cerebral infarction, from some intercurrent disease, or from cardiac infarction (Baker et al., 1968).

TREATMENT

When a patient is comatose or semicomatose as the result of an ischaemic stroke, the usual measures necessary in the management of the unconscious patient are required [p. 1170]. Recent evidence suggests that in severe strokes in which it can be presumed that the infarct is associated with oedema of the affected hemisphere, treatment with steroids (dexamethasone 5 mg four times daily) as employed in cerebral oedema due to any cause [p. 291] may reduce mortality and improve the prognosis (Patten et al., 1972). Other workers (Meyer et al., 1971 a) suggest, again in severe cases, that intravenous (1·2 g per kg body weight) or oral (1·5 g per kg) glycerol may have a similar effect. Vasodilator drugs have been widely employed in the treatment of stroke but it is generally agreed that they have little if any observable effect if given after a single episode of cerebral infarction. However, cyclandelate 200 mg four times daily given over a four-month period was shown to produce a significant improvement in mental function and brain circulation time in elderly patients many of whom were presumed to have diffuse cerebral vascular disease (Ball and Taylor, 1967) and this drug was shown to increase blood flow in patients with cerebrovascular disease by O'Brien and Veall (1966). Hexobendine, which is a potent cerebral vasodilator in animals has been shown, when given in a dosage of 15–40 mg intravenously, to produce a significant increase in regional cerebral blood flow and also to give some clinical improvement in patients with ischaemic cerebrovascular disease (Meyer et al., 1971 b; McHenry et al., 1972); the effect of oral medication with this remedy is still uncertain, but the view that such agents are worthless is no longer tenable (McHenry, 1972).

The role of anticoagulant therapy in cerebral ischaemic disorders has been a source of controversy for many years (Marshall and Shaw, 1959; Hill et al., 1960; Carter, 1964; Marshall, 1968; Toole and Patel, 1974). It is now generally agreed that these drugs are of no value in the treatment of a completed stroke, and although some workers continue to use them in cases of 'stroke-in-evolution', in an attempt to restrict extension of the thrombotic process and thus of the infarct, in such cases, too, their use has been largely abandoned. The principal risk is that of mistaking a small haemorrhage or a haemorrhagic infarct for an ischaemic infarct as it is only in the latter type of case that these drugs would be likely to be successful. Even after full investigation including CSF examination (in an attempt to detect red cells), angiography, and/or an EMI scan, diagnosis cannot always be certain. However, there is still general agreement that anticoagulant therapy, given for a minimum of six months and more often for two years or more, is effective in many cases of transient cerebral ischaemia, both in abolishing the attacks and in preventing a completed stroke (Millikan, 1971; Whisnant et al., 1973 b; Toole and Patel, 1974). Hence this treatment is to be recommended in patients with transient ischaemic attacks in whom an arterial stenosis inaccessible to surgery has been demonstrated or in whom no evident cause has been found; even in such cases the treatment is only likely to be successful if micro-emboli of platelets and not cholesterol are causing the attacks. Heparin is not usually required for long-term treatment; the drugs most commonly employed are phenindione or warfarin, and the dose must be regulated in order to reduce the prothrombin to about 10 per cent of normal. Aspirin 600 mg daily, which has an anticoagulant effect, has been shown to reduce attacks of amaurosis fugax (Harrison *et al.*, 1971); the role of drugs such as dipyridamole, 25–50 mg three times daily, which reduce platelet aggregation, has yet to be evaluated in such cases. When there is hypercholesterolaemia, clofibrate 500 mg three times a day may be of theoretical benefit but rarely gives clinical improvement.

There is also general agreement that hypotensive drugs are of little value in the immediate management of the acute stroke, although the potential risk of increasing ischaemia by sudden lowering of the blood pressure has probably been overestimated, and if the pressure is reduced gradually, the CVR [p. 316] is reduced and the CBF rises (Meyer *et al.*, 1968). There is, however, good evidence that the effective control of hypertension substantially improves the prognosis in stroke survivors (Carter, 1970; Beevers *et al.*, 1973; Hutchinson and Acheson, 1975).

Within recent years, operations upon the large arteries in the neck have been carried out increasingly, sometimes in an attempt to relieve the effects of a completed stroke, but much more often in order to relieve transient ischaemic attacks. Without doubt surgical disobliteration of the occluded segment of the affected subclavian artery will abolish the symptoms of the 'subclavian steal' syndrome, and carotid endarterectomy, first performed by Rob and Eastcott (Eastcott *et al.*, 1954) in a case of recurring amaurosis fugax and contralateral hemiparesis, has been widely used in the treatment of stenosis of the internal carotid artery, especially when there is a circumscribed atheromatous plaque close to the bifurcation (Edwards *et al.*, 1960; Edwards and Gordon, 1962; Dickinson *et al.*, 1964; Morris, 1968). Crawford and de Bakey (1963) reported impressive results following operation upon the carotid, innominate, subclavian, and vertebral arteries in over 1,000 cases. However, few controlled series have been reported, and those that have have not shown the results of surgical treatment to be immeasurably superior to those achieved by other methods (Fields *et al.*, 1970; *The Lancet*, 1974). However, in skilled hands, the mortality and morbidity of endarterectomy is small and while operation now seems to be contra-indicated in cases of completed stroke, the removal of accessible stenotic lesions in patients with frequent transient ischaemic attacks is in general preferable to long-term anticoagulant therapy in most cases though each must be considered individually in the light of the patient's age, general condition, and clinical presentation.

Finally, the invaluable role of physiotherapy, occupational therapy, and other methods of rehabilitation must be stressed (Hurwitz and Adams, 1972; Millard, 1973). Exercise, re-education, the provision where appropriate of walking aids, toe-raising springs or calipers and other appliances, adaptation to the home and domestic environment, speech therapy in the aphasic, anticonvulsant drugs in the management of post-hemiplegic epilepsy, antibiotics for the management of complications, attention to diet and vitamin intake in the confused elderly subject and instruction of relatives and home-helps, all these and many more are invaluable. With appropriate and intensive treatment, many patients with strokes, of whatever age, can be helped to resume a useful life in society despite residual disability. Many problems may require to be resolved relating to employment, driving of motor vehicles, hostel or hospital residential care, and the like, but can only be determined in the light of the patient's progress and the doctor's experience of similar cases.

CEREBRAL EMBOLISM

AETIOLOGY AND PATHOLOGY

Embolism of a cerebral artery is a complication of many disorders which possess in common the opportunity for blood clot, or, less frequently, other material, to enter the circulation in such a way that it can reach the brain. Retracing the circulation backwards from the brain we find that the nearest sources of a thrombus are the internal carotid, vertebral, and common carotid arteries. In rare cases of thrombosis of the right subclavian artery due to pressure by a cervical rib, the thrombus has extended into the right common carotid and a detached portion has been carried to the brain (Symonds, 1927). A clot may come also from an aneurysm of the innominate artery or of the aorta or from mural thrombosis on an atheromatous ulcer in this vessel and cholesterol emboli may be dislodged during cardiac surgery (Price and Harris, 1970). A vegetation may become detached from the aortic or mitral valves in bacterial endocarditis. The left ventricle may be the source of an embolus, following coronary thrombosis, when a clot forms on the endocardium over the infarcted area or when aneurysm of the ventricle results. In auricular fibrillation, whether due to mitral stenosis or to some other cause, a clot may form in the atrium and in such cases detachment of the clot may occur spontaneously or may follow the restoration of the normal cardiac rhythm by means of quinidine. This may also occur in auricular flutter or after mitral valvulotomy. Even in cases of rheumatic heart disease without endocarditis, transient visual obscurations presumed to be due to micro-embolism, perhaps from small thrombi on a roughened valve, have been described (Swash and Earl, 1970) and embolism may also result from 'mute' juvenile endocarditis (Reske-Nielsen et al., 1965). An important but rare cause of cerebral embolism, usually occurring in young women, is atrial myxoma (Maroon and Campbell, 1969; Price et al., 1970; Schwarz et al., 1972); in such cases the presence of a cardiac murmur which varies with time and with changing body position is a useful sign and it is important to be aware of this possibility as many myxomas can be removed surgically. Episodes of cerebral embolism of undetermined origin have also been described in young women taking oral contraceptives (Enzell and Lindemalm, 1973) and as a consequence of a prolapsing mitral valve.

The source of the thrombus may be in the lung, when thrombosis of a pulmonary vein occurs. Infected emboli from the lungs are the cause of cerebral abscess complicating pulmonary infection, and tumour cells may pass in the same way from the lung to the brain. The lung capillaries constitute a filter which protects the general circulation from emboli of any size derived from the systemic veins. Fat globules, however, may pass through the pulmonary circulation and so reach the brain after fracture of one of the long bones (Larson, 1968). A patent interatrial septum short-circuits the pulmonary capillary filter and provides a route by which emboli from the systemic veins can in very exceptional circumstances reach the brain—*paradoxical embolism*.

The arteries of the left side of the brain are the site of embolism more frequently than those of the right, and the left middle cerebral is the vessel most often affected. The point at which the embolus lodges depends upon its size. A large clot may be arrested in the internal carotid. A small one may pass to a cortical branch of one of the main arteries. Following the lodgement of an embolus thrombosis usually occurs in the vessel and may spread distally, or less frequently proximally, and infarction occurs in the area of brain deprived of its blood supply [see p. 327]. When the embolus is infected, meningitis or cerebral abscess may subsequently develop, or, when the infection is of low virulence, embolism may be followed by infective softening of the vessel wall and aneurysm formation. Such mycotic aneurysms may rupture into the subarachnoid space or into the brain [see pp. 356–7].

SYMPTOMS

The onset of the symptoms of cerebral embolism with blood clot is usually extremely sudden, the lodgement of the embolus occurring more rapidly than either cerebral haemorrhage or thrombosis. However, cases of less sudden onset, resembling that of 'stroke-in-evolution', have been described (Fisher and Pearlman, 1967). Loss of consciousness is not very common, but the patient is usually somewhat dazed. A convulsion may occur at the onset, and there is sometimes headache. The nature of the focal symptoms depends upon the vessel in which the embolus becomes impacted [see p. 331]. After the onset of embolism there may be a gradual increase in the severity of the symptoms due to spasm of the vessel or the development of oedema or the proximal extension of thrombosis. On the other hand, symptoms may diminish in severity owing to the embolus becoming dislodged and passing on peripherally.

Fat Embolism. Fat embolism causes symptoms after a latent interval lasting from hours to days following the injury. Restlessness, tachycardia, precordial pain, and dyspnoea are the symptoms of fat embolism of the lungs, and when the fat reaches the brain insomnia, disorientation, and delirium occur, passing into stupor or coma, with signs of cortical irritation or paralysis. The patient is usually pyrexial, petechial haemorrhages may be present, especially on the chest and neck, and fat may be found in the urine.

DIAGNOSIS

See page 337.

PROGNOSIS

The immediate mortality of cerebral embolism is 7–10 per cent. There is always the risk that embolism of other organs may occur and the prognosis of the condition causing the embolism must be taken into consideration. As shock passes off and the oedema of the infarcted area of the brain diminishes, the extent and severity of the symptoms grow less, and the patient is finally left with such disabilities as result from destruction of the region of the brain supplied by the obstructed artery. Epilepsy is a not uncommon sequel.

TREATMENT

Hypotension, if present, should be treated. Wright and McDevitt (1954) stress the prophylactic value of anticoagulants for patients with heart disease who are liable to embolism, otherwise treatment of the cerebral lesion is the same as that of cerebral infarction from any cause. Carter (1957) also found anti-coagulants of value [see p. 340] but they should not be used when the embolus is due to infective endocarditis. Adams *et al.* (1974) in a long-term follow-up of cases of mitral stenosis over 20 years have shown conclusively that long-term anticoagulant therapy greatly reduces the risks of recurrent cerebral embolism.

When the source of emboli can be identified with confidence and when the causal condition can be eradicated, appropriate treatment (often surgical) is indicated as soon as the patient's condition permits. Phenoxybenzamine 1 mg per kg body weight intravenously or other vasodilator drugs have been recommended in the acute stage and this treatment, combined with intravenous low molecular weight dextran and surface cooling (hypothermia) have been recommended in cases of fat embolism, combined with assisted positive pressure respiration when necessary (Larson, 1968).

REFERENCES

(Cerebral atheromatosis, Syndromes of the cerebral arteries, Cerebral embolism.)

ACHAR, V. S., COE, R. P. K., and MARSHALL, J. (1966) Echoencephalography in the differential diagnosis of cerebral haemorrhage and infarction, *Lancet*, **i**, 161.

ACHESON, J., BOYD, W. N., HUGH, A. E., and HUTCHINSON, E. C. (1969) Cerebral angiography in ischemic cerebrovascular disease, *Arch. Neurol. (Chic.)*, **20**, 527.

ACHESON, R. M., and FAIRBAIRN, A. S. (1970) Burden of cerebrovascular disease in the Oxford area in 1963 and 1964, *Brit. med. J.*, **2**, 621.

AD HOC COMMITTEE, NATIONAL ADVISORY COUNCIL OF THE NATIONAL INSTITUTE OF NEUROLOGICAL DISEASES AND BLINDNESS (1958) *Neurology (Minneap.)*, **8**, Supplement.

ADAMS, G. F., and HURWITZ, L. J. (1963) Mental barriers to recovery from strokes, *Lancet*, **ii**, 533.

ADAMS, G. F., and MERRETT, J. W. (1961) Prognosis and survival in the aftermath of hemiplegia, *Brit. med. J.*, **1**, 309.

ADAMS, G. F., MERRETT, J. D., HUTCHINSON, W. M., and POLLOCK, A. M. (1974) Cerebral embolism and mitral stenosis: survival with and without anticoagulants, *J. Neurol. Neurosurg. Psychiat.*, **37**, 378.

ADAMS, R. D. (1954) Mechanisms of apoplexy as determined by clinical and pathological correlation, *J. Neuropath. exp. Neurol.*, **13**, 1.

ANDERSON, A. G., LOCKHART, R. D., and SOUTER, W. C. (1931) Lateral syndrome of the medulla, *Brain*, **54**, 460.

ANDERSON, T. W., and MacKAY, J. S. (1968) A critical reappraisal of the epidemiology of cerebrovascular disease, *Lancet*, **i**, 1137.

AUSTIN, J. H., and SAJID, M. H. (1966) Direct thermometry in ophthalmic-internal carotid blood flow, *Arch. Neurol. (Chic.)*, **15**, 376.

AUSTIN, J. H., and STEARS, J. C. (1971) Familial hypoplasia of both internal carotid arteries, *Arch. Neurol. (Chic.)*, **24**, 1.

BAKER, R. N., RAMSEYER, J. C., and SCHWARTZ, W. (1968) Prognosis in patients with transient cerebral ischemic attacks, *Neurology (Minneap.)*, **18**, 1157.

BALL, J. A. C., and TAYLOR, A. R. (1967) Effect of cyclandelate on mental function and cerebral blood flow in elderly patients, *Brit. med. J.*, **3**, 525.

BAUER, R. B., SHEEHAN, S., and MEYER, J. S. (1961) Arteriographic study of cerebrovascular disease. II. Cerebral symptoms due to kinking, tortuosity and compression of carotid and vertebral arteries in the neck, *Arch. Neurol. (Chic.)*, **4**, 119.

BEEVERS, D. G., FAIRMAN, M. J., HAMILTON, M., and HARPUR, J. E. (1973) Antihypertensive treatment and the course of established cerebral vascular disease, *Lancet*, **i**, 1407.

BICKERSTAFF, E. R. (1964) Aetiology of acute hemiplegia in childhood, *Brit. med. J.*, **2**, 82.

BICKERSTAFF, E. R. (1975) *Neurological Complications of Oral Contraceptives*, Oxford.

BIEMOND, A. (1951) Thrombosis of the basilar artery and vascularization of the brain stem, *Brain*, **74**, 300.

BRICE, J. G., DOWSETT, D. J., and LOWE, R. D. (1964) Haemodynamic effects of carotid artery stenosis, *Brit. med. J.*, **2**, 1363.

BULL, J. W. D., MARSHALL, J., and SHAW, D. A. (1960) Cerebral angiography in the diagnosis of the acute stroke, *Lancet*, **i**, 562.

CAMERON, W. J., and WRIGHT, I. S. (1964) Subclavian steal syndrome with olfactory hallucinations, *Ann. intern. Med.*, **61**, 128.

CARTER, A. B. (1957) The immediate treatment of cerebral embolism, *Quart. J. Med.*, **26**, 335.

CARTER, A. B. (1964) *Cerebral Infarction*, Oxford.

CARTER, A. B. (1970) Hypotensive therapy in stroke survivors, *Lancet*, **i**, 485.

CRAWFORD, E. S., and DE BAKEY, M. E. (1963) *Surgical Treatment of Stroke by Arterial Reconstructive Operation*, in *Clinical Neurosurgery*, ed. Mosberg, W. H., p. 150, London.

CRITCHLEY, M. (1929) Arteriosclerotic Parkinsonism, *Brain*, **52**, 23.

CROSS, J. N., CASTRO, P. O., and JENNETT, W. B. (1968) Cerebral strokes associated with pregnancy and the puerperium, *Brit. med. J.*, **3**, 214.

DALAL, P. M., SHAH, P. M., AIYAR, R. R., and KIKANI, B. J. (1968) Cerebrovascular diseases in West Central India. A report on angiographic findings from a prospective study, *Brit. med. J.*, **3**, 769.

DAVID, N. J., KLINTWORTH, G. K., FRIEDBERG, S. J., and DILLON, M. (1963) Fatal atheromatous cerebral embolism associated with bright plaques in the retinal arterioles, *Neurology (Minneap.)*, **13**, 709.

DAVISON, C., GOODHART, S. P., and SAVITSKY, N. (1935) The syndrome of the superior cerebellar artery and its branches, *Arch. Neurol. Psychiat. (Chic.)*, **33**, 1143.

DENNY-BROWN, D. (1951) The treatment of recurrent cerebrovascular symptoms and the question of 'vasospasm', *Med. Clin. N. Amer.*, **35**, 1457.

DENNY-BROWN, D. (1960) Recurrent cerebro-vascular episodes, *Arch. Neurol. (Chic.)*, **2**, 194.

DICKINSON, P. H., HANKINSON, J., and MARSHALL, M. (1964) Internal carotid artery stenosis, *Brit. J. Surg.*, **51**, 703.

EASTCOTT, H. H. G., PICKERING, G. W., and ROB, C. G. (1954) Reconstruction of internal carotid artery in a patient with intermittent attacks of hemiplegia, *Lancet*, **ii**, 994.

EDWARDS, C. H., and GORDON, N. S. (1962) Surgical treatment of narrowing of the internal carotid artery, *Brit. med. J.*, **1**, 1289.

EDWARDS, C. H., GORDON, N. S., and ROB, C. G. (1960) The surgical treatment of internal carotid artery occlusion, *Quart. J. Med.*, **29**, 67.

EISENBERG, H., MORRISON, J. T., SULLIVAN, P., and FOOTE, F. M. (1964) Cerebrovascular accidents, *J. Amer. med. Ass.*, **189**, 883.

ENZELL, K., and LINDEMALM, G. (1973) Cryptogenic cerebral embolism in women taking oral contraceptives, *Brit. med. J.*, **4**, 507.

FIELDS, W. S., MASLENIKOV, V., MEYER, J. S., HASS, W. K., REMINGTON, R. D., and MACDONALD, M. (1970) Joint study of extracranial arterial occlusion, *J. Amer. med. Ass.*, **211**, 1993.

FISHER, C. M. (1957) Cranial bruit associated with occlusion of the internal carotid artery, *Neurology (Minneap.)*, **7**, 299.

FISHER, C. M. (1959) Observations of the fundus oculi in transient monocular blindness, *Neurology (Minneap.)*, **9**, 333.

FISHER, C. M. (1967) A lacunar stroke: the dysarthria-clumsy hand syndrome, *Neurology (Minneap.)*, **17**, 614.

FISHER, C. M. (1969) The arterial lesions underlying lacunes, *Acta neuropath. (Berl.)*, **12**, 1.

FISHER, C. M. (1970 a) Facial pulses in internal carotid artery occlusion, *Neurology (Minneap.)*, **20**, 476.

FISHER, C. M. (1970 b) Occlusion of the vertebral arteries causing transient basilar symptoms, *Arch. Neurol. (Chic.)*, **22**, 13.

FISHER, C. M., and CAMERON, D. G. (1953) Case report: concerning cerebral vasospasm, *Neurology (Minneap.)*, **3**, 468.

FISHER, C. M., and CAPLAN, L. R. (1971) Basilar artery branch occlusion: a cause of pontine infarction, *Neurology (Minneap.)*, **21**, 900.

FISHER, C. M., MOHR, J. P., and ADAMS, R. D. (1974) in *Harrison's Principles of Internal Medicine*, 7th ed., p. 1749, New York.

FISHER, C. M., and PEARLMAN, A. (1967) The nonsudden onset of cerebral embolism, *Neurology (Minneap.)*, **17**, 1025.

FREEMON, F. R. (1971) Akinetic mutism and bilateral anterior cerebral artery occlusion, *J. Neurol. Neurosurg. Psychiat.*, **34**, 693.

GRAHAM, D. I., and ADAMS, H. (1972) 'Idiopathic' thrombosis in the vertebrobasilar artery system in young men, *Brit. med. J.*, **1**, 26.

GROSS, M., and POPHAM, M. (1969) Thermography in vascular disorders affecting the brain, *J. Neurol. Neurosurg. Psychiat.*, **32**, 484.

GUNNING, A. G., PICKERING, G. W., ROBB-SMITH, A. H. T., and RUSSELL, R. (1964) Mural thrombosis of the internal carotid artery and subsequent embolism, *Quart. J. Med.*, **33**, 155.

HARRISON, M. J. G., MARSHALL, J., MEADOWS, J. C., and RUSSELL, R. W. R. (1971) Effect of aspirin in amaurosis fugax, *Lancet*, **ii**, 743.

HARTMAN, J. D., YOUNG, I., BANK, A. A., and ROSENBLATT, S. A. (1971) Fibromuscular hyperplasia of internal carotid arteries. Stroke in a young adult complicated by oral contraceptives, *Arch. Neurol. (Chic.)*, **25**, 295.

HEYMAN, A., KARP, H. R., and BLOOR, B. M. (1957) Determination of retinal artery pressures in diagnosis of carotid artery occlusion, *Neurology (Minneap.)*, **7**, 97.

HILL, A. B., MARSHALL, J., and SHAW, D. A. (1960) A controlled clinical trial of long-term anticoagulant therapy in cerebro-vascular disease, *Quart. J. Med.*, **29**, 597.

HUGHES, J. T., and BROWNELL, B. (1968) Traumatic thrombosis of the internal carotid artery in the neck, *J. Neurol. Neurosurg. Psychiat.*, **31**, 307.

HUGHES, W. (1965) Origin of lacunes, *Lancet*, **ii**, 19.

HÜHN, A. (1969) in *Die zerebralen Durchblutungsstörungen des Erwachsenenalters*, p. 303, Stuttgart.

HUMPHREY, J. G., and NEWTON, T. H. (1960) Internal carotid occlusion in young adults, *Brain*, **83**, 565.

HURWITZ, L. J., and ADAMS, G. F. (1972) Rehabilitation of hemiplegia: indices of assessment and prognosis, *Brit. med. J.*, **1**, 94.

HUTCHINSON, E. C., and ACHESON, E. J. (1975) *Strokes: Natural History, Pathology and Surgical Treatment*, London.

HUTCHINSON, E. C., and YATES, P. O. (1956) The cervical portion of the vertebral artery: a clinico-pathological study, *Brain*, **79**, 319.

INMAN, W. H. W., and VESSEY, M. P. (1968) Investigation of deaths from pulmonary, coronary, and cerebral thrombosis and embolism in women of child-bearing age, *Brit. med. J.*, **2**, 193.

JOHNSON, K. G., YANO, K., and KATO, H. (1967) Cerebral vascular disease in Hiroshima, Japan, *J. Chron. Dis.*, **20**, 545.

KANE, W. C., and ARONSON, S. M. (1969) Cerebrovascular disease in an autopsy population. I. Influence of age, ethnic background, sex, and cardiomegaly upon frequency of cerebral hemorrhage, *Arch. Neurol. (Chic.)*, **20**, 514.

KEMPER, T. L., and ROMANUL, F. C. A. (1967) State resembling akinetic mutism in basilar artery thrombosis, *Neurology (Minneap.)*, **17**, 74.

KENDELL, R. E., and MARSHALL, J. (1963) Role of hypotension in the genesis of transient focal cerebral ischaemic attacks, *Brit. med. J.*, **2**, 344.

KUBIK, C. S., and ADAMS, R. D. (1946) Occlusion of the basilar artery—a clinical and pathological study, *Brain*, **69**, 73.

KUDO, T. (1968) Spontaneous occlusion of the circle of Willis. A disease apparently confined to Japanese, *Neurology (Minneap.)*, **18**, 485.

KURTZKE, J. F. (1969) *Epidemiology of Cerebrovascular Disease*, Berlin, Heidelberg, New York.

THE LANCET (1974) Carotid endarterectomy and T.I.A.s, *Lancet*, **i**, 51.

LARSON, A. G. (1968) Treatment of cerebral fat-embolism with phenoxybenzamine and surface cooling, *Lancet*, **ii**, 250.

LASCELLES, R. G., and BURROWS, E. H. (1965) Occlusion of the middle cerebral artery, *Brain*, **88**, 85.

LEHRICH, J. R., WINKLER, G. D., and OJEMANN, R. G. (1970) Cerebellar infarction with brain stem compression: diagnosis and surgical treatment, *Arch. Neurol. (Chic.)*, **22**, 490.

LHERMITTE, F., GAUTIER, J. C., DEROUESNÉ, C., and GUIRAUD, B. (1968) Ischemic accidents in the middle cerebral artery territory: a study of the causes in 122 cases, *Arch. Neurol. (Chic.)*, **19**, 248.

McALLEN, P. M., and MARSHALL, J. (1973) Cardiac dysrhythmia and transient cerebral ischaemic attacks, *Lancet*, **i**, 1212.

McBRIEN, D. J., BRADLEY, R. D., and ASHTON, W. (1963) The nature of retinal emboli in stenosis of the internal carotid artery, *Lancet*, **i**, 697.

McHENRY, L. C. (1972) Cerebral vasodilator therapy in stroke, *Stroke*, **3**, 686.

McHENRY, L. C., JAFFE, M. E., WEST, J. W., COOPER, E. S., KENTON, E. J., KAWAMURA, J., OSHIRO, T., and GOLDBERG, H. I. (1972) Regional cerebral blood flow and cardiovascular effects of hexobendine in stroke patients, *Neurology (Minneap.)*, **22**, 217.

MANNOCK, J. A., SUTER, L. G., and HUME, D. M. (1961) The 'subclavian steal' syndrome, *J. Amer. med. Ass.*, **182**, 254.

MAROON, J. C., and CAMPBELL, R. L. (1969) Atrial myxoma: a treatable cause of stroke, *J. Neurol. Neurosurg. Psychiat.*, **32**, 129.

MARQUARDSEN, J. (1969) The natural history of acute cerebrovascular disease. A retrospective study of 769 patients, *Acta neurol. scand.*, suppl. **38**.

MARSHALL, J. (1968) *The Management of Cerebrovascular Disease*, 2nd ed., London.

MARSHALL, J. (1971) Angiography in the investigation of ischaemic episodes in the territory of the internal carotid artery, *Lancet*, **i**, 719.

MARSHALL, J., and SHAW, D. A. (1959) Anticoagulant therapy in cerebrovascular disease, *Proc. roy. Soc. Med.*, **52**, 547.

MAWDSLEY, C., SAMUEL, E., SUMERLING, M. D., and YOUNG, G. B. (1968) Thermography in occlusive cerebrovascular diseases, *Brit. med. J.*, **3**, 521.

MERRITT, H., and FINLAND, M. (1930) Vascular lesions of the hindbrain (lateral medullary syndrome), *Brain*, **53**, 290.

MEYER, J. S., CHARNEY, J. Z., RIVERA, V. M., and MATHEW, N. T. (1971 *a*) Treatment with glycerol of cerebral oedema due to acute cerebral infarction, *Lancet*, **ii**, 993.

MEYER, J. S., KANDA, T., SHINOHARA, Y., FUKUUCHI, Y., SHIMAZU, K., ERICSSON, A. G., and GORDON, W. H. (1971 *b*) Effect of hexobendine on cerebral hemispheric blood flow and metabolism. Preliminary clinical observations concerning its use in ischemic cerebrovascular disease, *Neurology (Minneap.)*, **21**, 691.

MEYER, J. S., SAWADA, T., KITAMURA, A., and TOYODA, M. (1968) Cerebral blood flow after control of hypertension in stroke, *Neurology (Minneap.)*, **18**, 772.

MEYER, J. S., STOICA, E., PASCU, I., SHIMAZU, K., and HARTMANN, A. (1973) Catecholamine concentrations in CSF and plasma of patients with cerebral infarction and haemorrhage, *Brain*, **96**, 277.

MILLARD, J. B. (1973) Medical rehabilitation and hemiplegia, *Proc. roy. Soc. Med.*, **66**, 1003.

MILLIKAN, C. H. (1971) Reassessment of anticoagulant therapy in various types of occlusive cerebral vascular disease, *Stroke*, **2**, 201.

MILLIKAN, C. H., SIEKERT, R. G., and SHICK, R. N. (1955) Studies in cerebrovascular disease. III. Use of anticoagulant drugs in treatment of insufficiency or thrombosis within basilar arterial system, *Mayo Clin. Proc.*, **30**, 116. V. Use of anticoagulant drugs in treatment of intermittent insufficiency of internal carotid system, *Mayo Clin. Proc.*, **30**, 578.

MILLIKAN, C. H., SIEKERT, R. G., and WHISNANT, J. P. (1959) The syndrome of occlusion of the labyrinthine division of the internal auditory artery, *Trans. Amer. Neurol. Ass.*, **84,** 11.

MINDERHOUD, J. M. (1971) Diagnostic significance of symptomatology in brain stem ischaemic infarction, *Europ. Neurol.*, **5,** 343.

MORRIS, W. R. (1968) Long-term results of carotid artery surgery. A report of 65 cases, *Guy's Hosp. Rep.*, **117,** 225.

NORTH, R. R., FIELDS, W. S., DE BAKEY, M. E., and CRAWFORD, E. S. (1962) Brachio-basilar insufficiency syndrome, *Neurology (Minneap.)*, **12,** 810.

O'BRIEN, M. D., and VEALL, N. (1966) Effect of cyclandelate on cerebral cortex perfusion-rates in cerebrovascular disease, *Lancet*, **ii,** 729.

PATEL, A., and TOOLE, J. F. (1965) Subclavian steal syndrome—reversal of cephalic blood flow, *Medicine*, **44,** 289.

PATTEN, B. M., MENDELL, J., BRUUN, B., CURTIN, W., and CARTER, S. (1972) Double-blind study of the effects of dexamethasone on acute stroke, *Neurology (Minneap.)*, **22,** 377.

PEARCE, J., and AZIZ, H. (1969) Uric acid and plasma lipids in cerebrovascular disease. Part 1: Prevalence of hyperuricaemia, *Brit. med. J.*, **4,** 78.

PEARCE, J., and AZIZ, H. (1970) Uric acid and serum lipids in cerebrovascular disease. Part 2: Uric acid–plasma lipid correlations, *J. Neurol. Neurosurg. Psychiat.*, **33,** 88.

PHILLIPS, B. M. (1964) Temporal lobe changes associated with the syndromes of basilar vertebral insufficiency: an electroencephalographic study, *Brit. med. J.*, **2,** 1104.

POÓR, G., and GÁCS, G. (1974) The so-called 'Moyamoya disease', *J. Neurol. Neurosurg. Psychiat.*, **37,** 370.

PRICE, D. L., and HARRIS, J. (1970) Cholesterol emboli in cerebral arteries as a complication of retrograde aortic perfusion during cardiac surgery, *Neurology (Minneap.)*, **20,** 1209.

PRICE, D. L., HARRIS, J. L., NEW, P. F. J., and CANTU, R. C. (1970) Cardiac myxoma: a clinicopathologic and angiographic study, *Arch. Neurol. (Chic.)*, **23,** 558.

RESKE-NIELSEN, E., SVENDSEN, K., and SØGAARD, H. (1965) Cerebral emboli as a result of 'mute' juvenile endocarditis, *Acta path. microbiol. scand.*, **63,** 321.

ROWLANDS, R. A., and WAKELEY, C. P. G. (1941) Fat embolism, *Lancet*, **i,** 502.

RUSSELL, R. W. R. (1961) Observations on the retinal blood vessels in monocular blindness, *Lancet*, **ii,** 1422.

RUSSELL, R. W. R. (1963) Atheromatous retinal embolism, *Lancet*, **ii,** 1354.

RUSSELL, R. W. R., and GREEN, M. (1971) Mechanisms of transient cerebral ischaemia, *Brit. med. J.*, **1,** 646.

SCHOENBERG, B. S., WHISNANT, J. P., TAYLOR, W. F., and KEMPERS, R. D. (1970) Strokes in women of childbearing age: a population study, *Neurology (Minneap.)*, **20,** 181.

SCHWARZ, G. A., SCHWARTZMAN, R. J., and JOYNER, C. R. (1972) Atrial myxoma: cause of embolic stroke, *Neurology (Minneap.)*, **22,** 1112.

SEGARRA, J. M. (1970) Cerebral vascular disease and behavior. I. The syndrome of the mesencephalic artery (basilar artery bifurcation), *Arch. Neurol. (Chic.)*, **22,** 408.

SILVERSTEIN, A., GILBERT, H., and WASSERMAN, L. R. (1962) Hemiplegic complications of polycythaemia, *Ann. intern. Med.*, **57,** 909.

SOLOMON, G. E., HILAL, S. K., GOLD, A. P., and CARTER, S. (1970) Natural history of acute hemiplegia of childhood, *Brain*, **93,** 107.

SÖRNÄS, R., ÖSTLUND, H., and MÜLLER, R. (1972) Cerebrospinal fluid cytology after stroke, *Arch. Neurol. (Chic.)*, **26,** 489.

SWASH, M., and EARL, C. J. (1970) Transient visual obscurations in chronic rheumatic heart-disease, *Lancet*, **ii,** 323.

SYMONDS, C. P. (1927) Cervical rib: thrombosis of subclavian artery. Contralateral hemiplegia of sudden onset, probably embolic, *Proc. roy. Soc. Med.*, **20,** 1244.

SYMONDS, C. P., and MACKENZIE, I. (1957) Bilateral loss of vision from cerebral infarction, *Brain*, **80,** 415.

TAKEUCHI, K. (1961) Occlusive diseases of the carotid artery. Recent advances, *Res. nerv. Syst.*, **5**, 511.

TOMKIN, G., COE, R. P. K., and MARSHALL, J. (1968) Electrocardiographic abnormalities in patients presenting with strokes, *J. Neurol. Neurosurg. Psychiat.*, **31**, 250.

TOMLINSON, B. E. (1959) Brain changes in ruptured intracranial aneurysms, *J. clin. Path.*, **12**, 391.

TOOLE, J. F., JANEWAY, R., CHOI, K., CORDELL, R., DAVIS, C., JOHNSTON, F., and MILLER, H. S. (1975) Transient ischemic attacks due to atherosclerosis: a prospective study of 160 patients, *Arch. Neurol.* (*Chic.*), **32**, 5.

TOOLE, J. F., and PATEL, A. N. (1974) *Cerebrovascular Disorders*, 2nd ed., New York.

TOOLE, J. F., and TUCKER, S. H. (1960) Influence of head position upon cerebral circulation, *Arch. Neurol.* (*Chic.*), **2**, 616.

WEIBEL, J., and FIELDS, W. S. (1969) *Atlas of Arteriography in Occlusive Cerebrovascular Disease*, Philadelphia.

WHISNANT, J. P., FITZGIBBON, J. P., KURLAND, L. T., and SAYRE, G. P. (1971) Natural history of stroke in Rochester, Minnesota, 1945 through 1954, *Stroke*, **2**, 11.

WHISNANT, J. P., MATSUMOTO, N., and ELVEBACK, L. R. (1973 a) Transient cerebral ischaemic attacks in a community, Rochester, Minnesota, 1955 through 1969, *Mayo Clin. Proc.*, **48**, 194.

WHISNANT, J. P., MATSUMOTO, N., and ELVEBACK, L. R. (1973 b) The effect of anticoagulant therapy on the prognosis of patients with transient cerebral ischemic attacks in a community, Rochester, Minnesota, 1955 through 1969, *Mayo Clin. Proc.*, **48**, 844.

WILLIAMS, A. O., RESCH, J. A., and LOEWENSON, R. B. (1969) Cerebral atherosclerosis—a comparative autopsy study between Nigerian Negroes and American Negroes and Caucasians, *Neurology* (*Minneap.*), **19**, 205.

WILLIAMS, D., and WILSON, T. G. (1962) The diagnosis of the major and minor syndromes of basilar insufficiency, *Brain*, **85**, 741.

WOLINTZ, A. H., JACOBS, L. D., CHRISTOFF, N., SOLOMON, M., and CHERNIK, N. (1969) Serum and cerebrospinal fluid enzymes in cerebrovascular disease: creatine phosphokinase, aldolase, and lactic dehydrogenase, *Arch. Neurol.* (*Chic.*), **20**, 54.

WRIGHT, I. S., and McDEVITT, E. (1954) Cerebral vascular diseases, *Ann. intern. Med.*, **41**, 682.

YATES, P. O., and HUTCHINSON, E. C. (1961) Cerebral infarction: the role of stenosis of the extracranial vessels, *Spec. Rep. Ser. med. Res. Coun.* (*Lond.*), No. 300, H.M.S.O.

ZIEGLER, D. K., ZILELI, T., DICK, A., and SEBAUGH, J. L. (1971) Correlation of bruits over the carotid artery with angiographically demonstrated lesions, *Neurology* (*Minneap.*), **21**, 860.

HYPERTENSIVE ENCEPHALOPATHY

Definition. An acute and transitory disturbance of cerebral function which occurs in association with high blood pressure, in acute and chronic glomerulonephritis, malignant hypertension, and eclampsia. The cardinal symptoms are convulsions and focal disturbances, such as amaurosis, aphasia, and hemiplegia.

AETIOLOGY AND PATHOLOGY

The term hypertensive encephalopathy was first used by Oppenheimer and Fishberg (1928) to describe a form of cerebral disturbance occurring in disorders which differ in their pathology but possess a common tendency to cause arterial hypertension. Byrom (1954) has shown that it is the result of constriction of the cerebral arterioles. The commonest pathological finding is oedema of the brain, but this is not always present and since oedema of the brain when due to other causes, such as intracranial tumour, does not necessarily lead to symptoms like those of hypertensive encephalopathy, it seems likely that it is itself a by-product of the pathological process and not the cause of the symptoms. Lead encephalopathy in general resembles hypertensive encephalopathy and may be associated with hypertension, and there is experimental evidence that lead produces vasoconstriction by acting directly upon the smooth muscles of the vessels. Attacks have been described as a consequence of the ingestion of tyramine-containing foods such as cheese in patients taking aminoxidase inhibitors for the treatment of depression and may also occur in paroxysms of hypertension in cases of phaeochromocytoma (see Toole and Patel, 1974).

The age incidence of hypertensive encephalopathy is that of the causal disorders. Acute glomerulonephritis is commonest in childhood, adolescence, and early adult life; chronic glomerulonephritis in the second and third decade; eclampsia during the early part of the child-bearing period; and malignant hypertension in the thirties and forties, though it may occur in childhood or late middle age.

SYMPTOMS

The onset of symptoms is usually subacute, the patient complaining of head-aches of increasing severity, which are often associated with vomiting. Epileptiform convulsions are common and may be followed either by mental confusion or coma. Impairment of vision, or even complete blindness, may occur. This is cortical in origin, for the retina may be normal and during recovery of vision one homonymous pair of visual half-fields may recover before the other. Other focal disturbances include aphasia and hemiparesis.

Arterial hypertension is present in every case, but the blood pressure may not be greatly raised in acute nephritis and eclampsia. A rise in an already high blood pressure frequently heralds the encephalopathy. The retinae usually show bilateral papilloedema with or without the exudative changes of hypertensive retinopathy, depending upon the causal condition. Cervical rigidity, tachycardia, and fever sometimes occur. Jellinek et al. (1964) noted that transient blindness of cortical type was common and pointed out that during this stage the EEG often showed diffuse slow activity, loss or impairment of the alpha rhythm, and absence of the normal 'following' response to photic stimulation. Both renal function and the composition of the urine may be normal except when the encephalopathy complicates acute or chronic renal damage. The pressure of the cerebrospinal fluid is usually increased but its composition is generally normal.

DIAGNOSIS

Hypertensive encephalopathy must be distinguished from uraemia, cerebral vascular lesions such as haemorrhage and thrombosis, and intracranial tumour. In uraemia convulsive phenomena consist usually of myoclonic twitches rather than of epileptiform attacks and amaurosis is rare. Cerebral vascular lesions do not produce such a diffuse picture of cerebral disturbance and are never as transient as the symptoms of encephalopathy. The diagnosis from intracranial tumour may be difficult in the presence of papilloedema, since cerebral tumour may occur in a patient who also has hypertension. When gamma-encephalography and/or an EMI scan are inconclusive, ventriculography may be needed to exclude neoplasm or benign intracranial hypertension, but the symptoms of hypertensive encephalopathy are usually so transient that this is rarely necessary. Examination of the urine and blood pressure will enable convulsions due to encephalopathy complicating acute nephritis in childhood to be distinguished from epilepsy, and in doubtful cases examination of the cerebrospinal fluid will exclude meningitis.

PROGNOSIS

Alarming though the symptoms are, the outlook in hypertensive encephalopathy is on the whole good as to recovery from the cerebral disturbance, though the ultimate outlook depends upon the underlying cause. Most patients recover from encephalopathy complicating acute nephritis and from eclampsia. Even in malignant hypertension the patient may recover from an attack if hypertension is vigorously treated. Severe and frequent convulsions are a bad sign. Recovery from the amaurosis, aphasia, and other focal symptoms is usually complete in a few days.

TREATMENT

Hypotensive drugs may bring an attack of encephalopathy to an end, and usually produce dramatic relief within hours. Intravenous pentolinium (20–200 mg/l) or trimetaphan camsylate (*Arfonad*) (100 mg/l) given by slow intravenous infusion with constant monitoring of the blood pressure, preferably in an intensive care unit, are recommended by Toole and Patel (1974). Impairment of consciousness is due probably to diffuse cerebral arteriolar spasm with resultant cerebral ischaemia but also to cerebral oedema. Thus reduction of oedema with appropriate drugs (e.g. steroids or powerful diuretics such as frusemide, see p. 291) may also be helpful. If the convulsions prove intractable barbiturates or intravenous diazepam are indicated. The treatment appropriate to the causal condition will also be required.

REFERENCES

BYROM, F. B. (1954) The pathogenesis of hypertensive encephalopathy, *Lancet*, **i**, 201.
BYROM, F. B. (1968) The calibre of the cerebral arteries in experimental hypertension, *Proc. roy. Soc. Med.*, **61**, 605.
FINNERTY, F. A. (1972) Hypertensive encephalopathy, *Amer. J. Med.*, **52**, 672.
JELLINEK, E. H., PAINTER, M., PRINEAS, J., and ROSS RUSSELL, R. (1964) Hypertensive encephalopathy with cortical disorders of vision, *Quart. J. Med.*, **33**, 239.
KUNG, P. C., LEE, J. C., and BAKAY, L. (1968) Electron microscopic study of experimental acute hypertensive encephalopathy, *Acta neuropath. (Berl.)*, **10**, 263.
THE LANCET (1965) Pressor attacks during treatment with monoamine-oxidase inhibitors, *Lancet*, **i**, 945.
OPPENHEIMER, B. S., and FISHBERG, A. M. (1928) Hypertensive encephalopathy, *Arch. intern. Med.*, **41**, 264.
SKINHØJ, E., and STRANDGAARD, S. (1973) Pathogenesis of hypertensive encephalopathy, *Lancet*, **i**, 461.
TOOLE, J. F., and PATEL, A. N. (1974) *Cerebrovascular Disorders*, 2nd ed., New York.

INTRACRANIAL ANEURYSM

Definition. A localized dilatation of an intracranial artery which may cause symptoms either through localized pressure upon neighbouring structures, especially cranial nerves, or by sudden rupture leading to subarachnoid haemorrhage.

ANEURYSM OF CONGENITAL ORIGIN
'BERRY' OR SO-CALLED 'CONGENITAL' ANEURYSMS

PATHOLOGY

A congenital abnormality is an important factor in the aetiology of intra-cranial aneurysm. 'Congenital' aneurysms appear to arise, as Turnbull (1914–15) and Forbus (1930) have shown, at a point where there is a deficiency in the media at the point of junction of two of the components of the circle of Willis or at a bifurcation of one of the cerebral arteries. It is now apparent, however, that a medial defect alone is not sufficient to cause aneurysmal formation and that there must be an acquired lesion which breaches the internal elastic

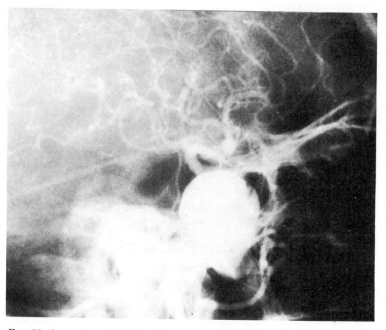

FIG. 80. A very large infraclinoid aneurysm of the right internal carotid artery shown by angiography to be within the cavernous sinus

lamina at the same point, as the latter alone will withstand more than twice the highest recorded arterial blood pressure. This acquired lesion is atheroma which explains why, despite the ubiquity of congenital medial defects in cerebral arteries, aneurysms usually appear and produce their clinical effects in middle life (Carmichael, 1950; Walton, 1956). These aneurysms may be single or multiple, as many as eight having been present in the same individual. They are most frequently encountered on the intracranial course of the internal carotid artery, on the middle cerebral artery, and at the junction of the anterior com-municating with the anterior cerebral arteries, but may occur on any superficial cerebral artery. Only about 10 per cent are in the posterior fossa. They range in size from smaller than a pin's head to 30 mm or more in diameter [FIG. 80]. Microscopically the media is extremely narrow and fibrous, and the elastic and muscular elements are absent. 'Congenital' intracranial aneurysms have occurred in more than one member of the same family (Beumont, 1968; Bannerman *et al.*, 1970) and subarachnoid haemorrhage resulting from the rupture of almost identical aneurysms has been reported in identical twins (Fairburn, 1973). They may be found at any age, even in infancy (Thompson and Pribram, 1969), but more than half first cause symptoms between the ages of 40 and 55 (Fearnsides, 1916) [FIG. 84, p. 358], and they occur almost equally in the two sexes with perhaps a slight predominance in females. Sooner or later most aneurysms rupture, and the extravasated blood may pass into the subarachnoid space or into the substance of the brain, even reaching the ventricles. Rupture into the subdural space (Clarke and Walton, 1953) and even externally to the dura has been observed. Subarachnoid haemorrhage accounts for about 8 per cent of all cases of cerebral vascular disease, and occurs about as often as intracerebral haemorrhage.

The effects of rupture of an aneurysm on the brain have been studied by Tomlinson (1959) and Crompton (1964 *a* and *b*), who stress the frequency of cerebral infarction and of damage to the hypothalamus (Crompton, 1963). 'Congenital' aneurysm often occurs in the absence of raised blood pressure, though it is likely that a rise of blood pressure in later life may be responsible, if not for the formation of the aneurysm, at least for its rupture.

Other congenital vascular abnormalities, such as congenital heart disease, aneurysm or defects of the media of abdominal arteries leading to intraperitoneal haemorrhage, coarctation of the aorta, and cutaneous naevi, have occasionally been observed in patients suffering from intracranial aneurysm which may also co-exist with an intracranial angioma. Intracranial aneurysms are also commonly found in patients with renal polycystic disease.

SYMPTOMS

The symptoms of congenital intracranial aneurysm differ according to whether the patient is observed (1) before rupture, (2) immediately after rupture, or (3) after recovery from the immediate effects of rupture, and (4) angiography may show abnormalities [FIG. 80].

Symptoms before Rupture of the Aneurysm

It is often impossible to diagnose an intracranial aneurysm before rupture occurs, since it may be too small to produce symptoms by compressing structures in its neighbourhood. However, if such symptoms occur, it is frequently possible to make a correct diagnosis. Unless the aneurysm is very large (Bull, 1969), symptoms of increased intracranial pressure do not occur at this stage. Some 25 per cent of patients suffer from recurrent headaches—about half of these from typical migraine. The diagnosis of aneurysm rests upon evidence of focal pressure fairly sharply localized and only slowly, if at all, progressive. The nature of such focal symptoms depends upon the situation of the aneurysm. Aneurysms placed anteriorly in the circle of Willis may compress the optic nerve, leading to unilateral impairment of vision, which may be fluctuating and cause transitory attacks of blindness in one eye, superficially resembling migraine. In such cases optic atrophy and rarely slight papilloedema may be found in the affected eye and exophthalmos may be present. Hemianopia may result from compression of one optic tract, or the chiasm may be compressed (Jefferson, 1937, 1938). Paralysis of the third, fourth, or sixth cranial nerves may occur with or without exophthalmos and pain, sometimes of sudden onset, often with anaesthesia in the cutaneous area supplied by the first division of the trigeminal nerve. This is the characteristic picture which may result from an aneurysm of the internal carotid artery within the cavernous sinus [FIG. 80] (an infraclinoid aneurysm) (Barr *et al.*, 1971) and if sudden expansion occurs there is pain behind the eye. Aneurysms situated on the cortical course of the middle cerebral artery occasionally cause monoplegia or hemiplegia either through direct pressure if they are very large or through ischaemia in the distribution of their parent vessel, and this is the only situation in which an aneurysm is likely to cause convulsions. Aneurysm of the posterior part of the circle of Willis, for example the posterior communicating artery, usually causes paralysis of the third nerve and possibly hemianopia due to compression of the optic tract. An isolated third nerve palsy is not infrequently produced by pressure from an enlarging aneurysm of the internal carotid artery above the cavernous sinus (a supraclinoid aneurysm—FIG. 81). Aneurysms in this situation may rarely cause Raeder's paratrigeminal syndrome (ocular sympathetic

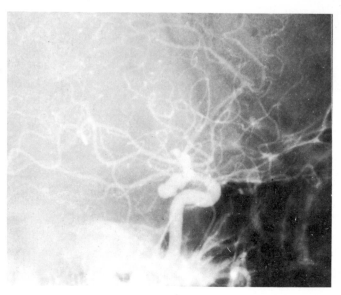

FIG. 81. A supraclinoid aneurysm arising at the junction of the right internal carotid and posterior communicating arteries

paralysis as in Horner's syndrome but without anhidrosis) (Law and Nelson, 1968) or even hypopituitarism if the sella is invaded (Cartlidge and Shaw, 1972). Aneurysm of the posterior cerebral artery may cause crossed hemianopia, owing to coincident thrombosis of the vessel. Aneurysm of the basilar artery [FIG. 82] usually causes conspicuous localizing signs early. There is often a crossed hemiplegia with paresis of some of the cranial nerves originating from the pons on one side, and of the limbs on the opposite side. A somewhat similar picture may be produced by aneurysm of the vertebral artery which, however, is less common; aneurysms on the vertebrobasilar system may produce effects either as a result of direct pressure or by causing ischaemia in the distribution of small arterial branches. Aneurysms of the cerebellar arteries [FIG. 83] rarely give rise to localizing signs.

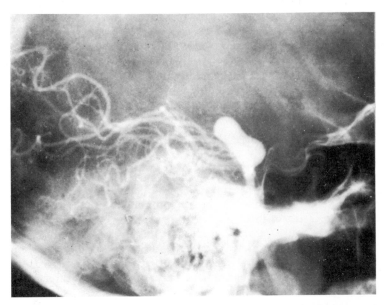

FIG. 82. A large aneurysm at the bifurcation of the basilar artery demonstrated
by vertebral angiography

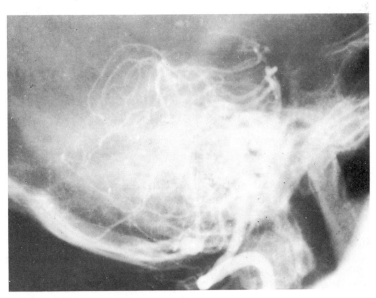

FIG. 83. An aneurysm of a posterior inferior cerebellar artery shown by vertebral
angiography

It may be concluded that whereas large or expanding intracranial aneurysms, and particularly those at the base of the brain (Bull, 1969) may produce localizing signs due to compression of the brain, brain stem, or cranial nerves, many are asymptomatic prior to rupture. Unruptured aneurysms may develop intramural calcification which may be seen on skull radiographs but angiography is necessary for diagnosis and localization (Bull, 1962). Surgical treatment of large aneurysms is often both difficult and unrewarding. Rupture of an aneurysm is the commonest cause of subarachnoid haemorrhage, which is considered on pages 357–67.

EMBOLIC INTRACRANIAL ANEURYSM

Embolic or 'mycotic' aneurysms are rare. They are due to the impaction in a cerebral vessel of an embolus, bearing organisms of low virulence. The aneurysm is the result of infective softening of the vessel wall. More virulent organisms usually cause cerebral abscess or meningitis. The embolus usually lodges in a cortical branch of one or other middle cerebral artery, the right and left being involved with equal frequency. Less often the main trunk of the middle cerebral artery or the anterior cerebral artery is affected. Embolic aneurysms elsewhere in the intracranial circulation are rare. Subacute bacterial endocarditis is the commonest cause of embolic aneurysm, which may rarely result from other chronic forms of septicaemia and pyaemia, including brucellosis. In most cases the aneurysm subsequently ruptures in the same manner as a congenital aneurysm giving subarachnoid haemorrhage.

The lodgement of the embolus often causes a 'stroke' giving hemiplegia or monoplegia. The signs of subacute bacterial endocarditis or of some other pyaemic source for the embolus are usually evident and emboli may occur elsewhere in the body. Treatment of rupture is the same as in subarachnoid haemorrhage due to rupture of a 'berry' aneurysm but in embolic aneurysm the underlying infective condition will also need treatment.

CAROTID CAVERNOUS-SINUS ANEURYSM OR FISTULA

Arteriovenous aneurysm produced by rupture of the internal carotid artery into the cavernous sinus may arise spontaneously or follow head injury with or without skull fracture. Hamby (1966) thinks that 'the majority of spontaneous fistulas develop as a result of rupture of pre-existing aneurysms'. However, many cases follow cranial trauma and angiography fails to demonstrate evidence of any predisposing cause for arterial rupture. The resulting clinical picture is distinctive, consisting of unilateral pulsating exophthalmos, with oedema of the eyelids, conjunctivae, and cornea, and sometimes papilloedema. There is a loud systolic murmur, audible to the patient and on auscultation over the eye and temporal region, and suppressible by compression of the ipsilateral carotid artery. There is complete or partial ophthalmoplegia of the affected eye. The other eye may become involved, blood at arterial pressure being carried by the circular sinus to the opposite cavernous sinus. Common carotid ligation is the method of treatment usually employed and, though not without risk it is generally successful. Some fistulae heal spontaneously.

OTHER CAUSES OF INTRACRANIAL ANEURYSM

Other causes of intracranial aneurysms are extremely rare, though examples undoubtedly due to polyarteritis nodosa, to atheroma, and to syphilis have occasionally been described. An atheromatous aneurysm is usually a fusiform dilatation of the internal carotid or basilar artery. The characteristic syphilitic change of the small elastic and muscular arteries, to which group the intra-cranial vessels belong, is an obliterative endarteritis, a fact which probably explains the rarity of syphilitic intracranial aneurysm. Most of the veri-fied syphilitic aneurysms have been situated upon the basilar artery; in these cases, which are now very rare, the usual treatment for syphilis will be required.

SUBARACHNOID HAEMORRHAGE

AETIOLOGY

Subarachnoid haemorrhage may occur as the result of any condition in which there is rupture of one or more blood vessels so placed that the extravasated blood can reach the subarachnoid space. The bleeding may be arterial, capillary, or venous, and its site of origin single or multiple. Head injury, including birth injury, may thus cause subarachnoid haemorrhage. Capillary damage leading to haemorrhage may be present in exceptionally acute forms of encephalitis or encephalopathy, and subarachnoid haemorrhage may occur as a symptom of haemorrhagic diseases including thrombotic microangiopathy (Heron et al., 1974) or during the use of anticoagulants. Rarely it may be the result of septic or aseptic venous sinus thrombosis or of an intracranial tumour (angioblastic meningioma, glioma, pituitary adenoma, intracranial metastases—particularly of malignant melanoma, Walton, 1956). Choroid plexus papilloma is another rare cause (Ernsting, 1955). It has also been described as a result of an acute hypertensive reaction following the ingestion of cheese in a patient receiving tranylcypromine, one of the group of amine-oxidase inhibitor drugs (Espir and Mitchell, 1963). It has been reported in so-called Moyamoya disease in Chinese patients, secondary to carotid occlusion (Lee and Cheung, 1973). Intracerebral haemorrhage, due to vascular degeneration associated with high blood pressure, may reach the subarachnoid space either by rupture into the ventricular system or, more rarely, to the surface of the brain, or the haemorrhage which enters the subarachnoid space may also invade the brain from an aneurysm or angioma. The chief causes of intracranial subarachnoid haemorrhage are intracranial aneurysm [see p. 351] and angioma [see p. 243], the former being nine or ten times as common as the latter. In a series of 3,042 cases Richardson (1969) found an aneurysm in 1,571, an angioma in 142, a primary intracerebral, cerebellar, or brain stem haemorrhage in 725, and 604 were unexplained. In a small proportion of cases no cause can be found even at autopsy. Spontaneous spinal subarachnoid haemorrhage usually results from an angioma of the spinal cord (Henson and Croft, 1956) or less often from a tumour such as a neurofibroma or an ependymoma of the filum terminale (Walton, 1956; Nassar and Correll, 1968).

Subarachnoid haemorrhage was found in 15 per cent of 200 patients suffering from cerebral vascular disease: its age incidence, and that of its two principal causes, is shown in FIGURE 84. Females are affected slightly more often than males, and about 50 per cent of the patients are normotensive.

In addition to blood in the subarachnoid space, secondary haemorrhages may occur in the brain stem, and spasm of the artery on which the aneurysm is situated may lead to oedema or infarction of the part of the brain which it supplies. Infarction may also result from compression, tearing, or distortion of arteries resulting from subarachnoid haematoma formation within sulci (Tomlinson, 1959).

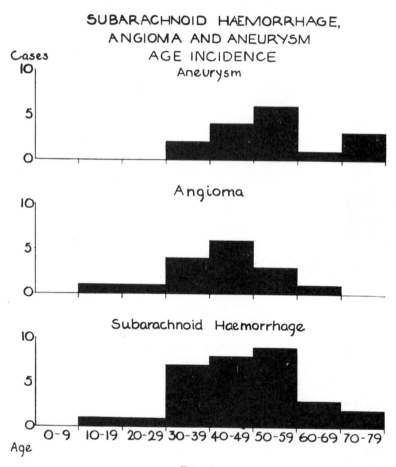

FIG. 84

SYMPTOMS AND SIGNS

When subarachnoid haemorrhage is due to head injury, acute encephalitis or encephalopathy, or rupture of an intracerebral haemorrhage, it usually constitutes a minor part of the total clinical picture. When it is caused by an aneurysm or an angioma it is usually the most prominent and sometimes the sole obvious disturbance. The following account of its symptomatology will therefore be limited to such cases.

The symptoms of cerebral subarachnoid haemorrhage may be divided into: (1) those due to rapidly increasing intracranial pressure with meningeal irritation; (2) focal symptoms; (3) changes in the CSF; and (4) radiographic evidence.

1. The intensity of the symptoms of increasing intracranial pressure varies according to the rapidity and persistence of the haemorrhage. The onset or ictus may occur during physical exertion but in many cases it arises during sleep and it seems likely that effort or a rise in blood pressure may simply precipitate bleeding from an aneurysm or angioma which was about to rupture spontaneously (Walton, 1956). Loss of consciousness occurs rapidly when the leakage is considerable. Vomiting is not uncommon at the onset; convulsions occasionally occur. When coma is deep, the breathing is usually irregular and the pulse slow. The patient may present a picture of profound shock with generalized flaccidity and there may be no cervical rigidity. In less severe cases the patient may not lose consciousness completely, but may pass into a semi-stuporose state, lying in an attitude of general flexion, resenting interference, and confused and irritable when roused. Headache is severe, and the presence of blood in the subarachnoid space produces signs of meningeal irritation, such as cervical rigidity and Kernig's sign. Moderate pyrexia is common at this stage.

Changes are often found in the fundus oculi. Papilloedema is sometimes present, though slight in amount. Unilateral or bilateral retinal haemorrhages occur in some cases and may be accompanied by subhyaloid or vitreous haemorrhages. These have been attributed to the passage of blood from the subarachnoid space of the optic nerves into the eye, but it is more probable that the haemorrhages occur in the eye as the result of acute compression of the central vein of the retina by the blood in the optic sheaths. Fundal changes may be absent when the leaking aneurysm is remote from the optic nerves.

Other signs of subarachnoid haemorrhage include diminution or loss of the tendon reflexes, and of the abdominal reflexes, and extensor plantar responses in the absence of paralysis. Albuminuria and glycosuria occasionally occur while hyperpyrexia and severe transient arterial hypertension may result from damage to hypothalamic centres. Adipsia and hypothermia have been described (Spiro and Jenkins, 1971) as well as other disturbances of hypothalamic-pituitary-adrenal function (Jenkins et al., 1969), and a delay and/or deficiency of thromboplastin generation has been reported (Uttley and Buckell, 1968). A fall in CSF pH, presumed to be due to an increase in CSF lactic acid, is associated with a poor prognosis and there is often evidence of salt and water depletion (Sambrook et al., 1973a and b). Changes in the ECG are common, including peaking of the P and T waves, a short PR interval, a long Q-Tc and tall U waves, and have been shown to be associated with increased urinary catecholamine excretion; excess catecholamine production may be associated with the frequent evidence of arterial spasm found in subarachnoid haemorrhage (Cruickshank et al., 1974). The blood leucocyte count is often raised and a persistent rise in the WBC's to above 10,000/mm³ is associated with a less good prognosis (Neil-Dwyer and Cruickshank, 1974).

2. Focal symptoms are due to compression of neighbouring cranial nerves by blood clot or to invasion of the cerebral hemisphere by the haemorrhage or to cerebral infarction. Visual field defect may occur as a result of compression of the optic nerves, chiasm, or tracts. The third, fourth, and sixth cranial nerves are likely to be compressed if an aneurysm is near the cavernous sinus. Haemorrhage from an aneurysm at the junction of the anterior cerebral and anterior

communicating arteries is apt to invade the frontal lobe and may cause mental impairment, incontinence or, less commonly, urinary retention (Andrew *et al.*, 1966), hemiparesis, and, if on the left side, expressive aphasia. Leakage from an aneurysm on the cortical course of the middle cerebral may cause epileptiform convulsions, and a monoplegia; and rupture of an aneurysm on the cortical course of the posterior cerebral may cause a crossed homonymous hemianopia as a result of haemorrhage into the substance of the occipital lobe or thrombosis of the artery. Leakage from an aneurysm of the basilar artery may lead to quadriplegia or to one of the various forms of 'crossed paralysis'; and head retraction is likely to be conspicuous when the haemorrhage is derived from an aneurysm in the posterior fossa.

Haemorrhage from an intracranial angioma may pass into the neighbouring brain tissue, or into the subarachnoid space, or into both. Subarachnoid haemorrhage seems more likely to occur from a small cortical angioma which has given rise to no other disturbance than from the massive malformations which extend widely and deeply into the white matter. Herpes zoster is an occasional sequel of subarachnoid haemorrhage.

Spinal subarachnoid haemorrhage usually begins with pain in the lower back and lower limbs and sphincter disturbances, with rigidity of the spine and Kernig's sign. Later there may be flaccid weakness of the lower limbs with sensory loss and loss of reflexes. Extension of the haemorrhage to the cerebral subarachnoid space causes headache, cervical rigidity, and other symptoms of intracranial subarachnoid haemorrhage.

3. *The Cerebrospinal Fluid.* Subarachnoid haemorrhage causes characteristic changes in the cerebrospinal fluid, the pressure of which is raised at first. In the first week or more red cells are present, and the supernatant fluid exhibits a yellow coloration which persists for from two to three weeks. The faint coloration of the supernatant fluid which appears within 4–6 hours is due to oxyhaemoglobin while bilirubin first appears within 36–48 hours (Barrows *et al.*, 1955; Roost *et al.*, 1972). The protein content of the fluid is raised, though rarely above 0·1 g per cent. Irritation of the meninges by the extravasated blood leads to a pleocytosis consisting usually of mononuclear cells, though rarely polymorphonuclear cells may be present when the substance of the brain has been invaded. In some cases the colloidal gold curve is 'paretic' in type after a severe haemorrhage. Red cells may disappear from the fluid within a few days but may persist, with xanthochromia, depending upon the severity of the haemorrhage, for as long as 4–6 weeks (Walton, 1956). Metabolic acidosis in the fluid due to presence of red cells (Shannon *et al.*, 1972; Sambrook *et al.*, 1973 *a*) may cause systemic respiratory alkalosis and altered consciousness.

4. *Angiography.* Plain X-rays rarely show evidence of the source of a subarachnoid haemorrhage, though there may be X-ray signs of an angioma [see p. 257] or very rarely an aneurysm may show calcification in its wall [FIG. 85]. Angiography is obligatory in such cases unless the patient's level of consciousness, age, general condition, or neurological status would make surgery impracticable even if the causal lesion were demonstrated. Except in the comatose patient, therefore, bilateral carotid arteriography should be performed as soon as possible after the ictus and if this fails to demonstrate an aneurysm or angioma, vertebral angiography is then indicated. Even if an aneurysm on one carotid tree is shown, it may still be wise to carry out vertebral injection, depending upon the condition of the patient, as many individuals have multiple aneurysms. When multiple lesions are shown, the presence of

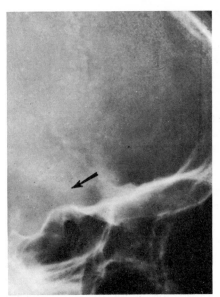 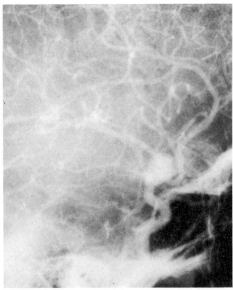

FIG. 85. A lateral radiograph of skull (left) showing curvilinear calcification in the wall of an aneurysm of one middle cerebral artery later demonstrated by angiography (on the right)

arterial spasm may be a valuable guide in indicating which has bled, but this is not always possible and the EEG, though relatively imprecise, may help (Binnie *et al.*, 1969; Margerison *et al.*, 1970). Even with improved radiological techniques, including the use of oblique views, magnification and image intensification, in about 20 per cent of cases no causal lesion is demonstrated though some of these later prove to have aneurysms at autopsy (Richardson, 1969).

DIAGNOSIS

The essence of the clinical picture of subarachnoid haemorrhage is the acute or subacute onset of symptoms of meningeal irritation associated with the presence of blood in the cerebrospinal fluid demonstrated by lumbar puncture. To this extent the diagnosis is usually easy. Meningitis rarely comes on so acutely, and is readily distinguished by examination of the fluid. A lumbar puncture, again, usually enables subarachnoid haemorrhage to be distinguished from other conditions causing coma. But the presence of subarachnoid haemorrhage having been established, it is still necessary to decide its origin. Subarachnoid haemorrhage is occasionally found in exceptionally acute forms of encephalitis, but in such states the blood is likely to be present only in small amounts, and there will be evidence of diffuse lesions of the nervous system. Traumatic subarachnoid haemorrhage is usually easily recognized through the history. Intracerebral haemorrhage, due to vascular degeneration associated with hypertension, may reach the subarachnoid space either by rupture into the ventricular system, or, more rarely, to the surface of the brain. Such patients usually exhibit hemiplegia, which is less common in subarachnoid haemorrhage from an intracranial aneurysm, and a raised blood pressure and arterial degeneration which are not necessarily associated with it. When, however, a cerebral aneurysm bleeds both into the subarachnoid space and into the substance of one hemisphere the clinical picture may be indistinguishable from that of a primary intracerebral haemorrhage which has ruptured into the ventricle. In such a case angiography will often settle the diagnosis by demonstrating the presence, or absence, of an aneurysm. Rupture of an embolic aneurysm may lead to a clinical picture indistinguishable from that which occurs when a congenital aneurysm is responsible for the haemorrhage. The former, however, is usually associated with subacute infective endocarditis, and its embolic origin is often indicated by the sudden development of hemiplegia some time before the onset of the haemorrhage. An angioma is a much less common cause of subarachnoid haemorrhage than an aneurysm; there may be a cranial bruit and angiography will again be diagnostic. The possibility of the rarer causes mentioned on page 357 should also be borne in mind. Finally, in about 20 per cent of all cases of spontaneous subarachnoid haemorrhage, the source of the haemorrhage is not found.

PROGNOSIS

The prognosis of subarachnoid haemorrhage depends upon a number of factors—the size and site of the leakage and whether it can be found and treated surgically, the age of the patient and the condition of the cardiovascular system, especially the presence or absence of hypertension and cerebral athero-sclerosis.

In a review of the literature and an analysis of 312 personal cases not treated surgically, Walton (1956) found a mortality of 45 per cent in the first 8 weeks; about 15 per cent of patients died within the first 48 hours, 15 per cent within 7–14 days as a result of the initial haemorrhage, and 15 per cent from recurrent bleeding of which the peak incidence was in the second week. About 20 per cent of those who survived for 8 weeks subsequently died of recurrent bleeding, half within the first 6 months; of the survivors most were able to pursue some useful activity but about a third were disabled by hemiplegia, epilepsy, headache, or severe neurotic symptoms and fear of recurrence. In general the immediate prognosis of angiomal bleeding is better than that of aneurysmal rupture as many angiomas tend to bleed little and often, except for small angiomas in children which may cause a fatal intracerebral haematoma (Henderson and Gomez, 1967). Sahs et al. (1969), in a national co-operative study in the U.S.A., found that the prognosis was adversely influenced by increasing age, hypertension, the presence of hemiplegia or of other focal neurological signs indicating bleeding into the brain, or concomitant infarction and loss of consciousness. They and Alvord et al. (1972) found that a method of clinical grading of cases was useful in predicting the outcome; thus patients in coma or semicoma consistently did worse, as did those subjected to angiography or surgery too early when vasospasm was often severe and widespread (Weir et al., 1975). Thus it is generally unwise to operate upon a comatose patient except in order to remove an intracerebral haematoma and the time of operation must be carefully judged in each case; if the aneurysm is accessible it is often best to operate (see below) at about 7–14 days when vasospasm is diminishing and if possible before the period when the risk of recurrent bleeding is at its peak.

A rare complication of chronic or recurrent subarachnoid bleeding is super-ficial haemosiderosis of the nervous system which often gives deafness, dementia, cerebellar ataxia, and other progressive neurological signs (Tomlinson and Walton, 1964; Hughes and Oppenheimer, 1967).

TREATMENT

In the medical treatment of subarachnoid haemorrhage it is necessary first to relieve headache with appropriate analgesics such as pethidine 100 mg by mouth or injection as required, and often combined with phenothiazine drugs such as chlorpromazine 50 mg or haloperidol 1-2 mg, which have the effect of sedating the patient while at the same time reducing body temperature, transient hypertension, and cerebral metabolism. Unconscious patients should be treated in the usual way [p. 1170]; antibiotics are often needed to prevent respiratory infection, catheterization may be needed and the airway must be kept patent, but it is rarely, if ever, justifiable to begin assisted respiration if spontaneous breathing ceases as this usually implies irreversible brain-stem damage. Induced hypotension and/or hypothermia have had a vogue but are no longer widely employed because of the risk of infarction (Walton, 1956). However, there is recent evidence that the use of epsilon-aminocaproic acid (0·1 g/kg body weight by mouth or intravenous infusion every four hours) may reduce the risk of recurrent bleeding by inhibiting fibrinolysis (*Today's Drugs*, 1967); tranexamic acid (15-20 mg/kg four hourly in an intravenous infusion) seems to be even more effective (Andersson *et al.*, 1965; Melander *et al.*, 1965; Tovi *et al.*, 1972; Tovi, 1972). Surviving patients, depending upon their disability, often require speech therapy, physiotherapy, and occupational therapy; epilepsy will require appropriate anticonvulsant drugs.

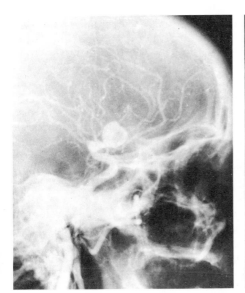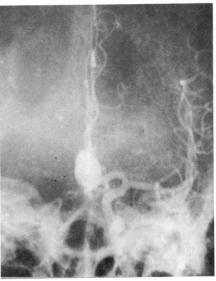

FIG. 86. An aneurysm of the anterior communicating artery

Although it has proved impossible to compare directly the results of surgical treatment of ruptured aneurysms with those of conservative management (Walton, 1956; McKissock and Paine, 1959) a vast literature has now accumulated which indicates without reasonable doubt that whereas surgical treatment carries an appreciable mortality and morbidity, the prognosis of the condition is considerably improved by the judicious application of operative treatment. Carotid ligation or temporary clamping of the vessel (Atkinson, 1975) is often employed in the management of aneurysms on the internal carotid artery (McKissock and Walsh, 1956) but in the acute phase it carries a considerable risk of infarction and may not prevent further bleeding (McKissock *et al.*, 1960; Sahs *et al.*, 1969). Direct intracranial attack upon accessible aneurysms is generally preferred with clipping of the neck (Paterson, 1968). A variety of other surgical techniques have been used including investment of the aneurysm with plastic (Dutton, 1959). The results are better, in experienced hands, in aneurysms on the internal carotid and middle cerebral arteries (McKissock *et al.*, 1962) than in those in the region of the anterior communicating [FIG. 86], and even some aneurysms on the vertebral, basilar and cerebellar vessels can be treated successfully (Dimsdale and Logue, 1959; Drake, 1968); however, satisfactory results have been reported with anterior communicating aneurysms (Logue, 1956; Sengupta, 1975).

Relatively few arteriovenous angiomas can be removed, if these are small and situated in comparatively 'silent' areas of the brain (Paterson and McKissock, 1956), but very rarely these lesions may resolve spontaneously (Levine *et al.*, 1973), presumably due to thrombosis.

REFERENCES

ALVORD, E. C., LOESER, J. D., BAILEY, W. L., and COPASS, M. K. (1972) Subarachnoid haemorrhage due to ruptured aneurysms. A simple method of estimating prognosis, *Arch. Neurol. (Chic.)*, **27**, 273.

ANDERSSON, L., NILSSON, I. M., NILÉHN, J. E., HEDNER, U., GRANSTRAND, B., and MELANDER, B. (1965) Experimental and clinical studies on AMCA, the antifibrinolytically active isomer of p-aminomethyl cyclohexane carboxylic acid, *Scand. J. Haemat.*, **2**, 230.

ANDREW, J., NATHAN, P. W., and SPANOS, N. C. (1966) Disturbances of micturition and defaecation due to aneurysms of anterior communicating or anterior cerebral arteries, *J. Neurosurg.*, **24**, 1.

ATKINSON, W. J. (1975) New approach to management of intracranial aneurysms, *Lancet*, **i**, 5.

BANNERMAN, R. M., INGALL, G. B., and GRAF, C. J. (1970) The familial occurrence of intracranial aneurysms, *Neurology (Minneap.)*, **20**, 283.

BARR, H. W. K., BLACKWOOD, W., and MEADOWS, S. P. (1971) Intracavernous carotid aneurysms. A clinical–pathological report, *Brain*, **94**, 607.

BARROWS, L., HUNTER, T., and BANKER, B. (1955) The nature and clinical significance of pigments in cerebrospinal fluid, *Brain*, **78**, 59.

BEUMONT, P. J. V. (1968) The familial occurrence of berry aneurysm, *J. Neurol. Neurosurg. Psychiat.*, **31**, 399.

BINNIE, C. D., MARGERISON, J. H., and McCAUL, I. R. (1969) Electroencephalographic localization of ruptured intracranial aneurysms, *Brain*, **92**, 679.

BULL, J. W. D. (1962) Contribution of radiology to the study of intracranial aneurysms, *Brit. med. J.*, **2**, 1701.

BULL, J. W. D. (1969) Massive aneurysms at the base of the brain, *Brain*, **92**, 535.

CARMICHAEL, R. (1950) The pathogenesis of non-inflammatory cerebral aneurysms. *J. Path. Bact.*, **62**, 1.

CARTLIDGE, N. E. F., and SHAW, D. A. (1972) Intrasellar aneurysm with subarachnoid hemorrhage and hypopituitarism: case report, *J. Neurosurg.*, **36**, 640.

CLARKE, E., and WALTON, J. N. (1953) Subdural haematoma complicating intracranial aneurysm and angioma, *Brain*, **76**, 378.

CROMPTON, M. R. (1963) Hypothalamic lesions after rupture of cerebral aneurysms, *Brain*, **86**, 301.

CROMPTON, M. R. (1964 *a*) Cerebral infarction following the rupture of cerebral berry aneurysms, *Brain*, **87**, 263.

CROMPTON, M. R. (1964 b) The pathogenesis of cerebral infarction following the rupture of cerebral berry aneurysms, *Brain*, **87**, 491.

CRUICKSHANK, J. M., NEIL-DWYER, G., and BRICE, J. (1974) Electrocardiographic changes and their prognostic significance in subarachnoid haemorrhage, *J. Neurol. Neurosurg. Psychiat.*, **37**, 755.

DANDY, W. E. (1944) *Intracranial Arterial Aneurysms*, Ithaca, N.Y.

DIMSDALE, H., and LOGUE, V. (1959) Ruptured posterior fossa aneurysms and their surgical treatment, *J. Neurol. Neurosurg. Psychiat.*, **22**, 202.

DRAKE, C. G. (1968) The surgical treatment of aneurysms of the basilar artery, *J. Neurosurg.*, **29**, 436.

DUTTON, J. (1959) Acrylic investment of intracranial aneurysms, *Brit. med. J.*, **2**, 597.

ERNSTING, J. (1955) Choroid plexus papilloma causing spontaneous subarchnoid haemorrhage, *J. Neurol. Neurosurg. Psychiat.*, **18**, 134.

ESPIR, M. L. E., and MITCHELL, L. (1963) Tranylcypromine and intracranial haemorrhage, *Lancet*, **ii**, 639.

FAIRBURN, B. (1973) 'Twin' intracranial aneurysms causing subarachnoid haemorrhage in identical twins, *Brit. med. J.*, **1**, 210.

FALCONER, M. A. (1951) The surgical treatment of bleeding intracranial aneurysms, *J. Neurol. Neurosurg. Psychiat.*, **14**, 153.

FEARNSIDES, E. G. (1916) Intracranial aneurysms, *Brain*, **39**, 224.

FORBUS, W. D. (1930) On the origin of miliary aneurysms of the superficial cerebral arteries, *Bull. Johns Hopk. Hosp.*, **47**, 239.

HAMBY, W. B. (1966) *Carotid-cavernous Fistula*, Springfield, Ill.

HENDERSON, W. R., and GOMEZ, R. DE R. L. (1967) Natural history of cerebral angiomas, *Brit. med. J.*, **4**, 571.

HENSON, R. A., and CROFT, P. B. (1956) Spontaneous spinal subarachnoid haemorrhage, *Quart. J. Med.*, **25**, 53.

HERON, J. R., HUTCHINSON, E. C., BOYD, W. N., and ABER, G. M. (1974) Pregnancy, subarachnoid haemorrhage, and the intravascular coagulation syndrome, *J. Neurol. Neurosurg. Psychiat.*, **37**, 521.

HUGHES, J. T., and OPPENHEIMER, D. R. (1967) Superficial siderosis of the central nervous system: a report on nine cases with autopsy, *Acta neuropath. (Berl.)*, **13**, 56.

JEFFERSON, G. (1937) Compression of the chiasma, optic nerves and optic tracts by intracranial aneurysms, *Brain*, **60**, 444.

JEFFERSON, G. (1938) On the saccular aneurysms of the internal carotid artery in the cavernous sinus, *Brit. J. Surg.*, **26**, 267.

JENKINS, J. S., BUCKELL, M., CARTER, A. B., and WESTLAKE, S. (1969) Hypothalamic-pituitary-adrenal function after subarachnoid haemorrhage, *Brit. med. J.*, **4**, 707.

LAW, W. R., and NELSON, E. R. (1968) Internal carotid aneurysm as a cause of Raeder's paratrigeminal syndrome, *Neurology (Minneap.)*, **18**, 43.

LEE, M. L. K., and CHEUNG, E. M. T. (1973) Moyamoya disease as a cause of subarachnoid haemorrhage in Chinese, *Brain*, **96**, 623.

LEVINE, J., MISKO, J. C., SERES, J. L., and SNODGRASS, R. G. (1973) Spontaneous angiographic disappearance of a cerebral arteriovenous malformation: third reported case, *Arch. Neurol. (Chic.)*, **28**, 195.

LOGUE, V. (1956) Surgery in spontaneous subarachnoid haemorrhage. Operative treatment of aneurysms on the anterior cerebral and anterior communicating artery, *Brit. med. J.*, **1**, 473.

MCKISSOCK, W., and PAINE, K. W. E. (1959) Subarachnoid haemorrhage, *Brain*, **82**, 356.

MCKISSOCK, W., RICHARDSON, A., and WALSH, L. (1960) Posterior communicating aneurysms, *Lancet*, **ii**, 1203.

MCKISSOCK, W., RICHARDSON, A., and WALSH, L. (1962) Middle cerebral aneurysms, *Lancet*, **ii**, 417.

MCKISSOCK, W., and WALSH, L. (1956) Subarachnoid haemorrhage due to intracranial aneurysms: results of treatment of 249 verified cases, *Brit. med. J.*, **2**, 559.

MARGERISON, J. H., BINNIE, C. D., and McCAUL, I. R. (1970) Electroencephalographic signs employed in the location of ruptured intracranial arterial aneurysms, *Electroenceph. clin. Neurophysiol.*, **28**, 296.

MELANDER, B., GLINIECKI, G., GRANSTRAND, B., and HANSHOFF, G. (1965) Biochemistry and toxicology of Amikapron; the anti-fibrinolytically active isomer of AMCHA (a comparative study with ε-aminocaproic acid), *Acta pharmacol. toxicol.*, **22**, 340.

NASSAR, S. I., and CORRELL, J. W. (1968) Subarachnoid hemorrhage due to spinal cord tumors, *Neurology (Minneap.)*, **18**, 87.

NEIL-DWYER, G., and CRUICKSHANK, J. (1974) The blood leucocyte count and its prognostic significance in subarachnoid haemorrhage, *Brain*, **97**, 79.

PATERSON, A. (1968) Direct surgery in the treatment of posterior communicating aneurysms, *Lancet*, **ii**, 808.

PATERSON, J. H., and McKISSOCK, W. (1956) A clinical survey of intracranial angiomas with special reference to their mode of progression and surgical treatment: a report of 110 cases, *Brain*, **79**, 233.

RICHARDSON, A. (1969) Subarachnoid haemorrhage, *Brit. med. J.*, **4**, 89.

RIDDOCH, G., and GOULDEN, C. (1925) On the relationship between subarachnoid and intraocular haemorrhage, *Brit. J. Ophthal.*, **9**, 209.

ROOST, K. T., PIMSTONE, N. R., DIAMOND, I., and SCHMID, R. (1972) The formation of cerebrospinal fluid xanthochromia after subarachnoid haemorrhage. Enzymatic conversion of hemoglobin to bilirubin by the arachnoid and choroid plexus, *Neurology (Minneap.)*, **22**, 973.

SAHS, A. L., PERRET, G. E., LOCKSLEY, H. B., and NISHIOKA, H. (1969) *Intracranial Aneurysms and Subarachnoid Hemorrhage. A Co-operative Study*, p. 296, Philadelphia and London.

SAMBROOK, M. A., HUTCHINSON, E. C., and ABER, G. M. (1973 a) Metabolic studies in subarachnoid haemorrhage and strokes. I. Serial changes in acid-base values in blood and cerebrospinal fluid, *Brain*, **96**, 171.

SAMBROOK, M. A., HUTCHINSON, E. C., and ABER, G. M. (1973 b) Metabolic studies in subarachnoid haemorrhage and strokes. II. Serial changes in cerebrospinal fluid and plasma urea electrolytes and osmolality, *Brain*, **96**, 191.

SCHMIDT, M. (1930) Intracranial aneurysms, *Brain*, **53**, 489.

SENGUPTA, R. (1975) Quality of survival following direct surgery of anterior communicating aneurysms, *J. Neurosurg.*, **43**, 58.

SHANNON, D. C., SHORE, N., and KAZEMI, H. (1972) Acid-base balance in hemorrhagic cerebrospinal fluid, *Neurology (Minneap.)*, **22**, 585.

SPIRO, S. G., and JENKINS, J. S. (1971) Adipsia and hypothermia after subarachnoid haemorrhage, *Brit. med. J.*, **3**, 411.

SYMONDS, C. P. (1924–5) Spontaneous subarachnoid haemorrhage, *Quart. J. Med.*, **18**, 93.

THOMPSON, R. A., and PRIBRAM, H. F. W. (1969) Infantile cerebral aneurysm associated with ophthalmoplegia and quadriparesis, *Neurology (Minneap.)*, **19**, 785.

TODAY'S DRUGS (1967) Epsilon aminocaproic acid, *Brit. med. J.*, **4**, 725.

TOMLINSON, B. E. (1959) Brain changes in ruptured intracranial aneurysm, *J. clin. Path.*, **12**, 391.

TOMLINSON, B. E., and WALTON, J. N. (1964) Superficial haemosiderosis of the central nervous system, *J. Neurol. Neurosurg. Psychiat.*, **27**, 332.

TOVI, D. (1972) Studies on fibrinolysis in the central nervous system with special reference to intracranial haemorrhages and to the effect of antifibrinolytic drugs, *Umea University Medical Dissertations*, No. 8.

TOVI, D., NILSSON, I. M., and THULIN, C. A. (1972) Fibrinolysis and subarachnoid haemorrhage. Inhibitory effect of tranexamic acid, *Acta neurol. scand.*, **48**, 393.

TURNBULL, H. M. (1914–15) Alterations in arterial structure, and their relation to syphilis, *Quart. J. Med.*, **8**, 201.

TURNBULL, H. M. (1918) Intracranial aneurysms, *Brain*, **41**, 50.

UTTLEY, A. H. C., and BUCKELL, M. (1968) Biochemical changes after spontaneous subarachnoid haemorrhage. Coagulation and lysis with special reference to recurrent haemorrhage, *J. Neurol. Neurosurg. Psychiat.*, **31**, 621.

WALTON, J. N. (1956) *Subarachnoid Haemorrhage*, Edinburgh.

WECHSLER, I. S., GROSS, S. W., and COHEN, I. (1951) Arteriography and carotid artery ligation in intracranial aneurysm and vascular malformation, *J. Neurol. Neurosurg. Psychiat.*, **14**, 25.

WEIR, B., ROTHBERG, C., GRACE, M., and DAVIS, F. (1975) Relative prognostic significance of vasospasm following subarachnoid hemorrhage, *Canad. J. neurol. Sci.*, **2**, 109.

WOLF, G. A., GOODELL, H., and WOLFF, H. G. (1945) Prognosis of subarachnoid hemorrhage, *J. Amer. med. Ass.*, **129**, 715.

CEREBRAL HAEMORRHAGE

AETIOLOGY AND PATHOLOGY

Intracranial haemorrhage may be venous, capillary, or arterial. Bleeding from ruptured veins traversing the subdural space is the usual cause of subdural haematoma [p. 395] which is generally a consequence of trauma to the head though it sometimes seems to develop spontaneously, especially in patients with liver disease or in those receiving anticoagulants. We are concerned here with haemorrhage into the substance of the brain; bleeding from venous sources is rare but may occur in pyaemia (Alpers and Gaskill, 1944) or in venous sinus thrombosis [p. 380]. Capillary or petechial haemorrhages are found in toxic and infective conditions, for example in acute encephalitis, in septicaemia, and in severe anaemia, leukaemia, and thrombocytopenic purpura. Acute brain purpura due to anaphylaxis or to other forms of acute hypersensitivity reaction is similar. Haemorrhage may occur into a cerebral tumour, for example a glioma, or one of the vessels composing an angioma may bleed, either into the substance of the brain or into the subarachnoid space. Severe trauma, especially if it involves fracture of the skull or penetration of the brain by a missile, is also likely to cause haemorrhage. In a series of 108 cases of cerebral haemorrhage Richardson and Einhorn (1963) found that 77 were due to hypertension, 10 were unexplained, 7 were due to neoplasms, 6 to blood disease, 3 to arteritis, 2 to anticoagulants, and 3 resulted from other miscellaneous causes.

Arterial haemorrhage may be extradural, rarely subdural, subarachnoid, or intracerebral. The first three are described elsewhere. The commonest cause of intracerebral arterial haemorrhage is rupture of an atheromatous artery in an individual suffering from high blood pressure. The rise in blood pressure is usually due to primary hypertension, much less frequently to chronic nephritis or polycystic kidney. As already mentioned, hypertension causes medial hypertrophy in small arteries and arterioles. The hypertrophied media undergoes degeneration, and atheroma of the intima often occurs as well. The result is a thickened but brittle vessel. Miliary aneurysms have often been described on the cerebral vessels in arteriosclerosis, and Russell (1963) has shown that they are much commoner in hypertensive than in normotensive subjects.

There are thus two factors in the causation of arterial cerebral haemorrhage, the degeneration of the vessel and the raised blood pressure. The former in the absence of the latter is likely to lead to thrombosis rather than haemorrhage, while haemorrhage does not necessarily occur even when the blood pressure is very high, unless vascular hypertrophy has given place to degeneration. As in subarachnoid haemorrhage, spontaneous bleeding into the brain substance may also result from angiomal rupture and from rare causes such as bleeding diseases (haemophilia, Christmas disease, thrombocytopenic purpura, thrombotic microangiopathy, etc.), leukaemia, collagen disease, and septic embolism.

Most cases of cerebral haemorrhage are found in late middle life. Freytag (1968) found that 11 per cent of her cases were under 40 years of age, 36 per cent over 60. It is comparatively rare in younger hypertensives and the vascular changes of old age more often lead to thrombosis and cerebral softening. Males are more frequently affected than females. A familial incidence is common.

While cerebral haemorrhage may occur in any situation, Freytag (1968) in a study of 393 cases found that 42 per cent were in the region of the internal capsule and corpus striatum, 16 per cent in the pons, 15 per cent in the thalamus, 12 per cent in the cerebellum, and 10 per cent in the cerebral white matter. Seventy-five per cent ruptured into the ventricles, 15 per cent through the cortex into the subarachnoid space, and 6 per cent into the subdural space. Secondary pressure haemorrhages were present in the midbrain and pons in 54 per cent of cases with supratentorial haematomas.

After a large intracerebral haemorrhage the affected hemisphere is enlarged and the gyri are flattened. The site of haemorrhage is occupied by a red clot and the surrounding tissues are compressed and may be oedematous. Later the clot is absorbed and may be replaced by a neuroglial scar or by a cavity containing a yellow serous fluid. During absorption of the clot, gliosis occurs in the walls of the cavity with phagocytosis of destroyed neural tissue by compound granular corpuscles. Multiple haemorrhages sometimes occur.

SYMPTOMS

The occurrence of cerebral haemorrhage is always sudden, but the patient may be known to have a high blood pressure and there may have been premonitory symptoms, such as transitory speech disturbances or attacks of weakness of a limb. The actual rupture of the vessel may be brought about by mental excitement or physical effort, or may occur during rest or sleep. Usually the patient complains of sudden severe headache and may vomit. He becomes dazed, and in all but the mildest cases loses consciousness in a few minutes. Convulsions may occur at the onset, but are exceptional. The physical signs produced by a cerebral haemorrhage depend upon its situation and its size.

Haemorrhage in the region of the Corpus Striatum and Internal Capsule

The patient is usually unconscious, but the depth of coma depends upon the size of the haemorrhage and the extent of pressure upon or of secondary haemorrhage in the brain stem. Slight pyrexia is usually present. The pulse rate is generally slow—50 to 60—and the pulse full and bounding. The respirations are deep and stertorous, and the respiratory rate may be either slow or quickened or exhibit irregularity, for example Cheyne-Stokes respiration. An unconscious patient is unable to swallow. The head is usually rotated and the eyes are deviated towards the side of the lesion. This is due to paralysis of rotation of the head and of conjugate deviation of the eyes to the opposite side and the consequent unbalanced action of the undamaged cerebral hemisphere. The fundi are likely to show arteriosclerosis of the retinal vessels, but the discs are usually normal, though slight papilloedema is not uncommon. The pupils may be unequal, but react to light unless the patient is deeply comatose. A divergent squint is common, and the eyes often exhibit irregular, jerky movements. The corneal reflexes are often lost when coma is profound. A capsular haemorrhage causes paralysis of the opposite side of the body, but the comatose patient cannot be asked to carry out voluntary movements. It is therefore necessary to resort to indirect methods of demonstrating paralysis.

Flattening of the nasolabial furrow may be evident on the paralysed side, and the cheek is often distended more on the paralysed than on the normal side during expiration. If the patient is not deeply comatose he may also be seen to move the limbs spontaneously on the normal but not on the paralysed side. Spasticity takes two or three weeks to develop in the paralysed limbs after a capsular haemorrhage. Before this the limbs are flaccid, and this flaccidity is one of the most valuable signs of hemiplegia in a comatose patient. The arm and the leg if lifted up fall to the bed inertly, whereas even in deep coma the normal arm and leg subside much more gradually. Painful stimuli may be used to demonstrate the presence of paralysis. Pricking with a pin in a semicomatose patient usually causes contraction of the muscles of the face and withdrawal of the limb which is pricked. These movements do not occur on the paralysed side. Their absence, however, may also be due to hemianalgesia. This may often be demonstrated by the fact that reflex contraction of the facial muscles occurs when the patient is pricked on one side of the body, the normal side, but not when he is pricked on the analgesic side. The tendon reflexes are variable. They may be much diminished or abolished on the paralysed side; sometimes they are exaggerated. The plantar reflex on the affected side is extensor; on the other side it may be flexor or extensor. The abdominal reflexes are often lost on both sides in coma. Retention or incontinence of urine and faeces is the rule as long as the patient is unconscious.

Thalamic Haemorrhage

Like a capsular or putaminal haemorrhage (see above), a thalamic haemorrhage also produces a hemiplegia due to pressure on the internal capsule but the sensory deficit is usually prominent. There may be a transient hemianopia and aphasia if the dominant hemisphere is involved (Ciemins, 1970). Extension medially or into the subthalamus may cause paralysis of vertical gaze, occasionally skew deviation with downward displacement of the contralateral eye, ipsilateral ptosis and miosis, and even hemiballismus; mutism has been described in non-dominant thalamic lesions (Fisher *et al.*, 1974).

Pontine Haemorrhage

If the patient is seen soon after the onset of the haemorrhage, the signs may be those of a unilateral lesion of the pons, namely facial paralysis on the side of the lesion with flaccid paralysis of the limbs on the opposite side. Owing to paralysis of conjugate ocular deviation and of rotation of the head to the side of the lesion the patient often lies with his head and eyes turned towards the side of the paralysed limbs. Even when the signs at the outset are those of a unilateral lesion of the pons, extension of the haemorrhage soon involves the opposite side, or the signs may be bilateral from the beginning. When both sides of the pons are thus affected there is paralysis of the face and limbs on both sides, with bilateral extensor plantar reflexes and sometimes decerebrate rigidity. Marked contraction of the pupils, 'pinpoint pupils', the result of bilateral destruction of the ocular sympathetic fibres, is characteristic of a pontine haemorrhage. Moreover, destruction of the pons cuts off the body from the control of the heat-regulating centres in the hypothalamus, and the patient becomes poikilothermic so that hyperpyrexia is common. Absence of nystagmus induced by cold water injected into one or both auditory meati may be useful in distinguishing the condition from cerebral haemorrhage.

Haemorrhage into the Ventricles

It is not uncommon for a haemorrhage in the region of the internal capsule to burst into the lateral ventricle. If the patient is not seen until after this has occurred it may be difficult to differentiate ventricular from pontine haemorrhage. After ventricular haemorrhage coma deepens and signs of a corticospinal lesion are usually present on both sides of the body. There is often a tendency for the upper limbs to adopt a posture of rigid extension. The temperature frequently exhibits a terminal rise, also seen in pontine haemorrhage.

The symptoms of cerebral haemorrhage in other situations are those of a massive focal lesion of sudden onset and are similar to the focal symptoms of a tumour in the same region.

Cerebellar Haemorrhage

Cerebellar haemorrhage is usually sudden, and in some cases consciousness is lost sooner or later, but in one series of 56 patients, two-thirds were responsive on admission to hospital (Ott et al., 1974). Occipital headache and vomiting are common at the onset. Only a minority of patients show localizing signs: in many of the remainder the clinical picture suggests a cerebrovascular accident without clear evidence as to its site (McKissock et al., 1960). Repeated vomiting and intense vertigo at the onset in a conscious patient who is ataxic and complains of headache but may have no classical 'cerebellar signs' should always suggest this diagnosis as a possibility. Ocular signs such as paralysis of conjugate gaze to the side of the lesion, a sixth nerve palsy or 'skew deviation' are seen in some cases. If the haemorrhage is not evacuated, coma due to brain stem compression supervenes. A similar picture may result from small cerebellar angiomas in children (Erenberg et al., 1972).

Investigations

Lumbar puncture is not entirely innocuous in cases of cerebral haemorrhage because of the risk of cerebellar or tentorial herniation with consequent increased brain stem compression and/or secondary haemorrhage. Nevertheless the risk may have to be taken when diagnosis is in doubt.

The cerebrospinal fluid after cerebral haemorrhage is under increased pressure and its protein content may be somewhat raised. The presence of blood visible to the naked eye in the fluid indicates usually that the haemorrhage has ruptured into the ventricular system, less frequently that it has come to the surface of the brain and ruptured into the subarachnoid space. Even when no blood can be seen with the naked eye, red cells may be seen microscopically. There is often a slight leucocytosis and the sedimentation rate is raised.

The heart is usually enlarged and the blood pressure raised. Albuminuria may be present, and glycosuria may be a result of the cerebral lesion.

An EMI scan may be successful in localizing and identifying the lesion. Angiography is rarely indicated unless the patient is relatively young, loss of consciousness is not profound and surgical treatment (especially in the case of cerebellar haemorrhage) would be contemplated if the lesion were accurately localized; ventriculography may be needed to localize cerebellar haematomas (Norris et al., 1969; Freeman et al., 1973; Ott et al., 1974).

DIAGNOSIS

In the majority of cases an intracerebral haemorrhage leads to impairment or loss of consciousness, sometimes very rapidly, sometimes more gradually. In such cases it has to be distinguished from other conditions causing coma. This is discussed on page 1158. Important diagnostic points are the association of the impairment of consciousness with the physical signs of a focal cerebral lesion of acute or subacute onset, the presence of factors predisposing to a cerebral vascular lesion, particularly hypertension and atheroma, and the presence of blood, visible either microscopically or macroscopically, in the cerebrospinal fluid.

A cerebral vascular lesion having been diagnosed, it is necessary to decide whether it is haemorrhagic or ischaemic in origin. Ischaemic lesions are either embolic, or due to atheroma or other conditions of arterial degeneration or inflammation, with or without thrombosis. An embolic lesion usually comes on suddenly and presents the neurological picture of obstruction of a particular artery. Moreover, the source of the embolus is usually evident. Ischaemic infarction due to atheroma is usually more gradual than haemorrhage. There may have been previous recurrent episodes with complete or partial recovery, or the onset is insidious over a period of 24 to 48 hours. Exceptionally, however, it is as sudden as a haemorrhage. Unconsciousness is less common and when it occurs usually less profound. The blood pressure is less frequently raised, and there may be evidence of pre-existing disease leading to vascular damage, for example, diabetes.

The cerebrospinal fluid is often helpful. The presence of red blood cells will usually suggest haemorrhage, while after infarction the fluid is more likely to be free from red cells but may contain a raised protein.

Primary subarachnoid haemorrhage is distinguished from intracerebral haemorrhage by the prominence of signs of meningeal irritation, i.e. cervical rigidity and Kernig's sign, and the absence of signs of a cerebral lesion. It may, however, be impossible to distinguish on clinical grounds between an intracerebral haemorrhage reaching the ventricle or subarachnoid space, and a subarachnoid haemorrhage from an aneurysm invading one cerebral hemisphere. Angiography, however, should settle the question, and is also useful, as is the EMI scan, in doubtful cases in distinguishing between a primary intracerebral haemorrhage and infarction due to narrowing or occlusion of a major artery.

An intracranial tumour rarely simulates a cerebral vascular lesion unless it is itself the site of a haemorrhage or of rapidly developing oedema. The true nature of the lesion may be difficult to recognize if there have been no preceding symptoms of increased intracranial pressure. However, the occurrence of what appears to be a cerebral haemorrhage in a patient without hypertension may suggest the possibility of a cerebral tumour, and the need for appropriate investigation. The 'congestive attacks' of general paresis or hemiplegia due to meningo-vascular syphilis may simulate a cerebral haemorrhage closely owing to the rapid onset of hemiplegia with loss of consciousness but are now rare.

PROGNOSIS

The immediate problem in the case of cerebral haemorrhage is whether or not the haemorrhage will prove fatal. Death may occur from medullary compression or brain stem haemorrhage as a result of continued bleeding. Even if the bleeding stops, the destruction of brain tissue and rise of intracranial pressure may cause the patient to remain unconscious so long that he dies of exhaustion or from an intercurrent infection, such as pneumonia. When haemorrhage continues, death may occur rapidly, though rarely in less than a few hours, usually during the first two days. The patient may linger in a comatose condition for as long as a week. If the haemorrhage is continuing there is a progressive deepening of the coma, indicated by inability to rouse a formerly responsive patient, and loss of the corneal and pupillary reflexes; the pulse tends to become rapid and irregular; the respiratory rate is often irregular and finally becomes rapid and shallow, and both the temperature and the blood pressure tend to rise.

Bilateral paralysis of limbs is a sign of bad prognostic import, because it indicates either ventricular or pontine haemorrhage, both of which are usually fatal. A visibly blood-stained cerebrospinal fluid usually means a ventricular haemorrhage. If the patient shows no signs of recovery from coma 48 hours after the onset of the haemorrhage the chances of recovery are poor, even though the haemorrhage may have stopped. McKissock *et al.* (1961) in their series of 180 cases had an over-all mortality of 51 per cent and it was about twice as high in men as in women. Freytag (1968) found that almost all patients with pontine haemorrhage died within 24 hours, while the immediate mortality of haemorrhage in the cerebral white matter was 48 per cent.

When the patient recovers consciousness he is naturally anxious to know whether he is likely to suffer from permanent disability. This depends upon the situation of the haemorrhage, and the extent of the resulting destruction of brain tissue. It must be remembered that neural shock and oedema of surrounding areas of brain usually cause a more severe depression of function than is actually due to the destructive effect of the lesion. Some improvement may therefore be expected in most cases. The mental efficiency of the patient is rarely as good after a cerebral haemorrhage as before. Apart from lesions grossly impairing functions of intelligence and speech, there is usually diminished power of concentration and memory, together with irritability and emotional instability.

Haemorrhage in the region of the posterior part of the inferior frontal gyrus on the left side may cause for a time total expressive aphasia, but in these cases considerable recovery of speech usually occurs in time, and improvement may continue for many months. The speech defect which follows a capsular haemorrhage is more often dysarthria and usually improves rapidly. Damage to the corticospinal tract by a haemorrhage in the region of the internal capsule causes spastic hemiplegia on the opposite side, the signs of which are described elsewhere [see p. 20]. Some return of power always occurs in the lower limb, so that the patient is likely to be able to walk. If the upper limb exhibits returning power at the end of a month after the onset a considerable degree of recovery of movement at the larger joints will probably occur in it. If, however, there is no improvement at the end of 3 months the paralysis is likely to be permanent. When the posterior part of the capsule is involved, sensory loss and homonymous hemianopia on the side opposite to the lesion may be added to the paralysis. Improvement may occur in respect of these disorders, but is often incomplete. Pain on the paralysed side of the body may occur after a capsular haemorrhage, and is of thalamic origin. If it develops it is likely to be persistent. Involuntary movements sometimes occur after cerebral haemorrhage, but only when paralysis of the limbs is incomplete. They usually appear several weeks or months after the onset, with the return of voluntary power, and are always more marked in the upper than in the lower limb. Simple tremor may develop and is most evident on voluntary movement. Less often there is tremor of the Parkinsonian type which occurs when the limb is at rest. Athetosis is also sometimes seen. All these movements tend to be persistent, though some improvement may occur, especially in the tremor. They are probably due to involvement of the corpus striatum. Choreiform movements or even frank hemiballismus may occur as a result of haemorrhage in the region of the subthalamic nucleus. This lesion is often fatal, though improvement and even recovery may take place. Trophic changes are common in the paralysed limbs and post-hemiplegic epilepsy is not uncommon.

TREATMENT

Continuing cerebral haemorrhage causes death from brain stem compression or secondary haemorrhage in this region. The objects of treatment are, therefore, to stop the haemorrhage and to reduce the intracranial pressure. Steroids may be helpful as in all cases of raised intracranial pressure [pp. 228 and 291].

Surgical evacuation of the clot is a rational procedure but is rarely practicable or beneficial. It should, however, be considered when cerebral haemorrhage occurs before middle life, in view of the possibility of haemorrhage from a congenital vascular abnormality which it may be possible to demonstrate by angiography (Small et al., 1953). McKissock et al. (1959) compared surgical and conservative treatment in a series of 244 cases of primary intracerebral haemorrhage. They concluded that with the possible exception of normotensive subjects no group of patients fared better with operation than with conservative treatment. However, there is good evidence to suggest that surgical evacuation of the intracerebellar haematoma in cases of primary cerebellar haemorrhage will often save life and lessen morbidity (McKissock et al., 1960; Ott et al., 1974). Hypotensive therapy appears to be of no value in the acute stage.

Lumbar puncture should be used only when absolutely necessary for diagnostic purposes as it may be dangerous because of the risk of tentorial or cerebellar herniation.

The usual treatment of the unconscious patient should be carried out [see p. 1170]. After recovery from the immediate effects of the haemorrhage the principles of rehabilitation are the same as in cerebral infarction [p. 341].

REFERENCES

ALPERS, B. J., and GASKILL, H. S. (1944) The pathological characteristics of embolic or metastatic encephalitis, J. Neuropath. exp. Neurol., **3**, 210.

BAGLEY, C., Jun. (1932) Spontaneous cerebral hemorrhage, Arch. Neurol. Psychiat. (Chic.), **27**, 1133.

CHASE, W. H. (1937) Hypertensive apoplexy and its causation, Arch. Neurol. Psychiat. (Chic.), **38**, 1176.

CIEMINS, V. A. (1970) Localized thalamic hemorrhage: a cause of aphasia, Neurology (Minneap.), **20**, 776.

CRAIG, W. McK., and ADSON, A. W. (1936) Spontaneous intracerebral hemorrhage, Arch. Neurol. Psychiat. (Chic.), **35**, 701.

ERENBERG, G., RUBIN, R., and SHULMAN, K. (1972) Cerebellar haematomas caused by angiomas in children, J. Neurol. Neurosurg. Psychiat., **35**, 304.

FIELDS, W. S. (1961) Pathogenesis and Treatment of Cerebrovascular Disease, Springfield, Ill.

FISHER, C. M., MOHR, J. P., and ADAMS, R. D. (1974) Cerebrovascular diseases, in Harrison's Principles of Internal Medicine, 7th ed., chap. 326, New York.

FREEMAN, R. E., ONOFRIO, B. M., OKAZAKI, H., and DINAPOLI, R. P. (1973) Spontaneous intracerebellar hemorrhage: diagnosis and surgical treatment, *Neurology (Minneap.)*, **23**, 84.

FREYTAG, E. (1968) Fatal hypertensive intracerebral haematomas: a survey of the pathological anatomy of 393 cases, *J. Neurol. Neurosurg. Psychiat.*, **31**, 616.

MCKISSOCK, W., RICHARDSON, A., and TAYLOR, J. (1961) Primary intracerebellar haemorrhage, *Lancet*, **ii**, 221.

MCKISSOCK, W., RICHARDSON, A., and WALSH, L. (1959) Primary intracerebral haemorrhage: results of surgical treatment in 244 consecutive cases, *Lancet*, **ii**, 683.

MCKISSOCK, W., RICHARDSON, A., and WALSH, L. (1960) Spontaneous cerebellar haemorrhage, *Brain*, **83**, 1.

MURPHY, J. P. (1954) *Cerebrovascular Disease*, Chicago.

NORRIS, J. W., EISEN, A. A., and BRANCH, C. L. (1969) Problems in cerebellar hemorrhage and infarction, *Neurology (Minneap.)*, **19**, 1043.

OTT, K. H., KASE, C. S., OJEMANN, R. G., and MOHR, J. P. (1974) Cerebellar hemorrhage: diagnosis and treatment, *Arch. Neurol. (Chic.)*, **31**, 160.

RICHARDSON, J. C., and EINHORN, R. W. (1963) in *Clinical Neurosurgery*, ed. Mosberg, Wilf, p. 114, London.

RIISHEDE, J. (1957) Cerebral apoplexy, *Acta psychiat. (Kbh.)*, **32**, Supp. 118.

RUSSELL, R. W. R. (1963) Observations on intracranial aneurysms, *Brain*, **86**, 425.

SMALL, J. M., HOLMES, J. M., and CONNOLLY, R. C. (1953) The prognosis and role of surgery in spontaneous intracranial haemorrhage, *Brit. med. J.*, **2**, 1072.

STERN, K. (1938) The pathology of apoplexy, *J. Neurol. Psychiat.*, N.S. **1**, 26.

VASCULAR DISEASES WITHOUT CHANGES IN THE BRAIN AND STROKES OF UNDETERMINED AETIOLOGY

These categories of cerebral vascular disease were included by the *ad hoc* Committee of NINDB (1958) [see p. 326] in their classification simply in order to indicate that the pathologist may find evidence of extensive atherosclerosis and/or arteriolosclerosis at autopsy in patients without symptoms of cerebral ischaemia and without pathological evidence of disease in the cerebral parenchyma. Similarly it must be noted that despite extensive clinical and pathological study it may still be impossible, using techniques at present available, to determine the cause of certain strokes.

REFERENCE

AD HOC COMMITTEE, NATIONAL ADVISORY COUNCIL OF THE NATIONAL INSTITUTE OF NEUROLOGICAL DISEASES AND BLINDNESS (1958) A classification and outline of cerebrovascular diseases, *Neurology (Minneap.)*, **8**, Supplement.

INFLAMMATORY DISEASES OF INTRACRANIAL ARTERIES

POLYARTERITIS NODOSA (Periarteritis Nodosa)

This disorder is characterized by multiple focal lesions in the arteries. These begin with necrosis of the media and the internal elastic lamina, which is followed by extension of the inflammation to the adventitia, and periarteritis. Proliferation of the intima produces gradual narrowing of the lumen of the vessels. Secondary aneurysm formation is exceptional. The nervous system is said to be involved in 8 per cent of cases; and lesions may occur in the meninges, cerebral cortex, medulla, spinal cord, and peripheral nerves due to occlusion of vasa nervorum.

Cerebral lesions may lead to headache, convulsions, hemiplegia, mental dullness, and coma. Pupillary changes may be present. The symptoms of involvement of the peripheral nerves are often those of multiple interstitial neuritis ('mononeuritis multiplex') rather than symmetrical polyneuritis. Pain and muscular weakness may develop in the course of a few hours. Tenderness of the nerve trunks and muscles with muscular wasting and weakness, loss of reflexes, and sensory loss are irregularly distributed according to the distribution of the spinal roots and peripheral nerves affected. The spinal fluid may be under increased pressure and there may be xanthochromia and a polymorphonuclear leucocytosis in the fluid.

Changes are often present in the ocular fundi. There may be choroidal exudate in the form of perivascular hillocks resembling choroidal tubercles. Detachment of the retina may occur, and in the later stages hypertensive retinopathy.

The general symptoms include fever and loss of weight, and focal visceral symptoms depending upon the situation of the lesions, which tend to involve especially the kidneys, heart, liver, and gastro-intestinal tract. The spleen may be enlarged, and radiographically the lungs may show a characteristic infiltration. There is often a leucocytosis in the blood and occasionally an eosinophilia. Asthma is common. Hypertension and albuminuria usually occur in the later stages. Muscle infarcts may occur and a biopsy may show the characteristic vascular lesion. Many patients improve when treated with steroid drugs, a few recover after long-term treatment and in some the disease appears to become 'burnt-out' but there is still an appreciable mortality.

REFERENCES

KERNOHAN, J. W., and WOLTMAN, H. W. (1938) Periarteritis nodosa. A clinico-pathologic study with special reference to the nervous system, *Arch. Neurol. Psychiat. (Chic.)*, **39**, 665.

MILLER, H. G., and DALEY, R. (1946) Clinical aspects of polyarteritis nodosa, *Quart. J. Med.*, **15**, 255.

SYSTEMIC LUPUS ERYTHEMATOSUS

Symptoms and signs of cerebral ischaemia have been reported as an uncommon manifestation of systemic lupus erythematosus; the manifestations are often those of a restricted brain-stem stroke but cerebral hemisphere lesions, often resulting from small areas of perisulcal softening, occasionally occur and focal spinal cord lesions have also been described (Johnson and Richardson, 1968; Berry, 1971). The clinical manifestations of cerebral involvement are diverse, including not only manifestations of focal ischaemia but also epileptiform seizures, cranial nerve palsies, chorea and arachnoiditis in some cases (Glaser, 1952; *British Medical Journal*, 1975). Optic neuritis has also been described (Hackett *et al.*, 1974) and a progressive spinal cord syndrome resembling multiple sclerosis (Fulford *et al.*, 1972), while symmetrical sensori-motor polyneuropathy is also relatively common. Kurland *et al.* (1969) have assessed the relative incidences of systemic lupus and of other collagen or connective tissue diseases which may involve the nervous system.

REFERENCES

BERRY, R. G. (1971) Lupus erythematosus, in *Pathology of Nervous System*, ed. Minckler, J., Vol. 2, pp. 1482–8, New York.

BRITISH MEDICAL JOURNAL (1975) Cerebral lupus, *Brit. med. J.*, **1**, 537.

FULFORD, K. W. M., CATTERALL, R. D., DELHANTY, J. J., DONIACH, D., and KREMER, M. (1972) A collagen disorder of the nervous system presenting as multiple sclerosis, *Brain*, **95**, 373.

GLASER, G. H. (1952) Lesions of the central nervous system in disseminated lupus erythematosus, *Arch. Neurol. Psychiat. (Chic.)*, **67**, 745.

HACKETT, E. R., MARTINEZ, R. D., LARSON, P. F., and PADDISON, R. M. (1974) Optic neuritis in systemic lupus erythematosus, *Arch. Neurol. (Chic.)*, **31**, 9.

JOHNSON, R. T., and RICHARDSON, E. P. (1968) The neurological manifestations of systemic lupus erythematosus, *Medicine (Baltimore)*, **47**, 337.

KURLAND, L. T., HAUSER, W. A., FERGUSON, R. H., and HOLLEY, K. E. (1969) Epidemiologic features of diffuse connective tissue disorders in Rochester, Minn., 1951 through 1967, with special reference to systemic lupus erythematosus, *Mayo Clin. Proc.*, **44**, 649.

BUERGER'S DISEASE

It has been suggested in the past that thromboangiitis obliterans may sometimes involve cerebral vessels, but it is now generally agreed, on the basis of pathological evidence, that most cases so diagnosed have resulted either from atheroma or from granulomatous arteritis (Fisher, 1957; Bruetsch, 1971; Hutchinson and Acheson, 1975).

REFERENCES

BRUETSCH, W. L. (1971) Cerebral thromboangiitis obliterans, in *Pathology of the Nervous System*, ed. Minckler, J., vol. 2, chap. XVII, Section 108, New York.

FISHER, C. M. (1957) Cerebral thromboangiitis obliterans, *Medicine (Baltimore)*, **36**, 169.

HUTCHINSON, E. C., and ACHESON, E. J. (1975) *Strokes: Natural History, Pathology and Surgical Treatment*, London.

TEMPORAL (GIANT CELL) ARTERITIS

The disorder originally described as temporal, or cranial, arteritis is now recognized to be a generalized vascular disease which attacks elderly patients, being rare before the age of 60 years. The pathological features are those of a subacute inflammation, spreading probably by the vasa vasorum to the media of the arteries with a tendency to spread longitudinally along the vessels in contrast to the lesion in polyarteritis nodosa. The intima becomes hypertrophied, and thrombosis is a common sequel. Stress has been laid upon the presence of giant cells, and the disorder has been described as giant cell arteritis. The characteristic pathological changes have been found in many large and small vessels (Crompton, 1959), including the aorta and the retinal arteries. Biopsy of an affected portion of a superficial temporal artery will establish the diagnosis.

The characteristic physical signs are anorexia, loss of weight, joint and muscle pains, fever and sweating, painful arterial thrombosis, and severe headache. Sometimes diffuse muscular pain is the presenting symptom, resembling polymyalgia rheumatica [p. 1015]. The superficial temporal arteries are intensely tender during the acute stage and may become thrombosed through part or the whole of their length. Papilloedema may occur, and unilateral or bilateral loss of vision is common. Indeed, in a survey of 80 personal cases Meadows (1966) found that unilateral or bilateral blindness due to central retinal artery occlusion occurred in over half and diplopia in 15 per cent. Sudden unilateral blindness in an elderly patient, even when other evidence of arteritis is unobtrusive, should always raise the possibility of this condition and an erythrocyte sedimentation rate estimation (this is invariably raised in the untreated case) is the single most useful investigation. Treatment with steroid drugs (prednisone 30–40 mg daily in the first instance) is mandatory as this may be the only means of preserving remaining vision. The disease usually burns itself out in 1–2 years when treatment can gradually be withdrawn. Cerebral symptoms due to involvement of the carotid and vertebral arteries are occasionally seen and brain stem strokes are not uncommon, though intracranial vessels are rarely involved (Wilkinson and Russell, 1972).

REFERENCES

COOKE, W. T., CLOAKE, P. C. P., GOVAN, A. D. T., and COLBECK, J. C. (1946) Temporal arteritis: a generalized vascular disease, *Quart. J. Med.*, **15**, 47.
CROMPTON, M. R. (1959) The visual changes in temporal (giant-cell) arteritis. Report of a case with autopsy findings, *Brain*, **82**, 377.
MEADOWS, S. P. (1966) Temporal or giant-cell arteritis, *Proc. roy. Soc. Med.*, **59**, 329.
WILKINSON, I. M. S., and RUSSELL, R. W. R. (1972) Arteries of the head and neck in giant cell arteritis. A pathological study to show the pattern of arterial involvement, *Arch. Neurol. (Chic.)*, **27**, 378.

GRANULOMATOUS ANGIITIS

Within the last few years a number of cases have been described in adults of all ages and both sexes of a disorder presenting with symptoms of focal or generalized cerebral dysfunction, epileptic seizures, and evidence of spinal cord involvement which may precede symptoms of cerebral disease and in which a diffuse granulomatous angiitis of small intracerebral and meningeal arteries has been discovered at autopsy. The pathological changes, with giant cells in the inflammatory lesions of the affected vessels, resemble in some degree those of sarcoidosis and in other respects those of temporal arteritis, with which condition earlier cases of this disorder were confused (McCormick and Neubuerger, 1958), although, as mentioned above, the latter condition affects mainly larger extracranial vessels. The CSF is usually under increased pressure and contains an excess of protein and lymphocytes; the aetiology of the disorder is unknown; most cases have proved to be fatal within months or exceptionally a few years, but in rare instances where cerebral biopsy has established the diagnosis, steroid treatment has been thought to be helpful (Kolodny et al., 1968; Nurick et al., 1972).

REFERENCES

KOLODNY, E. H., REBEIZ, J. J., CAVINESS, V. S., and RICHARDSON, E. P. (1968) Granulomatous angiitis of the central nervous system, *Arch. Neurol. (Chic.)*, **19**, 510.
McCORMICK, H. M., and NEUBUERGER, K. T. (1958) Giant-cell arteritis involving small meningeal and intracerebral vessels, *J. Neuropath. exp. Neurol.*, **17**, 471.
NURICK, S., BLACKWOOD, W., and MAIR, W. G. P. (1972) Giant cell granulomatous angiitis of the central nervous system, *Brain*, **95**, 133.

PULSELESS DISEASE

Episodes of cerebral ischaemia or infarction in patients with absent or reduced pulses, especially in the upper limbs, have been recognized for many years to occur in young Japanese women with that form of obliterative arteritis of the brachiocephalic branches of the aortic arch first described by Takayashu (1908) and often now called Takayashu's disease. This condition, though rare, has been described in racial groups other than the Japanese, but in Western countries 'pulseless disease' more often results from atherosclerotic occlusion of major vessels, though it has been described in systemic lupus erythematosus (Lessof and Glynn, 1959).

REFERENCES

LESSOF, M. H., and GLYNN, L. E. (1959) The pulseless syndrome, *Lancet*, **i,** 799.
TAKAYASHU, M. (1908) A case with peculiar changes of the central retinal vessels, *Acta Soc. ophthal. Jap.*, **12,** 554.

THROMBOTIC MICROANGIOPATHY

Thrombotic microangiopathy (thrombotic thrombocytopenic purpura), often now called the 'disseminated intravascular coagulation syndrome', is a fulminating disorder involving small blood vessels which become inflamed and in which platelet thrombi form resulting in widespread small vessel occlusion in many organs. Fever, haemolytic anaemia, renal damage and variable and fleeting neurological manifestations including confusion, pareses, subarachnoid haemorrhage (Heron *et al.*, 1974), and convulsions are seen; the response to steroid drugs is variable and most cases are fatal. It should also be noted that disseminated intravascular coagulation, possibly due to the release of thromboplastin from damaged brain tissue, has been thought to be a rare consequence or primary cerebral lesions (Preston *et al.*, 1974).

REFERENCES

HERON, J. R., HUTCHINSON, E. C., BOYD, W. N., and ABER, G. M. (1974) Pregnancy, subarachnoid haemorrhage, and the intravascular coagulation syndrome, *J. Neurol. Neurosurg. Psychiat.*, **37,** 521.
McKAY, D. G. (1965) *Disseminated Intravascular Coagulation*, New York.
PRESTON, F. E., MALIA, R. G., SWORN, M. J., TIMPERLEY, W. R., and BLACKBURN, E. K. (1974) Disseminated intravascular coagulation as a consequence of cerebral damage, *J. Neurol. Neurosurg. Psychiat.*, **37,** 241.
SYMMERS, W. ST. C. (1952) Thrombotic microangiopathic haemolytic anaemias (thrombotic microangiopathy), *Brit. med. J.*, **2,** 897.
SYMMERS, W. ST. C. (1956) Thrombotic microangiopathy (thrombotic thrombocytopenic purpura) associated with acute haemorrhagic leucoencephalitis and sensitivity to oxophenarsine, *Brain*, **79,** 511.

THE CEREBRAL VENOUS CIRCULATION

THE VENOUS SINUSES

The intracranial venous sinuses are spaces lying between layers of the dura mater and are lined with endothelium. They receive blood from the veins of the brain and directly or indirectly drain into the internal jugular vein. They communicate with the meningeal veins, and by emissary veins with the veins of the scalp.

The following sinuses are unpaired:

The Superior Sagittal Sinus. The superior sagittal sinus begins anteriorly at the crista galli where it communicates through the foramen caecum with the nasal veins, and passes upwards, backwards, and finally downwards at the convex upper margin of the falx. It ends at the level of the internal occipital protuberance by turning, usually to the right, into the right transverse sinus. Occasionally it turns into the left transverse sinus. It possesses a terminal dilatation—the confluence of the sinuses—from which a communicating channel passes to the junction of the straight sinus and the left transverse sinus. The superior sagittal sinus receives the superior group of superficial cerebral veins and thus drains the upper part of the cerebral hemispheres.

The Inferior Sagittal Sinus. The inferior sagittal sinus lies in the free lower border of the falx for its posterior two-thirds and terminates posteriorly by joining the great cerebral vein to form the straight sinus, which passes between layers of the dura along the line of junction of the falx with the tentorium. Posteriorly it turns to the left at the level of the internal occipital protuberance to become the left transverse sinus.

The following sinuses are paired:

The Transverse Sinuses. The transverse sinuses arise posteriorly, the right from the superior sagittal sinus, the left from the straight sinus, and pass laterally and forwards in the attached border of the tentorium, lying in a groove in the occipital bone. Each then turns downwards on the inner surface of the mastoid process and leaves the skull by the jugular foramen, to enter the internal jugular vein.

The Cavernous Sinuses. The cavernous sinuses lie one on either side of the body of the sphenoid. They begin anteriorly at the inner end of the superior orbital fissure, where they receive the ophthalmic veins, and terminate posteriorly at the apex of the petrous portion of the temporal bone by dividing into the superior and inferior petrosal sinuses. In the lateral wall of the cavernous sinus lie the internal carotid artery with its sympathetic plexus, the third and fourth nerves, and first and second divisions of the fifth nerve, and the sixth nerve.

The Superior Petrosal Sinuses. The superior petrosal sinuses run backwards and laterally along the attached edge of the tentorium, to end in the transverse sinuses.

The Inferior Petrosal Sinuses. The inferior petrosal sinuses run backwards, outwards, and downwards in the posterior fossa, to join the internal jugular veins by passing through the jugular foramina.

The Cerebral Veins. The venous sinuses receive as tributaries the cerebral veins. The superficial cerebral veins are divided into two groups—the superior, which run upwards to the superior sagittal sinus and drain the upper halves of the hemispheres, and the inferior, which drain the lower halves of the hemispheres and run downwards to join the venous sinuses of the base. The most important of the deep cerebral veins is the great cerebral vein of Galen, which drains the choroid plexuses of the third and lateral ventricles and the basal ganglia, and terminates by joining the inferior sagittal sinus to form the straight sinus. Much new information about the cerebral venous system, identifying specific veins not previously named in anatomical texts, has been derived in recent years from angiographic studies (Newton and Potts, 1974).

The Diploic Veins. The venous channels in the bones of the skull, the diploic veins, drain either into the venous sinuses or into the superficial veins of the scalp.

THROMBOSIS OF THE INTRACRANIAL VENOUS SINUSES AND VEINS

AETIOLOGY

Thrombosis of the intracranial venous sinuses is usually the result of the extension of infection from neighbouring structures or of direct injury. Rarely it occurs in the absence of any evident local cause. These two varieties of sinus thrombosis are rather unsatisfactorily distinguished as 'secondary' and 'primary' respectively.

'Primary' sinus thrombosis is rare and is most frequently seen at the extremes of life, especially during the first year. It occurs in wasted, debilitated infants, especially as a complication of congenital heart disease or gastrointestinal infections, and later in life in individuals suffering from severe anaemia, exhausting infections such as enteric fever, or emaciating diseases such as carcinoma and tuberculosis. It has also been described as a complication of oral contraceptive medication (Bickerstaff, 1975) and in pregnancy and the puerperium (Carroll *et al.*, 1966). The principal predisposing factors of 'primary' sinus thrombosis appear to be anaemia, increased coagulability of the blood, low blood pressure, and dehydration. It may form part of the picture of thrombophlebitis migrans.

'Secondary' sinus thrombosis may be the result of direct injury of a sinus through fracture of the skull or surgical operation in its vicinity, or puncture of the superior sagittal sinus in infancy for therapeutic purposes. Infection may spread to the sinuses from an area of osteitis of one of the cranial bones. The transverse sinus may thus become infected from mastoiditis, or through the jugular vein from the fauces. Infection may spread from the transverse to the superior sagittal sinus. The latter and the cavernous sinus may be directly infected from frontal sinusitis or from infection of the other nasal air sinuses. Owing to the comparatively free communication between the intracranial venous sinuses and the superficial veins of the face and scalp, cutaneous sepsis may cause intracranial sinus thrombosis. The cavernous sinus is especially liable to become infected as a result of pyogenic infections in the neighbourhood of the upper lip.

Though sinus thrombosis may be the only manifestation of infection, it may be associated with extradural or subdural abscess, intracerebral abscess, or localized or diffuse leptomeningitis.

PATHOLOGY

The affected sinus contains a reddish clot, which tends in time to become paler and adherent to the sinus wall. In sinus thrombophlebitis due to pyogenic organisms the clot may become purulent. It may extend into tributary veins or into other sinuses. The internal jugular vein is frequently involved by extension from the transverse sinus. The area of brain drained by the affected sinus exhibits congestive oedema and in some cases softening and haemorrhage, and the development of some degree of collateral venous circulation causes congestion of neighbouring veins. Obstruction of a large sinus, such as the superior sagittal, may so impede the absorption of cerebrospinal fluid that hydrocephalus results. Involvement of the Galenic vein causes softening of the central areas of the brain. Extension of infection from the sinus may cause localized or diffuse leptomeningitis or intracerebral abscess, while the liberation of organisms or of fragments of infected clot into the general circulation may lead to pyaemia and pyaemic abscesses, especially in the lungs. The pathology of the condition, as well as its clinical features, have been reviewed by Kalbag and Woolf (1967).

SYMPTOMS

The symptoms in intracranial venous sinus thrombosis consist of symptoms of the predisposing condition; symptoms of obstruction to the venous drainage of tissues adjacent to the sinus; in the case of infective thrombophlebitis, symptoms of extension of the infection to neighbouring structures and of its dissemination in the blood stream; and in some cases hydrocephalus due to defective absorption of cerebrospinal fluid. Conditions predisposing to intracranial sinus thrombosis have already been mentioned. The symptoms due to obstructed venous drainage differ according to the sinus affected.

Thrombosis of the Cavernous Sinus

Pain is severe and is located in the eye and forehead on the affected side and is usually associated with hyperpathia over the cutaneous distribution of the ophthalmic division of the trigeminal nerve. There is conspicuous oedema of the eyelids, the cornea, and the root of the nose, associated with exophthalmos due to congestion of the orbital veins. Papilloedema is sometimes present, but in some cases the optic disc is normal and vision unimpaired. Since the third, fourth, and sixth cranial nerves lie in the lateral wall of the sinus, ocular palsies are usually present and there may be complete internal and external ophthalmoplegia. Cavernous sinus thrombosis is usually unilateral at the outset, but thrombophlebitis readily extends through the circular sinus to the cavernous sinus of the opposite side, the signs then becoming bilateral.

Thrombosis of the Transverse Sinus

Thrombosis of the transverse sinus is almost always the result of an extension of infection from the mastoid. The patient complains of headache and of pain in the ear, which tends to be intensified by moving the head. Vomiting may occur. Venous congestion may be observed in the neighbourhood of the mastoid process and extension of the phlebitis to the jugular vein causes tenderness in the neck. The vein is rarely palpable as a tender cord. Papilloedema is sometimes present, but is usually slight and may be confined to the eye of the affected side. Focal cerebral symptoms include convulsions and contralateral hemiparesis. Aphasia may be present when the left transverse sinus is affected.

Thrombosis of the Superior Sagittal Sinus

Thrombosis of the superior sagittal sinus usually leads to a considerable rise of intracranial pressure. The earliest symptoms consist of headache, vomiting, delirium, and in some cases convulsions. There is rarely congestion of the scalp and external nasal veins, and in infants the fontanelle is tense. Papilloedema is sometimes present, and squint may occur. Since the superior sagittal sinus receives the superior cortical veins which drain the upper half of the hemi-spheres, and since the lower limbs are represented in the areas of the precentral gyrus nearest the vertex, thrombosis of this sinus may cause symptoms of bilateral corticospinal lesions, which are most marked in, and may be confined to, the lower limbs. Focal symptoms may be unilateral, e.g. Jacksonian epilepsy and hemiplegia, or even absent. Subarachnoid haemorrhage has been described (Walton, 1956). The symptoms may be mainly or exclusively those of hydro-cephalus, as in so-called 'otitic hydrocephalus' [see p. 227].

Thrombosis of other Sinuses

Thrombophlebitis may spread from the transverse sinus to the superior petrosal sinus and so reach the cerebral veins draining the lower part of the precentral gyrus causing faciobrachial monoplegia. Thrombophlebitis of the inferior petrosal sinus may explain Gradenigo's syndrome (Symonds, 1944) and involvement of the posterior group of cranial nerves.

Thrombophlebitis in Pregnancy

According to Carroll *et al.* (1966) the presenting symptoms in order of frequency are severe headache, convulsions, speech disturbances, and drowsi-ness and confusion.

The cerebrospinal fluid is usually under increased pressure, but may be otherwise normal. In thrombosis of the superior sagittal sinus, however, it is not uncommon to find red blood cells in considerable numbers, with a corresponding rise in the protein content, and even a xanthochromic fluid. The presence of a slight excess of leucocytes, usually both polymorphonuclear and mononuclear, is not uncommon and indicates a localized extension of the infection to the neighbouring leptomeninges. When one transverse sinus is filled with clot the pressure of the cerebrospinal fluid may fail to show the normal rise when the jugular vein on the affected side is compressed alone in Queckenstedt's test, but the sinus may be infected without being obstructed.

Other Investigations

Carotid angiography, with particular attention being paid to the venous phase, is the definitive investigation and frequently demonstrates occlusion of, or filling defects in, the affected sinus or sinuses [FIG. 87].

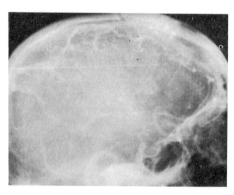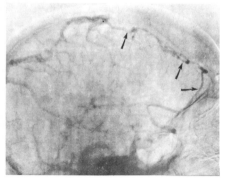

FIG. 87. Occlusion of the superior sagittal sinus in the frontal region demonstrated by carotid angio-graphy (on the left). A subtraction film (on the right) shows the anastomotic venous arcade (arrows)

Intracranial sinus thrombosis of infective origin often leads to *general symptoms* resulting from septicaemia. The patient is extremely ill, with a swinging temperature and rapid pulse, and rigors are common. Detachment of fragments of clot with resulting pulmonary embolism is most likely to occur in the case of transverse sinus thrombosis with extension to the jugular vein. This event is indicated by a sudden pain in the chest, associated with dyspnoea and sometimes with haemoptysis, followed by the development of signs of pulmonary consolidation and frequently a pleural rub. Pulmonary abscess may follow. The commonest intracranial extension of the infection is to the leptomeninges, resulting in many cases in a diffuse leptomeningitis, characterized by an increase in the severity of the headache, the development of cervical rigidity, the presence of Kernig's sign and other symptoms of meningitis, together with a marked polymorphonuclear pleocytosis with or without organisms in the cerebrospinal fluid. In many cases, however, thrombophlebitis of cranial sinuses develops insidiously, or after the acute phase of the infection has passed.

DIAGNOSIS

Cavernous sinus thrombosis may occasionally be confused with other lesions in the neighbourhood of the superior orbital fissure. Similar local symptoms may be produced by carotico-cavernous fistula due to trauma or aneurysmal rupture [p. 356]. Pulsation is present in the eye and a bruit is audible to the patient and often to the observer. Symptoms of infection are absent. The symptoms of retro-orbital or orbital tumour are of gradual onset and unassociated with symptoms of infection. Unilateral exophthalmos due to Graves's disease, mucocele of the ethmoid sinus, or orbital pseudotumour (*British Medical Journal*, 1974) may occasionally give rise to diagnostic difficulty, as may the syndrome of painful ophthalmoplegia [p. 169].

Thrombosis of the superior sagittal sinus, when it occurs in infancy, may be difficult to distinguish from other causes of hydrocephalus, to which it often gives rise. The selective paralysis of the lower limbs, when this is present, is the most useful distinctive feature. Examination of the cerebrospinal fluid will enable sinus thrombosis to be distinguished from meningitis.

Transverse sinus thrombosis may be difficult to distinguish from other intracranial complications of mastoiditis, especially extradural, subdural, and intracerebral abscess, with any of which it may coexist. When any of these conditions is suspected, however, the region of the transverse sinus should be explored and the dura and the sinus itself inspected.

PROGNOSIS

Antibiotic chemotherapy has entirely changed the prognosis of infective thrombophlebitis, and recovery usually now occurs even from cavernous sinus thrombosis which was formerly often fatal. The outlook is good in transverse sinus thrombosis treated by aural surgery combined with antibiotic treatment. Hydrocephalus due to thrombosis of the superior sagittal sinus usually responds to appropriate treatment. Cranial nerve palsies usually recover. Some permanent loss of function is likely to occur after cortical venous thrombosis and this may be followed by epilepsy as a late sequel. The mortality rate in thrombophlebitis of pregnancy is 33 per cent and 19 per cent of the survivors are left with permanent neurological deficits (Carroll *et al.*, 1966).

TREATMENT

When sinus thrombosis is infective in origin the source of infection must be treated with appropriate antibiotics. Ligature of the jugular vein, once commonly used in transverse sinus thrombosis, is now rarely if ever required. The value of anticoagulants is controversial because of the risk of haemorrhage: they are most likely to be useful if given in cases of primary thrombophlebitis before venous infarction has occurred. Intravenous infusion of low molecular weight dextran is sometimes employed. Meningitis will call for appropriate treatment. Otherwise treatment is symptomatic; dexamethasone in high dosage [p. 228] is useful in reducing cerebral oedema, especially when there are symptoms and signs of hydrocephalus.

REFERENCES

(The cerebral venous circulation, Thrombosis of the intracranial venous sinuses and veins.)

BAILEY, O. T., and HASS, G. M. (1937) Dural sinus thrombosis in early life, *Brain*, **60**, 293.

BICKERSTAFF, E. R. (1975) *Neurological Complications of Oral Contraceptives*, Oxford.

BRITISH MEDICAL JOURNAL (1974) Pseudotumours of the orbit, *Brit. med. J.*, **2**, 5.

CARROLL, J. D., LEAK, D., and LEE, H. A. (1966) Cerebral thrombophlebitis in pregnancy and the puerperium, *Quart. J. Med.*, **35**, 347.

FRENCKNER, P. (1936) Sinography: a method of radiography in the diagnosis of sinus thrombosis, *Proc. roy. Soc. Med.*, **30**, 413.

HOLMES, G., and SARGENT, P. (1915) Injuries of the superior longitudinal sinus, *Brit. med. J.*, **2**, 493.

KALBAG, R. M., and WOOLF, A. L. (1967) *Cerebral Venous Thrombosis*, London.

LANGWORTHY, H. G. (1916) Anatomic relations of the cavernous sinus to other structures, with consideration of various pathologic processes by which it may become involved, *Ann. Otol. (St. Louis)*, **25**, 554.

MARTIN, J. P., and SHEEHAN, H. L. (1941) Primary thrombosis of cerebral veins (following childbirth), *Brit. med. J.*, **1**, 349.

NEWTON, T. H., and POTTS, D. F. (1974) *Radiology of the Skull and Brain, Volume 2 (Angiography)*, St. Louis.

SYMONDS, C. P. (1937) Hydrocephalic and focal cerebral symptoms in relation to thrombophlebitis of the dural sinuses and cerebral veins, *Brain*, **60**, 531.

SYMONDS, C. P. (1944) Venous thrombosis in the central nervous system, *Proc. roy. Soc. Med.*, **37**, 387.

WALTON, J. N. (1956) *Subarachnoid Haemorrhage*, Edinburgh.

WEILL, G. (1929) De la thrombo-phlébite du sinus caverneux, *Rev. Oto-neuro-ophthal.*, **7**, 737.

5

NON-PENETRATING INJURIES OF THE BRAIN

AETIOLOGY

DURING recent years head injuries have occurred with increasing frequency, owing to the high speed of modern life. In civil life most head injuries are due to direct violence resulting from motor and industrial accidents. Less frequently they are produced by indirect violence after falls on the feet or buttocks. Penetrating wounds of the brain are comparatively rare. There is no direct parallelism between the severity of an injury to the skull and the extent to which the brain is damaged. Though severe fractures of the skull are often associated with severe cerebral injury, the brain may be extensively damaged without skull fracture and, on the other hand, fracture may occur without severe damage to the brain. Compound fractures of the skull, especially those involving the base and extending into the nasopharynx, nasal air sinuses, middle ear, and mastoid, assume additional importance as being liable to lead to infection of the intracranial contents and thus to cause meningitis or intracranial abscess. Apart from this risk, however, the crucial question after a head injury is the state of the brain rather than the state of the skull, and this alone will be considered here. For the physics of brain injury, and the characteristics of fractures of the skull and their treatment, see Gurdjian and Webster (1958), Rowbotham (1964), and Feiring (1974).

PATHOLOGY

The factors operating upon the brain in head injury are multiple and complex, and their results are often equally so. As Gurdjian *et al.* (1966) recently put it, 'compression, acceleration, and deceleration may occur during the traumatic episode. Tissues are injured by compression, tension, and shear. All of these modes of injury may occur simultaneously or in succession in the same accident.' These factors and their effects on the brain were described and discussed by Greenfield and Russell (1963) and by Tomlinson (1964). More recent work has shown that these factors, of which shearing forces may well be the most important, may give widespread microscopic lesions throughout the brain and brain stem (Oppenheimer, 1968), microglial clusters (Clark, 1974), and ischaemic or haemorrhagic lesions of the anterior hypothalamus (Crompton, 1971). Ommaya and Gennarelli (1974) suggest that rotational and accelerative forces produce a graded centripetal progression of diffuse cortical–subcortical disconnection phenomena maximal at the periphery and enhanced at junctions between grey and white matter. Studies of cerebral blood flow and angiography have shown that after severe closed head injury there is widespread vascular spasm and slowing of the cerebral circulation (Macpherson and Graham, 1973) but these changes do not invariably correlate with the pathological finding of widespread ischaemic lesions which were found in 55 per cent of a series of cases of fatal head injury (Graham and Adams, 1971). Unexplained haemorrhages in spinal posterior root ganglia may also be found (Spicer and Strich, 1967).

Concussion

Concussion was defined by Trotter as 'a condition of widespread paralysis of the functions of the brain which comes on as an immediate consequence of a blow on the head, has a strong tendency to spontaneous recovery, and is not necessarily associated with any gross organic change in the brain substance'. Here the stress is upon the reversibility of the process and in clinical terminology, concussion means a reversible impairment of consciousness of comparatively brief duration. It is now clear, however, that this cannot occur without damage to nerve cells and fibres and it is now doubtful if any physiological or anatomical distinction can be drawn between concussion as just defined and more prolonged states of unconsciousness resulting from head injury (Symonds, 1962). We know that consciousness is dependent upon the integrity of the ascending reticular alerting formation, and there is evidence that 'this system can be reversibly blocked by acceleration concussion' (Ward, 1966). The brain stem, attached above to the massive cerebral hemispheres and passing through an opening in the tentorium may well be especially vulnerable to brief displacements of the cranial contents. This fact led to the view that head injuries producing a decerebrate state or prolonged unconsciousness probably resulted from primary brain stem injury (Maciver *et al.*, 1958 *a*) but it is now clear that brain stem injury does not exist in isolation but is only one aspect of diffuse brain damage (Mitchell and Adams, 1973; Ommaya and Gennarelli, 1974). A persistent vegetative state after head injury may be due to diffuse damage to the cortex, to subcortical structures, or to the brain stem, but often to all three areas (Jennett and Plum, 1972).

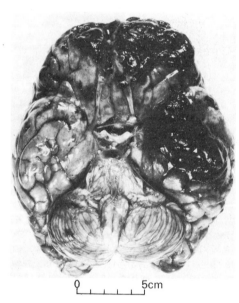

FIG. 88. The brain in a case of fatal closed head injury showing extensive areas of superficial haemorrhage over both frontal poles and in the left temporal region

0   5cm

Cerebral Contusion

The term cerebral contusion has traditionally been used to identify bruising of the brain, or a diffuse state more severe than concussion characterized by diffuse nerve cell and axonal damage, multiple punctate haemorrhages and oedema but, as indicated above, it is doubtful whether it is now useful to distinguish this condition from concussion, as the pathological changes in the two conditions are similar, differing only in degree and depending upon the severity of the injury. Larger areas of intracerebral haemorrhage are sometimes found, either in the cortex beneath the site of the blow, or in the contralateral hemisphere where the cortex has been driven forcibly against the interior of the skull vault (*contre-coup* injury). Superficial haemorrhages are often found in one or both frontal, temporal, or occipital poles [FIG. 88] and may sometimes occur even after relatively minor injury, especially in the elderly. Diffuse degeneration of the cerebral white matter is an important sequel of severe injury (Strich, 1956; Tomlinson, 1964).

Hydrocephalus

The cerebral oedema which usually accompanies severe head injury generally causes a substantial rise in intracranial pressure (Johnston et al., 1970) with an accompanying increase in the pressure of the cerebrospinal fluid in the ventricles and lumbar theca but arachnoidal adhesions may subsequently form resulting in disturbances of CSF formation and flow and even communicating hydrocephalus; rarely rupture of the arachnoid may allow CSF to enter the subdural space, producing a subdural hygroma.

Cerebral Laceration

'Cerebral laceration' is the term used when a cerebral contusion is sufficiently severe to cause a visible breach in the continuity of the brain substance. This may occur either immediately beneath the site of the blow or by *contre-coup* on the opposite side of the brain.

Intracranial Haemorrhage

Traumatic intracranial haemorrhage may be either intracerebral, sub-arachnoid, subdural, or extradural. An intracerebral haematoma may develop immediately after the injury but is rarely delayed, giving symptoms after an asymptomatic interval of hours or days, especially in older patients (Baratham and Dennyson, 1972). Bleeding into the subarachnoid space is generally associated with contusion of the cerebral cortex. Acute subdural haemorrhage is usually the result of a severe laceration, which may either involve the surface of the hemisphere or cause a large cavity filled with blood within its substance. Less often acute subdural haemorrhage is due to rupture of venous tributaries of the superior sagittal sinus or to laceration of one of the venous sinuses. Chronic subdural haematoma [p. 395] usually develops after a latent interval following minor trauma but sometimes arises spontaneously. Extradural haemorrhage is almost invariably the result of tearing of the middle meningeal artery or one of its branches due to a fracture of the skull vault crossing the groove in which it lies.

SYMPTOMS

Concussion and Contusion

After a slight injury the patient may be merely dazed or unconscious for a few seconds only, but his higher mental functions may subsequently be impaired for a period lasting up to several hours, during which he may carry out complicated activities in an automatic fashion, afterwards remembering nothing of these events. This is the period of *post-traumatic amnesia* (Russell, 1971) which is best measured from the injury to the time of the beginning of continuous awareness. This loss of memory may also extend to incidents which occurred before the accident, and is then known as *retrograde amnesia*. For example, a patient who sustains a head injury in an aeroplane crash may remember nothing that happened after he left the ground; or one injured in a motor accident may forget the incidents of a long drive [see p. 1147]; retrograde amnesia does not occur without post-traumatic amnesia (Yarnell and Lynch, 1970; Wolpaw, 1971).

In cases of more severe injury unconsciousness is more prolonged, and in addition the patient often exhibits signs of brain stem dysfunction. The pupils may be dilated and may fail to react to light, and the cutaneous and tendon reflexes may be lost, the musculature being flaccid; in severe cases a decerebrate or decorticate state is present. The blood pressure is low and the pulse is slow, or, in some cases, rapid and feeble, or imperceptible. Respiration may stop or may be shallow and sighing. Death may occur in severe cases from medullary paralysis.

Recovery is manifest first in an improvement of visceral function; the volume of the pulse increases, respiration becomes deeper, and the pupils again react to light. Vomiting is common at this stage. On recovering consciousness the patient may be delirious, restless, and irritable, and almost always complains of headache. In cases of mild concussion, however, these symptoms, with the possible exception of headache, usually disappear within a few days, though even after mild injury, the post-concussional syndrome (see below) may develop, especially in a compensation setting.

Traumatic Encephalopathy

Focal brain damage may occur in the absence of clinical manifestations of concussion or contusion, especially when a localized blow causes a depressed fracture of the skull, when consciousness is often retained (Miller and Jennett, 1968); the severity of the underlying damage to the brain may be dependent upon whether or not the dura is penetrated. In such cases, infection, haemorrhage, and focal neurological symptoms and signs are the most important complications. In moderate or severe closed head injury, with or without linear skull fracture, however, consciousness is usually lost immediately. In the most severe cases the depth of coma steadily increases, and the patient dies from medullary paralysis within a few hours. In less severe cases the patient, after recovering from concussion, passes into a state of stupor or confusion. He is usually drowsy and presents the picture long known as 'cerebral irritation', but better described as traumatic delirium, lying in a flexed attitude, resenting interference, confused and disorientated when roused, and at times noisy and violent. This condition may last for days or even weeks with a corresponding duration of post-traumatic amnesia, and in favourable cases gradually passes away. Or the patient may remain in a state of stupor (persistent vegetative state—Jennett and Plum, 1972) for many months. Symptoms of a focal lesion of the brain are usually absent, but focal convulsions, hemiparesis, or aphasia (Luria, 1970; Heilman et al., 1971) may follow a contusion involving the cortex; injury to the basal ganglia may cause mutism and extrapyramidal syndromes, and damage to the midbrain may cause quadriplegia, tonic convulsions, and in less severe cases ocular palsies, diplopia, and nystagmus; other cranial nerve palsies may be present (see below); and diabetes insipidus and disorders of hypothalamic function (Byrne, 1951) are rare complications.

Though a patient may recover rapidly and completely from a cerebral contusion, persistent disabling symptoms are extremely common. The three cardinal late symptoms are headache, giddiness, and mental disturbances, and they usually develop out of the symptoms of the acute stage. Headache tends to be severe and to occur in paroxysms which may last several hours, often against a background of continuous pain. It is brought on or exacerbated by activities such as stooping, sneezing, physical exertion, noise, and excitement. The giddiness is not always a sense of rotation, but a feeling of instability, though transitory vertigo and staggering on sudden head movement are common. Post-traumatic vertigo induced by change of posture is probably due to damage to the utricle and saccule of the internal ear and is accompanied by nystagmus which can be recorded in the electronystagmogram (Cartlidge and Shaw, 1977).

The commonest mental symptoms are inability to concentrate, fatigability and impairment of memory, together with nervousness and anxiety, and intolerance of alcohol. There are often symptoms of mild dementia of traumatic origin and all grades are encountered between the common milder cases and the less frequent more severe examples. In the latter the patient passes from the initial stupor into a stage of profound disorientation and confusion with defects of perception and disorganization of speech, and then sometimes into a stage resembling Korsakow's psychosis with gross defects of memory for recent events and sometimes confabulation (Friedman and Brenner, 1945). The final picture depends on many factors, especially the psychological constitution of the patient. Residual intellectual impairment is not uncommon: severe dementia is uncommon but not as rare as has been suggested (Fahy et al., 1967). Moods of excitement or depression are not infrequent in cyclothymic individuals while after severe head injury with prolonged unconsciousness paranoid and other psychotic manifestations have been reported (Fahy et al., 1967).

There has been considerable dispute as to whether the so-called *post-concussional* or *post-traumatic syndrome* as described above, when occurring in a setting which may involve financial compensation (e.g. in industrial accidents or road accidents) is largely an organic disorder or an 'accident neurosis' (Miller, 1961). Unquestionably headache, giddiness, impaired concentration, and the other symptoms described above occurring after moderate or severe head injury are the result of organic brain damage and may take between one and three years to recover, if indeed they ever do so. These symptoms tend to be directly proportional in severity and duration to the duration of the post-traumatic amnesia (Steadman and Graham, 1970) but may sometimes occur after relatively minor head injury (Gronwall and Wrightson, 1974). Unquestionably, however, neurotic and hysterical manifestations may cloud the clinical picture, especially when prolonged disability follows minor or even trivial injury and even frank malingering may be difficult to recognize (Miller and Cartlidge, 1972). Considerable experience is necessary in the assessment of such cases; detailed psychometric testing may be needed but reliable objective measures are few and it may only be possible to talk of 'the balance of probabilities'.

'*Punch-drunkenness*' is a chronic traumatic encephalopathy which may occur in professional boxers. It leads to deterioration of the personality, impairment of memory, dysarthria, tremor, Parkinsonian features, and ataxia (Critchley, 1957; Neubuerger et al., 1959; Royal College of Physicians, 1969; The Lancet, 1973). Pneumoencephalography in such cases often shows not only cortical atrophy but absence or cavitation of the septum pellucidum (Harvey and Davis, 1974).

Acute Traumatic Cerebral Compression

Cerebral compression leads to progressively deepening unconsciousness, indicated by the failure of the patient to respond to stimuli which have previously been capable of rousing him, and by loss of corneal reflexes. Deepening coma is of special importance when it follows a lucid interval after concussion. Ocular symptoms are important, the pupil on the side of the haemorrhage being first contracted and later dilated and failing to react to light, the same sequence of events subsequently occurring on the opposite side (Hutchinson pupil). These signs are due to tentorial herniation causing pressure upon the trunk of one or both third cranial nerves. Papilloedema is usually absent, though the optic discs and fundi may exhibit venous congestion. These symptoms must always raise the possibility of an extradural haematoma which is a neurosurgical emergency, but similar symptoms may result from an acute subdural haematoma, an intra-cerebral haemorrhage, or even severe unilateral cerebral oedema associated with contusion or laceration, a fact which underlines the importance of skilled neurosurgical assessment and management of such cases. Symptoms and signs of a progressive lesion of the affected hemisphere, focal convulsions or a flaccid hemiparesis are more likely to be due to an intracerebral lesion but rarely occur in extradural haemorrhage. Medullary symptoms are prominent, especially in the later stages of cerebral compression. The pulse at first is slow and full, later rapid, thready, and irregular. The blood pressure may be subnormal or may exhibit a steady rise. The respirations are at first slow and deep, later irregular, e.g. of the Cheyne-Stokes type, and finally rapid and shallow. The temperature is often somewhat raised. Sugar may be present in the urine.

Cranial Nerve Palsies

Cranial nerve palsies may be due to injury of the brain stem or of the nerves, either in their intracranial or in their extracranial course. Bilateral anosmia [p. 154] is a common complication due to tearing of the olfactory nerve filaments as they pass through the cribriform plate of the ethmoid; ageusia [p. 206] is much less common. Contusion of the midbrain may leave permanent paresis of ocular movement, usually in the vertical plane, either unilaterally or bilaterally, resulting in diplopia and often associated with nystagmus. Intracranial injuries of the nerves are usually the result of fracture of the base of the skull. After the olfactory, the seventh is the nerve most frequently affected and then the eighth, sixth, second, third, and fourth in this order (Sherren, 1908). The effects of injuries of these nerves are described in the sections dealing with the cranial nerves. The facial nerve, or its branches, and branches of the trigeminal may be divided or contused as a result of wounds and blows upon the face. Traumatic cranial nerve palsies are usually permanent, but recovery occasionally occurs when intra-cranial or extracranial nerve trunks have been contused rather than divided.

Cerebrospinal Fluid

Examination of the cerebrospinal fluid may yield information of value, but lumbar puncture is not free from risk after head injury because of the risk of herniation of swollen brain. It should not be performed, therefore, unless absolutely necessary for diagnostic purposes. It is rarely necessary in the acute stage if the EMI scan and angiography and other appropriate investigations are available, but may be necessary to exclude meningitis. Blood is present in the fluid immediately after the accident in most cases of cerebral contusion and of more serious injury. The number of red cells present is not always pro-portionate to the severity of the injury; the protein content of the fluid is proportionate to the number of red cells. The supernatant fluid is xantho-chromic. The red cells tend to disappear in four or five days, but the xantho-chromia may remain for two or three weeks. Recording of the intracranial pressure is done more safely by inserting extradural transducers through a burr-hole, but repeated lumbar punctures may sometimes still be needed in less sophisticated centres in order to monitor the response of cerebral oedema to treatment.

Electroencephalography

Suppression of the normal frequencies, widespread abnormally slow waves, and outbursts of high voltage 2 to 3 Hz waves are seen in the acute stage. In the chronic post-traumatic state generalized low voltage 2 to 7 Hz waves, sometimes seen in one or both temporal regions, are the rule and the disturbance is on the whole proportional to the severity of the injury and the persistence of symptoms (Williams, 1941 a and b). However, the EEG may be surprisingly normal after severe brain injury and is often disappointing in predicting which patients will and which will not develop post-traumatic epilepsy (Walton et al., 1964).

Radiography

Radiography during the acute stage may show an unsuspected fracture of the skull, which often proves of greater medico-legal than clinical importance. Echo-encephalography may show a space-occupying lesion. Angiography may demonstrate, and help to locate, an acute haematoma, either within the brain or in the subdural or extradural space. The EMI scan has proved to be a major advance in identifying and localizing intracranial lesions complicating head injury.

Variations from the normal encephalogram have been described in 80 per cent of cases in the late stages. The commonest abnormality is a slight diffuse enlargement of the lateral ventricles or focal or generalized pooling of air over the cortex due to cortical atrophy, while an extensive cortical scar may lead to the formation of a diverticulum from one cerebral ventricle (traumatic porencephaly). Enlargement of the Sylvian aqueduct may indicate midbrain damage (Boller et al., 1972). Communicating hydrocephalus due to meningeal adhesions is an occasional late complication. Isotope encephalography [p. 148] may be needed to identify sites of CSF leakage following skull fracture.

Other Investigations

Inspection and palpation of the scalp and skull form part of the routine examination of cases of head injury, the presence of haematomas being noted and the bones carefully examined for depressed fracture. Bleeding from the nasopharynx and ears in the absence of external injury is an important sign of fracture of the base of the skull, and inquiry should always be made as to the discharge of cerebrospinal fluid, which may be recognized by its sugar content. The urinary output should be measured from the beginning because of the risk of renal failure (Taylor, 1957). As profound disturbances of hydration and acid–base balance readily occur in patients with head injury (Vapalahti, 1970) and as pulmonary complications leading to cerebral anoxia are also common (Maciver et al., 1958 b) regular monitoring of the blood urea and serum electrolytes and of the blood gases (oxygen and carbon dioxide) is necessary in the unconscious patient.

DIAGNOSIS

Although in most cases the injury to the head is clearly the cause of the patient's symptoms, it is necessary to bear in mind the possibility that a pre-existing illness, especially a cerebral vascular lesion or intoxication with alcohol or other drugs, may have led to an accident in which the head has been injured, in which case the symptoms may not be due to the injury. When this source of confusion has been eliminated it is necessary to decide the nature of the injury to the brain. If after a head injury the patient remains unconscious for more than a few minutes, or if after recovery of consciousness he remains confused or exhibits other symptoms of cerebral disturbance, it is reasonable to conclude that he has suffered concussion or cerebral contusion. The symptoms which distinguish acute traumatic cerebral compression from cerebral contusion have already been described. The occurrence of cerebral fat embolism in a patient also suffering from a head injury may give rise to difficulty. The existence of a latent interval, pulmonary symptoms and signs, and cutaneous haemorrhages may enable the correct diagnosis to be made. The onset of meningitis is to be suspected, in a patient with known traumatic subarachnoid haemorrhage, when the patient develops increasing cervical rigidity and pyrexia, and is confirmed by the presence of a polymorphonuclear leucocytosis, with or without pyogenic organisms, in the cerebrospinal fluid.

When confusion and drowsiness increase in severity the possibility of intracranial haemorrhage or increasing oedema must be considered. When these are present the symptoms tend to get worse, whereas in concussion or contusion the early symptoms tend to improve. Progressive symptoms in the later stages may suggest chronic subdural haematoma and render further investigation advisable.

PROGNOSIS

Concussion is rarely fatal and, when the patient survives the immediate effects of the injury, is followed by complete recovery within a few weeks or months, provided it is not severe or complicated by contusion or more serious injuries. The post-concussional syndrome has been discussed above.

Traumatic encephalopathy, when severe, may prove fatal, usually within a few hours, from medullary paralysis. However, in Lewin's (1966 a) series of 7,000 patients with non-missile injuries admitted to hospital, the mortality rate was only 48 per cent. After severe injury some patients remain comatose for days or weeks and subsequently die from respiratory infection or other complications, but with modern nursing and medical care this is relatively uncommon and many enter, after a few weeks, a 'persistent vegetative state' (Jennett and Plum, 1972), showing periods of apparent wakefulness, random eye movements, and primitive postural and reflex motor activity. Most remain in this state for months or even years but a few ultimately regain limited speech and volitional motor activity and all have severe residual intellectual and neurological deficits. Among the factors which have been shown to have an adverse influence upon prognosis are age (children often recover remarkably from severe injuries), decerebrate rigidity or extensor spasms, prolonged coma, hypertension, a low arterial $p(CO_2)$, a high respiratory minute volume, and a temperature persistently above 39 °C. (Vapalahti and Troupp, 1971; Overgaard et al., 1973). In comatose patients, careful neurological examination with particular attention being paid to caloric, oculocephalic, and other brain stem reflexes and to the respiratory pattern may give valuable prognostic clues (Plum and Posner, 1972). Jennett and Bond (1975) have devised a useful five-point scale for assessing the ultimate outcome, namely: (1) death; (2) persistent vegetative state; (3) severe disability (conscious but disabled); (4) moderate disability (disabled but independent); (5) good recovery. Miller and Stern (1965) reviewed the condition of 100 consecutive cases of severe head injury at a mean interval of 11 years. Approximately half were closed head injuries. Eight patients had died, 21 out of 25 with spastic pareses showed unexpectedly good recovery, 19 had developed epilepsy, and 16 had persisting psychiatric symptoms, of whom 10 had dementia.

Acute traumatic cerebral compression is fatal in many cases, the outlook being worse in acute subdural haemorrhage (which usually implies severe underlying cortical damage) than in extradural or intracerebral haematoma, provided surgical treatment is undertaken early. After successful evacuation of a clot, many patients recover completely but others are left with a variable degree of disability.

Prophylactic chemotherapy has much reduced the incidence of meningitis, and lessened its dangers if it occurs. Late results of head injury, which include aphasia, persisting symptoms of injuries to the hypothalamus and midbrain (such as diplopia and diabetes insipidus), cranial nerve palsies, intracranial aerocele, cerebrospinal rhinorrhoea, subdural haematoma, and traumatic epilepsy, are described elsewhere.

TREATMENT

The usual treatment of the unconscious patient should be carried out [see p. 1170]. If there is respiratory embarrassment this should be treated by suction or tracheostomy. Oxygen should be administered by nasal tube or tracheostomy catheter. Hypothermia should be used if necessary to control pyrexia and may be useful in other severe cases. Hyperosmolarity of the blood may require intravenous fluid and other disorders of acid–base balance will require appropriate treatment. Convulsions, if severe, may need to be controlled by intravenous diazepam or thiopentone. Traumatic cerebral oedema responds well to steroids such as dexamethasone [see p. 228].

For details of surgical treatment the reader is referred to neurosurgical texts (Rowbotham, 1964; Northfield, 1973). The most important principles are first, to maintain an adequate airway and pulmonary ventilation from the outset, secondly to reduce cerebral oedema and thus the intracranial pressure, and thirdly to be prepared to operate on suspicion that an expanding intracranial haematoma may be present.

The broad outlines of rehabilitation are now well defined; they were well set out by Jefferson (1942), Cairns (1942), Symonds (1942), Lewis (1942), and Goldstein (1942) and have been reviewed by Tobis *et al.* (1957), Trethowan (1970), and Feiring (1974). It is essential to ascertain and take into account the personality of the patient before the accident. Explanation of symptoms and reassurance play an important part as soon as consciousness is regained. The present practice is to shorten the stay in bed and to let the patient get up as soon as he feels able to do so. After getting up activity is increased, beginning with walking, games, and light exercises, and going on to more strenuous exercises. Supervised occupation should begin as early as possible and occupational therapy should gradually merge into therapeutic occupation. Throughout convalescence the patient's mental attitude must be kept constantly in mind. Psychological tests are of value for discovering specific disabilities, but the patient's emotional attitude to his difficulties is of equal importance, and explanation and encouragement are necessary throughout. During the later stages of convalescence the patient should be encouraged to go into a town, to the cinema, etc., to test his reactions to noise and bustle. In cases uncomplicated by focal lesions absence from work is likely to last from six weeks to many months according to the severity of the injury. Persistent disabilities may make it impossible for him to return to his pre-accident occupation. Special disabilities, especially speech disturbances, require prolonged treatment by experts.

TRAUMATIC PNEUMOCEPHALUS

Synonym. Intracranial aerocele.

Definition. The presence of air within the skull as a result of head injury.

AETIOLOGY AND PATHOLOGY

Trauma is the commonest cause of the pathological presence of air within the skull; this is usually due to a fracture of the skull affording communication between an air-containing cranial cavity and the interior of the cranium. It may occur as the result of a fracture which involves the frontal, ethmoidal, or sphenoidal sinuses or the mastoid air cells or, rarely, after operation on a nasal sinus. Occasionally, however, air enters the skull as a result of erosion of bone from within, for example by intracranial tumour, abscess, or hydrocephalus.

Within the cranial cavity the collection of air may be external to the brain. Both subdural and subarachnoid collections have been described, but as the arachnoid is often torn, it is difficult to differentiate these. The air sometimes penetrates one cerebral hemisphere, in which it becomes encysted.

SYMPTOMS

Cerebrospinal rhinorrhoea, a discharge of cerebrospinal fluid from the nose, is usually an accompaniment of traumatic pneumocephalus. It may, however, occur when the base of the skull is eroded from within by intracranial tumour, abscess, or internal hydrocephalus. The volume of the discharge is variable: it may be small or there may be enough to necessitate the use of a number of handkerchiefs. The discharge is usually influenced by change of posture and may occur, for example, only when the patient sits up and leans forward. It often affords relief from headache and other symptoms. The presence of sugar in the fluid can be demonstrated by appropriate tests and is a useful diagnostic point. The presence of air within the skull may occasionally be demonstrated by means of a tympanitic note on percussion, more frequently by a succussion splash audible to the patient and to the observer on shaking the patient's head. This last symptom implies the presence of both air and fluid within the same part of the cranial cavity.

Air within the skull may lead to focal symptoms, especially when it has invaded one cerebral hemisphere. They may include mental confusion, convulsions, aphasia, hemiparesis, and a grasp reflex. They tend to fluctuate in severity and may be relieved by an attack of cerebrospinal rhinorrhoea. Symptoms of increased intracranial pressure, for example headache and papilloedema, may also be present. In severe cases coma may develop.

X-ray examination of the skull is the most valuable single method of diagnosis, the situation of the air being exactly demonstrated. When fluid is also present within the cavity it may be demarcated from the air by a horizontal line which varies in position in relation to gravity.

DIAGNOSIS

Diagnosis offers little difficulty. All cases of serious head injury should be X-rayed and the air is then demonstrated. Isotope ventriculography is valuable in localizing the point of leakage in cerebrospinal rhinorrhoea [p. 149].

PROGNOSIS

Two factors influence the prognosis: the risks of a focal lesion of the brain associated with increased intracranial pressure and the risks of meningitis due to infection entering the skull through the opening in the bone.

Air in the ventricles and in the subarachnoid space is normally absorbed in from ten days to a fortnight. It is doubtful, however, whether absorption occurs when the air is encysted by brain tissue. The risk of infection is high and in most cases of head injury with cerebrospinal rhinorrhoea meningitis supervenes in the absence of prophylactic antibiotic therapy and/or operative interference.

TREATMENT

In order to diminish the risks both of further entry of air within the skull and of meningeal infection, the patient should be kept flat and should be told to avoid forcibly blowing his nose. Prophylactic chemotherapy should be employed. In Lewin's view 'operative repair is the treatment of choice for all cases of paranasal sinus fracture with cerebral fluid rhinorrhoea, whether this is of early or late onset, of brief or long duration' (Lewin, 1966 b).

SUBDURAL HAEMATOMA

Definition. An encysted collection of blood between the dura mater and the arachnoid, sometimes traumatic, but also occurring in the absence of recognized injury.

PATHOLOGY

Acute subdural haematoma is common in fatal cases of head injury: an extensive but thin layer of haemorrhage may raise the intracranial pressure enough to cause herniation of the uncus, or midbrain haemorrhages.

In chronic subdural haematoma blood slowly accumulates in the subdural space. It is usually the result of a minor head injury causing rupture of veins which traverse the subdural space. Russell and Cairns (1934) in four cases of metastatic carcinoma of the dura complicated by subdural haematoma attributed the bleeding to engorgement and rupture of the capillaries of the areolar layer. In most cases the collection of blood, which may attain a large size, lies over the frontal and parietal lobes, and in nearly half of all cases the haematoma is bilateral. Subdural bleeding in the posterior fossa is rare. The blood is encysted between an outer wall consisting of a layer of highly vascularized granulation tissue slightly adherent to the dura ('the membrane'), and a thinner, inner wall of fibrous tissue with a single layer of mesothelium on the side next to the arachnoid. It is mostly fluid, though a coagulum may be present. Subdural hygroma is a collection of cerebrospinal fluid, which eventually becomes xanthochromic, and is indistinguishable before operation from a subdural haematoma.

AETIOLOGY

Males are affected more often than females in the ratio of three to one. Subdural haematoma may occur at any age. It is sometimes seen in infancy, when it has been attributed to birth injury but is sometimes due to postnatal trauma (Yashon et al., 1968) as in the 'battered baby syndrome'. Subdural effusions may, however, develop as a complication of meningitis in infancy (Rabe et al.,

1968). In adult life it is commonest in the elderly, usually resulting from trauma which may be trivial. However, it is also an uncommon complication of aneurysmal rupture, especially recurrent bleeding, when the aneurysm may rupture directly into the subdural space (Golden et al., 1953; Clarke and Walton, 1953). It may also follow air encephalography (Robinson, 1957) or whiplash injury to the neck (Ommaya and Yarnell, 1969) and has been reported during haemodialysis (Leonard et al., 1969). Other causes include chronic alcoholism, liver disease, neurosyphilis, streptococcal infections, blood diseases such as scurvy and thrombocytopenic purpura, treatment with anticoagulants, and carcinoma of the dura; in such cases there is rarely any history of injury.

SYMPTOMS

The symptoms of subdural haematoma may follow an injury immediately. Alternatively there is a latent interval lasting weeks or months, less often more than a year, rarely of many years. During the latent interval the patient may be free from symptoms or may feel vaguely unwell (Scheinberg and Scheinberg, 1964). After the latent interval there is a gradual onset of headache, drowsiness, and, often, confusion: epilepsy is rare. These symptoms often fluctuate greatly in severity but headache is often severe, paroxysmal and induced by bending or coughing. As is usually the case when the brain is compressed from without, focal cerebral symptoms may be lacking or slight, considering the size of the haematoma. When present they are likely to consist of hemiparesis, with aphasia when the lesion is left-sided. The grasp reflex may be present. Papilloedema is often absent. Transient ocular paralysis may occur. Inequality of the pupils is often present, the larger pupil, together with slight ptosis, being found on the side of the haematoma.

In infants the onset occurs during the first year. Enlargement of the head may be the first abnormality to be noticed, but convulsions, irritability, and vomiting are common and pyrexia may be present (Till, 1968). The head is found to be enlarged, with a bulging anterior fontanelle and frequently separation of the sutures. The veins of the scalp are often dilated. Papilloedema and retinal and subhyaloid haemorrhages are usually present, leading in the later stages to optic atrophy. The symptoms are therefore those of increased intracranial pressure with cortical irritation, and paralysis of the limbs is usually absent. The cerebrospinal fluid may be blood stained or xanthochromic with considerable excess of protein, and is rarely normal. The diagnosis is established by subdural puncture, carried out at the lateral margin of the anterior fontanelle, xanthochromic or blood-stained fluid being withdrawn from the subdural space.

DIAGNOSIS

The diagnosis of subdural haematoma offers little difficulty when there is a clear history of recent head injury. In the absence of this the clinical picture may simulate that of intracranial tumour, especially when papilloedema is present. The fluctuating character of the drowsiness and confusion, however, may suggest the true diagnosis. In an elderly patient with a history of head injury it may be difficult to distinguish subdural haematoma from a cerebral vascular accident. Chronic alcoholism in its later stages may lead to confusion and drowsiness, and, since it is a predisposing cause of subdural haematoma, and may also lead to accidents which involve head injury, may give rise to difficulties in diagnosis. The cerebrospinal fluid is usually normal, but the protein may be increased, and the fluid may be xanthochromic. The pressure is usually raised but may be subnormal. There may be a pleocytosis. Spectrophotometry of the fluid (Kjellin and Steiner, 1974) can be very helpful. Angiography shows a characteristic displacement of arteries, with an avascular area beneath the skull vault [FIG. 89] and the EMI scan also gives a diagnostic appearance. Calcification has occasionally been observed radiographically in a haematoma of very long standing, and Bull (1951) has shown that the floor of the middle fossa may be excavated. The EEG may be helpful. In doubtful cases burr-hole exploration is necessary.

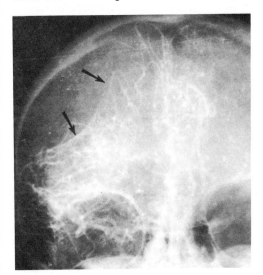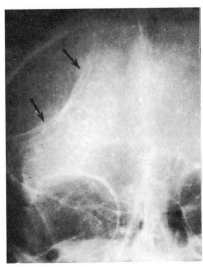

FIG. 89. A right-sided chronic subdural haematoma demonstrated by carotid angiography; arterial phase on the left, capillary phase on the right

PROGNOSIS

The prognosis of subdural haematoma is good, provided the diagnosis is made sufficiently early, for operation to be performed before the patient's general condition has deteriorated seriously. In such cases complete recovery is the rule. In other cases, however, the patient fails to respond to drainage of the haematoma. Echlin *et al.* (1956) reported a mortality rate of 39 per cent in 300 cases. McKissock *et al.* (1960), dividing their cases into acute, subacute, and chronic had a mortality rate of 57 per cent in the acute, 24 per cent in the subacute, and 6 per cent in the chronic group. The prognosis is worst in the aged.

TREATMENT

Treatment consists in the surgical evacuation of the blood clot. The fact that the haematoma is bilateral in nearly 50 per cent of cases must always be borne in mind. Occasionally in chronic cases, craniotomy and removal of the membrane is required. Among others, Bender and Christoff (1974) have advised non-surgical treatment, but this view has received little acceptance.

TRAUMATIC EPILEPSY

AETIOLOGY AND PATHOLOGY

Our knowledge of the factors influencing the development of epileptic attacks after head injury is mainly derived from observation of cases of gunshot wound of the head. Such injuries are not strictly comparable with the head injuries of civil life, since they include a much higher proportion of penetrating wounds and a much smaller proportion of cases of simple concussion and fracture of the base of the skull.

The frequency with which epilepsy follows head injury has been variously estimated at from $4\frac{1}{2}$ per cent (Sargent) to 25 per cent (Rawling), 34 per cent (Ascroft, 1941), and 36 per cent (Watson, 1947) of cases of gunshot wound of the head. The incidence in 500 closed head injuries in soldiers was 6 per cent (Phillips, 1954). Probably under 5 per cent represents the average incidence in civil life.

The latent period between the injury and the onset of fits is extremely variable. In a small proportion of cases fits occur immediately after the injury, or in the first week (Jennett, 1969), and status epilepticus has been described after relatively minor injury in childhood (Grand, 1974). These usually cease, and if convulsions subsequently develop they do so only after an interval of freedom. There is some evidence (Whitty, 1947; Jennett, 1965, 1969) that early attacks predispose to late ones. Apart from these early attacks, attacks may develop within a month or two of the injury, or they may be delayed for many years. A patient of Brain's, with a retained metallic foreign body, had his first attack 27 years after being wounded. The commonest time of onset is between six and twelve months after the injury (Watson), but figures vary. Jennett (1965) found that half the patients had their first attack within a year of the injury but both in missile wounds (Adeloye and Odeku, 1971) and in closed head injury there is a substantial, though declining, subsequent risk which can be calculated by actuarial methods (Jennett et al., 1973). However, the majority who become epileptic do so within two years (Miller and Stern, 1965).

The severity of the injury is important in relation to the likelihood of the development of convulsions. Wagstaff (1928) found that when the injury caused penetration of the dura the incidence of epilepsy was 18 per cent, whereas in all cases of less severe injury it was only 2 per cent. This fact acquires significance from Foerster and Penfield's observation (1930) of the part played by scar tissue in the aetiology of traumatic epilepsy. It would appear that epilepsy is most likely to occur when vascularized scar tissue unites the surface of the brain to the dura, and this is obviously most likely to occur when the dura has been penetrated. Jennett (1965) found that late epilepsy was commoner in patients with depressed fracture and that, except in children, it was rare with a duration of post-traumatic amnesia of less than 24 hours. Epilepsy following trivial head injury in adult life is rare, but certainly occurs in childhood (Small and Woolf, 1957). A family history of epilepsy is sometimes present, so it is probable that inherited predisposition plays a part in the aetiology of traumatic epilepsy in some cases. The site of the injury in the hemisphere is relatively unimportant, but posterior frontal and parietal lesions seem the most likely to cause epilepsy (Watson, 1947; Russell, 1947).

SYMPTOMS

Traumatic epileptic attacks may be focal or generalized. Focal attacks often occur immediately after the injury. Their character and the nature of the aura, if any, depends upon the situation of the lesion. Even when the early attacks are focal there is a tendency for subsequent attacks, if they occur, to be major or sometimes minor, of the 'temporal lobe' type [pp. 1104–5]. Radiography, especially encephalography, is often of diagnostic value, since air may fail to reach the area of cortex adherent to the dura and it may be possible to demonstrate a 'traction diverticulum', the lateral ventricle being drawn towards the lesion by atrophy of the white matter and by the scar. The electroencephalogram may be normal between the attacks (Walter, 1938; Walton et al., 1964; Jennett and van de Sande, 1975).

DIAGNOSIS

For the diagnosis of epilepsy see page 1111. Post-traumatic syncope and hysterical 'faints' may give rise to particular difficulty, especially in a setting involving financial compensation. Eye-witness descriptions of the attacks may be particularly important. The traumatic origin of genuine epilepsy can usually only be established when there is a history of injury, and this should be especially inquired for, since the patient may not realize its importance when the attacks do not begin until several years later. It must be remembered that a previous head injury is not necessarily the cause of the attacks, but its aetiological significance is reinforced if the fits have a focal onset, if there are persistent signs of a focal cerebral lesion, and if the radiographic abnormalities already described are present.

PROGNOSIS

The factors which influence the prognosis of idiopathic epilepsy apply equally to traumatic cases, but it appears that when a gross focal lesion of the brain is present the prognosis as to recovery is worse than in epilepsy not thus complicated. The attacks ceased in one-third of Ascroft's cases. The prognosis is best when they begin within two weeks of the injury, worst when the latent interval is over two years. The life expectancy of patients with post-traumatic epilepsy is slightly reduced (Walker et al., 1971).

TREATMENT

Patients with traumatic epilepsy should receive medical treatment on the same lines as cases of idiopathic epilepsy. Only when this fails to yield satisfactory results should operation be considered. The surgical treatment of traumatic epilepsy has been carried out for many years, but has fallen into comparative disrepute. It was revived by Foerster and Penfield (1930) and Penfield and Erickson (1941) claimed good results in selected cases. If it is to be successful the presence of a focal lesion of the brain must be established by the methods already described, and it should be possible to find electrocorticographic abnormalities on the exposed cortex in the affected area. Treatment consists in a free excision of the scar tissue (Rasmussen and Gossman, 1963).

Other sequels of head injury, which are described in their respective sections, include meningitis, intracranial abscess, diabetes insipidus, and a Parkinsonian syndrome.

REFERENCES

ADELOYE, A., and ODEKU, E. L. (1971) Epilepsy after missile wounds of the head, *J. Neurol. Neurosurg. Psychiat.*, **34,** 98.

ASCROFT, P. B. (1941) Traumatic epilepsy after gunshot wounds of the head, *Brit. med. J.,* **i,** 739.

BARATHAM, G., and DENNYSON, W. G. (1972) Delayed traumatic intracerebral haemorrhage, *J. Neurol. Neurosurg. Psychiat.*, **35,** 698.

BENDER, M. B., and CHRISTOFF, N. (1974) Nonsurgical treatment of subdural haematomas, *Arch. Neurol. (Chic.)*, **31,** 73.

BIELSCHOWSKY, P. (1928) Störungen des Liquorsystems bei Schädeltraumen, *Z. ges. Neurol. Psychiat.*, **117,** 55.

BOLLER, F. C., ALBERT, M. L., LeMAY, M., and KERTESZ, A. (1972) Enlargement of the Sylvian aqueduct: a sequel of head injuries, *J. Neurol. Neurosurg. Psychiat.*, **35,** 463.

BULL, J. W. D. (1951) Diagnostic radiology, in *Modern Trends in Neurology*, 1st series, ed. Feiling, A., London.

BYRNE, E. A. J. (1951) Post-traumatic disturbance of hypothalamic function. *Brit. med. J.,* **i,** 850.

CAIRNS, H. (1937) Injuries of the frontal and ethmoidal sinuses with special reference to cerebrospinal rhinorrhoea and aerocele, *J. Laryng.*, **52,** 589.

CAIRNS, H. (1941–2) Rehabilitation after injuries to the central nervous system, *Proc. roy. Soc. Med.*, **35,** 299.

CARTLIDGE, N. E. F., and SHAW, D. A. (1977) *Head Injury*, London.

CLARK, J. M. (1974) Distribution of microglial clusters in the brain after head injury, *J. Neurol. Neurosurg. Psychiat.*, **37,** 463.

CLARKE, E., and WALTON, J. N. (1953) Subdural haematoma complicating intracranial aneurysm and angioma, *Brain*, **76,** 378.

CRITCHLEY, M. (1957) Medical aspects of boxing, *Brit. med. J.*, **i,** 357.

CROMPTON, M. R. (1971) Hypothalamic lesions following closed head injury, *Brain*, **94,** 165.

DANDY, W. E. (1925) Pneumocephalus (intracranial pneumatocele or aerocele), *Arch. Surg.*, **12,** 949.

DENNY-BROWN, D., and RUSSELL, W. R. (1941) Experimental cerebral concussion, *Brain*, **64,** 93.

ECHLIN, F. A., SORDILLO, S. V. R., and GARVEY, T. Q. (1956) Acute, subacute and chronic subdural haematoma, *J. Amer. med. Ass.*, **161,** 1345.

FAHY, T. J., IRVING, M. H., and MILLAC, P. (1967) Severe head injuries, *Lancet*, **ii,** 475.

FEIRING, E. H. (1974) *Brock's Injuries of the Brain and Spinal Cord and Their Coverings*, 5th ed., New York.

FOERSTER, O., and PENFIELD, W. (1930) The structural basis of traumatic epilepsy and results of radical operation, *Brain*, **53,** 99.

FRIEDMAN, A. P., and BRENNER, C. (1945) Amnestic-confabulatory syndrome (Korsakoff psychosis) following head injury, *Amer. J. Psychiat.*, **102,** 61.

GOLDEN, J., ODOM, G. L., and WOODHALL, B. (1953) Subdural hematoma following subarachnoid hemorrhage, *Arch. Neurol. Psychiat. (Chic.)*, **69,** 486.

GOLDSTEIN, K. (1942) *After-effects of Brain Injuries in War*, London.

GRAHAM, D. I., and ADAMS, J. H. (1971) Ischaemic brain damage in fatal head injuries, *Lancet*, **i,** 265.

GRAND, W. (1974) The significance of post-traumatic status epilepticus in childhood, *J. Neurol. Neurosurg. Psychiat.*, **37,** 178.

GREENFIELD, J. G., and RUSSELL, D. S. (1963) Traumatic lesions of the central and peripheral nervous systems, in *Greenfield's Neuropathology*, ed. Blackwood, W., McMenemey, W. H., Meyer, A., Norman, R. M., and Russell, D. S., 2nd ed., p. 441, London.

GRONWALL, D., and WRIGHTSON, P. (1974) Delayed recovery of intellectual function after minor head injury, *Lancet*, **ii,** 605.

GURDJIAN, E. S., LISSNER, H. R., HODGSON, V. R., and PATRICK, L. M. (1966) Mechanism of head injury, in *Clinical Neurosurgery*, p. 112, Baltimore.

GURDJIAN, E. S., and WEBSTER, J. E. (1958) *Head Injuries*, London.

HARVEY, P. K. P., and DAVIS, J. N. (1974) Traumatic encephalopathy in a young boxer, *Lancet*, **ii**, 928.

HEILMAN, K. M., SAFRAN, A., and GESCHWIND, N. (1971) Closed head trauma and aphasia, *J. Neurol. Neurosurg. Psychiat.*, **34**, 265.

HUNT, F. C. (1930) Internal hemorrhagic pachymeningitis in young children, *Amer. J. Dis., Childn.*, **39**, 84.

JEFFERSON, G. (1941–2) Rehabilitation after injuries to the central nervous system, *Proc. roy. Soc. Med.*, **35**, 295.

JENNETT, W. B. (1965) Predicting epilepsy after blunt head injury, *Brit. med. J.*, **1**, 1215.

JENNETT, W. B. (1969) Early traumatic epilepsy: definition and identity, *Lancet*, **i**, 1023.

JENNETT, W. B., and BOND, M. (1975) Assessment of outcome after severe brain damage: a practical scale, *Lancet*, **i**, 480.

JENNETT, W. B., and PLUM, F. (1972) Persistent vegetative state after brain damage: a syndrome in search of a name, *Lancet*, **i**, 734.

JENNETT, W. B., TEATHER, D., and BENNIE, S. (1973) Epilepsy after head injury. Residual risk after varying fit-free intervals since injury, *Lancet*, **ii**, 652.

JENNETT, W. B., and VAN DE SANDE, J. (1975) EEG prediction of post-traumatic epilepsy, *Epilepsia*, **16**, 251.

JOHNSTON, I. H., JOHNSTON, J. A., and JENNETT, W. B. (1970) Intracranial-pressure changes following head injury, *Lancet*, **ii**, 433.

KAPLAN, A. (1931) Chronic subdural haematoma: a study of eight cases with special reference to the state of the pupil, *Brain*, **54**, 430.

KJELLIN, K. G., and STEINER, L. (1974) Spectrophotometry of cerebrospinal fluid in subacute and chronic subdural haematomas, *J. Neurol. Neurosurg. Psychiat.*, **37**, 1121.

THE LANCET (1973) Boxing brains, *Lancet*, **ii**, 1064.

LEONARD, C. D., WEIL, E., and SCRIBNER, B. H. (1969) Subdural haematomas in patients undergoing haemodialysis, *Lancet*, **ii**, 239.

LEWIN, W. (1966 a) Nonsurgical treatment of patients with head injuries, in *Clinical Neurosurgery*, p. 75, Baltimore.

LEWIN, W. (1966 b) Cerebrospinal fluid rhinorrhea in nonmissile head injuries, in *Clinical Neurosurgery*, p. 237, Baltimore.

LEWIS, A. (1941–2) Differential diagnosis and treatment of post-contusional states, *Proc. roy. Soc. Med.*, **35**, 607.

LURIA, A. R. (1970) *Traumatic Aphasia: Its Syndromes, Psychology and Treatment*, The Hague.

MACIVER, I. N., FREW, I. J. C., and MATHESON, J. G. (1958 b) The role of respiratory insufficiency in the mortality of severe head injuries, *Lancet*, **i**, 390.

MACIVER, I. N., LASSMAN, L. P., THOMSON, C. W., and McLEOD, I. (1958 a) Treatment of severe head injuries, *Lancet*, **ii**, 544.

MACPHERSON, P., and GRAHAM, D. I. (1973) Arterial spasm and slowing of the cerebral circulation in the ischaemia of head injury, *J. Neurol. Neurosurg. Psychiat.*, **36**, 1069.

McKISSOCK, W., RICHARDSON, A., and BLOOM, W. H. (1960) Subdural haematoma, *Lancet*, **i**, 1365.

McLAURIN, R. M. (1966) Metabolic changes accompanying head injury, in *Clinical Neurosurgery*, p. 143, Baltimore.

MILLER, H. (1961) Accident neurosis, *Brit. med. J.*, **1**, 919, 992.

MILLER, H., and CARTLIDGE, N. (1972) Simulation and malingering after injuries to the brain and spinal cord, *Lancet*, **i**, 580.

MILLER, H., and STERN, G. (1965) The long-term prognosis of severe head injury, *Lancet*, **i**, 225.

MILLER, J. D., and JENNETT, W. B. (1968) Complications of depressed skull fracture, *Lancet*, **ii**, 991.

O

MITCHELL, D. E., and ADAMS, J. H. (1973) Primary focal impact damage to the brainstem in blunt head injuries. Does it exist?, *Lancet*, **ii**, 215.

NEUBUERGER, K. T., SINTON, D. W., and DENST, J. (1959) Cerebral atrophy associated with boxing, *Arch. Neurol. Psychiat. (Chic.)*, **81**, 403.

NORTHFIELD, D. W. C. (1973) *The Surgery of the Central Nervous System*, Oxford.

OMMAYA, A. K., and GENNARELLI, T. A. (1974) Cerebral concussion and traumatic unconsciousness, *Brain*, **97**, 633.

OMMAYA, A. K., and YARNELL, P. (1969) Subdural haematoma after whiplash injury, *Lancet*, **ii**, 237.

OPPENHEIMER, D. R. (1968) Microscopic lesions in the brain following head injury, *J. Neurol. Neurosurg. Psychiat.*, **31**, 229.

OVERGAARD, J., CHRISTENSEN, S., HVID-HANSEN, O., HAASE, J., LAND, A. M., HEIM, O., PEDERSEN, K. K., and TWEED, W. A. (1973) Prognosis after head injury based on early clinical examination, *Lancet*, **ii**, 631.

PENFIELD, W., and ERICKSON, T. C. (1941) *Epilepsy and Cerebral Localization*, London.

PHILLIPS, G. (1954) Traumatic epilepsy after closed head injury, *J. Neurol. Neurosurg. Psychiat.*, **17**, 1.

PLUM, F., and POSNER, J. B. (1972) *The Diagnosis of Stupor and Coma*, 2nd ed., Philadelphia.

RABE, E. F., FLYNN, R. E., and DODGE, P. R. (1968) Subdural collections of fluid in infants and children: a study of 62 patients with special reference to factors influencing prognosis and the efficacy of various forms of therapy, *Neurology (Minneap.)*, **18**, 559.

RAND, C. W. (1930) Traumatic pneumocephalus, *Arch. Surg.*, **20**, 935.

RAND, C. W., and COURVILLE, C. B. (1936) Histologic studies of the brain in cases of fatal injury to the head, *Arch. Neurol. Psychiat. (Chic.)*, **36**, 1277.

RASMUSSEN, T., and GOSSMAN, H. (1963) Epilepsy due to gross destructive brain leasions: results of surgical therapy, *Neurology (Minneap.)*, **13**, 659.

ROBINSON, R. G. (1957) Subdural haematoma in an adult after air encephalography, *J. Neurol. Neurosurg. Psychiat.*, **20**, 131.

ROWBOTHAM, G. F. (1964) *Acute Injuries of the Head*, 4th ed., Edinburgh.

ROYAL COLLEGE OF PHYSICIANS (1969) *Report on the Medical Aspects of Boxing*, London.

RUSSELL, D. S., and CAIRNS, H. (1934) Subdural false membrane or haematoma (pachymeningitis interna haemorrhagica) in carcinomatosis and sarcomatosis of the dura mater, *Brain*, **57**, 32.

RUSSELL, W. R. (1947) The anatomy of traumatic epilepsy, *Brain*, **70**, 225.

RUSSELL, W. R. (1971) *The Traumatic Amnesias*, London.

SCHEINBERG, S. C., and SCHEINBERG, L. (1964) Early description of chronic subdural hematoma: etiology, symptomatology and treatment, *J. Neurosurg.*, **21**, 445.

SHERREN, J. (1908) *Injuries of Nerves and Their Treatment*, London.

SHERWOOD, D. (1930) Chronic subdural hematoma in infants, *Amer. J. Dis. Childh.*, **39**, 980.

SMALL, J. M., and WOOLF, A. L. (1957) Fatal damage to the brain by epileptic convulsions after a trivial injury to the head, *J. Neurol. Neurosurg. Psychiat.*, **20**, 293.

SPICER, E. J. F., and STRICH, S. J. (1967) Haemorrhages in posterior-root ganglia in patients dying from head injuries, *Lancet*, **ii**, 1389.

STEADMAN, J. H., and GRAHAM, J. G. (1970) Head injuries: an analysis and follow-up study, *Proc. roy. Soc. Med.*, **63**, 23.

STRICH, S. J. (1956) Diffuse degeneration of the cerebral white matter in severe dementia following head injury, *J. Neurol. Psychiat.*, **19**, 163.

SYMONDS, C. P. (1941–2) Rehabilitation after injuries to the central nervous system, *Proc. roy. Soc. Med.*, **35**, 601.

SYMONDS, C. P. (1960) Concussion and contusion of the brain and their sequelae, in *Injuries of the Brain and Spinal Cord*, ed. Brock, S., p. 69, London.

SYMONDS, C. P. (1962) Concussion and its sequelae, *Lancet*, **i**, 1.

TAYLOR, W. H. (1957) Management of acute renal failure following surgical operation and head injury, *Lancet*, **ii**, 703.

TILL, K. (1968) Subdural haematoma and effusion in infancy, *Brit. med. J.*, **3**, 400.

TOBIS, J. S., LOWENTHAL, M., and MARINGER, S. (1957) Evaluation and management of the brain-damaged patient, *J. Amer. Med. Ass.*, **165**, 2035.

TOMLINSON, B. E. (1964) Pathology, in *Acute Injuries of the Head*, 4th ed., ed. Rowbotham, G. F., Edinburgh.

TRETHOWAN, W. H. (1970) Rehabilitation of the brain injured: the psychiatric angle, *Proc. roy. Soc. Med.*, **63**, 32.

VAPALAHTI, M. (1970) *Intracranial Pressure, Acid-Base Status of Blood and Cerebrospinal Fluid, and Pulmonary Function in the Prognosis of Severe Brain Injury*, Helsinki.

VAPALAHTI, M., and TROUPP, H. (1971) Prognosis for patients with severe brain injuries, *Brit. med. J.*, **iii**, 404.

WAGSTAFFE, W. W. (1928) The incidence of traumatic epilepsy after gunshot wounds of the head, *Lancet*, **ii**, 861.

WALKER, A. E., LEUCHS, H. K., LECHTAPE-GRÜTER, H., CAVENESS, W. F., and KRETSCHMAN, C. (1971) Life expectancy of head injured men with and without epilepsy, *Arch. Neurol. (Chic.)*, **24**, 95.

WALTER, W. G. (1938) The technique and applications of electroencephalography, *J. Neurol. Psychiat.*, N.S. **1**, 359.

WALTON, J. N., BARWICK, D. D., and LONGLEY, B. P. (1964) The electroencephalogram in brain injury, in *Acute Injuries of the Head*, 4th ed., ed. Rowbotham, G. F., Edinburgh.

WARD, A. A. (1966) The physiology of concussion, in *Clinical Neurosurgery*, p. 95, Baltimore.

WATSON, C. W. (1947) The incidence of epilepsy following craniocerebral injury, *Res. Publ. Ass. nerv. ment. Dis.*, **26**, 516.

WHITTY, C. W. M. (1947) Early traumatic epilepsy, *Brain*, **70**, 416.

WILLIAMS, D. (1941 *a*) The EEG in acute head injuries, *J. Neurol. Psychiat.*, N.S. **4**, 107.

WILLIAMS, D. (1941 *b*) The EEG in chronic post-traumatic states, *J. Neurol. Psychiat.*, N.S. **4**, 131.

WOLPAW, J. R. (1971) The aetiology of retrograde amnesia, *Lancet*, **ii**, 356.

YARNELL, P. R., and LYNCH, S. (1970) Retrograde memory immediately after concussion, *Lancet*, **i**, 863.

YASHON, D., JANE, J. A., WHITE, R. J., and SUGAR, O. (1968) Traumatic subdural hematoma of infancy: long-term follow-up of 92 patients, *Arch. Neurol. (Chic.)*, **18**, 370.

INTRACRANIAL BIRTH INJURIES

AETIOLOGY AND PATHOLOGY

Normal labour involves considerable compression of the fetal head and probably in many cases slight intracranial damage, as is indicated by the presence of red blood cells in the cerebrospinal fluid in a proportion of normal newly-born infants. It is not surprising, therefore, that serious intracranial injury may result from excessive or otherwise abnormal compression due to abnormal presentations or contracted pelvis or difficult forceps delivery. The most serious intracranial birth injuries are tears of the dura involving rupture of important venous sinuses with consequent haemorrhage. As Holland (1922 *a* and *b*) showed, the most important aetiological factor is excessive longitudinal stress leading to abnormal tension on the falx, which is anchored postero-inferiorly to the tentorium; as a result the tentorium may be torn or the internal cerebral vein ruptured. Large basal haemorrhages occur in such cases. In Holland's series of 167 fresh fetuses the tentorium was torn in 81 (48 per cent) and the falx in 5. Subdural haemorrhages occurred in all but 6. Over-riding of the parietal bones may lead to rupture of the superior sagittal sinus or of one or more of its venous tributaries, with the production of a supracortical subdural haemorrhage, which is usually confined to, or predominates upon, one side. Abnormal longitudinal stress is most likely to occur in breech presentations, which are, therefore fraught with special danger to the child. In such presentations, moreover, the thorax may be subjected to considerable compression, thus leading to intra-cranial venous congestion, oedema, and petechial haemorrhages. Prematurity appears to predispose to intracranial haemorrhage, perhaps because the intra-cranial vessels are more delicate in the premature than in the full-term child. Bilateral subependymal haemorrhages may be found in the lateral ventricles and are commonly associated with severe asphyxia.

The borderline between brain damage resulting from direct trauma to the head during delivery and that which may result from perinatal hypoxia, acidosis, hypoglycaemia, and cerebral ischaemia due to vascular distortion and com-pression (Norman et al., 1957; Norman, 1963; Courville, 1971) is indistinct. Whereas traumatic haemorrhage per se is also rarely the direct cause of cerebral palsy in the usual sense of spastic diplegia (Ingram, 1964), there can be little doubt that most of the syndromes of cerebral palsy result from a combination of the factors referred to above, often identified by the inclusive term 'peri-natal trauma', though various cerebral malformations also play a part (Menkes, 1974). Among the consequent pathological changes resulting from these complex factors are ulegyria (atrophic sclerosis of gyri), porencephaly, cystic degeneration of the central white matter (Benda, 1952), periventricular encephalomalacia, especially in premature infants (Banker and Larroche, 1962), communicating hydrocephalus, and état marbré of the corpus striatum. Localized damage to the cerebellum is sometimes seen (Courville, 1971).

SYMPTOMS

After a severe intracranial haemorrhage the child may be stillborn. If it is living it is likely to exhibit 'white asphyxia' due to medullary paralysis. If it recovers from this, it may be cyanosed, breathing slowly and irregularly. The pulse may be slow or rapid and feeble. The child cries feebly and is difficult to feed. Generalized rigidity with head retraction is common, and local or general convulsions may occur. A supracortical haemorrhage is likely to lead to hemiplegia. Papilloedema and retinal haemorrhages may be present, and in some cases exophthalmos, inequality of the pupils, squint, and nystagmus occur. The fontanelles may be bulging and non-pulsating. The cerebrospinal fluid is likely to be blood stained and under increased pressure, and when the haemorrhage is supracortical it may be possible to withdraw blood by subdural puncture at the lateral angle of the anterior fontanelle.

In some cases the signs of injury are absent at birth but develop gradually in the course of the first four or five days.

DIAGNOSIS

There is usually little doubt about the diagnosis, though the effects of hypoxia, hypercarbia, acidosis, and hypoglycaemia which may occur in various combinations, giving cerebral oedema (Menkes, 1974) may be similar, but in these disorders the CSF contains only a few red cells and sometimes a raised protein. A high CSF bilirubin is a useful indication of intracranial haemorrhage (Menkes, 1974).

PROGNOSIS

In most cases in which the symptoms are sufficiently severe to enable an intracranial birth injury to be diagnosed, death occurs, if not before or immediately after birth, within three or four days. Infants who survive may suffer from infantile hemiplegia, epilepsy, mental defect, or congenital hydrocephalus. The various forms of cerebral palsy are considered on pages 626–37.

TREATMENT

Maintenance of an adequate airway, oxygen, the treatment of respiratory infection, the correction of metabolic abnormalities, steroids to reduce cerebral oedema, and the provision of adequate fluid and nutrition are all important. A subdural haematoma may require surgical evacuation.

REFERENCES

BANKER, B. Q., and LARROCHE, J. C. (1962) Periventricular leukomalacia of infancy, *Arch. Neurol. (Chic.)*, **7**, 386.

BENDA, C. E. (1952) *Developmental Disorders of Mentation and Cerebral Palsies*, New York.

BYERS, R. K. (1920) Late effects of obstetrical injuries at various levels of the nervous system, *New Engl. J. Med.*, **203**, 507.

CHRISTENSEN, E., and MELCHIOR, J. (1967) *Cerebral Palsy, A Clinical and Neuropathological Study*, Clinics in Developmental Medicine, No. 25, London.

COURVILLE, C. B. (1971) *Birth and Brain Damage*, Pasadena.

DAVISON, G., and SNAITH, L. M. (1964) Cerebral birth injury, in *Acute Injuries of the Head*, 4th ed., ed. Rowbotham, G. F., Edinburgh.

FORD, F. R., CROTHERS, B., and PUTNAM, M. C. (1927) *Birth Injuries of the Central Nervous System*, London.

HOLLAND, E. (1922 *a*) *The Causation of Foetal Death*, Ministry of Health Reports, No. 7.

HOLLAND, E. (1922 *b*) Cranial stress in the foetus during labour and on the effects of excessive stress on the intracranial contents; with an analysis of eighty-one cases of torn tentorium cerebelli and subdural cerebral haemorrhage, *J. Obstet. Gynaec. Brit. Emp.*, **29**, 549.

INGRAM, T. T. S. (1964) *Paediatric Aspects of Cerebral Palsy*, Edinburgh.

IRVING, F. C. (1930) The obstetrical aspect of intracranial hemorrhage, *New Engl. J. Med.*, **203**, 499.

MENKES, J. H. (1974) *Textbook of Child Neurology*, Philadelphia.

MUNRO, D. (1930) Symptomatology and immediate treatment of cranial and intracranial injury in the new-born, *New Engl. J. Med.*, **103**, 502.

NORMAN, R. M. (1963) Cerebral birth injury, in *Greenfield's Neuropathology*, ed. Blackwood, W., McMenemey, W. H., Meyer, A., Norman, R. M., and Russell, D. S., p. 382, London.

NORMAN, R. M., URICH, H., and McMENEMEY, W. H. (1957) Vascular mechanisms of birth injury, *Brain*, **80**, 49.

SCHWARTZ, P. (1965) Parturitional injury of the newborn as a cause of mental deficiency, in *Medical Aspects of Mental Retardation*, ed. Carter, C. H., Springfield, Ill.

SHARPE, W., and MACLAIRE, A. S. (1925) Further observations of intracranial hemorrhage in the new-born, *Surg. Gynec. Obstet.*, **41**, 583.

6

DISEASES OF THE MENINGES

THE ANATOMY OF THE MENINGES

THE brain and spinal cord are covered by three membranes or meninges named, from without inwards, the dura mater, the arachnoid, and the pia mater.

The *dura mater* is thick and fibrous and serves as the internal periosteum of the bones of the skull, to which it is closely applied. The inner surface is covered with a layer of endothelial cells. Sheaths of dura mater extend outwards for a short distance as a covering for the cranial nerves as they pass through their respective foramina. Certain fibrous processes of the dura, or septa, partially separate the cranial cavity into compartments. These are the falx, the tentorium, the falx cerebelli, and the diaphragma sellae. The falx descends from the cranial vault in the midline lying between the cerebral hemispheres in the longitudinal fissure. It is attached anteriorly to the crista galli and posteriorly to the tentorium. At its superior attached border it splits into two layers to contain the superior sagittal sinus, and its lower free border similarly splits to contain the inferior sagittal sinus. The tentorium cerebelli forms a partition between the posterior and middle fossae of the skull, its free border surrounding the midbrain, and its attached border being fixed to the occipital and parietal bones and to the superior border of the petrous portion of the temporal bone. The posterior part of its attached border splits to enclose the transverse sinus, and the anterior part similarly encloses the superior petrosal sinus. The falx cerebelli lies in the midline between the tentorium and the internal occipital protuberance, to both of which it is attached, and its free border separates the cerebellar hemispheres posteriorly. The diaphragma sellae forms a roof to the sella turcica and contains an opening, through which passes the infundibulum.

The *pia mater* is a delicate membrane lined with endothelial cells, which intimately clothes the surface of the brain, dipping into the sulci.

The *arachnoid* is a similar membrane, lying between the dura mater and the pia mater and bridging over the sulci. The space between the arachnoid and the pia mater, which is known as the subarachnoid space, contains the cerebro-spinal fluid. Its expansions are known as the subarachnoid cisterns. The cerebello-medullary cistern lies between the inferior surface of the cerebellum and the posterior surface of the medulla. The cisterna pontis, continuous with this, lies anteriorly to the pons and is continued upwards into the cisterna inter-peduncularis. This in turn is continued forwards into a cistern lying in front of the optic chiasm—the cisterna chiasmatis. The subarachnoid space and its continuations into the substance of the nervous system—the perivascular spaces—have been described in the section on the cerebrospinal fluid [p. 121]. Between the dura mater and the arachnoid lies a potential space, the subdural space.

The spinal meninges are described in the section on the spinal cord [p. 715].

The dura mater is sometimes called the pachymeninx, the arachnoid and the pia mater the leptomeninges. Inflammation of the dura has been called pachymeningitis, but this term is now rarely used; inflammation of the pia and arachnoid is sometimes called leptomeningitis, but more often simply meningitis.

TUMOURS OF THE MENINGES

See Intracranial Tumour, page 230.

CALCIFICATION OF THE FALX

Calcification of the falx is usually discovered accidentally in routine radiographs of the skull. It is best seen in postero-anterior radiograms as a well-defined linear opacity in the midline. The calcification is much less evident in lateral views, in which it appears as scattered opaque flecks, most evident immediately above the crista galli and extending backwards for a variable distance. Little is known as to its cause, but it is of no pathological significance.

PACHYMENINGITIS

This term is now outmoded but syphilitic pachymeningitis was commonly described in the older literature [p. 46]. Suppuration between the dura and the skull (extradural abscess) usually results from cranial osteitis; subdural abscess [p. 434] usually complicates paranasal sinusitis. Subdural haematoma was once identified by the obsolete term pachymeningitis interna haemorrhagica.

ACUTE LEPTOMENINGITIS

Definition. Acute inflammation of the leptomeninges.

AETIOLOGY

Infection may reach the leptomeninges by the following routes:

1. *Direct spread from without.* This may occur as a result of fracture of the skull, either in the case of penetrating wounds of the cranial vault or fractures of the base, when organisms may spread to the meninges from the nasopharynx. In the latter case the fracture may be unsuspected until meningitis develops. Other external sources of meningitis are osteitis of the cranial bones, especially mastoiditis, infection of the nasal air sinuses, especially the frontal sinus, and of the soft tissues of the scalp, and thrombophlebitis of the intracranial venous sinuses. Organisms may be introduced by lumbar puncture.

2. *Direct spread from within* may occur when the meninges are breached by a brain abscess or in tuberculous meningitis secondary to a cerebral tuberculoma.

3. *Infection through the blood stream.* In such cases meningitis follows bacteraemia. It may be the only or the principal manifestation, as in so-called 'primary' pneumococcal meningitis, meningococcal meningitis, acute lymphocytic meningitis, or the infection of the meninges may be secondary to focal infection elsewhere in the body, for example, pneumonia, empyema, osteomyelitis, erysipelas, typhoid fever, etc., in which case the bacteraemia may or may not be associated with endocarditis due to the infecting organism. Tuberculous meningitis may thus be a manifestation of miliary tuberculosis.

4. *Meningitis complicating encephalitis and myelitis.* Meningeal inflammation often plays a subordinate part in the picture of encephalitis or myelitis. Polio-myelitis is one example of such a meningo-encephalomyelitis, and meningeal inflammation similarly occurs in other viral encephalitides. In such conditions meningeal symptoms may be prominent or slight, but the cerebrospinal fluid yields evidence of meningeal inflammation.

5. *Other forms of meningitis.* Subarachnoid haemorrhage excites an inflam-matory reaction in the leptomeninges, though organisms are absent. Aseptic meningitis may also result from the release of other irritative substances (e.g. air, cholesterol, keratin, spinal anaesthetics) into the subarachnoid space. The term 'serous meningitis' has no constant meaning and is outmoded. 'Meningism' occurs as a complication of acute infections, especially in childhood. Symptoms of meningeal irritation are associated with a rise in CSF pressure, often due to cerebral oedema.

Meningitis arising in, and at first limited to, the spinal canal (spinal menin-gitis) is rare; it may result from vertebral osteitis but has been described in tuberculosis (Wadia and Dastur, 1969; Dastur and Wadia, 1969) and is a rare consequence of staphylococcal infection.

The organisms commonly responsible for meningitis are the *Neisseria meningitidis, Diplococcus pneumoniae, Haemophilus influenzae, Listeria mono-cytogenes* (particularly in neonates), streptococcus, staphylococcus, *Escherichia coli*, all of which cause pyogenic meningitis; the *Mycobacterium tuberculosis*; and various viruses which cause 'lymphocytic meningitis'. Other organisms less frequently the cause of meningitis are *Salmonella typhosa, Bacillus anthracis, Brucella abortus, Pseudomonas aeruginosa*, leptospira, and yeasts such as *Crypto-coccus neoformans (Torula histolytica)*. Mixed infections may occur.

ACUTE PYOGENIC MENINGITIS
PATHOLOGY

Whatever the causative organism the pathological changes in acute pyogenic meningitis are similar in all cases. Whether the organism reaches the meninges by direct spread or through the blood stream, inflammation spreads rapidly through the whole subarachnoid space of the brain and spinal cord. The space between the pia mater and the arachnoid becomes filled with purulent exudate, which may cover the whole cerebral cortex or may be occasionally confined to the sulci. In cases of cranial osteitis and cerebral abscess the pus may be most evident near the source of the infection. The cortical veins are congested, and the gyri are often flattened owing to internal hydrocephalus. Microscopically the leptomeninges show inflammatory cell infiltration which in the early stages consists wholly of polymorphonuclear cells, though in the later stages lympho-cytes and plasma cells are present [FIG. 90]. In acute cases the cerebral hemi-spheres show little change except for perivascular inflammatory infiltration in the cortex. In pneumococcal meningitis, in particular, greenish-yellow pus is particularly evident over the vertex and at the base of the brain. Indolent meningitis due to staphylococcus albus has been described in cases of hydro-cephalus treated by shunting procedures (Holt, 1969). If a purulent infection becomes subacute, due to an inadequate response to treatment, or in meningitis due to *H. influenzae*, which tends to run a subacute course, especially in children, there may be diffuse degeneration and even sometimes necrosis with glial proliferation in the superficial areas of the cerebral and cerebellar cortex and spinal cord (toxic encephalomyelopathy) and in the cranial nerves (especially the second and eighth, giving visual loss and/or deafness, but sometimes also in the third, fourth, sixth, and seventh). Similar changes may occur in the hypothalamus and corpora mammillaria, with perivascular cellular infiltration around subependymal veins, and thrombosis of subarachnoid veins and even of the venous sinuses (Adams and Kubik, 1947); subdural empyema is a rare

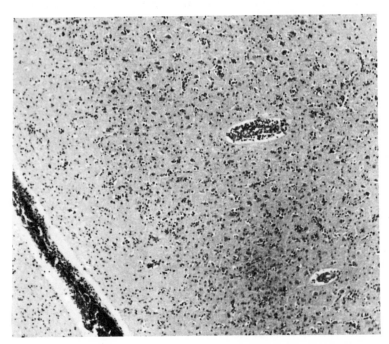

FIG. 90. Suppurative meningitis; a dense collection of inflammatory cells is present in the subarachnoid space and there is a superficial encephalitis with cellular infiltration of the cortex, especially around venules and capillaries, H & E, ×64

complication. Hydrocephalus results in part from inflammatory adhesions in the basal cisterns and foramina of the fourth ventricle, in part from impairment of absorption of CSF due to blockage of arachnoidal villi. In tuberculous meningitis and other granulomatous meningitides, and occasionally in pyogenic meningitis (Smith *et al.*, 1957), there may be endarteritis of the circle of Willis and its branches as additional complications, giving cerebral ischaemia or infarction.

SYMPTOMS

All forms of acute meningitis, whatever their cause, possess a number of symptoms in common. The onset may be fulminating, acute, or, less commonly, insidious. Headache, increasing in severity, is usually the initial symptom.

The general symptoms of an infection are usually conspicuous. Fever is the rule, though the degree of pyrexia varies. The temperature is usually between 37·8 °C. and 38·9 °C. though hyperpyrexia may occur, especially in the terminal stages. The pulse rate is also variable. It is sometimes slow in the early stages, for example between 50 and 60, but always rises as the disease progresses and at the end is usually very rapid and often irregular. The respiratory rate is usually slightly increased, and various forms of irregularity of respiration, especially Cheyne-Stokes breathing, occur in the later stages. Headache is a prominent symptom and is usually very severe, possessing a 'bursting' character. It may be diffuse or mainly frontal, and usually radiates down the neck and into the back, being associated with pain in the spine which radiates to the limbs, especially the lower. Vomiting may occur, especially in the early stages. Convulsions are common in children, especially in influenzal meningitis (Menkes, 1974) but rare in adults. The patient tends to lie in an attitude of general flexion, curled up under the bed-clothes and resenting interference. There may be a high-pitched 'meningeal' cry in infants.

Signs of Meningeal Irritation

The following signs are of special value.

Cervical Rigidity. Cervical rigidity is present at an early stage in almost every case. It is elicited by the observer's placing his hand beneath the patient's occiput and endeavouring to cause passive flexion of the head so as to bring the chin towards the chest. In a normal individual this can be accomplished with ease and without pain. In meningitis there is resistance due to spasm of the extensor muscles of the neck, and an attempt to overcome this causes pain.

Head Retraction. Head retraction is an extreme degree of cervical rigidity brought about by spasm of the extensor muscles. Flexion of the neck causes a rise in the tension of the cerebrospinal fluid in the cerebellomedullary cistern. When the meninges are inflamed this is painful, and cervical rigidity and head retraction are examples of reflex protective spasm. Cervical rigidity is usually associated with some rigidity of the spine at lower levels.

Kernig's and Brudzinski's Signs. To elicit Kernig's sign one knee is extended with the hip fully flexed; when positive there is pain and spasm of the hamstrings. Brudzinski's sign consists first of spontaneous flexion of the knees and hips on attempted neck flexion and secondly spontaneous flexion of one leg when the other is flexed passively. Both signs are due to the presence of inflammatory exudate around roots in the lumbar theca; these signs are sometimes present in subarachnoid haemorrhage.

Other Signs

The mental state of the patient varies according to the stage and progress of the disease. Delirium is common in the early stages, but tends, when the disease is progressive, to give place to drowsiness and stupor, which is followed by coma. Photophobia is frequently present. The ocular fundi may be normal or may show venous congestion or, sometimes, papilloedema. The pupils are often unequal and may react sluggishly. In the later stages they tend to be dilated and fixed. Ptosis is common, and squint and diplopia are often present. Any of the ocular muscles may be paralysed, most frequently one or both lateral recti. Facial paresis is not rare. Difficulty in swallowing may occur in the later stages. Muscular power in the limbs is usually well preserved, though slight incoordination and tremor are common and there is considerable muscular hypotonia. A general flaccid paralysis is a terminal event. The tendon reflexes are usually sluggish and often are soon lost; the abdominal reflexes also disappear early; the plantar reflexes are usually flexor at first, though later one or both may become extensor. Sensory loss does not usually occur. True paralysis of sphincter control occurs only late, but the mental state of the patient may lead to retention or incontinence of urine early in the illness. *Tache cérébrale* is often elicitable, but is not pathognomonic of meningitis.

Meningitis localized for a time to one hemisphere may cause Jacksonian convulsions, hemiparesis, and even hemianopia. The toxic encephalomyelopathy referred to above, and/or hydrocephalus and cranial nerve involvement may give rise to dementia, amnesia, epilepsy, paresis of the limbs, ataxia, blindness and deafness, paraplegia, and many other complications depending upon the site of maximal pathological change, but with the increasingly effective control of meningitis with antibiotics these late complications are becoming much less common. Persistent pyrexia, and increased intracranial pressure, along with vomiting, convulsions, and focal neurological signs present 72 hours after the start of treatment in infants should make one suspect the presence of a subdural effusion (Rabe *et al.*, 1968; Menkes, 1974).

The Cerebrospinal Fluid

The cerebrospinal fluid is under increased pressure. Its appearance depends upon the number of leucocytes present, and ranges from slight turbidity to frank purulence. When the fluid is turbid the deposit is yellow, and when macroscopic pus is present the supernatant fluid is frequently xanthochromic. The spontaneous formation of a fine coagulum is not uncommon. The cells are predominantly polymorphonuclear and these may be present in very large numbers, amounting to many thousands per mm^3. There is frequently a small proportion of large mononuclear cells. The protein is increased, and in frankly purulent fluids may reach a high level—0·5 g/100 ml or more. A reduction in chloride is usually secondary to vomiting and is of no diagnostic value. Glucose rapidly disappears from the fluid. IgA and IgG levels in the fluid are increased in all forms of meningitis, less so in the viral varieties, but in purulent meningitis the most striking increase occurs in IgM, a finding which may be used for diagnostic purposes (Smith *et al.*, 1973). Lactic dehydrogenase (Beaty and Oppenheimer, 1968), aminotransferase (GOT) (Belsy, 1969), and creatine phosphokinase (Katz and Liebman, 1970) may all be raised in the fluid, as may acid phosphatase and betaglucuronidase, especially in chronic meningitis (Shuttleworth and Allen, 1968). Lange's colloidal gold curve is of the meningitic type. Organisms may be demonstrated in the films or on culture. Meningococci may be difficult to find and to culture but other cocci and *H. influenzae* are usually present in profusion. Tubercle bacilli should be sought, using the Ziehl–Neilsen stain, on centrifuged deposits of CSF [p. 135]. Special methods are needed to isolate or culture viruses and yeasts.

Electrolyte Disturbances

About 6 per cent of patients show hyponatraemia, sometimes with inappropriate secretion of antidiuretic hormone, giving hypervolaemia and oliguria with symptoms of water intoxication (restlessness, irritability, and convulsions) and requiring restriction of water intake and the administration of sodium.

DIAGNOSIS

Acute pyogenic leptomeningitis must be distinguished from: (1) general infections associated with toxaemia, especially those of which headache is a prominent symptom; (2) meningism; (3) acute cerebral infections, including various forms of encephalitis and intracranial abscess; (4) subarachnoid haemorrhage; (5) other forms of meningitis and meningeal irritation.

1. *Acute general infections* which most commonly simulate meningitis are influenza, pneumonia, typhoid fever, and various viral infections. These are distinguished from meningitis by the presence of the characteristic local and general symptoms of the infection and by the absence of signs of meningeal irritation, especially cervical rigidity and Kernig's sign. It must be remembered, however, that acute infections may lead to meningism or may be complicated by meningitis, and in either case signs of meningeal irritation will be present. When the diagnosis is in doubt, therefore, lumbar puncture should be performed.

2. *Meningism* is a state of meningeal irritation complicating acute infections. It is usually encountered in association with the acute specific fevers and pneumonia in childhood, but may occur in adults with typhoid fever (Osuntokun *et al.*, 1972). Cervical rigidity and Kernig's sign are present, but the cerebrospinal fluid, though under increased pressure, is normal in composition.

3. Symptoms of meningeal irritation may be present in *acute meningo-encephalomyelitis* in childhood and in *acute disseminated encephalomyelitis* complicating the specific fevers, and are almost constant in the early stages of *poliomyelitis*. The diagnosis of these disorders is based upon the presence of signs of involvement of the nervous system, especially the grey matter of the midbrain in meningo-encephalitis and of the corticospinal tracts in the various forms of acute disseminated encephalomyelitis. In acute poliomyelitis the stage of meningeal irritation precedes the development of atrophic paralysis. In meningo-encephalitis and acute disseminated encephalomyelitis the cerebrospinal fluid usually shows a modest mononuclear pleocytosis. In acute poliomyelitis the fluid contains an excess of cells, which during the first few days are both polymorphonuclear cells and lymphocytes. After the first week lymphocytes alone are found. The presence of large numbers of lymphocytes and of a normal glucose content of the fluid differentiates the condition from acute pyogenic leptomeningitis, and the normal glucose content distinguishes it from tuberculous meningitis. *Intracranial abscess* may simulate meningitis when it gives rise to cervical rigidity, which, however, is not usually severe unless meningitis coexists. In cases of abscess the cerebrospinal fluid usually contains an excess of cells, though not often more than 100 per mm^3, the majority being lymphocytes. The protein may be disproportionately increased. The sugar content of the fluid is undiminished and organisms are absent.

4. *Subarachnoid haemorrhage*, since it leads to meningeal irritation, may closely simulate meningitis. Its onset, however, is usually more rapid, and the true diagnosis is readily established by the demonstration of blood in the cerebrospinal fluid.

5. *Other forms of meningitis.* A localized meningitis may occur as a complication of pyogenic infection in the neighbourhood of the meninges, especially in mastoiditis, subdural abscess, and intracranial thrombophlebitis. In such cases the cerebrospinal fluid is usually under increased pressure and exhibits a slight excess of cells, which may be either polymorphonuclear, mononuclear, or mixed. Organisms are absent. *Virus meningitis* should be suspected in cases

of meningitis of acute onset running a benign course, in which no focal source of infection can be detected, in which there is a lymphocytic pleocytosis in the fluid and organisms cannot be demonstrated on repeated examination by ordinary methods. *Tuberculous meningitis* usually develops much more insidiously than meningitis due to pyogenic organisms, and symptoms of meningeal irritation, for example cervical rigidity and Kernig's sign, are often slight and may be absent. The cerebrospinal fluid contains an excess of cells, consisting usually of polymorphonuclear and mononuclear cells in varying proportions. The glucose content is diminished, usually to between 10 and 40 mg per 100 ml. Tubercle bacilli may be demonstrable in the fluid or on culture, and there is usually tuberculous infection elsewhere in the body. *Syphilitic meningitis* is occasionally sufficiently acute to lead to confusion with pyogenic meningitis. In such cases the cerebrospinal fluid contains an excess of cells which are usually mononuclear, but in the most acute cases polymorphonuclear cells may also be present. The Wassermann or V.D.R.L. reactions are usually positive in the fluid and also in the blood. A subacute or chronic picture of meningitis with an excess of cells in the cerebrospinal fluid may be due to *brucellosis, cysticercosis*, infection with *Cryptococcus neoformans, Behçet's disease, sarcoidosis, carcinomatosis of the meninges*, or Mollaret's benign recurrent meningitis (Mollaret, 1952; Bruyn and Straathof, 1961).

PROGNOSIS

The prognosis of acute pyogenic leptomeningitis depends upon the nature of the invading organism, the number of organisms present in the cerebrospinal fluid, the possibility of removing the source of infection, and the effectiveness of chemotherapy. The introduction of the sulphonamide group of drugs, which pass readily into the cerebrospinal fluid and exert a strong bacteriostatic action there, of penicillin and streptomycin and other newer antibiotics revolutionized the prognosis of many forms of meningitis. In the past pneumococcal meningitis was almost invariably fatal and streptococcal meningitis was fatal in more than 90 per cent of cases. Recent work suggests that a recovery rate of 90 per cent or over may be expected in cases of 'primary' pneumococcal meningitis and meningitis due to *H. influenzae*. In meningitis complicating surgical conditions the mortality rate is still likely to be between 10 and 20 per cent. In uncomplicated meningococcal meningitis treated early the mortality rate is now usually less than 5 per cent. Early and effective treatment of pyogenic meningitis should lead to recovery without residual symptoms. In any form of pyogenic meningitis treated late or inadequately, permanent damage may lead to mental defect, epilepsy, deafness, blindness, or spastic weakness.

TREATMENT

See page 421.

SPECIAL FEATURES OF MENINGOCOCCAL MENINGITIS

AETIOLOGY

Neisseria meningitidis is usually obtainable from the secretions of the nasopharynx of both patients and 'carriers', and in the early stages of the infection can often be isolated from the patient's blood. Meningococcal meningitis occurs both in epidemics and sporadically. It occurs in the tropics and temperate zone, in which the period of epidemic prevalence is the spring. Since antibiotics came to be widely used for minor infections, epidemics have become less frequent. Group A organisms were once the commonest but have been superseded by Groups B and C which are less sensitive to sulphonamides. Sporadic cases occur at any time of year.

The disease, although contagious, is only slightly so, and it is exceptional for multiple cases to occur in a single household or for the infection to spread in hospital. It is spread by droplet infection, mainly through 'carriers'. These are usually individuals who have been in contact with a patient and who harbour the meningococcus in the nasopharynx for a period which usually lasts only two or three weeks. Such 'carriers', who greatly outnumber overt cases, may infect other persons without themselves developing the disease, or after a period of apparently good health may develop meningitis. An important cause of epidemics is overcrowding, and the disease is thus especially prevalent among school-children, and soldiers who are crowded together. Catarrhal disorders of the nose and throat may predispose to the infection. Both sexes are affected equally, and the age of greatest susceptibility is from infancy to ten years, the highest incidence being in the first year of life. It is rare after the age of 40. The incubation period varies from one to seven days and is usually about four days.

The route by which the meningococci, having been implanted in the naso-pharynx, reach the meninges is still unsettled. Probably they are carried by the blood stream, though direct spread along the lymphatics of the olfactory nerves cannot be excluded.

PATHOLOGY

The pathology of meningitis is described on page 408. Some of the toxic changes in the brain found in severe cases are probably due to meningococcal endotoxin in the CSF (Ducker and Simmons, 1968) while endotoxaemia may give increased peripheral vascular resistance, decreased visceral perfusion, and other manifestations of shock (Lillehei et al., 1964). In the 'adrenal type', there is haemorrhage in both adrenals.

SYMPTOMS

Several clinical types of infection are recognized, viz. (1) the average meningitic type, (2) the fulminating cerebral type, (3) the adrenal type, and (4) ameningitic meningococcal septicaemia. The symptoms of the average meningitic type are described on page 409.

The Skin

Several types of rash may occur, the most characteristic being a purpuric eruption which may take the form of petechiae, which are purple at first, fading to a brownish colour, and do not disappear on pressure. They are especially liable to occur on regions subjected to pressure. The purpuric patches may be larger, even measuring 2 cm in diameter, but these are found only in very severe cases. The purpuric eruption may appear during the first 24 hours and is usually present before the third day. It is seen in about one-third of all cases. A maculopapular rash is present somewhat less frequently, usually appearing before the fourth day, first on the trunk and later on the extensor surfaces of the thighs and forearms. Erythematous rashes may occur at any stage of the disease, and facial herpes febrilis is common.

The Blood

A well-marked polymorphonuclear leucocytosis occurs in the blood. Meningococci can sometimes be cultured from the blood in the early stages, but rarely after the signs of meningitis have appeared. In meningococcal septicaemia the petechiae (as described above) may be due to small bacterial emboli; rarely there is extensive bruising with intravascular coagulation similar to the Schwartzman phenomenon (Margaretten and McAdams, 1958).

The Cerebrospinal Fluid

The changes in the fluid are those of pyogenic meningitis [see p. 411].

Meningococci can sometimes be demonstrated in the fluid but are often difficult to find. Usually they are present in smears made from the centrifuged deposit. Most are intracellular, lying within the polymorphonuclear leucocytes; a large number of extracellular meningococci is believed to be indicative of a severe infection. If meningococci are not demonstrable on the first day they can usually be cultured.

It may be desirable to examine ventricular or cisternal fluid if internal hydrocephalus develops or if, in spite of improvement in the condition of the lumbar spinal fluid, symptoms of infection persist. In infants showing such a picture, subdural tap is indicated [pp. 396 and 411].

Other Symptoms

Slight cardiac dilatation may occur as a result of the toxaemia, the cardiac apex being displaced outwards and the apical first sound soft or muffled. Albuminuria may also occur. A catarrhal inflammation of the upper respiratory tract is also common. Rapid flushing of the skin in response to a light scratch (*tache cérébrale*), is often present, but is not pathognomonic.

Complications of Meningococcal Origin

The symptoms already described are those attributable to the meningitis and the bacteraemia which precedes it. We may describe as complications manifestations of the infection which are inconstant and in some instances rare. Neurological complications of all forms of meningitis, including hydrocephalus, deafness and blindness, toxic encephalomyelopathy, and paraparesis, have already been described. They were once relatively common sequelae of meningococcal meningitis but have become rare since effective chemotherapy and antibiotic treatment were introduced.

The Eye. Conjunctivitis is a fairly common complication. More severe ocular lesions, such as keratitis or panophthalmitis, are fortunately rare (Williams and Geddes, 1970).

The Heart. Fibrinopurulent pericarditis is a rare complication in severe cases but myocarditis is commonly found at autopsy in fatal cases (Hardman and Earle, 1969). Bacterial endocarditis is rare.

Arthritis. This used to occur in from 10 to 15 per cent of cases in epidemics but is now much less common. Purulent meningococcal arthritis was once the rule, but aseptic joint effusions are now seen more often. The knee- and shoulder-joints are most frequently affected, but almost any joint may be involved.

Genito-urinary System. Albuminuria is common. Rarely a focal nephritis develops, often with haematuria, presumably due to septicaemia and bacterial embolism. Epididymitis and orchitis are rare complications.

Non-Meningococcal Complications

Though bronchopneumonia may very rarely be due to the meningococcus, it is more often the result of a secondary infection. Infection of the urinary tract may occur, especially when frequent catheterization is necessary. Bed sores are a risk in chronic cases.

Other Clinical Types

In the *fulminating cerebral type*, presumed to be due to severe meningococcal septicaemia and endotoxaemia, the onset is sudden and the patient may rapidly become comatose. Death may occur in a few hours without signs of meningeal irritation and with a clear cerebrospinal fluid. In less acute cases there is slight cervical rigidity and the fluid is turbid and contains meningococci.

In the *adrenal type*—the Waterhouse-Friderichsen syndrome—the characteristic features are grave hypotension and cyanosis (circulatory collapse), with the biochemical changes characteristic of acute adrenal failure. There is a petechial rash with some larger purpuric elements. The affected patients (usually children) are generally alert and signs of meningitis are usually absent as the condition is due to septicaemia.

Chronic Posterior Basic Meningitis. This is a chronic form of meningococcal meningitis occurring in infants, usually between the ages of 4 months and $2\frac{1}{2}$ years. It was once relatively common, due either to failure to recognize the nature of the initial infection, or to inadequate treatment, but is now infrequent. The onset is usually acute with fever, which, however, tends to subside at the end of the first week. Head retraction is usually well marked, often with opisthotonos and hydrocephalus soon develops.

Chronic Meningococcaemia. While acute meningococcal septicaemia usually gives the more explosive clinical features described above, chronic septicaemia may give mild recurrent fever, fleeting maculopapular rashes, joint pains and swelling, and meningococci may be cultured from the blood. Spontaneous recovery may occur but a few patients ultimately develop meningitis.

PROPHYLAXIS

Since meningococcal meningitis is spread chiefly by droplet infection from carriers, hygienic measures should be taken to ensure adequate ventilation and to avoid overcrowding in institutions and communities exposed to infection. The detection of carriers by swabbing the nasopharynx is impracticable on a large scale but may be of value in communities in which infection has occurred. A carrier should be isolated from children and young persons. Sulphadiazine, 2 g, has been said to free carriers of the organism within 24 hours, and sulphadiazine given prophylactically for two days in individuals exposed to infection may terminate an epidemic (Kuhns *et al.*, 1943); but since meningococci of groups B and C are not sensitive to sulphonamides, penicillin G is now preferred.

LISTERIAL MENINGITIS

Diffuse infection with *Listeria monocytogenes* may be found in aborted, premature, and stillborn children or in neonates dying soon after birth. Listerosis is, however, one of the commonest causes of pyogenic meningitis occurring within the first four weeks of life and cannot be differentiated from other forms of pyogenic meningitis except by culture of the organism, which is, however, readily mistaken for a diphtheroid bacillus. Listerial meningitis has also been reported rarely in adults, and particularly in elderly subjects suffering from debilitating diseases (Ford *et al.*, 1968). The organism is very sensitive to penicillin and to sulphonamides, chloramphenicol and erythromycin, so that prompt recognition of the condition in neonates is important, as is treatment of genital listerosis in the pregnant female, as treatment may prevent infection of the fetus.

The other organism which commonly causes neonatal meningitis is *E. coli*.

TUBERCULOUS MENINGITIS

AETIOLOGY

Tuberculous meningitis may be a consequence of miliary tuberculosis, especially in children. Rich and McCordock (1933) and MacGregor and Green (1937), however, showed that in most cases the infection spreads to the meninges from a haematogenous caseous focus in the brain in contact with either the subarachnoid space or the ventricles. In children the condition most often arises as a consequence of primary or miliary tuberculosis, but in adults it usually develops in individuals with known tuberculosis elsewhere, especially in the lung. In Lincoln's (1947) series 50 per cent of patients were known sufferers from tuberculosis and 57 per cent had tuberculous contacts. While about a quarter of all cases used to be due to the bovine bacillus (MacGregor and Green, 1937), most now result from the human organism. Once a disease mainly of childhood, it is now seen at any age and is equally frequent in adults. The pattern of tuberculous infection of the nervous system is changing (Kocen and Parsons, 1970); thus some patients with symptoms of meningitis may show no pleocytosis in the spinal fluid, at least initially, others may show a transient aseptic meningitis which recovers spontaneously, despite culture of *M. tuberculosis* from the fluid (Emond and McKendrick, 1973). Some, especially after BCG inoculation, may present a clinical picture of a mild meningitic illness strongly suggestive of benign lymphocytic meningitis, and others may present with symptoms and signs of a chronic spinal meningitis with evidence of spinal cord compression but with, at least initially, no evidence of intracranial spread (Wadia and Dastur, 1969; Dastur and Wadia, 1969; Kocen and Parsons, 1970). Meningitis may also occur in patients with intracranial tuberculomas which may initially give symptoms of an intracranial space-occupying lesion.

PATHOLOGY

In acute cases, macroscopically, the brain is usually pale and the gyri are somewhat flattened. A yellowish gelatinous exudate is found matting together the leptomeninges at the base and extending along the lateral sulci. Miliary tubercles may be visible on the leptomeninges, being most conspicuous along the vessels, especially the middle cerebral artery and its branches. In many cases, however, careful sectioning of the brain is needed in order to demonstrate the causal focus. Microscopically the tubercles consist of collections of round cells, chiefly mononuclear [FIG. 91], often with central caseation. Giant cells are rare. Hydrocephalus, toxic encephalomyelopathy, involvement of cranial nerves, endarteritis [FIG. 91B] with consequent cerebral infarction (Smith and Daniel, 1947), and other complications of subacute or chronic meningitis [p. 409] are especially common in tuberculous meningitis.

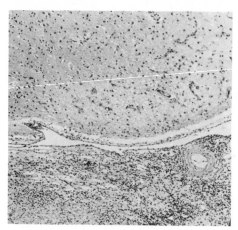

A. Lymphoid and epithelioid cells in the meninges with neuronal loss and gliosis in the cortex, H & E, ×64

c. Collections of lymphoid and epithelioid cells in the subarachnoid space, H & E, ×400

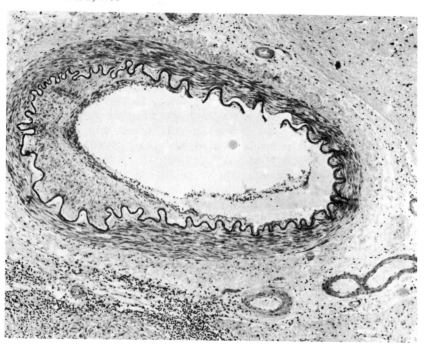

B. Endarteritis in tuberculous meningitis, H & E, ×64

FIG. 91. Tuberculous meningitis.

SYMPTOMS

The onset of symptoms is insidious, and there is almost always a prodromal phase of vague ill health. In children lassitude, anorexia, loss of weight, and intermittent vomiting are prominent. In adults mental changes may be conspicuous, and symptoms of a confusional psychosis may precede those of meningitis. This prodromal phase usually lasts two or three weeks, and is followed by the development of symptoms of meningeal irritation. The pulse, which was previously rapid, becomes slow and irregular. Fever, if previously absent, usually now appears but is rarely high. The temperature, which is often markedly irregular, does not usually rise much above 38·9 °C. Headache and vomiting make their appearance and convulsions may occur. The patient becomes drowsy and at times delirious, but the occurrence of lucid intervals, even up to a late stage of the illness, is a characteristic feature. Signs of meningeal irritation are usually slighter than in pyogenic meningitis. There is usually slight cervical rigidity, but this may be absent and actual head retraction is rare. Kernig's sign is usually present. The patient frequently lies in a flexed attitude, resenting interference, and in the early stages often exhibits photophobia. Children sometimes utter what has been called a 'meningeal cry', a high-pitched scream.

Papilloedema is inconstant and when present develops only in the late stages of the illness. Choroidal tubercles are present in up to 20 per cent of patients and are visible ophthalmoscopically as rather ill-defined rounded or oval yellowish bodies about half the size of the disc. The pupils are usually contracted at first, but later become dilated and fixed. In subacute, chronic, or inadequately treated cases, involvement of the cranial nerves may give ptosis, diplopia, facial weakness, deafness, or dysphagia. Endarteritis leading to cerebral infarction may give a hemiplegia while if hydrocephalus and diffuse arachnoiditis develop, there may be paresis and spasticity of all four limbs with extensor rigidity or even opisthotonus. Often in the early stages the tendon reflexes in the lower limbs are depressed but later they often become increased and the plantars extensor. Retention of urine is often followed by incontinence of urine, less often of faeces. The *tache cérébrale* is common. In the uncommon spinal form, back pain and rigidity and progressive paraparesis with early urinary retention are usual; girdle or root pains are frequent.

Tuberculous lesions are usually discoverable outside the nervous system. In one series radiography of the chest showed miliary dissemination in the lungs in 27 per cent, and enlarged hilar glands or active primary complex in 25 per cent; 13 per cent showed other lesions in lung, skin, or bone. The Mantoux text is positive in 85 per cent of cases (Lincoln, 1947; Lincoln and Sewell, 1963).

The Cerebrospinal Fluid

The cerebrospinal fluid is under increased pressure. It is clear, but a fine 'cobweb' clot frequently forms on standing. There is an increase in the number of cells, usually to the number of about 100 per mm^3 but varying from 10 to 1,000. These may be all mononuclear or a mixture of mononuclear and polymorphonuclear, the former predominating. There is a moderate increase in the protein, up to about 0·1–0·4 g per 100 ml but increasing to 1·0 g per 100 ml or more in the presence of severe arachnoidal adhesions or in the spinal form. The chloride content of the fluid is usually much reduced, on an average to 510 mg per 100 ml, but it now seems that this is simply an index of the severity of the vomiting which occurs in most cases. There is a diminution in the glucose content of the fluid, usually to below 50 mg per 100 ml, and Lange's colloidal gold curve is of the meningitic type. The frequency with which tubercle bacilli are found in the fluid varies in the hands of different workers. Some report that they are almost invariably demonstrable: others find them less often. Consequently, though their presence clinches the diagnosis, their absence is of less significance. The organism should be cultured and its sensitivity to streptomycin tested; guinea-pig inoculation should be used in doubtful cases.

The bromide test, in which serum and cerebrospinal fluid bromide concentrations are measured after 3 days of oral bromide administration or a single intravenous dose of 2–4 g in 10 ml of sterile distilled water, is valuable in diagnosis, as in tuberculous meningitis the cerebrospinal fluid:serum ratio approaches unity, whereas in normal individuals it is about 1:3 (Taylor et al., 1954). The test is also positive in many cases of carcinomatosis of the meninges.

DIAGNOSIS

Now that we possess an effective method of treatment, early diagnosis is of the utmost importance. The general diagnosis of meningitis is discussed on page 412. Owing to the importance of the examination of the cerebrospinal fluid, lumbar puncture should be carried out without delay in any doubtful case, especially in any patient known to be tuberculous who develops symptoms or signs of meningitis. If a patient with meningitis is found to have a mononuclear pleocytosis in the cerebrospinal fluid with a glucose content below 50 mg per 100 ml, and if no malignant cells are detected by cytological examination of a centrifuged deposit of the fluid, it is wise to treat him for tuberculous meningitis even though there may be no mycobacteria discoverable.

PROGNOSIS

Before the introduction of streptomycin and other antituberculous drugs, tuberculous meningitis was almost invariably fatal in from 1 to 4 weeks after the onset of meningeal symptoms, though recovery was very occasionally reported after tubercle bacilli had been demonstrated in the cerebrospinal fluid and still occurs in the transient aseptic meningitis which has been occasionally reported as a consequence of tuberculosis (Emond and McKendrick, 1973).

It is still too early to estimate what proportion of patients it may be possible to cure by means of modern treatment. Hitherto recoveries have been claimed in between 10 per cent and 50 per cent in different centres. Cairns and Taylor (1949) reported a fatality rate of 20 out of 49 patients, but a review by Miller et al. (1963) showed that whereas up to 1952 a mortality of about 30 per cent was usual, the introduction of isoniazid has transformed the situation so that nowadays the mortality should be less than 10 per cent and recurrence after adequate treatment is rare. As would be expected, the earlier the patient is treated the better the prognosis, and it is generally agreed that if he is already comatose when first seen the outlook is almost hopeless. Otherwise, the treated disease may run one of several courses, though the reasons for these variations are not yet understood. In cases which are ultimately fatal the patient may show no response to treatment and deteriorate rapidly and die within the period expected of untreated cases, or there may be a slow progressive deterioration with no period of improvement. Others show a short initial period of improvement, followed by progressive deterioration, others again improve for so long that they appear to be going to recover, when they relapse and progressively deteriorate. Those who survive show an equal variability. Some improve uninterruptedly from the beginning; others only after an initial stationary or deteriorating period. Some recover in spite of a relapse, and some after a long period of deterioration remain in a stationary condition with evidence of gross cerebral lesions. Broadly, among patients treated early the mortality-rate should be under 10 per cent and of those who survive 70 per cent should be free from sequelae.

THE TREATMENT OF MENINGITIS

The Choice of Drug

The appropriate treatment of meningitis depends upon the isolation of the organism and tests of its sensitivity to the various available chemotherapeutic and antibiotic agents. The chemotherapy of meningitis is a field in which, owing to the rapidity with which advances are being made, techniques have changed rapidly. This is particularly evident at the moment in the chemotherapy of tuberculous meningitis, where new developments may render older methods out of date. All that can be done in a textbook, therefore, is to provide an up-to-date summary of the methods which, at the time of writing, are generally regarded as the best. Valuable reviews are given by Garrod et al. (1973) and by Menkes (1974) who point out that the policy of administering immediately 10,000 units (6 mg) of benzylpenicillin in 10 ml saline intrathecally as soon as turbid fluid is found on lumbar puncture has much to commend it. Until a bacteriological diagnosis is made ampicillin, 150 mg/kg body weight per day, is the most satisfactory initial systemic treatment.

The principles involved in the specific treatment of meningitis are that the infecting organism shall be sensitive to the agent used, and that this shall be used in such a way as to reach the organism in sufficient strength. The application of these principles will be considered in relation to particular varieties of meningitis.

Pyogenic Meningitis

Some authorities believe that by giving massive systemic doses of antibiotics most cases of pyogenic meningitis, especially in meningococcal infection, can be satisfactorily treated without intrathecal injections. This may often be true; nevertheless there are cases in which the response to a combination of intrathecal and systemic therapy is more rapid than that of systemic therapy alone, and others in which the latter does not completely eradicate the infection which may smoulder on in the meninges and involve the substance of the brain or spinal cord. Hence it is wise to use both routes of administration at least initially.

When a tentative diagnosis of meningitis has been made no treatment should be given until a lumbar puncture has been performed, since the administration of antibiotics at that stage may make it impossible to identify the causal organism. If the fluid is turbid it may be assumed that the meningitis is pyogenic. Ten ml in two consecutive portions of 5 ml each should be removed for examination and culture. Testing the sensitivity of the organism takes time and valuable time may be lost if treatment is delayed until this has been reported upon. Hence in all cases of pyogenic meningitis it is wise to begin treatment at once with an intrathecal injection of benzylpenicillin (penicillin G) at the initial puncture, once fluid for examination has been obtained. The dose for an adult is 10,000 units (6 mg) mixed with 10 ml of saline or of the patient's cerebrospinal fluid, that for a child being calculated in proportion to its weight; 600 mg of penicillin should also be given intramuscularly. If the infection proves to be pneumococcal, treatment should be continued with 4-hourly intramuscular injections of 1·2 g of penicillin for an adult and daily intrathecal injections of 10,000 units (6 mg) of benzylpenicillin should be given until the infection is well under control (usually for about one week). Streptococcal and staphylococcal infections should be treated in the same way, but substituting ampicillin, or another drug, for penicillin should the organism be penicillin-resistant.

TABLE 6.1

CHOICE OF ANTIBIOTIC IN MENINGITIS*

Organism	Drug of choice
Aerobacter	Gentamicin or kanamycin
Bacteroides	Gentamicin
Clostridium	Penicillin G
Corynebacterium	Penicillin G
Diplococcus pneumoniae	Penicillin G
Escherichia coli	Gentamicin or kanamycin
Haemophilus influenzae	Ampicillin or chloramphenicol
Klebsiella	Gentamicin or kanamycin
Listeria monocytogenes	Penicillin G
Neisseria meningitidis ·	Penicillin G
Neisseria gonorrhoeae	Penicillin G
Proteus mirabilis (indole negative)	Ampicillin
Proteus morganii (indole positive)	Gentamicin or kanamycin
Pseudomonas	Gentamicin, colistin, or polymyxin
Salmonella	Ampicillin, gentamicin, or chloramphenicol
Staphylococci-penicillinase negative	Penicillin G
Staphylococci-penicillinase positive	Methicillin
Streptococci	Penicillin G
Unknown	Ampicillin, gentamicin, or kanamycin, methicillin if question of staphylococcal infection

* From Menkes, J. H. (1974) *Child Neurology*, p. 219, New York.

While recommendations relating to the use of chemotherapeutic agents and antibiotics in cases of meningitis change rapidly from year to year, and while no simple guide can be comprehensive, taking account of all eventualities in the light of varying sensitivity of organisms to different remedies, Table 6.1 (Menkes, 1974) presents the current position clearly, and a useful review is also given by Garrod *et al.* (1973). Sulphadiazine, used as the drug of choice in meningococcal infections and also often given in influenzal and *E. coli* meningitis even 10 years ago, has now been virtually discarded in favour of the antibiotics.

Ampicillin is normally given by mouth in a dose of 250 mg 6-hourly to an adult, 125 mg 6-hourly to a child, but can also be given by intravenous injection in a dose of 200–400 mg/kg body weight in children. It is particularly recommended for infections with *H. influenzae, Streptococcus viridans*, and enterococci.

Methicillin (100–200 mg/kg daily in four to six divided doses in a child or 1 g four times daily in an adult) or erythromycin (250–500 mg four times daily in an adult) are recommended for staphylococcal infections with penicillinase-producing organisms. Gentamicin is a wide-spectrum antibiotic, effective in most coccal infections, including those with methicillin-resistant staphylococci, but also of particular value in infections with *Aerobacter*, *Bacteroides*, *B. proteus*, *E. coli*, and *Pseudomonas*; the dose is 0·8–1·2 mg/kg daily in two to four equally divided doses in childhood and 60–80 mg 8-hourly in adults. Kanamycin is another antibiotic of value in infections with *Aerobacter*, *B. proteus*, and *E. coli*, but also with *Klebsiella*; the dose is 5–15 mg/kg intramuscularly in divided daily doses in children, 250–500 mg 6-hourly by mouth in adults. Both gentamicin and kanamycin must be used cautiously if there is evidence of impaired renal function and both may cause labyrinthine damage if high blood levels are maintained for more than a week.

Polymyxin B (1·5–2·5 mg/kg daily in four equally divided doses) or colistin (2·5–5·0 mg/kg) are especially recommended for pseudomonas infections but may occasionally be useful in other infections; streptomycin, once widely used in infection with *H. influenzae*, *E. coli*, and *Pseudomonas*, is now used as a rule only in tuberculous meningitis. Chloramphenicol, too (75–100 mg/kg daily in children, 250 mg four times daily in adults), is now little used in meningitis because of the risk of bone marrow suppression, unless the organism responsible is not sensitive to any other available antibiotic. Lincomycin (500 mg three times daily) is another useful antibiotic, effective in infections with gram-positive pathogens. Most of the remedies listed can also be given, if need be, by intra-muscular injection; the reader is referred to the manufacturer's instructions for details.

The question as to whether intrathecal as well as systemic treatment is necessary has been mentioned above. While penicillin and some other anti-biotics mentioned above normally cross the blood-brain barrier, when given systemically, in very small amounts, all cross the inflamed meninges in adequate concentration to deal with meningeal infections. Nevertheless it is clear that meningitis is controlled more rapidly if intrathecal therapy is given. In meningo-coccal meningitis, a single intrathecal injection followed by systemic treatment will usually suffice, but in other infections it is usual to give an intrathecal injection daily or every other day for the first one or two weeks, depending upon the condition of the patient, until the infection is under control. Among drugs which can be given intrathecally are benzylpenicillin (penicillin G), 10,000 units (6 mg), streptomycin, 5–10 mg, polymyxin, 2 mg in children, 5 mg in adults, ampicillin, 3–5 mg for children, 10–20 mg for adults, methicillin, 3–5 mg for children, 10 mg for adults, and gentamicin, 1 mg; all should be given well diluted in 10 ml of saline or CSF. Systemic antibiotic therapy should be given for about one week after the fluid has become sterile and relatively free from cells and after all clinical evidence of infection has subsided.

In all cases of pyogenic meningitis other than meningococcal, a careful search should be made for a source of infection, especially in the ears or paranasal sinuses, and the possibility of a coexistent intracranial abscess should be borne in mind.

Tuberculous Meningitis

Each introduction of a new antibiotic effective against the tubercle bacillus has been followed by an improvement in the recovery rate from tuberculous meningitis. The routine treatment, therefore, consists of the systemic administration of isoniazid and streptomycin in the following doses for an adult: isoniazid, 100 mg thrice daily by mouth, and streptomycin, 1 g daily by intramuscular injection. PAS is also given in a dosage of 18–20 g daily. The doses in childhood are isoniazid, 20 mg/kg, streptomycin 20 mg/kg, and PAS 200 mg/kg daily. Even after clinical recovery treatment should probably be continued for six to twelve months. As in the case of pyogenic infections, some workers believe that tuberculous meningitis can be adequately treated without intrathecal injections. This is true in some cases, but there still appears to be a place for intrathecal injections, particularly in advanced cases and if a patient is not otherwise responding well. The intrathecal dose of streptomycin is from 20 to 50 mg daily or every other day for ten injections. The routine administration of steroid drugs (e.g. prednisone, 40 mg daily at first and later 30 mg or 20 mg daily) during the first few weeks probably helps to reduce complications such as adhesive arachnoiditis and communicating hydrocephalus and is now recommended in virtually all cases by most authorities. When a rise in cerebrospinal fluid protein and a fall in its pressure suggests that a spinal subarachnoid block is developing, an intrathecal dose of 10–25 mg of hydrocortisone, repeated daily if necessary for a week, is often valuable. Pyridoxine in doses of 40 mg daily should be given to prevent the development of isoniazid neuropathy, and anticonvulsants are needed in some cases. Now that more strains of tubercle bacilli resistant to isoniazid and streptomycin are emerging, newer remedies such as ethambutol, ethionamide, pyrazinamide, or cycloserine may be needed in some cases. The development of hydrocephalus calls for surgical intervention and sometimes for the administration of streptomycin into the ventricles.

The main index of a good response to treatment is the disappearance of tubercle bacilli from the cerebrospinal fluid. In favourable cases these usually disappear within the first fortnight. Of the chemical constituents the glucose level is the most useful but is of little help after streptomycin has been given intrathecally. The protein content may rise considerably in response to treatment, and a high protein content with a falling cell count has been regarded as a good sign, though both ultimately fall. A high cell count, mainly polymorphonuclear, may be a reaction to the streptomycin.

A relapse is indicated by a gradual or sudden deterioration in the condition of the patient who has previously been making good progress. Fever, vomiting, increase in headache, irritability, and apathy are the chief symptoms of a relapse, while the cerebrospinal fluid is likely to show a fall in the glucose content, a rising cell count, and a reappearance of the organism in films or cultures. This calls for a prolongation of intrathecal treatment, or a return to it if it has already been stopped. The development of resistance to streptomycin by the organism is fortunately rare. Details of treatment and of prognosis are given by Miller *et al.* (1963).

Toxic effects of the streptomycin include vertigo, which is often transitory, and possibly an ataxic gait in the convalescent, which also usually disappears after re-education. Deafness is a more serious complication, since when it occurs it is likely to be permanent.

After an illness involving many months in bed convalescence must necessarily be prolonged, and the after-care should be that of any form of chronic tuberculosis.

General Measures

Good nursing is of the utmost importance and in severe cases the long illness, often with relapses, and the need for repeated lumbar punctures, make heavy demands upon the skill and patience of the nurses. Nasal feeding or the administration of fluids by intravenous drip will be required when swallowing is difficult. An indwelling catheter is often needed for a time. Sedatives will usually be needed to control restlessness and in some cases convulsions. Ounsted (1951) stressed the dangers of status epilepticus. In childhood especially prophylactic anticonvulsant therapy with phenobarbitone 30 mg twice daily or sodium phenytoin 50 mg twice daily is often wise. Repeated convulsions in children or adults may require intravenous diazepam as given in the treatment of status epilepticus [p. 1124].

REFERENCES

PYOGENIC MENINGITIS

ADAMS, R. D., and KUBIK, C. (1947) The effects of influenzal meningitis on the nervous system, *N.Y. St. J. Med.*, **47**, 2676.

BANKS, H. S. (1948) Meningococcosis, *Lancet*, **ii**, 635.

BANKS, H. S., and McCARTNEY, J. E. (1943) Meningococcal adrenal syndromes and lesions, *Lancet*, **i**, 771.

BEATY, H. N., and OPPENHEIMER, S. (1968) Cerebrospinal fluid lactic dehydrogenase and its isoenzymes in infections of the central nervous system, *New Engl. J. Med.*, **279**, 1197.

BELSY, M. A. (1969) CSF glutamic oxaloacetic transaminase in acute bacterial meningitis, *Amer. J. Dis. Child.*, **117**, 288.

BRUYN, G. W., and STRAATHOF, L. J. A. (1961) La méningite endothélioleucocytaire multirécurrente bénigne de Mollaret, *Presse Méd.*, **69**, 1741.

DUCKER, T. B., and SIMMONS, R. L. (1968) The pathogenesis of meningitis. Systemic effects of meningococcal endotoxin within the cerebrospinal fluid, *Arch. Neurol. (Chic.)*, **18**, 123.

FORD, P. M., HERZBERG, L., and FORD, S. E. (1968) *Listeria monocytogenes*: six cases affecting the central nervous system, *Quart. J. Med.*, **37**, 281.

GARROD, L. P., LAMBERT, H. P., and O'GRADY, F. (1973) *Antibiotic and Chemotherapy*, 4th ed., Edinburgh.

HAGGERTY, R. J., and ZIAI, M. (1960) Acute bacterial meningitis in children, *Pediatrics*, **25**, 742.

HARDING, J. W., and BRUNTON, G. B. (1962) *Listeria monocytogenes* meningitis in neonates, *Lancet*, **ii**, 484.

HARDMAN, J. M., and EARLE, K. M. (1969) Myocarditis in 200 fatal meningococcal infections, *Arch. Path.*, **87**, 318.

HOEPRICH, P. D. (1958) Infection due to *Listeria monocytogenes*, *Medicine (Baltimore)*, **37**, 142.

HOLT, R. (1969) The classification of staphylococci from colonized ventriculo-atrial shunts, *J. Clin. Path.*, **22**, 475.

KATZ, R. M., and LIEBMAN, W. (1970) Creatine phosphokinase activity in central nervous system disorders and infections, *Amer. J. Dis. Child.*, **120**, 543.

KREMER, M. (1945) Meningitis after spinal analgesia, *Brit. med. J.*, **2**, 309.

KUHNS, D. M., NELSON, C. T., FELDMAN, H. A., and KUHN, L. R. (1943) The prophylactic value of sulfadiazine in the control of meningococcic meningitis, *J. Amer. med. Ass.*, **123**, 335.

LILLEHEI, R. C., LONGERBEAM, J. K., BLOCH, J. H., and MANAX, W. G. (1964) The modern treatment of shock based on physiologic principles, *Clin. Pharmacol. Ther.*, **5**, 63.

LONG, P. H. (1959) Use of antibiotics in central nervous infections, *Res. Publ. Ass. nerv. ment. Dis.*, **37**, 16.

McKENDRICK, G. D. W. (1954) Pyogenic meningitis, *Lancet*, **ii**, 510.

McKENDRICK, G. D. W. (1954) Pneumococcal meningitis, *Lancet*, **ii**, 512.

MARGARETTEN, W., and McADAMS, A. J. (1958) An appraisal of fulminant meningo-coccemia with reference to the Schwartzman phenomenon, *Amer. J. Med.*, **25**, 868.

MENKES, J. H. (1974) *Textbook of Child Neurology*, Philadelphia.

MOLLARET, P. (1952) Benign recurrent pleocytic meningitis and its presumed causative virus, *J. Nerv. Ment. Dis.*, **116**, 1072.

OSUNTOKUN, B. O., BADEMOSI, O., OGUNREMI, K., and WRIGHT, S. G. (1972) Neuro-psychiatric manifestations of typhoid fever in 959 patients, *Arch. Neurol. (Chic.)*, **27**, 7.

OUNSTED, C. (1951) Significance of convulsions in children with purulent meningitis, *Lancet*, **i**, 1245.

RABE, E. F., FLYNN, R. E., and DODGE, P. R. (1968) Subdural collections of fluid in infants and children: a study of 62 patients with special reference to factors influencing prognosis and the efficacy of various forms of therapy, *Neurology (Minneap.)*, **18**, 559.

SHUTTLEWORTH, E. C., and ALLEN, N. (1968) Early differentiation of chronic meningitis by enzyme assay, *Neurology (Minneap.)*, **18**, 534.

SMITH, H., BANNISTER, B., and O'SHEA, M. J. (1973) Cerebrospinal-fluid immunoglobulins in meningitis, *Lancet*, **ii**, 591.

SMITH, H. V., NORMAN, R. M., and URICH, H. (1957) The late sequelae of pneumococcal meningitis, *J. Neurol. Neurosurg. Psychiat.*, **20**, 250.

WILLIAMS, D. N., and GEDDES, A. M. (1970) Meningococcal meningitis complicated by pericarditis, panophthalmitis, and arthritis, *Brit. med. J.*, **2**, 93.

TUBERCULOUS MENINGITIS

ASHBY, M., and GRANT, H. (1955) Tuberculous meningitis treated with cortisone, *Lancet*, **i**, 65.

BHAGWATI, S. N. (1971) Ventriculo-atrial shunt in tuberculous meningitis with hydro-cephalus, *J. Neurosurg.*, **35**, 309.

CAIRNS, H. (1951) Neurosurgical methods in the treatment of tuberculous meningitis, *Arch. Dis. Childh.*, **26**, 373.

CAIRNS, H., SMITH, H. V., and VOLLUM, R. L. (1950) Tuberculous meningitis, *J. Amer. med. Ass.*, **144**, 92.

CAIRNS, H., and TAYLOR, M. (1949) Streptomycin in tuberculous meningitis, *Lancet*, **i**, 148.

CATHIE, I. A. B. (1949) Streptomycin-streptokinase treatment of tuberculous meningitis, *Lancet*, **i**, 441.

DASTUR, D. K., and WADIA, N. H. (1969) Spinal meningitides with radiculo-myelopathy. Part 2: Pathology and pathogenesis, *J. neurol. Sci.*, **8**, 261.

DRURY, M. I., O'LOCHLAINN, S., and SWEENEY, E. (1968) Complications of tuberculous meningitis, *Brit. med. J.*, **1**, 842.

EMOND, R. T. D., and McKENDRICK, G. D. W. (1973) Tuberculosis as a cause of transient aseptic meningitis, *Lancet*, **ii**, 234.

FREIMAN, I., and GEEFHUYSEN, J. (1970) Evaluation of intrathecal therapy with strepto-mycin and hydrocortisone in tuberculous meningitis, *J. Pediat.*, **76**, 895.

ILLINGWORTH, R. S., and WRIGHT, T. (1948) Tubercles of the choroid, *Brit. med. J.*, **2**, 365.

KOCEN, R. S., and PARSONS, M. (1970) Neurological complications of tuberculosis: some unusual manifestations, *Quart. J. Med.*, **39**, 17.

THE LANCET (1959) Treatment of tuberculous meningitis, **i**, 214.

LINCOLN, E. M. (1947) Tuberculous meningitis in children, with special reference to serous meningitis, *Am. Rev. Tuberc.*, **56**, 75.

LINCOLN, E. M., and SEWELL, E. M. (1963) *Tuberculosis in Children*, New York.

LORBER, J. (1960) Treatment of tuberculous meningitis, *Brit. med. J.*, **1**, 1309.

MacGregor, A. R., and Green, C. A. (1937) Tuberculosis of the central nervous system, with special reference to tuberculous meningitis, *J. Path. Bact.*, **45**, 613.

Menkes, J. H. (1974) *Textbook of Child Neurology*, Philadelphia.

Miller, F. J. W., Seal, R. M. E., and Taylor, M. D. (1963) *Tuberculosis in Children*, London.

Rich, A. R., and McCordock, H. A. (1933) The pathogenesis of tuberculous meningitis, *Bull. Johns Hopk. Hosp.*, **52**, 5.

Smellie, J. M. (1954) The treatment of tuberculous meningitis without intrathecal therapy, *Lancet*, **ii**, 1091.

Smith, H. V., and Daniel, P. (1947) Some clinical and pathological aspects of tuberculosis of the central nervous system, *Tubercle (Lond.)*, **28**, 64.

Smith, H. V., and Vollum, R. L. (1950) Effects of intrathecal tuberculin and streptomycin in tuberculous meningitis, *Lancet*, **ii**, 275.

Taylor, L. M., Smith, H. V., and Hunter, G. (1954) The blood-cerebrospinal fluid barrier to bromide in the diagnosis of tuberculous meningitis, *Lancet*, **i**, 700.

Wadia, N. H., and Dastur, D. K. (1969) Spinal meningitides with radiculo-myelopathy. Part 1: Clinical and radiological features, *J. neurol. Sci.*, **8**, 239.

LEPTOSPIRAL MENINGITIS

Infection with either *Leptospira icterohaemorrhagica* or *Leptospira canicola* may manifest itself solely or mainly as a meningitis. *L. icterohaemorrhagica* is excreted in the urine of infected rats and is transmitted to human beings who come in contact with media contaminated by rats' urine. Fish-workers, coal-miners, sewer-workers, and farm-labourers are exposed to the risk of infection by their occupations. The other chief source is accidental immersion or bathing in contaminated water, and the meningitic form of Weil's disease is particularly likely to follow infection while bathing (Buzzard and Wylie, 1947). *L. canicola* is transmitted to man from dogs, in which it may cause diarrhoea, but which may harbour the organism while remaining apparently in normal health.

The clinical picture of the meningeal form of both diseases is very similar. The usual symptoms and signs of meningitis are present, often in a benign form, though in Weil's disease the meningitis may be severe. Symptoms and signs of involvement of the cerebral hemispheres or brain stem rarely occur (Alston and Broom, 1958). The fundi are often congested and there may be papilloedema. The cerebrospinal fluid is under increased pressure and contains a considerable excess of cells. In Weil's disease polymorphonuclear cells predominate at the outset, later giving place to lymphocytes, while in canicola fever a lymphocytosis seems to be characteristic. The number of cells ranges from 50 to over 1,000 per mm³ and the protein content of the fluid may be normal or as high as 400 mg per 100 ml.

Though in either disease meningitis may be associated with the characteristic general symptoms, these may be absent. The most distinctive sign outside the nervous system appears to be ciliary congestion. In canicola fever there may be a morbilliform rash and the spleen may be enlarged. In Weil's disease jaundice may be absent, and there may be no haemorrhages or severe renal damage.

The clinical picture may thus be that of so-called acute aseptic meningitis, and the only clues pointing to the cause may be the ciliary congestion, the occupation of the patient, a history of recent bathing, or of a fall into water. The diagnosis is confirmed by a rising serum-agglutination titre to the infecting organism and by the demonstration by appropriate techniques of leptospirae in the blood, urine, or conjunctival secretion.

When the clinical picture is purely or predominantly meningeal the prognosis is good and complete recovery is the rule. Penicillin is often given systemically, but its value is doubtful.

REFERENCES

ALSTON, J. M., and BROOM, J. C. (1958) *Leptospirosis in Man and Animals*, Edinburgh.
BUZZARD, E. M., and WYLIE, J. A. H. (1947) Meningitis leptospirosa, *Lancet*, **ii,** 417.
DAVIDSON, L. S. P., and SMITH, J. (1939) Weil's disease in the north-east of Scotland, *Brit. med. J.*, **2,** 753.
EDWARDS, G. A., and DOMM, B. M. (1960) Human leptospirosis, *Medicine (Baltimore)*, **39,** 117.
LAURENT, L. J. M., NORRIS, T. ST. M., STARKS, J. M., BROOM, J. C., and ALSTON, J. M. (1948) Four cases of leptospira canicola infection in England, *Lancet*, **ii,** 48.
MACKAY-DICK, J., and WATTS, R. W. E. (1949) Canicola fever in Germany, *Lancet*, **i,** 907.
WEETCH, R. S., KOLQUHOUN, J., and BROOM, J. D. (1949) Fatal human case of canicola fever, *Lancet*, **i,** 906.

ACUTE LYMPHOCYTIC CHORIOMENINGITIS AND ACUTE ASEPTIC MENINGITIS

[See page 512.]

BRUCELLOSIS

Any of the three organisms *Brucella melitensis*, *Brucella abortus*, and *Brucella suis*, may directly or indirectly affect the nervous system. There are now many recorded cases of meningo-encephalitis due to these organisms. To the naked eye, there are greyish-white 'tubercles' in the meninges, which histologically consist of hyalinized connective tissue infiltrated with chronic inflammatory cells, with, in places, necrosis. The meninges themselves are invaded by lymphocytes, plasma cells, and a few polymorphonuclear cells.

The clinical picture may consist predominantly of a subacute or chronic meningitis, or there may be symptoms of increased intracranial pressure suggesting a tumour, or the picture may be that of focal encephalitis. Epilepsy, aphasia, mental confusion or deterioration, and spastic weakness of the limbs have all been observed. Myelitis is rare. Polyneuritis is uncommon. The cerebrospinal fluid contains an excess of mononuclear cells, usually below 100 per mm³. The protein is raised as a rule, but is sometimes disproportionately high, and the fluid may be xanthochromic. In one reported case it was blood-stained, owing to rupture of a mycotic aneurysm.

Headache, fatigability, irritability, and toxic confusional states may occur as symptoms of the toxaemia in the absence of direct involvement of the nervous system. Brucellosis may lead to spondylitis, and neurological symptoms may be secondary to this, lumbar spondylitis, for example, leading to sciatica.

The clinical picture of meningeal irritation associated with a lymphocytosis of the cerebrospinal fluid may lead to confusion with tuberculous meningitis or meningitis due to *Cryptococcus neoformans*. The diagnosis rests upon the appropriate serological tests for brucellosis, reinforced by the isolation of the organism, which may be obtained from the cerebrospinal fluid. These organisms are largely resistant to antibiotics but some strains are sensitive to gentamicin or kanamycin.

REFERENCES

DALRYMPLE-CHAMPNEYS, W. (1960) *Brucella Infection and Undulant Fever in Man*, London.
HARRIS, H. J. (1950) *Brucellosis (Undulant Fever)*, New York.
HUDDLESON, I. F. (1943) *Brucellosis in Man and Animals*, New York.

MENINGITIS DUE TO *CRYPTOCOCCUS NEOFORMANS (TORULA HISTOLYTICA)*

Cryptococcus neoformans, also known as *Torula histolytica*, is a fungus consisting of a round or oval body surrounded by a thick polysaccharide capsule. It appears to be of world-wide distribution, but most cases have occurred in the more southern parts of the United States and in Australia (Edwards *et al.*, 1970). It has also been found in Great Britain. Its usual portal of entry appears to be the lung where it forms lesions not unlike those of pulmonary tuberculosis, though rarely undergoing cavitation. The brain, however, is the most important site of infection. There it forms an irregular granulomatous thickening of the meninges which are infiltrated with lymphocytes and occasional plasma cells. Multinucleated giant cells are also present. Capsulated cryptococci are scattered throughout the meninges. To the naked eye the brain shows a diffuse or more localized opacity of the meninges with flattening of the gyri and other evidence of increased intracranial pressure. Other organs besides the nervous system and the lungs may be involved, including the kidneys, spleen, and the lymph nodes. The histological changes in lymph nodes have been likened to those of Hodgkin's disease but there is evidence that Hodgkin's disease may predispose to the infection with the cryptococcus as may carcinomatosis and other debilitating diseases.

Clinically there is an insidious onset of symptoms with a history varying from weeks to years, but usually measured in months. The symptoms of meningitis are usually present, including cervical rigidity and Kernig's sign, but the presence of papilloedema and symptoms of a focal lesion of the nervous system may suggest an intracranial tumour. The cerebrospinal fluid is very variable. It may be clear with only a small excess of cells and protein, or may contain a considerable excess of cells, usually lymphocytes and occasionally polymorphonuclears, with or without a high protein. A paretic colloidal gold curve is rather characteristic. Cryptococci may be present in the fluid or may be cultured on Sabouraud's medium: special stains are required to stain the capsule. The condition must be distinguished from other forms of subacute or chronic meningitis, sarcoidosis, intracranial tumour, and carcinomatosis of the meninges. The presence of a characteristic pulmonary lesion may be helpful, with fever and hepatosplenomegaly, but these features are rarely present. Spinal arachnoiditis giving signs of cord compression has been described (Davidson, 1968).

Amphotericin B given intravenously in a dosage of 0·25 mg, increasing to 1·0 mg/kg body weight daily by slow infusion, is an effective treatment but may be toxic, giving renal damage. The same drug given intrathecally has been shown to be effective (McIntyre, 1967). Steroids, given in combination with amphotericin B, may have an adjuvant value; given alone they cause exacerbation of the condition and have been used as a provocative diagnostic test in doubtful cases, since after the administration of prednisone, 30 mg daily for 48 hours, the cryptococcus may be found for the first time in the cerebrospinal fluid. 5-fluorocytosine, 100–200 mg per kg body weight, given by mouth for 6–8 weeks, may be more effective than amphotericin B and is usually less toxic (Watkins *et al.*, 1969).

REFERENCES

BUTLER, W. T., ALLING, D. W., SPICKARD, A., and UTZ, J. (1964) Diagnostic and prognostic value of clinical and laboratory findings in cryptococcal meningitis, *New Engl. J. Med.*, **270**, 59.

DAVIDSON, S. (1968) Cryptococcal spinal arachnoiditis, *J. Neurol. Neurosurg. Psychiat.*, **31**, 76.

EDWARDS, V. E., SUTHERLAND, J. M., and TYRER, J. H. (1970) Cryptococcosis of the central nervous system: epidemiological, clinical, and therapeutic features, *J. Neurol. Neurosurg. Psychiat.*, **33**, 415.

GREENFIELD, J. G. (1958) in *Neuropathology*, by Greenfield, J. G., Blackwood, W., McMenemey, W. H., Meyer, A., and Norman, R. M., p. 149, London.

McINTYRE, H. B. (1967) Cryptococcal meningitis. A case successfully treated by cisternal administration of amphotericin B with a review of recent literature, *Bull. Los Angeles neurol. Soc.*, **32**, 213.

ROSE, F. C., GRANT, C., and JEANES, A. L. (1958) Torulosis of the central nervous system in Britain, *Brain*, **81**, 542.

WATKINS, J. S., GARDNER-MEDWIN, D., INGHAM, H. R., and MURRAY, I. G. (1969) Two cases of cryptococcal meningitis, one treated with 5-fluorocytosine, *Brit. med. J.*, **3**, 29.

AMOEBIC MENINGOENCEPHALITIS

Primary amoebic meningoencephalitis, due to the amoebae *Naegleria* and *Hartmannella*, acquired by bathing in infected water, has been reported to cause either a mild meningitic illness or a fatal meningoencephalitis in children in Australia (Fowler and Carter, 1965), the United States (Duma *et al.*, 1969), and in Great Britain (Symmers, 1969); amphotericin B appears to be an effective treatment (Apley *et al.*, 1970).

REFERENCES

APLEY, J., CLARKE, S. K. R., ROOME, A. P. C. H., SANDRY, S. A., SAYGI, G., SILK, B., and WARHURST, D. C. (1970) Primary amoebic meningoencephalitis in Britain, *Brit. med. J.*, **1**, 596.

DUMA, R. J., FERRELL, H. W., NELSON, E. C., and JONES, M. M. (1969) Primary amebic meningoencephalitis, *New Engl. J. Med.*, **281**, 1315.

FOWLER, M., and CARTER, R. F. (1965) Acute pyogenic meningitis probably due to *Acanthamoeba* sp.: a preliminary report, *Brit. med. J.*, **2**, 740.

SYMMERS, W. ST. C. (1969) Primary amoebic meningoencephalitis in Britain, *Brit. med. J.*, **4**, 449.

OTHER RARE FUNGAL INFECTIONS

Other rare fungal infections include aspergillosis (multiple brain abscesses and vascular thrombosis), blastomycosis and cephalosporium infection (both giving meningitis), mucormycosis (thrombosis of cerebral and meningeal arteries), and nocardiosis (meningitis, multiple abscesses) (see Menkes, 1974). Most of these also respond to amphotericin B.

REFERENCE

MENKES, J. H. (1974) *Textbook of Child Neurology*, Philadelphia.

7

SUPPURATIVE ENCEPHALITIS:
INTRACRANIAL ABSCESS

PATHOLOGY

INTRACRANIAL abscess may be (1) extradural, (2) subdural, (3) subarachnoid, or (4) intracerebral. (1) Extradural abscess is secondary to osteitis of one of the cranial bones. The infection passes through the bone, but as its further advance is arrested by the dura, the accumulating pus strips the dura from the bone. (2) In subdural abscess the infection has penetrated the dura and the pus lies between this membrane and the brain surface. (3) Subarachnoid abscess is a rare form of abscess in which the pus is limited to the subarachnoid space and spreads along the surface of the brain. (4) Intracerebral abscess may follow the spread of infection from the surface of the brain, or may be haematogenous. In the former case it usually, but not necessarily, possesses a track communicating with the surface. Intracerebral abscesses are usually single, but may be multilocular, or, less commonly, multiple. The developing intracerebral abscess passes through three stages. The first is an acute encephalitis without pus formation. In the second stage pus appears, but the abscess is not well defined from surrounding tissue. In the third stage a definite wall is formed, and the abscess is localized [FIG. 92]. The localization of the abscess depends upon various factors, of which the resistance of the patient to the organism is one of the most important. In some rapidly fatal cases the condition remains one of a spreading suppurative encephalitis.

Abscesses of otitic origin are usually situated in the middle or posterior part of the temporal lobe or in the cerebellum, the former situation being about twice as common as the latter. An otitic cerebellar abscess usually occupies the antero-superior part of the lateral lobe and is adherent to the posterior part of the petrous bone (Pennybacker, 1948). Much more rarely such abscesses occur in the pons, frontal, or parietal lobes. In otitic cases the brain may become infected as a result of (1) purulent thrombosis of the transverse sinus, or (2) osteomyelitis of the tympanic wall, or (3) by spread along the adventitial spaces of perforating blood vessels (Evans, 1931). The anterior part of the frontal lobe is the usual seat of abscess following frontal sinusitis. Haematogenous abscesses may occur in any situation, but are nearly always above the tentorium. The left hemisphere is more often affected than the right, and in most cases the abscess lies in the area supplied by the middle cerebral artery and rather superficially.

Microscopically an intracerebral abscess consists of an inner layer of pus cells, outside which is a layer of granulation tissue containing new blood vessels and hyperplastic fibrous tissue. Outside this is a layer of glial reaction, mainly cellular in the early stages, mainly fibrous later. Fat-granule cells, plasma cells, and polymorphonuclear leucocytes are plentiful, especially in the middle layer. Inflammatory reactions are present in the overlying meninges, and in extradural and subdural abscess granulation tissue is present on the surface of the dura.

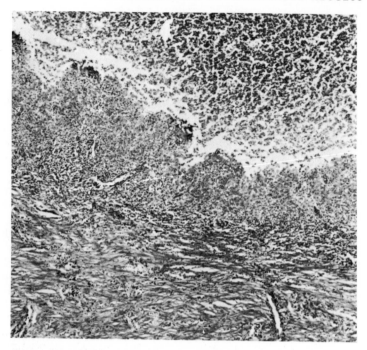

FIG. 92. The wall of a chronic pyogenic cerebral abscess with pus cells above, a line of granulation tissue in the centre and the fibroglial capsule below, Mallory's PTAH, ×40

AETIOLOGY

The causes of intracranial abscess in approximate order of frequency are: (1) infection of the middle ear, mastoid, and nasal sinuses; (2) pyaemia or bacteraemia; (3) metastasis from intrathoracic suppuration; and (4) head injury. In Evans's (1931) series of 194 cases, 121 were due to infection in the ear or paranasal sinuses, 24 to pyaemia, 22 to pulmonary suppuration; even today up to 40 per cent of cases in adults, but even more in children (Nestadt *et al.*, 1960), result from ear or sinus infection, but in about 20 per cent the source of infection may never be traced (Pennybacker and Sellors, 1948; Beller *et al.*, 1973).

1. Infection of the middle ear and mastoid is from four to nine times as common a cause of cerebral abscess as infection of the nasal sinuses, of which the frontal sinus is most often involved, and the sphenoidal sinus next.

2. Pyaemia is now rare, following the widespread use of antibiotics, but a cerebral abscess may still arise as a consequence of acute infective endocarditis; it rarely results from subacute bacterial endocarditis in view of the low virulence of the infecting organism. Unsuspected bacteraemia occurring in acute osteomyelitis and in other pyogenic infections including even simple boils or cutaneous sepsis is sometimes the cause.

3. When intracranial abscess is secondary to localized infection elsewhere, the thorax is usually the source, and most cases are complications of bronchiectasis, empyema, or lung abscess. Rarely the primary abscess is elsewhere, for example in the liver. There is a clear association between cerebral abscess and cyanotic

congenital heart disease (Maronde, 1950; Campbell, 1957; Nestadt *et al.*, 1960; Matson and Salem, 1961).

4. Fracture of the skull is liable to cause abscess when the injury leads to free communication between the surface of the body and the brain, especially when fragments of bone, clothing, or a missile penetrate the latter.

Any of the common pyogenic organisms may be responsible for intracranial abscess, the commonest being *Staphylococcus aureus*, streptococci, and pneumococci. Friedländer's bacillus and organisms of the *E. coli* group are also found. The causal agent may be a streptothrix, as in actinomycotic abscess, and amoebic abscess of the brain sometimes occurs. In certain parts of South-East Asia, chronic cerebral abscess due to paragonimiasis is relatively common and may be associated with recurrent episodes of low-grade meningitis (Oh, 1969).

SYMPTOMS

Mode of Onset

The history of the development of the symptoms of an intracranial abscess may be of greater diagnostic importance than the physical signs, which are often slight at the stage at which treatment is most likely to be effective.

When abscess follows fracture of the skull it usually develops soon after the injury, though when a missile penetrates the brain there may be a latent interval. These cases, however, offer little difficulty. The history is particularly important when abscess is secondary to otitis media or mastoiditis. In some such cases the onset is acute or subacute. After an exacerbation of a pre-existing otitis media, or a temporary suppression of aural discharge, or the operation of mastoidectomy, the patient rapidly develops headache, vomiting, delirium, and other symptoms to be described. In other cases there is a 'latent interval' which may last weeks or even months before the *signs* of abscess appear. The existence of *symptoms* during this period may suggest that all is not well. There may be attacks of headache, loss of appetite and weight, occasional unexplained pyrexia, and a change in temperament leading to lassitude, depression, and irritability.

Abscess of haematogenous origin may develop slowly and insidiously, in which case, unless the primary infective focus is discovered, it may be clinically indistinguishable from an intracranial tumour. It is comparatively rare, since the virtual disappearance of pyaemia, to obtain a history of an acute episode corresponding to the lodgement of the infected embolus in the brain. Even so, in occasional cases there may be a history of sudden headache with perhaps some impairment of consciousness, and weakness of a limb, followed by a remission of these symptoms for weeks or months before those of the abscess develop.

The symptoms of intracranial abscess may be conveniently divided into (1) general symptoms of infection; (2) symptoms of increased intracranial pressure; (3) focal symptoms; and (4) changes in the cerebrospinal fluid.

General Symptoms

The severity of the general symptoms is usually proportionate to the acuteness of the abscess, and is therefore most marked in the cases best described as acute suppurative encephalitis. In the acute cases an irregular pyrexia is the rule; in chronic cases the temperature may be intermittently raised but not invariably. In both there may be a polymorphonuclear leucocytosis in the blood.

P

Symptoms of Increased Intracranial Pressure

The incidence of symptoms of increased intracranial pressure differs some-what in abscess from that found in intracranial tumour. Headache is usually present. In chronic abscess it is paroxysmal, is increased by stooping and exer-tion, and presents the other features of headache due to increased intracranial pressure. In more acute cases headache may be persistent and very severe. Papilloedema is a late sign and is often absent or slight. When present it is some-times more marked upon the side of the lesion. Bradycardia is commoner in abscess than in tumour, but is not constant, and when it occurs usually indicates a rapid increase in the severity of the condition. In severe cases delirium, somno-lence, stupor, and coma develop. Exceptionally the signs of increased intra-cranial pressure are slight or lacking, even when a large abscess is present.

Focal Symptoms

Extradural Abscess. This is difficult to diagnose because, unless the abscess is very large, focal symptoms are absent, except for headache radiating from the ear and mastoid process or from the infected sinus towards the vertex. Increasing local headache with tenderness and/or oedema of the scalp in the region of the infected ear or sinus when surgical drainage appears adequate are suspicious signs.

Subdural Abscess or Empyema. This condition is almost always a complica-tion of frontal sinusitis but rarely develops as a result of sphenoidal sinusitis or otitis media. A layer of pus forms in the subdural space over one frontal lobe (or rarely over the temporal lobe). The clinical manifestations usually consist of high fever, fits (either focal or generalized), and a rapidly-developing hemiplegia with aphasia if the major hemisphere is involved (Farmer and Wise, 1973). Early surgical evacuation of the pus and irrigation of the subdural space with a weak solution of an appropriate antibiotic is imperative; thrombosis of cortical veins is an important complication which may lead to a substantial residual disability even if appropriate treatment is given.

Intracerebral Abscess. 1. *Temporal Lobe Abscess.* An abscess in this position, if situated on the left side in a right-handed individual, may cause aphasia, usually of the nominal or amnestic type, that is, a difficulty in naming objects. A patient who can name familiar objects accurately often shows hesitation, or misnames less familiar articles. Abscess on either side may produce a defect of the visual fields, an especially valuable localizing sign. It usually consists of a homonymous upper quadrantic defect on the opposite side due to involve-ment of the lower fibres of the optic radiation. Damage to the corticospinal tract is usually slight, and weakness is most marked in the face and tongue. The opposite plantar reflex may be extensor. Oculomotor paralyses may result from pressure upon the third or sixth cranial nerves.

2. *Cerebellar Abscess.* Headache in cerebellar abscess is often predominantly suboccipital. It may radiate down the neck and be associated with some cervical rigidity. The head may be flexed to the side of the lesion or retracted. Signs of cerebellar deficiency vary in severity and may be slight. The most important are—nystagmus, most marked on conjugate deviation to the side of the lesion, the slow phase being centripetal; hypotonia and inco-ordination in the limbs on the affected side, with an inability to carry out rapid alternating movements as well with the upper limb on the affected side as on the normal side. Pressure upon the brain stem may occur, leading to compression of cranial nerves, especially

the sixth and seventh, on the side of the abscess, and slight signs of corticospinal defect on the opposite side. Pass-pointing outwards with the affected hand and a tendency to deviate or fall to the side of the lesion when walking are additional signs which may be present.

3. *Frontal Abscess.* Headache, drowsiness, apathy, and impairment of memory and attention are usually conspicuous, but focal signs are often lacking. A large abscess or much oedema may cause aphasia or hemiparesis. Unilateral anosmia and slight exophthalmos may be present.

4. *Abscesses in other Situations.* These require no special description, the focal symptoms depending upon the position of the abscess, and usually resembling those of tumour in the same situation.

Subarachnoid Abscess. This rather rare condition may be suspected when the signs point to abscess of otitic origin, though neither of the clinical pictures just described is present. Convulsions may occur with a superficial abscess of the cerebral hemisphere. When the signs have pointed to involvement of the cerebellum but no abscess can be found in the cerebellum itself, search should be made for a superficial abscess in the cerebellopontine angle.

The Cerebrospinal Fluid

Examination of the cerebrospinal fluid is often of great diagnostic value, but lumbar puncture may be dangerous because of the risk of tentorial or cerebellar herniation and is better avoided if an abscess is strongly suspected (Garfield, 1969). As long as the abscess remains localized, the fluid is clear. Its pressure may be increased. There is usually an excess of cells, though not often more than 100 per mm^3, the majority of which are lymphocytes, the remainder being polymorphonuclear: the protein is somewhat raised. A protein of perhaps 200 mg/100 ml with relatively few cells is particularly suggestive. There is no diminution in the chloride or sugar content, and organisms are absent. If meningitis develops, the changes are those of pyogenic meningitis [p. 411].

OTHER METHODS OF INVESTIGATION

The EEG may yield valuable evidence as to the site of an abscess, demonstrating a striking focus of high amplitude slow delta activity. Echoencephalography may indicate displacement of the midline as in the case of an intracranial tumour. Isotope encephalography may accurately localize an abscess (Planiol, 1963). Angiography has been shown to localize the lesion in 90 per cent of cases and to suggest its character in 61 per cent (Beller *et al.*, 1973) but computerized transaxial tomography (the EMI scan) seems likely to be even more successful. Ventriculography is also useful if doubt remains and is sometimes more reliable than angiography (Garfield, 1969) but should only be performed as a preliminary to surgery. Once an abscess has been diagnosed and localized, if aspiration is preferred to excision, it is usual to inject contrast medium into the cavity [FIG. 93] in order to observe its subsequent shrinkage.

DIAGNOSIS

Intracranial abscess is occasionally encountered without an evident source of infection. It is then usually exposed at an operation for a supposed intracranial tumour. The diagnosis of such cases from tumour is difficult and often impossible. Pyrexia, leucocytosis in the blood, and an excess of cells in the cerebrospinal fluid, however, may suggest the correct diagnosis, as may the gamma scan

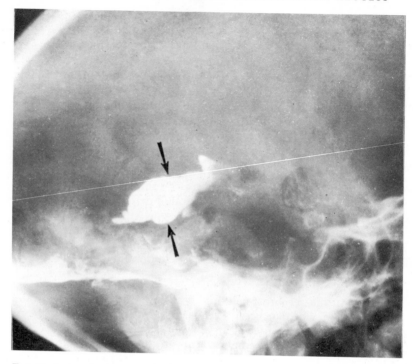

FIG. 93. A chronic abscess cavity into which contrast medium (*Steripaque*) has been injected; some of the medium has leaked out into the subarachnoid space

or EMI scan When the causal infective focus is obvious, it is necessary to distinguish abscess from other pyogenic intracranial complications. Generalized meningitis, which may coexist with abscess, is distinguished by the prominence of signs of meningeal irritation, cervical rigidity, Kernig's sign, and the changes in the cerebrospinal fluid already described. Transverse sinus thrombosis causes few cerebral symptoms, though it may cause slight papilloedema, more marked on the affected side, and slight signs of corticospinal tract defect on the opposite side. The signs of pyaemia are usually conspicuous with swinging temperature and rigors. A useful but inconstant sign may be demonstrated in cases of the latter type by Queckenstedt's test. The rise of cerebrospinal fluid pressure may be slight or absent when the jugular vein on the affected side is compressed alone, because the blocked transverse sinus prevents communication of the raised jugular pressure to the cranial cavity. Acute 'labyrinthitis' may be confused with cerebellar abscess, with which it may coexist. In the former vertigo is more, and headache less, intense than in the latter. Hypotonia is in favour of a cerebellar lesion. Papilloedema and changes in the cerebrospinal fluid indicate that the infection has passed beyond the internal ear.

PROGNOSIS

Very rarely an intracranial abscess becomes quiescent and is found accidentally at post-mortem, surrounded by a thick layer of gliosis. Recovery by spontaneous drainage may also occur. These occurrences, however, are too exceptional to have any bearing upon prognosis, which may be regarded as uniformly fatal in the absence of surgical interference. Spreading encephalitis, rupture of the abscess into the ventricular system, meningitis, and sinus thrombosis are the usual terminations. Even after surgical drainage or excision these complications may occur, and the mortality rate is high, but with modern surgical methods and antibiotics it should probably be no more than 20 per cent though it was 40 per cent in a recent large series (Garfield, 1969). Thoracogenic and otitic cerebellar abscesses are the most serious. Epilepsy is an important sequel, occurring in between 50 and 72 per cent of cases (Jooma *et al.*, 1951; Legg *et al.*, 1973), usually within 12 months.

TREATMENT

Treatment is surgical, the choice lying between primary excision, and repeated aspiration followed by the instillation of penicillin or other appropriate antibiotics, with secondary excision in reserve if this treatment fails. Excision is attended by the lowest mortality (Jooma *et al.*, 1951) but is not always practicable and much depends upon the situation of the lesion. Antibiotics should be given as for meningitis [see p. 421], but intrathecal penicillin should not be given unless there is also meningitis and then not until the abscess has been dealt with surgically. In the early stages, dexamethasone may be useful in reducing cerebral oedema, provided antibiotic cover is adequate.

REFERENCES

BELLER, A. J., SAHAR, A., and PRAISS, I. (1973) Brain abscess: review of 89 cases over a period of 30 years, *J. Neurol. Neurosurg. Psychiat.*, **36**, 757.

CAMPBELL, M. (1957) Cerebral abscess in cyanotic congenital heart disease, *Lancet*, **i**, 111.

EVANS, W. (1931) The pathology and aetiology of brain abscess, *Lancet*, **i**, 1231 and 1289.

FARMER, T. W., and WISE, G. R. (1973) Subdural empyema in infants, children and adults, *Neurology (Minneap.)*, **23**, 254.

GARFIELD, J. (1969) Management of supratentorial intracranial abscess: a review of 200 cases, *Brit. med. J.*, **2**, 7.

JOOMA, O. V., PENNYBACKER, J., and TUTTON, G. K. (1951) Brain abscess, aspiration, drainage or excision?, *J. Neurol. Psychiat.*, **14**, 308.

KERR, F. W. L., KING, R. B., and MEAGHER, J. N. (1958) Brain abscess, *J. Amer. med. Ass.*, **168**, 868.

LEGG, N. J., GUPTA, P. C., and SCOTT, D. F. (1973) Epilepsy following cerebral abscess— a clinical and EEG study of 70 patients, *Brain*, **96**, 259.

MARONDE, R. F. (1950) Brain abscess and congenital heart disease, *Ann. intern. Med.*, **33**, 602.

MATSON, D. D., and SALEM, M. (1961) Brain abscess in congenital heart disease, *Pediatrics*, **27**, 772.

NESTADT, A., LOWRY, R. B., and TURNER, E. (1960) Diagnosis of brain abscess in infants and children, *Lancet*, **ii**, 449.

NORTHFIELD, D. W. C. (1942) The treatment of brain abscess, *J. Neurol. Psychiat.*, N.S. **5**, 1.

OH, S. J. (1969) Cerebral paragonimiasis, *J. neurol. Sci.*, **8**, 27.

PENNYBACKER, J. (1948) Cerebellar abscess, *J. Neurol. Neurosurg. Psychiat.*, N.S. **11**, 1.

PENNYBACKER, J., and SELLORS, T. H. (1948) Treatment of thoracogenic brain abscess, *Lancet*, **ii**, 90.

PLANIOL, T. (1963) La gamma-encéphalographie, *Rev. Prat. (Paris)*, **13**, 3625.

SCHILLER, F., CAIRNS, H., and RUSSELL, D. S. (1948) Treatment of purulent pachymeningitis and subdural suppuration with particular reference to penicillin, *J. Neurol. Psychiat.*, **11**, 143.

SPERL, M. P., MacCARTY, C. S., and WELLMAN, W. E. (1959) Observations on current therapy of abscess of the brain, *Arch. Neurol. Psychiat. (Chic.)*, **81**, 439.

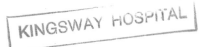

8

NERVOUS COMPLICATIONS
OF MISCELLANEOUS INFECTIONS

ACUTE TOXIC ENCEPHALOPATHY

Synonyms. Acute toxic encephalitis; acute serous encephalitis.

Definition. An acute cerebral disturbance occurring chiefly in children, not uncommonly in small epidemics and characterized pathologically by toxic changes in the nervous system, and clinically by delirium or coma and convulsions, variable pareses of the limbs, and symptoms of meningeal irritation.

PATHOLOGY

The changes in the nervous system distinguish this disorder both from viral encephalitis and from post-infective encephalomyelitis. Pathologically there is an acute degeneration of the ganglion cells of the brain with hyperaemia and conspicuous perivascular and pericellular oedema, and focal collections of glial cells and round cells. Ring haemorrhages have been described, and 'acute brain purpura', in which multiple punctate haemorrhages with a perivascular distribution are conspicuous in the nervous system, is probably an intense variety of this disorder.

AETIOLOGY

The pathological changes are thought to be due to a toxaemia which varies in the severity of its effects upon nerve cells and the blood vessels, so producing varying degrees of neural degeneration, oedema, and haemorrhage. In some cases the source of the toxaemia is an acute systemic infection and it can occur in children with burns (Warlow and Hinton, 1969). In others it is unknown and this applies to the small epidemics which sometimes attack young children during the summer months. It is not very common in infancy, most cases occurring between the ages of two and ten years.

SYMPTOMS

The onset of the illness is usually acute and may be fulminating. It is sometimes preceded by sore throat or gastro-intestinal disturbance. Severe headache, vomiting, and convulsions are common and the latter may be predominantly unilateral. The child when conscious is usually delirious, but may later pass into coma. There is usually high fever. Meningeal symptoms are often conspicuous. Involvement of the cerebral hemispheres may lead to aphasia, monoplegia, hemiplegia, or double hemiplegia. Optic neuritis may occur; pupillary abnormalities are inconstant. Trismus may occur and facial paresis is frequently present. The tendon reflexes are sometimes diminished or lost, but may be exaggerated, and the plantar reflexes extensor on one or both sides. Retention and incontinence of urine are common when consciousness is clouded. The symptoms may be predominantly meningeal, cerebral, or spinal. The cerebro-spinal fluid is usually normal in composition though under increased pressure. Exceptionally there is a pleocytosis or a rise of protein content. Rarely in those cases characterized pathologically by acute haemorrhagic lesions in the brain, haematuria or albuminuria may occur and a purpuric rash has been described.

DIAGNOSIS

The fact that the cerebrospinal fluid is usually normal in composition, and the early involvement of the substance of the nervous system, distinguishes acute toxic encephalopathy from the various forms of meningitis, encephalitis, and poliomyelitis. Lead encephalopathy must also be excluded.

PROGNOSIS

The prognosis varies in different groups of reported cases. In some small epidemics almost all the affected individuals have died. In others almost all have recovered. The condition accounted for 6 per cent of all infants and children coming to autopsy at the Massachusetts General Hospital in one decade (Lyon et al., 1961). In fatal cases death usually occurs within two or three days of the onset, coma having supervened within a few hours. In those who survive, the dangers are persistent mental defect, aphasia, hemiplegia, or epilepsy. Sometimes the patient recovers consciousness, and hemiparesis clears up in a few days. In other cases improvement is slower but recovery is often surprisingly complete.

TREATMENT

Treatment is symptomatic. Repeated lumbar puncture has been advocated and anticonvulsant drugs may be required to control the convulsions. Cerebral oedema may be treated by dexamethasone, 2–5 mg three times daily in the acute stage, depending upon the age of the patient.

REYE'S SYNDROME

This condition, also called acute toxic encephalopathy with fatty degenera-tion of the viscera, is a disorder of childhood in which a toxic encephalopathy as described above is associated with hypoglycaemia and with fatty degeneration of the liver giving symptoms and signs of hepatic dysfunction; similar degenera-tive changes have been described in the kidney (Reye et al., 1963). The mortality is as high as 85 per cent; hyperkalaemia, hyperpnoea, and haematemesis are unfavourable signs, but if the patient survives two or three days, recovery may be complete. While the condition has been described in association with various viral infections (Jenkins et al., 1967) and has been attributed to chemical toxins (Glasgow and Ferris, 1968), the aetiology is unknown. An association with type I vaccine-like poliovirus has been described (Brunberg and Bell, 1974) and the EEG has been found to be of some value in assessing prognosis (Aoki and Lombroso, 1973). Treatment must be directed to controlling cerebral oedema and manifestations of hepatic dysfunction, including a rising blood ammonia (Menkes, 1974).

REFERENCES

AOKI, Y., and LOMBROSO, C. T. (1973) Prognostic value of electroencephalography in Reye's syndrome, Neurology (Minneap.), 23, 333.

BRAIN, W. R., and HUNTER, D. (1929) Acute meningo-encephalomyelitis of childhood, Lancet, i, 221.

BRITISH MEDICAL JOURNAL (1973) Clinical diagnosis of Reye's syndrome, *Brit. med. J.*, **iii**, 308.

BROWN, C. L., and SYMMERS, D. (1925) Acute serous encephalitis; a newly recognized disease of children, *Amer. J. Dis. Child.*, **29**, 174.

BRUNBERG, J. A., and BELL, W. E. (1974) Reye syndrome. An association with type I vaccine-like poliovirus, *Arch. Neurol. (Chic.)*, **30**, 304.

GLASGOW, J. F. T., and FERRIS, J. A. J. (1968) Encephalopathy and visceral fatty infiltration of probable toxic aetiology, *Lancet*, **i**, 451.

GRINKER, R. R., and STONE, T. T. (1928) Acute toxic encephalitis in childhood, *Arch. Neurol. Psychiat. (Chic.)*, **20**, 244.

JENKINS, R., DVORAK, A., and PATRICK, J. (1967) Encephalopathy and fatty degeneration of the viscera associated with chickenpox, *Pediatrics*, **39**, 769.

LOW, A. A. (1930) Acute toxic (non-suppurative) encephalitis in children, *Arch. Neurol. Psychiat. (Chic.)*, **23**, 696.

LYON, G., DODGE, P. R., and ADAMS, R. D. (1961) The acute encephalopathies of obscure origin in infants and children, *Brain*, **84**, 680.

MENKES, J. H. (1974) *Textbook of Child Neurology*, Philadelphia.

REYE, R. D., MORGAN, G., and BARAL, J. (1963) Encephalopathy and fatty degeneration of the viscera. A disease entity in childhood, *Lancet*, **ii**, 749.

WARLOW, C. P., and HINTON, P. (1969) Early neurological disturbances following relatively minor burns in children, *Lancet*, **ii**, 978.

SCARLET FEVER

Nervous complications of scarlet fever are rare. Although focal vascular lesions have been reported, the pathological changes in most cases have been those of acute haemorrhagic encephalitis. Ferraro (1944) suggested that post-scarlatinal encephalitis, like glomerulonephritis, may have an allergic basis. Meningism is not uncommon, symptoms of meningeal irritation coexisting with a normal cerebrospinal fluid. True meningitis occurs less frequently and is usually secondary to otitis or other complications; in a few cases the *Streptococcus scarlatinae* has been isolated from the fluid. Hydrocephalus has been reported in a few instances as a sequel of meningitis. Cerebral abscess may occur without otitis. Hemiplegia, however, is the commonest complication resulting from vascular occlusion; Rolleston collected 66 cases from the literature. Hypertensive encephalopathy due to renal damage may be responsible for cerebral symptoms. A few cases of localized and multiple neuritis have been reported. Optic neuritis is rare but chorea is a not uncommon sequel. Hemiplegia of vascular origin is usually permanent, but symptoms due to hypertensive encephalopathy disappear if the patient recovers.

REFERENCES

FERRARO, A. (1944) Allergic brain changes in post-scarlatinal encephalitis, *J. Neuropath. exp. Neurol.*, **3**, 239.

FORBERS, J. G. (1926) Post-scarlatinal meningitis, *Lancet*, **ii**, 1207.

MILLER, H. G., STANTON, J. B., and GIBBONS, J. L. (1956) Para-infectious encephalomyelitis and related syndromes, *Quart. J. Med.*, **25**, 427.

NEAL, J. B., and JONES, A. (1927) Streptococcic meningitis following scarlet fever recovery, *Arch. Pediat.*, **44**, 395.

NEURATH, R. (1912) Die Rolle des Scharlachs in der Ätiologie der Nervenkrankheiten, *Ergebn. inn. Med. Kinderheilk.*, **9**, 103.

ROLLESTON, J. D. (1927-8) Hemiplegia following scarlet fever, *Proc. roy. Soc. Med.*, **21**, 213.

SOUTHARD, E. E., and SIMS, F. R. (1904) A case of cortical hemorrhages following scarlet fever, *J. Amer. med. Ass.*, **43**, 789.
TOOMEY, J. A., DEMBO, L. H., and MCCONNELL, G. (1923) Acute hemorrhagic encephalitis: report of a case following scarlet fever, *Amer. J. Dis. Child.*, **25**, 98.

WHOOPING COUGH

The pathogenesis of nervous symptoms in whooping cough is varied. Some are due to focal vascular lesions, especially haemorrhages. Jarke (1896) described multiple patches of softening of the cerebral hemispheres and Askin and Zimmerman (1929) reported a case of encephalitis with focal collections of inflammatory cells. Convulsions are not uncommon in whooping cough, especially in young children. Though they may sometimes be due to encephalitis, in other cases the changes are those of an encephalopathy, possibly resulting from the mechanical effects of venous congestion due to repeated coughing. Focal symptoms, which include aphasia, unilateral or bilateral hemiplegia, blindness, and deafness, are probably the result of focal haemorrhage or softening. Patients who have severe and frequent convulsions usually die. Of the group with focal lesions approximately one-fifth die, two-fifths are incapacitated by residual symptoms, and two-fifths recover.

An encephalopathy has been described as a sequel to pertussis inoculation, usually occurring within one to three days after the injection (Byers and Moll, 1948; Berg, 1958; Ström, 1960). Convulsions leading to coma are common; most patients survive but many are left with permanent mental retardation, variable neurological signs of diffuse brain damage, and recurrent seizures.

REFERENCES

ASKIN, J. A., and ZIMMERMAN, H. M. (1929) Encephalitis accompanying whooping-cough: clinical history and report of postmortem examination, *Amer. J. Dis. Child.*, **38**, 97.
BERG, J. M. (1958) Neurological complications of pertussis immunization, *Brit. med. J.*, **2**, 24.
BYERS, R. K., and MOLL, F. C. (1948) Encephalopathies following prophylactic pertussis vaccine, *Pediatrics*, **1**, 437.
DUBOIS, R., LEY, R. A., and DAGNELIE, J. (1932) Protocoles anatomo-cliniques de huit cas de complications nerveuses de la coqueluche, *J. Neurol. (Brux.)*, **32**, 645.
ELLISON, J. B. (1934) Whooping-cough eclampsia, *Lancet*, **i**, 227.
FONTEYNE, P., and DAGNELIE, J. (1932) Action de l'endotoxine coquelucheuse sur les centres nerveux (Recherches expérimentales), *J. Neurol. (Brux.)*, **32**, 660.
JARKE, O. (1896) Ein Fall von acuter symmetrischer Gehirnerweichung bei Keuchhusten, *Arch. Kinderheilk.*, **20**, 212.
MIKULOWSKI, V. (1929) Pertussis-encephalitis im Kindesalter, *Jb. Kinderheilk.*, **124**, 103.
MILLER, H. G., STANTON, J. B., and GIBBONS, J. L. (1956) Para-infectious encephalo-myelitis and related syndromes, *Quart. J. Med.*, **25**, 427.
STRÖM, J. (1960) Is universal vaccination against pertussis always justified?, *Brit. med. J.*, **2**, 1184.

TYPHOID FEVER

Mental symptoms are common, those most frequently encountered being acute toxic confusional states during the febrile period and post-typhoid psychosis or amnesia; psychotic reactions of schizophrenic type may be particularly common in the African (Osuntokun *et al.*, 1972). Meningeal symptoms may be due to meningism, the cerebrospinal fluid being normal. Much more rarely true typhoid meningitis occurs [p. 408]. Suppurative meningitis may also result from infection with other pyogenic organisms, with or without the *Salmonella typhosa*. The substance of the nervous system is less often involved than the meninges, but focal symptoms, especially hemiplegia, with or without aphasia, convulsions, myoclonus, or Parkinsonian features, may occur (Osuntokun *et al.*, 1972). Optic neuritis is rare. Cerebral abscess may occur either by extension from otitis media or by metastasis from a focus of pyogenic infection elsewhere. Such abscesses are usually due to a secondary invader, but may be caused by the *S. typhosa*. Occasionally spinal symptoms predominate, yielding a picture of transverse myelitis or of ascending paralysis of the Landry type. Neuritis is a rare sequel, polyneuritis involving the feet and causing tenderness of the toes being the commonest form. Similar complications may occur in paratyphoid fever, but much less frequently than in typhoid.

Meningitis occurring in typhoid fever is usually fatal, and cerebral abscess is a serious complication which usually terminates fatally, but the use of chloramphenicol has probably improved the prognosis. Focal lesions do not threaten life to the same extent, but frequently cause permanent disability, e.g. hemiplegia.

REFERENCES

LAROCHE, G., and PEJU, G. (1920) Méningite typhique bénigne au cours d'une septicémie typhique à rechute, *Bull. Soc. méd. Hôp. Paris*, **44**, 150.
MELCHIOR, E. (1911) Über Hirnabscesse und sonstige umschriebene intrakranielle Eiterungen im Verlauf und Gefolge des Typhus abdominalis, *Zbl. GrGeb. Med. Chir.*, **14**, 49.
OSUNTOKUN, B. O., BADEMOSI, O., OGUNREMI, K., and WRIGHT, S. G. (1972) Neuropsychiatric manifestations of typhoid fever in 959 patients, *Arch. Neurol. (Chic.)*, **27**, 7.
ROLLESTON, J. D. (1929) *Acute Infectious Diseases*, 2nd ed., London.
SMITHIES, F. (1907) Hemiplegia as a complication in typhoid fever, with report of a case, *J. Amer. med. Ass.*, **49**, 389.

TYPHUS FEVER

The classical or European epidemic form of typhus fever is transmitted to man through the body-louse; the murine type is endemic all over the world and is passed on by rat fleas; Brill's disease is the name given to a form of recurrent typhus often seen in the past in European immigrants to the U.S.A., but now very rare (Woodward, 1959).

Nervous symptoms may occur in typhus fever, and there is abundant evidence that they are usually due to infection of the nervous system by the causative organism. Histologically microscopic nodules in the walls of the very small blood vessels—typhus nodules—have frequently been observed in the nervous system, where they consist of perivascular collections of glial, endothelial, and other mononuclear cells (Aschoff, Wolbach, Spielmeyer, and others). Thrombosis frequently occurs in the affected vessel. *Rickettsia prowazeki*, the causal organism of typhus, has been seen in the endothelium of the cerebral vessels and sometimes in the typhus nodules.

Headache, delirium, and insomnia, which are common during the febrile stage of the illness, are probably toxic in origin and do not necessarily indicate invasion of the nervous system. Focal nervous symptoms indicative of the latter usually occur during the last few days of the febrile period or within a few days afterwards. Meningeal symptoms may occur, and any part of the nervous system may be involved (Herman, 1949). Cerebral symptoms may indicate multiple lesions, a disseminated encephalitis, but hemiplegia is the commonest symptom. An acute cerebellar ataxia occurs in a small proportion of cases, and multiple bulbar foci may occur, leading to dysphagia and dysarthria. Lesions are sometimes confined to the spinal cord, yielding the clinical picture of a myelitis. The cranial and peripheral nerves frequently suffer. Optic neuritis may occur. Facial paralysis is particularly common, and deafness may develop. In the peripheral nerves the symptoms may be those of a focal mononeuritis, associated with pain and tenderness, or of a polyneuritis.

Changes are frequently present in the cerebrospinal fluid, which is sometimes xanthochromic and may exhibit a lymphocytosis. The albumin content of the fluid is usually little raised, but an excess of globulin is present in 50 per cent of cases and may persist for from two to eight months after the acute stage.

The occurrence of severe nervous symptoms naturally adds to the gravity of the prognosis. In patients who survive, cerebral symptoms usually recover but Grodzki (1929) described chronic encephalitis following typhus.

OTHER RICKETTSIAL INFECTIONS

Q fever and trench fever are both due to rickettsiae but do not as a rule give neurological manifestations. However, in tick-borne Rocky mountain spotted fever (or Colorado fever) which is due to the *Rickettsia ricketsii* and which is similar to many other rickettsial illnesses seen in other parts of the world (e.g. Kenya fever, Brazilian spotted fever), neurological complications similar to those of typhus are quite common (Horsfall and Tamm, 1965; Miller and Price, 1972). The same is true of scrub typhus (Tsutsugamushi disease) (Ripley, 1946) in which the ulcerated lesion on the skin where bitten by the mite may give a useful clue to the diagnosis.

REFERENCES

ARKWRIGHT, J. A., and FELIX, A. (1930) Typhus fever, in *A System of Bacteriology*, vol. vii, ch. xxxiv, p. 393, London.

FELDMANN, P. M. (1926) Über Erkrankungen des zentralen Nervensystems beim Fleck-fieber, *Arch. Psychiat. Nervenkr.*, **77**, 357.

GRODZKI, A. B. (1929) Über einige Formen der Flecktyphusenzephalitis, *Münch. med. Wschr.*, **76**, 709.

HERMAN, E. (1949) Neurological syndromes in typhus fever, *J. Nerv. Ment. Dis.*, **109**, 25.

HORSFALL, F. J., and TAMM, I. (1965) *Viral and Rickettsial Infections of Man*, 4th ed., Philadelphia.

MILLER, J. Q., and PRICE, T. R. (1972) The nervous system in Rocky mountain spotted fever, *Neurology (Minneap.)*, **22**, 561.

RIPLEY, H. S. (1946) Neuropsychiatric observations on Tsutsu-gamushi fever (scrub typhus), *Arch. Neurol. Psychiat. (Chic.)*, **56**, 42.

STRONG, R. P., SHATTUCK, G. C., et al. (1920) *Typhus Fever, with Particular Reference to the Serbian Epidemic*, Cambridge, Mass.

WOODWARD, T. E. (1959) Rickettsial diseases in the United States, *Med. Clin. N. Amer.*, **43**, 1507.

MALARIA

Acute nervous symptoms in malaria, cerebral malaria, occur chiefly in infections with the malignant tertian parasite, blackwater fever, and are due to sporulation of the parasite in the cerebral capillaries. Sections of nerve tissue exhibit macroscopically a smoky grey appearance with oedema, hyperaemia, and punctate haemorrhages. Histologically, the chief abnormality is more or less complete blocking of capillaries with parasitized red cells, leading to thrombosis, oedema, and petechial haemorrhages. The leptomeninges exhibit a perivascular infiltration with small, round cells. Malarial nodules (granulomas) have been observed. These consist of a central capillary filled with parasitized red cells and surrounded by a perivascular necrotic area, with glial proliferation (Thompson and Annecke, 1926).

Acute cerebral malaria is characterized by hyperpyrexia and rapidly developing coma, with or without precedent convulsions. Symptoms of meningeal irritation may occur, especially in children. In such cases the prognosis is always very grave. Focal manifestations include hemiplegia, aphasia, and cerebellar ataxia, which are usually transitory. Paraplegia has been described. Optic neuritis and retinal haemorrhages are often seen, and complete external ophthalmoplegia may occur. In the acute stage, the response to dexamethasone may be dramatic (Woodruff and Dickinson, 1968).

Chronic nervous symptoms in malaria are probably toxic in origin and are usually due to neuropathy. Trigeminal neuralgia, facial palsy, mononeuritis, and polyneuritis may all occur.

REFERENCES

AUSTREGESILO, A. (1927) Des troubles nerveux dans quelques maladies tropicales, *Rev. neurol.*, **34**, 1.

MANSON-BAHR, P. H. (1972) *Manson's Tropical Diseases*, 19th ed., London.

PERWUSCHIN, G. W. (1924) Malaria und Erkrankungen des Nervensystems, *Z. ges. Neurol. Psychiat.*, **93**, 446.

THOMPSON, J. G., and ANNECKE, S. (1926) Pathology of the central nervous system in malignant tertian malaria, *J. trop. Med. Hyg.*, **29**, 343.

WOODRUFF, A. W., and DICKINSON, C. J. (1968) Use of dexamethasone in cerebral malaria, *Brit. med. J.*, **3**, 31.

TRYPANOSOMIASIS

African trypanosomiasis is transmitted to man by the bite of the tsetse fly. After an incubation period of about two weeks a local erythematous nodule may form at the site of the bite and this may be followed by insomnia, impaired concentration, formication, and deep muscular aching. The parasites may not enter the central nervous system for several years; the onset may then be explosive with convulsions, coma, and death within a few days but more often there is a chronic fluctuating illness characterized by progressive drowsiness, apathy, dysarthria, and involuntary movements ('sleeping sickness'). The condition is usually fatal within a few months. The cerebrospinal fluid shows a mononuclear pleocytosis and a rise in protein with a 'tabetic' type of colloidal gold curve. Tryparsamide by intravenous injection or pentamidine intramuscularly may be effective in treatment of such cases.

South American trypanosomiasis (Chagas's disease) is acquired as a result of a bite from an affected bug. Meningo-encephalitis may occur, particularly in childhood but diffuse myositis with swelling of the face (pseudomyxoedema) is more common in the adult although central nervous system involvement may result in convulsions and paralysis.

REFERENCES

Bogaert, L. van, and Vansen, P. (1957) Contribution à l'étude de la neurologie et neuro-pathologie de la trypanosomiase humane, *Ann. Soc. Belge med. Trop.*, **37**, 380.

Chagas, C. (1922) Descoberta do tripanozomia cruzi e verificação da Tripanozomiase americana, *Mem. Inst. Oswaldo Cruz*, **15**, 67.

Manson-Bahr, P. (1972) *Manson's Tropical Diseases*, 19th ed., London.

INFLUENZA

Nervous symptoms are frequently attributed to influenza, but the diagnosis is usually speculative and, except in cases occurring during epidemics, should always be received with caution. *H. influenzae* is one cause of pyogenic meningitis but clinical influenza is a virus infection. Acute haemorrhagic encephalitis has been ascribed to influenza, and Greenfield reported two cases of acute dis-seminated encephalomyelitis characterized by perivascular demyelination which followed a febrile illness diagnosed as 'influenza'. Small epidemics of encephalitis and polyneuritis have been observed to coincide with epidemics of influenza. Proof, however, is lacking that these forms of encephalitis are actually due to influenza, since a precedent febrile illness, when it occurs, may well be due to invasion by the organism which is responsible for the nervous symptoms. Alternatively, influenza may be one of many specific and non-specific infections which can, from time to time, be followed by a post-infective encephalitis or myelitis, or both, due to an allergic or hypersensitivity phenomenon. Thus, during certain influenza epidemics, especially the pandemic of 1957, cases of acute, sometimes fulminating, encephalomyelitis occurred (Kapila *et al.*, 1958; McConkey and Daws, 1958; Flewett and Hoult, 1958; Thiruvengadam, 1959). In the most acute cases the pathology was that of an acute haemorrhagic encephalomyelitis, and it seems likely that these were cases of acute disseminated encephalomyelitis [see p. 529] complicating influenza. Other neurological manifestations affecting predominantly the spinal cord and roots and giving a transverse myelopathy as the principal complication have been described by Wells (1971). Influenza A virus may certainly cause a fatal encephalitis in mice (Bell *et al.*, 1971); the fact that the virus has been isolated from the brain in human subjects is not incompatible with the hypersensitivity theory and it is still uncertain whether this is the cause of neurological complications or whether they are due to a direct effect of the virus itself.

REFERENCES

Bell, T. M., Narang, H. K., and Field, E. J. (1971) Influenzal encephalitis in mice. A histopathological and electron microscopical study, *Arch. ges. Virusfors.*, **34**, 157.

Dunbar, J. M., Jamieson, W. M., Langlands, H. M., and Smith, G. H. (1958) Encephalitis and influenza, *Brit. med. J.*, **1**, 913.

Flewett, T. H., and Hoult, J. G. (1958) Influenzal encephalopathy and post-influenzal encephalitis, *Lancet*, **i**, 11.

GREENFIELD, J. G. (1930) Acute disseminated encephalomyelitis as a sequel to 'influenza', *J. Path. Bact.*, **33**, 453.

KAPILA, C. C., KAUL, S., KAPUR, S. C., KALAYANAIN, T. S., and BANERJEE, D. (1958) Neurological and hepatic disorders associated with influenza, *Brit. med. J.*, **2**, 1311.

McCONKEY, B., and DAWS, R. A. (1958) Neurological disorders associated with Asian influenza, *Lancet*, **ii**, 15.

RIDDOCH, G. (1928-9) Discussion on disseminated encephalomyelitis, *Proc. roy. Soc. Med.*, **22**, 1260.

THIRUVENGADAM, K. V. (1959) Disseminated encephalomyelitis after influenza, *Brit. med. J.*, **2**, 1233.

WELLS, C. E. C. (1971) Neurological complications of so-called 'influenza': a winter study in south-east Wales, *Brit. med. J.*, **1**, 369.

INFECTIVE HEPATITIS

Serious nervous complications of infective hepatitis and serum hepatitis (types A and B) are uncommon, though mild cerebral, meningeal, and neuritic symptoms have been observed in epidemics. Brain saw one case with unilateral convulsions and hemiplegia, and another with myelitis and neuritis. Byrne and Taylor (1945) reported five cases, one with myelitis. The nervous symptoms usually develop four or five days before the jaundice appears. Jaundice, however, may coexist with nervous symptoms in other diseases—with meningitis in leptospirosis icterohaemorrhagica, and with encephalitis in St. Louis and equine encephalomyelitis, while the influenza virus may cause hepatitis (Kapila *et al.*, 1958). Neurological symptoms due to focal lesions of the nervous system in infective hepatitis must be distinguished from those of hepatic failure [see p. 829].

REFERENCES

BYRNE, E. A. J., and TAYLOR, G. F. (1945) An outbreak of jaundice with signs in the nervous system, *Brit. med. J.*, **1**, 477.

KAPILA, C. C., KAUL, S., KAPUR, S. C., KALAYANAM, T. S., and BANERJEE, D. (1958) Neurological and hepatic disorders associated with influenza, *Brit. med. J.*, **2**, 1311.

NEWMAN, J. L. (1942) Infective hepatitis: the history of an outbreak in the Lavant valley, *Brit. med. J.*, **1**, 61.

SHERLOCK, S. (1975) *Diseases of the Liver and Biliary System*, 5th ed., Oxford.

WALSHE, J. M. (1951) Observations on the symptomatology and pathogenesis of hepatic coma, *Quart. J. Med.*, **20**, 421.

INFECTIOUS MONONUCLEOSIS

Nervous complications of infectious mononucleosis are not uncommon. The clinical picture may be meningitic, encephalitic, myelitic, or polyneuritic. Anosmia, optic neuritis, ophthalmoplegia, facial palsy, and acute cerebellar ataxia (Lascelles *et al.*, 1973) have been described. Poliomyelitis may be simulated, or the Guillain–Barré type of polyneuritis. The cerebrospinal fluid may contain an excess of lymphocytes.

Dolgopol and Husson (1949) reviewed the literature and reported a fatal case, dying of respiratory paralysis. There was selective degeneration of the nerve cells of the third and fourth cranial nerves, of the Purkinje cells of the cerebellum, and of the ventral portion of the inferior reticular nucleus, together with recent haemorrhages in the grey matter of the spinal cord. In the polyneuritic type of cases mononuclear cell infiltration of the spinal roots and nerves has been described. Gautier-Smith (1965) drew attention to the occurrence of mononeuritis (of cranial or peripheral nerves) in certain cases and gave reasons for supposing that in some cases there is direct viral invasion of the central nervous system; however, in some patients with encephalomyelitis the aetiology of the nervous manifestations may be allergic. When the visceral symptoms and blood changes are typical no difficulty in diagnosis arises, but the nervous symptoms may come first, and the diagnosis may then depend upon the positive heterophile antibody test. Antibodies to the causal Epstein–Barr virus may be discovered in both the serum and CSF (Lascelles *et al.*, 1973).

REFERENCES

DOLGOPOL, V. B., and HUSSON, G. S. (1949) Infectious mononucleosis with neurologic complications, *Arch. intern. Med.*, **83**, 179.
GAUTIER-SMITH, P. C. (1965) Neurological complications of glandular fever (infectious mononucleosis), *Brain*, **88**, 323.
LASCELLES, R. G., LONGSON, M., JOHNSON, P. J., and CHIANG, A. (1973) Infectious mononucleosis presenting as acute cerebellar syndrome, *Lancet*, **ii**, 707.

SARCOIDOSIS

It is now recognized that lesions of Boeck's sarcoidosis may involve any level of the nervous system and the muscles (see Colover, 1948; Jefferson, 1957; and Matthews, 1965). The meninges or peripheral nerves may be infiltrated with endothelioid cells, giant cells, lymphocytes, plasma cells, and mononuclear leucocytes. Associated with the meningo-encephalitis there may be tumour-like masses in the dura mater. Adhesive arachnoiditis may cause hydrocephalus and the hypothalamus may be involved. The eyes may suffer in various ways. There may be papilloedema or retinal lesions, uveitis, and sometimes exophthalmos while paresis of the third or sixth nerves is not uncommon. Facial paralysis on one or both sides, with or without loss of taste, is common, and the glossopharyngeal and vagus nerves may also suffer. The limbs may be the site of polyneuritis or of a focal mononeuritis. An affected peripheral nerve may be palpably thickened. The characteristic lesions of sarcoidosis are likely to be found elsewhere in the body, e.g. the lymph nodes, liver, and spleen and phalanges. The combination of iridocyclitis with parotitis and polyneuritis was the first neurological manifestation of this disorder to be recognized. Crompton and MacDermot (1961) reported three cases of sarcoidosis of muscle without other clinical manifestations of the disease, and presenting with progressive muscular wasting and weakness (sarcoid myopathy). The condition tends to run an indolent course, sometimes with relapses and remissions (James and Sharma, 1967; Wells, 1967), but many cases ultimately prove fatal (Douglas and Maloney, 1973), although temporary or sustained remission is often produced by large doses of steroids with maintenance therapy of as much as 30–40 mg of prednisone daily, given for several years.

REFERENCES

COLOVER, J. (1948) Sarcoidosis with involvement of the nervous system, *Brain*, **71**, 451.
CROMPTON, M. R., and MacDERMOT, V. (1961) Sarcoidosis associated with progressive muscular wasting and weakness, *Brain*, **84**, 62.

DOUGLAS, A. C., and MALONEY, A. F. J. (1973) Sarcoidosis of the central nervous system, *J. Neurol. Neurosurg. Psychiat.*, **36**, 1024.

FEILING, A., and VINER, G. (1921-2) Iridocyclitis-parotitis-polyneuritis: a new clinical syndrome, *J. Neurol. Psychiat.*, **2**, 353.

GARCIN, R. (1960) Les atteintes neurologiques et musculaires dans la maladie de Besnier-Boeck–Schaumann, *Psychiat. Neurol. Neurochir.* (*Amst.*), **63**, 285.

JAMES, D. G., and SHARMA, O. P. (1967) Neurosarcoidosis, *Proc. roy. Soc. Med.*, **60**, 1169.

JEFFERSON, M. (1957) Sarcoidosis of the nervous system, *Brain*, **80**, 540.

MATTHEWS, W. B. (1965) Sarcoidosis of the nervous system, *J. Neurol. Psychiat.*, **28**, 23.

WELLS, C. E. C. (1967) The natural history of neurosarcoidosis, *Proc. roy. Soc. Med.*, **60**, 1172.

TOXOPLASMOSIS

Toxoplasmosis is the result of infection with toxoplasma, an organism found in animals, birds, and reptiles and conveyed to man from domestic animals, rats, or mice. The toxoplasma is a crescentic organism 2 to 4 μm wide and 4 to 7 μm long, which is found intracellularly and extracellularly in the central nervous system, retina, heart muscle, kidneys, and endocrine glands. Pathologically it leads to disseminated encephalomyelitis with areas of yellow necrotic softening of the cerebral cortex and a contiguous leptomeningitis (Sabin, 1941; Cowen *et al.*, 1942; Remington *et al.*, 1960). Miliary granulomata are found. The spinal cord may also show softening and necrosis (Wyllie and Fisher, 1950).

Campbell and Clifton (1950) recognized the following clinical types—congenital infantile, acquired infantile, acquired adult, and latent. In the congenital infantile type the cerebral symptoms are present at or soon after birth. The head is large and the eyes are often abnormally small. The fundi show characteristic choroidoretinitis and there may be hemiplegia or diplegia. In the acquired forms the patient is likely to complain of headache and vomiting and joint pains, and may exhibit a rash and fever. Choroidoretinitis is less common than in the congenital form, but papilloedema or optic atrophy may be present together with nerve deafness and the symptoms of a meningo-encephalitis. The spleen may be enlarged and the blood may show an eosinophilia. Toxoplasmic polymyositis has been described (Rowland and Greer, 1961). The cells and protein in the cerebrospinal fluid are likely to be increased and it may be possible to isolate the organism from the fluid. A skin test and various serological tests may be helpful as are the characteristic X-ray changes which have been described by Sutton (1951). Calcification is observed in the brain in the form of multiple subcortical flakes and linear or granular areas in the basal ganglia.

REFERENCES

BLACKWOOD, W., MCMENEMEY, W. H., MEYER, A., and NORMAN, R. M. (1963) *Greenfield's Neuropathology*, 2nd ed., London.

CAMPBELL, A. M. G., and CLIFTON, F. (1950) Adult toxoplasmosis in one family, *Brain*, **73**, 281.

COWEN, D., WOLF, A., and PAIGE, B. H. (1942) Toxoplasmic encephalomyelitis, *Arch. Neurol. Psychiat.* (*Chic.*), **48**, 689.

REMINGTON, J. S., JACOBS, L., and KAUFMAN, H. E. (1960) Toxoplasmosis in the adult, *New Engl. J. Med.*, **262**, 180.

ROWLAND, L. P., and GREER, M. (1961) Toxoplasmic polymyositis, *Neurology* (*Minneap.*), **11**, 367.

SABIN, A. B. (1941) Toxoplasmic encephalitis in children, *J. Amer. med. Ass.*, **116**, 801.
SUTTON, D. (1951) Intracranial calcification in toxoplasmosis, *Brit. J. Radiol.*, **24**, 31.
WYLLIE, W. G., and FISHER, H. J. W. (1950) Congenital toxoplasmosis, *Quart. J. Med.*, N.S. **19**, 57.

BENIGN MYALGIC ENCEPHALOMYELITIS
(EPIDEMIC NEUROMYASTHENIA)

Benign myalgic encephalomyelitis is the term applied to a puzzling disorder which has occurred often in small epidemics, especially in institutions, and has been recognized during recent years in many parts of the world. An epidemic in the Royal Free Hospital, London, some years ago led to its being sometimes called the Royal Free Disease. Its puzzling features are the severity of the symptoms in relation to the slightness of the physical signs, its selective incidence upon females, and the absence of any evidence as to its cause. Its mode of spread in institutions is unknown. Sporadic cases undoubtedly occur.

The onset is usually that of a febrile illness, sometimes accompanied by sore throat, upper respiratory or gastro-intestinal symptoms, and often a generalized lymphadenopathy. Jaundice is occasionally seen. In many cases there is no evidence of involvement of the nervous system and the patient recovers completely in a few days. When the nervous system is involved—in 10 out of 48 cases in an outbreak in Newcastle (Pool *et al.*, 1961)—psychological disturbances are prominent, particularly depression, disturbances of sleep, and reactions commonly described as hysterical. The limbs are prominently affected with flaccid weakness, muscle pain and tenderness, and paraesthesiae, hyperaesthesia, or relative analgesia of irregular distribution. The tendon jerks may be normal, but are sometimes slightly exaggerated or slightly depressed. The plantar reflexes are usually flexor, but occasionally extensor. Cranial nerve palsies are sometimes observed, but are rare. A characteristic feature of the muscular weakness is the intermittency of muscular contraction, confirmed by electromyography (see below). Objective sensory changes are uncommon.

The cerebrospinal fluid is usually normal, the only abnormalities found on laboratory investigation being the occurrence of an abnormal appearance in the large lymphocytes of the blood. Changes which are believed to be characteristic have been found on electromyography, in particular a characteristic grouping of motor-unit activity with brief silent intervals between groups of two or three motor-unit potentials.

The disease is never fatal and therefore its pathology is unknown. Major persistent disability is rare. A striking feature is the tendency for relapses to occur during the months, and in some cases even years, after the infection. The condition may easily be regarded as hysterical, and indeed some believe that its regular occurrence in closed communities (such as colleges and nurse-training schools) indicate that it is due to a 'mass' hysterical reaction in a community afflicted by an epidemic due to a benign non-neurotropic virus. As Pool *et al.* say, 'the condition should be borne in mind in any patient suffering from a relapsing illness characterised by muscular weakness and by emotional lability'.

REFERENCES

ACHESON, E. D. (1959) The clinical syndrome variously called benign myalgic encephalomyelitis, Iceland disease and epidemic neuromyasthenia, *Amer. J. Med.*, **26**, 569–95.
FIELDS, W. S., and BLATTNER, R. J. (1958) *Viral Encephalitis*, Springfield, Ill.

POOL, J. H., WALTON, J. N., BREWIS, E. G., ULDALL, P. R., WRIGHT, A. E., and GARDNER,
    P. S. (1961) Benign myalgic encephalomyelitis in Newcastle upon Tyne, *Lancet*,
    i, 733.
PRICE, J. L. (1961) Myalgic encephalomyelitis, *Lancet*, **i,** 737.
An Outbreak of Encephalomyelitis in the Royal Free Hospital Group, London, in 1955.
    By the Medical Staff of the Royal Free Hospital, *Brit. med. J.* (1957), **2,** 895.

BEHÇET'S DISEASE

Behçet's disease is an obscure disorder characterized by ulceration of the mouth and genitalia and involvement of the eyes, particularly with iritis, and running a remittent course characteristically with attacks three or four times a year.

The nervous system may also be involved, the characteristic lesions being disseminated encephalomyelitic lesions with low-grade perivascular inflammatory exudates in the meninges and cortex, but more particularly in the white matter, foci of softening in relation to the blood vessels, and extensive and patchy areas of cortical infarction. The lesions may be widespread, but seem to show a predilection for the upper brain stem. Evans *et al.* (1957) record the isolation of a virus, but even if a virus is the primary cause this does not exclude the possibility that the lesions in the nervous system are allergic in nature, as McMenemey and Laurence (1957) and Kawakita *et al.* (1967) point out. The relationship of Behçet's syndrome to Reiter's disease is unknown, but in Reiter's disease, too, ocular lesions may be associated with a meningo-encephalitis or with radiculitic or neuritic symptoms (Oates and Hancock, 1959).

When the nervous system is involved in Behçet's disease headache is often a common symptom. Progressive mental deterioration, Parkinsonian features, ophthalmoplegia leading to diplopia, and spastic weakness of the limbs have all been observed. During an active phase the cerebrospinal fluid frequently contains an excess of cells, usually lymphocytes. They rarely number more than a hundred per mm^3, but occasionally much larger numbers have been observed with a high proportion of polymorphonuclears. Aphthous ulceration of the mouth and ulceration of the vagina or scrotum are characteristic. The iritis may lead to hypopyon, and other ocular lesions include conjunctivitis, keratitis, retinitis, retrobulbar neuritis, retinal haemorrhage, and thrombophlebitis. Permanent blindness may occur. Thrombophlebitis of small or large veins elsewhere is said to occur in 25 per cent of cases. Remissions may occur, but the mortality rate varies from about 21 per cent in Japan to almost 50 per cent in Western countries (Kawakita *et al.*, 1967).

Diagnostic difficulty is likely to arise only if the mouth and skin lesions are small or overlooked. Then the neurological manifestations may be confused with tuberculous meningitis, but the fact that in Behçet's syndrome the sugar in the cerebrospinal fluid is normal is stressed by Wadia and Williams (1957). Alternatively the subacute development of spastic weakness of the limbs may suggest multiple sclerosis, but the cell count in the cerebrospinal fluid is likely to be considerably larger than is commonly found in that disease.

No certainly effective treatment is known, but benefit has been claimed in some cases to result from ACTH or prednisone.

REFERENCES

Evans, A. D., Pallis, C. A., and Spillane, J. D. (1957) Involvement of the nervous system in Behçet's syndrome, *Lancet*, **ii**, 349.

Kawakita, H., Nishimura, M., Satoh, Y., and Shibata, N. (1967) Neurological aspects of Behçet's disease: a case report and clinico-pathological review of the literature in Japan, *J. neurol. Sci.*, **5**, 417.

McMenemey, W. H., and Laurence, B. J. (1957) Encephalomyelopathy in Behçet's disease, *Lancet*, **ii**, 353.

Oates, J. K., and Hancock, J. A. H. (1959) Neurological symptoms and lesions occurring in the course of Reiter's disease, *Amer. J. med. Sci.*, **238**, 79.

Pallis, C. A., and Fudge, B. J. (1956) The neurological complications of Behçet's syndrome, *Arch. Neurol. Psychiat. (Chic.)*, **75**, 1.

Viane, A. (1957) La méningo-myélo-encéphalite dans la maladie de Behçet, *Acta neurol. belg.*, **57**, 599.

Wadia, N., and Williams, E. (1957) Behçet's syndrome with neurological complications, *Brain*, **80**, 59.

[For neurological sequelae and complications of prophylactic inoculation and of childhood exanthemata, mumps, and some other common viral infections, see CHAPTERS 10 and 11.]

METAZOAL INFECTIONS

TAENIA SOLIUM (CYSTICERCOSIS)

Cysticercosis is the infestation of man with the encysted larval stage of the human tapeworm, *Taenia solium*, resulting from the ingestion of the ova. The embryos are carried to all parts of the body, and may invade the nervous system and the muscles. Most cases seen in Great Britain were the result of infection of British soldiers serving in India. Dixon and Lipscomb (1961) stated that the incidence of clinical cysticercosis was between 1·2 and 2·0 per thousand men serving in that country.

In man, the cysts grow for a time, but the larvae die, and the cysts then tend to become calcified. This happens more frequently in the muscles than in the brain. In the brain, the cysts usually measure about 1 cm in diameter, and are found in the subarachnoid space, in the cerebral cortex, and to a lesser extent in the white matter. A racemose form is encountered particularly in the fourth ventricle and basal cisterns, where there is a cluster of grape-like cystic bodies with thin, perhaps translucent, walls containing colourless fluid.

The incubation period between infection and the development of symptoms varies from less than one year to 30 years, the average interval being about 5 years. The commonest symptom is epilepsy, which occurred in 91·8 per cent of patients in Dixon and Lipscomb's series. The epilepsy may consist of generalized or focal attacks. All other neurological symptoms are relatively rare, mental disorder occurring in 8·7 per cent of Dixon and Lipscomb's series, intracranial hypertension in 6·4 per cent, and focal nervous lesions of the brain in 2·7 per cent, and in the spinal cord in 0·2 per cent. Intracranial hypertension may be the result of hydrocephalus produced by the racemose type of cysticercosis, while occasional patients demonstrate the characteristic triad of occipital headache, postural vertigo, and morning vomiting which can result from lesions in the fourth ventricle (Bickerstaff *et al.*, 1956; Kuper *et al.*, 1958).

Exceptionally, the clinical picture may be that of a subacute meningo-encephalitis or recurrent lymphocytic meningitis. In chronic cases, there may be a moderate excess of protein and a moderate lymphocytic pleocytosis in the fluid, and sometimes a paretic or meningitic colloidal gold curve.

Subcuticular nodules are found in approximately half of all cases, and exceptionally a nodule may be seen in the eye or in the tongue. The muscular lesions are usually asymptomatic but in over 90 per cent of cases, calcified cysts can be demonstrated by X-raying the muscles. Calcification of intracranial cysts occurs in only about one-third of all cases, and then very rarely less than 10 years after infection. Biopsy of a subcuticular nodule may be helpful in diagnosis.

According to Dixon and Lipscomb, the annual death rate ranges between 3·3 and 5·8 per thousand cases per annum, death being due usually to status epilepticus or intracranial hypertension. Epilepsy should be treated along the usual lines: this is often successful in diminishing and sometimes in abolishing the attacks. Intracranial hypertension calls for surgical investigation and treatment.

MULTICEPS MULTICEPS (COENURUS CEREBRALIS)

In some countries, especially South Africa, *Multiceps multiceps* is the common tapeworm of dogs, and human infection may lead to the presence of cysts in the ventricles or in the posterior fossa, the clinical picture being predominantly that of intracranial hypertension.

REFERENCES

BICKERSTAFF, E. R., SMALL, J. M., and WOOLF, A. L. (1956) Cysticercosis of the posterior fossa, *Brain*, **79**, 622.
DIXON, H. B. F., and LIPSCOMB, F. M. (1961) Cysticercosis: an analysis and follow-up of 450 cases, *Spec. Rep. Ser. med. Res. Coun. (Lond.)*, No. 299.
KUPER, S., MENDELOW, H., and PROCTOR, N. S. F. (1958) Internal hydrocephalus caused by parasitic cysts, *Brain*, **81**, 235.

TOXOCARA INFECTION

In children who have a history of frequent contact with dogs or cats or of eating dirt (pica) a syndrome of recurrent wheezy bronchitis or pneumonitis may be accompanied by fleeting urticarial rashes and convulsions. The condition is due to the ingestion of larvae of the dog roundworm *Toxocara canis* or *Toxocara cati* which may produce a widespread granulomatous reaction in liver, lungs, skeletal muscle and brain. Focal epilepsy in an adult has been reported (Brain and Allan, 1964), and uveitis or endophthalmitis may occur (Ashton, 1960). There is often a striking eosinophilia and a skin test may be diagnostic (Duguid, 1961). Diethylcarbamazine is probably an effective treatment.

REFERENCES

ASHTON, N. (1960) Larval granulomatosis of the retina due to *Toxocara*, *Brit. J. Ophthal.*, **44**, 129.
BRAIN, W. R., and ALLAN, B. (1964) Encephalitis due to infection with Toxocara cania, *Lancet*, **i**, 1355.
DUGUID, I. M. (1961) Chronic endophthalmitis due to *Toxocara*, *Brit. J. Ophthal.*, **45**, 705, 789.

TRICHINOSIS

This condition develops in man as a consequence of the ingestion of pork infected with *Trichinella spiralis*. Usually the condition gives rise to fever, periorbital oedema, and widespread muscle pain due to myositis, but the central nervous system is involved in between 10 and 24 per cent of cases (Kramer and Aita, 1972). In the brain larvae become impacted in cerebral capillaries giving petechial haemorrhages, perivascular cellular infiltration, and/or granulomatous nodules. The clinical manifestations include confusion, delirium, and focal neurological signs such as hemiparesis (Gould, 1945; Dalessio and Wolff, 1961); unilateral lateral rectus palsy has been described (Kramer and Aita, 1972). Treatment with steroids and thiabendazole 2 g daily is recommended.

REFERENCES

DALESSIO, D., and WOLFF, H. G. (1961) Trichinella spiralis infection of the central nervous system, *Arch. Neurol. (Chic.)*, **4**, 407.
GOULD, S. E. (1945) *Trichinosis*, Springfield, Ill.
KRAMER, M. D., and AITA, J. F. (1972) Trichinosis with central nervous system involvement, *Neurology (Minneap.)*, **22**, 485.

SCHISTOSOMIASIS (BILHARZIA)

This condition, which is common in the Middle East and Orient, is due to bathing in infested water. The ova of the trematodes may be deposited in the bladder wall, giving haematuria, and in the lungs. Involvement of the nervous system is comparatively uncommon, but *S. japonicum* shows a predilection for the cerebral hemispheres (Blankfein and Chirico, 1965), *S. haematobium* and *S. mansoni* for the spinal cord (Bird, 1964). Cerebral involvement may give oedema and papilloedema, headache, convulsions, and focal neurological signs; when the spinal cord is involved the signs are generally those of an incomplete transverse myelopathy. The CSF may show an increase in both cells and protein. Skin and complement fixation tests and/or rectal biopsy and eosinophilia are helpful in diagnosis. Antimony preparations such as fuadin, given intravenously, are effective in controlling the condition.

REFERENCES

BIRD, A. V. (1964) Acute spinal schistosomiasis, *Neurology (Minneap.)*, **14**, 647.
BLANKFEIN, R. J., and CHIRICO, A. M. (1965) Cerebral schistosomiasis, *Neurology (Minneap.)*, **15**, 957.

ECHINOCOCCOSIS (HYDATID CYSTS)

Rarely, and especially in sheep-rearing countries, man may become the intermediate host of the *Echinococcus granulosus*. Hydatid cysts are most common in the liver and lungs but rarely occur in the brain (Araná-Iniguez and San Julian, 1955) where they are usually single and present as space-occupying lesions; even more rarely they may be found in the spine, giving spinal cord compression (Malloch, 1965).

REFERENCES

ARANÁ-INIGUEZ, R., and SAN JULIAN, J. (1955) Hydatid cysts of the brain, *J. Neurosurg.*, **12**, 323.
MALLOCH, J. D. (1965) Hydatid disease of the spine, *Brit. med. J.*, **1**, 633.

GNATHOSTOMA INFECTION

Human infection by *Gnathostoma spinigerum* is usually characterized by painless migratory cutaneous swellings, but in Thailand cases of eosinophilic meningoencephalomyelitis due to this infection have been described causing either a subacute meningoencephalitis, often with cranial nerve palsies, or an acute painful myelitis with paraparesis (Punyagupta *et al.*, 1968 *a* and *b*).

REFERENCES

PUNYAGUPTA, S., JUTTIJUDATA, P., BUNNAG, T., and COMER, D. S. (1968 *a*) Two fatal cases of eosinophilic myeloencephalitis: a newly recognized disease caused by *Gnathostoma spinigerum*, *Trans. roy. Soc. trop. Med. Hyg.*, **62,** 801.
PUNYAGUPTA, S., LIMTRAKUL, C., VICHIPANTHU, P., KARNCHANACHETANEE, C., and NYE, S. W. (1968 *b*) Radiculomyeloencephalitis associated with eosinophilic pleo-cytosis, *Amer. J. trop. Med. Hyg.*, **17,** 551.

WHIPPLE'S DISEASE

The cause of this condition, which usually gives progressive weight loss, malabsorption, and polyarthritis, is unknown though the possibility that it could be due to viral infection has been considered. Neurological complications associated with subependymal granulomatous lesions containing the characteristic sickleform particle-containing (SPC) cells have been described in about 6 per cent of cases (Tengström and Werner, 1966). Trigeminal neuralgia, myoclonus, and ophthalmoplegia were the clinical features in a case shown at autopsy to have a nodular encephalitis (Stoupel *et al.*, 1969).

REFERENCES

STOUPEL, N., MONSEU, G., PARDOE, A., HEIMANN, R., and MARTIN, J. J. (1969) Encephalitis with myoclonus in Whipple's disease, *J. Neurol. Neurosurg. Psychiat.*, **32,** 338.
TENGSTRÖM, B., and WERNER, I. (1966) Whipple's disease. A report of two cases and a review of the literature, *Acta Soc. Med. upsalien.*, **71,** 237.

9

SYPHILIS OF THE NERVOUS SYSTEM

AETIOLOGY

SYPHILIS is growing less common and less dangerous as a result of modern treatment. The Registrar General's Annual Statistical Review shows that in England and Wales the mortality from general paresis declined by 94 per cent between 1916 and 1954 and that from tabes dorsalis by 86·2 per cent in the same period. Headache and palsies were attributed to syphilis in the Middle Ages, but there was little exact knowledge of neurosyphilis before the nineteenth century. Bayle described general paralysis in 1822, though the term was first used by Delaye in 1824, and the first adequate account of tabes was given by Romberg in 1846, and amplified by Duchenne and Charcot. Argyll Robertson described the pupillary abnormalities which bear his name in 1869. Fournier, also in 1869, described congenital syphilis. The discovery of the causal organism in the spirochaete *Treponema pallidum* by Schaudinn and Hoffmann in 1903 and the elaboration of the Bordet–Wassermann reaction (1901–7) were other important landmarks. The Wassermann reaction has recently been supplanted by more modern serological tests of which the V.D.R.L. and treponema immobilization tests are those most commonly used. Some laboratories also use the fluorescent treponemal antibody absorption test (FTA-ABS) which may ultimately become the standard technique because of its greater specificity and sensitivity. There are still, however, many unsolved problems in the aetiology and classification of neurosyphilis.

Although the earliest manifestation of acquired syphilitic infection is the primary chancre, spirochaetes may obtain access to the blood and be present in the spleen within ten days of infection and before the chancre appears. There is also evidence that in the secondary stage spirochaetes have reached the nervous system in a large proportion of persons infected, though they may not then give rise to symptoms. The secondary stage is usually followed by a period of latency, but even within a year, frequently within two or three years, symptoms of the tertiary stage may develop. Latent syphilis (an asymptomatic patient, not previously treated for syphilis, who shows no clinical abnormality but has a positive treponemal antibody test for syphilis or gives birth to a child with congenital syphilis) may, however, last for several years. Asymptomatic neurosyphilis is a term often applied to patients with latent syphilis who show no neurological abnormality but in whom the cerebrospinal fluid shows a pleocytosis or a positive V.D.R.L. test.

On clinical grounds a distinction has long been drawn between two groups of tertiary or late manifestations of neurosyphilis, one of which has been known as meningovascular or cerebrospinal syphilis, the other, which comprises tabes and general paresis, being distinguished as parenchymatous syphilis. In meningovascular or cerebrospinal syphilis symptoms may occur within a few years of infection, tend to be focal, and on the whole respond well to treatment. Tabes and general paresis, on the other hand, exhibit a longer latent interval, are characterized by diffuse or systematized pathological changes, and respond less satisfactorily to treatment. McIntosh and Fildes (1914) suggested that in cerebrospinal or meningovascular syphilis the essential lesion is limited to the blood vessels and the mesoblastic tissues and that the parenchyma of the nervous system suffers secondarily, while in tabes and general paresis there is invasion of the nervous tissue itself by spirochaetes in addition to a mesoblastic reaction. This hypothesis justifies the use of meningovascular syphilis as a convenient term for the more benign form of tertiary neurosyphilis, and parenchymatous neurosyphilis for tabes and general paresis.

Clinical neurosyphilis occurs in only a small proportion—about 10 per cent—of persons infected with the *Treponema pallidum*. In patients with untreated asymptomatic neurosyphilis, the cumulative probability of progression to clinical neurosyphilis is about 20 per cent in the first 10 years and increases with the passage of time, being greatest in those with substantial CSF pleocytosis and elevation of protein (Holmes, 1974). There is no convincing evidence to confirm the view once widely held that any single strain of *T. pallidum* is specifically neurotropic. There is, however, evidence that in populations more recently exposed to syphilitic infection, acute secondary and tertiary manifestations of the infection (meningoencephalitis, meningovascular manifestations, and gumma) are commoner, whereas in those communities long exposed to the disease, such as the North American Indian, neurosyphilis (which some prefer to call quaternary rather than tertiary syphilis) occurs more frequently. Before penicillin intensive methods of treatment of syphilis were blamed as a cause of the subsequent development of neurosyphilis, and it was suggested that such treatment might diminish the patient's natural powers of resistance to the organism or permit the development of resistant strains of spirochaetes in the nervous system. This theory, however, has not received general support, and in any case the early and intensive treatment of infected persons, by diminishing their infectivity, is certainly reducing the prevalence of neurosyphilis.

Out of every twelve patients with neurosyphilis approximately five have general paresis, four meningovascular syphilis, and three tabes.

SECONDARY NEUROSYPHILIS

PATHOLOGY

Spirochaetes may reach the nervous system during the primary stage and before the development of the cutaneous exanthem. Nicolau found a lymphocytosis in the cerebrospinal fluid in 9 per cent of cases at this stage and Cutler *et al.* (1954) positive serological reactions in 1·5 per cent. In the secondary stage abnormalities, which may be transitory, have been found in the fluid in from 36 to 80 per cent of cases in different series. Cutler *et al.* (1954) found serological abnormalities in 6 per cent. Such pathological changes as are present in the nervous system are those of a lymphocytic meningitis.

SYMPTOMS

There may be no symptoms referable to the nervous system in spite of the presence of slight changes in the cerebrospinal fluid, or the symptoms may be no more severe than the headache and pains in the back and limbs commonly associated with the secondary stage of syphilis. An acute meningitic illness occurs in 1–2 per cent of cases with headache, neck stiffness, and a marked CSF pleocytosis; meningoencephalitis is rare as an initial manifestation of secondary syphilis but may occur if the untreated condition, as it may, appears to remit spontaneously with a subsequent relapse. While fever, malaise, anorexia, skin eruptions including condylomata, lymphadenopathy, uveitis, hepatitis, and nephritis may all occur in this stage, when meningoencephalitis does occur, the headache, papilloedema, convulsions, and confusion or coma which can result may be similar in their effects to those of tertiary meningovascular syphilis.

The Cerebrospinal Fluid

In patients in the secondary stage who show no symptoms of involvement of the nervous system the changes in the fluid are usually slight and consist of a slight increase in the number of mononuclear cells or of protein or of both. The V.D.R.L. reaction is negative in the fluid but may be positive or negative in the blood, according to whether the patient has received treatment. Patients with nervous symptoms show more marked changes in the fluid, and these are usually proportional to their severity. When clinical evidence of meningitis is present, pressure of the fluid is usually raised and the cell content is increased and may be as high as 1,000 per mm³. The cells are usually mononuclear, but in some acute cases polymorphonuclear cells may also be present. CSF gamma globulin, especially the IgM and IgG fractions are increased and the V.D.R.L. reaction is usually positive in the fluid. It is also generally positive in the blood, but may be negative if the patient has been treated.

For **Diagnosis, Prognosis,** and **Treatment,** see pages 460–4.

TERTIARY MENINGOVASCULAR SYPHILIS

CEREBRAL SYPHILIS

PATHOLOGY

The essential pathological changes in tertiary syphilis involving the brain are first subacute meningitis, secondly vascular and perivascular inflammation involving large- and medium-sized arteries, and thirdly gumma formation. **Cranial pachymeningitis** involving the dura is sometimes secondary to syphilitic osteitis of the cranium; though often described in the past, it is now very rare. **Subacute leptomeningitis** is comparatively common in the basal meninges and over the convexity of the hemispheres; the changes are those of a granulomatous process, frequently involving cranial nerves and giving adhesive arachnoiditis, sometimes with communicating hydrocephalus, rarely arachnoid cyst formation.

The principal arterial lesion is an **obliterative endarteritis**; the intima is thickened so that the vessel may be occluded either by such thickening or consequent thrombosis, causing cerebral infarction or even infarction of cranial nerves due to involvement of vasa nervorum. The walls of the affected vessels are infiltrated with lymphocytes and plasma cells and there is perivascular fibroplastic proliferation.

A gumma is a syphilitic granuloma, often with central necrosis which may be around a small vessel, surrounded by mononuclear and epithelioid cells, occasional giant cells, and an outer layer of fibroblasts and connective tissue.

T. pallidum can only rarely be isolated from gummas and from the inflamed blood vessels and meninges described above. Gummas may be small and multiple or large and single, up to several centimetres in diameter. Though they are commonest in skin and bone and abdominal viscera, they may occur in the dura and the meninges though they, like all manifestations of tertiary syphilis, are becoming very rare in Western countries.

SYMPTOMS

Meningovascular syphilis may cause symptoms within a few months of infection or at any subsequent period in the patient's life. In most cases, however, symptoms develop between 5 and 10 years after infection. Symptoms are very varied on account of the multiplicity and different sites of the lesions. Frequently symptoms of both cerebral and spinal syphilis are present in the same patient.

Asymptomatic Neurosyphilis

As already mentioned, in some patients abnormalities are found in the cerebrospinal fluid though the nervous system appears normal. This is known as asymptomatic neurosyphilis.

Cranial Pachymeningitis

This rare condition may give no symptoms other than headache, but if the dura is adherent to the cortical meninges there are likely to be symptoms of cortical irritation, such as focal convulsions and paresis of the limbs.

Cerebral Leptomeningitis

The symptoms of syphilitic meningitis may be relatively diffuse or sharply focal, for example, limited to one cranial nerve. When the lesions are diffuse the onset of symptoms is usually insidious. Headache is frequently severe, with nocturnal exacerbations, and papilloedema may occur. Mental changes are common with impairment of memory and intellectual capacity. The patient becomes inefficient at his work and if, as is not uncommon, he exhibits anxiety and nervousness, the condition may be mistaken for neurosis. In more severe cases there is apathy and dementia, or the mental state may resemble that of Korsakow's psychosis. Aphasia may be present, and loss of sphincter control is common. The patient may finally pass into a state of semi-stupor. When the meninges over the convexity of the cerebral hemispheres are involved, convulsions may occur. These may be Jacksonian attacks without loss of consciousness, or generalized attacks in which consciousness is lost. Paresis and inco-ordination of the limbs on one or both sides are common. Basal meningitis frequently involves the chiasmal region and may thus lead to optic atrophy with defects in the visual fields. Hypothalamic involvement may cause obesity, diabetes insipidus, transient glycosuria, or narcolepsy. Hydrocephalus occasionally occurs. Reflex iridoplegia is almost constant and cranial nerve palsies are common, the nerves being involved in inflammation in the subarachnoid space. They may be affected singly or in association with adjacent nerves, and usually unilaterally. The third nerve is most often affected, and painless third-nerve palsy is a common isolated symptom. The paralysis of the intrinsic and extrinsic ocular muscles supplied by the nerve may be incomplete. Its onset is usually rapid. Next in frequency the sixth, seventh, and fifth cranial nerves are liable to be attacked. Thus facial paralysis clinically indistinguishable from

Bell's palsy is rarely syphilitic. When the fifth nerve suffers, sensory disturbances are more common than motor weakness. Neuralgic pain referred to the distribution of one or more of its branches may be associated with either hyperalgesia or analgesia, and sometimes with ophthalmic herpes zoster or neuropathic keratitis. Syphilitic lesions of the eighth nerve may cause vertigo and deafness. The nerves arising from the medulla may be involved, the twelfth suffering more frequently than the tenth and eleventh, but any of the three may be affected either alone or in combination with the others.

Cerebral Endarteritis

Any cerebral artery may be involved. Before occlusion is complete there are frequently premonitory motor or sensory symptoms due to ischaemia. Finally, thrombosis leads to symptoms of infarction which are described elsewhere [p. 327]. The middle cerebral artery or its branches and the posterior cerebral are most frequently the site of syphilitic thrombosis, but the anterior cerebral or vertebro-basilar system may be involved.

Hemiplegia is the commonest manifestation and may occur as a result of occlusion of the middle cerebral artery itself or of one of its basal branches supplying the internal capsule. It usually occurs within two or three years of infection. Its onset is rapid and associated with headache, but not often with loss of consciousness. Syphilitic hemiplegia is rarely bilateral. Once a common cause of hemiplegia in young adults, syphilis is now rarely responsible; atheromatous occlusion of the internal carotid is much commoner. Parkinsonian features rarely occur in syphilitic mesencephalitis.

Cerebral Gumma

Small gummatous lesions are often found in the meninges in syphilitic meningitis but a large gumma causes the symptoms of an intracranial tumour, situated usually subcortically in one cerebral hemisphere. The syphilitic origin of the tumour can only be inferred from the history of infection, signs of syphilis elsewhere, and a positive V.D.R.L. reaction in the blood or cerebrospinal fluid. Cerebral gumma is very rare, however, whereas both intracranial neoplasm and syphilitic infection are common, and may be present in the same individual. A positive V.D.R.L. reaction, therefore, must not be interpreted as indicating that a space-occupying lesion within the skull is necessarily, or even probably, a gumma.

The Cerebrospinal Fluid

In meningovascular syphilis the V.D.R.L. reaction is positive in the blood in 60 or 70 per cent of cases. The treponema immobilization and FTA-ABS tests are even more specific, a positive result invariably being indicative of syphilitic infection. The pressure of the cerebrospinal fluid may be either normal or increased. There is usually an excess of cells ranging between 20 and 100 per mm^3. The cells are mononuclear. The protein content of the fluid is usually increased and lies between 0·05 and 0·15 g per 100 ml. An increase in gamma-globulin (IgG and IgM) is almost invariable, and the V.D.R.L. reaction is positive in from 90 to 100 per cent of cases when 1 ml of fluid is used. In cases of syphilitic cerebral thrombosis, the V.D.R.L. reaction may be positive in the blood and negative in the fluid. Lange's colloidal gold test yields either a 'paretic' curve, e.g. 5542210000, or a 'luetic' curve—1355421000.

DIAGNOSIS

Cerebral syphilis is so protean in its manifestations that its diagnosis covers a large field of neurology. Fortunately, serological tests come to the aid of clinical observation. It is rare that the V.D.R.L. reaction is negative in the cerebrospinal fluid in active cerebral syphilis, and still more rare to find the reaction negative in both the cerebrospinal fluid and the blood. Any suspicion of syphilis should, therefore, lead to the examination of both.

The mental changes associated with cerebral syphilis require to be distinguished from other mental disorders and in their milder forms from neurosis. A clue to their true nature is usually afforded by the presence of abnormalities in the nervous system, especially in the pupils and their reactions.

When meningovascular syphilis is associated with papilloedema it may be confused with other conditions causing increased intracranial pressure, especially intracranial tumour. Focal symptoms of subacute onset in syphilis, however, are relatively uncommon (except in the rare gumma), and if such are present the possibility of a tumour should not be too readily dismissed, even if the V.D.R.L. reaction is positive, since it is not very rare for a tumour to develop in a patient with syphilis.

Cerebral thrombosis of syphilitic origin usually occurs at an earlier age than thrombosis due to atheroma, but otherwise it can be distinguished from the latter only when a history of infection or other signs of syphilis are present, or, in their absence, by serological tests.

Meningovascular syphilis, since it frequently causes multiple cerebral lesions, may be confused with encephalitis, other causes of granulomatous meningitis, and multiple sclerosis. In encephalitis, impairment of consciousness is often more profound and pupillary changes are uncommon; nevertheless diagnosis ultimately rests upon serological tests in blood and CSF. These too are important in distinguishing meningovascular syphilis from sarcoidosis, carcinomatosis of the meninges, and cryptococcosis, all of which may give the clinical picture of subacute meningitis with multiple cranial nerve palsies. In multiple sclerosis it is very rare for the pupillary reflexes to be affected, while nystagmus and inco-ordination of the limbs in the absence of sensory loss are rare in syphilis. In multiple sclerosis the tendon jerks are exaggerated, in neurosyphilis they are more often diminished or lost.

PROGNOSIS

The prognosis of cerebral syphilis is on the whole good, and excellent results are often obtained from energetic treatment. When severe mental symptoms have occurred, however, despite marked improvement, the patient may be left with some impairment of memory, intellectual capacity, and emotional stability. The results of vascular occlusion are permanent, and though some improvement is usual as in cerebral infarction however caused, variable permanent disability persists, while the hemianopia resulting from posterior cerebral thrombosis remains unaltered. Relapses are not uncommon, especially in patients who have abandoned treatment. They are unlikely to occur in those who are thoroughly treated and kept under regular observation.

TREATMENT

See page 463.

SPINAL SYPHILIS

PATHOLOGY

The lesions of meningovascular syphilis have already been described.

Spinal Pachymeningitis

Syphilitic inflammation of the spinal dura mater may follow spread of infection from syphilitic osteitis of the spine or may occur independently but is now very rare. The cervical region is usually involved—pachymeningitis cervicalis hypertrophica—the dura mater is thickened and adherent to the arachnoid and pia. The vessels and nerve roots entering and leaving the cord are involved in the inflammation, and the cord becomes ischaemic, and may contain a central cavity. Destruction of the long tracts is followed by ascending and descending degeneration.

Meningomyelitis

As in cerebral syphilis the meninges and blood vessels are both involved, though often unequally. When leptomeningitis predominates, degenerative changes in the cord itself may be superficial, as in syphilitic amyotrophy. When the vessels also suffer severely, lesions of the cord substance are more extensive. Though the lesions are chronic, thrombosis of an important vessel may precipitate acute changes leading to an acute or subacute transverse lesion of the cord ('Erb's syphilitic spastic paraplegia'). In such cases the leptomeninges are adherent to the cord, which is visibly softened. Microscopically the vessels show endarteritis and perivascular cellular infiltration, and the meninges are also infiltrated. Within the cord there is degeneration of both myelin sheaths and axis cylinders. The ganglion cells exhibit chromatolysis, and ascending and descending degeneration are to be found. Syphilitic myelitis usually involves the dorsal region and, though the leptomeninges may be extensively infiltrated, the area of softening is usually limited to two or three segments.

Spinal Endarteritis

As in the brain, endarteritis of one of the spinal arteries or of its branches may be followed by thrombosis leading to a circumscribed area of softening within the cord, corresponding to the area of supply of the obstructed vessel.

Radiculitis

The spinal roots may be involved in syphilitic inflammation spreading inwards from the meninges.

SYMPTOMS

Cervical Pachymeningitis

The earliest symptom is pain due to strangulation of the spinal nerves; it radiates round the neck, over the shoulders, and down the upper limbs. The pain is followed by progressive atrophy of the corresponding muscles. Finally, compression and ischaemia of the cord lead to progressive spastic paraplegia with sensory loss below the level of the lesion.

Meningomyelitis

Myelitis is frequently an early symptom of meningovascular syphilis and may occur within three to five years of infection. The dorsal region of the cord is usually affected but when the cervical region is involved, and the course of the illness is subacute, pain in the neck and upper limbs may be followed by amyotrophy and sensory loss in the upper extremities due to root involvement. When sensory loss is slight or absent, the clinical picture of lower motor neurone involvement in the upper limbs and upper motor neurone signs in the lower (syphilitic amyotrophy) may mimic that of motor neurone disease (amyotrophic lateral sclerosis). Motor symptoms resulting from a dorsal lesion are generally preceded by pain in the back and in girdle distribution. Weakness of the lower limbs develops between a few days and several weeks after the onset of the pains. In some cases complete flaccid paraplegia develops rapidly, with retention of urine and impairment or loss of all forms of sensibility below the level of the lesion. Sometimes the onset is more gradual and the functions of the cord are less severely affected. In such cases the patient develops spastic paraplegia-in-extension; control over the bladder is less severely impaired and sensory loss may be slight ('Erb's syphilitic spastic paraplegia'). In flaccid paraplegia the reflexes in the lower limbs may at first be lost; extensor plantar responses shortly appear, however, and as spinal shock passes off, severe flexor spasms are likely to develop.

Spinal Endarteritis

Endarteritis and arterial thrombosis play an important part in syphilitic myelitis. Exceptionally thrombosis of the anterior or posterior spinal arteries comparable with syphilitic cerebral thrombosis occurs. Rarely the picture of complete anterior spinal artery occlusion is seen [p. 784]. When a lateral branch of the anterior spinal artery is occluded there is a sudden onset of weakness, followed by wasting of the muscles innervated by the affected spinal segment. The spinothalamic tract on the same side is frequently damaged, giving hemi-analgesia and hemi-thermo-anaesthesia on the opposite side of the body, with an upper level a few segments below that involved in the lesion. When thrombosis of one posterior spinal artery occurs this is usually limited to a few segments. All forms of sensibility are then impaired in the corresponding cutaneous segments owing to destruction of the posterior horn of grey matter. The posterior columns and the corticospinal tract on the same side are also the site of softening, so that position and joint sense and vibration sense are lost below the level of the lesion on the same side, and there is also spastic paralysis below the lesion on the side affected.

Radiculitis

Syphilitic radiculitis usually affects the dorsal roots and causes pain and hyperpathia or analgesia in the corresponding segmental distribution. Herpes zoster is a not uncommon complication. When the ventral roots are also affected, weakness and wasting develop in the muscles which they supply.

The Cerebrospinal Fluid

In spinal syphilis the changes in the cerebrospinal fluid are generally the same as those found in cerebral syphilis [p. 459]. After a subacute lesion, such as meningomyelitis, there is frequently a considerable excess of protein and of mononuclear cells; in this condition and in syphilitic pachymeningitis meningeal adhesions may obstruct the subarachnoid space giving a spinal block [p. 128]. There is usually an excess of cells, however, and the V.D.R.L. reaction is positive. A vascular lesion of the spinal cord is rarely associated with a normal spinal fluid, but the V.D.R.L. reaction is usually positive in the blood.

DIAGNOSIS

Spinal syphilis has to be differentiated from other conditions causing paraplegia or irritation of spinal roots, especially from spinal tumour, cervical spondylosis, motor neurone disease, and multiple sclerosis. The diagnosis is not as a rule difficult. A history of infection is usually obtainable. Signs of cerebral syphilis, especially irregularity of the pupils and impairment of their reaction to light may be present and characteristic changes, especially a positive V.D.R.L. reaction, are found in the cerebrospinal fluid. Nevertheless, myelography may still be necessary to exclude cord compression.

PROGNOSIS

Spinal syphilis may respond well to treatment, the determining factor in prognosis being the extent to which irreparable damage has been done to the spinal cord. Even when myelitis has led to complete paraplegia, improvement can occur as shock passes off and oedema of the cord disappears. Complete recovery, however, is not to be expected and this is especially the case after cord infarction. The prognosis is naturally worse in patients who have developed urinary infection or other serious complications. In amyotrophy the progress of the muscular wasting can sometimes be arrested and slight improvement may occur, but much of the disability will be permanent. Root pains can usually be relieved, but are sometimes intractable.

TREATMENT OF MENINGOVASCULAR SYPHILIS

Before treatment is begun, the blood V.D.R.L. reaction should be examined and a complete investigation of the cerebrospinal fluid should be carried out for comparison with future findings. The object of treatment is the destruction of all the spirochaetes in the body. Until the introduction of penicillin few were sanguine enough to believe that this could be accomplished, at least unless treatment was begun within a few weeks of infection but penicillin can achieve a complete cure. Before penicillin the most important spirochaeticidal drugs were bismuth and the arsenobenzene derivatives. The action of the first was gradual, that of arsenic more intense but less enduring, so that the best results were obtained by using them in combination. Iodide also helped to promote absorption of inflammatory products. However, these preparations have now been supplanted by penicillin and, where necessary, other antibiotics.

Penicillin

Experience showed that the smaller doses of penicillin at first given were inadequate and the dose now employed is 600 mg of benzylpenicillin (penicillin G) or procaine penicillin daily. Dattner et al. (1947) gave an intramuscular injection every 3 hours, Nicol and Whelen (1947) only once a day. Most workers are now agreed that a single daily injection of 600 mg of procaine penicillin for 20 days is all that is required. However, occasional untoward allergic reactions to penicillin continue to occur (Beerman et al., 1962) and chloramphenicol and chlortetracycline are also effective. Erythromycin, 500 mg four times daily for 10–15 days, is now probably the drug of choice in patients known to be allergic to penicillin (Thomas, 1964; Brown, 1971; Holmes, 1974).

THE ROUTINE OF TREATMENT

It is generally agreed that penicillin is the foundation of treatment. To diminish the risk of Herxheimer reactions some authorities have advised beginning with small doses of penicillin which are then gradually increased but there is now general agreement that this is no longer necessary. After the initial course of 12 g, no other treatment should be necessary for 6 months, when the blood V.D.R.L. reaction and the cerebrospinal fluid are re-examined. The first favourable change in the fluid is a fall in the cell count, the protein falls next, sometimes after an initial rise, and changes in the immunoglobulins and V.D.R.L. reaction occur last. If the fluid shows improvement at the end of 6 months and the patient's clinical condition is satisfactory he can safely be left without treatment for a further 6 months, when the blood and cerebrospinal fluid are examined again; continuing evidence of activity in the fluid is an indication for a further course of treatment. If, however, the abnormality of the fluid is much less, the blood V.D.R.L. reaction should be examined every 6 months and the cerebrospinal fluid once a year. The object to be aimed at is primarily the relief of symptoms and the arrest of the progress of the disease. The latter can only be regarded as having been achieved when the cerebrospinal fluid is normal, with a negative V.D.R.L. reaction, and the V.D.R.L. reaction in the blood is also negative. When this has taken place the patient should be examined clinically and the blood V.D.R.L. reaction tested once a year for 5 years, but it is unnecessary to examine the CSF again unless fresh symptoms appear. Somtimes, however, patients in whom the clinical course of the disease appears to be arrested continue to manifest a positive V.D.R.L. reaction in the blood or in the fluid or in both. Such patients may benefit from further penicillin; fever treatment, once widely used, is no longer necessary. If, in spite of several courses of treatment given over two or three years, the patient remains 'V.D.R.L.-fast' and his clinical condition is satisfactory, further treatment is inadvisable.

GENERAL PARESIS

Synonyms. Dementia paralytica; general paralysis of the insane (G.P.I.).

AETIOLOGY

General paresis was recognized as a clinical entity about a hundred years ago, though, as its name 'general paralysis of the insane' implies, it was at first regarded as a form of paralysis supervening in persons who had already become insane. In the latter half of the last century its relationship to syphilitic infection was established, though syphilis was then regarded as predisposing to general paresis rather than as actually causing it, hence it was termed a 'parasyphilitic' or 'metasyphilitic' disorder. Noguchi, however, in 1911, first demonstrated the presence of spirochaetes in the brains of sufferers from general paresis.

As McIntosh and Fildes (1914) were the first to show, the effects of tertiary meningovascular syphilis upon the nervous parenchyma are secondary to granulomatous inflammatory changes in the blood vessels and meninges, while in general paresis the spirochaetes actually invade the substance of the brain and spinal cord and themselves attack the cortical neurones. As previously mentioned, populations and races long exposed to syphilis (North America and Europe) are more liable to develop quaternary neurosyphilis (general paresis and tabes) while those which have acquired the infection comparatively recently (e.g. in many tropical countries) tend to develop the more florid secondary and tertiary manifestations (gummas and meningovascular syphilis).

General paresis is the disorder present in about five out of 12 sufferers from neurosyphilis. Males are more liable to it than females in the proportion of four to one. It usually develops between 10 and 15 years after infection, though the interval may be much shorter, and exceptionally 30 or more years may elapse. It is rare, however, that the incubation period is more than 20 years. The first symptoms usually appear between the ages of 40 and 50 but a congenital form is known to occur rarely [see p. 478].

PATHOLOGY

Macroscopically the brain is shrunken, the gyri being unusually well defined, and there is a compensatory hydrocephalus, both external and internal, but the atrophy is confined to the anterior two-thirds of the hemispheres. The pia-arachnoid is usually more opaque than normal, and the walls of the ventricles present a granular appearance due to ependymitis.

Microscopic changes are predominantly cortical and are found in the meninges, blood vessels, and neurones. The leptomeninges show a diffuse infiltration with lymphocytes and plasma cells. Similar cells occupy the peri-vascular spaces of the small vessels and capillaries of the cerebral cortex, and there is usually evidence of new formation of capillaries. The ganglion cells of the cortex show a varying degree of degeneration, going on to complete dis-appearance. These changes are most marked in the molecular layer and the layers of small- and medium-sized pyramidal cells. The deeper layers, including the large pyramidal cells, show slighter or sometimes more acute alterations. Demyelination of cortical and subcortical fibres is also present, frequently with a focal distribution. There is widespread gliosis and giant astrocytes and activated microglial cells are sometimes seen. Perivascular and microglial haemosiderin is often present.

These cortical changes are always diffuse, but the frontal and temporal regions usually suffer most severely. Similar changes may be found in the basal ganglia and in the cerebellar cortex. There appears to be no relationship between the severity of the cortical degeneration and the degree of infiltration of the over-lying leptomeninges. Spirochaetes are demonstrable in the cortex in some 50 per cent of cases, especially in the frontal region, and have sometimes been found within ganglion cells. In the 'Lissauer type' of general paresis, localized cortical atrophy, a 'spongy state' and patchy demyelination of the white matter are found. The pathological changes of tabes may coexist with general paresis (taboparesis). Aortitis is almost invariably present.

SYMPTOMS

Mental Symptoms

The earliest symptoms are usually mental, and in the early stages are fre-quently so slight as to be apparent only to those who know the patient well. It is important, therefore, to obtain a history from a relative or friend. The earliest change is usually an impairment of intellectual efficiency. The patient is unable to do his work as well as before. He loses the power to concentrate, and his memory becomes untrustworthy. His business inefficiency is often apparent to others but not to himself, though exceptionally anxiety may be prominent, and together with the other symptoms described may lead to a mistaken diagnosis of neurosis. As the condition progresses, the patient's behaviour becomes more abnormal, and he is apt to become careless about dress and personal appearance,

Q

and about money, as a result of which he may throw away large sums in extravagance or in ill-judged speculations. Alcoholic excess and sexual aberrations are common at this stage. These are the symptoms of dementia [see also p. 1181], and this form of the disorder is sometimes described as the 'simple dementing type'.

The form taken by the mental disorder, however, doubtless depends upon the patient's mental constitution, and thus other clinical pictures occur. The grandiose form, though frequently regarded as typical, is less common than simple dementia. These patients are euphoric, and develop delusions in which they figure as exceptional persons endowed with superhuman strength, immense wealth, or other magnificent attributes. They readily act on these delusions, and may order large quantities of goods or write a cheque for a million pounds, and see no discrepancy between their imaginary attributes and their debilitated and unfortunate actual condition. Other emotional states may dominate the picture, leading to so-called depressed, agitated, and maniacal, types. Sometimes the condition closely resembles Korsakow's syndrome. As the patient becomes worse, however, the symptoms of dementia become more prominent, and in the terminal stage there is little evidence of any mental activity, and the sufferer, bedridden, incontinent, and dirty, leads a vegetative existence.

Speech exhibits a degradation parallel with that of other mental activities and suffers both in its receptive and expressive functions. Difficulty in naming objects is common. Echolalia may occur.

Physical Symptoms and Signs

Epileptiform attacks occur in about 50 per cent of cases. They may take the form of localized convulsions, without loss of consciousness; generalized attacks, in which consciousness is lost; or minor seizures, in which brief impairment or loss of consciousness occurs without a convulsion. Status epilepticus is sometimes seen.

Apoplectiform episodes, so-called 'congestive attacks', sometimes occur and may bring the patient under observation. The resulting symptoms, of which hemiplegia is the commonest, but which include aphasia, apraxia, and hemianopia, are always transitory and the associated loss of consciousness is usually brief. Recovery is often complete in a week or two.

Although in most cases physical abnormalities are present when the patient first comes under observation, it is important to recognize that physical signs may be absent when mental changes are conspicuous. The expression is often vacant or fatuously smiling, sometimes somewhat mask-like. The pupils are usually contracted and irregular and react sluggishly to light. Typical Argyll Robertson pupils are often found. Optic atrophy is not uncommon, but is rarely severe enough to cause marked loss of visual acuity.

Voluntary power becomes progressively impaired, and weakness is usually associated with tremor, which is most conspicuous on voluntary movement, and is best seen in the facial muscles, especially the lips and the tongue, and in the outstretched fingers. The slow slurred speech is highly characteristic. In addition, inco-ordination usually develops during the later stages, rendering the gait unsteady, and the movements of the upper limbs ataxic.

Owing to bilateral degeneration of the corticospinal tracts, the tendon reflexes are usually exaggerated, the abdominal reflexes diminished or lost, and the plantar reflexes extensor. When tabes is associated with general paresis—so-called 'taboparesis'—the tendon reflexes are lost. Except in taboparesis, when the sensory changes characteristic of tabes are present, sensation is unimpaired in general paresis. Loss of control over the sphincters is common at a comparatively early stage, but is then the result of the cerebral lesions and not of a disorder of innervation at lower levels.

Syphilitic aortitis is common, but rarely causes symptoms. There is usually a progressive loss of weight.

The Cerebrospinal Fluid

The CSF exhibits characteristic changes of great diagnostic importance. The pressure is frequently somewhat increased. There is usually an excess of cells, which are mononuclear, but the cell count rarely exceeds 100 per mm^3. The protein content is also increased and usually lies between 0·05 and 0·10 g per 100 ml. Marked increase of globulin is found and of the total globulin, more than 25 per cent may be found to be gamma-globulin with a considerable increase in IgG and IgM. Lange's colloidal gold curve is of the paretic type, e.g. 5554311000 or even 5555555444. Exceptionally, though the curve remains of this type, precipitation is not quite complete, and the highest figure is 4. The V.D.R.L. reaction is positive in the cerebrospinal fluid in 100 per cent of cases, and in the blood in from 90 to 100 per cent. The treponema immobilization test is even more specific, being invariably positive in the fluid in the untreated case.

DIAGNOSIS

The constancy of serological abnormalities in the blood and cerebrospinal fluid in general paresis is of the utmost diagnostic importance, as it frequently confirms a diagnosis which on clinical grounds alone might be doubtful. In all cases, therefore, in which general paresis is a possibility these tests should be carried out.

The mental symptoms in the early stage may simulate neurosis or manic-depressive psychosis. Neither of these conditions, however, is associated with signs of organic disease in the nervous system.

General paresis must be distinguished from the presenile and senile dementias and from arteriosclerotic dementia in which tremor, spasticity, and extensor plantar responses may be present. In such cases the diagnosis can be made only after an examination of the blood and cerebrospinal fluid. Alcoholic dementia— 'alcoholic pseudoparesis'—may closely simulate general paresis and may again be distinguishable only by serological tests.

It is often difficult to distinguish general paresis from meningovascular syphilis when this condition is associated with severe mental changes, since the V.D.R.L. reaction may be positive in both blood and cerebrospinal fluid in both conditions. When the colloidal gold curve in the fluid is of the luetic type this is a point in favour of meningovascular syphilis, but a paretic curve is not pathognomonic of general paresis.

PROGNOSIS

Before the introduction of malarial treatment general paresis was invariably fatal, and it was exceptional for a patient to survive more than three years. Exceptionally the disease ran a rapid course and proved fatal within a year. Remissions, which, however, are only temporary, occur spontaneously in from 10 to 20 per cent of cases. Malarial treatment considerably improved the outlook, but penicillin is much more effective (Hahn *et al.*, 1958). Arrest can usually be achieved, hence the earlier the stage at which the diagnosis is made and treatment is begun, the better the outlook. Nevertheless, complete cure is unusual and in a series of 100 cases followed up for 10 years after initial treatment, 31 per cent developed new neurological manifestations (Wilner and Brody, 1968).

TREATMENT

Penicillin

Penicillin is the treatment of choice or other antibiotics as in the treatment of meningovascular syphilis [pp. 463–4].

Malarial Therapy

The introduction of infection with malaria by Wagner-Jauregg in 1917 was a great advance in the treatment of general paresis. Histologically, after treatment with malaria spirochaetes disappeared from the brain and the inflammatory exudate diminished. The parasite of benign tertian malaria (*P. vivax*) was generally employed (Rudolf, 1927; Meagher, 1929), being inoculated by the bite of an infected mosquito or by injection of infected donor blood. Other methods of inducing pyrexia were sometimes used. Though malarial and/or fever therapy was still used, especially in resistant cases, in some centres until a few years ago, all authorities now agree that it is no longer necessary if adequate antibiotic therapy is given.

General Measures

Early cases of general paresis, especially those characterized by simple dementia, can usually be treated at home, if suitable attention is available, or in a general hospital. Those with more severe mental symptoms will require to be treated in a mental hospital. Adequate medical supervision is necessary for a long time in those who do well, and patients who return to positions of responsibility must be carefully watched, and the cerebrospinal fluid examined annually for evidence of deterioration. A relapse may be treated in the same way as the first attack, but the results are usually not as good as after the first treatment.

TABES DORSALIS

Synonym. Locomotor ataxia.

AETIOLOGY

Tabes was first recognized as a clinical entity by Romberg and Duchenne. Its association with syphilis was first suspected by Fournier, and was established by the introduction of the Wassermann reaction and the discovery of spirochaetes in the brain and spinal cord of affected individuals by Noguchi and by Marinesco and Minea. Tabes, like general paresis, differs from meningovascular syphilis with respect to the systematized character of the spinal lesions and less satisfactory response of advanced cases to treatment.

As in the case of general paresis, it is not uncommon to find that tabetic patients deny having had a primary chancre and the secondary manifestations of syphilis. These indications of infection may, therefore, be absent or so slight as to pass unnoticed. Tabes affects males much more frequently than females in the ratio of at least 4 to 1, and is the disorder present in 3 out of 12 cases of neurosyphilis. Although trauma has sometimes been blamed for precipitating the onset it seems more likely that the patient in whom tabes is developing may be able to compensate for his ataxia until he is confined to bed by an injury, when he temporarily loses this power, so that inco-ordination is conspicuous when he gets up. Tabetic symptoms usually appear between 8 and 12 years after infection. Exceptionally they may develop within 3 years, or may be delayed until after 20 years or even longer. The age of onset usually lies between 35 and 50 years.

PATHOLOGY

Macroscopically there is evidence of atrophy of the dorsal spinal roots, especially of those in the lower thoracic and lumbosacral regions. The posterior columns of the spinal cord are flat or even sunken; hence the name tabes dorsalis or dorsal wasting. On section of the cord the posterior columns appear grey and translucent, in contrast to the normal appearance of the rest of the white matter.

Microscopically the essential lesion is a degeneration of the exogenous fibres of the cord, that is, of the central processes of the dorsal root ganglion cells, which themselves are usually little affected. Since the only exogenous fibres which possess a long course within the cord are situated in the posterior columns, these

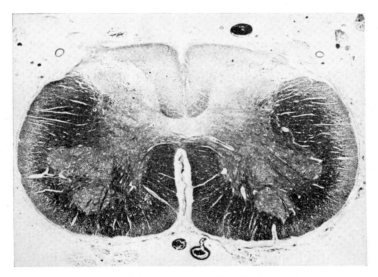

FIG. 94. Tabes dorsalis. Section of spinal cord

exhibit a selective degeneration and their demyelination is conspicuous when stained by myelin stains [FIG. 94]. The endogenous fibres in the cornu-commissural zone, the region of the posterior columns lying just posterior to the grey commissure, usually escape. The incoming fibres earliest affected are those which in the thoracic region constitute the middle-root zone of the posterior columns or the bandelette of Pierret. Since the lower thoracic and lumbosacral roots are first attacked and their fibres entering the posterior columns shift towards the midline as they ascend the cord, the fasciculus gracilis suffers earlier than the fasciculus cuneatus in the cervical region. The latter, however, is affected later. In early cases the intraspinal portion of the posterior roots may be infiltrated with lymphocytes and plasma cells (Merritt *et al.*, 1946); later there is secondary gliosis in the posterior columns and the overlying pia mater is thickened. Exceptionally degeneration of anterior horn cells may occur in certain segments, in which case there is atrophy of the fibres of the corresponding ventral roots.

Many theories have been proposed in explanation of the selective character of the degenerative lesions of tabes in the spinal cord. The view of the older pathologists, and that adopted by Spielmeyer, was that tabes is due to a primary degeneration of the exogenous fibres within the cord. Obersteiner and Redlich (1894-5) believed that degeneration is due to compression of the dorsal root fibres by meningeal constriction at the point at which they pass through the pia mater and this view is still generally favoured, though Nageotte (1894) and Richter (1921) felt that the primary lesion was in the radicular nerve, closer to the dorsal root ganglion.

Optic atrophy is common and occurs in two forms, the degeneration of the nerve fibres being either primary or secondary to syphilitic inflammation of the interstitial tissues [see p. 162]. The Argyll Robertson pupil has been variously explained [see p. 93]. Sensory fibres of the cranial nerves, especially the trigeminal and glossopharyngeal, like those of the dorsal roots, may exhibit degeneration as they approach the brain stem, and degenerative changes have also been described in the afferent fibres of the sympathetic. The pathological changes of meningovascular syphilis may be associated with tabes, and those of general paresis may also be found ('taboparesis').

Tabes is an important cause of trophic arthropathy—Charcot's joints. According to Moritz (1928), the earliest change in the joint is a hyperplasia of the cartilage. Later, destruction of the cartilage and erosion of the epiphyses occur and are often associated with the development of osteophytic outgrowths. There is an increase in the volume of the synovial fluid, and subluxation of an affected joint is not uncommon. Trauma frequently plays a part in the production of arthropathy. Syphilitic aortitis is a common complication of tabes.

SYMPTOMS

The principal symptoms of tabes are readily interpreted as a result of the degeneration of the afferent fibres of the dorsal roots. Pain and paraesthesiae are attributable to irritation of the degenerating sensory fibres. Sensory loss, i.e. analgesia and impairment of postural sensibility and vibration sense, are due to interruption of the corresponding sensory fibres. Ataxia is due in part to impaired appreciation of posture and passive movement, in part to interruption of afferent fibres conveying impulses concerned in co-ordination which do not reach consciousness. Diminution and loss of the tendon reflexes are due to interruption of their reflex arcs on the afferent side. Impotence and sphincter disturbances are the result of a similar loss of afferent impulses concerned in sexual function and in the evacuation of the bladder and rectum.

Mode of Onset

The onset of tabes is usually insidious, but exceptionally it is rapid and the patient may become grossly ataxic within three months. Usually sensory symptoms, especially pain, precede ataxia by months or years (the pre-ataxic stage), but ataxia may develop early. Frequently the early sensory symptoms are so slight that the patient does not come for treatment until a more serious symptom develops. Hence the symptom which brings him to the doctor may be pain, ataxia, vomiting, impotence, disorder of micturition, failing vision, diplopia, or even arthropathy.

Sensory Symptoms

Pain is the most characteristic early symptom and usually takes the form of so-called 'lightning pains'. These pains, which are stabbing in character, occur in brief paroxysms in the lower limbs and may be very severe. As a rule they do not radiate longitudinally along the limb, but are localized to one spot, where the patient experiences a sensation as though a sharp object were being driven into the limb. Each attack lasts only a few seconds, but attacks may recur repeatedly in the same place, or may shift from place to place in the limb. A fresh attack of lightning pains may be precipitated by a change in the weather. Intercurrent illness may lead to a severe exacerbation. It is not uncommon to find hyperalgesia, and vasodilatation of the skin in the region to which the pains are referred, and in severe cases ecchymosis may occur. Similar severe paroxysmal pains may occur in the upper limbs or in the distribution of the trigeminal nerve. Other forms of pain may be experienced, such as burning or tearing pains in the feet, pain in the distribution of the sciatic nerve, and a constricting pain around the chest or abdomen—'root pains' or 'girdle pains'.

Paraesthesiae are not uncommon, especially in the lower limbs. The patient may complain that the feet feel numb or cold, and a sensation as of walking on wool is a common complaint. The skin of the trunk and lower limbs is frequently hypersensitive to touch and to heat and cold. The patient may be aware that certain parts of the body are anaesthetic. Thus he may be unable to feel the chair upon which he sits, and he may notice that he is unaware when his bladder is full, and that he is unconscious of the act of defaecation.

Objective Sensory Changes

The forms of sensibility which are first impaired are usually those mediated by the posterior columns. Appreciation of vibration suffers early, and usually before recognition of posture and passive movement. As a rule the lower limbs are affected before the upper, though exceptionally the upper limbs suffer first—so-called 'cervical tabes'.

Painful sensibility is also impaired early, the deep tissues becoming insensitive to pain before the skin. Forcible compression of the muscles and the tendo calcaneus evokes no pain, and testicular sensation is frequently lost. Cutaneous painful sensibility is not uniformly impaired, but is usually lost first on the side of the nose, the ulnar border of the arm and forearm, the region of the trunk between the nipples and the costal margin, the outer border of the leg and dorsum and sole of the foot, and the region surrounding the anus. In these regions, even when pin-prick is appreciated as painful, there is often a long delay, which may reach several seconds, between the application of the stimulus and its perception. Cutaneous sensibility to light touch, heat, and cold is usually unimpaired at first, but finally there may be a diffuse loss of all forms of sensibility, extending over the whole of the body.

Ataxia

Ataxia is due partly to loss of postural sensibility and partly to loss of 'unconscious' afferent impulses concerned in the regulation of posture and movement. The importance of the latter factor is well seen in patients who exhibit considerable ataxia of the lower limbs without detectable impairment of position and joint sense. Ataxia usually begins in the lower limbs with slight unsteadiness in walking and turning. Since the patient is able to some extent to compensate by means of vision for the deficit, his ataxia becomes worse in the dark or when he closes his eyes, whence arises the characteristic symptom of falling into the basin when the eyes are closed in washing the face. As the ataxia increases, movements of the lower limbs become increasingly incoordinate. The patient walks with a wide base; the feet are lifted too high and brought down to the ground too violently. Walking becomes impossible without a stick, and finally he can only walk supported on both sides. The ataxia is equally evident when the patient is lying in bed in the heel-knee test. Voluntary movement of the lower limbs against resistance is jerky and irregular, and when the patient is lying at rest irregular, jerky, involuntary movements can often be observed, especially in the feet and toes ('pseudoathetosis').

In the early stages ataxia of the lower limbs is best demonstrated by asking the patient to stand with the toes and heels together and the eyes closed, and watching whether he sways—Romberg's test—or by asking him to walk along a line placing one heel in front of the opposite toe.

In severe cases the trunk muscles also become ataxic and the patient may then be unable to sit up in bed without support. Ataxia of the upper limbs is manifest in the clumsiness with which fine movements of the fingers are performed. The defective maintenance of posture may often be demonstrated in the outstretched fingers by asking the patient to close his eyes. When the posture of the fingers is no longer controlled by vision they either droop or wander in space ('pseudoathetosis').

Muscle Tone

Partial deafferentation leads to muscular hypotonia, as a result of which exaggerated passive movements of the joints may become possible.

The Reflexes of the Limbs and Trunk

Degeneration of afferent fibres of the reflex arc leads to depression of tendon reflexes and ultimately to their disappearance. The ankle-jerks are thus affected before the knee-jerks, and it is not uncommon to find the reflexes unequal on the two sides. The tendon-jerks of the upper limbs are usually diminished at an early stage, but are finally lost only after those of the lower limbs have disappeared. The plantar reflexes usually remain elicitable and are flexor, except in taboparesis, when they are extensor. The abdominal reflexes are also obtainable, and are frequently unusually brisk.

Sphincter Disturbances

Disturbances in bladder control may occur early when the sacral roots are involved. When lumbar roots suffer first, considerable ataxia of the lower limbs may precede bladder symptoms. The patient may complain either of difficulty of micturition or of incontinence. The bladder is large and atonic; catheterization often reveals the presence of several ounces of residual urine, and complete retention may occur. Infection of the urinary tract develops sooner or later, and ascending pyelonephritis may develop. Constipation is the rule, but faecal incontinence may occur, especially when the patient is unconscious of the act of defaecation. Impotence is sometimes an early symptom but is not invariable.

Ocular Symptoms

Pupillary abnormalities are present in many patients when they come under observation and in more than 90 per cent at some time in the course of the disease. The pupils are usually contracted and frequently irregular. Exceptionally they are moderately or even widely dilated, especially in congenital neurosyphilis. Somewhat more frequently one is moderately dilated and the other contracted. The pupillary reaction to light is at first impaired and later lost, while that on accommodation-convergence is retained. The iris is pale and atrophic. The complete Argyll Robertson pupil [p. 93], however, is often a late manifestation, and in the early stages it is commoner to find that the reaction of the pupil to light is present but reduced in amplitude, exhibits a latent period which is longer than normal, and is ill-sustained. The light reflex is often brisker in one eye than in the other, and the consensual reaction may be brisker than the direct. Rarely the pupil dilates in response to light. The contracted pupil fails to dilate in response to a scratch upon the skin of the neck, and both the myosis and the loss of this ciliospinal reflex are probably due to degeneration of the fibres of the oculosympathetic. A moderate degree of ptosis, probably also due to oculosympathetic paralysis, is common, and the compensatory action of the frontalis muscle by wrinkling the brow contributes to the characteristic facies. Diplopia occurs in about 20 per cent of cases; in the early stages it is often transitory, but nuclear ophthalmoplegia or permanent paralysis of the third or sixth nerve may develop.

Optic atrophy is of the 'primary' variety [see p. 162]. The optic disc is small and pale, the physiological cup is preserved, and the lamina cribrosa is often visible. The fundal vessels are usually reduced in calibre. Optic atrophy in tabes may be slight and non-progressive, with little or no subjective impairment of visual acuity, being discovered only on routine examination. When, however, the patient complains of failing vision the atrophy is likely to progress and to terminate in blindness. Usually acuity deteriorates first in the periphery of the visual fields; less often there is a central scotoma.

Other Cranial Nerves

Pain and analgesia in the distribution of the trigeminal nerve have already been described. Loss of smell and taste occasionally occurs. Degeneration of the eighth nerve may lead to deafness, and involvement of the vestibular fibres may cause vertigo. Exceptionally, degeneration of part of the nucleus ambiguus causes bilateral paralysis of the abductors of the larynx, and paralysis of the accessory and hypoglossal nerves is occasionally observed.

Trophic Changes

Arthropathies—Charcot's joints—are common; symptoms not infrequently appear after an injury. The onset of the joint change is frequently rapid, and there is considerable swelling, with increase in the synovial fluid. The skin may appear hot, but pain is almost invariably absent. Later, osteophytic outgrowths frequently develop around the joint, which thus becomes much enlarged, and considerable disorganization with subluxation may occur. Radiograms show as a rule marked erosion of the joint surfaces with formation of new bone at the articular margins or from the adjacent part of the shaft [FIG. 95]. The knee is most frequently affected, and after that the hip. The shoulder, tarsal joints, elbow, ankle, small joints of the fingers and toes and spine are involved in approximately this order of frequency. The long bones are brittle, and fractures may occur as a result of slight trauma.

The commonest trophic change in the skin is the perforating ulcer, which is usually seen beneath the pad of the great toe or at other pressure-points on the sole [FIG. 96]. The first stage is an epithelial thickening resembling a corn, and, either spontaneously or as a result of attempts to cut it away, an indolent ulcer develops. Sometimes a sinus extends deeply as far as the underlying bone, and bony disorganization and deformity may then result. Other trophic changes include cutaneous ecchymoses, brittleness, and loss of hair, and even occasionally of the teeth. Symptomatic herpes zoster may occur, as in other conditions affecting spinal dorsal roots.

Tabetic Crises

Paroxysmal painful disorders of function of various viscera occur in tabes, and have been called crises. The gastric crisis is the commonest. It is characterized by attacks of epigastric pain associated with severe vomiting, and may last from a few hours to several days. Laryngeal crises consist of attacks of dyspnoea associated with cough and inspiratory and expiratory stridor, and appear to be associated with laryngeal paralyses. Rectal crises, characterized by tenesmus, and vesical crises, characterized by pain in the bladder or penis and strangury, may also occur, and renal and other crises have been described. The feature common to most tabetic crises appears to be increased motility of a hollow viscus, presumably the result of a disorder of autonomic afferent impulses.

The Cerebrospinal Fluid

The pressure is normal or only slightly increased. There is usually an excess of cells, which are mononuclear and do not often exceed 70 per mm^3. The protein may be normal or slightly increased. There is an excess of gamma-globulin in 90 per cent of cases. The colloidal gold curve is usually of the 'luetic' type. A 'paretic' curve, even in the absence of signs of general paresis, suggests the possibility that this may develop later. The V.D.R.L. reaction is positive in both blood and cerebrospinal fluid in 65 per cent of cases, positive in the fluid alone in 10 per cent, in the blood alone in 5 per cent, and negative in both in 20 per cent. The treponema immobilization test is positive in the fluid in about 60 per cent of the cases but is almost invariably positive in the blood (Duperrat and Cayol, 1962). The V.D.R.L. reaction may be negative in the fluid in spite of an excess of cells, protein, and globulin, and a negative reaction in both blood and fluid or indeed a completely normal fluid may be found in a patient in whom the disease is progressive.

Complications

Symptoms of meningovascular syphilis, including muscular wasting, may coexist with those of tabes, though this is unusual. A tabetic patient may, after a lapse of years, develop general paresis, or the symptoms of tabes may be present in an individual who comes under observation on account of symptoms of the latter disorder. Apart from general paresis, psychotic reactions, often with a paranoid trend, may occur in long-standing cases of tabes. Syphilitic aortitis

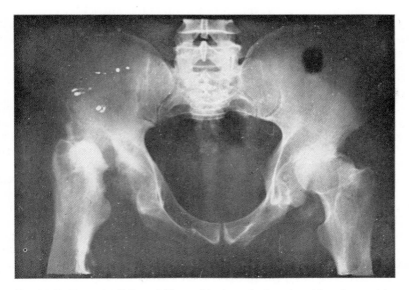

FIG. 95. Radiograph of bilateral Charcot hips in a tabetic patient. Note the opacities due to bismuth injections in the right buttock

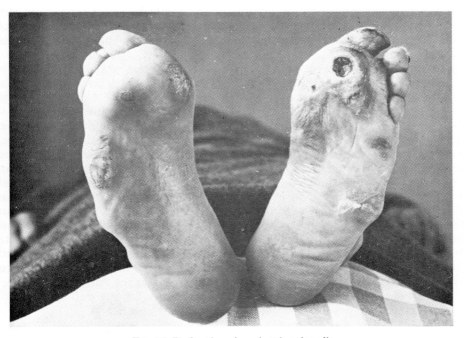

FIG. 96. Perforating ulcers in tabes dorsalis

is often present, but rarely gives rise to symptoms. However, even after the apparently successful treatment of neurosyphilis with penicillin, cardiovascular manifestations of syphilis, and particularly signs of aortitis, may appear several years later. Chronic gastric ulcer occurs more often than can be explained by chance, and the symptoms may be mistaken for gastric crises.

DIAGNOSIS

When the patient has reached the ataxic stage, diagnosis usually presents little difficulty, for the characteristic physical signs are by then well developed, and the matter is clinched by investigation of the blood and cerebrospinal fluid. In multiple sclerosis ataxia of the lower limbs is associated with spasticity, exaggerated tendon reflexes, and extensor plantar responses. Friedreich's ataxia resembles tabes in the association of ataxia of the lower limbs with diminution or loss of the ankle-jerks, but this disorder usually begins at an early age and is differentiated from tabes clinically by the presence of nystagmus, dysarthria, extensor plantar responses, scoliosis, and pes cavus. Polyneuritis may simulate tabes when there is pronounced ataxia of the lower limbs. In alcoholic polyneuritis the pupillary reactions may be sluggish, the tendon reflexes are diminished or lost, the lower limbs are frequently ataxic, pains occur in the limbs, and there is an impairment of postural sensibility. In this condition, however, weakness of the peripheral muscles of the limbs is conspicuous and wrist- and foot-drop are often present, and the deep tissues, especially the muscles, are tender on pressure and not, as in tabes, analgesic. However, some patients with diabetic polyneuropathy may experience pain in the limbs and on examination show pupillary changes, areflexia, and peripheral impairment of pain sensation ('diabetic pseudotabes'); even if the patient has been diabetic for some time the coincidental association of tabes dorsalis may have to be excluded by serological tests and motor nerve conduction velocity measurements which are usually abnormal in diabetic neuropathy and normal in tabes. Argyll Robertson pupils have been described in cases of peroneal muscular atrophy (Charcot–Marie–Tooth disease), but in this condition the peripheral amyotrophy is diagnostic.

When ataxia is absent the prominence of some other symptom may lead to a mistake in diagnosis; for example, pains in the limbs may be attributed to arthritis, root pains in the trunk to lesions of underlying viscera, gastric crises to ulceration of the stomach or duodenum, disturbances of the vesical sphincter to enlarged prostate or lesions of the bladder, arthropathy to arthritis, facial pain to trigeminal neuralgia, and optic atrophy to toxic amblyopia. These mistakes can be avoided only by systematic examination of the nervous system, special stress being laid upon the pupillary reflexes and upon diminution, absence, or inequality of the tendon reflexes in the lower limbs, especially the ankle-jerks. In doubtful cases the blood and cerebrospinal fluid should be examined. It must always be borne in mind that tabes may coexist with other disorders. All patients suspected of gastric crisis should have a barium meal, as the failure to diagnose a gastric ulcer in a tabetic may be more disastrous for the patient than to mistake a gastric crisis for an organic lesion of the stomach.

PROGNOSIS

Tabes is extremely variable in its rate of progress and in the extent to which it responds to treatment. A rapidly progressive course with the development of ataxia in a few months is rare. Usually the duration of the pre-ataxic stage is from 2 to 5 years. In some cases overt ataxia never develops and one encounters abortive forms with signs such as Argyll Robertson pupils and absent knee- and ankle-jerks, but no symptoms. The rate at which ataxia is likely to increase can be roughly assessed from the duration of the pre-ataxic stage. The longer this is, the slower is likely to be the subsequent deterioration. The response to treatment is equally variable. Sometimes considerable improvement occurs and the disorder seems to be arrested. Other patients go downhill rapidly or slowly in spite of all treatment. Optic atrophy is not necessarily progressive, but when the patient complains of failing vision it often terminates in blindness. Early treatment may be expected to arrest its progress in about 50 per cent of cases. Gastric crises often respond satisfactorily to the general treatment of tabes, and perforating ulcers which are not too far advanced can usually be induced to heal. No improvement can be expected in the bony changes associated with arthropathy. Improvement frequently occurs in sphincter control, and impotence, though often permanent, is not necessarily so, for sexual power may return after treatment. In fatal cases death usually occurs from intercurrent infection, often of the urinary tract, or from cardiovascular complications.

TREATMENT
General Treatment

Special attention should be paid to the care of the bladder and bowels, to the treatment of secondary infections, and the care of the feet.

Vigorous antisyphilitic treatment must be carried out along the lines indicated for meningovascular syphilis [pp. 463–4]. Various appliances, including walking sticks, supporting bandages for neuropathic joints, and even spinal corsets are sometimes needed.

Treatment of Special Symptoms

Pain. Tabetic pains are often ameliorated by simple analgesics; sometimes chlorpromazine is also helpful. When lightning pains are more severe and frequent, systemic steroids (Moore, 1953) or intrathecal prednisone (Bertini, 1958) have been recommended, but the most successful drug seems to be carbamazepine (*Tegretol*) given in a dosage of 400–800 mg daily (Ekbom, 1972).

Ataxia. Co-ordination of the limbs may be improved by suitable re-educational exercises on the lines of those first suggested by Frenkel.

The Bladder. Precipitancy of micturition may be relieved by propantheline, 15 mg three times daily, or similar remedies. The atonic bladder should not be treated surgically unless either there is impairment of renal function or there is an infection of the urinary tract which has failed to respond to chemotherapy. The choice will then lie between suprapubic cystostomy, and transurethral division of the internal sphincter. Catheterization should always be carried out to determine whether there is any residual urine. The patient should be instructed to pass urine at four-hourly intervals whether he feels the need to micturate or not. Even when the bladder has become overdistended it is probably best treated in this way, with the addition of drugs of the acetylcholine group such as carbamylcholine. Catheterization should not be carried out unnecessarily, and surgical intervention should be postponed as long as possible.

Crises. Patients subject to gastric crises should take a bland, non-irritating diet, together with alkalies. A crisis can frequently be cut short by an injection of pethidine hydrochloride, 100 mg. If this fails, morphine and atropine may be tried. In severe recurrent cases benefit has followed section of the lower thoracic spinal dorsal roots, and very rarely bilateral upper cervical cordotomy may be necessary.

Perforating Ulcer. Tabetic patients should wear well-fitting shoes and should be warned against cutting their corns, on account of the risk that a perforating ulcer may follow a slight injury. Regular attention from a skilled chiropodist is recommended. When an ulcer has developed, rest and appropriate antibiotic dressings often promote healing.

Arthropathy. The object of treatment is to relieve the strain on the damaged joint. The knee and ankle may be supported by a firm elastic support. When the hip or knee is affected a walking caliper may be required. Spinal arthropathy necessitates a leather corset or spinal brace. When there is much fluid in the joint this may be aspirated. Excision of an arthropathic joint or the insertion of prostheses should not be attempted, since the results are uniformly unsatisfactory.

Optic Atrophy. No treatment other than penicillin or other appropriate antibiotics is of any value; surgical decompression of the optic nerves is ineffective (Bruetsch, 1948).

CONGENITAL NEUROSYPHILIS

Active neurosyphilis occurs in from 8 to 10 per cent of congenitally syphilitic children, males being affected slightly more often than females (Jeans and Cooke, 1930). Neither in its pathological nor in its clinical features does congenital neurosyphilis differ in any essential respects from the acquired form except for the fact that fixed dilated pupils rather than those of the typical Argyll Robertson type are more common in the congenital variety. Both meningovascular and parenchymatous neurosyphilis occur. The intra-uterine infection of the nervous system with the spirochaete may lead to actual developmental arrest so that the cerebral hemispheres are unusually small. Gross disappearance of Purkinje cells with gliosis of the cerebellar cortex is rather characteristic of juvenile general paresis.

SYMPTOMS

The meningovascular form is much commoner than the parenchymatous. Both mental deficiency (Schachter, 1959) and convulsions are common. Slight hydrocephalus is not rare and appears always to be of the communicating type. Pupillary abnormality is the most frequent sign of cranial nerve involvement. The pupils are often large, irregular, and unequal and the reaction to light is sluggish or absent. Optic atrophy is often present and may arise in several ways. It may be secondary to choroidoretinitis or to involvement of the optic nerves or chiasm in basal syphilitic meningitis, or be associated with congenital general paresis or tabes. Facial weakness is frequently seen. Deafness, a common manifestation of congenital syphilis, is due in most cases to a lesion within the temporal bone and not to involvement of the eighth nerve in its intracranial course. Destruction of corticospinal fibres may lead to diplegia or hemiplegia. Moderate degrees of infantilism are not uncommon. Narcolepsy and diabetes insipidus are rare manifestations.

Parenchymatous neurosyphilis is rare. Stewart (1933) estimated that general paresis occurs in 1 per cent of congenital syphilitics. The child may be mentally defective from birth, but symptoms usually develop during the first half of the second decade of life. The symptoms are similar to those of the acquired form, though the mental symptoms are usually less florid and are those of acquired mental subnormality. Grandiose delusions, if present, are puerile in type; for example, a boy stated that he owned all the sweet shops in the country. The course of the disorder is somewhat slower than in the adult, and the untreated patient may live for ten or more years.

Congenital tabes usually develops somewhat later in life than congenital general paresis, and may not make its appearance until early adult life but tabo-paresis may occur in adolescence (Joffe et al., 1968). Optic atrophy is common in both, and in both the pupils are often widely dilated and fixed.

The blood V.D.R.L. reaction is usually positive and the treponema immobilization test is always so when congenital neurosyphilis is progressive, but the V.D.R.L. test is sometimes negative in latent or arrested cases. The cerebrospinal fluid usually shows the changes associated with the acquired disorders, but in some cases of congenital meningovascular syphilis the V.D.R.L. reaction is negative in the fluid, even when the cells and protein are increased.

DIAGNOSIS

The diagnosis is usually easy when it is considered, since other signs of congenital syphilis are generally present, and is confirmed by the serological reactions of the child and its parents. However, juvenile general paresis or taboparesis, when presenting, as it may with fits, dementia and even akinetic mutism, with or without areflexia and sphincter disturbance, may be mistaken for encephalitis or polyradiculitis.

PROGNOSIS

The response to treatment is disappointing in patients who come under observation on account of the presence of nervous symptoms, especially in congenital general paresis and tabes. Hence it is important that the cerebrospinal fluid should be examined in all congenitally syphilitic children at an early age, in order that latent neurosyphilis may be detected.

TREATMENT

Treatment should be carried out on the same lines as for acquired syphilis.

REFERENCES

ADAMS, R. D., and MERRITT, H. H. (1944) Meningeal and vascular syphilis of the spinal cord, Medicine (Baltimore), 23, 181.

BEERMAN, H., NICHOLAS, L., SCHAMBERG, I. L., and GREENBERG, M. S. (1962) Syphilis: review of the recent literature, 1960–1, Arch. intern. Med., 109, 323.

BERTINI, F. (1958) Terapia cortisonica a scopo antalgico nella tabe dorsale, Gazz. med. ital., 117, 417.

BOGAERT, L. VAN, and VERBRUGGE, J. (1928) The pathogenesis and the surgical treatment of gastric crisis of tabes: neuroramisectomy, Surg. Gynec. Obstet., 47, 543.

BROWN, W. J. (1971) Status and control of syphilis in the United States, J. infect. Dis., 124, 428.

BRUETSCH, W. L. (1948) Surgical treatment of syphilitic primary atrophy of the optic nerves (syphilitic optochiasmatic arachnoiditis), Arch. Ophthal., 38, 735.

CLARK, E. G., and DANBOLT, N. (1964) The Oslo study of the natural course of untreated syphilis, *Med. Clin. N. Amer.*, **48**, 613.

CURTIS, A. C., KRUSE, W. T., and NORTON, D. H. (1950) Neurosyphilis. IV. Post-treatment evaluation 4–5 years following penicillin and penicillin plus malaria, *Amer. J. Syph.*, **24**, 554.

CUTLER, J. C., BAUER, T. J., PRICE, E. V., and SCHWIMMER, B. H. (1954) Comparison of spinal fluid findings among syphilitic and nonsyphilitic individuals, *Amer. J. Syph.*, **38**, 447.

DATTNER, B. (1948 *a*) Neurosyphilis and the latest methods of treatment, *Med. Clin. N. Amer.*, **32**, 707.

DATTNER, B. (1948 *b*) Treatment of neurosyphilis with penicillin alone, *Amer. J. Syph.*, **32**, 399.

DATTNER, B., KAUFMAN, S. S., and THOMAS, E. W. (1947) Penicillin in treatment of neurosyphilis, *Arch. Neurol. Psychiat. (Chic.)*, **58**, 426.

DATTNER, B., THOMAS, E. W., and WEXLER, S. (1944) *The Management of Neurosyphilis*, New York.

DUPERRAT, B., and CAYOL, J. (1962) Le test de Nelson dans les tabès, *Bull. Soc. Méd. Paris*, **113**, 556.

EKBOM, K. (1972) Carbamazepine in the treatment of tabetic lightning pains, *Arch. Neurol. (Chic.)*, **26**, 374.

FOIX, C., CRUSEM, L., and NACHT, S. (1926) Sur l'anatomo-pathologie de la syphilis médullaire en général et en particulier des paraplégies syphilitiques progressives, *Ann. Méd.*, **20**, 81.

GILLESPIE, E. J., and BROWN, B. C. (1964) New laboratory methods in the diagnosis of syphilis and other treponematoses, *Med. Clin. N. Amer.*, **48**, 731.

GOLDMAN, D. (1945) Treatment of neurosyphilis with penicillin, *J. Amer. med. Ass.*, **128**, 274.

HAHN, R. D. (1951) The treatment of neurosyphilis with penicillin and with penicillin plus malaria, *Amer. J. Syph.*, **35**, 433.

HAHN, R. D., CUTLER, J. C., CURTIS, A. C., GAMMON, G., HEYMAN, A., JOHNWICK, E., STOKES, J. H., SOLOMON, H., THOMAS, E., TIMBERLAKE, W., WEBSTER, B., and GLEESON, G. (1956) Penicillin treatment of asymptomatic central nervous system syphilis, A and II, *Arch. Derm.*, **74**, 355, 367.

HAHN, R. D., WEBSTER, B., WEICKHARDT, G., THOMAS, E., TIMBERLAKE, W., SOLO-MON, H., STOKES, J. H., HEYMAN, A., GAMMON, G., GLEESON, G. A., CURTIS, A. C., and CUTLER, J. C. (1958) The results of treatment in 1,086 general paralytics the majority of whom were followed for more than five years, *J. chron. Dis.*, **7**, 209.

HASSIN, G. B. (1929) Tabes dorsalis, *Arch. Neurol. Psychiat. (Chic.)*, **21**, 311.

HOFF, H., and KAUDERS, O. (1926) Über die Malariabehandlung der Tabes dorsalis, *Z. ges. Neurol. Psychiat.*, **104**, 306.

HOLMES, K. K. (1974) Syphilis, in *Harrison's Principles of Internal Medicine*, 7th ed., ed. Wintrobe, M. M., Thorn, G. W., Adams, R. D., Braunwald, E., Isselbacher, K. J., and Petersdorf, R. G., Chapter 159, p. 876, New York.

HURIEZ, C., AGACHE, P., and SOUILLART, F. (1963) Panorama actuel des syphilis viscérales, *Vie méd.*, **44**, 369.

JAUREGG, W. (1929) La malariathérapie de la paralysie générale et des affections syphilitiques du système, *Rev. neurol.*, **36**, 889.

JEANS, P. C., and COOKE, J. V. (1930) *Prepubescent Syphilis* (Clin. Pediatrics, xvii), New York.

JOFFE, R., BLACK, M. M., and FLOYD, M. (1968) Changing clinical picture of neurosyphilis: report of seven unusual cases, *Brit. med. J.*, **1**, 211.

KENNEY, J. A., and CURTIS, A. C. (1953) The treatment of syphilitic optic atrophy by penicillin with and without therapeutic malaria, *Amer. J. Syph.*, **37**, 449.

LÉRI, A. (1925) Sur certaines pseudo-scléroses latérales amyotrophiques syphilitiques, *Rev. neurol.*, **32**, 827.

LHERMITTE, J. (1933) La syphilis diencéphalique et les syndromes végétatifs qu'elle conditionne—étude clinique, *Ann. Méd.*, **33**, 272.

McINTOSH, J., and FILDES, P. (1914-15) A comparison of the lesions of syphilis and 'parasyphilis', together with evidence in favour of the identity of these two conditions, *Brain*, **37**, 141.

McINTOSH, J., and FILDES, P. (1914) The demonstration of *Spirochœta pallida* in chronic parenchymatous encephalitis (dementia paralytica), *Brain*, **37**, 401.

MARTIN, J. P. (1925) Amyotrophic meningo-myelitis, *Brain*, **48**, 153.

MARTIN, J. P. (1948) Treatment of neurosyphilis with penicillin, *Brit. med. J.*, **1**, 922.

MEAGHER, E. T. (1929) *General Paralysis and its Treatment by Induced Malaria* (Board of Control), London.

MERRITT, H. H., ADAMS, R. D., and SOLOMON, H. C. (1946) *Neurosyphilis*, New York.

MERRITT, H. H., and MOORE, M. (1935) Acute syphilitic meningitis, *Medicine (Baltimore)*, **14**, 119.

MONTGOMERY, C. H., and KNOX, J. M. (1959) Antibiotics other than penicillin in the treatment of syphilis, *New Engl. J. Med.*, **261**, 277.

MOORE, J. E. (1932) The syphilitic optic atrophies, *Medicine (Baltimore)*, **11**, 263.

MOORE, J. E. (1953) The effect of adrenocortical hormones on the lightning pains and visceral crises of tabes dorsalis, *Amer. J. Syph.*, **37**, 226.

MORITZ, A. R. (1928) Tabische Arthropathie, *Virchows Arch. path. Anat.*, **267**, 746.

NAGEOTTE, J. (1894) La lésion primitive du tabes, *Bull. Soc. Anat. de Paris*, **69**, 808.

NELSON, R. A., and DUNCAN, L. (1945) Acute syphilitic meningitis treated with penicillin, *Amer. J. Syph.*, **29**, 141.

NICOL, W. D. (1948) Neurosyphilis, *Postgrad. med. J.*, **24**, 25.

NICOL, W. D., and WHELEN, M. (1947) Penicillin in the treatment of neurosyphilis, *Proc. roy. Soc. Med.*, **40**, 684.

NIELSEN, A., and IDSOE, O. (1962) *Evaluation of the Fluorescent Treponemal Antibody Test (FTA)*, W.H.O. Monograph No. 102.

OBERSTEINER, H., and REDLICH, E. (1894-5) Ueber das Wesen und Pathogenese der tabischen Hinterstrangs Degeneration, *Arbeiten aus dem Hirnanatomischen Institut*, **2**, 158, and **3**, 192.

RICHTER, H. (1921) Zur Histogenese der Tabes, *Z. ges. Neurol. Psychiat.*, **67**, 1.

RIMBAUD, P. (1958) Le traitement des syphilis sérologiques asymptomatiques, *Sem. méd. (Paris)*, **34**, 1209.

ROSE, A. S., and CARMEN, L. R. (1951) Clinical follow-up studies of 130 cases of long-standing paretic neurosyphilis treated with penicillin, *Amer. J. Syph.*, **35**, 278.

RUDOLF, G. DE M. (1927) *Therapeutic Malaria*, London. (Contains nearly 400 references.)

SCHACHTER, M. (1959) Etude clinique-psychologique d'un cas de paralysie generale juvenile chez une debile mentale, *Giornale di Psichiatria e di Neuropatologia*, **4**, 1149.

SPITZER, H. (1926) Zur Pathogenese der Tabes dorsalis, *Arb. neurol. Inst. Univ. Wien*, **28**, 227.

STERN, R. O. (1932) Certain pathological aspects of neurosyphilis, *Brain*, **55**, 145.

STEWART, R. M. (1933) Juvenile types of general paralysis, *J. ment. Sci.*, **79**, 602.

THOMAS, E. W. (1964) Some aspects of neurosyphilis, *Med. Clin. N. Amer.*, **48**, 699.

WILKINSON, A. E. (1963) The fluorescent treponemal antibody test in the serological diagnosis of syphilis, *Proc. roy. Soc. Med.*, **56**, 478.

WILNER, E., and BRODY, J. A. (1968) Prognosis of general paresis after treatment, *Lancet*, **ii**, 1370.

WILSON, S. A. K., and COBB, S. (1924-5) Mesencephalitis syphilitica, *J. Neurol. Psychopath.*, **5**, 44.

10

VIRUS INFECTIONS OF THE NERVOUS SYSTEM

GENERAL CONSIDERATIONS

THE NATURE OF VIRUSES

THE term 'neurotropic virus' has been used to describe minute filterable pathogenic agents which attack the nervous system. The first neurotropic virus, the causal organism of rabies, was discovered by Pasteur in 1884, and poliomyelitis was shown to be due to a neurotropic virus in 1909. During recent years the causal organisms of many other nervous diseases, both in man and in animals, have been found to be neurotropic viruses. Recent work has, however, shown that the distinction between neurotropic and non-neurotropic viruses according to whether or not the nervous system is the primary or secondary site of attack by the disease process is largely artificial (Harter, 1973). Most viruses which attack the nervous system do so after multiplying in other organs; involvement of the nervous system results from haematogenous spread or retrograde dissemination along nerve fibres after endocytosis at axonal terminals (Blinzinger and Anzil, 1974).

Viruses have been classified according to their nucleic acid content, size, sensitivity to lipid solvents, morphology, and method of development in cells. Most consist of a single form of nucleic acid associated with a protein coat; if the nucleic acid is DNA, the virus is usually double-stranded, like herpes simplex, if RNA it is single-stranded like poliovirus. DNA virus replication is like that of any cellular organism and these viruses act by transcription to messenger RNA and then translation to polypeptides and protein. RNA virus replication may be direct, by the formation of a complementary RNA strand, or indirect, by reverse transcription to a DNA provirus template from which identical RNA strands are then transcribed; RNA viruses act directly as messenger RNA (Legg, 1975). Viruses of virtually every known animal group have caused neurological illness in animals or man [see TABLE 10.1]. Their effects vary depending upon the nature of the virus, the human or experimental conditions relating to infection, and various complex immunological responses. They have been known to produce neoplastic transformation (as in Burkitt's lymphoma in man and brain tumours in various animals), a variety of developmental abnormalities if infection is prenatal or neonatal, including microcephaly, cerebellar hypoplasia, and aqueduct stenosis leading to hydrocephalus (Johnson, 1968; Raine and Fields, 1973) as well as the more typical acute inflammatory changes normally associated with viral infections. Most viruses appear to be obligatory intracellular parasites so that they damage the nervous system by attacking ganglion cells or, sometimes, glial cells; some show an affinity for specific cells or areas of the nervous system, so that poliovirus attacks principally motor neurones, herpes simplex virus the temporal and frontal lobes, and some myxoviruses attack ependymal cells (Harter, 1973). Pathologically they pro-

TABLE 10.1

VIRAL INFECTIONS OF THE NERVOUS SYSTEM
(modified from Harter, 1973)

	Some representative viruses causing neurological disease in man and animals
RNA viruses	
Picornavirus	Poliovirus
	Coxsackie virus
	ECHO viruses
Arbovirus	Equine encephalomyelitis
	St. Louis encephalitis
	Japanese B encephalitis
	California encephalitis
	Tick-borne encephalitis (including louping-ill)
Myxovirus	Influenza
Paramyxovirus	Measles (and subacute sclerosing panencephalitis)
	Mumps
	Canine distemper
Arenavirus	Lymphocytic choriomeningitis
Rhabdovirus	Rabies
Unclassified	Rubella
DNA viruses	
Herpes viruses	Herpes simplex
	Varicella-zoster
	Cytomegalovirus
	Epstein–Barr virus (infectious mononucleosis)
Papova virus	Progressive multifocal leucoencephalopathy
Poxvirus	Vaccinia
Unidentified presumed viral illnesses	Encephalitis lethargica
	Kuru
	Creutzfeld–Jakob disease
	Scrapie

duce chromatolysis followed by necrosis and neuronophagia, microglial pro-liferation, perivascular cellular infiltration, meningeal inflammation, and inclusion bodies in nerve or glial cells in various combinations.

Most epidemic forms of viral encephalomyelitis are due to picornaviruses (enteroviruses) or arboviruses; the latter multiply in mosquitoes or ticks before infecting man [see TABLE 10.1]. Neurological disease due to viruses of other groups usually occurs sporadically as part of a viral disorder involving primarily other organs or systems. Thus it has been known for some time that the neuro-logical complications of mumps are due to invasion of the nervous system by the causal virus; however, it has long been thought that encephalomyelitis com-plicating other childhood exanthemata (e.g. measles) or following vaccination against smallpox is due to an allergic or hypersensitivity reaction of the nervous system so that these disorders have been classified traditionally with the demyelinating diseases, as in this volume (CHAPTER 11). However, the recent isolation of measles virus from the brain of a patient with measles encephalitis (ter Meulen *et al.*, 1972) has suggested that these disorders, too, may ultimately prove to be due to viral invasion rather than hypersensitivity.

Much interest has been aroused in recent years by the concept of 'slow virus' infections. Thus it is now evident that subacute sclerosing panencephalitis is due to the long persistence of measles virus in the brain for many years after the initial infection. Kuru, a progressive and fatal disorder of the nervous system seen in the eastern highlands of New Guinea, is due to an unidentified transmissible agent, presumably viral, which shows some affinities with those responsible for subacute spongiform encephalopathy (Creutzfeld–Jakob disease) and for scrapie, a disease of sheep; all three disorders have a long incubation period after initial inoculation. Progressive multifocal leukoencephalopathy (due to polyoma virus) and cytomegalic inclusion body disease are other slow virus infections.

Viral infections can be diagnosed by a variety of serological tests involving complement fixation, haemagglutination–inhibition or antibody neutralization reactions, or by the inoculation of blood, nasopharyngeal exudates, faeces, or cerebrospinal fluid into animals or tissue culture systems. If a viral agent is isolated, final identification depends upon neutralization of specific antiserum. Immunofluorescent techniques for the identification of specific antibodies can be applied to brain biopsy sections or to cells isolated from the cerebrospinal fluid (Dayan and Stokes, 1973; Lindeman *et al.*, 1974; Legg, 1975).

REFERENCES

BLINZINGER, K., and ANZIL, A. P. (1974) Neural route of infection in viral diseases of the central nervous system, *Lancet*, **ii**, 1374.

DAYAN, A. D., and STOKES, M. I. (1973) Rapid diagnosis of encephalitis by immunofluorescent examination of cerebrospinal fluid cells, *Lancet*, **i**, 177.

FARKAS, E. (1970) Encephalitides and encephalopathies arising in the course of virus infections; anatomical considerations, chap. 6 in *Clinical Virology*, ed. Debré, R., and Celers, J., Philadelphia.

FERRER, F., and WHITE, D. O. (1970) *Medical Virology*, New York.

FIELDS, W. S., and BLATTNER, R. J. (1958) *Viral Encephalitis*, Springfield, Ill.

GEAR, J. (1949) Virus diseases of the central nervous system, *J. Neurol. Neurosurg. Psychiat.*, **12**, 66.

HARTER, D. (1973) Viral infections, in *A Textbook of Neurology*, by Merritt, H. H., 5th ed., New York.

HORSFALL, F. L., and TAMM, I. (1965) *Viral and Rickettsial Infections of Man*, 4th ed., Philadelphia.

JOHNSON, R. T. (1968) Mumps virus encephalitis in the hamster: studies of the inflammatory response and noncytopathic infection of neurons, *J. Neuropath. exp. Neurol.*, **27**, 80.

LEGG, N. (1975) How viruses affect the nervous system, in *Modern Trends in Neurology—6*, ed. Williams, D., London.

LINDEMANN, J., MÜLLER, W. K., VERSTEEG, J., BOTS, G. T. A. M., and PETERS, A. C. B. (1974) Rapid diagnosis of meningoencephalitis, encephalitis, *Neurology (Minneap.)*, **24**, 143.

TER MEULEN, V., MÜLLER, D., KÄCKELL, Y., KATZ, M., and MEYERMANN, R. (1972) Isolation of infectious measles virus in measles encephalitis, *Lancet*, **ii**, 1172.

MILLER, J. D., and ROSS, C. A. C. (1968) Encephalitis: a four-year survey, *Lancet*, **i**, 1121.

RAINE, C. S., and FIELDS, B. N. (1973) Neurotropic viruses and the developing brain, *N.Y. State J. Med.*, **73**, 1169.

EPIDEMIC ENCEPHALITIS LETHARGICA

Synonyms. Epidemic encephalitis, type A; 'sleepy sickness'.

Definition. An epidemic disease probably due to a neurotropic virus with an acute, subacute, or insidious onset and in most cases a chronic course, and characterized pathologically by inflammatory and degenerative changes, especially in the grey matter of the midbrain, and clinically in the acute stage by disturbance of the sleep rhythm, especially lethargy, and pupillary abnormalities, and in the chronic stage by the Parkinsonian syndrome.

AETIOLOGY

Encephalitis lethargica was first described by von Economo in May 1917, and about the same time by Cruchet, Moutier, and Calmette. It seems to have made its first appearance in 1915, though some authorities believe that previous epidemics can be recognized in medical historical texts. During the next decade widespread epidemics occurred, but now an illness with all the characteristic clinical features is virtually unknown. It affects the sexes equally and no age is exempt, though it is commonest in early adult life. There was a seasonal incidence, most cases occurring in the first quarter of the year. The disease was clearly contagious, though only feebly so. There was no evidence for its transmission by non-human agencies. Numerous attempts to isolate a causative organism have failed, but there is little doubt that it is due to a virus. Outbreaks of epidemic hiccup sometimes coincided with epidemics of encephalitis lethargica, and it is possible that both were due to the same organism.

PATHOLOGY

The macroscopic changes in the nervous system were slight, consisting, in the acute stage, of congestion, oedema, and sometimes petechial haemorrhages. Microscopically [FIGS. 97 and 98] perivascular changes were conspicuous. The smaller vessels exhibited perivascular cuffs or sleeves of inflammatory cells, chiefly lymphocytes and plasma cells. In addition the nerve tissue was diffusely infiltrated with mononuclear cells, and the nerve cells themselves showed degenerative changes. In the chronic stages there was little evidence of inflammatory reaction, but degeneration of nerve cells continued. In the acute stage the principal changes were in the grey matter of the upper midbrain, the region of the oculomotor nuclei, and the substantia nigra. The basal ganglia, the pons, and medulla were affected next in frequency. No part of the nervous system was exempt, and the spinal cord was sometimes affected. In the chronic stage also the degenerative changes were diffuse. The substantia nigra usually suffered severely, but the grey matter of the cerebral cortex and basal ganglia was involved. The Parkinsonian syndrome, a common sequel of encephalitis lethargica, was largely the result of damage to the substantia nigra.

SYMPTOMS

The symptoms of encephalitis lethargica have changed remarkably in 60 years. When it first appeared it was an acute disease, often with a fulminating onset. After several years the acute stage became less severe and the chronic stage more prominent. It is now doubtful if acute cases ever occur, and fresh cases of post-encephalitic Parkinsonism are probably the outcome of infection acquired in the past, possibly even 40 or more years ago. Many authorities

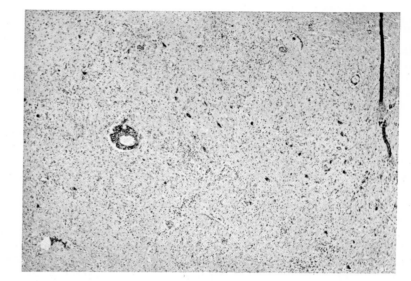

FIG. 97. Encephalitis lethargica. Substantia nigra showing perivascular and
diffuse inflammatory infiltration. H & E, ×36

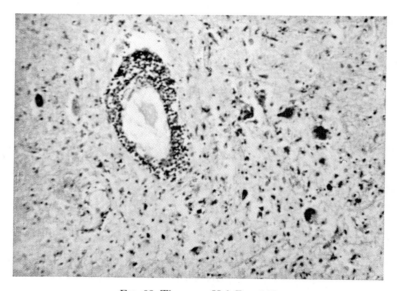

FIG. 98. The same. H & E, ×145

believe that the disease has died out, although sporadic cases showing some features of the condition are rarely seen. Espir and Spalding (1956) reported three possible cases of the disease occurring in British soldiers serving in Western Germany. Bojinov (1971) described 11 cases of an encephalitis causing an acute Parkinsonian syndrome developing in patients aged from 4 to 33 years of age. The illness developed acutely with the symptoms reaching maximum severity in one to three weeks; four patients died and autopsy revealed bilateral inflammatory necrosis of the substantia nigra, but the other seven improved, four recovering completely. In most patients there was a mild lymphocytic pleocytosis in the cerebrospinal fluid but attempts to isolate a causal virus and serological tests were all negative. Whether this illness could be construed as being due to a virus akin to that of encephalitis lethargica which has become modified in its clinical effects can only be a matter of speculation. If it is true that the disease no longer exists, then no new cases of post-encephalitic Parkinsonism are likely to be seen in the future.

Symptoms of the Acute Stage

The onset was sudden or gradual. In the early epidemics it was often fulminating and characterized by headache, vertigo, delirium, convulsive and apoplectic phenomena, and severe pain in the trunk or limbs. Later the onset became more gradual. The three most constant symptoms of the acute stage were headache, disturbance of sleep rhythm, and visual abnormalities, such as blurred vision or diplopia. The headache was not usually severe and was occasionally accompanied by vomiting or by pain in the back or limbs. The characteristic disturbance of sleep rhythm was lethargy by day with insomnia or restlessness at night. The lethargy was sufficiently constant to contribute the epithet 'lethargica' to the name of the disease. The patient could always be roused, except when lethargy passed into coma. Neither lethargy by day nor insomnia by night was present in all cases. Either might dominate the picture throughout the 24 hours. Delirium and fever occurred only in the more severe cases.

Visual disturbances were common; papilloedema and optic atrophy were rare but the pupils were often abnormal, frequently being irregular and unequal. The reaction on accommodation was more often lost than that to light. Ptosis was frequent but usually slight. External ophthalmoplegia was common, the sixth nerve being most often affected. Nuclear and supranuclear ophthalmoplegias were less common, but all forms of conjugate ocular palsy were seen. Blurred vision, a common complaint, was usually due either to paresis of accommodation or diplopia.

Facial weakness was common and usually transitory, as were vertigo and nystagmus due to damage to vestibular nuclei. Bulbar symptoms were rare as were aphasia and hemiplegia, though slight corticospinal tract damage, indicated by unilateral or bilateral extensor plantar responses without gross weakness, was frequently encountered.

Extrapyramidal disturbances so typical of the chronic stage could also appear in the acute. A Parkinsonian facies was often seen, but the muscles were usually hypotonic and rarely rigid. Rigidity, when present, was catatonic: true Parkinsonian rigidity was never present in the acute stage. Choreiform movements were often seen between 1916 and 1922, as was myoclonus, of which hiccup was perhaps a special form. More often myoclonic jerks at any frequency from 10 to 80 contractions a minute occurred in the abdominal muscles but sometimes synchronous and painful myoclonus affected several limbs and the trunk. Static or intention tremor sometimes occurred; sensory loss was rare but a unilateral thalamic syndrome was reported. Signs of cerebellar or spinal cord dysfunction were also rare but a transverse myelitic form was described, as was polyneuropathy.

The tendon reflexes were often diminished in the acute stage. There was usually no sphincter disturbance unless the patient was comatose, when retention or incontinence of urine and faeces might occur.

Signs of meningeal irritation were rare and the cerebrospinal fluid was usually normal, though a slight excess of lymphocytes and a modest increase in protein and globulin was sometimes found. There was no constant abnormality of the colloidal gold curve.

After passing through the acute stage the disease sometimes became arrested or persisted as a chronic and slowly progressive disorder. The chronic progressive form of the disease could follow an acute attack, or else it developed insidiously, without being preceded by any acute symptoms. It seems probable that in these cases the infection persisted in a chronic form in some ways comparable to other 'slow virus' infections.

Symptoms of the Chronic Stage

Parkinsonism. This is described in CHAPTER 12, pages 579–600.

Sleep Disturbances. Lethargy or insomnia, or both, frequently outlasted the acute attack with persistent reversal of the sleep rhythm.

Mental Symptoms. Though dementia was reported in only 27 per cent of cases, if less severe degrees of impairment of mental efficiency were included this figure would have been much higher. In adults, nervousness, fatigability, inability to concentrate, anxiety, and depression often persisted for long periods. Behaviour disorders were common in children, who often became restless and unstable and exhibited abnormalities ranging from mere naughtiness to stealing, cruelty, acts of violence, and sexual offences, which often brought them into the hands of the police.

Ocular Abnormalities. Gross abnormalities, such as nystagmus, squint, and diplopia, persisted in only a few cases, but the patient often complained of blurred vision, due to defective muscle balance or weakness of accommodation. These symptoms were usually associated with slight inequality of the pupils and an impairment of pupillary reactions on accommodation, and less frequently to light. Oculogyric crises, one of the most striking sequelae, are described in the section on Parkinsonism.

Involuntary Movements. (1) Choreiform movements were at one time common in the acute stage but were rare in chronic cases. (2) Bradykinesias. This term was applied to slow, regular, rhythmical movements of large amplitude, involving the limbs and trunk. Other involuntary movements included (3) myoclonus, (4) tremor, and (5) dyskinesias, or complex co-ordinated rhythmical movements of the jaw, lips, tongue, and palate, and (6) torticollis.

Respiratory Disturbances. In chronic cases, disorders of respiratory rate and rhythm were common.

Metabolic and Endocrine Disorders. Metabolic and endocrine disorders due to hypothalamic involvement were rare but included obesity, genital atrophy, diabetes insipidus, and hyperthyroidism.

Epileptiform Convulsions. Epileptiform convulsions were an uncommon sequel of encephalitis lethargica.

DIAGNOSIS

Encephalitis lethargica was distinguished from other forms of encephalitis and from poliomyelitis and acute multiple sclerosis by the characteristic disturbance of sleep rhythm, the prominence of the ocular symptoms, and the rarity of convulsions and paralysis of the limbs; and from meningitis by the absence of cervical rigidity and Kernig's sign and frequently of an excess of cells in the cerebrospinal fluid. For the diagnosis of encephalitis from other conditions causing coma see page 1170, and for that of encephalitic Parkinsonism see pages 587–8.

PROGNOSIS

When it first made its appearance epidemic encephalitis lethargica was an acute illness. Today, if it occurs at all, the acute stage may pass unnoticed. The mean death-rate in one large series of over 2,000 cases was 38·2 per cent. Most patients who died in the acute stage did so during the first month, and fourteen days was the commonest length of a fatal attack. The mortality rate during the acute stage was highest in the first year of life and after the age of 70, and lowest between the ages of 20 and 30.

Complete recovery occurred in only about 25 per cent of cases. The remainder who survived the acute stage were more or less severely disabled, most of them being unable to carry on their usual occupations. Even after apparent recovery from an acute attack, the patient could suffer from relapses at intervals of a year or two before passing into the chronic stage; this could occur after an interval of twenty years or more after the acute attack.

The prognosis in Parkinsonism is described in CHAPTER 12, page 588.

TREATMENT

The Matheson Commission reported upon seventy-five methods of treating encephalitis lethargica, none of which influenced the course of the illness. All treatment was therefore symptomatic. Treatment in the chronic stage was also very disappointing but modern remedies may ameliorate post-encephalitic Parkinsonism [p. 593]. The treatment of mental sequelae of encephalitis in adults followed the usual lines. Children suffering from mental abnormality often required institutional treatment.

REFERENCES

BOJINOV, S. (1971) Encephalitis with acute Parkinsonian syndrome and bilateral inflammatory necrosis of the substantia nigra, *J. neurol. Sci.*, **12**, 383.

EAVES, E. C., and CROLL, M. M. (1930) The pituitary and hypothalamic region in chronic epidemic encephalitis, *Brain*, **53**, 56.

EBAUGH, F. G. (1923) Neuropsychiatric sequelae of acute epidemic encephalitis in children, *Amer. J. Dis. Child.*, **25**, 89.

VON ECONOMO, C. (transl. Newman, K. O.) (1931) *Encephalitis Lethargica: Its Sequelae and Treatment*, London.

ESPIR, M. L. E., and SPALDING, J. M. K. (1956) Three recent cases of encephalitis lethargica, *Brit. med. J.*, **1**, 1142.

HALL, A. J. (1924) *Epidemic Encephalitis*, Bristol.

HALL, A. J. (1931) Chronic epidemic encephalitis with special reference to the ocular attacks, *Brit. med. J.*, **2**, 833.

HALL, A. J., and YATES, A. G. (1926) Clinical report. Report of sub-committee on the Sheffield outbreak of epidemic encephalitis in 1924, *Spec. Rep. Ser. med. Res. Coun. (Lond.)*, No. 108, p. 29.

HOLT, W. L., Jun. (1937) Epidemic encephalitis. A follow-up study of two hundred and sixty-six cases, *Arch. Neurol. Psychiat. (Chic.)*, **38**, 1135.

LEVADITI, C. (1929) Etiology of epidemic encephalitis, its relation to herpes, epidemic poliomyelitis, and post-vaccinal encephalopathy, *Arch. Neurol. Psychiat. (Chic.)*, **22**, 767.

PARSONS, A. C. (1928) Report of an enquiry into the after-histories of persons attacked by encephalitis lethargica, *Min. Hlth Rep. publ. Hlth*, No. 49, London.

REIMOLD, W. (1925) Über die myoklonische Form der Encephalitis, *Z. ges. Neurol. Psychiat.*, **95**, 21.

RISER, M., and MERIEL, P. (1931) Les 'séquelles' neurologiques de l'encéphalite épidémique, *Rev. Oto-neuro-ophtal.*, **9**, 297, 323.

TURNER, W. A., and CRITCHLEY, M. (1925) Respiratory disorders in epidemic encephalitis, *Brain*, **48**, 72.

TURNER, W. A., and CRITCHLEY, M. (1927–8) The prognosis and the late results of post-encephalitic respiratory disorders, *J. Neurol. Psychopath.*, **8**, 191.

WIMMER, A. (1924) *Chronic Epidemic Encephalitis*, London.

Epidemic Encephalitis. Report of a survey by the Matheson Commission, New York, 1929.

Epidemic Encephalitis. Second report by the Matheson Commission, New York, 1932.

EPIDEMIC ENCEPHALITIS: JAPANESE TYPE B, ST. LOUIS TYPE, AND MURRAY VALLEY TYPE

Definition. These three varieties of epidemic encephalitis, one occurring in Japan and other Asian countries, another in the United States of America, and the third in Australia, have been shown to be due to neurotropic viruses. These viruses are distinct because no cross-immunity exists between them, but the epidemiology and the pathological and clinical features of the three diseases are so similar that they can conveniently be considered together.

AETIOLOGY

These diseases are all caused by arthropod-borne arboviruses which measure 60–75 mm in diameter. Of the large group of arboviruses, relatively few are encephalitogenic. The reservoir of these viruses in nature is probably in mammals, birds, or arthropods and the virus is usually transmitted to man by the bite of a mosquito or tick.

The Japanese encephalitis type B is caused by a virus which was first transmitted to monkeys by Hayashi. Kawamura and his fellow workers transmitted the virus to mice and monkeys and proved that it was filterable (Inada, 1937 *a* and *b*). These workers also showed that it was immunologically distinct from the virus of the St. Louis epidemic which was also transmitted to monkeys and mice by Muckenfuss *et al.* (1933) and Webster and Fite (1935). Russian autumnal encephalitis is now generally regarded as identical with Japanese type B encephalitis while the Murray Valley type (Australian X disease) which occurs in Australia and New Guinea is clinically indistinguishable from the Japanese variety and is due to a very similar but nevertheless distinctive virus. Also closely related are the so-called Russian tick-borne complex including Russian spring-summer encephalitis, West Nile encephalitis, and louping-ill (which is the only disease of this group to occur in Great Britain (Webb *et al.*, 1968) and in which the reservoir of infection is in the sheep).

EPIDEMIOLOGY

Eight epidemics of encephalitis occurred in Japan in various summers between 1871 and 1919, since when outbreaks have occurred every few years, and in 1935 there were 5,000 cases. The St. Louis epidemic occurred in 1933 when there were over 1,000 cases in the neighbourhood during the late summer. There were smaller outbreaks in other cities in the United States, including one in Toledo in 1934. In St. Louis relatively more cases occurred in the county than in the city. Multiple cases in the same family were not common. The incubation period appeared usually to be between 9 and 14 days. There was a marked preponderance of susceptibility among the elderly and aged, and a relatively small incidence in children but children are more commonly affected by the Japanese and Murray Valley types. Though mosquitoes have been demonstrated to be carriers both in the United States and in Japan, there is also evidence that the disease may be spread by human carriers and that the route of infection is the nose, from which the virus travels to the brain by the olfactory nerves. It has been shown that mosquitoes may infect patients with the viruses of St. Louis and Western equine encephalitis at the same time (Hammon, 1941).

PATHOLOGY

The pathological picture in the three diseases is identical except that Japanese observers have described small patches of softening in the brain which were not observed in the American epidemics, and in the Japanese B and Murray Valley types selective damage to Purkinje cells is seen. All levels of the nervous system may be affected, and severe inflammation is always observed in the brain stem, the basal ganglia, and the white matter of the hemispheres. The inflammatory changes are diffuse, involving the basilar part of the pons, the entire width of the medulla, the cortex and white matter of the cerebellum, the basal ganglia, and also the cerebral cortex (Löwenberg and Zbinden, 1936; Robertson, 1952). The brain shows ganglion-cell degeneration, diffuse, microglial and macroglial proliferation, and perivascular cuffing. Perivascular microglial nodes are common. Intranuclear inclusion bodies have been found in the cells of the tubular epithelium of the kidney.

SYMPTOMS

Several workers classify cases as (1) abortive, (2) mild, and (3) severe, including the fulminating cases. Abortive cases, with fever, headache, malaise, and recovery in a few days are occasionally seen in epidemics but are uncommon. The onset of the disease is usually acute with high fever, 40–40·6 °C, headache and stiffness of the neck, and within a few hours many patients develop mental confusion and tremor of the lips, tongue, and hands, Rigidity may involve the upper limbs or the whole body. Drowsiness is common but the patient may be hyperexcitable. In severe cases coma develops early. The optic discs are usually normal as are the pupils and their reactions. Nystagmus, facial palsy, monoparesis, and spastic tetraparesis are not infrequent.

The cerebrospinal fluid is usually clear and under increased pressure. There is an excess of cells, usually between 50 and 500 per mm³, predominantly lymphocytes. The globulin content is increased but the sugar is normal. The blood usually exhibits a moderate or striking polymorphonuclear leucocytosis.

DIAGNOSIS

Clinical diagnosis depends mainly upon recognition of an encephalitic illness in an endemic area after exposure to an insect vector. Laboratory diagnosis depends upon the recognition of complement-fixing and neutralizing antibodies which appear at about the seventh day (MacCallum, 1967; Hannoun *et al.*, 1970).

PROGNOSIS

In the St. Louis epidemic the mortality rate was 20 per cent. In the Japanese and Murray Valley epidemics it has been much higher, usually 50 to 60 per cent. The mortality rate increases after the age of 50. In favourable cases recovery is often rapid and complete. Many patients in the St. Louis epidemic had apparently recovered completely in from 10 to 14 days, but the disease sometimes ran a protracted course. A study by Bredeck *et al.* (1938) of survivors of the 1933 St. Louis epidemic showed that 66 per cent had made a complete recovery and only 6·3 per cent were physically unfit for work. Finley (1958) made similar observations in a follow-up of 350 cases.

PROPHYLAXIS AND TREATMENT

Prophylaxis consists of measures to eliminate insect vectors. Attempts to prepare specific protective vaccines have to date been unsuccessful. No specific treatment is known, and it is therefore purely symptomatic.

REFERENCES

BECKMANN, J. W. (1935) Neurologic aspects of the epidemic of encephalitis in St. Louis, *Arch. Neurol. Psychiat. (Chic.)*, **33**, 732.

BREDECK, J. F., BROUN, G. O., HEMPELMANN, T. C., McFADDEN, J. F., and SPECTOR, H. I. (1938) Follow-up studies of the 1933 St. Louis epidemic of encephalitis, *J. Amer. med. Ass.*, **111**, 15.

FINLEY, K. H. (1958) in *Viral Encephalitis*, ed. Fields, W. S., and Blattner, R. J., Springfield, Ill.

HAMMON, W. M. (1941) Encephalitis in Yakima valley: mixed St. Louis and Western equine types, *J. Amer. med. Ass.*, **117**, 161.

HANNOUN, C., SHIRAKI, H., and OSETOWSKA, E. (1970) Encephalitides due to arboviruses, in *Clinical Virology*, ed. Debré, R., and Celers, J., Philadelphia.

HORSFALL, F. L., Jun., and TAMM, I. (1965) *Viral and Rickettsial Infections of Man*, 4th ed., Philadelphia.

INADA, R. (1937 *a*) Recherches sur l'encéphalite épidémique du Japon, *Presse méd.*, **45**, 99.

INADA, R. (1937 *b*) Du mode d'infection dans l'encéphalite épidémique, *Presse méd.*, **45**, 386.

KAWAKITA, Y. (1939) Cultivation *in vitro* of the virus of Japanese encephalitis, *Jap. J. exp. Med.*, **17**, 211.

LÖWENBERG, K., and ZBINDEN, T. (1936) Epidemic encephalitis (St. Louis type) in Toledo, Ohio, *Arch. Neurol. Psychiat. (Chic.)*, **36**, 1155.

MACCALLUM, F. O. (1967) Arboviruses, in *Virus and Rickettsial Diseases of Man*, ed. Bedson, S., Downie, A. W., MacCallum, F. O., and Stuart-Harris, C. H., 4th ed., London.

MUCKENFUSS, R. S., ARMSTRONG, C., and McCORDOCK, H. A. (1933) Encephalitis: studies on experimental transmission, *Publ. Hlth Rep. (Wash.)*, **48**, 1341.

ROBERTSON, E. G. (1952) Murray Valley encephalitis: pathological aspects, *Med. J. Aust.*, **i**, 107.

ROBERTSON, E. G., and McLORINAN, H. (1952) Murray Valley encephalitis: clinical aspects, *Med. J. Aust.*, **i**, 103.

WEBB, H. E., CONNOLLY, J. H., KANE, F. F., O'REILLY, K. J., and SIMPSON, D. I. H. (1968) Laboratory infections with louping-ill with associated encephalitis, *Lancet*, **ii**, 255.

WEBSTER, L. T., and FITE, G. L. (1935) Experimental studies on encephalitis, *J. exp. Med.*, **61**, 103.

WOLSTENHOLME, G. E. W., and CAMERON, M. P. (1960) *Virus Meningoencephalitis*, Ciba Foundation Study Group No. 7, London.

EQUINE ENCEPHALOMYELITIS

Equine encephalomyelitis has been known in the United States for many years. In 1931 a neurotropic virus was first identified as the cause of an outbreak among mules in California, and a few years later a virus was isolated from an epizootic occurring in the Eastern states. These viruses, though similar, are immunologically distinct, and are known as the Western and Eastern strains; like those responsible for the disorders considered above and like those of Venezuelan encephalitis and a number of other disorders (see MacCallum, 1967; Hannoun et al., 1970) they belong to the arbovirus group. Numerous cases of human infection with these viruses have been observed, and in 1941 an epidemic of infection with the Western virus affected at least 1,700 persons in Minnesota and North Dakota with 150 deaths. It has been proved that various species of bird constitute a reservoir of infection, that a wood-tick also harbours the virus, and that mosquitoes can transmit it to man.

Pathological changes differ somewhat in the two forms. In the Western type the vessels of the nervous system are always much congested, and petechial haemorrhages may or may not be present. Both neutrophil and mononuclear inflammatory cells are present in the perivascular spaces and as focal or diffuse infiltrations. Small, discrete patches of demyelination are scattered irregularly throughout the entire brain. The nervous elements appear to suffer secondarily to these changes. The spinal cord may show disseminated involvement, mainly in the central grey matter. The meninges show little change as a rule.

In the Eastern variety, on the other hand, there is widespread involvement of nerve cells, ranging from early nuclear changes to complete disappearance. Polymorphonuclear infiltration of the brain is conspicuous and there is an inflammatory infiltration of the meninges, lymphocytes predominating.

The clinical features of the two diseases also differ. In the Western form the onset is sudden, with generalized headache, nausea, elevation of temperature, and lethargy. Focal signs of nervous involvement are usually absent, but there are stiffness of the neck, muscular weakness, and diminution of tendon reflexes. The spinal fluid shows a moderate, predominantly mononuclear, pleocytosis. The mortality rate is about 10 per cent. Most patients make a complete recovery in a week or two, but mental defect, epilepsy, and spastic palsies have been observed as sequels, especially in infants after perinatal infection and in young children (Finley, 1958; Aguilar et al., 1968). These features may be due to the effect of the virus upon cerebral development (Raine and Fields, 1973).

In the Eastern form, which chiefly attacks children, the onset is very abrupt with severe general symptoms; lethargy soon appears, passing into stupor or coma. Cervical rigidity and Kernig's sign are present. Aphasia, diplopia, and paralyses indicate damage to the brain. The spinal fluid contains many cells, often more than 1,000 per mm³, and polymorphonuclears may predominate.

There is a mortality rate of 65 per cent, and severe sequels are common in those who survive.

Prophylaxis is directed to the destruction of mosquitoes and protection from their bites. Treatment is symptomatic.

REFERENCES

AGUILAR, M. J., CALANCHINI, P. R., and FINLEY, K. H. (1968) Perinatal arbovirus encephalitis and its sequelae, chap. 13 in *Infections of the Nervous System*, ed. Zimmerman, H. M., A.R.N.M.D., vol. 94, Baltimore.

BAKER, A. B., and NORAN, H. H. (1942) Western variety of equine encephalitis in man, *Arch. Neurol. Psychiat. (Chic.)*, **47**, 565.

DAVID, W. A. (1940) A study of birds as hosts for the virus of Eastern equine encephalomyelitis, *Amer. J. Hyg.*, **32**, 45.

FINLEY, K. H. (1958) in *Viral Encephalitis*, ed. Fields, W. S., and Blattner, R. J., Springfield, Ill.

FOTHERGILL, N. D., DINGLE, J. H., FARBER, S., and CONNERLEY, M. L. (1938) Human encephalitis caused by the virus of the Eastern variety of equine encephalomyelitis, *New Engl. J. Med.*, **219**, 411.

HAMMON, W. H. (1941) Encephalitis in Yakima Valley: mixed St. Louis and Western equine types, *J. Amer. med. Ass.*, **117**, 161.

HANNOUN, C., SHIRAKI, H., and OSETOWSKA, E. (1970) Encephalitides due to arboviruses, in *Clinical Virology*, ed. Debré, R., and Celers, J., Philadelphia.

MACCALLUM, F. O. (1967) Arboviruses, in *Virus and Rickettsial Diseases of Man*, ed. Bedson, S., Downie, A. W., MacCallum, F. O., and Stuart-Harris, C. H., 4th ed., London.

RAINE, C. S., and FIELDS, B. N. (1973) Neurotropic viruses and the developing brain, *N.Y. State J. Med.*, **73**, 1169.

SYVERTON, J. T., and BERRY, G. P. (1941) Hereditary transmission of the Western type of equine encephalitis by the wood tick, Dermacentor Andersoni Stiles, *J. exp. Med.*, **73**, 507.

SUBACUTE SCLEROSING PANENCEPHALITIS

First described by Dawson (1933) and subsequently by van Bogaert (1945), who entitled the condition subacute sclerosing leuco-encephalitis, this condition became widely known as subacute inclusion body encephalitis as Dawson (1933) and subsequently Brain et al. (1948), Greenfield (1950), Foley and Williams (1953), and many others found characteristic acidophilic intranuclear and cytoplasmic inclusion bodies within affected neurones and glial cells. The distinctive pathological changes are first widespread degeneration of neurones with associated inflammatory changes, and secondly extensive gliosis. Connolly et al. (1967) found that antibody titres to measles virus rose in the serum during the course of the illness, while Dayan et al. (1967) and Lennette et al. (1968) demonstrated myxovirus-like particles in the brain of affected patients and Saunders et al. (1969) found lymphocyte transformation in response to measles antigen in such a case. Subsequently Horta-Barbosa et al. (1969) isolated measles virus from brain cell cultures of two patients and there is now general agreement that the condition is due to the long persistence of this virus in the brain after an attack of measles (Brody et al., 1972; Detels et al., 1973) though there are still a good many complex and unanswered virological and immunological problems to be resolved (*The Lancet*, 1972; Legg, 1975). It is also apparent that a similar clinical picture can rarely be due to the rubella virus (Townsend *et al.*, 1975; Weil *et al.*, 1975).

The disease runs a slowly progressive course of from 2 to 18 months in which three stages can be recognized. First the mood changes and there is some intellectual deterioration, sometimes accompanied by epileptic attacks or more often by recurrent myoclonic jerking. This is followed by progressive dementia leading to akinetic mutism often with complex involuntary movements. The third stage is one of decortication. The cerebrospinal fluid may show mild pleocytosis, a rise in protein, a paretic colloidal gold curve with increased gamma-globulin, and characteristic EEG changes have been described taking the form of complex generalized slow-wave complexes, recurring repetitively and often in time with the myoclonic jerks and separated by intervals of comparative electrical silence in the record (Cobb and Hill, 1950). Synthesis of oligoclonal IgG and measles antibody activity within the central nervous system have been shown by Link *et al.* (1973) and Mehta *et al.* (1975) have demonstrated measles-specific IgG in the serum of such cases. The disease has been reproduced in dogs (Notermans *et al.*, 1973), hamsters (Lehrich *et al.*, 1970; Raine *et al.*, 1974), and the ferret (Mehta *et al.*, 1975) by inoculation of brain material from human subjects.

The disease usually terminates fatally, but may become arrested and occasional cases of possible spontaneous recovery have been reported (Pearce and Barwick, 1964; Cobb and Morgan-Hughes, 1968). No treatment is known to be of value. Amantadine hydrochloride has been shown to be unsuccessful (Haslam *et al.*, 1969).

HERPES SIMPLEX ENCEPHALITIS

It has been known for many years that herpes simplex may occasionally cause an acute and fatal illness in neonates with encephalitic and multiple necrotic lesions in brain, liver, kidneys, adrenals, and other organs (Legg, 1975). The virus implicated is usually herpes simplex type II which is often found in the female genital tract (Pettay *et al.*, 1972) but occasionally a similar illness due to the type I strain which is responsible for oral and labial herpes is seen.

For many years occasional cases of acute necrotizing encephalitis have been reported in adults (Greenfield, 1950; Crawford and Robinson, 1957) and some such cases have been called limbic encephalitis because of selective and severe damage to the temporal lobes and often to other parts of the limbic system. However, some cases of so-called limbic encephalitis (Brierley *et al.*, 1960), especially when occurring in association with carcinoma (Corsellis *et al.*, 1968), have run a chronic course with severe and persistent loss of recent memory or sometimes severe dementia. Nevertheless, it has become clear in the last few years that most cases of acute necrotizing encephalitis with necrosis of one or both temporal lobes are due to herpes simplex virus Type I. The illness is usually explosive with coma, hyperpyrexia, convulsions, and often hemiparesis with other features suggesting a temporal lobe lesion. Often intracerebral haemorrhage or cerebral abscess is suspected and angiography may suggest a space-occupying lesion. The EEG sometimes shows periodic sharp wave discharges (Upton and Gumpert, 1970) but the changes are not pathognomonic (Illis and Taylor, 1972). Diagnosis may be confirmed by serological tests but for rapid confirmation brain biopsy followed by identification of the virus by immunofluorescence (Johnson, 1964), culture (Johnson *et al.*, 1972), or electron microscopy (Harland *et al.*, 1967; Joncas *et al.*, 1976) is more reliable. The mortality rate is high but more patients are now recovering with the aid of dexamethasone 5 mg four times daily to reduce oedema, and surgical decompression. The role of antiviral agents such as idoxuridine (80–200 mg/kg body weight daily by intravenous infusion) (Meyer *et al.*, 1970; Illis and Merry, 1972) and cytosine arabinoside (Sarubbi *et al.*, 1973) is still controversial; some believe that they have been of value (Marshall, 1967), others that they are of little value and have unacceptable toxic side-effects (Johnson *et al.*, 1972; Joncas *et al.*, 1976). In patients who recover, variable defects of memory and focal neurological signs may persist (Rennick *et al.*, 1973), but a few recover completely. Rarely a similar clinical picture may be due to Coxsackie B5 virus infection (Heathfield *et al.*, 1967), while it has also been reported that milder subacute encephalitic illnesses and even chronic limbic encephalitis may on occasion be due to herpes simplex (Corsellis *et al.*, 1975).

REFERENCES

BOGAERT, L. VAN (1945) Une leuco-encéphalite sclérosante subaigue, *J. Neurol. Neurosurg. Psychiat.*, **8**, 101.

BRAIN, W. R., GREENFIELD, J. G., and RUSSELL, D. (1948) Subacute inclusion encephalitis (Dawson type), *Brain*, **71**, 365.

BRIERLEY, J. B., CORSELLIS, J. A. N., HIERONS, R., and NEVIN, S. (1960) Subacute encephalitis of later adult life, mainly affecting the limbic areas, *Brain*, **83**, 357.

BRODY, J. A., DETELS, R., and SEVER, J. L. (1972) Measles-antibody titres in sibships of patients with subacute sclerosing panencephalitis and controls, *Lancet*, **i**, 177.

COBB, W. A., and HILL, D. (1950) Electroencephalogram in subacute progressive encephalitis, *Brain*, **73**, 392.

COBB, W. A., and MORGAN-HUGHES, J. A. (1968) Non-fatal subacute sclerosing leuco-encephalitis, *J. Neurol. Neurosurg. Psychiat.*, **31**, 115.

CONNOLLY, J. H., ALLEN, I. V., HURWITZ, L. J., and MILLAR, J. H. D. (1967) Measles-virus antibody and antigen in subacute sclerosing panencephalitis, *Lancet*, **i**, 542.

CORSELLIS, J. A. N., GOLDBERG, G. J., and NORTON, A. R. (1968) 'Limbic encephalitis' and its association with carcinoma, *Brain*, **91**, 481.

CORSELLIS, J. A. N., JANOTA, I., and HIERONS, R. (1975) A clinicopathological study of long-standing cases of limbic encephalitis. Paper presented to the Association of British Neurologists.

CRAWFORD, A. R., and ROBINSON, F. L. J. (1957) Necrotizing encephalitis, *Brain*, **80**, 209.

DAWSON, J. R. (1933) Cellular inclusions in cerebral lesions of lethargic encephalitis, *Amer. J. Path.*, **9**, 7.

DAYAN, A. D., GOSTLING, J. V. T., GREAVES, J. L., STEVENS, D. W., and WOODHOUSE, M. A. (1967) Evidence of a pseudomyxovirus in the brain in subacute sclerosing leucoencephalitis, *Lancet*, **i**, 980.

DETELS, R., BRODY, J. A., McNEW, J., and EDGAR, A. H. (1973) Further epidemiological studies of subacute sclerosing panencephalitis, *Lancet*, **ii**, 11.

FOLEY, J., and WILLIAMS, D. (1953) Inclusion encephalitis and its relation to subacute sclerosing leuco-encephalitis, *Quart. J. Med.*, **22**, 157.

GOSTLING, J. V. T. (1967) Herpetic encephalitis, *Proc. roy. Soc. Med.*, **60**, 693.

GREENFIELD, J. G. (1950) Encephalitis and encephalomyelitis in England and Wales during the last decade, *Brain*, **73**, 141.

HARLAND, W. A., ADAMS, J. H., and McSEVENEY, D. (1967) Herpes-simplex particles in acute necrotizing encephalitis, *Lancet*, **ii**, 581.

HASLAM, R. H. A., McQUILLEN, M. P., and CLARK, D. B. (1969) Amantadine therapy in subacute sclerosing panencephalitis: a preliminary report, *Neurology (Minneap.)*, **19**, 1080.

HAYMAKER, W., SMITH, M. G., BOGAERT, L. VAN, and DE CHENAN, L. (1958) Inclusion body encephalitis, in *Viral Encephalitis*, ed. Fields, W. S., and Blattner, R. J., Springfield, Ill.

HEATHFIELD, K. W. G., PILSWORTH, R., WALL, B. J., and CORSELLIS, J. A. N. (1967) Coxsackie B5 infections in Essex, 1965, with particular reference to the nervous system, *Quart. J. Med.*, **36**, 579.

HORTA-BARBOSA, L., FUCCILLO, D. A., LONDON, W. T., JABBOUR, J. T., ZEMAN, W., and SEVER, J. L. (1969) Isolation of measles virus from brain cell cultures of two patients with subacute sclerosing panencephalitis, *Proc. Soc. exp. Biol. Med.*, **132**, 272.

ILLIS, L. S., and MERRY, R. T. G. (1972) Treatment of herpes simplex encephalitis, *J. Roy. Coll. Phycns. Lond.*, **7**, 34.

ILLIS, L. S., and TAYLOR, F. M. (1972) The electroencephalogram in herpes-simplex encephalitis, *Lancet*, **i,** 718.

JOHNSON, K. P., ROSENTHAL, M. S., and LERNER, P. I. (1972) Herpes simplex encephalitis. The course in five virologically proven cases, *Arch. Neurol. (Chic.)*, **27**, 103.

JOHNSON, R. T. (1964) The pathogenesis of herpes virus encephalitis. I: Virus pathways to the nervous system of suckling mice demonstrated by fluorescent antibody stain, *J. exp. Med.*, **119**, 343.

JONCAS, J. H., BERTHIAUME, L., MCLAUGHLIN, B., and GRANGER-JULIEN, M. (1976) Herpes encephalitis: rapid diagnosis and treatment with antiviral drugs, *J. neurol. Sci.*, **28**, 203.

THE LANCET (1972) What's new in S.S.P.E.?, *Lancet*, **ii,** 263.

LEGG, N. (1975) How viruses affect the nervous system, in *Modern Trends in Neurology—6*, ed. Williams, D., London.

LEHRICH, J. R., KATZ, M., RORKE, L. B., BARBANTI-BRODANO, G., and KOPROWSKI, H. (1970) Subacute sclerosing panencephalitis: encephalitis in hamsters produced by viral agents isolated from human brain cells, *Arch. Neurol. (Chic.)*, **23**, 97.

LENNETTE, E. H., MAGOFFIN, R. L., and FREEMAN, J. N. (1968) Immunological evidence of measles virus as an etiologic agent in subacute sclerosing panencephalitis, *Neurology (Minneap.)*, **18**, 21.

LINK, H., PANELIUS, M., and SALMI, A. A. (1973) Immunoglobulins and measles antibodies in subacute sclerosing panencephalitis. Demonstration of synthesis of oligoclonal IgG with measles antibody activity within the central nervous system, *Arch. Neurol. (Chic.)*, **28, 23.**

MARSHALL, W. J. S. (1967) Herpes simplex encephalitis treated with idoxuridine and external decompression, *Lancet*, **ii,** 579.

MEHTA, P. D., TETLEY, A. J., and THORMAR, H. (1975) Measles antibodies and immunoglobulins in sera from patients with subacute sclerosing panencephalitis (SSPE) and from an infected ferret, *J. neurol. Sci.*, **26**, 283.

MEYER, J. S., BAUER, R. B., RIVERA-OLMOS, V. M., NOLAN, D. C., and LERNER, A. M. (1970) Herpesvirus hominis encephalitis. Neurological manifestations and use of idoxuridine, *Arch. Neurol. (Chic.)*, **23**, 438.

NOTERMANS, S. L. H., TIJL, W. F. J., WILLEMS, F. T. C., and SLOOFF, J. L. (1973) Experimentally induced subacute sclerosing panencephalitis in young dogs, *Neurology (Minneap.)*, **23**, 543.

PEARCE, J. M. S., and BARWICK, D. D. (1964) Recovery from presumed subacute inclusion-body encephalitis, *Brit. med. J.*, **2**, 611.

PETTAY, O., LEINIKKI, P., DONNER, M., and LAPINLEIMU, K. (1972) Herpes simplex virus infection in the newborn, *Arch. Dis. Childh.*, **47**, 97.

RAINE, C. S., BYINGTON, D. P., and JOHNSON, K. P. (1974) Experimental subacute sclerosing panencephalitis in the hamster: ultrastructure of the chronic disease, *Lab. Invest.*, **31**, 355.

RENNICK, P. M., NOLAN, D. C., BAUER, R. B., and LERNER, A. M. (1973) Neuropsychologic and neurologic follow-up after herpesvirus hominis encephalitis, *Neurology (Minneap.)*, **23**, 42.

R

SARUBBI, F. A., SPARLING, P. F., and GLEZEN, W. P. (1973) Herpesvirus hominis encephalitis. Virus isolation from brain biopsy in seven patients and results of therapy, *Arch. Neurol. (Chic.)*, **29**, 268.

SAUNDERS, M., KNOWLES, M., CHAMBERS, M. E., CASPARY, E. A., GARDNER-MEDWIN, D., and WALKER, P. (1969) Cellular and humoral responses to measles in subacute sclerosing panencephalitis, *Lancet*, **i**, 72.

TOWNSEND, J. J., BARINGER, J. R., WOLINSKY, J. S., MALAMUD, N., MEDNICK, J. P., PANITCH, H. S., SCOTT, R. A. T., OSHIRO, L. S., and CREMER, N. E. (1975) Progressive rubella panencephalitis: late onset after congenital rubella, *New Engl. J. Med.*, **292**, 990.

UPTON, A., and GUMPERT, J. (1970) Electroencephalography in diagnosis of herpes-simplex encephalitis, *Lancet*, **i**, 650.

WEIL, M. L., ITABASHI, H., CREMER, N. E., OSHIRO, L. S., LENNETTE, E. H., and CARNAY, L. (1975) Chronic progressive panencephalitis due to rubella virus simulating SSPE, *New Engl. J. Med.*, **292**, 994.

POLIOMYELITIS

Synonyms. Infantile paralysis; Heine-Medin disease.

Definition. An acute infective disease due to a virus with a predilection for the anterior horn cells of the spinal cord and the motor nuclei of the brain stem, destruction of which causes muscular paralysis and atrophy.

PATHOLOGY

In the acute stage naked-eye examination yields evidence of a general reaction to the infection in parenchymatous degeneration of the liver and kidneys, and a general enlargement of the lymphoid tissue of the body, including the lymph nodes of the alimentary canal. The spinal cord is congested, soft, and oedematous, and minute haemorrhages may be visible in the grey matter.

Histologically the changes in the nervous system are usually most marked in the grey matter of the spinal cord and medulla. The basal ganglia and cerebral cortex are little affected. In the cord the changes consist of degeneration of the anterior horn cells and an inflammatory reaction with small haemorrhages in the grey matter. The ganglion cells of the anterior horns show changes varying from slight chromatolysis to complete destruction with neuronophagia. The inflammatory reaction consists of perivascular cuffing, mainly with lymphocytes but with a smaller number of polymorphonuclear cells, and a diffuse infiltration of the grey matter, with similar cells and cells of neuroglial origin [FIG. 99]. The white matter may also show some perivascular infiltration. The meninges share in the inflammatory reaction, exhibiting infiltration with lymphocytes and endothelial cells.

Cortical lesions are similar but more focal, and inflammatory changes have been observed in the spinal dorsal roots and in the peripheral nerves. Rarely the brunt of the infection falls upon the brain stem (polioencephalitis). Focal necroses are found in the liver, and an inflammatory hyperplasia of the lymphoid tissue. The virus has been demonstrated in the walls of the pharynx, the small and large intestines and mesenteric lymph nodes, as well as in the nervous system.

Recovery from the acute stage is attended by restoration to normal of ganglion cells which have not been too severely damaged. Others disappear completely, and sections therefore show a paucity of cells in the anterior horns in the affected regions with secondary degeneration in the corresponding ventral roots and peripheral nerves. The affected muscles show varying degrees of neurogenic atrophy with a relative increase of connective tissue and fat.

AETIOLOGY

Our knowledge of the causative organism of poliomyelitis dates from the observation of Landsteiner and Popper in 1909 that the disease could be transmitted to monkeys, and it has since been shown to be an enterovirus. Detailed reviews of the virology and epidemiology have been given by MacCallum (1967), Cohen (1969), and Drouhet *et al.* (1970). Three strains of virus have now been isolated, known as 'Brunhilde' (Type 1), 'Lansing' (Type 2), and 'Leon' (Type 3). The virus was first grown in tissue culture by Enders *et al.* (1949). It is a spherical particle measuring 30 nm in diameter. The virus can

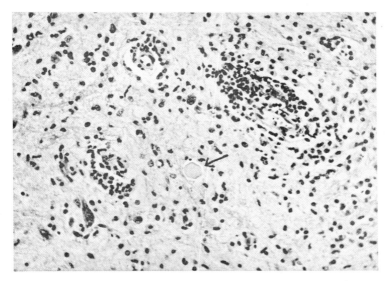

FIG. 99. Poliomyelitis. Anterior horn showing inflammatory infiltration and advanced chromatolysis of neurone (arrow). H & E, ×215

be obtained from the nasopharyngeal mucous membranes of patients in the acute stage, healthy contacts, and convalescents, and also from the stools. Monkeys can be successfully inoculated by direct intracerebral injection or by injection subcutaneously, intraperitoneally, into the lymph nodes, or into a nerve trunk, but the usual route of infection in man is from the alimentary tract, and it has been suggested that the virus reaches the nervous system by way of the autonomic nerves (Howe and Bodian, 1941 *a* and *b*, 1942). Fairbrother and Hurst (1930) showed that the virus travels along axis cylinders both in the peripheral nerves and in the central nervous system. However, it is now thought that spread by the blood or lymphocytic system is also common (Horstmann, 1952; Bodian, 1952) and that the pharynx is also a common portal of entry, especially from the raw tonsillar bed after tonsillectomy (Aycock and Luther, 1929). There is good evidence also that physical exertion during the stage of incubation may predispose to paralysis, particularly of those muscles which have been most used and paralysis may also develop in a limb which has been traumatized as by an injection. For these reasons prophylactic inoculations and tonsillectomy are generally abandoned during an epidemic and physical exercise is unwise in those unprotected individuals who have been exposed to infection (Russell, 1956). The virus is highly resistant to chemical agents, but sensitive to heat and to desiccation. It can readily be cultured in HeLa cells or monkey kidney cells, and a series of specific serological tests, including complement-fixing and antibody neutralization methods are available. Coxsackie A7 virus may produce a clinical illness indistinguishable from paralytic poliomyelitis.

EPIDEMIOLOGY

In Great Britain and the United States poliomyelitis occurs for the most part sporadically, but considerable epidemics occurred in the past. Wickman (1909) found that the spread of the disease could often be traced to an apparently healthy individual who had been in contact with a paralytic case but never himself developed it. Such healthy carriers and abortive cases, in which recovery occurs before the paralytic stage is reached, greatly outnumber the paralytic cases and are probably mainly responsible for the spread of the infection, though it can certainly be acquired from a paralytic case. There is evidence that most members of a household have been infected by the time a paralytic case appears, though multiple paralytic cases in a household occur in less than 10 per cent of infected families. For every person with symptoms there may be 10 to 100 infected individuals with no obvious illness. Infectivity is probably greatest in the viraemic phase. Some strains of virus have seemed much more virulent than others, as shown by the high incidence of paralysis and fatality in British and American troops in India and in the Philippines in 1944-5. Type I virus is generally more virulent than Types II and III. The virus has been demonstrated in the pharyngeal secretions and in the faeces of patients, in sewage, and in flies caught in the neighbourhood of infected cases. Personal contact and the faecal contamination of food appear to be the principal modes of transmission.

The seasonal incidence in the late summer and early autumn may be explained by these facts. Infants under the age of 1 year are rarely attacked. In a country where hygiene is poor most sufferers are between the ages of 2 and 4 years. After the age of 5 susceptibility rapidly diminishes, and after the age of 25 the disease is rare. During and after the Second World War in the U.S.A. and in Great Britain the age incidence rose steadily. In Massachusetts in 1907, 7 per cent of those affected were over the age of 15, in 1945, 25 per cent; and cases in adults became commoner (Horstmann, 1948). The incidence in adult white immigrants to South Africa was shown to be much higher than in the South African-born population of all races (Dean and Malk, 1967). Males suffer somewhat more frequently than females. The incubation period appears to be usually from 7 to 14 days, but may be as long as 5 weeks.

The last 20 years has seen a dramatic decline in the incidence of the disease in all countries in which campaigns of prophylactic inoculation have been carried out using first injections of the Salk (Salk, 1960) and British vaccines and subsequently the Sabin type oral attenuated live vaccine (Sabin, 1959). It seems probable that within the next decade the disease will virtually disappear.

SYMPTOMS

There are four possible ways in which a person may react to infection by the virus of poliomyelitis. (1) Exposure to the virus may lead to the development of immunity without any symptoms of illness. This may be termed subclinical or inapparent infection. (2) There are patients in whom the symptoms in the phase of viraemia are those of a mild general infection without involvement of the nervous system. These may be termed abortive cases. (3) Many patients, in some epidemics as many as 75 per cent, develop fever, headache, malaise, and often meningism, and at this stage show an excess of cells in the cerebrospinal fluid yet never develop paralysis. The infection is overcome in the pre-paralytic stage and these are called meningitic or non-paralytic cases. (4) Only in a minority does the infection run its full course and cause paralysis.

(1) Patients with subclinical infection have no symptoms. (2) Symptoms of the abortive type are indistinguishable from those of any other general infection unless serological tests are positive or the virus can be isolated. There remain to be considered the symptoms of: (3) the pre-paralytic stage; and (4) the stage of paralysis.

The Pre-paralytic Stage

In this stage two phases can often be recognized. The first symptoms of infection are fever, malaise, headache, drowsiness or insomnia, sweating, flushing, faucial congestion, and often gastro-intestinal disturbances such as anorexia, vomiting, and diarrhoea. This phase, the 'minor illness', which lasts one or two days, is sometimes followed by temporary improvement with remission of fever for 48 hours, or it may merge into the second phase, 'the major illness', in which headache is more severe and associated with pain in the back and limbs sometimes with muscle tenderness. The symptoms closely resemble those of other forms of viral meningitis.

Delirium may occur. The patient is often tremulous, and cervical rigidity and Kernig's sign may be observed. In the absence of such signs of meningeal irritation the 'spinal sign' is of occasional diagnostic value; attempted passive flexion of the spine may be prevented by pain. Convulsions may occur in infants in either of the first two phases.

In non-paralytic cases the patient recovers after exhibiting in mild or more severe form either or both of the phases of the pre-paralytic stage.

The Cerebrospinal Fluid

In the second phase the cerebrospinal fluid shows the changes of mild meningitis. The pressure is increased and there is an excess of cells, usually 50 to 250 mm^3. At first both polymorphonuclear cells and lymphocytes are present, but after the first week lymphocytes alone are found. The protein and globulin show a moderate increase, but the glucose content of the fluid is normal. During the second week the protein may rise to between 100 and 200 mg.

The Paralytic Stage

Spinal Form. The onset of paralysis, which is often ushered in by muscular fasciculation, usually follows rapidly upon the pre-paralytic stage, and is attended by considerable pain in the limbs and tenderness of the muscles on pressure. Exceptionally the pre-paralytic phase may last for a week or even two. The paralysis may be widespread or localized. In severe cases the muscles of the neck, trunk, and all four limbs may be powerless, except for a feeble movement here and there. When the paralysis is less extensive its asymmetry and patchy character are conspicuous features, and some muscles may be severely affected on one side of the body and escape on the other. Usually paralysis reaches its maximum within the first 24 hours, but less often it is progressive. In the ascending form it gradually spreads upwards from the legs, and endangers life through respiratory paralysis. A descending form is described. Sometimes the infection seems to smoulder on and fresh weakness may appear a week or more after the onset. The lower limbs are more often affected than the upper. In the former the quadriceps and the muscles below the knee suffer most, especially the peronei and the anterior tibial group. In the latter the small muscles of the hands are frequently involved. Movement of the intercostals and the diaphragm must be observed carefully. A useful test for early respiratory paralysis is to ask the patient to count aloud without taking a breath; if he cannot count beyond 12 to 15 there is serious respiratory insufficiency and appropriate measurements of forced expiratory volume should be carried out in order to confirm the probability that assisted respiration will be needed urgently.

Fortunately it is the rule that only a proportion of the muscles affected at the outset remain permanently paralysed. The disease produces temporary loss of function in many anterior horn cells which ultimately recover. Improvement usually begins at the end of the first week after the onset of paralysis. Like other causes of lower motor neurone paralysis, poliomyelitis leads to wasting of, and loss of cutaneous and tendon reflexes subserved by, the affected muscles, though tendon reflexes may be exaggerated briefly at the onset. Complete paralysis of the muscles around a joint may permit subluxation to occur. When opposing muscle groups are unequally affected, contractures are apt to occur in the stronger muscles, restricting movement at the joint. In the upper limb this most often happens at the shoulder after paralysis of the deltoid; in the lower limb, in the calf muscles, after paralysis of the peronei and anterior tibial group. Talipes equinovarus results from contracture of the calf. Asymmetrical palsy of spinal muscles causes scoliosis. The affected limbs are blue and cold and may be the site of oedema or chilblains. Fasciculation may continue for years in partially paralysed muscles. Bone growth is retarded in the paralysed limbs (Ring, 1957, 1958), and the bones show atrophy and rarefaction radiographically (Walton and Warrick, 1954).

Rarely the inflammation extends to the white matter of the lateral columns of the cord. Involvement of the spinothalamic tracts then causes impaired appreciation of pain, heat, and cold, and damage to the corticospinal tracts spastic paralysis. Except in such cases sphincter disturbance is rare and sensory loss is absent.

Brain Stem Form (Polioencephalitis). In a small percentage of cases the brunt of the infection falls upon the brain stem, leading to facial, pharyngeal, laryngeal, lingual, or very rarely ocular paralysis. Vertigo and nystagmus may occur and there is grave danger of involvement of the cardiac and respiratory centres. It is of great practical importance to distinguish embarrassment of respiration caused by the accumulation of saliva and mucus in pharyngeal paralysis from true paralysis of the muscles of respiration.

DIAGNOSIS

Diagnosis is rarely possible in the stage of constitutional disturbance, except in an epidemic. Even then suspicion cannot be confirmed until changes in the cerebrospinal fluid indicate that the nervous system is invaded. At this stage in sporadic cases the disease has to be distinguished from other causes of meningitis. In the acute pyogenic forms the glucose content of the spinal fluid is reduced, and the cells are exclusively polymorphonuclear. Mumps meningitis, which is also lymphocytic, is not likely to cause confusion if parotitis is present. Tuberculous meningitis may be difficult to distinguish but in this condition the onset is usually more gradual. The diagnosis, however, rests upon the examination of the spinal fluid, which in both may contain an excess of cells, both polymorphonuclear and lymphocytes, and an excess of protein. In poliomyelitis the sugar content of the fluid is normal; in tuberculous meningitis the sugar is invariably diminished. Tubercle bacilli if present are, of course, conclusive.

The spinal form of the disease in the paralytic stage is usually easy to diagnose. When the pain and tenderness are severe it may be confused with acute rheumatism and acute osteomyelitis. In these, however, the tenderness is more localized than in poliomyelitis and is in or near a joint. Moreover, the tendon reflexes are not lost as in poliomyelitis.

In adults poliomyelitis may need to be distinguished from acute transverse myelitis and from the Guillain–Barré syndrome, but in the former condition flaccid paralysis of the legs is associated with extensor plantar reflexes, sensory loss, and loss of sphincter control, and in the latter weakness is usually proximal and asymmetrical and the cerebrospinal fluid shows an increase in protein but rarely any pleocytosis.

When the patient is seen years after the acute attack the presence of muscular wasting may suggest motor neurone disease, syringomyelia, or myopathy. The fact that the wasting is not usually progressive, however, excludes all these alternatives. The absence of fasciculation also helps to distinguish it from the first named, and the absence of sensory loss from the second, while the wasting is usually too patchy and asymmetrical to simulate myopathy very closely.

The bulbar form must be distinguished from other forms of encephalitis. In encephalitis complicating the exanthemata and vaccination the primary cause is usually obvious, and the long tracts, both motor and sensory, are likely to be involved. Diagnosis from other viral encephalitides will usually depend upon serological tests and virus isolation.

PROGNOSIS

The mortality has varied in different epidemics from under 5 per cent to over 25 per cent. The cause of death is usually respiratory paralysis due to direct involvement of the respiratory centre in the bulbar form or to ascending paralysis involving the intercostals and diaphragm; mortality has been much lower since the introduction of refined methods of assisted respiration.

When the progress of the paralysis has ceased, it is safe to predict that considerable recovery will occur (Russell and Fischer-Williams, 1954). Favourable indications are the presence of voluntary movement, of reflex responsiveness, and of a muscular contraction evoked by nerve stimulation persisting three weeks after the onset of the paralysis. Improvement once begun may be expected to continue for at least a year and in some cases for even longer. The nature and extent of the remaining disability will, of course, depend upon the distribution of the residual paralysis; disability often increases to the extent of impairing mobility and employability solely as a consequence of the superimposition of the effects of ageing (Jennekens et al., 1971; Anderson et al., 1972). Late onset respiratory failure is also an uncommon sequel, often accentuated by kyphoscoliosis and sometimes heralded by prolonged alveolar hypoventilation (Lane et al., 1974). Second attacks, though very rare, are well authenticated but are usually due to a different strain of virus (Cohen, 1969).

Motor neurone disease is a rare sequel of acute anterior poliomyelitis, which it may follow after many years, the progressive wasting usually beginning in the region originally affected (Campbell *et al.*, 1969).

TREATMENT

General Management

Immediate and complete rest should be insisted on in every suspected case, however mild, since physical activity in the pre-paralytic stage increases the risk of severe paralysis (Russell, 1949, 1955).

Three categories of paralytic case require to be distinguished because in each form the treatment needed is different. These are: (1) the patient with neither respiratory nor bulbar paralysis; (2) the patient with respiratory paralysis with or without bulbar paralysis; and (3) the patient with bulbar paralysis.

The Treatment of a Patient without Respiratory and Bulbar Paralysis

During the acute stage plenty of fluid should be given. Lumbar puncture may be needed for diagnostic purposes and may help to relieve headache and backache. Aspirin in doses of 300–600 mg and sedatives, such as diazepam, will be required for the relief of pain and restlessness. Gentle passive movements are the only form of physical treatment which is permissible at this stage. Antibiotics are of no value except as a prophylactic against pneumonia in patients with respiratory paralysis, and immune globulin is valueless because as soon as the virus has reached the nervous system it is beyond the reach of antibodies.

For purposes of treatment the course of the disease after the onset of paralysis is divided into: (1) An acute stage, during which pain and tenderness of the muscles persist. This usually lasts for three or four weeks. (2) A convalescent stage, during which improvement in muscular power continues. This may last from six months to two years. (3) A chronic stage in those left with permanent paralysis after the maximum recovery has occurred.

The principal object in the treatment of the muscular paralysis in the acute stage is to prevent stretching of the paralysed muscles and contracture of their antagonists. If great care is not taken, damage may be done in a few days which it will take months to repair. The patient should be nursed on a firm bed and the limbs kept in the positions in which the paralysed muscles are relaxed (but not stretched) by means of sandbags and pillows.

During the stage of convalescence prolonged rest in bed will be necessary in severe cases, contractures being prevented by suitable splints if necessary. Passive movements should be carried out from the beginning so far as the patient will tolerate them. Except when the trunk muscles are severely paralysed the patient should as soon as possible be allowed to stand for a few minutes daily, but paralysis of spinal muscles requires prolonged recumbency or suitable spinal supports if severe spinal deformity is to be prevented. During convalescence active exercises are of great importance. They may need to be assisted or carried out in baths or in a sling-suspension apparatus. Passive movement is also necessary. The affected parts should be put through a full range of movement at least once, and if possible twice, a day. Adequate instrumental support for the spine and limbs may be required and both the physiotherapist and occupational therapist play an important role (Taylor, 1955). In the later stages contractures and deformities may require tenotomy or other surgical treatment, but these may often be avoided by adequate care during the acute stage.

In the chronic stage when oedema, cyanosis, and chilblains are trouble-some in the feet, lumbar sympathectomy may be helpful in improving the circulation.

Treatment of Respiratory Paralysis (with or without Bulbar Paralysis)

A patient suffering from respiratory paralysis needs to be treated by some method of artificial respiration which may be required for weeks, or even for months and occasionally indefinitely. As Beaver (1962) pointed out, the proper handling of respiratory failure is now so rewarding that it must be instituted as soon as respiratory insufficiency threatens. This is the case when the $p(CO_2)$ and $p(O_2)$ can be kept within normal limits only by excessive effort which may soon become exhausting. It was customary in the past when respiratory paralysis was not accompanied by pharyngeal paralysis, so that the patient could swallow his own secretions, to use either a cuirass or cabinet respirator. The cuirass applies external positive and negative pressure directly to the chest wall (Kelleher et al., 1952) while the cabinet, in which the entire patient other than the head is enclosed, works by applying negative pressure to the chest so that air is sucked into the lungs. The use of these respirators, once widely employed with excellent results, requires considerable skill (Bourdillon et al., 1950; Russell, 1956), but nowadays they have been largely abandoned in favour of intermittent positive pressure respiration applied either through a nasal or oral endotracheal tube through which the lungs are inflated (when respiratory paralysis is unlikely to last more than two or three days at the most) or through a cuffed tube inserted via a tracheostomy (Lassen, 1953; Smith et al., 1954; Beaver, 1962). Occasionally, when respiratory insufficiency is slight, and the patient can survive the hours of sleep without becoming dangerously hypoxic or hypercapnic, intermittent diurnal inflation of the lungs via a Bird type respirator with the nose occluded, via a mouthpiece held between the closed lips, is sufficient. Sometimes even simpler devices suffice (Lane et al., 1974). Whenever possible, assisted ventilation, if likely to be prolonged, should be carried out under expert supervision in an intensive care unit with regular monitoring of the blood gases in order to avoid under- or over-ventilation.

The great advantage of intermittent positive pressure respiration is that if pharyngeal (bulbar) paralysis is also present, the cuffed intratracheal tube effectively prevents the passage of pharyngeal secretions into the lungs and also prevents the inhalation of food and vomit. Infection is an important complication which requires the frequent use of appropriate antibiotics; pulmonary collapse may necessitate bronchoscopy and suction; acute dilatation of the stomach, once a common accompaniment of respiratory failure, is rare now that gastric intubation is routine. Patients on artificial respiration also require the usual care of the skin, bladder (often including catheterisation), and bowels.

Treatment of Bulbar Paralysis Alone

Russell (1956) and Lassen (1956) did much to clarify the treatment of bulbar paralysis in poliomyelitis. When this occurs in the absence of respiratory paralysis the danger to the patient arises from his inability to prevent fluids, or secretions in the pharynx, from being sucked into the lungs with inspiration. Vomiting, for example, may be followed by fatal inhalation. The dysphagia also leads to difficulty in feeding. The proper posture of the patient is all-important. He should be nursed in the semi-prone position, being turned from one side to the other every few hours, while the foot of the cot or bed should be raised to make an angle of 15 degrees with the horizontal. This posture should be relaxed for nursing or other purposes only for short periods under close supervision. Tracheostomy in such cases is rarely necessary except in the presence of bilateral abductor paralysis of the vocal cords. A mechanical sucker is required to remove pharyngeal secretions. After about 24 hours of starvation feeding should be carried out by an oesophageal catheter, preferably passed through the nose.

PROPHYLAXIS

Since the nasopharyngeal secretions, the urine, and the faeces of the patient may contain the virus barrier nursing is wise. Virus is present in the stools 3 weeks after the onset in 50 per cent of patients and 5–6 weeks after the onset in 25 per cent. It is not easy to say how long the patient remains infectious, but he should be isolated for at least 6 weeks.

During an epidemic residential schools should not be closed. For reasons given earlier it is uncertain whether closure of a school will modify the spread of the disease among those already exposed to it, and there is a risk that this course might disseminate the infection among younger and therefore more susceptible children. Children in an affected household should be isolated from other children for three weeks after the isolation of the patient. Modern techniques of immunization are so successful in halting epidemics that measures which were once traditional (e.g. the closure of swimming baths) are no longer needed. Operations on the ear, nose, and throat and inoculations should not be carried out during an epidemic, and dental extractions should be avoided if possible.

The protective value of the Salk vaccine was well established between 1950 and 1960. Three doses, which give 90 per cent protection, were given as a routine, and a fourth was often added later in special circumstances. Immunity induced by injection did not prevent colonization of the gut by wild virus; hence an immune person could still be a carrier. On the other hand, attenuated live vaccine, given orally, by multiplying in the gut blocks the entry of wild virus (Koprowski, 1960). Its capacity to confer immunity is now established and the Sabin type vaccine, given as one or two drops on a sugar lump, appears to confer almost total immunity for three years or more. In the United States it has been customary to give Type I vaccine first followed by a combination of Types II and III 6–8 weeks later, but tritypic vaccine is preferred in Great Britain and the latter type should certainly be used during an epidemic or after exposure to a paralytic case in an endemic area. In children and young adults, 'booster' doses at regular intervals are recommended.

REFERENCES

AFFELDT, J. E. (1954) Recent advances in the treatment of poliomyelitis, *J. Amer. med. Ass.*, **156**, 12.

ANDERSON, A. D., LEVINE, S. A., and GELLERT, H. (1972) Loss of ambulatory ability in patients with old anterior poliomyelitis, *Lancet*, **ii**, 1061.

AYCOCK, W. L., and LUTHER, E. H. (1929) The occurrence of poliomyelitis following tonsillectomy, *New Engl. J. Med.*, **200**, 164.

BEAVER, R. (1962) The management of respiratory failure, in *Modern Trends in Neurology*, vol. 3, ed. Williams, D., London.

BODIAN, D. (1952) A reconsideration of the pathogenesis of poliomyelitis, *Amer. J. Hyg.*, **55**, 414.

BOURDILLON, R. B., DAVIES-JONES, E., STOTT, F. D., and TAYLOR, L. M. (1950) Respiratory studies in paralytic poliomyelitis, *Brit. med. J.*, **2**, 539.

CAMPBELL, A. M. G., WILLIAMS, E. R., and PEARCE, J. (1969) Late motor neuron degeneration following poliomyelitis, *Neurology (Minneap.)*, **19**, 1101.

COHEN, A. (1969) *Textbook of Medical Virology*, Oxford and Edinburgh.

COX, H. R., CABASSO, V. J., MARKHAM, F. S., MOSES, M. J., MAYER, A. W., ROCA-GARCIA, M., and RUEGSEGGER, J. M. (1959) Immunological response to trivalent oral poliomyelitis vaccine, *Brit. med. J.*, **2**, 591.

DANE, D. S., DICK, G. W. A., McALISTER, J. J., and NELSON, R. T. (1960) Epidemic control of poliomyelitis with inactive virus vaccines, *Lancet*, **i**, 835.

DEAN, G., and MALK, M. (1967) Poliomyelitis among white immigrants to South Africa, *S.A. med. J.*, **41**, 294.

DROUHET, V., DEBRÉ, R., and CELERS, J. (1970) Laboratory diagnosis of enterovirus infections. Poliomyelitis: pathophysiology, and Poliomyelitis: prophylaxis, in *Clinical Virology*, ed. Debré, R., and Celers, J., Philadelphia.

ENDERS, J. F., WELLER, T. H., and ROBBINS, F. C. (1949) Cultivation of the Lansing strain of poliomyelitis virus in tissue culture, *Science*, **109**, 85.

FAIRBROTHER, R. W., and HURST, E. W. (1930) The pathogenesis of, and propagation of the virus in, experimental poliomyelitis, *J. Path. Bact.*, **33**, 17.

HALE, J. H., DORAISINGHAM, M., KANAGARATNAM, K., LEONG, K. W., and MONTEIRO, E. S. (1959) Large scale use of Sabin type 2 attenuated poliomyelitis vaccine in Singapore during a type 1 poliomyelitis epidemic, *Brit. med. J.*, **1**, 1541.

HORSTMANN, D. M. (1948) Problems in the epidemiology of poliomyelitis, *Lancet*, **i**, 273.

HORSTMANN, D. M. (1952) Poliomyelitis virus in blood of orally infected monkeys and chimpanzees, *Proc. Soc. exp. Biol. (N.Y.)*, **79**, 417.

HOWE, H. A., and BODIAN, D. (1941 a) The pathology of early, arrested and nonparalytic poliomyelitis, *Bull. Johns Hopk. Hosp.*, **69**, 135.

HOWE, H. A., and BODIAN, D. (1941 b) Poliomyelitis in the chimpanzee: a clinical-pathological study, *Bull. Johns Hopk. Hosp.*, **69**, 149.

HOWE, H. A., and BODIAN, D. (1942) *Neural Mechanisms in Poliomyelitis*, New York.

HURST, E. W. (1930) A further contribution to the pathogenesis of experimental poliomyelitis: inoculation into the sciatic nerve, *J. Path. Bact.*, **33**, 1133.

HURST, E. W. (1932) Further observations on the pathogenesis of experimental poliomyelitis: intrathecal inoculation of the virus, *J. Path. Bact.*, **35**, 41.

JENNEKENS, F. G. I., TOMLINSON, B. E., and WALTON, J. N. (1971) Histochemical aspects of five limb muscles in old age: an autopsy study, *J. neurol. Sci.*, **14**, 259.

KELLEHER, W. H., WILSON, A. B. K., RUSSELL, W. R., and STOTT, F. D. (1952) Notes on cuirass respirators, *Brit. med. J.*, **2**, 413.

KOPROWSKI, H. (1960) Historical aspects of the development of live virus vaccine in poliomyelitis, *Brit. med. J.*, **2**, 85.

KRAMER, S. D., HOSKWITH, B., and GROSSMAN, L. H. (1939) Detection of virus of poliomyelitis in nose and throat and gastro-intestinal tract of human beings and monkeys, *J. exp. Med.*, **59**, 49.

LANE, D. J., HAZLEMAN, B., and NICHOLS, P. J. R. (1974) Late onset respiratory failure in patients with previous poliomyelitis, *Quart. J. Med.*, **43**, 551.

LASSEN, H. C. A. (1953) A preliminary report on the 1952 epidemic of poliomyelitis in Copenhagen, *Lancet*, **i**, 37.

LASSEN, H. C. A. (1956) *Management of Life-Threatening Poliomyelitis*, Edinburgh and London.

MacCALLUM, F. O. (1967) Poliomyelitis, in *Virus and Rickettsial Diseases of Man*, ed. Bedson, S., Downie, A. W., MacCallum, F. O., and Stuart-Harris, C. H., 4th ed., London.

MURPHY, D. P., DRINKER, C. K., and DRINKER, P. (1931) The treatment of respiratory arrest in the Drinker respirator, *Arch. intern. Med.*, **47**, 424.

PAUL, J. R., TRASK, J. W., BISHOP, M. B., MELNICK, J. L., and CASEY, A. E. (1941) The detection of poliomyelitis virus in flies, *Science*, **94**, 395.

RING, P. A. (1957) Shortening and paralysis in poliomyelitis, *Lancet*, **ii**, 980.

RING, P. A. (1958) Prognosis of limb inequality following paralytic poliomyelitis, *Lancet*, **ii**, 1306.

RUSSELL, W. R. (1949) Paralytic poliomyelitis, *Brit. med. J.*, **1**, 465.

RUSSELL, W. R. (1955) The management of acute poliomyelitis, in *W.H.O. Monograph Series* No. 26, p. 137, Geneva.

RUSSELL, W. R. (1956) *Poliomyelitis*, 2nd ed., London.

RUSSELL, W. R., and FISCHER-WILLIAMS, M. (1954) Recovery of muscular strength after poliomyelitis, *Lancet*, **i**, 330.

SABIN, A. B. (1959) Present position of immunization against poliomyelitis with live virus vaccines, *Brit. med. J.*, **1**, 663.

SALK, J. E. (1960) Persistence of immunity after administration of formalin-treated poliovirus vaccine, *Lancet*, **ii**, 715.

SEDDON, H. J. (1947) The early treatment of poliomyelitis, *Brit. med. J.*, **2**, 319.

SMITH, A. C., SPALDING, J. M. K., and RUSSELL, W. R. (1954) Artificial respiration by intermittent positive pressure in poliomyelitis and other diseases, *Lancet*, **i**, 939.

TAYLOR, R. A. R. (1955) *Poliomyelitis and Polioencephalitis*, London.

TRASK, J. D., VIGNEC, A. J., and PAUL, J. R. (1938) Poliomyelitis virus in human stools, *J. Amer. med. Ass.*, **111**, 6.

WALTON, J. N., and WARRICK, C. K. (1954) Osseous changes in myopathy, *Brit. J. Radiol.*, **27**, 1.

WICKMAN, I. (1909) *Beitrage zur Kenntnis der Heine-Medinschen Krankheit*, Berlin.

WORLD HEALTH ORGANIZATION EXPERT COMMITTEE ON POLIOMYELITIS, First Report (1954) *Wld Hlth Org. techn. Rep. Ser.*, No. 81.

RABIES

Synonym. Hydrophobia.

Definition. An infection of the nervous system due to a virus communicated to man by the bite of an infected animal. The resulting encephalitis, which is almost always fatal, is distinguished by the characteristic pharyngeal spasm evoked by the attempt to drink.

AETIOLOGY

Rabies is due to a virus which is difficult to classify but is probably of the RNA type, is about 80–150 nm in diameter, and shows some resemblance to the myxoviruses. It is not strictly neurotropic as it is commonly found in mucus-secreting glands (such as the salivary glands) (MacCallum, 1967), but its most devastating effects are upon the central nervous system. It is communicated to man by the bite of an infected animal which carries the virus in its saliva. Most cases of human infection are due to dog bites, though bites of jackals, cats, and wolves are occasionally responsible. The bites of rabid horses and cattle hardly ever communicate the disease. An epidemic in Trinidad has been attributed to vampire bats which are believed to carry the infection from cattle to man. The virus of rabies has been isolated from a fatal case occurring in a human epidemic of encephalitis in Japan. The risk of infection is influenced by the severity of the bite and is much diminished when the individual is bitten through clothes, which to some extent free the animal's teeth from saliva. The virus, having entered the body, is transmitted only along the nerve trunks, moving in both directions.

PATHOLOGY

The pathological changes in the nervous system are in part those usually associated with virus infection. Severe degenerative changes are found in the ganglion cells of the cerebrospinal and sympathetic ganglia. The small vessels are narrowed with swollen endothelial cells, and marked perivascular round-cell infiltration. The ganglion-cell degeneration is more diffuse than the inflammatory reaction, and the ganglion cells of the cortex may be extensively affected. There is considerable microglial reaction and collections of inflammatory and glial cells known as Babes' nodes. The Negri body is of diagnostic importance. It is an acidophil inclusion body contained within the cytoplasm or protoplasmic processes of the ganglion cells. These bodies are most often found in the ganglion cells of the hippocampus, but are seen less often in the cortical pyramidal cells, the cerebellar Purkinje cells, and ganglion cells elsewhere. Negri bodies are not constantly present in human rabies nor in experimental infection in animals.

The pathological picture resulting from complications of rabies vaccination is different [see p. 532].

SYMPTOMS
Rabies in Animals

The first symptoms of rabies in the dog are a change in behaviour associated with perversion of appetite. The animal will gnaw and swallow paper, sticks, earth, and other unusual substances. This stage is followed by excitement, in which it will snap at and bite other animals. There is a flow of saliva from the mouth, and the bark often becomes high-pitched. After one or two days paralysis develops, beginning first in the hind limbs and spreading to the forelimbs and jaw. Muscular spasms may occur affecting the whole body. Emaciation is marked and death is almost invariable. In other animals, especially rodents and herbivora, the stage of excitement does not occur, and the symptoms are paralytic from the beginning; this paralytic form occurs in a small number of dogs.

Rabies in Man

The incubation period in man depends upon the distance of the infected lesion from the central nervous system. When the bite is on the head it is about 27 days, when on the arm 32 days, when on the leg 64 days, but these periods are liable to wide variation. During the incubation period there are no symptoms. Local pain in the bitten limb is often the first symptom. The first general symptom is depression, often associated with apprehension, and disturbed sleep. The next is pharyngeal spasm brought on by an attempt to drink and rapidly extending to involve both the ordinary and the accessory muscles of respiration, and later all the muscles of the body, often producing opisthotonus. When this stage is at its height not only the attempt to drink but the sound and even the thought of water will bring on the spasm, which may also be excited by other external stimuli, even a current of air. Salivation is excessive, and vomiting is common. A horror of water develops and hallucinations may appear. Even so, the human patient does not as a rule exhibit the impulse to bite characteristic of the rabid dog. Later the symptoms of excitement and the spasm diminish and may give place to terminal paralysis. Fever is usually present, and terminal hyperpyrexia may occur. Death may take place during the spasmodic stage from respiratory or cardiac failure, or the patient may die paralysed and in coma.

Rarely the spasms and mental excitement are absent and the symptoms are paralytic from the beginning, as in certain animals. An epidemic of paralytic rabies occurred in Trinidad in 1931. In such cases the clinical picture is that of ascending paralysis associated with loss of sphincter control. The upper limbs may or may not be affected and sensory loss is inconstant. Finally, bulbar paralysis leads to dysphagia, and death occurs from respiratory paralysis.

DIAGNOSIS

The diagnosis of typical rabies is usually easy on account of the history of the bite and the presence of the distinctive pharyngeal spasm. The condition must be distinguished from tetanus, the incubation period of which is shorter. The symptoms of tetanus unmodified by the injection of serum usually begin within 14 days of the injury and almost invariably within 3 weeks. Trismus is an early symptom and pharyngeal spasm is usually absent.

Hysteria may simulate hydrophobia in a patient who has been bitten by a dog thought to be rabid. In hysteria, however, true pharyngeal spasm does not occur and the condition is usually amenable to drugs and suggestion.

The paralytic form of rabies should offer no diagnostic difficulty when there is a history of a bite, but in cases such as those in Trinidad, when the mode of infection is obscure, the diagnosis may be established only by means of animal inoculation. More recently, it has been shown that the diagnosis may be confirmed by finding specific fluorescence in corneal impression smears, skin or brain biopsies, or by detecting fluorescent antibody in serum (*British Medical Journal*, 1975).

PROGNOSIS

The risk of contracting rabies is estimated at about 5 per cent of individuals bitten by animals supposed to be rabid. Adequate prophylactic treatment reduces this incidence to about 1·5 per cent. The mortality rate is almost 100 per cent, but very occasional patients treated with curarisation and assisted ventilation have recovered (Hattwick *et al.*, 1972).

PROPHYLAXIS AND TREATMENT

The prophylactic treatment of rabies introduced by Pasteur is still carried out, though it has been modified in various details. It consists of successive doses of a vaccine derived from animals which have been infected with the virus. The vaccine may consist of living or dead virus from the cord or brain of infected animals and may be given alone or combined with antiserum. The Semple vaccine prepared from rabbit brain is still widely used. A vaccine free from brain tissue and prepared in duck embryos was introduced in the United States and is given in a course of 14 daily injections to the individual exposed to infection. The indications for vaccine treatment were set out in the report of the W.H.O. Committee (1966). The administration should be begun as early as possible after the bite. The long incubation period of rabies permits the development of an acquired immunity after infection. The prophylactic vaccine treatment of rabies is thus analogous to the vaccination of individuals after exposure to smallpox. The risk of producing acute or subacute demyelinating encephalomyelitis as a complication of the treatment [p. 532] should be borne in mind and treatment interrupted if this is suspected. Though complications have been most frequent following the use of vaccines prepared in brain or spinal cord tissue (Gibbs *et al.*, 1961), a case of transverse myelitis following the use of the duck embryo vaccine has been described (Prussin and Katabi, 1964) and other neurological complications have been reported, including an illness resembling the Guillain–Barré syndrome (MacCallum, 1967; Mozer *et al.*, 1973). The Flury vaccine made from living but attenuated virus is successful in protecting animals (Koprowski and Cox, 1948) but has not been thought safe enough for use in man; passive immunity conferred by hyper-immune gamma-globulin is now given as a rule with vaccine but only gives short-term protection. Newer vaccines are now being developed; the inactivated vaccine grown in the human diploid strain WI-38 (Wiktor *et al.*, 1964) seems likely to be the safest and most effective yet produced and is being progressively refined (Wiktor *et al.*, 1973). It has been shown to be safe, acceptable, and effective in human volunteers (Aoki *et al.*, 1975). The bite itself should be treated, though cauterization has little influence in preventing the development of the disease. When rabies has developed, treatment is purely symptomatic, its principal object being to diminish the spasms. Total paralysis with curare and assisted respiration may be the only hope. The paralytic form of the disease will require the usual treatment of paraplegia.

REFERENCES

AOKI, F. Y., TYRRELL, D. A. J., HILL, L. E., and TURNER, G. S. (1975) Immunogenicity and acceptability of a human diploid-cell culture rabies vaccine in volunteers, *Lancet*, **i,** 660.

BALTAZARD, M. (1970) Rabies, in *Clinical Virology*, ed. Debré, R., and Celers, J., Philadelphia.

BRITISH MEDICAL JOURNAL (1975) Diagnosis and management of human rabies, *Brit. med. J.*, **3,** 721.

GIBBS, F. A., GIBBS, E. L., CARPENTER, P. R., and SPIES, H. W. (1961) Comparison of rabies vaccines grown on duck embryo and on nervous tissue, *New Engl. J. Med.*, **265,** 1002.

HATTWICK, A. W., WEIS, T. T., STECHSCHULTE, J., BAER, G. M., and GREGG, M. B. (1972) Recovery from rabies; a case report, *Ann. intern. Med.*, **76,** 931.

HILDRETH, E. A. (1963) Prevention of rabies, or the decline of Sirius, *Ann. intern. Med.*, **58,** 883.

HURST, E. W., and PAWAN, J. L. (1931) An outbreak of rabies in Trinidad without history of bites and with the symptoms of acute ascending myelitis, *Lancet*, **ii,** 622.

HURST, E. W., and PAWAN, J. L. (1932) A further account of the Trinidad outbreak of acute rabic myelitis. Histology of the experimental disease, *J. Path. Bact.*, **35,** 301.

KNUTTI, R. E. (1929) Acute ascending paralysis and myelitis due to the virus of rabies, *J. Amer. med. Ass.*, **93,** 754.

KOPROWSKI, H., and COX, H. R. (1948) Studies in chick embryo adapted rabies virus, *J. Immunol.*, **60,** 533.

KORITSCHONER. (1923) Ueber die Ueberimpfung des Enzephalitisvirus auf Hunde, *Wien. klin. Wschr.*, **36,** 385.

MACCALLUM, F. O. (1967) Rabies, in *Virus and Rickettsial Diseases of Man*, ed. Bedson, S., Downie, A. W., MacCallum, F. O., and Stuart-Harris, C. H., 4th ed., London.

MOZER, H. N., FINNIGAN, F. B., PETZOLD, H., SPITTER, L. E., EMMONS, R. W., and ROTHENBERG, B. (1973) Myelopathy after duck embryo rabies vaccine, *J. Amer. med. Ass.*, **224,** 1605.

PRUSSIN, G., and KATABI, G. (1964) Dorsolumbar myelitis following antirabies vaccination with duck embryo vaccine, *Ann. intern. Med.*, **60,** 114.

SCHÜKRI, I., and SPATZ, H. (1925) Über die anatomischen Veränderungen bei der menschlichen Lyssa und ihre Beziehungen zu denen der Encephalitis epidemica, *Z. ges. Neurol. Psychiat.*, **97**, 627.

VIETS, H. R. (1926) A case of hydrophobia with Negri bodies in the brain, *Arch. Neurol. Psychiat.* (*Chic.*), **15**, 735.

WIKTOR, T. J., FERNANDES, M. V., and KOPROWSKI, H. (1964) Cultivation of rabies virus in human diploid cell strain WI-38, *J. Immunol.*, **93**, 353.

WIKTOR, T. J., PLOTKIN, S. A., and GRELLA, D. W. (1973) Human cell culture rabies vaccine. Antibody response in man, *J. Amer. med. Ass.*, **224**, 1170.

WORLD HEALTH ORGANIZATION EXPERT COMMITTEE ON RABIES (1966) *Wld Hlth Org. techn. Rep. Ser.*, No. 321.

VIRUS MENINGITIS

Synonyms. Acute benign lymphocytic meningitis; epidemic serous meningitis; acute aseptic meningitis.

AETIOLOGY

There is no clearcut distinction between encephalitis and meningitis, as is shown by the term meningo-encephalitis. Nevertheless, a number of virus infections may present the clinical picture of an acute meningitis with a pleocytosis in the cerebrospinal fluid, and little or no evidence of involvement of the substance of the nervous system. These viruses include those of acute lymphocytic choriomeningitis, mumps, infectious mononucleosis, some of the Coxsackie and Echo viruses, poliomyelitis, psittacosis, and louping-ill.

Recent observations suggest that benign lymphocytic meningitis accounts for about 50 per cent of all cases of infectious meningitis seen in hospital. Mumps is one of the commonest causes in Britain, being found in 26 per cent of a recent series of cases in Glasgow in which Echo 9 virus accounted for 61 per cent and other enteroviruses for 13 per cent; lymphocytic choriomeningitis was uncommon in this series (Grist, 1967).

Some of the commoner of these will now be discussed separately.

ACUTE LYMPHOCYTIC CHORIOMENINGITIS

The disorder occurs sporadically and also in small epidemics. Children are usually affected, but it may also occur in adults. The work of Armstrong and Lillie (1934), Findlay *et al.* (1936), and others showed that it is caused by a filterable virus, now classified as an arenavirus; it has been recovered from the cerebrospinal fluid of patients and transmitted to mice and monkeys. Mice are subject to the disease in the wild state and may be the source of the human disease, which has been encountered in Europe, North America, New Zealand, and Malaya.

PATHOLOGY

Animals infected experimentally show intense lymphocytic infiltration of the leptomeninges, the ependyma of the ventricles, and the choroid plexuses. Viets and Warren (1937) reported similar changes in a fatal case together with degeneration of the ganglion cells of the brain, which in the midbrain showed cytoplasmic inclusion bodies. Perivascular infiltration with round cells was seen in both the brain and the spinal cord. Fatal cases of bulbar paralysis, ascending paralysis, and acute meningoencephalitis due to this virus have been reported by Adair *et al.* (1953) and Warkel *et al.* (1973).

SYMPTOMS

The onset is acute, and symptoms of meningeal irritation usually develop rapidly but there may be prodromal manifestations of a general infection followed by a remission before nervous symptoms occur. The symptoms resemble those of any acute meningitis [see p. 409]. Papilloedema may occur, and squint and nystagmus are common. Apart from the occasional occurrence of facial paralysis, the other cranial nerves are normal. Paraplegia and retention of urine have been described, but symptoms of invasion of the substance of the nervous system are rare. There is usually high fever at the onset, and as a rule the temperature falls by lysis in about a week. Pneumonitis—'atypical pneumonia'—may occur (Smadel et al., 1942), and it is probable that a general infection without meningitis is the commonest form of the disease (Farmer and Janeway, 1942).

The cerebrospinal fluid is under increased pressure and may be clear or turbid. The albumin and globulin are increased and a 'cobweb clot' has occurred in some cases. There is an excess of cells ranging from 50 to 1,500 per mm^3; about half show over 1,000 at some stage. These may be mainly mononuclear from the onset, but in a minority of cases polymorphonuclear cells predominate at the beginning, giving place to mononuclear cells in the course of the first week. The sugar of the fluid is usually little, if at all, depressed. The pleocytosis in the cerebrospinal fluid is often remarkably persistent, and a considerable excess of mononuclear cells may be present for many weeks after the disappearance of symptoms, when the patient has apparently been in normal health.

DIAGNOSIS

For the diagnosis of meningitis see page 412.

Acute lymphocytic choriomeningitis is most likely to be confused with tuberculous meningitis, and since the absence of tubercle bacilli from the cerebrospinal fluid cannot be held to exclude the latter, the two conditions may be difficult to distinguish. A low sugar content in the fluid, however, is against the benign disorder. A bromide partition test using bromine-82 has been shown to be of some value (Crook et al., 1960) in identifying the abnormal serum/CSF bromide ratio which is suggestive of tuberculous meningitis. The acute onset of symptoms in lymphocytic choriomeningitis may help to distinguish this condition from the tuberculous form, and the white cell count in the blood and Paul–Bunnell test from meningitis due to infectious mononucleosis. Mumps meningitis is very similar, and cannot be distinguished clinically in the absence of parotitis or orchitis. It may be possible to transmit the disease to mice or hamsters from the cerebrospinal fluid, to demonstrate antibodies in the blood, or to find specific immunofluorescence in cells isolated from CSF. Serum complement-fixing antibodies may be found within 2 weeks, neutralizing antibodies within 6–8 weeks.

PROGNOSIS

The prognosis is good and complete recovery is the rule, though rare fatal cases have been reported (Warkel et al., 1973). Relapses occasionally occur. Paraplegia, however, may be permanent and diffuse arachnoiditis has been described as a sequel.

TREATMENT

Treatment is purely symptomatic; appropriate analgesics should be given for the relief of headache; chemotherapy is of no value.

REFERENCES

ADAIR, C. V., GOULD, R. L., and SMADEL, J. E. (1953) Aseptic meningitis: a disease of diverse etiology, *Ann. intern. Med.*, **39**, 675.

ARMSTRONG, C., and LILLIE, R. D. (1934) Experimental lymphocytic choriomeningitis of monkeys and mice, *Publ. Hlth Rep. (Wash.)*, **49**, 1019.

BAIRD, R. D., and RIVERS, T. M. (1938) Relation of lymphocytic choriomeningitis to acute aseptic meningitis (Wallgren), *Amer. J. publ. Hlth*, **28**, 47.

CROOK, A., DUNCAN, H., GUTTERIDGE, B., and PALLIS, C. (1960) Use of ^{82}Br in differential diagnosis of lymphocytic meningitis, *Brit. med. J.*, **i**, 704.

FARMER, T. W., and JANEWAY, C. A. (1942) Infections with the virus of lymphocytic choriomeningitis, *Medicine (Baltimore)*, **21**, 1.

FINDLAY, G. M., ALCOCK, N. S., and STERN, R. O. (1936) The virus aetiology of one form of lymphocytic meningitis, *Lancet*, **i**, 650.

GRIST, N. R. (1967) Acute viral infections of the nervous system, *Proc. roy. Soc. Med.*, **60**, 696.

KREIS, B. (1937) *La maladie d'Armstrong: chorio-méningite lymphocytaire*, Paris.

MACCALLUM, F. O., and FINDLAY, G. M. (1939) Lymphocytic choriomeningitis. Isolation of the virus from the nasopharynx, *Lancet*, **i**, 1370.

SMADEL, J. E., GREEN, R. H., PALTAUF, R. M., and GONZALES, T. A. (1942) Lymphocytic choriomeningitis: two human fatalities following an unusual febrile illness, *Proc. Soc. exp. Biol. (N.Y.)*, **49**, 683.

VIETS, H. R., and WARREN, S. (1937) Acute lymphocytic meningitis, *J. Amer. med. Ass.*, **108**, 357.

WARKEL, R. L., RINALDI, C. F., BANCROFT, W. H., CARDIFF, R. D., HOLMES, G. E., and WILSNACK, R. E. (1973) Fatal acute meningoencephalitis due to lymphocytic choriomeningitis virus, *Neurology (Minneap.)*, **23**, 198.

NERVOUS COMPLICATIONS OF MUMPS

AETIOLOGY

The experimental work of Gordon (1927) showed that mumps is due to infection with a virus which possesses potential neurotropic propensities. He produced meningitis in monkeys by the intracerebral injection of a filtrate of the saliva of patients suffering from mumps. The commonest nervous complication of mumps is meningitis, and in such cases the mumps virus has been recovered from the cerebrospinal fluid. While many other neurological manifestations including hemiplegia, quadriplegia, blindness, and deafness have been described, encephalomyelitis is much less common, occurring in 9 of a recent series of 64 cases with neurological involvement (Levitt *et al.*, 1970); the remaining 55 patients had meningitis alone. The observation of Johnson *et al.* (1967) that the inoculation of mumps virus into suckling hamsters produced hydrocephalus and aqueduct stenosis may eventually prove to be of importance in relation to the aetiology of similar lesions in man.

PATHOLOGY

Mumps meningitis is rarely fatal; in encephalomyelitis the pathological changes are those of any viral encephalomyelitis with meningeal infiltration with inflammatory cells and perivascular demyelination and inflammatory cell infiltration within the substance of the nervous system (Miller *et al.*, 1956; Bistrian *et al.*, 1972).

SYMPTOMS

Nervous symptoms may occur at the onset or during the first stage of the disease, but usually develop somewhat later, in the adult male immediately before the appearance of orchitis. They may occur without parotitis but with orchitis or may be the sole manifestation of the infection. The symptoms are usually those of an acute meningitis, but encephalomyelitis may occur and in rare cases aphasia and hemiplegia or paraplegia have been described. Optic neuritis and optic atrophy are rare complications. Deafness, either unilateral or bilateral, is commoner.

A few cases of polyneuritis occurring in association with mumps have been recorded, usually developing 2 or 3 weeks after the onset of the primary symptoms. In all the reported cases there has been a flaccid paralysis of all four limbs, and in some cases cranial nerve paralyses have occurred, most frequently facial paralysis. Isolated facial palsy occurs rarely.

The cerebrospinal fluid usually exhibits a marked lymphocytosis. Monod first pointed out that this is frequently present in mumps in the absence of any meningeal symptoms, and it may also occur in contacts who never develop other symptoms of the disease.

DIAGNOSIS

The parotitis usually renders the diagnosis easy. In cases of meningitis associated with lymphocytosis of the cerebrospinal fluid for which no cause can be found, inquiry should always be made whether symptoms of parotitis or orchitis have been present, as this may not have been mentioned spontaneously. Tests for complement-fixing antibodies in paired sera (Enders and Cohen, 1942; Kane *et al.*, 1945) are usually sufficient to confirm the diagnosis and occasionally the virus can be isolated from the cerebrospinal fluid (Bistrian *et al.*, 1972).

PROGNOSIS

Recovery from mumps meningitis is the rule, but the condition is occasionally fatal. Patients with polyneuritis usually recover, though slowly, and recovery may be incomplete. The mortality rate of encephalomyelitis is about 20 per cent (Russell and Donald, 1958).

TREATMENT

Treatment is purely symptomatic. Specific mumps immune globulin may be used to protect susceptible adolescents and adults during an epidemic and active immunization with a vaccine may confer temporary immunity.

REFERENCES

BIEN, G. (1913) Encephalitis und Mumps, *Jb. Kinderheilk.*, **78,** 619.

BISTRIAN, B., PHILLIPS, C. A., and KAYE, I. S. (1972) Fatal mumps meningoencephalitis, *J. Amer. med. Ass.*, **222,** 478.

COLLENS, W. S., and RABINOWITZ, M. A. (1928) Mumps polyneuritis; quadriplegia with bilateral facial paralysis. *Arch. intern. Med.*, **41,** 61.

ENDERS, J. F., and COHEN, S. (1942) Detection of antibodies by complement-fixation in sera of man and monkey convalescent from mumps, *Proc. Soc. exp. Biol.*, **1,** 180.

FINKLESTEIN, H. (1938) Meningo-encephalitis in mumps, *J. Amer. med. Ass.*, **111,** 17.

GORDON, M. H. (1927) Experimental production of the meningo-encephalitis of mumps, *Lancet*, **i,** 652.

GRIST, N. R. (1967) Acute viral infections of the nervous system, *Proc. roy. Soc. Med.*, **60**, 696.

HARRIS, W., and BETHELL, H. (1938) Meningo-encephalitis and orchitis as the only symptoms of mumps, *Lancet*, **ii**, 422.

JOHNSON, R. T., JOHNSON, K. P., and EDMONDS, C. J. (1967) Virus-induced hydrocephalus: development of aqueductal stenosis in hamsters after mumps infection, *Science*, **157**, 1066.

KANE, L. W., COHEN, S., and LEVENS, J. H. (1945) Immunity in mumps, *J. exp. Med.*, **81**, 93.

LENNETTE, E. H., CAPLAN, G. E., and MAGOFFIN, R. L. (1960) Mumps virus infection simulating paralytic poliomyelitis, *Pediatrics*, **25**, 788.

LEVITT, L. P., RICH, T. A., KINDE, S. W., LEWIS, A. L., GATES, E. H., and BOND, J. O. (1970) Central nervous system mumps: a review of 64 cases, *Neurology (Minneap.)*, **20**, 829.

MILLER, H. G., STANTON, J. B., and GIBBONS, J. L. (1956) Para-infectious encephalomyelitis and related syndromes, *Quart. J. Med.*, **25**, 427.

PITRES, A., and MARCHAND, L. (1922) Polynévrite post-ourlienne quadriplégique à forme pseudo-tabétique, *Progr. méd. (Paris)*, **35**, 397.

RUSSELL, R. R., and DONALD, J. C. (1958) The neurological complications of mumps, *Brit. med. J.*, **ii**, 27.

THE COXSACKIE VIRUSES

Following the isolation in Coxsackie, New York, of a virus which could produce paralysis in mice, the term Coxsackie or C. viruses has been applied to a group which now includes a number of viruses. In infant mice some strains attack the muscles, and some the nervous system also. In man the chief clinical manifestations so far recognized are: (1) Aseptic meningitis. The cerebrospinal fluid does not usually contain more than 100 cells per mm³, and the percentage of polymorphonuclears ranges from 10 to 50. The febrile period lasts on an average five days, and recovery is complete as a rule. However, there is now good evidence that the Coxsackie A7 virus, which closely resembles that of poliomyelitis, may on occasion cause paralysis which is generally less severe than that of poliomyelitis. However, this infection can occur in individuals immunized against poliomyelitis. In a recent series of hospital cases diagnosed neurologically over an 8-year period, paralysis was found in 70 per cent of poliovirus infections and in 19 per cent of Coxsackie A7 virus infections (Grist, 1966). (2) Encephalomyelitis. Coxsackie virus of types B3 and B5 was cultured from throat swabs or faeces obtained from 10 patients suffering from encephalitis in Essex in 1965; one patient had a fatal necrotizing encephalitis and the B5 virus was isolated from her cerebrospinal fluid (Heathfield *et al.*, 1967). (3) Epidemic myalgia or pleurodynia. It is now established that the clinical picture of Bornholm disease is usually caused by Coxsackie B5 virus and some patients also have pericarditis (Heathfield *et al.*, 1967). Epidemic myalgia and acute aseptic meningitis may both occur in the same patient. (4) Herpangina. This is a febrile illness with pharyngitis characterized by vesicular or ulcerative lesions. Vomiting and abdominal pain may be present. (5) Encephalomyocarditis of the new-born.

The diagnosis depends upon the isolation of one of the Coxsackie viruses from the faeces, from oropharyngeal swabs, or from cerebrospinal fluid, and the appearance of or an increase in neutralizing antibodies against the virus in the patient's serum at appropriate intervals.

C. virus has often been recovered from the faeces of patients suffering from poliomyelitis, but there is no evidence that either virus influences the patient's reaction to the other.

No specific treatment is known.

REFERENCES

GIUNCHI, G. (1960) Clinical aspects of Coxsackie viruses, in *Virus Meningo-encephalitis*, ed. Wolstenholme, G. E. W., and Cameron, M. P., London.

GRIST, N. R. (1966) *Tenth Symposium of the European Association against Poliomyelitis and Allied Diseases*, p. 275, Brussels.

HEATHFIELD, K. W. G., PILSWORTH, R., WALL, B. J., and CORSELLIS, J. A. N. (1967) Coxsackie B5 infections in Essex, 1965, with particular reference to the nervous system, *Quart. J. Med.*, **36,** 579.

HUMMELEN, K., KIRK, D., and OSTAPICK, M. (1954) Aseptic meningitis caused by Coxsackie virus and isolation of virus from cerebrospinal fluid, *J. Amer. med. Ass.*, **156,** 676.

MELWICK, J. L., and CURWEN, E. C. (1952) in *Viral and Rickettsial Infections in Man*, ed. Rivers, T. M., p. 338, London.

THE ECHO VIRUSES

There are at present 28 distinct antigenic types of the Echo virus (enteric cytopathic human orphan). They infect the gastro-intestinal tract and are excreted mainly in the stools. They cause a febrile illness, sometimes with a rash. Some types cause an acute aseptic meningitis, and it has been suggested that they can cause a poliomyelitis-like illness but it now seems more probable that in such cases paralysis is caused by a concomitant infection with poliovirus or Coxsackie A7 virus as enterovirus infections are commonly multiple. In the meningitic cases there may be more than 500 cells per mm^3, usually mainly mononuclear. The virus may be isolated from the fluid or stools. Antibodies may be present in the blood.

REFERENCES

GRIST, N. R. (1961) Echo viruses, in *Virus Meningo-encephalitis*, ed. Wolstenholme, G. E. W., and Cameron, M. P., p. 17, London.

KAHLMETER, O. (1961) Clinical aspects of Echo viruses, in *Virus Meningo-encephalitis*, ed. Wolstenholme, G. E. W., and Cameron, M. P., p. 24, London.

ACUTE HAEMORRHAGIC CONJUNCTIVITIS (A.H.C.)

This picornavirus, closely related to the Coxsackie and Echo viruses, usually causes acute haemorrhagic conjunctivitis but has been shown in epidemics in India to cause a radiculomyelopathy in some cases (Wadia *et al.*, 1972; Bharucha and Mondkar, 1972); inoculation of the virus into monkeys caused an inflammatory myelopathy (Kono *et al.*, 1973).

REFERENCES

BHARUCHA, E. P., and MONDKAR, V. P. (1972) Neurological complications of a new conjunctivitis, *Lancet*, **ii,** 970.

Kono, R., Uchida, N., Sasagawa, A., Akao, Y., Kodama, H., Mukoyama, J., and Fujiwara, T. (1973) Neurovirulence of acute-haemorrhagic-conjunctivitis virus in monkeys, *Lancet*, **i**, 61.

Wadia, N. H., Irani, P. F., and Katrak, S. M. (1972) Neurological complications of a new conjunctivitis, *Lancet*, **ii**, 970.

HERPES ZOSTER

Synonym. Shingles.

Definition. An acute infection involving primarily the first sensory neurone and the corresponding area of skin.

PATHOLOGY

The pathological changes in the nervous system are those of an acute inflammation at some point in the course of the first sensory neurone. The dorsal root ganglia and the corresponding sensory ganglia of the cranial nerves are the commonest sites of the lesion, but the posterior horn of the grey matter of the spinal cord, the dorsal root, and the peripheral nerves may also be involved. One or more successive metameric segments may be affected, but it is very rare for the lesion to be bilateral. The microscopic changes in the acute stage consist of haemorrhages and infiltration with mononuclear and occasional polymorphonuclear leucocytes, especially in the form of perivascular cuffs, and degenerative changes in the nerve cells. Fibrosis and secondary degeneration follow in severe cases. Inflammatory changes are present in the neighbouring leptomeninges. In fatal cases of zoster meningo-encephalitis, chromatolysis of ganglion cells, and perivascular infiltration are found at all levels of the nervous system up to the cerebral cortex (Biggart and Fisher, 1938). Focal areas of necrosis may also be found with Type A intranuclear inclusion bodies in oligodendroglial cells and the causal virus has been isolated from and identified by electron microscopy in such lesions (McCormick *et al.*, 1969). The cutaneous lesions show inflammatory infiltration of the epidermis and dermis, with vesicle formation produced by serous exudation beneath the stratum corneum. Acidophil nuclear inclusion bodies have been described in the cells of the vesicle epithelium.

AETIOLOGY

These pathological changes are clearly infective, and the infective character of zoster is borne out by numerous facts. It often occurs in epidemics with a seasonal incidence, most cases occurring in the early summer and late autumn. The contagiousness of the infection is well established. It is now clear that the same virus causes zoster and varicella (chicken-pox) so that it is known as varicella-zoster (VZ) virus. Either may give rise to the other in contacts, though varicella follows exposure to zoster much more frequently than the reverse. It has been suggested that herpes zoster may be due to reactivation of varicella virus which is latent in the tissues (Gajdusek, 1965). The VZ virus is serologically distinct from that of herpes simplex but resembles it closely under the electron microscope (Kaplan, 1969; McCormick *et al.*, 1969); it is circular and between 196 and 218 nm in size (Nagler and Rake, 1948; Farrant and O'Connor, 1949).

Zoster may occur without any evident predisposing cause, or as a complication of some other disease or toxic state, especially when this causes damage to the first sensory neurone. These two groups are distinguished as 'idiopathic' and 'symptomatic' zoster, but the evidence indicates that both are due to the same virus. 'Symptomatic' zoster may be precipitated by intoxication with arsenic, carbon monoxide, and other poisons, and may occur in the course of infections such as pneumonia and tuberculosis or toxic states such as uraemia. It may complicate any lesion of the dorsal roots and may therefore follow fracture-dislocation of the spine, secondary carcinoma of the vertebral column, meningo-coccal and other forms of meningitis, subarachnoid haemorrhage, and spinal tumour. It occasionally follows quite a slight injury.

Zoster may occur at any age, but is rare in infancy and more frequent in the second half of life than in the first. It is most often seen in patients over 50.

The incubation period is from 7 to 24 days, and is usually about a fortnight.

SYMPTOMS

General Symptoms

The eruption is often preceded by malaise, anorexia, and sometimes by fever, and there is enlargement of the lymph nodes draining the affected area of skin. The general symptoms are usually slight but may be severe in the aged.

Zoster of the Limbs and Trunk

The first local symptom is usually pain in the segment or segments involved; it is burning or shooting in character and is often associated with hyperalgesia of the area of skin supplied by the affected roots. Three or four days after the onset of pain the eruption appears as a series of localized papules which develop into vesicles grouped together upon an erythematous base [FIG. 100]. The eruption

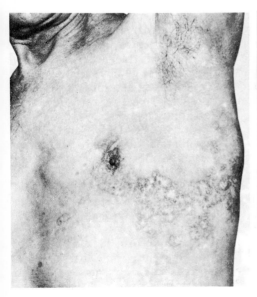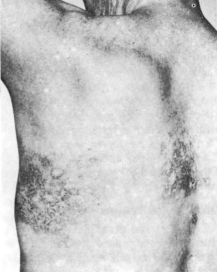

FIG. 100. Focal scarring and pigmentation due to herpes zoster in the mid-dorsal region on the left side (kindly provided by Dr. J. D. Spillane)

also possesses a segmental distribution. After a few days the eruption fades, the vesicles drying into crusts which separate, leaving small permanent scars in the skin. The skin in the affected area usually becomes partially or completely analgesic, though the pain may persist, the association of pain with sensory loss being sometimes described as anaesthesia dolorosa. Thermal and postural sensibility may also be impaired. Pain may persist for weeks or months or indefinitely after the eruption, and this 'post-herpetic neuralgia' is the more likely to occur the older the patient. Severe itching is sometimes a troublesome sequel.

Segmental Complications of Zoster

In addition to involving the first sensory neurone and the skin, zoster may cause a disturbance of function of other structures innervated by the spinal segment affected. Muscular wasting of segmental distribution is more common than generally realized and is probably due to an extension of the infection from the posterior to the anterior horns of grey matter in the spinal cord. Such wasting is easily overlooked when intercostal muscles are involved, zoster being commonest in the dorsal roots [Fig. 100], but is more readily identified when the infection involves the cervical or lumbar roots giving weakness in the upper or lower limb. These palsies are sometimes permanent but often recover slowly over a period of several months. Visceral manifestations of zoster may also occur. Arthritis is rare; it has been described only in the joints of the hand and wrist as a complication of zoster involving the upper limb. There is severe pain and peri-articular swelling with much limitation of movement, which is likely to be permanent. Radiographically the bones show rarefaction. Other visceral manifestations of zoster which have been reported include zoster of the pleura, and urinary bladder, and symptoms resembling those of duodenal ulceration.

Ophthalmic Zoster

When the zoster virus invades the trigeminal ganglion the eruption appears in some part of the cutaneous distribution of the trigeminal nerve, being usually confined to one division. When the ophthalmic division is involved vesicles usually appear on the forehead but the cornea may be attacked, usually only when the eruption also appears on the part of the nose supplied by the nasociliary branch, as Jonathan Hutchinson pointed out. The corneal lesion takes the form of small, round infiltrations in the more superficial layers of the substantia propria. Often there is severe swelling of the conjunctiva and eyelids. Other orbital structures may be involved, the most serious complication, fortunately a rare one, being optic neuritis, followed by atrophy and leading to blindness. Oculomotor paralyses may occur, the third nerve being more often affected than the fourth and sixth. Trigeminal zoster, like zoster elsewhere, may be either idiopathic or symptomatic. In the latter case it may follow any intracranial lesion of the fifth nerve, including alcoholic injection of the trigeminal ganglion.

Geniculate Zoster

Zoster of the geniculate ganglion was the explanation proposed by Ramsay Hunt (1915) for cases in which the vesicles are found in the auricle and less often on the anterior pillar of the fauces. There is pain in the ear and mastoid region radiating to the anterior pillar of the fauces and to the vertex. There may be a serosanguineous discharge from the ear. Taste may be lost on the anterior two-thirds of the tongue on the same side, the region innervated by the geniculate ganglion through the chorda tympani. Almost invariably the infection spreads to the trunk of the facial nerve and leads to facial paralysis, often associated with clonic facial spasm. The eighth nerve may become involved, with resulting deafness or vestibular disturbances and facial sensory loss on the same side is not uncommon. Some workers now doubt whether the geniculate ganglion is involved in all such cases (Denny-Brown *et al.*, 1944; O'Neill, 1945) and suggest that the seat of infection in such cases is more often in the brain stem but in a typical case subsequently examined at autopsy there were unequivocal pathological changes in the geniculate ganglion (Aleksic *et al.*, 1973).

Meningitis, Encephalitis, and Myelitis

Some degree of meningeal inflammation is the rule in zoster and is indicated by an excess of mononuclear cells and a raised protein content in the cerebrospinal fluid, almost constantly present. Less frequently clinical signs of meningitis may be observed, headache and cervical rigidity complicating zoster of the trigeminal ganglion, and pain in the lower limbs and Kernig's sign being associated with dorsal or lumbar zoster. Extension of the infection to the substance of the brain or the white matter of the spinal cord is less common. Nevertheless, zoster encephalitis and myelitis have been observed and necrosis of the cord resembling subacute necrotizing myelopathy was found in a fatal case (Rose *et al.*, 1964). When the cord is involved, myoclonus, intractable hiccup, and spastic monoparesis or paraparesis may all occur.

Generalized Zoster

Besides the segmental eruption, the patient may exhibit scattered vesicles. These may be few in number—'aberrant vesicles'—or a widespread eruption resembling varicella. Usually the generalized rash appears within three or four days of the outbreak of zoster, but the interval may be longer.

DIAGNOSIS

The diagnosis of herpes zoster offers little difficulty, as in no other condition is there a vesicular eruption associated with pain and hyperalgesia of a segmental distribution. Herpes febrilis is less painful, is usually situated in the proximity of a mucous membrane, is often bilateral, and leaves neither residual pain nor scarring. Post-herpetic neuralgia is distinguished from other types of root pain by the history of the eruption, the scars of which can usually be found. Diagnosis is difficult in the pre-eruptive stage, but the possibility of zoster should be suggested by root pains of sudden onset less than four days before examination.

PROGNOSIS

Most sufferers from zoster recover without residual symptoms, except for scarring of the skin. One attack usually confers permanent immunity but second or repeated attacks sometimes occur especially in the symptomatic form. Severe secondary infection of the vesicles is a rare complication. Zoster of the cornea may be followed by corneal ulceration, and the occurrence of optic atrophy has already been mentioned. Recovery from facial paralysis following geniculate zoster is often incomplete. Segmental muscular weakness due to anterior horn cell involvement (Thomas and Howard, 1972; Weiss *et al.*, 1975) usually recovers in a few months but various focal neurological signs, including spastic paresis, may persist after encephalomyelitis. The most troublesome sequel of zoster is persistent intractable pain, which may endure for years in elderly patients.

TREATMENT

In most cases the treatment of zoster is simple. Dusting powder and a dry dressing or collodion are all that are needed for the cutaneous eruption. Powerful analgesics are usually required. Dihydrocodeine or paracetamol may be sufficient in some cases but more often stronger remedies such as pethidine are required in the acute stage, particularly in ophthalmic cases. No antibiotic or antiviral agent has been shown to be of any value; amantadine hydrochloride had no significant effect in a double-blind trial carried out in general practice (Galbraith, 1973). Steroids are of no proven value. Persistent post-herpetic pain is a very troublesome complication which is very liable to occur in the elderly and aged. In severe cases analgesics are almost useless. It makes life a burden and may lead the patient to the verge of suicide. Morphine is contra-indicated owing to the risk of habit formation and carbamazepine (*Tegretol*) is only rarely helpful. Deep X-ray irradiation of the spinal cord and nerve roots or of the trigeminal ganglion has been tried and is occasionally successful but rarely has a lasting effect. Surgical division of sensory nerves or roots and alcohol or phenol injection of the Gasserian ganglion have also been advocated but relief is often temporary. The local application for up to 20 minutes three times a day of an electrical vibrator to the painful area (Russell *et al.*, 1957) or else repeated freezing of the skin segment involved with an ethyl chloride spray (Taverner, 1960), if continued for several weeks or months, may give lasting relief. Sometimes self-administered electrical cutaneous stimulation is even more successful (Nathan and Wall, 1974). Often dihydrocodeine and chlorpromazine three or four times daily must be given for as long as the local treatment is continued. The accompanying depression which is almost invariably present in severe cases must usually be treated with aminoxidase inhibitors or with amitriptyline or imipramine in appropriate dosage. Frequently it is best to admit the patient to hospital initially to teach him to use the vibrator, cooling spray, or stimulator, depending upon which is the more effective in the individual case.

REFERENCES

AITKEN, R. S., and BRAIN, R. T. (1933) Facial palsy and infection with zoster virus, *Lancet*, **i**, 19.

ALEKSIC, S. N., BUDZILOVICH, G. N., and LIEBERMAN, A. N. (1973) Herpes zoster oticus and facial paralysis (Ramsay-Hunt syndrome): clinicopathologic study and review of literature, *J. neurol. Sci.*, **20**, 149.

BIGGART, J. H., and FISHER, J. A. (1938) Meningo-encephalitis complicating herpes zoster, *Lancet*, **ii**, 944.

BRAIN, W. R. (1931) Zoster, varicella and encephalitis, *Brit. med. J.*, **1**, 81.

CHAUFFARD, A., and RENDU, H. (1907) Méningite zonateuse tardive dans un cas de zona ophthalmique, *Bull. Soc. méd. Hôp. Paris*, **24**, 141.

DENNY-BROWN, D., ADAMS, R. D., and FITZGERALD, P. J. (1944) Pathologic features of herpes zoster: a note on 'geniculate herpes', *Arch. Neurol. Psychiat. (Chic.)*, **51**, 216.

FARRANT, J. L., and O'CONNOR, J. L. (1949) Elementary bodies of varicella and herpes zoster, *Nature (Lond.)*, **163**, 260.

GAJDUSEK, D. C. (1965) in *Slow, Latent and Temperate Virus Infections*, N.I.N.D.B. Monograph No. 2, p. 3, Bethesda, Md.

GALBRAITH, A. W. (1973) Treatment of acute herpes zoster with amantadine hydrochloride (Symmetrel), *Brit. med. J.*, **4**, 693.

HEAD, H., and CAMPBELL, A. W. (1900) The pathology of herpes zoster and its bearing on sensory localisation, *Brain*, **23**, 353.

Hunt, J. R. (1915) The sensory field of the facial nerve: a further contribution to the symptomatology of the geniculate ganglion, *Brain*, **38**, 418.

Kaplan, A. S. (1969) *Herpes Simplex and Pseudorabies Viruses*, New York.

Levaditi, C. (1926) *L'herpès et le zona*, Paris.

Lidsky, M. D., Klass, D. W., McKenzie, B. F., and Goldstein, N. P. (1962) Herpes zoster encephalitis. Case report with electroencephalographic and cerebrospinal fluid studies, *Ann. intern. Med.*, **56**, 779.

McCormick, W. F., Rodnitzky, R. L., Schochet, S. S., and McKee, A. P. (1969) Varicella-zoster encephalomyelitis: a morphologic and virologic study, *Arch. Neurol. (Chic.)*, **21**, 559.

Nagler, F. P. O., and Rake, G. (1948) The use of the electron microscope in the diagnosis of variola, vaccinia and varicella, *J. Bact.*, **55**, 45.

Nathan, P. W., and Wall, P. D. (1974) Treatment of post-herpetic neuralgia by prolonged electric stimulation, *Brit. med. J.*, **3**, 645.

Netter, A., and Urbain, A. (1926) Les relations de zona et de la varicelle. Étude sérologique de 100 cas de zona, *C.R. Soc. Biol. (Paris)*, **94**, 98.

O'Neill, H. (1945) Herpes zoster auris ('geniculate' ganglionitis), *Arch. Otolaryng.* **42**, 309.

Rose, F. C., Brett, E. M., and Burston, J. (1964) Zoster encephalomyelitis, *Arch. Neurol. (Chic.)*, **11**, 155.

Russell, W. R., Espir, M. L. E., and Morganstern, F. S. (1957) Treatment of post-herpetic neuralgia, *Lancet*, **i**, 242.

Schiff, C. I., and Brain, W. R. (1930) Acute meningo-encephalitis associated with herpes zoster, *Lancet*, **ii**, 70.

Taverner, D. (1960) Alleviation of post-herpetic neuralgia, *Lancet*, **ii**, 671.

Thomas, J. E., and Howard, F. M. (1972) Segmental zoster paresis—a disease profile, *Neurology (Minneap.)*, **22**, 459.

Weiss, S., Streifler, M., and Weiser, H. J. (1975) Motor lesions in herpes zoster. Incidence and special features, *Europ. Neurol.*, **13**, 332.

Wohlwill, F. (1924) Zur pathologischen Anatomie des Nervensystems beim Herpes zoster (Auf Grund von zehn Sektionsfällen.), *Z. ges. Neurol. Psychiat.*, **89**, 171.

CYTOMEGALOVIRUS INFECTION

Cytomegalovirus is ubiquitous; the factors causing an infection which gives rise to clinical manifestations are unclear. The virus has an affinity for the subependymal cells which line the cerebral ventricles and, as infection of the fetus usually occurs in the third trimester of pregnancy, there is failure of brain growth with periventricular and intracerebral calcification (see Menkes, 1974). Intranuclear inclusion bodies are found in neurones and endothelial cells.

The typical clinical manifestations include persistent neonatal jaundice, hepatosplenomegaly, anaemia, and thrombocytopenia. Neurologically, microcephaly and microgyria, and, less often, hydrocephalus and other cerebral malformations occur. Variable ocular abnormalities include chorioretinitis, retinal calcification, cataract, and optic atrophy (Hanshaw, 1971). It has been suggested that mental retardation may be the result of less overt chronic infection (Stern *et al.*, 1969).

REFERENCES

Hanshaw, J. B. (1971) Congenital cytomegalovirus infection: a fifteen year perspective, *J. infect. Dis.*, **123**, 555.

Menkes, J. H. (1974) *Textbook of Child Neurology*, Philadelphia.

Stern, H., Elek, S. D., Booth, J. C., and Fleck, D. G. (1969) Microbial causes of mental retardation. The role of prenatal infections with cytomegalovirus, rubella virus, and toxoplasma, *Lancet*, **ii**, 443.

PROGRESSIVE MULTIFOCAL LEUCOENCEPHALOPATHY

This condition, due to papovavirus, occurring usually in association with reticulosis, is considered on page 866.

CONGENITAL RUBELLA

An acute encephalitis rarely occurs during the course of rubella [see p. 537] and there is evidence that this virus may rarely cause a clinical picture like that of subacute sclerosing panencephalitis [p. 494]. However, Gregg (1941) showed that maternal rubella was sometimes responsible for congenital cataract and it is now evident that many developmental anomalies may result from fetal infection, being more severe the earlier in pregnancy the maternal infection occurs. The commonest abnormalities are deafness, heart disease, and cataract, but chorioretinitis, mental retardation of varying severity, epilepsy, and spasticity have all been recorded, as have various cerebral malformations and spina bifida (Menkes, 1974).

REFERENCES

GREGG, N. (1941) Congenital cataract following German measles in the mother, *Trans. ophthal. Soc. Aust.*, **3**, 35.
MENKES, J. H. (1974) *Textbook of Child Neurology*, Philadelphia.

INFECTIOUS MONONUCLEOSIS

For the neurological complications of this disorder, due to infection with the Epstein–Barr virus, see page 446.

'SLOW VIRUS' INFECTIONS

KURU, SCRAPIE, AND CREUTZFELDT-JAKOB DISEASE

Kuru, a progressive and fatal disease of the nervous system which occurs in the Fore people of the Eastern highlands of New Guinea, has been shown to be due to a transmissible agent, presumably viral, though no virus has yet been identified. Commoner in young women, but also seen in male adults and very rarely in children, the condition is characterized by difficulty in walking, tremulous legs, headache, and pains in the legs in some cases and by disorders of mood, frequent dementia, and sometimes hyperreflexia. The condition is usually fatal within 6 to 24 months (Hornabrook, 1968); transmission from subject to subject has been thought to be due to cannibalism. The incubation period of the disease has been shown, following transmission to the chimpanzee by inoculation of brain material from affected subjects, to be a minimum of one and often several years (Beck *et al.*, 1973; Gajdusek, 1973; *The Lancet*, 1974). The histological changes in affected brains, showing spongiform change with loss of ganglion cells and fibrillary astrocytosis, closely resemble those of scrapie, a disorder of sheep also believed to be of viral origin, and also with a long incubation period (Hadlow, 1959; Alper, 1972). The pathological changes of Creutzfeldt–Jakob disease or subacute spongiform encephalopathy of man [p. 697] are also similar and this condition, too, has been transmitted to the chimpanzee and to New World monkeys, again with a very long incubation period (Gibbs *et al.*, 1968; Roos *et al.*, 1973). Virus-like particles and nucleoprotein-type filaments have been demonstrated by electron microscopy in brain tissue from two patients with the latter condition (Vernon *et al.*, 1970) but as yet the causal virus of this condition, too, has not been isolated.

REFERENCES

ALPER, T. (1972) The nature of the scrapie agent, *J. clin. Path. (Lond.)*, **25**, suppl. 154.

BECK, E., DANIEL, P. M., ASHER, D. M., GAJDUSEK, D. C., and GIBBS, C. J. (1973) Experimental kuru in the chimpanzee: a neuropathological study, *Brain*, **96**, 441.

GAJDUSEK, D. C. (1973) Kuru and Creutzfeldt–Jakob disease. Experimental models of noninflammatory degenerative slow virus disease of the central nervous system, *Ann. clin. Res.*, **5**, 254.

GIBBS, C. J., GAJDUSEK, D. C., ASHER, D. M., ALPERS, M. P., BECK, E., DANIEL, P. M., and MATTHEWS, W. B. (1968) Creutzfeldt–Jakob disease (spongiform encephalopathy): transmission to the chimpanzee, *Science (N.Y.)*, **161**, 388.

HADLOW, W. J. (1959) Scrapie and kuru, *Lancet*, **ii**, 289.

HORNABROOK, R. W. (1968) Kuru—a subacute cerebellar degeneration. The natural history and clinical features, *Brain*, **91**, 53.

THE LANCET (1974) Kuru, Creutzfeldt–Jakob, and scrapie, *Lancet*, **ii**, 1551.

ROOS, R., GAJDUSEK, D. C., and GIBBS, C. J. (1973) The clinical characteristics of transmissible Creutzfeldt–Jakob disease, *Brain*, **96**, 1.

VERNON, M. L., HORTA-BARBOSA, L., FUCCILLO, D. A., SEVER, J. L., BARINGER, J. R., and BIRNBAUM, G. (1970) Virus-like particles and nucleoprotein-type filaments in brain tissue from two patients with Creutzfeldt–Jakob disease, *Lancet*, **i**, 964.

11

DEMYELINATING DISEASES OF THE NERVOUS SYSTEM

CLASSIFICATION

A LARGE and important group of diseases of the nervous system possess, as a common pathological feature, foci in which the myelin sheaths of the nerve fibres are destroyed. These foci, which are mainly situated in the white matter, vary in size, shape, and distribution and also in the acuteness of the pathological process of which they are the result, but they are sufficiently similar in the different diseases to justify the application to the whole group of the name *demyelinating diseases of the nervous system*. However, it must be remembered that the axis cylinders often suffer in varying degree as well as their myelin sheaths and it is not certain that myelin destruction is always the primary change: it may be part of a more diffuse process. Moreover, as Lumsden (1961) points out, 'we mostly use the word "myelin" for a complex structural unit consisting of a formed sheath of myelin with satellite nutrient cells'. Not only does it not follow, but it is very unlikely, that destruction of myelin is always the result of the same process. Myelin has been the subject of much recent study (see Lumsden, 1957; Finean, 1961; Wright, 1961; Thompson, 1961; Robertson, 1965; Pette *et al.*, 1969; Field *et al.*, 1972; Adams, 1972; Lumsden, 1972). Much new information has been derived from studies involving the electron microscope and tissue culture of myelin, from biochemical studies of its composition (Eylar, 1971; Martenson *et al.*, 1971; Adams, 1972), from complex immunological investigations of demyelinating processes in animals and man (see Rowland, 1971; Field *et al.*, 1972; Lumsden, 1972) and from virological studies; these investigations will, where necessary, be considered when we comment upon individual disease entities within this group.

Apart from the fact that all but the most acute forms of demyelinating disease are sometimes familial, and that some of the most acute forms often follow acute infections, especially the exanthemata caused by viruses such as measles, smallpox, and vaccination, the aetiology of most of the demyelinating disorders remains obscure, though many seem to be due to a complex interrelationship of genetic, infective, immunological, and biochemical mechanisms. An aetiological classification is therefore impossible.

Any attempt to classify these conditions upon a pathological basis encounters the difficulty that although many pathological varieties have been distinguished, they merge into one another to form an almost continuous series. A purely clinical classification is equally unsatisfactory in that it fails to accommodate transitional forms exhibiting features common to two clinical varieties, which can usually clearly be distinguished. The best available classification is a clinico-pathological one, which is based upon the recognition that clinical and pathological features can often be closely correlated. Such a classification must be provisional and must be qualified by the recognition of transitional forms. Increased knowledge may well show that clinico-pathological distinctions do not correspond to aetiological differences, but that they are the outcome of differences in respect of the acuteness of the pathological process, which may be influenced by the patient's genetic constitution, his age, the nature of the precipitating factors, and also by immunological processes. There is growing evidence to indicate that some of these diseases are precipitated by viral or other infections and, as some now believe, that post-infectious encephalomyelitis may be due to a process initiated by actual viral invasion of the nervous system; others take the view that the primary pathological process is autoiummune, perhaps due to lymphocyte-mediated hypersensitivity, and that any virus present acts merely as the trigger which initiates the process. It is also becoming increasingly clear that many of the disorders traditionally embraced by the term diffuse sclerosis are due to specific metabolic defects which influence the formation or lipid composition of myelin and that they should be considered to be dysmyelinating disorders or so-called leukodystrophies [see pp. 638–55], i.e. disorders of myelin formation or composition, rather than demyelinating diseases in the traditional sense of the term. The confusion which has arisen over the use of the term Schilder's disease and through the use of 'diffuse sclerosis' to identify demyelinating as well as dysmyelinating disorders will be considered later in this chapter. It is uncertain, therefore, when a demyelinating disorder affects the brain and spinal cord, whether encephalitis or encephalopathy, myelitis or myelopathy is the more appropriate term. Encephalitis and myelitis are employed here as being less cumbersome and better known. The following is a convenient clinico-pathological classification:

Variety	Synonyms	Incidence	Distribution of lesion	Course
Acute disseminated encephalomyelitis following acute infections, e.g. measles, chickenpox, smallpox, vaccination against smallpox and rabies	Acute perivascular myelinoclasis	Sporadic, very rarely familial: usually in children or adolescents	Patchy in brain and spinal cord, tending especially to a perivenous distribution; rarely in optic nerves	Acute or subacute and self-limited
Acute haemorrhagic leuco-encephalitis	Acute necrotizing haemorrhagic leuco-encephalopathy	Sporadic, in all age groups	Patchy in white matter of brain, generally perivascular	Explosive, often fatal within 24–48 hours
Disseminated myelitis with optic neuritis	Neuromyelitis optica Ophthalmoneuromyelitis (Devic's disease)	Sporadic (once reported in twins), any age from childhood onwards	Massive in optic nerves and chiasm and spinal cord which may undergo softening and cavitation	Acute or subacute in onset; sometimes self-limited, sometimes relapsing and progressive
Multiple sclerosis	Insular sclerosis Disseminated sclerosis	Sporadic, occasionally familial; usually in the first half of adult life	Patchy in brain, optic nerves, and spinal cord, the lesions being multiple and successive	Progressive, ranging from acute to extremely chronic with a conspicuous tendency to remissions and relapses
Diffuse sclerosis	Encephalitis periaxialis diffusa (Schilder's disease)* Centrolobar sclerosis. Progressive degenerative subcortical encephalopathy Concentric demyelination (Baló's disease).	Sporadic, usually in infancy and adolescence, less often in adult life	Diffuse and massive, usually symmetrical, cerebral much more than spinal	Acute, subacute, and chronic, steadily progressive or intermittent
Central pontine myelinolysis	No synonyms at present	Sporadic, usually in alcoholic or malnourished patients or in those with chronic liver disease	Central in pons	Subacute, progressive

* The question as to whether X-linked recessive adrenoleucodystrophy is a demyelinating disease related to Schilder's disease or a dysmyelinating disorder is still uncertain but on the whole the latter seems more probable.

Demyelination may also be produced in man and animals by a variety of drugs and toxic agents. Thus it was described as an occasional complication of the arsphenamine treatment of syphilis and in animals it may result from cyanide intoxication (Adams and Leibowitz, 1969; Adams, 1972) and then shows some resemblance to the demyelination which is one feature of the pathological changes in the nervous system in human vitamin B_{12} deficiency. Demyelination may also be produced experimentally by diphtheria toxin (Weller, 1965; Hallpike and Adams, 1969) but in human diphtheria this change is, as a rule, confined to the peripheral nerves. Similarly, demyelination due to organophosphorus compounds (Cavanagh, 1954, 1963) is due to a 'dying-back' degeneration of the axon, again particularly in peripheral nerves, with secondary demyelination. Naturally occurring dysmyelinating disorders of animals, including swayback disease of sheep due to copper deficiency (Innes and Shearer, 1940; Howell et al., 1964) have been reviewed by Adams (1972); these disorders are now known to be quite different from any naturally occurring demyelinating disease which occurs in man. However, as will be seen below, several close analogies can be drawn between the experimental allergic encephalo-myelitis (EAE) (Raine et al., 1974) which can be produced in animals by the injection of encephalitogenic factor (EF) isolated from human brain (Field et al., 1963) on the one hand, and human encephalomyelitis on the other (Behan et al., 1968; Levine, 1971).

REFERENCES

ADAMS, C. W. M. (1972) Research on Multiple Sclerosis, Springfield, Ill.

ADAMS, C. W. M., and LEIBOWITZ, S. L. (1969) The general pathology of demyelinating diseases, in The Structure and Function of Nervous Tissue, ed. Bourne, G. H., vol. 3, p. 309, New York.

BEHAN, P. O., GESCHWIND, N., LAMARCHE, J. B., LISAK, R. P., and KIES, M. W. (1968) Delayed hypersensitivity to encephalitogenic protein in disseminated encephalo-myelitis, Lancet, ii, 1009.

CAVANAGH, J. B. (1954) The toxic effects of triorthocresyl phosphate on the nervous system—an experimental study in hens, J. Neurol. Neurosurg. Psychiat., 17, 163.

CAVANAGH, J. B. (1963) Organo-phosphorus neurotoxicity, a model 'dying-back' process comparable to certain human neurological disorders, Guy's Hosp. Rep., 112, 303.

EYLAR, E. H. (1971) Basic A1 protein of myelin: relationship to experimental allergic encephalomyelitis, in Immunological Disorders of the Nervous System (A.R.N.M.D. vol. XLIX), p. 50, ed. Rowland, L. P., Baltimore.

FERRARO, A. (1937) Primary demyelinating processes of the central nervous system, Arch. Neurol. Psychiat. (Chic.), 37, 100.

FIELD, E. J., BELL, T. M., and CARNEGIE, P. R. (1972) Multiple Sclerosis: Progress in Research, Amsterdam, London.

FIELD, E. J., CASPARY, E. A., and BALL, E. J. (1963) Some biological properties of a highly active encephalitogenic factor isolated from human brain, Lancet, ii, 11.

FINEAN, J. B. (1961) Electron microscopy of the myelin, Proc. roy. Soc. Med., 54, 19.

HALLPIKE, J. F., and ADAMS, C. W. M. (1969) Proteolysis and myelin breakdown: a review of recent histochemical and biochemical studies, Histochem. J., 1, 559.

HOWELL, J. McC., DAVISON, A. N., and OXBERRY, J. (1964) Biochemical and neuro-pathological changes in swayback, Res. Vet. Sci., 5, 376.

INNES, J. R. M., and SHEARER, G. D. (1940) Swayback, a demyelinating disease of lambs with affinities to Schilder's encephalitis in man, J. Comp. Neurol., 53, 1.

LEVINE, S. (1971) Relationship of experimental allergic encephalomyelitis to human disease, in *Immunological Disorders of the Nervous System* (A.R.N.M.D. vol. XLIX), p. 33, ed. Rowland, L. P., Baltimore.

LUMSDEN, C. E. (1950) Cyanide leucoencephalopathy in rats and observations on the vascular and ferment hypotheses of demyelinating diseases, *J. Neurol. Neurosurg. Psychiat.*, **13**, 1.

LUMSDEN, C. E. (1957) Aspects of the chemistry of myelin and the sheath cell complex, *and* Cell structure and cell physiology in relation to myelin, in *Modern Trends in Neurology*, ed. Williams, D., pp. 130, 148, London.

LUMSDEN, C. E. (1961) Consideration of multiple sclerosis in relation to the autoimmunity process, *Proc. roy. Soc. Med.*, **54**, 11.

LUMSDEN, C. E. (1972) The clinical pathology of multiple sclerosis, in *Multiple Sclerosis: A Reappraisal*, ed. McAlpine, D., Lumsden, C. E., and Acheson, E. D., Edinburgh, London.

MARTENSON, R. E., DEIBLER, G. E., and KIES, M. W. (1971) Microheterogeneity and species-related differences among myelin basic proteins, in *Immunological Disorders of the Nervous System* (A.R.N.M.D. vol. LXIX), p. 76, ed. Rowland, L. P., Baltimore.

PETTE, E., WESTPHAL, O., BURDZY, K., and KALLOS, P. (1969) *Pathogenesis and Etiology of Demyelinating Diseases*, Basel, New York.

RAINE, C. S., SNYDER, D. H., VALSAMIS, M. P., and STONE, S. H. (1974) Chronic experimental allergic encephalomyelitis in inbred guinea pigs—an ultrastructural study, *Lab. Invest.*, **31**, 369.

ROBERTSON, J. D. (1965) in *The Living Cell*, p. 45, Scientific American, San Francisco.

ROSE, A. S., and PEARSON, C. M. (1963) *Mechanisms of Demyelination*, New York.

ROWLAND, L. P. (1971) *Immunological Disorders of the Nervous System* (A.R.N.M.D. vol. XLIX), Baltimore.

THOMPSON, R. H. S. (1961) Myelinolytic mechanisms, *Proc. roy. Soc. Med.*, **54**, 30.

WELLER, R. O. (1965) Diphtheritic neuropathy in the chicken: an electron-microscopic study, *J. Path. Bact.*, **89**, 591.

WRIGHT, G. P. (1961) The metabolism of myelin, *Proc. roy. Soc. Med.*, **54**, 26.

See also Multiple sclerosis and the demyelinating diseases, *Res. Publ. Ass. nerv. ment. Dis.* (1958), **28**.

ACUTE DISSEMINATED ENCEPHALOMYELITIS

Synonym. Acute perivascular myelinoclasis.

Definition. An acute disorder characterized by demyelination of the nervous system, usually with a perivascular distribution, and by symptoms of damage to the brain and spinal cord, especially in the white matter, occurring in the course of infection with the causal virus of one of the exanthemata, such as measles, German measles, smallpox, mumps, chickenpox, as a sequel to vaccination against smallpox and rabies or banal infection, or spontaneously.

PATHOLOGY

Naked-eye changes consist merely of congestion and oedema of the nervous system. Microscopically [FIG. 101] there is marked perivascular infiltration of the brain and spinal cord with lymphocytes and plasma cells both within the perivascular spaces and still more conspicuously at a greater distance from the vessels. In the white matter the most striking feature is the presence of zones of demyelination, that is, loss of the myelin sheaths of the neurones, around the vessels, especially the veins. Activated microglial cells and fat-laden macrophages are common in the demyelinated areas and oligodendroglial cells are often pyknotic but the neurones usually remain intact, unlike the usual findings in viral

S

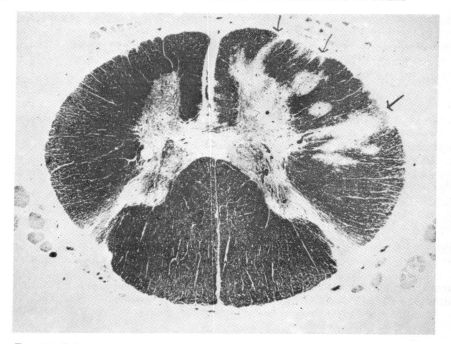

Fig. 101. Spinal cord in post-vaccinal encephalomyelitis. The arrows indicate patches of demyelination. (By courtesy of Dr. Urich.)

encephalomyelitis (Adams and Kubik, 1952; De Vries, 1960). The most intense changes are often found in the cerebral white matter and/or in the lumbar and upper sacral regions of the spinal cord, and in the pons. In the mid-brain the substantia nigra is the structure most affected. Inflammatory changes may be present throughout the whole length of the nervous system. Meningeal infiltration is relatively slight. Herkenrath (1935) reported a case of recovery from post-vaccinal encephalitis followed by death from another cause 18 months later. The nervous system showed no abnormality except for some fat-laden scavenger cells in the perivascular spaces of the cerebellum, pons, medulla, and spinal cord. It was inferred that the process which results in peri-vascular demyelination is capable of complete reversal resulting in clinical and anatomical recovery.

AETIOLOGY

It has been suggested that this form of encephalomyelitis may be due to direct invasion of the brain by the primary virus causing the exanthem; Shaffer *et al.* (1942) and Adams (1968) either isolated measles virus or identified cyto-plasmic and nuclear inclusion bodies suggestive of viral infection from the brains of patients with measles encephalitis. However, as stated above, the pathological picture of the condition differs in several important respects from that usually associated with viral encephalomyelitis, and direct inoculation of vaccinia and rabies virus into the nervous system of animals does not produce demyelination. It also seems inherently improbable that so many different viruses would produce this consistent pathological picture. An alternative theory once proposed that another virus capable of producing demyelination may be activated within the nervous system by a variety of different infections always seemed unlikely (Hurst, 1935) and now has few adherents.

Glanzmann (1927), van Bogaert (1932, 1933), and Finley (1937, 1938) were among the first to suggest that post-infectious encephalomyelitis might be due to an allergic response on the part of the nervous system to a variety of different infective agents, and this concept that the condition is due to hypersensitivity of the nervous system to viral multiplication or to the products of viral injury is now generally accepted. Since Rivers and Schwentker (1935) showed that experimental allergic encephalomyelitis (EAE) could be induced in animals by the injection of brain emulsion with Freund's adjuvant, much work has been done upon the animal model of the human disease (Kabat et al., 1947; Wolf et al., 1947; Lumsden, 1949 a and b; Kies and Alvord, 1959; Waksman, 1959; Field et al., 1963; Rauch and Griffin, 1969; dal Canto et al., 1975) and there is good evidence that the condition is due, at least in part, to lymphocyte-mediated delayed hypersensitivity; it may certainly be suppressed in the guinea-pig by treatment with antilymphocytic serum (Field, 1969). The fact that a similar disorder may occur in man after the inoculation of antirabic vaccine prepared in animal brain or spinal cord supports the analogy between the experimental disorder in animals and the naturally occurring human disease. The immuno-pathology of EAE has recently been reviewed in detail by Wisniewski (1975).

REFERENCES

ADAMS, J. M. (1968) Clinical pathology of measles encephalitis and sequelae, *Neurology (Minneap.)*, **18** (pt. 2), 52.

ADAMS, R. D., and KUBIK, C. S. (1952) The morbid anatomy of the demyelinative diseases, *Amer. J. Med.*, **12**, 510.

BOGAERT, L. VAN (1932) Essai d'interprétation des manifestations nerveuses observées au cours de la vaccination, de la maladie sérique et des maladies éruptives, *Rev. neurol. (Paris)*, **39**, 1.

BOGAERT, L. VAN (1933) Les manifestations nerveuses au cours des maladies éruptives, *Rev. neurol. (Paris)*, **40**, 150.

DAL CANTO, M. C., WISNIEWSKI, H. M., JOHNSON, A. B., BROSTOFF, S. W., and RAINE, C. S. (1975) Vesicular disruption of myelin in autoimmune demyelination, *J. neurol. Sci.*, **24**, 313.

DE VRIES, E. (1960) *Postvaccinal Perivenous Encephalitis*, Amsterdam.

FIELD, E. J. (1969) Antilymphocytic serum in experimental allergic encephalomyelitis, *Brit. med. J.*, **3**, 758.

FIELD, E. J., CASPARY, E. A., and BALL, E. J. (1963) Some biological properties of a highly active encephalitogenic factor isolated from human brain, *Lancet*, **ii**, 11.

FINLEY, H. K. (1937) Perivenous changes in acute encephalitis associated with vaccination, variola and measles, *Arch. Neurol. Psychiat. (Chic.)*, **37**, 505.

FINLEY, H. K. (1938) Pathogenesis of encephalitis occurring with vaccination, variola and measles, *Arch. Neurol. Psychiat. (Chic.)*, **39**, 1047.

GLANZMANN, E. (1927) Die nervösen Komplikationen der Varizellen, Variola und Vakzine, *Schweiz. med. Wschr.*, **8**, 145.

HERKENRATH, B. (1935) Pathologisch-anatomisch gesicherte Ausheilung eines Falles von Encephalitis post vaccinationem, *Z. ges. Neurol. Psychiat.*, **152**, 293.

HURST, E. W. (1935) The neurotropic virus diseases, *Lancet*, **ii**, 697, 758.

KABAT, E. A., WOLF, A., and BEZER, A. E. (1947) The rapid production of a demyelinating encephalomyelitis in Rhesus monkeys by injection of heterologous and homologous brain tissue with adjuvants, *J. exp. Med.*, **85**, 117.

KIES, M. W., and ALVORD, E. C., Jun. (1959) *Allergic Encephalomyelitis*, Springfield, Ill.

LUMSDEN, C. E. (1949 a) Experimental 'allergic' encephalomyelitis, *Brain*, **72**, 198.

LUMSDEN, C. E. (1949 b) Experimental 'allergic' encephalomyelitis: II. On the nature of the encephalitogenic agent, *Brain*, **72**, 517.

RAUCH, H. C., and GRIFFIN, J. (1969) Passive transfer studies in experimental allergic encephalomyelitis, in *Pathogenesis and Etiology of Demyelinating Diseases*, ed. Pette, E., Westphal, O., Burdzy, K., and Kallos, P., p. 387, Basel, New York.

RIVERS, T. M., and SCHWENTKER, F. F. (1935) Encephalomyelitis accompanied by myelin destruction experimentally produced in monkeys, *J. exp. Med.*, **61**, 689.

SHAFFER, M. F., RAKE, G., and HODES, H. L. (1942) Isolation of virus from a patient with fatal encephalitis complicating measles, *Amer. J. Dis. Child.*, **64**, 815.

WAKSMAN, B. H. (1959) *Experimental Allergic Encephalomyelitis and the 'Auto-allergic' Diseases*, Basle.

WISNIEWSKI, H. M. (1975) Morphogenesis of the demyelinating process, in *Multiple Sclerosis Research*, ed. Davison, A. N., Humphrey, J. H., Liversedge, L. A., McDonald, W. I., and Porterfield, J. S., London.

WOLF, A., KABAT, E. A., and BEZER, A. E. (1947) The pathology of acute disseminated encephalomyelitis produced experimentally in the rhesus monkey and its resemblance to human demyelinating disease, *J. Neuropath. exp. Neurol.*, **6**, 333.

ENCEPHALOMYELITIS FOLLOWING VACCINATION AGAINST RABIES

It now appears to be established that the nervous complications of antirabic inoculation, whose incidence varies from 1 in 1,000 to 1 in 4,000 persons treated with vaccines prepared in animal brain or spinal cord, are due to sensitization to the central nervous tissue contained in the vaccine and are therefore comparable with EAE (see above). The pathological changes are those of an acute disseminated encephalomyelitis (Uchimura and Shiraki, 1957). The clinical picture may be encephalitic, myelitic, or polyradiculitic. A clinical picture resembling that of the Guillain–Barré syndrome has been described (Adaros and Held, 1971). Retrobulbar neuritis, either unilateral or bilateral, may also occur in these cases. The death rate in the encephalitic and myelitic types of case is said to be 30 per cent. The incidence of these complications may be reduced by using vaccines grown in duck embryos or tissue culture [p. 510]. Lumsden (1961) in an analysis of the pathological findings in 9 fatal cases found that the changes were in certain respects different from those of multiple sclerosis on the one hand and from acute 'spontaneous' disseminated encephalomyelitis on the other.

REFERENCES

ADAROS, H. L., and HELD, J. R. (1971) Guillain–Barré syndrome associated with immunization against rabies: epidemiological aspects, in *Immunological Disorders of the Nervous System* (A.R.N.M.D. vol. XLIX), p. 178, ed. Rowland, L. P., Baltimore.

BASSOE, P., and GRINKER, R. R. (1930) Human rabies and rabies vaccine encephalomyelitis, *Arch. Neurol. Psychiat. (Chic.)*, **23**, 1138.

HURST, E. W. (1932) The effects of the injection of normal brain emulsion into rabbits with special reference to the paralytic accidents of antirabic treatment, *J. Hyg. (Lond.)*, **32**, 33.

LUMSDEN, C. E. (1961) The pathology and pathogenesis of multiple sclerosis, in *Scientific Aspects of Neurology*, ed. Garland, H., Edinburgh.

UCHIMURA, I., and SHIRAKI, H. (1957) A contribution to the classification and the pathogenesis of demyelinating encephalomyelitis, *J. Neuropath. exp. Neurol.*, **16**, 139.

POST-VACCINAL ENCEPHALOMYELITIS
AND ENCEPHALOPATHY

AETIOLOGY
See page 530.

PATHOLOGY
See page 529 and FIGURE 101.

EPIDEMIOLOGY

Nervous complications, for example hemiplegia, had been known to follow vaccination since 1860, but appeared to be isolated occurrences until 1922, since when epidemics of post-vaccinal encephalomyelitis occurred. Ninety-three cases were reported in England between November 1922 and November 1927, and 124 cases had been observed in Holland prior to the latter date. Cases were also observed elsewhere in Europe and the United States, though they were much rarer than in the countries mentioned. Post-vaccinal encephalomyelitis is a rare complication of vaccination. In Holland it has been estimated that one case occurred in over 5,000 persons vaccinated. It follows primary vaccination much more frequently than revaccination, the incidence in Holland being approximately one case in 2,300 primary vaccinations and one case in 50,000 revaccinations. It is practically unknown in infants vaccinated under the age of 1 year and most cases have occurred in children of school age. Though no age is exempt, it is rare after 30. Both sexes are affected equally.

The condition has occurred in epidemics which have coincided with an increase in the number of persons vaccinated owing to the prevalence of small-pox. In the English outbreak of 1923 the 51 cases reported were distributed across the country from Exeter in the south-west to Morpeth in the north-east, with an extension to London and the Home Counties. In the 1962 epidemic of smallpox in South Wales, Spillane and Wells (1964) record that of 800,000 individuals vaccinated, some 39 individuals (24 primary vaccinations, 15 re-vaccinations) suffered neurological complications. There were 11 cases of post-vaccinal encephalomyelitis, 3 of encephalopathy (convulsions and focal neurological signs in infants), 7 cases of meningism, 3 of epilepsy, 6 with focal lesions of brain or cord, 5 with polyneuritis, and 2 with brachial neuritis, while 2 patients with myasthenia gravis relapsed. De Vries (1965) also drew attention to the importance of encephalopathy as a cause of convulsions and coma in infancy, occurring as a sequel of vaccinations or other infections and pointed out that the pathological changes are different from those of encephalomyelitis. There is no evidence of spread of encephalomyelitis by contagion or by any other method of dissemination from one place to another, but it has been noticed that there are often proportionately more cases in small communities and rural areas than in large towns. In several cases two members of the same family who had been vaccinated at the same time both developed encephalomyelitis. The source of vaccine lymph does not appear to be of any aetiological significance.

SYMPTOMS
Incubation Period

In most cases the symptoms of encephalomyelitis develop between the tenth and the twelfth days after vaccination, though the onset has occurred as early as the second day or as late as the twenty-fifth. There is evidence that when the disorder follows revaccination the incubation period is less than when it occurs after primary vaccination.

The Clinical Picture

The onset is usually rapid and is characterized by headache, vomiting, drowsiness, fever, and in some cases convulsions. When fully developed, the clinical picture is usually that of meningeal irritation associated with widespread disturbance of function of the brain and spinal cord. In severe cases drowsiness passes into stupor and coma. Cervical rigidity and Kernig's sign are often present. The ocular fundi are usually normal, but transient papilloedema has occasionally been observed. The incidence of ocular abnormalities is variable. In some cases impairment of the pupillary reflexes and ocular palsies have been present. In others they have not been noted. Trismus has frequently been described, and more than one case has been mistaken for tetanus on account of this symptom. Flaccid paralysis of some or all of the limbs often develops, associated with loss of tendon reflexes and extensor plantar responses. Retention or incontinence of urine and faeces is the rule in severe cases. Sensory loss is inconstant, but may be marked when the spinal cord is severely affected. The CSF may be normal, though under increased pressure, but more often an excess of mononuclear cells and of protein is found. The cutaneous site of vaccination shows the usual inflammatory changes corresponding to the stage at which the patient comes under observation. Not uncommonly there is a severe local reaction, and in a few cases a generalized vaccinial rash has been observed.

DIAGNOSIS

The diagnosis is rarely difficult, since there is a history of recent vaccination and the cutaneous lesions are still visible. Otherwise, the clinical picture cannot be distinguished from other forms of acute disseminated encephalomyelitis or encephalopathy occurring spontaneously or complicating the exanthemata. The severe involvement of the substance of the nervous system indicated by flaccid paralysis distinguishes the condition from meningitis, while the presence of signs of meningeal irritation and the subsequent occurrence of convulsions, trismus, and paralysis of the limbs, together with the inconstancy of ocular abnormalities, distinguish it from encephalitis lethargica. Post-vaccinal encephalomyelitis is distinguished from poliomyelitis by the fact that the paralysis is upper rather than lower motor neurone in type, there is usually associated sensory loss and sphincter involvement and the plantar responses are generally extensor. Post-vaccinal encephalopathy is similar to that which may follow pertussis inoculation.

PROGNOSIS

The mortality rate is high, ranging from 30 per cent to over 50 per cent in different epidemics. In most fatal cases the patient dies in coma from medullary paralysis within a few days of the onset. Less frequently death is due to bronchopneumonia or urinary infection. If recovery occurs it is usually remarkably complete and residual symptoms are exceptional. In some cases, however, there may be some persistent loss of power or sensory loss or, in the case of young children, mental retardation.

PROPHYLAXIS

With the object of preventing post-vaccinal encephalomyelitis as far as possible, the British Ministry of Health made a number of recommendations contained in the Vaccination Order 1929, and the Memorandum on Vaccination against Smallpox (1956). Since the main incidence of post-vaccinal encephalomyelitis falls upon previously unvaccinated adolescents, the opinion was expressed that 'as long as the smallpox prevalent in this country retains its present mild character, it is not generally expedient to press for the vaccination of persons of these ages who have not previously been vaccinated, unless they have been in personal contact with a case of smallpox or directly exposed to smallpox infection'. In all ordinary cases of vaccination or revaccination the operation should be carried out in one insertion, preferably by the multiple pressure technique. With the rapid decline in incidence of smallpox throughout the world, it has been recommended that routine anti-smallpox vaccination should be discontinued in the United States (Brown, 1971).

TREATMENT

See page 541.

REFERENCES

Bastiaanse, F. S. van B. (1925) Encéphalite consécutive à la vaccination antivariolique, *Bull. Acad. Méd. (Paris)*, **94,** 815.

Brown, G. C. (1971) Is routine smallpox vaccination necessary in the United States?, *Amer. J. Epidemiol.*, **93,** 221.

Lucksch, F. (1924) Blatternimpfung und Encephalitis, *Med. Klin.*, **20,** 1170.

Lucksch, F. (1925) Die Vakzineencephalitis, *Med. Klin.*, **21,** 1377.

Ministry of Health. *Reports of the Committee on Vaccination*, London, 1928 and 1930.

Perdrau, J. R. (1928) The histology of post-vaccinal encephalitis, *J. Path. Bact.*, **31,** 17.

Pette, H. (1930) Infektion und Nervensystem, *Dtsch. Z. Nervenheilk.*, **110,** 221 (abs. *Arch. Neurol. Psychiat. (Chic.)*, **24,** 1064).

Spillane, J. D., and Wells, C. E. C. (1964) The neurology of Jennerian vaccination, *Brain*, **87,** 1.

Turnbull, H. M., and McIntosh, J. (1926) Encephalomyelitis following vaccination, *Brit. J. exp. Path.*, **7,** 181.

de Vries, E. (1965) The acute encephalopathic reaction in infants, *Psychiat. Neurol. Neurochir. (Amst.)*, **68,** 85.

Wiersma, D. (1929) Remarks on the etiology of encephalitis after vaccination, *Acta psychiat. (Kbh.)*, **4,** 75.

ENCEPHALOMYELITIS COMPLICATING SMALLPOX

The occurrence of nervous symptoms in smallpox has been known for many years, but is a rare event, having been observed in only about 2·5 per 1,000 cases. The investigations of Troup and Hurst (1930) and of McIntosh and Scarff (1928) showed that the pathological changes in the nervous system are indistinguishable from those of post-vaccinal encephalomyelitis. In some cases bulbar symptoms, especially dysarthria, are prominent, and are sometimes accompanied by paralysis of the limbs. In other cases paraplegia occurs, with or without sphincter disturbances and impairment of sensibility. Mental changes are sometimes present. Often recovery occurs and is strikingly complete, but the patient may die during the acute attack or subsequently from the complications of paraplegia.

REFERENCES

McINTOSH, J., and SCARFF, R. W. (1927–8) The histology of some virus infections of the central nervous system, *Proc. roy. Soc. Med.*, **21**, 705.

MARSDEN, J. P., and HURST, E. W. (1932) Acute perivascular myelinoclasis ('acute disseminated encephalomyelitis') in smallpox, *Brain*, **55**, 181.

TROUP, A. G., and HURST, E. W. (1930) Disseminated encephalomyelitis following smallpox, *Lancet*, **i**, 566.

TURNBULL, H. M., and McINTOSH, J. (1926) Encephalomyelitis following vaccination, *Brit. J. exp. Path.*, **7**, 181.

ENCEPHALOMYELITIS COMPLICATING MEASLES

According to Miller *et al.* (1956) neurological complications occur in less than 1 in 1,000 cases: 95 per cent are encephalitic or encephalomyelitic, less than 3 per cent myelitic, and less than 2 per cent polyradiculitic. The pathological picture ranges from congestion, perivascular infiltration, and occasional haemorrhages in the more acute cases to typical perivenous demyelination in the later stages. Aetiology and pathology are discussed on pages 529–30.

SYMPTOMS

Nervous complications of measles have been known for over a century, but appear to have become more common during recent years. The onset of symptoms is usually 4 to 6 days after the beginning of the illness when the fever has fallen and the rash is fading. Ford (1928) and Tyler (1957) have reviewed the literature and distinguished a number of clinical types. It is probable that acute disseminated encephalomyelitis is not the pathological basis of all the nervous complications of measles.

1. The nervous symptoms may be relatively mild and transient and present a clinical picture resembling 'meningism' or encephalopathy. In such cases headache, stupor, signs of meningeal irritation, and sometimes convulsions occur, but focal lesions of the substance of the nervous system are absent.

2. Multiple focal or diffuse lesions of the nervous system may occur, involving the cerebral cortex, basal ganglia, brain stem, cerebellum, optic nerves, and spinal cord in various combinations.

3. There may be a single focal cerebral lesion, hemiplegia and aphasia being the commonest.

4. The symptoms may be predominantly those of cerebellar deficiency.

5. The spinal cord may be mainly affected, the clinical picture being an acute ascending paralysis leading to paraplegia, with or without concurrent involvement of the brain. Neuromyelitis optica may be simulated.

6. Other nervous symptoms are rare, the clinical picture of polyradiculitis being the most important. The cerebrospinal fluid may be normal in cases of encephalopathy but in encephalomyelitis usually shows a moderate increase in lymphocytes and protein.

7. There is increasing evidence to indicate that subacute sclerosing panencephalitis is a late but rare sequel of measles infection [p. 494].

DIAGNOSIS

The diagnosis is usually easy, since the measles rash is generally present when the nervous symptoms develop. If the attack of measles has passed unnoticed the disorder cannot be distinguished from other forms of acute disseminated encephalomyelitis.

PROGNOSIS

The mortality rate is 10 to 20 per cent in different series, and probably about 50 per cent are left with residual symptoms, of which the most important are hemiplegia, ataxia, mental defect or change of personality, often with hyperkinesis and perceptual defects (Meyer and Byers, 1952), and epilepsy. Coma and convulsions are bad prognostic signs.

TREATMENT

See page 541.

REFERENCES

FERRARO, A., and SCHEFFER, I. H. (1931) Encephalitis and encephalomyelitis in measles, *Arch. Neurol. Psychiat. (Chic.)*, **25,** 748.

FERRARO, A., and SCHEFFER, I. H. (1932) Toxic encephalopathy in measles, *Arch. Neurol. Psychiat. (Chic.)*, **27,** 1209.

FORD, F. R. (1928) The nervous complications of measles with a summary of the literature and publication of 12 additional case reports, *Bull. Johns Hopk. Hosp.*, **43,** 140.

GREENFIELD, J. G. (1929) The pathology of measles encephalomyelitis, *Brain*, **52,** 171.

MALAMUD, N. (1937) Encephalomyelitis complicating measles, *Arch. Neurol. Psychiat. (Chic.)*, **38,** 1025.

MEYER, E., and BYERS, R. K. (1952) Measles encephalitis: a follow-up study of 16 patients, *Amer. J. Dis. Child.*, **84,** 543.

MILLER, H. G., STANTON, J. B., and GIBBONS, J. L. (1956) Para-infectious encephalomyelitis and related syndromes, *Quart. J. Med.*, **25,** 427.

TYLER, H. R. (1957) Neurological complications of rubeola (measles), *Medicine (Baltimore)*, **36,** 147.

ZIMMERMANN, H. M., and YANNET, H. (1930) Encephalomyelitis complicating measles, *Arch. Neurol. Psychiat. (Chic.)*, **24,** 1000.

ENCEPHALOMYELITIS COMPLICATING RUBELLA

Encephalomyelitis is a rare complication of rubella, occurring in about 1 in 5,000 cases (Sherman *et al.*, 1965). The clinical and pathological features are similar to those of measles encephalomyelitis; contrary to the common view, the illness tends to be more acute and severe than in either measles or varicella with a mortality of about 20 per cent. Coma and convulsions are common, and cerebellar involvement (Cantwell, 1957), myelitis, and polyradiculitis have been described but recovery is usually rapid and complete in surviving cases within two weeks (Margolis *et al.*, 1943).

REFERENCES

BRIGGS, J. F. (1935) Meningoencephalitis following rubella, *J. Pediat.*, **7,** 609.

CANTWELL, R. J. (1957) Rubella encephalitis, *Brit. med. J.*, **2,** 1471.

MARGOLIS, F. J., WILSON, J. L., and TOP, F. H. (1943) Post-rubella encephalomyelitis, *J. Pediat.*, **23,** 158.

MERRITT, H. H., and KOSKOFF, Y. D. (1936) Encephalomyelitis following German measles, *Amer. J. med. Sci.*, **191,** 690.

MILLER, H. G., STANTON, J. B., and GIBBONS, J. L. (1956) Para-infectious encephalomyelitis and related syndromes, *Quart. J. Med.*, **25,** 427.

SHERMAN, F. E., MICHAELS, R. H., and KENNY, F. M. (1965) Acute encephalopathy (encephalitis) complicating rubella, *J. Amer. med. Ass.*, **192,** 675.
SKINNER, H. O. (1935) Encephalitis complicating German measles, *J. Amer. med. Ass.*, **105,** 24.

ENCEPHALOMYELITIS COMPLICATING CHICKENPOX

Encephalitis and/or myelitis are rare complications of chickenpox (varicella).

PATHOLOGY

Owing to the relatively benign nature of this disorder there have been few opportunities of studying its pathology. On the whole the pathological picture appears to be the same as that found in measles encephalomyelitis though van Bogaert (1933) found foci of demyelination in the cerebral hemispheres of one case resembling early plaques of multiple sclerosis and Miget (1933) was impressed by the inflammatory cell infiltration of the meninges which he found in another.

SYMPTOMS

Symptoms of involvement of the nervous system develop in such cases between the fifth and the twentieth day after the appearance of the rash, usually during the first half of the second week. Encephalitis is said to occur in 90 per cent of cases, myelitis in 3 per cent, and polyradiculitis in 7 per cent (Miller et al., 1956). The onset is acute, and is characterized by fever, headache, vomiting, and giddiness, and sometimes by delirium. Coma and convulsions are less common than in other forms of post-infectious encephalomyelitis, occurring only in about 3 per cent of cases. The disturbance may be mainly meningeal, mainly cerebral, or mainly spinal but in addition some cases present with what appears to be an almost 'pure' cerebellar ataxia. The meningeal form is characterized by the usual symptoms of meningitis. In the 'cerebellar' cases, incoordination is the commonest symptom, occurring with or without involuntary movements. The ataxia is often so gross as to render the child incapable of walking. Tremor and choreic or choreo-athetoid movements sometimes occur. Signs of corticospinal tract lesions may be present, but diplegia and hemiplegia are rare. Ophthalmoplegia has been observed. The spinal lesion usually produces the picture of a dorsal transverse myelitis. The spinal fluid may be normal, or may show an excess of protein and cells, usually mononuclear.

DIAGNOSIS

The cause of the nervous symptoms is evident when the diagnosis of chickenpox has already been made. If, however, this has passed unnoticed, the encephalomyelitis cannot be distinguished from other forms of acute disseminated encephalomyelitis, except that the involvement of the cerebellum appears to be peculiarly frequent in encephalitis complicating chickenpox (Boughton, 1966).

PROGNOSIS

The prognosis is good, both as to life and as to recovery of function. The mortality rate in encephalitic cases is less than 10 per cent and sequelae are rare in those who survive.

TREATMENT

See page 541.

REFERENCES

BÉRODE, P. (1932), *Les Complications nerveuses de la varicelle (à propos des formes méningées)*, Thèse de Paris.

BOGAERT, L. VAN (1933) Les manifestations nerveuses au cours des maladies eruptives, *Rev. neurol.*, **1**, 150.

BOUGHTON, C. R. (1966) Neurological complications of varicella, *Med. J. Aust.*, **2**, 444.

BRAIN, W. R. (1931) Zoster, varicella, and encephalitis, *Brit. med. J.*, **1**, 81.

GLANZMANN, E. (1927) Die nervösen Komplikationen der Varizellen, Variola und Vakzine, *Schweiz. med. Wschr.*, **8**, 145.

GORDON, M. B. (1924) Acute hemorrhagic nephritis and acute hemorrhagic encephalitis following varicella, *Amer. J. Dis. Child.*, **28**, 589.

KRABBE, K. H. (1925) Varicella myelitis, *Brain*, **48**, 535.

MIGET, A. (1933) Les complications nerveuses de la varicelle, *Médecine*, **14**, 137.

MILLER, H. G., STANTON, J. B., and GIBBONS, J. L. (1956). Para-infectious encephalo-myelitis and related syndromes, *Quart. J. Med.*, **25**, 427.

WILSON, R. E., and FORD, F. R. (1927) The nervous complications of variola, vaccinia and varicella, with report of cases, *Bull. Johns Hopk. Hosp.*, **40**, 337.

ZIMMERMANN, H. M., and YANNET, H. (1931) Nonsuppurative encephalomyelitis accompanying chickenpox, *Arch. Neurol. Psychiat. (Chic.)*, **26**, 322.

SPONTANEOUS ACUTE DISSEMINATED ENCEPHALOMYELITIS AND ACUTE CEREBELLAR ATAXIA

A form of acute disseminated encephalomyelitis clinically and pathologically identical with that which follows the above-mentioned exanthems may occur spontaneously or as a complication of a febrile illness of an 'influenzal' type. Miller and Evans (1953) support the view that acute disseminated encephalo-myelitis represents a non-specific allergic reaction of the nervous system to various antigens, chiefly of bacterial or virus origin, in which case the 'spon-taneous' form of the disease may be a reaction to a banal infection, or may rarely follow an inoculation or the administration of antiserum.

The symptoms and signs of spontaneous acute disseminated encephalo-myelitis are indistinguishable from those of the post-exanthematous varieties described above. However, acute cerebellar ataxia of infancy and childhood has been identified as a distinctive syndrome, occurring usually in infants between 1 and 2 years of age and often following a non-specific infective illness (Weiss and Carter, 1959). As Menkes (1974) points out, the acute onset of cerebellar ataxia in childhood can be due to a variety of causes but in this distinctive syndrome which is characterized by severe truncal ataxia, nystagmus in most cases, and often by tremor of the head, trunk, and limbs (Brumlik and Means, 1969), there may be evidence of ECHO or Coxsackie or even poliovirus infec-tion, but most cases seem likely to be the result of an autoimmune response similar to that which occurs in other forms of encephalomyelitis. Ataxia may be so severe that the child cannot sit unsupported, and speech is often affected; the condition may last for two or more months, even though mildly affected children may recover in one or two weeks, and relapses may follow recurrent respiratory infection. Recovery is often complete but in up to a third of cases there is residual ataxia, dysarthria, and even mental retardation. The relation-ship between this condition and the so-called subacute myoclonic encephalo-pathy of infants described by Kinsbourne (1962) and by Dyken and Kolar

(1968) in which bizarre random eye movements (opsoclonus) and coarse irregular jerking movements of the extremities are also accompanied by variable ataxia is uncertain but the rapid response to treatment with ACTH in many of the latter group of cases suggests that the aetiology and pathogenesis are probably similar. In such cases the CSF may be normal but may sometimes show a modest lymphocytic pleocytosis and an increased protein count, particularly of immunoglobulins. In cases of encephalopathy in childhood, dexamethasone in appropriate dosage depending upon age may be preferred in order to reduce cerebral oedema in the acute stage.

DIAGNOSIS

The diagnosis of encephalomyelitis rests upon the occurrence of a febrile illness with evidence of subacute lesions of the white matter of the brain or spinal cord or both, usually in multiple foci, and with or without signs of meningeal irritation [see also p. 534]. The main difficulty lies in distinguishing acute disseminated encephalomyelitis from the acute lesions of multiple sclerosis.

McAlpine et al. (1972) have considered the differential diagnosis between acute disseminated encephalomyelitis and acute multiple sclerosis. They point out that whereas in the acute stage distinction between the two conditions may be impossible on clinical grounds, an acute attack of encephalomyelitis or myelitis may resolve completely and that subsequently the patient may remain free from relapse for many years. Pette (1928) first suggested that no clinical or pathological distinction could be made between the two conditions and this 'unitary' theory was later supported by Ferraro (1958) and Miller and Schapira (1959).

Van Bogaert (1950) pointed out that some cases diagnosed clinically as cases of acute encephalomyelitis are in every respect similar to those cases which occur after specific infectious fevers; others run a course typical of multiple sclerosis, while others recover and remain well. The encephalitic form is particularly common in children and young adults and may affect principally the cerebral hemispheres, brain stem or cerebellum, while the myelitic form may occur at any age (McAlpine et al., 1972).

After the acute stage has subsided, if the patient is found to have residual physical signs, the diagnosis from multiple sclerosis may be extremely difficult. It must be based upon the history of the onset and development of symptoms in the acute stage and the absence of any extension of the physical signs after the first few weeks of the illness.

PROGNOSIS

Although fresh lesions may occur within two or three weeks of the onset, acute disseminated encephalomyelitis is usually a self-limited disease, and relapses are uncommon, but Miller and Evans (1953) pointed out that recurrences may occur, especially when the nervous disorder follows a non-specific minor infection, usually of the upper respiratory tract, in which the development of lasting immunity is known to be exceptional, and in which repeated antigenic insults furnish a possible pathogenetic mechanism. In all acute demyelinating disorders a substantial degree of recovery of function can be expected, but if the initial disorder has been severe some residual disability is likely, and this may be added to if recurrences occur.

TREATMENT

When hyperpyrexia occurs in such cases, tepid sponging or other methods of cooling may be necessary. In comatose patients, tube-feeding, parenteral fluids, careful nursing care and even tracheostomy with or without assisted respiration may be required. Miller (1953) and Miller and Gibbons (1953) recommended corticotrophin (ACTH), 80 units daily, in the acute phase and it is now generally agreed that this drug is beneficial in limiting the spread of the inflammatory process. In cases of encephalopathy in childhood, dexamethasone in appropriate dosage depending upon age may be preferred in order to reduce cerebral oedema in the acute stage. Appropriate antibiotics are often needed to control secondary infections and anticonvulsants may also be required in selected cases to control convulsions.

REFERENCES

BOGAERT, L. VAN (1950) Post-infectious encephalomyelitis and multiple sclerosis, *J. Neuropath.*, **9**, 219.

BRUMLIK, J., and MEANS, E. D. (1969) Tremorine-tremor, shivering and acute cerebellar ataxia in the adult and child—a comparative study, *Brain*, **92**, 157.

DYKEN, P., and KOLAR, O. (1968) Dancing eyes, dancing feet: infantile polymyoclonia, *Brain*, **91**, 305.

FERRARO, A. (1958) Studies on multiple sclerosis, *J. Neuropath.*, **17**, 278.

KINSBOURNE, M. (1962) Myoclonic encephalopathy of infants, *J. Neurol. Neurosurg. Psychiat.*, **25**, 271.

McALPINE, D., LUMSDEN, C. E., and ACHESON, E. D. (1972) *Multiple Sclerosis: a Reappraisal*, 2nd ed., Edinburgh.

MENKES, J. H. (1974) *Textbook of Child Neurology*, Philadelphia.

MILLER, H. G. (1953) Acute disseminated encephalomyelitis treated with A.C.T.H., *Brit. med. J.*, **1**, 177.

MILLER, H. G., and EVANS, M. J. (1953) Prognosis in acute disseminated encephalomyelitis; with a note on neuromyelitis optica, *Quart. J. Med.*, N.S. **22**, 347.

MILLER, H. G., and GIBBONS, J. L. (1953) Acute disseminated encephalomyelitis and acute multiple sclerosis; results of treatment with ACTH, *Brit. med. J.*, **2**, 1345.

MILLER, H. G., and SCHAPIRA, K. (1959) Aetiological aspects of multiple sclerosis, *Brit. med. J.*, **1**, 737.

PETTE, H. (1928) Klinische und anatomische Studien über die Pathogenese der multiplen Sklerose, *Dtsch. med. Wschr.*, **84**, 2061.

WEISS, S., and CARTER, S. (1959) Course and prognosis of acute cerebellar ataxia in children, *Neurology (Minneap.)*, **9**, 711.

ACUTE HAEMORRHAGIC LEUCO-ENCEPHALITIS

Acute haemorrhagic leuco-encephalitis was first described by Hurst (1941) and subsequently by Henson and Russell in 1942. It is characterized pathologically by macroscopic oedema of the brain with numerous minute haemorrhages and microscopically by severe damage to the vessel walls, perivascular necrosis, perivascular and focal demyelination, intense polymorphonuclear exudation, and microglial reaction. Clinically there is a febrile illness characterized by headache, vomiting, deepening stupor with or without hemiparesis, and a leucocytosis in the blood. Hurst suggested, and Greenfield (1950) accepted, the view that the haemorrhagic lesions and the non-haemorrhagic areas of necrosis or demyelination represent different degrees of injury by a single noxious agent, and Russell (1955) agreed that acute haemorrhagic leuco-encephalitis is simply a hyperacute and explosive form of acute disseminated encephalomyelitis.

REFERENCES

GREENFIELD, J. G. (1950) Encephalitis and encephalomyelitis in England and Wales during the last decade, *Brain*, **73,** 141.

HENSON, R. A., and RUSSELL, D. S. (1942) Acute haemorrhagic leuco-encephalitis, *J. Path. Bact.*, **54,** 227.

HURST, E. W. (1941) Acute haemorrhagic leuco-encephalitis, a previously undefined entity, *Med. J. Aust.*, **2,** 1.

RUSSELL, D. S. (1955) The nosological unity of acute haemorrhagic leuco-encephalitis and acute disseminated encephalomyelitis, *Brain*, **78,** 369.

DISSEMINATED MYELITIS WITH OPTIC NEURITIS

Synonyms. Acute disseminated myelitis; diffuse myelitis with optic neuritis; neuromyelitis optica; ophthalmoneuromyelitis; Devic's disease.

Definition. A form of subacute encephalomyelitis characterized by massive demyelination of the optic nerves and spinal cord, sometimes running a self-limited and sometimes a progressive course.

PATHOLOGY

Both the optic nerves and spinal cord exhibit massive demyelination. Loss of myelin sheaths is found in the optic nerves and chiasm, and in the spinal cord may be limited to a few segments, usually in the lower cervical and upper dorsal region, or may be more diffuse, extending through the greater part of the cord's length. In severe cases cavitation may occur. Marked perivascular infiltration is not only present in the demyelinated areas but may be found throughout the nervous system. The infiltrating cells are principally mononuclear, but poly-morphonuclear cells may also be present. In the demyelinated areas there is a great multiplication of vessels surrounded by many fat-granule cells and also neuroglial cells, though with little formation of new neuroglial fibres. To the naked eye the affected areas are swollen, congested, and softened.

AETIOLOGY

The cause of Devic's disease is unknown. It is rare and affects both sexes at all ages from 12 to 60 years. McAlpine (1938) reported its occurrence in identical twins. While in the past the condition was generally regarded as an independent clinical and pathological entity, McAlpine *et al.* (1972) point out that there is a growing body of opinion which favours the view that it is simply a form of mul-tiple sclerosis. Even in Japan where it has proved to be very common, Okinaka *et al.* (1960) have reached a similar conclusion. Nevertheless, Scott (1961, 1967), who followed up cases seen in Edinburgh between 1937 and 1949, found that despite clear evidence of bilateral optic nerve involvement and variable signs of spinal cord disease, none of his patients had developed episodes of subsequent neurological illness to suggest recurring demyelination as would have been expected in multiple sclerosis and in general the ultimate prognosis was good.

SYMPTOMS

The clinical features were reviewed by Stansbury (1949) and Scott (1952), who pointed out that the illness often begins with a sore throat, cold in the head, or febrile disturbance. Either the ocular or the spinal lesion may develop first, and these events may be separated by days or weeks, or both may occur simultaneously. Usually one eye is first affected, to be followed by the other after an interval varying from a few hours to several weeks. Rarely the onset of the myelitis intervenes between the affection of the two eyes.

The ocular lesion may be a true optic neuritis or a retrobulbar neuritis, depending upon whether it is situated sufficiently anteriorly to involve the optic discs. In the former case papilloedema is present, though the swelling is usually slight; in the latter the discs are normal. The characteristic field defect is a bilateral central scotoma. In severe cases blindness may be complete or almost so. Homonymous field defects have been described. The two eyes are often unequally affected. Pain in the eyes is often severe and is accentuated by moving them and by pressure upon the globes.

The spinal cord lesion, the onset of which may be associated with severe pain in the back and limbs, leads to the usual symptoms of transverse myelitis, with paralysis of upper motor neurone type and loss of some or all forms of sensation below the level of the lesion and of sphincter control. When, as frequently happens, the cervical region of the cord is involved quadriplegia results.

The cerebrospinal fluid may show no abnormality or there may be an increase of protein and globulin and an excess of cells, which are usually mononuclear, though occasionally polymorphonuclear cells have been described. There is no characteristic colloidal gold curve but the gamma-globulin is usually raised.

It is probable that the disorder may abort after the development of optic neuritis and before the spinal symptoms appear and that the reverse may also occur, so that some cases of acute bilateral optic neuritis without other symptoms, and also some cases of acute transverse myelitis without optic neuritis, may belong to this group.

DIAGNOSIS

The presence of bilateral optic neuritis before symptoms of the lesion of the spinal cord appear, may suggest a diagnosis of intracranial tumour. In optic neuritis, however, the disc swelling is slight in proportion to the severity of the loss of vision and the characteristic field defect is bilateral central scotomas, in contrast to the peripheral constriction of the fields associated with papilloedema in increased intracranial pressure. Moreover, in cases of optic neuritis headache and vomiting are absent, though pain in the eyes may be severe.

PROGNOSIS

The mortality rate in the past was about 50 per cent, death occurring either from respiratory paralysis, or from infections complicating the paraplegia. If the patient survived, recovery was often remarkably complete. Cases occurring in the last 30 years have seemed often to be less severe and assisted respiration has greatly improved the outcome. Complete blindness may be followed by a considerable return of vision, though some degree of optic atrophy is likely to persist. Similarly, the functions of the spinal cord may be largely, if not completely, restored. Recovery, once achieved, may be permanent, but progressive and relapsing cases occur. These underline the close relationship of the disorder to multiple sclerosis.

TREATMENT

Corticotrophin (ACTH) 80 units daily at first, with subsequent reduction to 40 units daily, continuing until progressive clinical improvement is manifest and giving thereafter smaller maintenance doses for several weeks, is now generally recommended. The usual measures for the care of the skin, urinary and intestinal tracts, and musculature, which are required in paraplegia, will be necessary and assisted respiration may be required in severe cases with ascending paralysis.

REFERENCES

BRAIN, W. R. (1929–30) Critical review: disseminated sclerosis, *Quart. J. Med.*, **23**, 343.

GOULDEN, C. (1914) Optic neuritis and myelitis, *Trans. ophthal. Soc. U.K.*, **34**, 229.

HASSIN, G. B. (1937) Neuroptic myelitis versus multiple sclerosis, *Arch. Neurol. Psychiat.* (*Chic.*), **37**, 1083.

HOLMES, G. (1927) Discussion on diffuse myelitis associated with optic neuritis, *Brain*, **50**, 702.

LEJONNE, P., and LHERMITTE, J. (1909) De la nature inflammatoire de certaines scléroses en plaques, *Encéphale*, iv, i, 220.

MCALPINE, D. (1938) Familial neuromyelitis optica: its occurrence in identical twins, *Brain*, **61**, 430.

MCALPINE, D., LUMSDEN, C. E., and ACHESON, E. D. (1972) *Multiple Sclerosis: a Reappraisal*, 2nd ed., Edinburgh.

OKINAKA, S., MCALPINE, D., MIYAGAWA, K., SUWA, N., KUROIWA, Y., SHIRAKI, H., ARAKI, S., and KURLAND, L. T. (1960) Multiple sclerosis in Northern and Southern Japan, *Wld Neurol.*, **1**, 22.

SCOTT, G. I. (1952) Neuromyelitis optica, *Amer. J. Ophthal.*, **35**, 755.

SCOTT, G. I. (1961) Ophthalmic aspects of demyelinating diseases, *Proc. roy. Soc. Med.*, **54**, 38.

SCOTT, G. I. (1967) Optic disc oedema, *Trans. ophthal. Soc. U.K.*, **87**, 733.

STANSBURY, F. C. (1949) Neuromyelitis optica (Devic's disease), *Arch. Ophthal.* (*Chic.*), **42**, 292, 465.

SYMONDS, C. P. (1924) The pathological anatomy of disseminated sclerosis, *Brain*, **47**, 36.

MULTIPLE SCLEROSIS (MS)

Synonyms. Disseminated sclerosis; insular sclerosis.

Definition. A disease of unknown aetiology characterized pathologically by the widespread occurrence in the nervous system of patches of demyelination followed by gliosis. In many cases the early manifestations of the disease are followed by conspicuous improvement, so that remissions and relapses are a striking feature of the disorder, the course of which may thus be prolonged for many years. The early symptoms are often those of focal lesions of the nervous system, while the later clinical picture is one of progressive dissemination tending to produce the classical features of ataxic paraplegia.

PATHOLOGY

The first pathological accounts of the disease were given by Cruveilhier in 1835 and Carswell in 1838. The pathological 'unit' in MS is a circumscribed lesion in which the pathological process begins with destruction of the myelin sheaths of the nerve fibres and to a much lesser extent of the axis cylinders, and

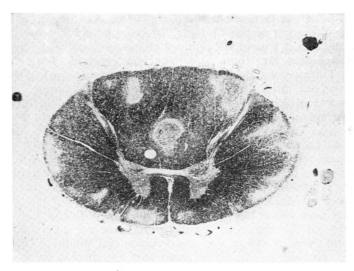

FIG. 102. Multiple sclerosis: spinal cord, T. 9

ends with the formation of a 'sclerotic plaque' [FIG. 102]. These plaques occur predominantly in the white matter of the brain and spinal cord. They are sometimes found in the grey matter of the cerebral cortex and in the cranial and spinal nerve roots, rarely in the grey matter of the spinal cord. Many writers have stressed their perivascular distribution, though Dawson (1916) pointed out that 'the changes appear within but do not coincide with the area of distribution of the arteries'. Putnam (1937) emphasized the relationship of the patches to cerebral venules, but Dow and Berglund (1942) reported many exceptions to this; and stated that thrombosis of a vein within a plaque, stressed by Putnam, is rare. The optic nerves and chiasm, the neighbourhood of the cerebral ventricles, and the subpial region of the spinal cord are favourite sites. In an extensive review, Lumsden (1970) showed that there is no evidence to indicate that venous thrombosis plays any part in pathogenesis, but immuno-fluorescent studies (Lumsden, 1971) have shown that immunoglobulins and complement accumulate in areas of active demyelination, and circulating immunoglobulin (antimyelin antibody) passing through the blood vessel wall may be important in pathogenesis. The part played by sensitized lymphocytes in this process is still uncertain (Caspary and Field, 1974; Webb et al., 1974). Electrophoretic studies of protein and analysis of proteolytic enzymes isolated from samples of cerebral white matter obtained from the brains of patients with MS (Riekkinen et al., 1970, 1971; Adams et al., 1971; Einstein et al., 1972) have shown consistent but as yet non-specific abnormalities and it is still uncertain as to whether sensitization to encephalitogenic factor (EF) plays a part in the human disease.

To the naked eye the sclerotic plaque appears slightly sunken, greyish, and more translucent than normal nervous tissue. In the acute stage the blood vessels are dilated, and the perivascular spaces contain fat-granule cells and frequently also lymphocytes and plasma cells. The myelin of the nerve sheaths degenerates, and the axis cylinders may show diffuse or irregular swellings.

Even at this stage, as Greenfield and King (1936) pointed out, there is a conspicuous proliferation of the fibroglia. In late plaques the myelin has been removed; the axis cylinders are reduced in number, some of those persisting show abnormalities, and there is a thick condensation of the original glial meshwork. Ultrastructural studies of plaques have confirmed that there is inflammatory cell infiltration and phagocytosis of myelin; several workers claim to have identified tubules and intranuclear inclusions resembling nucleocapsids of paramyxovirus (Narang and Field, 1973; Raine et al., 1974); the viral nature of these inclusions has been disputed (Dubois-Dalcq et al., 1973; Lampert and Lampert, 1975) although ter Meulen et al. (1972) isolated an infective agent related to group 1 parainfluenza virus from MS brain tissue studied in tissue culture. Mechanisms of remyelination, which may account for remission of symptoms, and the role of the oligodendroglia in this process have been reviewed by McDonald (1974 a and b).

There has been much dispute as to whether there is any pathological distinction between the lesions of acute disseminated encephalomyelitis on the one hand and those of MS on the other. Anton and Wohlwill (1912), Redlich (1927), and Spielmeyer (1923) believed that the two conditions could be differentiated and van Bogaert (1950) and Greenfield and Norman (1965) felt that despite the similarity of changes observed in the acute phase of both disorders, the chronic lesions of MS are distinctive. Many others, however, including Fraenkel and Jakob (1913), Ferraro (1937, 1958), and Alvord (1966) felt that the two conditions are pathologically indistinguishable. Lumsden (1970, 1972) is firmly of the opinion that the primary pathological process is identical in the two disorders but points out that in the chronic lesion of MS the appearances are such that it is impossible to determine what may have been the primary process. He points out that massive and widespread demyelination may well be the end result of several processes of varying aetiology and in his opinion acute disseminated encephalomyelitis, Devic's disease, MS, the concentric demyelination of Baló and Schilder's disease (see below) represent the differing end-stages of what is, in the first instance, the same essential pathological change.

AETIOLOGY

General Considerations

The aetiology of MS is still unknown. Earlier pathologists regarded the gliosis as the primary process, hence the word 'sclerosis', but it is now clear that the glial scar is simply the end-result of the initial inflammatory and demyelinating process. Earlier theories suggesting that the disease might be due to infection with a spirochaete or a rickettsial agent, that it was due to venular thrombosis, to the ingestion of heavy metals such as copper, or to excessive dietary fat have now been largely abandoned and the isolation of a specific virus claimed by Margulis et al. (1946) was never confirmed. Epidemiological studies (see below) have given some support to the possibility that the condition could prove to be due to a 'slow virus' infection while experimental work on recurrent rather than monophasic encephalomyelitis induced by EF and adjuvant (see Wisniewski, 1975) as well as much clinical, immunological, and genetic evidence suggests that the disease may be due to hypersensitivity. Field (1966) showed that the inoculation of brain biopsy material from a patient with MS ultimately produced the changes of scrapie in white mice but pointed out that his results were open to several interpretations and other transmission experiments have been unsuccessful (McAlpine *et al.*, 1972). However, many groups of workers have now reported the finding of significantly increased levels of measles antibodies in the serum and cerebrospinal fluid of such cases, and measles-specific immunoglobulin has been identified in CSF samples (Dowling *et al.*, 1968; Salmi *et al.*, 1972; Norrby *et al.*, 1974; *The Lancet*, 1974). In some cases, however, raised levels of antibodies to viruses as diverse as RSV virus, herpes simplex, mumps, varicella, and adenovirus have been found (Ross *et al.*, 1969; Sever *et al.*, 1971), and McDermott *et al.* (1974) have pointed out that EF and measles virus have similar antigenic determinants. An association postulated on epidemiological grounds between MS on the one hand and enterovirus infections such as poliomyelitis on the other (Poskanzer *et al.*, 1963) has not been supported by virological studies. Other viruses have been isolated from MS brains (Nemo *et al.*, 1974) and paramyxovirus-like inclusions have been identified by electron microscopy (see above), but recent antibody studies (Nemo *et al.*, 1974; Lehrich *et al.*, 1974) have not suggested that parainfluenza virus or any other viral agent plays a primary aetiological role (Brody, 1972). However, studies of histocompatibility antigens (see below) indicate that genetic predisposition may be of importance and the present consensus of opinion favours the view that MS is a disorder of the immune response of the nervous system, perhaps conditioned by inherited predisposition, to infection with a variety of viral agents, of which measles may be one; the infection may well have been acquired many years before the symptoms of MS first become manifest (Millar, 1971; Leibowitz and Alter, 1973). Recent work by Carp, Henle, and others supporting a viral aetiology has been reviewed by *The Lancet* (1976) and the *British Medical Journal* (1976).

The Role of Inherited Predisposition

Multiple cases of MS in the same family sometimes occur. Curtius in 1933 collected 84 references to this in the literature and the subject has been studied by Pratt *et al.* (1951) and by McAlpine *et al.* (1972). In most instances two sibs are affected. Affection of two successive generations is less common but conjugal cases rarely occur (Schapira *et al.* 1963) and the disease has been reported in the daughter of parents each of whom had MS (Gilbert, 1971).

McAlpine *et al.* (1972) have concluded that the risk that MS will develop in a first degree relative is about 15 times as great as in the general population. No definite pattern of inheritance emerges but much interest has been aroused by recent work showing that histocompatibility antigens HL-A 3 and 7 and W18 are significantly more common in patients with MS than in the general population (Lehrich *et al.*, 1974; Arnason *et al.*, 1974; Bertrams and Kuwert, 1972; Paty *et al.*, 1974). Since animal studies have shown that susceptibility to autoimmune disease and virus infection is linked to histocompatibility, this finding may help to explain the evidence for genetic predisposition.

Precipitating Factors

Many events may immediately precede the onset of the illness and have often been regarded as precipitating factors though their mode of operation is unknown. They include influenza and infections of the upper respiratory tract, the specific fevers, superficial sepsis, surgical operations, and the extraction of teeth. Recent investigation casts doubt on the danger of surgical operations (Miller, 1961) but relapses have been noted to occur after vaccination against smallpox (Miller *et al.*, 1967), and Currier *et al.* (1974) found a significantly increased incidence of infectious illness, trauma, and surgical operation before the age of 20 years in 60 MS patients when compared with matched control subjects. Cigarette smoking has no obvious aetiological influence (Simpson *et al.*, 1966) but may temporarily worsen the symptoms (McAlpine *et al.*, 1972) and Millar *et al.* (1959) believed that pregnancy did not influence the relapse rate, although Schapira *et al.* (1966) showed that relapses were particularly liable to occur in the 3 months after delivery. Relapse has also been described after emotional stress, as an allergic reaction to various drugs, including penicillin, after insect bites, blood transfusion, and as a result of exertion, fatigue, or exposure to high or low temperature (McAlpine *et al.*, 1972). In Switzerland, Wüthrich and Rieder (1970) showed that most relapses occurred in winter and in the spring months. McAlpine and Compston (1952) obtained a history of physical injury preceding the onset of symptoms by less than 3 months in 14·4 per cent of cases, but in only 5·2 per cent of controls, and there is some evidence for a relation between the site of the trauma and the site of the first symptom (Miller, 1964). Trauma may thus precipitate the onset of the disease or a relapse.

Distribution, Age, and Sex

MS is most prevalent in Northern Europe and Switzerland. It is less common in North America and is rare in Japan, in South Africa, and in tropical countries. A vast literature has now accumulated upon the incidence and prevalence of the disease, based upon careful population surveys carried out in many parts of the world and this has been reviewed in detail by Acheson (1972). In general the crude prevalence rate rises the further one moves north or south from the equator. Figures vary from 10 per 100,000 in New Orleans and 14 per 100,000 in rural Western Australia to 33 per 100,000 in Hobart, Tasmania, 41 per 100,000 in Boston, Massachusetts, 50 per 100,000 in Northumberland and Durham, England, and about 80 per 100,000 in south-eastern Norway and in the Orkney and Shetland islands, but there are many examples of a relatively high prevalence rate in isolated populations in low-risk areas and vice versa (Rinne *et al.*, 1968; McCall *et al.*, 1968; Panelius, 1969; Behrend, 1969; Kurtzke, 1975 *a* and *b*). There is also evidence that the clinical picture of the disease may be changing in some low-risk areas (Kuroiwa and Shibasaki, 1973; Shibasaki and Kuroiwa, 1973). Much work has also been done upon the incidence and prevalence of the disease in migrant populations (Leibowitz *et al.*, 1969; Dean and Kurtzke, 1971; Kurtzke *et al.*, 1971; Leibowitz and Alter, 1973) and in general this supports the view that migrants retain the risk associated with their mother country, a finding suggesting that, as Millar (1971) proposed, the environmental factor which is of aetiological importance, whatever its nature, may be acquired in childhood. Acheson (1972) concludes that the disease is neither a disorder of affluence nor one associated with malnutrition or atmospheric pollution. It is a disorder associated with particular localities rather than race and whatever agent or agents cause the disease is not freely transportable to other countries. In his view no particular factors other than latitude characterize low-risk and high-risk areas but Leibowitz and Alter (1973) suggest that hygiene and sanitation may be important. It remains to be determined whether epidemiological studies of the incidence of histocompatibility antigens in different populations may be shown to explain, at least in part, the unusual geographical distribution of the disease.

The disease principally attacks young adults. In two-thirds of all cases it begins between 20 and 40, rather more often in the third than the fourth decade.

Its occurrence below the age of 10 is doubtful, but it is occasionally seen in children between the ages of 12 and 15. During recent years the proportion of patients in whom the disease begins after the age of 50 has increased, but onset after 60 is very uncommon. In most published series males have been affected more often than females, but the disease often begins earlier and runs a more rapid course in females (Acheson, 1972).

SYMPTOMS AND SIGNS

The Clinical Picture

The disease produces a very varied clinical picture. In the early stages it is often that of a single focal lesion, acute or, during a remission, quiescent. As time goes on, the cumulative effects of earlier lesions constitute a persistent background of incapacity upon which fresh disabilities due to new lesions are superimposed. The early stages thus usually show long and often remarkably complete remissions, while later the patient's condition fluctuates only to the extent that fresh lesions temporarily regress. However, occasional severe cases beginning in early adult life and more indolent chronic cases of onset in middle life run a progressive course from the outset, without remission.

Mode of Onset

The disease usually begins with the rapid development, with a few hours or a day or two, of symptoms of a single focal lesion of the white matter of the nervous system. Much less often symptoms appear insidiously. In a series of 100 consecutive patients the first symptom noticed was as follows:

Weakness or loss of control over limbs	No.
Involving both lower limbs	18
Involving one lower limb	14
Involving one upper limb	9
Involving one upper and one lower limb	7
Involving all four limbs	2
	50

Visual symptoms	
'Blindness' in one eye	16
Double vision	8
'Dimness' of vision	4
Homonymous field defect	1
	29

Sensory symptoms	
Numbness and other painless paraesthesiae	11

Miscellaneous symptoms	
Vertigo	2
Tremor	2
Multiple symptoms	2
Ptosis	1
Loss of taste	1
Epilepsy	1
Impotence	1
	10

Thus weakness of one or both lower limbs is the first symptom in about one-third of all cases, and a disturbance of vision in almost one-third more. Sensory symptoms which cause no disability are often forgotten and probably occur more frequently than in 11 per cent. Patients who are carefully questioned at the time of onset often describe symptoms of multiple small lesions occurring within a period of a few weeks. Weakness of the lower limbs is the commonest presenting symptoms in patients in whom the disease develops insidiously, and in those in whom it begins after the age of 35.

Rarely the onset is fulminating, with an acute encephalitic, myelitic, or encephalomyelitic picture [see p. 554].

Motor Symptoms

Motor Weakness. Loss of power in the lower limbs is first manifest as fatigability or a feeling of heaviness, and later as spastic paraplegia; often patients with early spastic weakness complain of aching in the legs on exertion. Sometimes sudden weakness of one upper limb occurs, often associated with loss of postural sensibility in the fingers—the 'useless hand' of Oppenheim. Facial weakness and hemiplegia occur occasionally. Monoparesis of one lower limb occurs occasionally but even when the patient complains that only one leg is weak, signs of corticospinal tract dysfunction are often bilateral, if worse in the affected leg.

Muscular wasting is very rare owing to the infrequency of involvement of the anterior horn cells in the patches, but very occasional cases with amyotrophy, often in the small hand muscles, have been described.

Incoordination. This is frequently present. In the upper limbs it usually takes the form of *intention tremor*, a tremor occurring only on voluntary movement and increasing in intensity the greater the accuracy demanded of the movement. In touching the nose with the finger the tremor increases in amplitude as the finger approaches the nose. The same phenomenon is shown if the patient be asked to touch his own nose and the observer's finger alternately, and also in lifting a glass of water to the lips. Ataxia may, however, occur without intention tremor. In certain exceptionally severe cases cerebellar ataxia is so severe that the wild 'flinging' movements of the limbs which occur on attempted volitional activity make it virtually impossible for the patient to use the limbs for any purpose. In the lower limbs incoordination is evident in an ataxic gait and an abnormal heel-knee test. Tremor of the head is common in the late stages when evidence of cerebellar involvement is prominent.

Dysarthria. Dysarthria may be due either to spastic weakness or to ataxia of the muscles of articulation or to a combination of these factors. In the early stages articulation may be slurred, later it may become explosive and almost unintelligible. The 'syllabic' or 'scanning' speech, sometimes regarded as typical, is exceptional and only occurs when cerebellar ataxia dominates the clinical picture. Transitory aphasia is rare.

Sensory Symptoms

Paraesthesiae occur at some period of the disease in most cases, often in the form of numbness and tingling over one side of the face or one upper or both lower limbs. Impairment of position and joint sense and of the finer discriminative aspects of sensibility due to a lesion in the posterior columns of the spinal cord is often accompanied by sensations of apparent swelling of the limb and by feelings suggesting that tight strings or bandages have been applied to the trunk or extremities. When there is a patch in the posterior columns of the cervical cord a sensation resembling an electric shock may radiate down the back and limbs on flexing the cervical spine ('Lhermitte's sign'). Pain is uncommon except in spastic limbs with flexor spasms, but typical trigeminal neuralgia, which is sometimes bilateral, is occasionally encountered. Objective sensory loss is present in at least 50 per cent of cases. Defect of postural sensibility and of appreciation of vibration is the commonest disturbance, but cutaneous sensibility may also be impaired and transient unilateral facial sensory loss suggesting trigeminal neuropathy occasionally occurs. Inability to recognize objects placed in the hand may occur as the result of a plaque in the fasciculus cuneatus in the cervical region. There may be a sharply defined upper level of sensory loss on the trunk suggestive of myelitis or a spinal tumour and unilateral loss of pain and temperature sensation, often with contralateral spastic paresis (a partial Brown–Séquard syndrome) is another uncommon presentation. Sensory symptoms may be effectively localized and monitored by measurement of somatosensory evoked responses (Namerow, 1970).

Ocular Symptoms

Acute unilateral retrobulbar neuritis is one of the most important early symptoms of the disease. It occurs most often between the ages of 20 and 30. The vision of one eye becomes misty and in 24 or 48 hours is reduced to a perception of hand movement or of light only. The eye is painful on movement and tender on pressure, and there is a central scotoma larger for red and green than for white. The optic disc is usually normal in appearance during the acute stage, but if the lesion is near the disc papillitis may occur, though the swelling is usually slight. In a few weeks vision improves, but the residual damage to the nerve manifests itself in some degree of optic atrophy—pallor of the disc, especially in its temporal half—and often a persistent though smaller central scotoma. Enlargement of such a scotoma after exertion or a hot bath [p. 160] is well recognized (see McAlpine, 1972), and has been thought to be due to the effects of temperature upon axonal conduction (Davis, 1970). Permanent blindness is very rare. Simultaneous retrobulbar or optic neuritis in both eyes is uncommon in MS but undoubtedly occurs. The lesions of the optic nerves may be so insidious as to produce the characteristic temporal pallor of the disc, which is found in over 50 per cent of cases, without the patient's being aware of any impairment of vision. The measurement of the shape and latency of pattern-evoked, averaged, visual responses (Halliday et al., 1973; Asselman et al., 1975) and the assessment of delayed conduction in visual pathways using the Pulfrich pendulum (Rushton, 1975) have been shown to be capable of detecting visual lesions which were unsuspected clinically and are thus of considerable diagnostic value, say, in patients with undiagnosed spastic paraparesis. Lesions of the optic chiasm and optic tracts are uncommon, and when they occur cause distinctive defects of the visual fields.

Nystagmus. This is present in about 70 per cent of cases. It is usually absent on central fixation and appears on conjugate deviation laterally. The slow phase is towards the central fixation point and the quick phase away from it. A rotary element is sometimes present, especially on vertical fixation. Nystagmus on central fixation is rare in MS but pendular nystagmus and oscillopsia have been described (Aschoff et al., 1974).

Ocular Paralysis. Paralysis of conjugate ocular deviation may occur as the result of a plaque in the midbrain or pons, but is uncommon: paresis of single ocular muscles occurs in about 6 per cent of cases; but diplopia without objective ocular palsy is commoner (34 per cent of cases). Dissociation of lateral conjugate deviation may occur, the adducting eye being less completely deviated than the abducting. When this occurs (Harris' sign, a form of 'internuclear ophthalmo-plegia') nystagmus is often apparent only in the abducting eye (so-called 'ataxic' nystagmus); the lesion lies in the medial longitudinal fasciculus. The sign is almost pathognomonic of MS and is more common in this disease than other forms of internuclear ophthalmoplegia [p. 82]. Ptosis is rare, retraction of the upper lids slightly commoner.

Pupillary Abnormalities. The pupillary reactions are usually normal. Loss of the reaction to light with preservation of that to accommodation is occasionally observed and is more frequently unilateral than in syphilis. Total ophthalmo-plegia interna may occur. Paresis of the ocular sympathetic leading to ptosis, enopthalmos, and miosis may be seen as the result of a brain stem lesion.

Auditory and Vestibular Symptoms

Deafness is rare, but vertigo is a common and early symptom, usually as a mild sense of instability. Sometimes severe vertigo with vomiting and coarse nystag-mus occurs in attacks lasting for several days, but is usually accompanied by other signs indicating the presence of a pontine plaque involving vestibular nuclei and other contiguous structures.

Paroxysmal Symptoms

Paroxysmal symptoms occurring in MS include focal or generalized epilepti-form attacks which occur in about 2 per cent of cases (McAlpine, 1972), tonic seizures (brief and often painful episodes in which the limbs on one side adopt a posture reminiscent of tetany and which are often precipitated by movement or sensory stimulation) (Matthews, 1958; Shibasaki and Kuroiwa, 1974), paroxysmal dysarthria and ataxia (Osterman and Westerberg, 1975), and sensory symptoms or paresis of very brief duration. Matthews (1975) suggests that these attacks may be due to lateral spread of axonal excitation within demyelinated plaques.

Mental Symptoms

Some reduction in the intellectual efficiency of the patient is not uncommon, but emotional changes are more frequent. The characteristic sense of mental and physical well-being—euphoria—is well known. On the other hand, depres-sion and irritability are sometimes conspicuous. Some loss of control over emotional movements, leading to involuntary laughter and tears, is common, especially in the later stages of the illness. Delusional states are uncommon but dementia occurs relatively frequently, especially in the later stages. Kahana et al. (1971) found that cerebral manifestations (hemiparesis, hemianopia, aphasia, convulsions, and/or dementia) occurred in 10 per cent of their cases at the onset and in 34 per cent at some stage of the illness.

Reflex Changes

As corticospinal tract involvement is very common, the tendon reflexes are usually exaggerated in paretic limbs and generalized hyperreflexia with clonus as well as flexor or extensor spasms [p. 719] are frequently seen, especially in advanced cases. Occasionally spasticity is so great that the reflexes are difficult to elicit; loss of reflexes is uncommon but is occasionally seen, especially when sensory lesions are severe with interruption of the reflex arc. The abdominal reflexes are absent in at least two-thirds of all cases and may be lost at an early stage, and extensor plantar reflexes occur in from 80 to 90 per cent of cases in the later stages.

Other Symptoms

Sphincter control is frequently impaired. In the early stages urgency or precipitancy of micturition is common. Later, retention or reflex evacuation of both urine and faeces may occur. Occasionally acute retention of urine is the first symptom. Impotence is common and sweating is often impaired (Cartlidge, 1972). There is no consistent endocrine abnormality (Teasdale et al., 1967).

Pyrexia may develop during acute exacerbations of the disease, which is consequently sometimes described by the patient as having begun with an attack of 'influenza'. Headache sometimes occurs.

Cerebrospinal Fluid

Some abnormality is found in the cerebrospinal fluid in at least half of all cases. An excess of mononuclear cells is found in about 10 per cent. An abnormal colloidal gold curve was regarded in the past as the most characteristic change. This is usually of the 'paretic', less often of the 'luetic', type, one or the other occurring in from 50 to 75 per cent of cases. The protein is usually normal or only slightly raised but there may be an abnormally high gamma globulin estimated by paper electrophoresis (Kabat et al., 1942; Schapira and Park, 1961). Prineas et al. (1966) used a simple zinc sulphate precipitation method for estimating spinal fluid gamma globulin and found this to be raised to above 29 per cent of the total protein content in 44 per cent of patients with multiple sclerosis. Except for neurosyphilis and certain encephalitides, this figure was exceeded in less than 5 per cent of patients with other neurological diseases. Elevation of the immunoglobulins in the CSF is an even more specific finding when measured by electrophoresis or immunoelectrophoresis (Kolar and Zeman, 1967; Kolar et al., 1970; Schwartz et al., 1970; Link and Müller, 1971; Fischer-Williams and Roberts, 1971; Olsson and Link, 1973) or by electroimmunodiffusion (Schneck and Claman, 1969). The IgG is increased to more than 14 per cent of the total CSF protein in most patients with MS, and IgA, various complements and transferrin (Olsson and Link, 1973) may also be raised. Accompanying changes in the serum immunoglobulins suggest that the extracerebral lymphoreticular system may also be involved (Kolar et al., 1970). The CSF protein serine residue measured by quantitative chromatography (Poser et al., 1975) is closely correlated with the IgG level and may prove to be a more sensitive test. The CSF esterase, peptidase, and proteinase activity has been shown to be greatly increased, particularly in acute cases of MS. While all of these tests have added precision to diagnosis, none has yet been shown to be specific for MS as similar abnormalities may occur in other nervous diseases, particularly those associated with infection and an altered immune response, including various forms of meningitis and encephalitis.

Symptom Groups

The extreme variability of the clinical picture justifies the recognition of 'forms' of the disease due to the predominant involvement of different parts of the nervous system.

1. The classical triad of Charcot, namely nystagmus, intention tremor, and scanning speech, is comparatively rare, and occurs in under 10 per cent of cases.

2. The generalized form, common among younger patients, is characterized by temporal pallor of the optic discs, nystagmus, slight intention tremor, ataxia, weakness and spasticity of the lower limbs, and defective sphincter control.

3. Onset with ocular symptoms. Retrobulbar neuritis or a transient episode of diplopia may be the only symptom for many years.

4. The sensory form. In some patients recurrent episodes of paraesthesiae with loss of postural sensibility in one or more limbs indicative of a plaque in the posterior column of the cord may occur and often resolve after a few days or weeks only to recur months or years later in some other part of the body. This form often runs a benign course with long intervals between relapses before signs of corticospinal tract involvement appear.

5. The cerebral form. An onset with hemiplegia, hemianopia, aphasia, or epileptiform convulsions is uncommon; remission in a few weeks or months is usual but subsequently dementia often develops.

6. Spinal forms. (a) *Progressive spastic paraplegia* may occur with few if any other physical signs, especially in middle-aged patients. (b) *Unilateral spinal lesions* occur chiefly in the cervical cord. The posterior and lateral columns are usually involved. A partial Brown-Séquard syndrome developing in a young person is not uncommon in this disease and usually remits within a few months. (c) *Sacral form.* A plaque in the conus medullaris may lead to incontinence of urine and faeces, impotence, and anaesthesia in the region of the sacral cutaneous supply.

7. Cerebellar, vestibular, pontine, and bulbar forms are self-explanatory.

8. *Acute multiple sclerosis.* Rarely the illness may be of very acute onset, with clinical manifestations of any of the syndromes listed above. A fatal termination within a few months is known but is now very rare. In such acute cases fever may be present. Headache, vomiting, and giddiness are common at the onset, and delirium occurs in severe cases. The symptoms may be predominantly cerebral, predominantly spinal, or both brain and cord may be diffusely affected. There is a tendency for the affection to extend to hitherto unaffected parts of the nervous system after a lapse of days or even weeks. The symptoms of the cerebral type include mental changes, convulsions, aphasia, hemiplegia, hemianopia, nystagmus, vertigo, and ataxia of the upper limbs. However, aphasia and hemianopia are signs of exceptional rarity in this disease. Optic neuritis may occur, usually bilaterally. Cranial nerve palsies are comparatively uncommon, except for facial paresis, but diplopia, unilateral facial sensory loss, and nystagmus may all be seen when the brain stem is involved. Symptoms of meningeal irritation are usually absent. In the spinal type pains in the back and limbs or with a girdle distribution are common. Paraplegia of varying severity is usually present, associated with sensory loss, which may be confined either to postural sensibility and passive movement, or to appreciation of pain, heat, and cold. Bladder disturbances are present in the more severe cases of paraplegia. The

tendon reflexes may be exaggerated, but are not uncommonly diminished or lost in the acute stage of 'spinal shock'. The plantars are usually extensor and the clinical picture is indistinguishable from that of transverse myelitis.

DIAGNOSIS

MS must be distinguished from *diffuse sclerosis*, which has a more restricted age-range and often occurs in childhood. It is usually steadily progressive and by symmetrically destroying the white matter of the cerebral hemispheres leads to blindness, spastic tetraplegia, and dementia.

In *neuromyelitis optica* the symptoms of optic or retrobulbar neuritis are associated with those of transverse myelitis, both developing within a few weeks. Acute bilateral optic or retrobulbar neuritis may occur without myelitis, and also runs a benign course. Although both eyes may be successively the site of optic or retrobulbar neuritis in MS, it is rare for them both to be affected simultaneously and concurrently with spinal cord involvement in this disease. Nevertheless, many authorities now regard neuromyelitis optica as simply being one mode of presentation of MS (McAlpine *et al.*, 1972).

Meningovascular Syphilis. MS is distinguished from meningovascular syphilis by the rarity of pupillary changes and of diminution of the knee- and ankle-jerks in the former and the absence of a positive V.D.R.L. reaction and treponema immobilization test, which are present in the blood and spinal fluid in most cases of the latter. Nystagmus and signs of cerebellar dysfunction are very rare in neurosyphilis.

Tabes may to some extent be simulated by the ataxic gait of MS, but in the latter there is usually spasticity, the knee- and ankle-jerks are exaggerated and the plantar reflexes extensor, while the pupillary reflexes are normal.

Friedreich's ataxia causes, in common with many cases of MS, nystagmus, absent abdominal reflexes, ataxia of the lower limbs, loss of postural sensibility, and extensor plantar responses. In this disease, however, we find diminution or loss of the ankle-jerks, and later of the knee-jerks, scoliosis, and pes cavus, while the frequent onset in childhood, slow progressive course, and occurrence of multiple cases in one family are distinctive.

Other Familial Ataxias. Some forms of familial ataxia have been described of which individual cases have been indistinguishable from MS, e.g. the Drew family described by Ferguson and Critchley (1929). Differential points, however, are the familial incidence, the onset either earlier or later than is usual in MS, the steadily progressive course, and the occurrence of symptoms, e.g. marked ocular palsies, extrapyramidal signs, and extensive sensory loss, which are unusual in MS.

Subacute combined degeneration may lead to confusion as a cause of 'ataxic paraplegia'. It begins, however, later in life than do most cases of MS; paraesthesiae appear early and persist; the tendon reflexes in the lower limbs are often lost, and gastric achylia, megalocytic anaemia, and a low serum B_{12} activity are distinctive features.

Spinal Tumour. MS may closely simulate spinal tumour when it gives rise to progressive spastic paraplegia, with or without sensory loss up to a segmental level, and without evident physical signs above the spinal cord level. In any case of doubt myelography is an essential investigation.

Cervical spondylosis with myelopathy may lead to ataxic weakness of the upper limbs and spastic paraplegia, and so be confused with MS. Plain X-rays of the cervical spine and myelography will usually settle the diagnosis. However, the two conditions are so common that they not infrequently coexist.

Other Spinal Lesions. The neurological complications of Behçet's disease [p. 450] may give a similar picture to that of MS, especially if mucosal lesions in the mouth and genitalia are unobtrusive. An arteriovenous angioma of the spinal cord and subacute necrotic myelitis may also give symptoms and signs resembling those of MS but CSF examination and myelography are usually diagnostic.

Hysteria can be confused with MS only through neglect to make a thorough examination of the nervous system. Such early symptoms as giddiness, paraesthesiae, and paresis may superficially suggest hysteria, but these are rarely present without some sign of organic disease, and pallor of the optic discs, absent abdominal reflexes, and extensor plantar responses are unequivocal evidence of such a condition. It is not rare, however, for a patient to develop hysterical symptoms in addition to those of MS and an hysterical overlay present in the early stages when physical signs are minimal often causes difficulty in initial diagnosis.

PROGNOSIS

The extremely variable course renders prognosis difficult. The disease in its acute form may terminate fatally in three months or less, or the patient may still be able to work 50 years after the onset. When retrobulbar neuritis is the first symptom the next may not follow for many years. Among Brain's patients there were remissions of 13, 15, 17, and 19 years after an attack of retrobulbar neuritis, and of 20 and 25 years after another symptom, before the disease recurred. It is conceivable that a remission may last a lifetime and the patient recover permanently from his first attack (McAlpine *et al.*, 1972). McAlpine and Compston (1952) in their study of the course of the disease found the average number of fresh 'attacks' to be about 0·4 per year for patients of both sexes. It has often been said in the past that the disease is generally fatal within 5 to 25 years of the onset but there is now convincing evidence that many patients survive very much longer and that this is not simply due to the more effective treatment of intercurrent infection with antibiotics and of bedsores and other complications. Certainly patients presenting in early adult life with progressive ataxic paraparesis or signs of multiple lesions and especially those with severe cerebellar ataxia have a much worse prognosis than average (Leibowitz *et al.*, 1969). Even so, unexpectedly complete remission is sometimes seen and Kurtzke *et al.* (1973) found that most patients recovered from an initial severe episode especially if the symptoms and signs were predominantly sensory; prolonged but milder relapses recovered less completely. Kurtzke *et al.* (1970) found that 69 per cent of male patients lived more than 25, and 50 per cent more than 35 years after the onset and McAlpine *et al.* (1972) and others have also stressed the existence of benign forms of the disease (Percy *et al.*, 1971; *British Medical Journal*, 1972). Death from the disease seems to occur on average 10 years earlier in female than in male patients (Kurtzke, 1972), but for males the peak age at death is between 65 and 84 years.

This evidence that the disease often runs a benign course and that some patients remain mobile and unrestricted in their activity for 20 years or more and survive to a normal age does not, however, detract from the fact that in many severe cases the patient is confined to a wheelchair for many years or even, in the end, to bed. The terminal stages may be very distressing. An account is given by a sufferer who was also a graphic writer, W. N. P. Barbellion, in *The Diary of a Disappointed Man* and *Enjoying Life*. Ataxia, weakness, and spasticity confine the patient to bed and prevent him from carrying out the simplest actions for himself. Swallowing becomes difficult and speech almost unintelligible. Urinary or cutaneous infection or pneumonia finally releases the sufferer. In rare cases the last event is an acute exacerbation of the disease itself, taking the form of an acute myelitis or encephalomyelitis.

TREATMENT

General Measures

The management of the patient requires tact and judgement. Because of the public image of MS as a progressive and incurable disease, it is best in an early attack to use terms such as 'neuritis' to identify the condition, but when the condition enters upon a progressive course or if the patient asks 'Am I suffering from MS?' it is unjustifiable to withhold the diagnosis. Every effort should be made to keep the patient at his usual occupation as long as possible. The attachment of weights to an affected limb may lessen distressing intention tremor (Hewer *et al.*, 1972); when such tremor is very severe it may be abolished by stereotaxic ventrolateral thalamotomy but cases to be operated upon must be selected with the greatest care as the procedure may cause confusion or hasten the progression of incipient dementia. Measures designed to reduce the serum ionized calcium may cause temporary remission of symptoms and signs (Davis *et al.*, 1970). In the later stages encouragement and suggestion, and vigorous physiotherapy including active and passive movements and re-educational walking exercises may long postpone the bedridden state. Even though pregnancy may not influence the relapse rate it may accelerate deterioration in a moderately advanced case, so that contraceptive advice or even sterilization may be indicated. Spasticity may be relieved by drugs such as diazepam, 2–5 mg, dantrolene sodium 50–75 mg, or baclofen (5 mg initially, increasing to 15 mg), each given three or four times daily, while in selected cases intrathecal phenol or hypertonic saline injections are useful for the relief of flexor spasms. Carbamazepine, 200 mg three times daily, and other anticonvulsant drugs usually control paroxysmal symptoms such as tonic fits (Espir and Millac, 1970). Propantheline, 15 mg, may control urgency and incontinence of urine. Calipers and other mechanical aids are of value in appropriate cases. In the late stages the skin, bladder, and rectum will require special attention, as in paraplegia from any cause. In such patients investigation will often reveal residual urine and impaired renal efficiency.

Specific Treatment

Assessment of the effects of treatment upon the actual disease process is difficult in a condition like MS which remits and relapses spontaneously, and which is so variable in its clinical presentation and course. The number, duration, and severity of relapses occurring in a given period may be one helpful guide. Various scales or scores of disability assessment have been designed (see Kurtzke, 1955, 1970; McAlpine *et al.*, 1972) and Schumacher (1974) has defined the minimal acceptable criteria for assessing the effects of treatment. Earlier claims proposing treatment with intrathecal tuberculin (Smith *et al.*, 1957) or with a low fat diet (Swank, 1955, 1970) have not been substantiated and there is no indication that antirickettsial or other vaccines are helpful. However, there is some evidence that ACTH given in a dosage of 80 units daily for a week, every other day for 2 weeks and then twice weekly for 3 weeks may reduce the severity and duration of relapses (Rose *et al.*, 1970; McAlpine *et al.*, 1972) though long-term treatment with prednisone or ACTH is ineffective despite the occasional occurrence of patients who are apparently steroid-dependent (Miller *et al.*, 1961; Boman *et al.*, 1966; Millar *et al.*, 1967, 1970). Recent investigations with immunosuppressive agents (Neumann and Ziegler, 1972) have shown that 6-mercaptopurine or methotrexate alone are of no value; antilymphocyte globulin (ALG) has been thought to be effective in some hands (Seland *et al.*, 1974) but not in others (MacFadyen *et al.*, 1973), while the place of intensive immunosuppression with thoracic duct drainage, ALG, azathioprine, and prednisone (Brendel *et al.*, 1972; Ring *et al.*, 1974) has yet to be determined. There is no scientific evidence to support the use of a gluten-free diet, despite the publicity given to remission in one severe case on such a diet, but nutritional factors may yet prove to be significant (Alter *et al.*, 1974) and there is some evidence to support the use of linoleic acid in the form of sunflower seed oil 30 ml twice daily in MS though the results of this treatment obtained to date have been inconclusive (Millar *et al.*, 1973).

REFERENCES

ACHESON, E. D. (1972) The epidemiology of multiple sclerosis, in *Multiple Sclerosis: a Reappraisal*, ed. McAlpine, D., Lumsden, C. E., and Acheson, E. D., 2nd ed., Edinburgh.

ADAMS, C. W. M., HALLPIKE, J. F., and BAYLISS, O. B. (1971) Histochemistry of myelin. XIII. Digestion of basic protein outside acute plaques of multiple sclerosis, *J. Neurochem.*, **18**, 1479.

ALLISON, R. S. (1950) Survival in disseminated sclerosis, *Brain*, **73**, 103.

ALTER, M., YAMOOR, M., and HARSHE, M. (1974) Multiple sclerosis and nutrition, *Arch. Neurol. (Chic.)*, **31**, 267.

ALVORD, E. C., Jun. (1966) The relationship of hypersensitivity to infection, inflammation and immunity, *J. neuropath. exp. Neurol.*, **25**, 1.

ANTON, G., and WOHLWILL, F. (1912) Multiple nicht-eitrige Encephalomyelitis und multiple Sklerose, *Z. ges. Neurol. Psychiat.*, Orig. **12**, 31.

ARNASON, B. G. W., FULLER, T. C., LEHRICH, J. R., and WRAY, S. H. (1974) Histocompatibility types and measles antibodies in multiple sclerosis and optic neuritis, *J. neurol. Sci.*, **22**, 419.

ASCHOFF, J. C., CONRAD, B., and KORNHUBER, H. H. (1974) Acquired pendular nystagmus with oscillopsia in multiple sclerosis: a sign of cerebellar nuclei disease, *J. Neurol. Neurosurg. Psychiat.*, **37**, 570.

ASSELMAN, P., CHADWICK, D. W., and MARSDEN, C. D. (1975) Visual evoked responses in the diagnosis and management of patients suspected of multiple sclerosis, *Brain*, **98**, 261.

BEHREND, R. C. (1969) Multiple sclerosis in Europe, *Europ. Neurol.*, **2**, 129.

BERTRAMS, J., and KUWERT, E. (1972) HL-A antigen frequencies in multiple sclerosis. Significant increase of HL-A 3, HL-A 10 and W5, and decrease of HL-A 12, *Europ. Neurol.*, **7**, 74.

BOGAERT, L. VAN (1950) Post-infectious encephalomyelitis and multiple sclerosis, *J. neuropath. exp. Neurol.*, **9**, 219.

BOMAN, K., HOKKANEN, E., JARHO, L., and KIVALO, E. (1966) Double-blind study of the effect of corticotropin treatment in multiple sclerosis, *Ann. Med. Int. Fenn.*, **55**, 71.

BRAIN, W. R. (1929–30) Critical review. Disseminated sclerosis, *Quart. J. Med.*, **23**, 343.

BRENDEL, W., SEIFERT, J., and LOB, G. (1972) Effect of 'maximum immune suppression' with thoracic duct drainage, ALG, azathioprine and cortisone in some neurological disorders, *Proc. roy. Soc. Med.*, **65**, 531.

BRITISH MEDICAL JOURNAL (1972) Benign forms of multiple sclerosis, *Brit. med. J.*, **1**, 392.

BRITISH MEDICAL JOURNAL (1976) Multiple sclerosis, **ii**, 1030.

BRODY, J. A. (1972) Epidemiology of multiple sclerosis and a possible virus aetiology, *Lancet*, **ii**, 173.

CARTLIDGE, N. E. F. (1972) Autonomic function in multiple sclerosis, *Brain*, **95**, 661.

CASPARY, E. A., and FIELD, E. J. (1974) Lymphocyte sensitization to basic protein of brain in multiple sclerosis and other neurological diseases, *J. Neurol. Neurosurg. Psychiat.*, **37**, 701.

COURNAND, A. (1930) *La Sclérose en plaques aiguë: contribution à l'étude des encéphalo-myélites aiguës disséminées*, Paris.

CURRIER, R. D., MARTIN, E. A., and WOOLSEY, P. C. (1974) Prior events in multiple sclerosis, *Neurology (Minneap.)*, **24**, 748.

CURTIUS, F. (1933) *Multiple Sklerose und Erbanlage*, Leipzig.

DATTNER, B. (1937) Zur Pathogenese der multiplen Sklerose, *Wien, klin. Wschr.*, **50**, 87.

DAVIS, F. A. (1970) Axonal conduction studies based on some considerations of tempera-ture effects in multiple sclerosis, *Electroenceph. clin. Neurophysiol.*, **28**, 281.

DAVIS, F. A., BECKER, F. O., MICHAEL, J. A., and SORENSEN, E. (1970) Effect of intravenous sodium bicarbonate, disodium edetate (Na_2EDTA), and hyperventilation on visual and oculomotor signs in multiple sclerosis, *J. Neurol. Neurosurg. Psychiat.*, **33**, 723.

DAWSON, J. W. (1916) The histology of disseminated sclerosis, *Trans. roy. Soc. Edinb.*, **50**, 517.

DEAN, G., and KURTZKE, J. F. (1971) On the risk of multiple sclerosis according to age at immigration to South Africa, *Brit. med. J.*, **3**, 725.

DOW, R. S., and BERGLUND, G. (1942) Vascular pattern of lesions of disseminated sclerosis, *Arch. Neurol. Psychiat. (Chic.)*, **47**, 1.

DOWLING, P. C., KIM, S. U., MURRAY, M. R., and COOK, S. D. (1968) Serum 19s and 7s demyelinating antibodies in multiple sclerosis, *J. Immunol.*, **101**, 1101.

DUBOIS-DALCQ, M., SCHUMACHER, G., and SEVER, J. L. (1973) Acute multiple sclerosis: electron-microscopic evidence for and against a viral agent in the plaques, *Lancet*, **ii**, 1408.

EINSTEIN, E. R., CSEJTEY, J., DALAL, K. B., ADAMS, C. W. M., BAYLISS, O. B., and HALLPIKE, J. F. (1972) Proteolytic activity and basic protein loss in and around multiple sclerosis plaques: combined biochemical and histochemical observations, *J. Neurochem.*, **19**, 653.

ESPIR, M. L. E., and MILLAC, P. (1970) Treatment of paroxysmal disorders in multiple sclerosis with carbamazepine (Tegretol), *J. Neurol. Neurosurg. Psychiat.*, **33**, 528.

FERGUSON, F. R., and CRITCHLEY, M. (1929) A clinical study of an heredo-familial disease resembling disseminated sclerosis, *Brain*, **52**, 203.

FERRARO, A. (1937) Primary demyelinating processes of the central nervous system, *Arch. Neurol. Psychiat. (Chic.)*, **37**, 1, 100.

FERRARO, A. (1958) Studies on multiple sclerosis, *J. Neuropath. exp. Neurol.*, **17**, 278.

FIELD, E. J. (1966) Transmission experiments with multiple sclerosis: an interim report, *Brit. med. J.*, **2**, 564.

FISCHER-WILLIAMS, M., and ROBERTS, R. C. (1971) Cerebrospinal fluid proteins and serum immunoglobulins. Occurrence in multiple sclerosis and other neurological diseases: comparative measurement of γ-globulin and the IgG class, *Arch. Neurol. (Chic.)*, **25**, 526.

FRAENKEL, M., and JAKOB, A. (1913) Zur Pathologie der multiplen Sklerose mit besonderer Berücksichtigung der akuten Formen, *Z. ges. Neurol. Psychiat.*, **14**, 565.

GILBERT, G. J. (1971) Multiple sclerosis in the child of conjugal multiple sclerosis patients, *Neurology (Minneap.)*, **21**, 1169.

GREENFIELD, J. G., and KING, L. S. (1936) Histopathology of the cerebral lesions in disseminated sclerosis, *Brain*, **59**, 445.

GREENFIELD, J. G., and NORMAN, R. M. (1965) Demyelinating diseases, in *Greenfield's Neuropathology*, 2nd ed., London.

HALLIDAY, A. M., McDONALD, W. I., and MUSHIN, J. (1973) Visual evoked responses in diagnosis of multiple sclerosis, *Brit. med. J.*, **4**, 661.

HEWER, R. L., COOPER, R., and MORGAN, M. H. (1972) An investigation into the value of treating intention tremor by weighting the affected limb, *Brain*, **95**, 579.

KABAT, E. A., MOORE, D. H., and LANDOW, H. (1942) An electrophoretic study of the protein components in cerebrospinal fluid and their relationship to the serum proteins, *J. clin. Invest.*, **21**, 571.

KAHANA, E., LEIBOWITZ, U., and ALTER, M. (1971) Cerebral multiple sclerosis, *Neurology (Minneap.)*, **21**, 1179.

KOLAR, O. J., ROSS, A. T., and HERMAN, J. T. (1970) Serum and cerebrospinal fluid immunoglobulins in multiple sclerosis, *Neurology (Minneap.)*, **20**, 1052.

KOLAR, O. J., and ZEMAN, W. (1967) Immunoelectrophoretic changes of serum IgG during subacute inflammatory and demyelinating diseases of the central nervous system, *Zeitschrift für Immunitätsforschung*, **134**, 267.

KUROIWA, Y., and SHIBASAKI, H. (1973) Clinical studies of multiple sclerosis in Japan. I. A current appraisal of 83 cases, *Neurology (Minneap.)*, **23**, 611.

KURTZKE, J. F. (1955) A new scale for evaluating disability in multiple sclerosis, *Neurology (Minneap.)*, **5**, 580.

KURTZKE, J. F. (1970) Neurologic impairment in multiple sclerosis and the disability status scale, *Acta neurol. scand.*, **46**, 493.

KURTZKE, J. F. (1972) Multiple sclerosis death rates from underlying cause and total deaths, *Acta neurol. scand.*, **48**, 148.

KURTZKE, J. F. (1975 *a*) A reassessment of the distribution of multiple sclerosis—Part One, *Acta neurol. scand.*, **51**, 110.

KURTZKE, J. F. (1975 *b*) A reassessment of the distribution of multiple sclerosis—Part Two, *Acta neurol. scand.*, **51**, 137.

KURTZKE, J. F., BEEBE, G. W., NAGLER, B., AUTH, T. L., KURLAND, L. T., and NEFZGER, M. D. (1973) Studies on the natural history of multiple sclerosis. 7. Correlates of clinical change in an early bout, *Acta neurol. scand.*, **49**, 379.

KURTZKE, J. F., BEEBE, G. W., NAGLER, B., NEFZGER, M. D., AUTH, T. L., and KURLAND, L. T. (1970) Studies on the natural history of multiple sclerosis. V. Long-term survival in young men, *Arch. Neurol. (Chic.)*, **22**, 215.

KURTZKE, J. F., KURLAND, L. T., and GOLDBERG, I. D. (1971) Mortality and migration in multiple sclerosis, *Neurology (Minneap.)*, **21**, 1186.

LAMPERT, F., and LAMPERT, P. (1975) Multiple sclerosis: morphologic evidence of intra-nuclear paramyxovirus or altered chromatin fibers?, *Arch. Neurol. (Chic.)*, **32**, 425.

THE LANCET (1974) Measles and multiple sclerosis, *Lancet*, **i**, 247.

THE LANCET (1976) A milestone in multiple sclerosis, *Lancet*, **i**, 459.

LEHRICH, J. R., ARNASON, B. G. W., FULLER, T. C., and WRAY, S. H. (1974) Parainfluenza, histocompatibility, and multiple sclerosis. Association of parainfluenza antibodies and histocompatibility types in MS and optic neuritis, *Arch. Neurol. (Chic.)*, **30**, 327.

LEIBOWITZ, U., and ALTER, M. (1973) *Multiple Sclerosis: Clues to its Cause*, Amsterdam, London, New York.

LEIBOWITZ, U., KAHANA, E., and ALTER, M. (1969) Multiple sclerosis in immigrant and native populations of Israel, *Lancet*, **ii**, 1323.

LINK, H., and MÜLLER, R. (1971) Immunoglobulins in multiple sclerosis and infections of the nervous system, *Arch. Neurol. (Chic.)*, **25**, 326.

LUMSDEN, C. E. (1961) Consideration of multiple sclerosis in relation to the autoimmunity process, *Proc. roy. Soc. Med.*, **54**, 11.

LUMSDEN, C. E. (1970) The neuropathology of multiple sclerosis, in *Handbook of Clinical Neurology*, ed. Vinken, P. J., and Bruyn, G. W., Volume 9, Amsterdam.

LUMSDEN, C. E. (1971) The immunogenesis of the multiple sclerosis plaque, *Brain Research*, **28**, 365.

LUMSDEN, C. E. (1972) The clinical pathology of multiple sclerosis, in *Multiple Sclerosis: a Reappraisal*, ed. McAlpine, D., Lumsden, C. E., and Acheson, E. D., 2nd ed., Edinburgh.

McALPINE, D. (1931) Acute disseminated encephalomyelitis: its sequelae and its relationship to disseminated sclerosis, *Lancet*, **i**, 846.

McALPINE, D. (1972) Clinical studies, in *Multiple Sclerosis: a Reappraisal*, ed. McAlpine, D., Lumsden, C. E., and Acheson, E. D., 2nd ed., Edinburgh.

McALPINE, D., and COMPSTON, N. (1952) Some aspects of the natural history of disseminated sclerosis, *Quart. J. Med.*, **21**, 135.

McALPINE, D., COMPSTON, N., and LUMSDEN, C. E. (1955) *Multiple Sclerosis*, Edinburgh.

McALPINE, D., LUMSDEN, C. E., and ACHESON, E. D. (1972) *Multiple Sclerosis: a Reappraisal*, 2nd ed., Edinburgh.

McCALL, M. G., BRERETON, T. LE G., DAWSON, A., MILLINGEN, K., SUTHERLAND, J. M., and ACHESON, E. D. (1968) Frequency of multiple sclerosis in three Australian cities—Perth, Newcastle, and Hobart, *J. Neurol. Neurosurg. Psychiat.*, **31**, 1.

McDERMOTT, J. R., FIELD, E. J., and CASPARY, E. A. (1974) Relation of measles virus to encephalitogenic factor with reference to the aetiopathogenesis of multiple sclerosis, *J. Neurol. Neurosurg. Psychiat.*, **37**, 282.

McDONALD, W. I. (1974 *a*) Pathophysiology in multiple sclerosis, *Brain*, **97**, 179.

McDONALD, W. I. (1974 *b*) Remyelination in relation to clinical lesions of the central nervous system, *Brit. med. Bull.*, **30**, 186.

MacFADYEN, D. J., REEVE, C. E., BRATTY, P. J. A., and THOMAS, J. W. (1973) Failure of antilymphocytic globulin therapy in chronic progressive multiple sclerosis, *Neurology (Minneap.)*, **23**, 592.

MANDELBROTE, B. M., STANIER, M. W., THOMPSON, R. H. S., and THRUSTON, M. N. (1948) Studies on copper metabolism in demyelinating diseases of the nervous system, *Brain*, **71**, 212.

MARGULIS, M. S., SOLOVIEV, V. D., and SHUBLADZE, A. K. (1946) Aetiology and pathogenesis of acute sporadic encephalomyelitis and multiple sclerosis, *J. Neurol. Neurosurg. Psychiat.*, **9**, 63.

MATTHEWS, W. B. (1958) Tonic seizures in disseminated sclerosis, *Brain*, **81**, 193.

MATTHEWS, W. B. (1975) Paroxysmal symptoms in multiple sclerosis, *J. Neurol. Neurosurg. Psychiat.*, **38**, 617.

MILLAR, J. H. D. (1971) *Multiple Sclerosis: A Disease Acquired in Childhood*, Springfield, Ill.

MILLAR, J. H. D., ALLISON, R. S., CHEESEMAN, E. A., and MERRETT, J. D. (1959) Pregnancy as a factor influencing relapse in disseminated sclerosis, *Brain*, **82**, 417.

MILLAR, J. H. D., RAHMAN, R., VAS, C. J., NORONHA, M. J., LIVERSEDGE, L. A., and SWINBURN, W. R. (1970) Effect of withdrawal of corticotrophin in patients on long-term treatment for multiple sclerosis, *Lancet*, **i**, 700.

MILLAR, J. H. D., VAS, C. J., NORONHA, M. J., LIVERSEDGE, L. A., and RAWSON, M. D. (1967) Long-term treatment of multiple sclerosis with corticotrophin, *Lancet*, **ii**, 429.

MILLAR, J. H. D., ZILKHA, K. J., LANGMAN, M. J. S., WRIGHT, H. PAYLING, SMITH, A. D., BELIN, J., and THOMPSON, R. H. S. (1973) Double-blind trial of linoleate supplementation of the diet in multiple sclerosis, *Brit. med. J.*, **1**, 765.

MILLER, H. (1961) Aetiological factors in disseminated sclerosis, *Proc. roy. Soc. Med.*, **54**, 7.

MILLER, H. (1964) Trauma and multiple sclerosis, *Lancet*, **i**, 848.

MILLER, H., CENDROWSKI, W., and SCHAPIRA, K. (1967) Multiple sclerosis and vaccination, *Brit. med. J.*, **2**, 210.

MILLER, H., NEWELL, D. J., and RIDLEY, A. (1961) Multiple sclerosis. Trials of maintenance treatment with prednisolone and soluble aspirin, *Lancet*, **i**, 127.

MILLER, H., and SCHAPIRA, K. (1959) Aetiological aspects of multiple sclerosis, *Brit. med. J.*, **1**, 737, 811.

NAMEROW, N. S. (1970) Somatosensory recovery functions in multiple sclerosis patients, *Neurology (Minneap.)*, **20**, 813.

NARANG, H. K., and FIELD, E. J. (1973) Paramyxovirus like tubules in multiple sclerosis biopsy material, *Acta neuropath. (Berl.)*, **25**, 281.

T

NEMO, G. J., BRODY, J. A., and WATERS, D. J. (1974) Serological responses of multiple-sclerosis patients and controls to a virus isolated from a multiple-sclerosis case, *Lancet*, **ii**, 1044.

NEUMANN, J. W., and ZIEGLER, D. K. (1972) Therapeutic trial of immunosuppressive agents in multiple sclerosis, *Neurology (Minneap.)*, **22**, 1268.

NORRBY, E., LINK, H., and OLSSON, J.-E. (1974) Measles virus antibodies in multiple sclerosis: comparison of antibody titers in cerebrospinal fluid and serum, *Arch. Neurol. (Chic.)*, **30**, 285.

OLSSON, J.-E., and LINK, H. (1973) Immunoglobulin abnormalities in multiple sclerosis: relation to clinical parameters, *Arch. Neurol. (Chic.)*, **28**, 392.

OSTERMAN, P. O., and WESTERBERG, C.-E. (1975) Paroxysmal attacks in multiple sclerosis, *Brain*, **98**, 189.

PANELIUS, M. (1969) Studies on epidemiological, clinical and etiological aspects of multiple sclerosis, *Acta neurol. scand.*, **45**, suppl. 39.

PATY, D. W., MERVART, H., CAMPLING, B., RAND, C. G., and STILLER, C. R. (1974) HL-A frequencies in patients with multiple sclerosis, *Canad. J. neurol. Sci.*, **1**, 211.

PERCY, A. K., NOBREGA, F. T., OKAZAKI, H., GLATTRE, E., and KURLAND, L. T. (1971) Multiple sclerosis in Rochester, Minnesota—a 60-year appraisal, *Arch. Neurol. (Chic.)*, **25**, 105.

PETTE, H. (1928) Über die Pathogenese der multiplen Sklerose, *Dtsch Z. Nervenheilk.*, **105**, 76.

PETTE, H. (1929) Infektion und Nervensystem, *Dtsch Z. Nervenheilk.*, **110**, 221.

POSER, C. M., SYLWESTER, D. L., HO, B., and ALPERT, A. (1975) Amino acid residues of serum and CSF protein in multiple sclerosis: clinical application of statistical discriminant analysis, *Arch. Neurol. (Chic.)*, **32**, 308.

POSKANZER, D., MILLER, H., and SCHAPIRA, K. (1963) Epidemiology of multiple sclerosis in the counties of Northumberland and Durham, *J. Neurol. Psychiat.*, **26**, 368.

POSKANZER, D., SCHAPIRA, K., and MILLER, H. (1963) Multiple sclerosis and poliomyelitis, *Lancet*, **ii**, 917.

PRATT, R. T. C., COMPSTON, N. D., and McALPINE, D. (1951) The familial incidence of disseminated sclerosis and its significance, *Brain*, **74**, 191.

PRINEAS, J., TEASDALE, G., LATNER, A. L., and MILLER, H. (1966) Spinal fluid gamma-globulin and multiple sclerosis, *Brit. med. J.*, **2**, 922.

PUTNAM, T. J. (1937) Evidence of vascular occlusion in multiple sclerosis and 'encephalomyelitis', *Arch. Neurol. Psychiat. (Chic.)*, **37**, 1298.

RAINE, C. S., POWERS, J. M., and SUZUKI, K. (1974) Acute multiple sclerosis. Confirmation of 'paramyxovirus-like' intranuclear inclusions, *Arch. Neurol. (Chic.)*, **30**, 39.

REDLICH, E. (1927) Über ein gehäuftes Auftreten von Krankheitsfällen mit den Erscheinungen der Encephalomyelitis disseminata, *Mschr. Psychiat. Neurol.*, **64**, 152.

RIEKKINEN, P. J., CLAUSEN, J., and ARSTILA, A. U. (1970) Further studies on neutral proteinase activity of CNS myelin, *Brain Research*, **19**, 213.

RIEKKINEN, P. J., PALO, J., ARSTILA, A. U., SAVOLAINEN, H. J., RINNE, U. K., KIVALO, E. K., and FREY, H. (1971) Protein composition of multiple sclerosis myelin, *Arch. Neurol. (Chic.)*, **24**, 545.

RING, J., SEIFERT, J., LOB, G., COULIN, K., ANGSTWURM, H., FRICK, E., BRASS, B., MERTIN, J., BACKMUND, H., and BRENDEL, W. (1974) Intensive immunosuppression in the treatment of multiple sclerosis, *Lancet*, **ii**, 1093.

RINNE, U. K., PANELIUS, M., KIVALO, E., HOKKANEN, E., and MEURMAN, T. (1968) Multiple sclerosis in Finland: further studies on its distribution and prevalence, *Acta neurol. scand.*, **44**, 631.

ROSE, A. S., KUZMA, J. W., KURTZKE, J. F., NAMEROW, N. S., SIBLEY, W. A., and TOURTELLOTTE, W. W. (1970) Cooperative study in the evaluation of therapy in multiple sclerosis: ACTH vs. placebo, *Neurology (Minneap.)*, **20**, No. 5, Part 2.

Ross, C. A. C., Lenman, J. A. R., and Melville, I. D. (1969) Virus antibody levels in multiple sclerosis, *Brit. med. J.*, **3**, 512.

Rushton, D. (1975) Use of the Pulfrich pendulum for detecting abnormal delay in the visual pathway in multiple sclerosis, *Brain*, **98**, 283.

Salmi, A. A., Panelius, M., Halonen, P., Rinne, U. K., and Penttinen, K. (1972) Measles virus antibody in cerebrospinal fluids from patients with multiple sclerosis, *Brit. med. J.*, **1**, 477.

Schapira, K., and Park, D. C. (1961) Gamma globulin studies in multiple sclerosis and their application to the problem of diagnosis, *J. Neurol. Neurosurg. Psychiat.*, **24**, 121.

Schapira, K., Poskanzer, D. C., and Miller, H. (1963) Familial and conjugal multiple sclerosis, *Brain*, **86**, 315.

Schapira, K., Poskanzer, D. C., Newell, D. J., and Miller, H. (1966) Marriage, pregnancy and multiple sclerosis, *Brain*, **89**, 419.

Schneck, S. A., and Claman, H. N. (1969) CSF immunoglobulins in multiple sclerosis and other neurologic diseases: measurement by electroimmunodiffusion, *Arch. Neurol. (Chic.)*, **20**, 132.

Schumacher, G. A. (1974) Critique of experimental trials of therapy in multiple sclerosis, *Neurology (Minneap.)*, **24**, 1010.

Schwartz, S., Rieder, H. P., and Wüthrich, R. (1970) The protein fractions in cerebro-spinal fluid in the various states of multiple sclerosis, *Europ. Neurol.*, **4**, 267.

Seland, T. P., McPherson, T. A., Grace, M., Lamoureux, G., and Blain, J. G. (1974) Evaluation of antithymocyte globulin in acute relapses of multiple sclerosis, *Neurology (Minneap.)*, **24**, 34.

Sever, J. L., Kurtzke, J. F., Alter, M., Schumacher, G., Gilkeson, M. R., Ellenberg, J. H., and Brody, J. A. (1971) Virus antibodies and multiple sclerosis, *Arch. Neurol. (Chic.)*, **24**, 489.

Shibasaki, H., and Kuroiwa, Y. (1973) Clinical studies of multiple sclerosis in Japan. II. Are its clinical characteristics changing?, *Neurology (Minneap.)*, **23**, 618.

Shibasaki, H., and Kuroiwa, Y. (1974) Painful tonic seizure in multiple sclerosis, *Arch. Neurol. (Chic.)*, **30**, 47.

Simpson, C. A., Newell, D. J., and Schapira, K. (1966) Smoking and multiple sclerosis, *Neurology (Minneap.)*, **16**, 1041.

Smith, H. V., Espir, M. L. E., Whitty, C. W. M., and Russell, W. R. (1957) Abnormal immunological reactions in disseminated sclerosis, *J. Neurol. Psychiat.*, **20**, 1.

Spielmeyer, W. (1923) Der anatomische Befund bei einen zweiten Fall von Pelizaeus-Merzbacherscher Krankheit, *Z. ges. Neurol. Psychiat.*, **32**, 203.

Swank, R. L. (1955) Treatment of multiple sclerosis with low fat diet, *Arch. Neurol. Psychiat. (Chic.)*, **73**, 631.

Swank, R. L. (1970) Multiple sclerosis: twenty years on low fat diet, *Arch. Neurol. (Chic.)*, **23**, 460.

Teasdale, G. M., Smith, P. A., Wilkinson, R., Latner, A. L., and Miller, H. (1967) Endocrine activity in multiple sclerosis, *Lancet*, **i**, 64.

Ter Meulen, V., Koprowski, H., Iwasaki, Y., Käckell, Y. M., and Müller, D. (1972) Fusion of cultured multiple-sclerosis brain cells with indicator cells: presence of nucleocapsids and virions and isolation of parainfluenza-type virus, *Lancet*, **ii**, 1.

Turnbull, H. M. (1928) Encephalomyelitis in virus diseases and exanthemata, *Brit. med. J.*, **2**, 331.

Webb, C., Teitelbaum, D., Abramsky, O., Arnon, R., and Sela, M. (1974) Lymphocytes sensitised to basic encephalitogen in patients with multiple sclerosis unresponsive to steroid therapy, *Lancet*, **ii**, 66.

Wisniewski, H. M. (1975) Morphogenesis of the demyelinating process, in *Research in Multiple Sclerosis*, H.M.S.O., London.

Wüthrich, R., and Rieder, H. P. (1970) The seasonal incidence of multiple sclerosis in Switzerland, *Europ. Neurol.*, **3**, 257.

CENTRAL PONTINE MYELINOLYSIS

In 1959 Adams, Victor, and Mancall described four patients in whom autopsy studies revealed a single sharply outlined focus of myelin destruction in the rostral part of the pons, involving all fibre tracts indiscriminately but largely sparing nerve fibres and axis cylinders. The process appeared to begin centrally in the pons and to spread centrifugally. In two of their patients the clinical picture was one of a rapidly evolving flaccid paraplegia with facial and tongue weakness, dysphagia and anarthria; the clinical picture in the other two cases was less dramatic. Three of the patients were alcoholics, the other was severely malnourished. While the condition is provisionally classified at present in the demyelinating diseases it seems probable that it is of metabolic or nutritional origin. The condition has subsequently been described in association with Wernicke's encephalopathy, cirrhosis of the liver and Wilson's disease (Goebel and Herman-Ben Zur, 1972) and in leukaemia (Rosman et al., 1966), and as a complication of uraemia and haemodialysis (Tyler, 1965). Three cases occurring in childhood were all found to be suffering from severe liver disease which is one of the commonest associations (Valsamis et al., 1971), and recent ultrastructural studies support the view that the condition is due to an as yet unidentified toxic–metabolic process (Powers and McKeever, 1976), possibly affecting the oligodendroglia specifically (Tomlinson et al., 1976).

REFERENCES

ADAMS, R. D., VICTOR, M., and MANCALL, E. L. (1959) Central pontine myelinolysis, Arch. Neurol. Psychiat. (Chic.), 81, 154.
GOEBEL, H. H., and HERMAN-BEN ZUR, P. (1972) Central pontine myelinolysis—a clinical and pathological study of 10 cases, Brain, 95, 495.
POWERS, J. M., and McKEEVER, P. E. (1976) Central pontine myelinolysis: an ultrastructural and elemental study, J. neurol. Sci., 29, 65.
ROSMAN, N. P., KAKULAS, B. A., and RICHARDSON, E. P., Jun. (1966) Central pontine myelinolysis in a child with leukemia, Arch. Neurol. (Chic.), 14, 273.
TOMLINSON, B. E., PIERIDES, A. M., and BRADLEY, W. G. (1976) Central pontine myelinolysis, Quart. J. Med., 45, 373.
TYLER, H. R. (1965) Neurological complications of dialysis, transplantation, and other forms of treatment in chronic uremia, Neurology (Minneap.), 15, 1081.
VALSAMIS, M. P., PERESS, N. S., and WRIGHT, L. D. (1971) Central pontine myelinolysis in childhood, Arch. Neurol. (Chic.), 25, 307.

DIFFUSE SCLEROSIS (SCHILDER'S DISEASE)

Classification, Definition, Pathology, and Aetiology

As Poser (1973) and Menkes (1974) have pointed out, the term 'diffuse cerebral sclerosis' has been used for many years to identify a heterogeneous collection of diseases of the cerebral white matter, many of which are now known to be dysmyelinating disorders or leucodystrophies which are genetically determined disorders of myelin formation and metabolism [see p. 527] and not demyelinating diseases as the term is used in this chapter. Thus of the diseases which were classified by Bouman (1934) and Greenfield (1958) under this title, familial sudanophilic diffuse sclerosis, Pelizaeus–Merzbacher disease, Krabbe's diffuse sclerosis (globoid body disease) and metachromatic leucodystrophy, to name but a few of the many disorders which have been identified, are now known to belong to the leucodystrophies which are considered on pages 646-55. Binswanger's subcortical encephalopathy is now known to be an uncommon consequence of diffuse cerebral arteriosclerosis and is no longer accepted as an independent disease entity and Baló's concentric sclerosis (Baló, 1928) is now regarded as but one pathological manifestation of severe multiple sclerosis.

In 1912 Schilder described, under the title of 'encephalitis periaxalia diffusa', a brain in which there was extensive demyelination of the white matter, particularly in the posterior parts of both cerebral hemispheres with relative sparing of axons and comparative preservation of the cortex and of subcortical U fibres. Subsequently in 1924 he described another case in which the areas of demyelination had sharply demarcated borders, there was extensive glial proliferation and massive infiltration of lipid-laden phagocytes with some inflammatory cells. Recently it has been accepted that such a disorder may indeed occur sporadically in childhood and the term 'Schilder's disease' can reasonably be retained provided it is recognized that many cases of leucodystrophy of various types have been erroneously included under this title in the past. Poser and van Bogaert (1956) and Poser (1973) have identified two varieties of this disorder which they have called myelinoclastic diffuse sclerosis to differentiate it from the leucodystrophies; they distinguish between the severe and diffuse variety in which most of the central white matter is demyelinated and transitional diffuse sclerosis in which there are extensive areas of demyelination as well as smaller plaques resembling those of multiple sclerosis (MS). They point out that transitional diffuse sclerosis, like MS, usually occurs in early adult life, the more severe and diffuse variety, corresponding to Schilder's original description, being commoner in childhood. In fact many authors now adhere to the view that even classical Schilder's disease may well prove ultimately to be no more than an exceptionally severe and generalized variety of MS occurring in early life. In the absence of convincing aetiological evidence, however, this postulate is still unproven.

Pathologically, Schilder's diffuse sclerosis is characterized macroscopically by the conversion of the white matter of the posterior parts of both cerebral hemispheres into translucent, greyish, gelatinous areas. In fact, recent studies have shown that the subcortical U fibres are spared less often in this disease than in the leucodystrophies, though the cortex usually remains intact; on the other hand, the axons are generally spared whereas in leucodystrophy they are usually damaged early, while inflammatory cell infiltration is common in Schilder's disease, and rare in leucodystrophy. We know as little about the aetiology of the disease as we do about MS; the finding of a raised IgG in the CSF in such cases raises the possibility that autoimmune processes play an important role.

SYMPTOMS AND SIGNS

The condition usually begins in a previously healthy child between the age of 5 and 12 years with intellectual impairment and a disorder of gait. The onset of symptoms is sometimes rapid, sometimes insidious. Headache and giddiness may occur, but fever is exceptional. Visual impairment is often one of the earliest symptoms, but may be preceded by mental deterioration, epileptiform attacks, aphasia, or weakness and incoordination of the limbs. Visual failure is usually due to destruction of the optic radiations. When one occipital lobe is first involved, the first visual field defect is homonymous hemianopia on the opposite side, the remaining halves of the visual fields being subsequently gradually lost as the opposite occipital lobe becomes involved. More often both sides are involved symmetrically. In either case the end result is blindness. Sometimes visual impairment is due to demyelination of the optic nerves leading to retrobulbar or optic neuritis with bilateral central scotomas. In such cases there may be papillitis during the acute stage followed by optic atrophy. In acute cases widespread demyelination may cause cerebral oedema, raised intracranial pressure, and papilloedema rather than papillitis. Unless the optic nerves are thus involved the pupillary reactions are likely to be normal. Diplopia is not uncommon and is usually due to lateral rectus paralysis. Third-nerve palsy occurs much less frequently. Nystagmus is common. Loss of smell and taste, deafness, and tinnitus have been described.

Progressive spastic weakness of the extremities gradually develops. One side of the body may be affected before the other, but a spastic tetraplegia is the final state. Sensory loss is not uncommon and is usually of the cortical type, with loss of postural sensibility, appreciation of passive movement, and tactile discrimination, leading to astereognosis. When the internal capsules are involved, analgesia involving one or both halves of the body is added. General incoordination is common in the early stages. Aphasia may occur, but later tends to be masked by spastic dysarthria, while dysphagia due to pseudobulbar palsy is not uncommon. Mental changes are usually conspicuous and are those of a progressive dementia. Epileptiform attacks, which may be either generalized or Jacksonian, may occur at any stage of the disease. The cerebrospinal fluid may be normal, but slight mononuclear pleocytosis and an increase of protein and especially of gamma-globulin and IgG have been described.

DIAGNOSIS

In a typical case the early onset of blindness unattributable to a lesion of the optic nerves, together with progressive mental failure and spastic paralysis, constitute a distinctive clinical picture. When the symptoms of diffuse sclerosis are for a time predominantly unilateral and especially when papilloedema occurs, it may be confused with intracranial tumour. The EEG is often of considerable value in diagnosis from subacute encephalitis and lipidosis; it usually shows only diffuse slow activity and very rarely do recordings demonstrate changes in any way comparable to the recurrent bizarre complexes of subacute encephalitis or the irregular spike and wave discharges seen in cerebral lipidosis. Encephalography may help in the diagnosis by yielding evidence of cerebral atrophy, and the ultimate development in diffuse sclerosis of extensive involvement of both cerebral hemispheres will enable a tumour to be excluded. Diagnosis from the leucodystrophies may be difficult if not impossible on clinical grounds, especially if the family history is negative. In Krabbe's diffuse sclerosis the CSF is usually much more abnormal, while slowing of motor nerve conduction is common due to involvement of peripheral nerves; the latter is also true in cases of metachromatic leucodystrophy in which metachromatic granules may be detected in the urine and aryl-sulphatase estimation in leucocyte suspensions may be diagnostic [p. 648]. In the final analysis, however, diagnosis from some of the familial leucodystrophies may be dependent upon brain biopsy, a procedure which is frequently justified in cases of progressive dementia and paralysis in childhood, if only in order to determine the prognosis and to give the parents valid genetic counselling.

PROGNOSIS

The disease is invariably progressive and almost always terminates fatally, although exceptionally temporary remissions occur, and it may possibly sometimes become arrested. It may run an acute course, leading to death within one or two months, and few patients survive more than three years after the onset of the symptoms. Very rarely life may be prolonged for a number of years.

TREATMENT

The cause of the disease being unknown, treatment is empirical and none is known to arrest its course. ACTH and steroid drugs appear to be of no value. The usual anticonvulsant drugs should be employed to control the convulsions.

ADRENOLEUCODYSTROPHY (ADDISON-SCHILDER'S DISEASE)

This X-linked recessive disorder, manifest in males and transmitted by clinically unaffected carrier females, gives a clinical picture indistinguishable from that of Schilder's disease as described above (Siemerling and Creutzfeldt, 1923) save for the fact that the affected patients also show adrenal atrophy; some but not all develop the typical endocrinological and biochemical manifestations of Addison's disease. Estimation of the plasma ACTH, which is usually raised, may be helpful in diagnosis (Rees *et al.*, 1975) but adrenal biopsy is usually diagnostic, as ultrastructural studies of adrenal sections demonstrate membrane-like cytoplasmic inclusions which may also be found in brain tissue (Schaumburg *et al.*, 1974, 1975). Even though inflammatory changes are invariably found in the brains of affected individuals and even though intranuclear filamentous material resembling paramyxovirus has been found in the brains in some such cases (Raine *et al.*, 1975), it seems probable that this disease will ultimately prove to be a systemic metabolic disorder.

REFERENCES

BALÓ, J. (1928) Encephalitis periaxalis concentrica, *Arch. Neurol. Psychiat. (Chic.)*, **19**, 242.

BIELSCHOWSKY, M., and HENNEBERG, R. (1928) Über familiäre diffuse Sklerose. (Leukodystrophia Cerebri Progressiva Hereditaria), *J. Psychiat. Neurol.*, **36**, 131.

BOUMAN, L. (1934) *Diffuse Sclerosis*, Bristol.

COLLIER, J., and GREENFIELD, J. G. (1924) The encephalitis periaxalis of Schilder, *Brain*, **47**, 489.

FERRARO, A. (1937) Primary demyelinating processes of the central nervous system, *Arch. Neurol. Psychiat. (Chic.)*, **37**, 1100.

FOLCH-PI, J., and BAUER, H. (1963) *Brain Lipids and Lipoproteins and the Leucodystrophies*, Amsterdam.

GREENFIELD, J. G. (1958) Demyelinating diseases, in *Neuropathology*, 1st ed., ed. Greenfield, J. G., Blackwood, W., McMenemey, W. H., Meyer, A., and Norman, R. M., London.

GREENFIELD, J. G., and NORMAN, R. M. (1965) Demyelinating diseases, in *Greenfield's Neuropathology*, 2nd ed., ed. Blackwood, W., McMenemey, W. H., Meyer, A., Norman, R. S., and Russell, D. S., London.

MENKES, J. H. (1974) *Textbook of Child Neurology*, Philadelphia.

POSER, C. M. (1973) Diseases of the myelin sheath, in *A Textbook of Neurology*, ed. Merritt, H. H., Philadelphia.

Poser, C. M., and Bogaert, L. van (1956) Natural history and evolution of the concept of Schilder's diffuse sclerosis, *Acta Psychiat. Neurol. Scand.*, **31**, 285.

Raine, C. S., Schaumburg, H. H., Snyder, D. H., and Suzuki, K. (1975) Intranuclear 'paramyxovirus-like' material in multiple sclerosis, adreno-leukodystrophy and Kuf's disease, *J. neurol. Sci.*, **25**, 29.

Rees, L. H., Grant, D. B., and Wilson, J. (1975) Plasma corticotrophin levels in Addison–Schilder's disease, *Brit. med. J.*, **3**, 201.

Schaumburg, H. H., Powers, J. M., Raine, C. S., Suzuki, K., and Richardson, E. P., Jun. (1975) Adrenoleukodystrophy, *Arch. Neurol. (Chic.)*, **32**, 577.

Schaumburg, H. H., Powers, J. M., Suzuki, K., and Raine, C. S. (1974) Adreno-leukodystrophy (sex-linked Schilder disease), *Arch. Neurol. (Chic.)*, **31**, 210.

Schilder, P. (1912) Zur Kenntnis der sogenannten diffusen Sklerose, *Z. ges. Neurol. Psychiat.*, **10**, 1.

Schilder, P. (1924) Die Encephalitis periaxialis diffusa, *Arch. Psychiat. Nervenkr.*, **71**, 327.

Siemerling, E., and Creutzfeldt, H. G. (1923) Bronzenkrankheit und sklerosierende Encephalomyelitis, *Arch. Psychiat. Nervenkrank.*, **68**, 217.

Stewart, T. G., Greenfield, J. G., and Blandy, M. A. (1927) Encephalitis periaxalis diffusa. Report of three cases with pathological examinations, *Brain*, **50**, 1.

Symonds, C. P. (1928) A contribution to the clinical study of Schilder's encephalitis, *Brain*, **51**, 24.

12

EXTRAPYRAMIDAL SYNDROMES

THE BASAL GANGLIA

ANATOMY AND CONNECTIONS OF THE CORPUS STRIATUM AND OTHER PARTS OF THE BASAL GANGLIA

THE corpus striatum is, phylogenetically, the oldest part of the cerebrum. It lies deep in the substance of the cerebral hemisphere between the lateral ventricle and the insula. It consists of the caudate nucleus and the lentiform nucleus, the latter being divided into the putamen and the globus pallidus [FIGS. 4 [p. 18] and 103]. For recent comments upon its anatomy, see Denny-Brown (1962), Brodal (1969), Calne (1970), and Watkins (1972).

The Caudate Nucleus. The caudate nucleus is a pear-shaped mass of grey matter. Its head, the most anterior part of the corpus striatum, is on the lateral side of the anterior horn of the lateral ventricle, into which it bulges. Its tail runs backwards in the floor of the lateral ventricle, and then forwards and downwards in the roof of the descending horn.

The Putamen. This is separated from the insula by a narrow zone of grey matter, the claustrum, and another of white matter, the external capsule.

The Globus Pallidus. This lies medial to the putamen. It is separated from the thalamus and the caudate nucleus by the internal capsule, which also separates the head of the caudate from the anterior part of the putamen.

The caudate nucleus and putamen develop from the same mass of grey matter and show the same histological structure. They contain two types of ganglion cell, a small number of large cells among more frequent small ones. The globus pallidus contains only one type of ganglion cell. On account of their common origin and identical structure the caudate and putamen are grouped together by some writers as 'the striatum', the globus pallidus being distinguished as 'the pallidum'.

The corpus striatum contains numerous fibres which may be divided into (1) afferent, (2) internuncial, and (3) efferent [FIG. 103].

1. Afferent fibres reach it from the cerebral cortex, from the thalamus, and from the midbrain. They are distributed chiefly to the caudate nucleus and putamen. Recently evidence has also accumulated to confirm the existence of a nigrostriatal pathway arising in the substantia nigra and terminating in the corpus striatum, and particularly in the caudate nucleus (Mettler, 1968; Nauta and Mehler, 1969).

2. Internuncial fibres unite the caudate and the putamen, and also connect these fibres with the globus pallidus. It is thought that the afferent fibres terminate in relation with the small ganglion cells, and that the fibres connecting the striatum with the pallidum originate in the large ganglion cells.

3. Efferent fibres run from the striatum to the substantia nigra and from the globus pallidus by the ansa lenticularis to the thalamus, the red nucleus, the substantia nigra, and the subthalamic nucleus or corpus Luysii.

The Red Nucleus. The red nucleus lies in the tegmentum of the midbrain at the level of the superior colliculi. In addition to fibres from the corpus striatum it receives impulses from the opposite dentate nucleus of the cerebellum by the superior peduncle. It is divided into a large-celled and a small-celled portion.

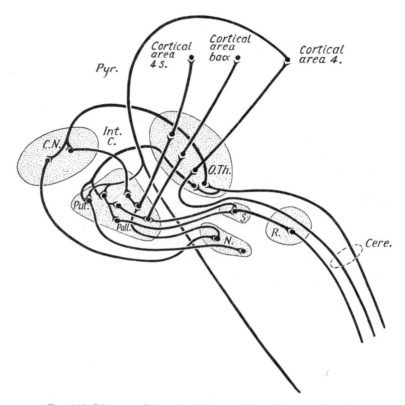

FIG. 103. Diagram of the principal connections of the basal ganglia

Abbreviations: Pyr., corticospinal tract; Int. C., internal capsule; C.N., caudate nucleus; Put., putamen; Pall., globus pallidus; O. Th., optic thalamus; S., subthalamic nucleus; N., substantia nigra; R., red nucleus; Cere., ascending cerebellar pathways

From the former the rubrospinal tract takes origin, and crossing the midline in the ventral tegmental decussation descends through the brain stem to the spinal cord. The small-celled portion gives rise to fibres which ascend to the frontal lobe.

The Thalamus. The structure and function of the thalamus which plays an important role in motor as in sensory function has been considered on pages 47–8.

The Substantia Nigra. The substantia nigra is a grey mass lying between the crus cerebri and tegmentum of the midbrain at the level of the superior colliculi.

It consists of a zona compacta lying dorsally and containing large melanin-bearing ganglion cells to which it owes its dark colour, and a zona reticulata lying under this and resembling in structure the globus pallidus. Besides incoming fibres from the corpus striatum it is said to receive a direct connection from the cortex of the frontal lobe, and it sends fibres to the red nucleus, to the subthalamic nucleus, and to lower regions of the brain stem. As mentioned above, recent work has also identified an important efferent pathway from the substantia nigra (not shown in FIGURE 103) to the corpus striatum.

The Subthalamic Nucleus. The subthalamic nucleus (corpus Luysii) is a small mass of grey matter on the dorsal aspect of the crus cerebri, to the lateral side of the substantia nigra. Besides receiving fibres from the globus pallidus, it communicates with the red nucleus and with the substantia nigra.

To sum up, the extrapyramidal pathways descend from the cortex to the striatum and thence to the substantia nigra, and also to the latter direct; some efferent fibres, as yet inadequately defined, also travel in the reverse direction. There is also a thalamo-pallido-rubral system. All three connect with the tegmental and pontine reticular substance and olives, from which the main spinal connections arise.

DISORDERS OF THE BASAL GANGLIA AND THEIR INTERPRETATION

The interpretation of disorders of the basal ganglia has proved difficult, and much still remains to be learned. Examination of this part of the brain using the classical methods of neuropathology has been disappointing in that relatively few clear-cut clinico-pathological correlations have emerged and the pathological substrate of disorders such as torsion dystonia, for instance, is still poorly defined. However, recent explosive developments in knowledge of catecholamine distribution and of the interplay of cholinergic and dopaminergic systems in this part of the brain have contributed much new information which has already thrown considerable light upon the pathogenesis of several disease states whose nature was until recently obscure. Nevertheless there are still many unanswered questions and it is still useful to consider the extent to which different symptoms and signs of basal ganglia dysfunction can be explained by known pathological and neuropharmacological and biochemical evidence.

SYMPTOMS OF STRIATAL AND OTHER EXTRA-PYRAMIDAL DISORDERS

In any consideration of the symptoms of striatal disorder, it is important to note at the outset that such symptoms are in a sense artificial abstractions from a larger whole. This is so for two reasons, first, because one individual symptom tends to merge into others, however clear-cut it may be in an individual patient. For example, there are intermediate forms between chorea and athetosis and between athetosis and dystonia. Similarly, Parkinsonian rigidity tends to merge into other types of muscular hypertonia. Hence a particular symptom of striatal disorder is to be regarded as part of a spectrum rather than as a completely isolated entity. The second reason is that although in some patients a symptom of striatal disease may remain virtually unchanged for years, in many others, suffering from a progressive disorder, the clinical picture itself changes in the course of time, moving as it were along the spectrum from one group of symptoms to another.

Athetosis

Athetosis is a term meaning instability of posture, and it is applied to a disturbance of both posture and voluntary movement resulting in involuntary movements. It may be unilateral or bilateral. In the upper limb, when, for example, the arm is outstretched, there is a characteristic alternation between two postures. The first is characterized by exaggerated flexion of the wrist and hyperextension of the fingers, particularly at the metacarpophalangeal joints, the forearm tending to be pronated. This is apt to change into a posture of flexion of the fingers, often with the thumb flexed beneath the remaining digits, and the wrist flexed and somewhat supinated. Rather characteristically, the change from extension to flexion occurs successively in one digit after another. The athetotic movements are less marked in the lower limb, where the characteristic picture is one of plantar flexion of the ankle and dorsiflexion of the great toe. Voluntary movement is impeded, and, in the upper limb particularly, wild excursions may occur at shoulder and elbow when it is attempted. The lips, jaw, and tongue are involved, particularly when the disorder is bilateral, and this leads to facial grimaces and dysarthria.

Chorea

As already mentioned, there is no sharp distinction between athetosis and chorea. Typical chorea, however, consists of a series of continuous involuntary movements involving the face, tongue and limbs, chiefly in their distal joints, and even the trunk and respiratory muscles. Choreic movements are rapid and are sometimes described as 'pseudo-purposive'. This means that they resemble fragmentary and disordered forms of emotional and voluntary movement, continually interrupted, and never proceeding to completion. As in athetosis, voluntary movement is grossly disturbed in the more severe forms of chorea by the involuntary movements. Associated movements are exaggerated in chorea. When a choreic patient is made to clench his fists, his whole body partakes in movements which are an exaggerated and disorganized form of the associated movements which normally accompany great muscular effort. The disorganization consists of a loss of reciprocal relaxation, and a loss or incoordination of the synergic muscular contractions necessary for orderly movement. Chorea is characterized by muscular hypotonia and impairment of the ability to maintain a posture. Many patients show a combination of the predominantly peripheral and relatively rapid movements of chorea with the slower, more proximal writhing movements of athetosis and are then said to demonstrate choreo-athetosis.

Hemiballismus

Hemiballismus is a somewhat uncommon form of involuntary movement related to chorea. It is limited to one side of the body, and differs from chorea chiefly in the greater involvement of the proximal joints of the limbs and a prominent tendency to rotation of the limbs. The wild 'flinging' and continuous character of the movement in severe cases may produce virtual exhaustion of the patient and excoriation of skin due to repeated trauma to the affected limbs.

Dystonia

Whereas in one direction athetosis merges into chorea, in the other direction it merges into dystonia. Dystonia is the term applied to the persistent maintenance of a posture by exaggerated muscle tone, the posture being usually not one intermediate between flexion and extension, as is the case in Parkinsonism, but an extreme degree of one or the other, usually extension in the lower limb and either extension or flexion in the upper limb. Dystonia frequently begins with an exaggerated plantar-flexion and inversion of the foot, or hyperextension of the fingers. In extreme cases, as Denny-Brown (1960, 1962) points out, the extremity becomes set in one of the postures of athetosis. The facial muscles and tongue may be involved. The disorder may be unilateral or bilateral, and the asymmetrical distribution of the hypertonia may lead to torsion of the trunk and torticollis. Some authorities believe that spasmodic torticollis is a fractional variety of torsion dystonia.

Rigidity

Rigidity is the muscular disorder characteristic of Parkinsonism. It is often described as a plastic rigidity, and it is characterized by a relatively constant resistance to passive stretching of the muscles, and approximately equal distribution to the flexors and extensors. It is usually evident in the flexors of the wrist and fingers, and pronators of the forearm. Denny-Brown points out that the plastic rigidity of Parkinsonism can be made to disappear if the limb is completely supported and the patient instructed to relax. In such a state of relaxation unimpeded passive movement is possible in either direction at any joint within a small range of 5 to 10 degrees. Movement of larger range, however, immediately sets up a contraction in the stretched muscle, demonstrating that the rigidity is a stretch reflex in each muscle concerned. Denny-Brown states that 'the plastic quality of Parkinsonian rigidity, that distinguishes it from spasticity, is due to a tendency of motor units recruited into a contraction by stretching, to drop out again one by one as others are recruited. . . . When a spastic muscle is stretched more and more motor units respond, and resistance to stretch mounts to a peak. At this point many units suddenly cease responding, and resistance to further stretch melts away ("lengthening reaction"). In plastic rigidity the lengthening reaction affects one motor unit after another from the beginning of stretch, so that resistance to stretch remains approximately constant.' So-called 'cog-wheel rigidity' is thought by some to be merely due to the combination of rigidity and tremor, the resistance to passive movement waxing and waning with the phases of contraction and relaxation of the muscle produced by the tremor. However, Lance et al. (1963) point out that cog-wheel rigidity may be present in patients without resting tremor and suggest that this phenomenon may be due to an exaggerated physiological tremor which has a different frequency from the resting tremor of Parkinsonism.

Tremor

Tremor is a rhythmical alternating contraction of opposing muscle groups (Yahr, 1972). Tremor is commonly associated with rigidity in Parkinsonism, but may occur independently of it. The typical tremor of Parkinsonism is present at rest (resting or static tremor) but it may also persist to some extent during voluntary movement. Postural or action tremor, present with the arms outstretched or throughout the entire range of movement, may be due to anxiety, thyrotoxicosis, drug intoxication, or many other causes but is also characteristic of so-called benign or essential tremor. Tremor which increases towards the end of movement as the limb approaches a target (intention tremor or kinetic tremor, sometimes erroneously called action tremor) is characteristic of disease of the cerebellar connections in the brain stem, less often of the cerebellum itself.

Abbe-Fessard *et al.* (1966) discuss the evidence, drawn from observations on man and monkeys, that a rhythmical activity capable of producing tremor originates in the thalamus. In Parkinsonian patients stereotaxic exploration has demonstrated thalamic rhythms corresponding to the tremor. It is suggested that the lesion responsible for Parkinsonism may damage the inhibitory nigro-striatal pathway, thus releasing an excitatory output from the striatum which in turn facilitates oscillatory activity in thalamic neurones (Calne, 1970).

THE RELATIONSHIP OF SYMPTOMS TO LESIONS OF THE BASAL GANGLIA

The precise correlation of particular striatal symptoms with pathological changes in particular regions is difficult. Many such disorders are diffuse and progressive, and it is therefore often not easy to say at autopsy which symptoms were due to individual components of the pathological change. On the other hand, acute lesions of the corpus striatum may also be diffuse, and tend to produce immediately clinical pictures otherwise associated only with very advanced stages of more slowly progressive disorders. We must be content, therefore, with certain established correlations which so far fill in only part of the picture.

Athetosis

The pathological evidence suggests that the lesion responsible for athetosis is situated in the outer segment of the putamen as in the *état marbré* responsible for congenital double athetosis.

Chorea

It is probable that experimental work in the past has not sufficiently distinguished between chorea and hemiballismus. True chorea appears to result from a lesion of the corpus striatum involving particularly the caudate nucleus. Hemiballismus appears almost always to be due to damage to the opposite subthalamic nucleus or to lesions which isolate it from the globus pallidus (Martin, 1957).

Dystonia

The close relationship between dystonia and athetosis has already been noted, so it is not surprising that the causative lesions may be in a similar situation. The putamen can be involved in both, but in dystonia the thalamus and cerebral cortex may possibly be involved as well though the neuropathology of dystonia is still undefined.

Parkinsonian Tremor and Rigidity

These two symptoms will be considered together, since they are closely related both clinically and physiologically, and it is not at present possible to distinguish their pathological basis. Indeed, the pathological basis of the Parkinsonian syndrome is still under dispute. The subject was discussed by Denny-Brown (1960, 1962). The older view attributed Parkinsonism to lesions of the globus pallidus. The importance of the substantia nigra, which suffers severely in encephalitis lethargica, was subsequently stressed (Greenfield, 1958). Pakkenberg and Brody (1965) found a significant reduction in the number of neurones and especially of those containing melanin in the brains of patients with Parkinsonism when compared with controls. Alvord (1958) and others have stressed the finding of Lewy bodies in the nigral neurones of patients with idiopathic paralysis agitans and the same cells are often the seat of Alzheimer's neurofibrillary change in post-encephalitic cases. Neurofibrillary tangles, granulovacuolar bodies, and 'rod-like' structures are especially common in the Guam Parkinsonism-dementia complex (Hirano *et al.*, 1968; Brody *et al.*, 1971). It is now generally agreed that the principal pathological abnormality in Parkinsonism lies in this structure and in the ascending nigrostriatal pathway (Stern, 1966; Calne, 1970). Nevertheless, Denny-Brown (1962) pointed out that extensive pathological changes may be present in the substantia nigra in patients who show no sign of Parkinsonism and it now seems that rigidity and tremor develop only when the nigral lesion is associated with damage to pathways which connect it with the globus pallidus, corpus striatum, and thalamus (Yahr, 1972).

Massive Lesions of the Basal Ganglia

Important light is thrown upon the functions of the corpus striatum by the clinical pictures which result from massive bilateral lesions of the putamen and caudate nucleus on the one hand, and of the globus pallidus on the other. Denny-Brown (1962), reviewing this question, noted that the characteristic effect of the former lesion is muscular rigidity with the upper limbs in flexion and the lower in extension, particularly evident when the patient is suspended in the air. The effect of symmetrical necrosis of the globus pallidus, commonly the result of carbon monoxide poisoning, is an akinetic mute state with generalized rigidity of all four limbs in a semi-flexed attitude. On the other hand, bilateral lesions of the substantia nigra produced experimentally in monkeys caused hypokinesia and immobility which was enhanced by additional lesions produced in the globus pallidus, but neither rigidity nor tremor developed (Stern, 1966); by contrast, Denny-Brown (1962) found that bilateral pallidal lesions *did* produce plastic rigidity.

THE PHYSIOLOGICAL NATURE OF DISORDERS OF THE BASAL GANGLIA

As Lance and McLeod (1975) and Lenman (1975) point out, the action of the extrapyramidal system on spinal motor neurones is largely mediated through reticulospinal pathways. The extrapyramidal system can be regarded as being made up of a succession of relatively short neurones which descend from the cortex through relay nuclei, often as multiple paths in parallel. At each relay the flow of caudally directed impulses is regulated by neurones which project rostrally from areas such as the subthalamic nucleus, substantia nigra, and midbrain reticular formation which provide a feedback control mechanism. There is a cortico-cortical current passing through the basal ganglia which regulates the cortical control of voluntary movement by a process of graded inhibition which assists in the smooth control of movement. Jung and Hassler (1960) also stressed that to consider the motor system in isolation from sensory input and control is to substitute a fiction for the reality. They and Denny-Brown (1962) agreed that the corpus striatum plays a fundamental part in the regulation of posture and point out that since man differs from animals in his assumption of the erect posture, neural centres concerned with posture and locomotion are likely to have functions in man which differ from those in quadrupeds. Denny-Brown (1962) suggested that many of the symptoms of lesions of the corpus striatum are due to abnormalities of the righting reflexes and pointed out that in many extrapyramidal syndromes the posture of the patient and his involuntary movements can be modified by changing the position of the body in space. Martin (1967) also stressed the disorder of postural reflexes which may occur in Parkinsonism and other extrapyramidal disorders, indicating in particular the way in which a patient with Parkinson's disease who is unable to initiate the act of walking (akinesia) can be made to walk if he leans forward, thus moving the centre of gravity of the body, an act which may initiate the walking reflex. He considers in detail the role of the globus pallidus in this 'starter function', pointing out, as have many others, that this nucleus is the main effector organ of the basal ganglia.

Much work has also been done upon the role of the basal ganglia in controlling the activity of the alpha and gamma motor neurones. Jung and Hassler (1960) suggested that there is a disorder of gamma innervation in Parkinson's disease. However, study of the Jendrassik manoeuvre (reinforcement of tendon reflexes) and of the H-reflex (the electrical analogue of the ankle jerk) in patients with Parkinsonism has given somewhat conflicting results relating to muscle spindle activity in Parkinsonism (Jung and Hassler, 1960; Gassel and Diamantopoulos, 1964; Yap, 1967; Calne, 1970; McLeod and Walsh, 1972; McLellan, 1973). The consensus of current opinion suggests that the basal ganglia are concerned with controlling the balance of alpha and gamma motor neurone activity and that in Parkinsonism there are two components responsible for rigidity; there is an enhancement of tonic stretch reflexes which depends upon both the alpha and gamma systems, and in addition there is, in advanced cases, a progressive flexion dystonia (responsible for the stooped posture) which results from increasing alpha neurone activity and which ultimately becomes irreversible (Lance and McLeod, 1975). The means by which the balance of reticulospinal activity is altered so as to increase the activity in static fusimotor and alpha motor neurones is, however, unknown. Recent neurophysiological studies have also confirmed that the typical static tremor of Parkinsonism is different in frequency from the action tremor which is seen in some cases and which is an exaggeration of physiological tremor; it is the latter, rather than the former, which accounts for the cog-wheel phenomenon. Akinesia appears to be due in part to a disorder of postural reflexes (Martin, 1967) and in part to flexion dystonia involving particularly the lower limbs (Andrews, 1973).

It is now generally accepted that the globus pallidus is the final efferent cell station in the basal ganglia and that its activity is regulated by an input from the cortex, caudate nucleus, putamen, substantia nigra, and subthalamic nucleus. The involuntary movements which result from diffuse partial lesions of the putamen and globus pallidus are due to impaired control of righting reflexes and of the incoming impulses which normally modify them; thus in a sense they are release phenomena, due to loss of normal inhibitory activity. Lesions of the putamen usually release the movements of athetosis, those of the caudate chorea, in which, in contrast to Parkinsonism, associated movements are increased while motor neurone excitability and the tonic stretch reflexes are often diminished. The subthalamic nucleus appears to be concerned with stabilization of the limbs on the opposite side of the body in relation to their resting posture and voluntary movement, so that a lesion of this structure leads to the violent uncontrolled movements of hemiballismus. As already mentioned, the patho-anatomical substrate of torsion dystonia is still undefined but in this disorder which gives fixed alterations in posture, the tonic stretch reflexes and alpha motor neurone activity are markedly enhanced.

Each of the extrapyramidal syndromes mentioned may thus be regarded as being due to a disturbance of a delicate physiological balance which normally exists in this intricate system. The fact that lesions produced surgically in the globus pallidus or ventrolateral nucleus of the thalamus may abolish contra-lateral tremor and reduce rigidity in Parkinsonism (Cooper, 1961) and that the same operation may be beneficial in abolishing hemiballismus or the intention tremor of cerebellar disease, while it is less effective in dystonia, chorea, and torticollis and almost totally ineffective in athetosis, is still difficult to explain convincingly. It is probably due to the fact that the lesion blocks the main efferent pathway from the globus pallidus which passes rostrally via the ventro-lateral nucleus of the thalamus. The question as to why the interruption of this output leaves the patient with little or no disability remains unanswered.

Some of these unsolved patho-physiological problems which remain un-resolved are becoming more easily understood as a result of recent neuro-pharmacological research. Ehringer and Hornykiewicz (1960) showed that the concentration of dopamine was reduced in the basal ganglia of patients with Parkinsonism and it is now known that the nigrostriatal tract is dopaminergic while striatal dopamine can be reduced by lesions of the substantia nigra induced experimentally in monkeys (Poirier and Sourkes, 1965). Strionigral neurones, by contrast, probably employ gamma-amino-butyric acid (GABA) as their transmitter (Hassler, 1972). Reserpine and the phenothiazines which may produce drug-induced Parkinsonism, act by depleting dopamine stores in the basal ganglia through inhibition of dopamine-stimulated adenylate cyclase activity (Steg, 1972; Calne et al., 1975). By giving levodopa, a precursor of dopamine, the dopamine stores can generally be repleted with amelioration of many of the symptoms of Parkinsonism [p. 594]. On the other hand, one important side-effect of levodopa therapy is the development of troublesome involuntary movements which sometimes resemble chorea or athetosis; similarly, phenothiazine derivatives are known on occasion to produce facial dyskinetic movements and postural changes resembling those of dystonia. There is also convincing evidence, reviewed fully by Calne (1970, 1971), that many neurones in the caudate nucleus and putamen are cholinergic, and that cholinergic activation aggravates the symptoms of Parkinsonism, a fact which almost certainly explains the beneficial effect of anticholinergic drugs in this disease. It may therefore be postulated that many of the symptoms of disease in the basal ganglia may well be due to an imbalance in the relative activities of cholinergic and dopaminergic neurones and their receptors. Much can be learned of these mechanisms by studying the concentration of metabolites of dopamine such as homovanillic acid (HVA) and of other catecholamines in the CSF and in the urine and there is no doubt that such studies will throw increas-ing light upon function and dysfunction of the basal ganglia within the next few years.

REFERENCES

ABBE-FESSARD, D., GUIOT, G., LAMARRE, Y., and ARFEL, G. (1966) Activation of thalamo-cortical projections related to tremorogenic processes, in *The Thalamus*, ed. Purpura, D. O., and Yahr, M. D., p. 237, New York.

ALVORD, E. C., Jun. (1958) Pathology of Parkinsonism, in *Pathogenesis and Treatment of Parkinsonism*, ed. Fields, W. S., Springfield, Ill.

ANDREWS, C. J. (1973) The influence of dystonia on the response to long-term L-dopa therapy, *J. Neurol. Neurosurg. Psychiat.*, **36**, 630.

BORIT, A., RUBINSTEIN, L. J., and URICH, H. (1975) The striatonigral degenerations—putaminal pigments and nosology, *Brain*, **98**, 101.

BRODAL, A. (1969) *Neurological Anatomy in Relation to Clinical Medicine*, 2nd ed., London.

BRODY, J. A., HIRANO, A., and SCOTT, R. M. (1971) Recent neuropathologic observations in amyotrophic lateral sclerosis and parkinsonism-dementia of Guam, *Neurology (Minneap.)*, **21**, 528.

CALNE, D. B. (1970) *Parkinsonism: Physiology, Pharmacology and Treatment*, London.

CALNE, D. B. (1971) Parkinsonism—physiology and pharmacology, *Brit. med. J.*, **3**, 693.

CALNE, D. B., CHASE, T. N., and BARBEAU, A. (1975) *Dopaminergic Mechanisms* (Advances in Neurology, vol. 9), New York.

COOPER, I. S. (1961) *Parkinsonism. Its Medical and Surgical Therapy*, Springfield, Ill.

DENNY-BROWN, D. (1960) Diseases of the basal ganglia, *Lancet*, **ii**, 1099, 1155.

DENNY-BROWN, D. (1962) *The Basal Ganglia and Their Relation to Disorders of Movement*, Oxford.

EHRINGER, H., and HORNYKIEWICZ, O. (1960) Verteilung von Noradrenalin und Dopamin (3-hydroxytyramin) im Gehirn des Menschen und ihr Verhalten bei Erkrankungen des extrapyramidalen Systems, *Klin. Wschr.*, **38**, 1236.

GASSEL, M. M., and DIAMANTOPOULOS, E. (1964) The Jendrassik maneuver. I. The pattern of reinforcement of monosynaptic reflexes in normal subjects and patients with spasticity or rigidity, *Neurology (Minneap.)*, **14**, 555.

GREENFIELD, J. G. (1958) in *Neuropathology*, by Greenfield, J. G., Blackwood, W., McMenemey, W. H., Meyer, A., and Norman, R. M., p. 530, London.

HASSLER, R. (1972) Physiopathology of rigidity, in *Parkinson's Disease*, ed. Siegfried, J., vol. 1, p. 20, Berne.

HIRANO, A., DEMBITZER, H. M., KURLAND, L. T., and ZIMMERMAN, H. M. (1968) The fine structure of some intraganglionic alterations: neurofibrillary tangles, granulo-vacuolar bodies and 'rod-like' structures as seen in Guam amyotrophic lateral sclerosis and Parkinsonism-dementia complex, *J. Neuropath. exp. Neurol.*, **27**, 167.

HORNYKIEWICZ, O. (1963) Die topische Lokalisation und das Verhallen von Noradrenaline und Dopamin im der Substantia der normallen und Parkinson Kranken Menschen, *Wien. Klin. Wschr.*, **75**, 309.

JUNG, R., and HASSLER, R. (1960) The extrapyramidal motor system, in *Handbook of Physiology*, vol. 2, p. 863, Washington.

LANCE, J. W., and McLEOD, J. G. (1975) *A Physiological Approach to Clinical Neurology*, London.

LANCE, J. W., SCHWAB, R. S., and PETERSON, E. A. (1963) Action tremor and the cogwheel phenomenon in Parkinson's disease, *Brain*, **86**, 95.

LENMAN, J. A. R. (1975) *Clinical Neurophysiology*, Oxford, London, Edinburgh, Melbourne.

McLELLAN, D. L. (1973) Dynamic spindle reflexes and the rigidity of Parkinsonism, *J. Neurol. Neurosurg. Psychiat.*, **36**, 342.

McLEOD, J. G., and WALSH, J. C. (1972) H reflex studies in patients with Parkinson's disease, *J. Neurol. Neurosurg. Psychiat.*, **35**, 77.

MARTIN, J. P. (1957) Hemichorea (hemiballismus) without lesions in the corpus Luysii, *Brain*, **80**, 1.

MARTIN, J. P. (1967) *The Basal Ganglia and Posture*, London.

METTLER, F. A. (1968) Anatomy of the basal ganglia, in *Diseases of the Basal Ganglia*

(Handbook of Clinical Neurology, vol. 6, ed. Vinken, P. J., and Bruyn, G. W., p. 1, Amsterdam.

NAUTA, W. H. J., and MEHLER, W. R. (1969) in *Psychotropic Drugs and Dysfunctions of the Basal Ganglia. A Multidisciplinary Workshop*, ed. Crane, G. E., and Gardner, R., Washington.

PAKKENBERG, H., and BRODY, H. (1965) The number of nerve cells in the substantia nigra in paralysis agitans, *Acta Neuropath. (Berl.)*, **5**, 320.

POIRIER, L. J., and SOURKES, T. L. (1965) Influence of the substantia nigra on the catecholamine content of the striatum, *Brain*, **88**, 181.

STEG, G. (1972) Biochemical aspects of rigidity, in *Parkinson's Disease*, ed. Siegfried, J., vol. 1, p. 48, Berne.

STERN, G. (1966) The effects of lesions in the substantia nigra, *Brain*, **89**, 449.

WATKINS, E. S. (1972) The basal ganglia, in *Scientific Foundations of Neurology*, ed. Critchley, M., O'Leary, J. L., and Jennett, B., London.

YAHR, M. D. (1972) Involuntary movements, in *Scientific Foundations of Neurology*, ed. Critchley, M., O'Leary, J. L., and Jennett, B., London.

YAP, C.-B. (1967) Spinal segmental and long-loop reflexes on spinal motorneurone excitability in spasticity and rigidity, *Brain*, **90**, 887.

THE PARKINSONIAN SYNDROME

Definition. The Parkinsonian syndrome, named after James Parkinson, who first described paralysis agitans in 1817, is a disturbance of motor function characterized chiefly by slowing and enfeeblement of emotional and voluntary movement, muscular rigidity, and tremor. Parkinsonism may be produced by a number of different pathological states and is usually ascribed to lesions involving the substantia nigra and its efferent pathways.

AETIOLOGY AND PATHOLOGY

Jakob and Ramsay Hunt considered that loss of the large ganglion cells of the corpus striatum was the essential cause of Parkinsonism, though the former placed the lesion principally in the caudate nucleus and putamen and the latter in the globus pallidus. However, as mentioned above [p. 575], it is now clear that the substantia nigra is the principal site of pathological change (Earle, 1968; Lewis, 1971).

The histological changes depend upon the nature of the causal pathological process. Greenfield and Bosanquet (1953) and Greenfield (1958) reviewed the pathology of idiopathic and encephalitic Parkinsonism, with special reference to the substantia nigra and the locus caeruleus. They described five types of cell change: (1) saccular distension with lipochrome granules; (2) vacuolation, and (3) binucleated cells—all changes found in post-encephalitic Parkinsonism; (4) Lewy's spherical concentric hyaline inclusions, found in idiopathic Parkinsonism [FIG. 104], and (5) neurofibrillary tangles, found in post-encephalitic cases and in the Parkinsonism–dementia complex. These changes are not affected by prior treatment with levodopa (Yahr et al., 1972). Den Hartog Jager (1969, 1970) suggests that the Lewy bodies contain sphingomyelin and found similar cytoplasmic inclusions in the adrenal medulla; he postulates that there is a disorder of lipid storage in this disease. On the other hand, Martin et al. (1971) suggested that juvenile Parkinsonism might be due to inherited tyrosine hydroxylase deficiency, and Barbeau et al. (1975), on the basis of studies of the uptake of dopamine by platelets, suggested that there is a diffuse defect of dopamine metabolism.

As mentioned above, there is now convincing evidence that in Parkinsonism there is depletion of dopamine stores in the cells of the substantia nigra; this is true of both the post-encephalitic and idiopathic varieties of the disease. In the former the condition is clearly a sequel of encephalitis lethargica but in the latter the cause of this depletion and of the accompanying pathological changes

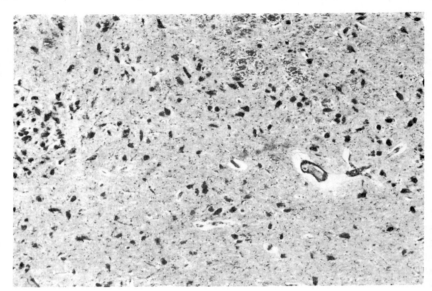

FIG. 104 *a*. The normal substantia nigra, H & E, × 40

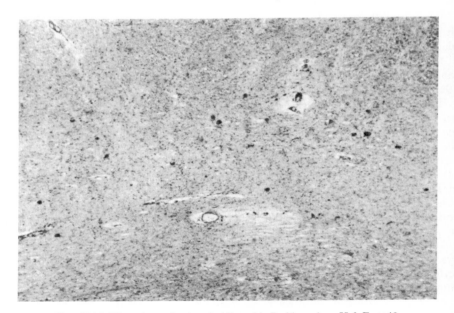

FIG. 104 *b*. The substantia nigra in idiopathic Parkinsonism, H & E, × 40

is unknown. The view that the idiopathic disorder may also be a sequel of sub-clinical lethargic encephalitis (Poskanzer *et al.*, 1969; Brown and Knox, 1972) is not generally accepted. Drug-induced Parkinsonism due to dopamine antagonists such as reserpine, haloperidol, tetrabenazine, and other pheno-thiazines is common (Ayd, 1961; Calne, 1970) but usually resolves when the offending drug is withdrawn.

So-called arteriosclerotic Parkinsonism differs from Parkinson's disease in several essential respects [see p. 589]; clinical features resembling those of Parkinsonism may also result from manganese intoxication, carbon monoxide poisoning, severe head injury, and the 'punch-drunk syndrome' of professional boxers. Parkinsonian features are also seen in various other degenerative diseases of the basal ganglia including progressive bulbar palsy, corticostriatonigral degeneration, progressive supranuclear palsy, progressive multisystem degeneration (the Shy–Drager syndrome), and the Parkinsonism–dementia complex which occurs on the island of Guam, but each of these disorders should be accepted as being distinct from Parkinson's disease in the accepted sense of the term.

The idiopathic disease occurs more often in more than one member of a family than can be accounted for by chance, and families suggesting dominant inherit-ance with incomplete penetrance have been described (Pratt, 1967; Kondo *et al.*, 1973). Polygenic inheritance of the disease, possibly related to an inherited deficiency of tyrosine hydroxylase, has been postulated (Martin *et al.*, 1973). There is some evidence that malignant disease occurs more often in patients with Parkinsonism than in a control population (Pritchard and Netsky, 1973). A prevalence rate of between 1 in 200 (Yahr, 1967) and 1 in 1,000 (Brewis *et al.*, 1966) has been reported; there is no convincing evidence of any specific racial

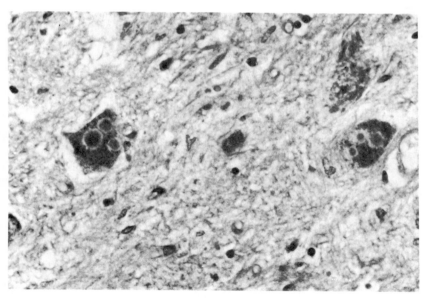

FIG. 104 *c*. Lewy bodies in the substantia nigra, H & E, × 400

(Illustrations kindly provided by Professor B. E. Tomlinson) or geographical incidence. The condition is slightly more common in males than in females (Calne, 1970) and the commonest age of onset is in the fifth and sixth decade with death occurring in from 1–33 years with a mean of 9 years after the development of symptoms, in the pre-levodopa era (Hoehn and Yahr, 1967). A very rare juvenile form, which is often familial, has been described as beginning in adolescence (Hunt, 1917; Martin *et al.*, 1973).

SYMPTOMS AND SIGNS

A general description of the symptoms of the Parkinsonian syndrome will first be given, and the distinctive features of the various forms of the disorder will then be considered separately. Their pathogenesis is discussed on page 575.

Facies and Attitude

The Parkinsonian facies is characteristic. The palpebral fissures may be wider than normal, and blinking is infrequent. The eyes have a staring appearance, due partly to these features and partly to the fact that spontaneous ocular movements are lacking or seldom occur. The glabellar tap reflex fails to habituate; thus in normal persons, tapping on the glabella produces blinking which ceases after the first few taps, whereas in many patients with Parkinsonism the blinking continues in time with the taps for as long as the stimulus is applied. Electrophysiological studies have shown that this reflex has two components of different latency (see Kugelberg, 1952; Rushworth, 1962, 1968; and page 52) and the abnormal reflex of Parkinsonism may be modified by treatment (Klawans and Goodwin, 1969; Penders and Delwaide, 1971). The facial muscles exhibit an unnatural immobility. The attitude of the limbs and trunk is one of moderate flexion with a typical 'stoop' [FIG. 105]. The spine is usually somewhat flexed, but is occasionally extended. There is little rotatory movement of the cervical spine. The limbs are moderately flexed and adducted, but the wrist is usually slightly extended. The fingers are flexed at the metacarpophalangeal, and extended or only slightly flexed at the interphalangeal, joints, and adducted. The thumb is usually adducted, and extended at the metacarpo- and interphalangeal joints.

Disorders of Movement (Akinesia and Bradykinesia)

Voluntary movement exhibits some impairment of power, but more striking are the difficulty in initiating movement (akinesia) and the slowness with which it is performed (bradykinesia). It is important to recognize that, in many cases, signs may initially be present on one side of the body and not on the other ('hemiplegic' Parkinsonism). In general, the movements which are carried out by small muscles suffer most. Hence the patient shows weakness of the ocular movements, especially convergence; of the facial movements, associated with tremor of the eyelids on closure of the eyes; and of movements concerned in mastication, deglutition, and articulation. The speech in severe cases is slurred, quiet, and monotonous, owing to defective pronunciation of consonants and lack of variation in pitch. Rarely palilalia occurs and occasionally in severe cases phonation and articulation are so impaired that the patient is virtually mute (Nakano *et al.*, 1973). Movements of the hands are also markedly affected, with resulting clumsiness and inability to perform fine movements, such as those used in needlework, dealing cards, and taking money from a pocket. Characteristically the range of movement, as in opposition of the thumb and individual fingers, is greatly reduced. Micrographia is common; the writing becomes pro-

Fig. 105. The characteristic posture of severe paralysis agitans (idiopathic Parkinsonism). Note the typical stoop and the flexion of the arms at the elbow. From *An Atlas of Clinical Neurology* 2nd ed., 1975 by J. D. Spillane, reproduced by kind permission of the author

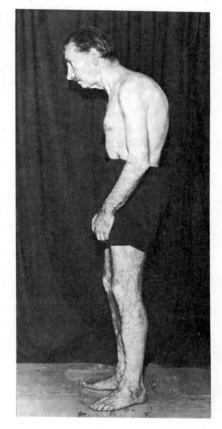

gressively smaller and may trail away to nothing. Certain associated and synergic movements suffer conspicuously. Swinging of the arms in walking is early diminished and later lost, and the synergic extension of the wrist, which is normally associated with flexion of the fingers, is also impaired. Various methods of analysing the defects of movement, using 'tracking tasks' and recording devices have been designed in order to assess the abnormality quantitatively (Calne, 1970; Angel *et al.*, 1970). Thoracic expansion in inspiration is reduced, but the contraction of the diaphragm may be increased in compensation. Emotional movements of the face are also reduced in amplitude, slow in developing, and unduly protracted.

Muscular Rigidity

Muscular rigidity does not always develop *pari passu* with the disorders of movement just described, which not uncommonly precede it. It differs from the hypertonia associated with corticospinal lesions in that it is present to an equal extent in opposing muscle-groups, for example, the flexors and extensors of the elbow; it is uniform throughout the whole range of movement at a joint. Sometimes the rigidity exhibits an interrupted character when tested by passive movement, the muscles yielding to tension in a series of jerks ('cog-wheel rigidity') while sometimes it is smooth and is of the so-called 'plastic' or 'lead-pipe' variety. Parkinsonian rigidity, like other Parkinsonian symptoms, is often unequal on the two sides of the body. In spite of it full passive movement is usually possible at all joints. Occasionally, however, contractures occur which limit such movement. This happens most frequently in the hands and the feet. The fingers may be so strongly flexed that a pad has to be used to prevent the nails being driven into the palm. Similar flexor deformity of the toes may occur, and talipes equinovarus may be produced.

Gait

The Parkinsonian gait is in part at least the outcome of the patient's attitude and rigidity. It is usually slow, shuffling, and composed of small steps (*marche à petits pas*). The patient is often unable to stop quickly when pushed forwards or backwards—propulsion and retropulsion. When propulsion occurs spontaneously during walking, the patient exhibits a 'festinating' gait, hurrying with small steps in a bent attitude as if trying to catch up his centre of gravity. Often there is difficulty in beginning to walk and the patient's feet seem to 'freeze' to the floor (akinesia); similarly, there may be great difficulty in getting out of a chair. Often the patient seems to 'mark time' on one spot and then takes a few short, shuffling steps before beginning to walk more normally. If the patient looks down at a line on the floor in front of him, or leans forward slightly on to a frame-type walking aid (Martin, 1967) the walking reflex may be initiated so that he walks without difficulty. A striking feature of Parkinsonism is the frequent ability of the patient to carry out rapid movements requiring considerable exertion better than slower and less energetic movements. Thus a patient who can walk only very slowly may be able to run quite fast. This phenomenon has been called 'kinesia paradoxa'.

Tremor

Tremor is the characteristic involuntary movement of Parkinsonism. Tremor, rigidity, and slowness and weakness of movement are, however, to a large extent independent variables. Tremor may be the first symptom, as it frequently is in paralysis agitans, and may precede rigidity by months or years. An onset with unilateral tremor often implies a benign course, especially in cases of early onset, i.e. at less than 40 years of age (Scott *et al.*, 1970; Scott and Brody, 1971); it usually begins in one hand and arm, later involves the leg, and may not spread to the other side of the body for many months or years. In post-encephalitic Parkinsonism rigidity more often precedes tremor. The head is involved late, if at all.

The tremor consists of rhythmic alternating movements of opposing muscle-groups [FIG. 106]. In the upper limb the hand is most affected. Movements of the fingers occur at the metacarpophalangeal joints and may be combined with movements of the thumb—the 'pill-rolling movement'. Movements at the wrist may be flexion and extension, lateral displacement, or pronation and supination. Often the tremor shifts from one to another group of muscles while the patient is under observation. Little movement usually occurs at the joints above the wrist. In the lower limb tremor is most marked at the ankle, at which flexion and extension occur. Either flexion and extension or a rotatory tremor of the head may occur. When the mandibular muscles are involved, rhythmical opening and closure of the mouth are observed, and the tongue is sometimes involved.

The frequency of the tremor is 4–8 Hz, being slower in paralysis agitans than in post-encephalitic Parkinsonism. It is present when the patient is at rest ('static' tremor), and is often temporarily or wholly suppressed when the limb is voluntarily moved. Action tremor, which is not uncommon [p. 573], is more rapid with a frequency of 7–12 Hz (Lance and McLeod, 1975). Tremor can often be inhibited for a time by conscious effort, but is liable to break from this control with increased intensity. It is increased by emotional excitement and almost always disappears during sleep.

Akithisia

This is a form of intolerable restlessness and associated discomfort, requiring continual changes of position, occasionally seen in Parkinsonism.

Sensory Symptoms

There is no loss of sensibility in Parkinsonism. Pain, however, is common, especially in the later stages, when most patients complain of cramp-like pains

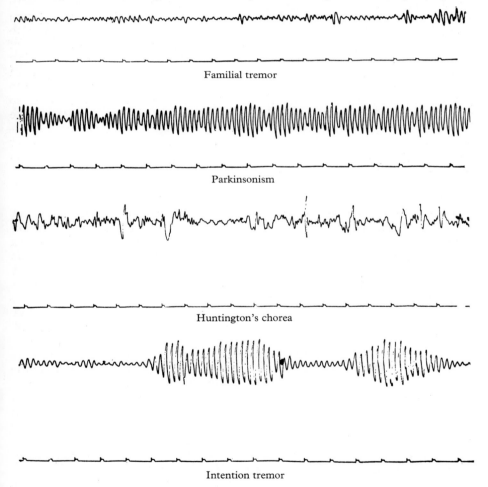

Familial tremor

Parkinsonism

Huntington's chorea

Intention tremor

FIG. 106. Recordings of four different types of tremor.
The intervals on the time marker are one second.
(By courtesy of Professor John Marshall.)

in the limbs and spine due to rigidity and the changes induced in the joints and ligaments by the abnormal posture. Even in early cases, aching discomfort in the affected limbs is occasionally the presenting symptom, especially when rigidity is unilateral.

The Reflexes

Parkinsonism does not involve any essential changes in the reflexes, though rigidity may render the tendon-jerks difficult to elicit and reduced in amplitude. However, in the early stages the reflexes may actually be increased in limbs showing early rigidity and in a case of 'hemiplegic' Parkinsonism this may give rise to diagnostic difficulty. The plantar reflexes are flexor in uncomplicated paralysis agitans, but it is not unknown for one or both to be extensor in post-encephalitic Parkinsonism or due to associated cervical spondylosis leading to myelopathy. Extensor plantar responses are common in so-called arterio-sclerotic 'Parkinsonism' and in the Parkinsonism–dementia complex; they are also seen in various forms of degenerative disease which show Parkinsonian features, including some types of presenile dementia, cortico-striatonigral degeneration, and progressive multisystem degeneration. Hence the finding of such responses should certainly cast doubt upon the diagnosis of idiopathic paralysis agitans.

Changes in the H-reflex excitability curve have been reported in such cases [see p. 576].

Autonomic Symptoms

Autonomic dysfunction is probably responsible for certain symptoms which often cause much discomfort. Flushing of the skin may occur accompanied by uncomfortable sensations of heat and sometimes by sweating. These symptoms may be limited to, or more marked upon, one side of the body; cutaneous sebum excretion has been shown to be increased (Burton and Shuster, 1970). Oedema and cyanosis of a limb are rare. Parkinsonian patients usually tolerate cold much better than heat; this fact, combined with their immobility, renders such patients particularly liable to suffer episodes of hypothermia, particularly if confined to bed in an unheated room in cold weather. Excessive salivation is also a feature in many cases. There is usually a gradual loss of weight.

The resting blood pressure is often low (Aminoff and Wilcox, 1972) and many patients also show orthostatic hypotension with an abnormal fall of pressure on tilting (Gross et al., 1972). In post-encephalitic cases particularly, but to a lesser extent in paralysis agitans, the resting respiratory rate is often increased with fewer variations in amplitude than in normal subjects (Kim, 1968). Retention of urine is relatively common, but is probably due as a rule to the effects of treatment with anticholinergic drugs rather than to the disease itself.

Mental State

Parkinsonism is not necessarily accompanied by any mental change, and the sufferer's intellectual capacity and emotional reactions may continue unimpaired behind the mask in which his disorder fixes his features. However, it has been known for many years that disorders of personality and mood are common sequelae of encephalitis lethargica and dementia is well-known to occur in many patients with post-encephalitic Parkinsonism. Depression, which may respond to appropriate drugs, is also accepted as a common accompaniment of paralysis agitans, occurring in up to 90 per cent of cases (Mindham, 1970). Psychotic episodes have often been attributed to the effects of treatment but are now known to occur spontaneously and there is growing evidence to indicate that progressive dementia occurs in idiopathic Parkinsonism much more frequently than has been appreciated in the past (Loranger *et al.*, 1972; *British Medical Journal*, 1973 *a*, 1974) and is often associated with progressive cerebral atrophy (Selby, 1968).

FORMS OF PARKINSONISM

PARALYSIS AGITANS

Synonyms. Parkinson's disease; shaking palsy.

PATHOLOGY AND AETIOLOGY

See page 579.

SYMPTOMS

Tremor is often the first symptom, beginning either unilaterally or bilaterally, but in many other patients stiffness and slowness of movement, sometimes beginning on one side, are the presenting features. Often, slight facial immobility, a stoop, early fatigue, and slowness of movement are thought by the patient and his family to be due simply to ageing and the early symptoms and signs of the illness may go unrecognized for months or years. As rigidity and akinesia increase, difficulty in getting out of a chair, bed, or bath or even in turning over in bed develop and in severe cases the patient is ultimately immobile and bed-ridden.

PROGNOSIS

The disease is always progressive, though cases differ considerably in the rate or progress. The symptoms may be confined to one limb for months or years, and the spread to other limbs when it occurs may be slow or fairly rapid. The prognosis in cases in which tremor in one upper limb is the only manifestation of the disease during the first two or three years is very much better than in the average case. The outlook is worse when the condition begins with akinesia and progressive rigidity leading to immobility, but even helpless patients may survive for many years. There is some evidence that levodopa therapy favourably influences the natural history (Stern *et al.*, 1972) but the long-term effect of treatment is still uncertain. The average duration of the disease is about ten years, but it is not uncommon for patients to live considerably longer (Hoehn and Yahr, 1967). Death occurs usually from complications such as pneumonia, vascular disease, or neoplasia (Calne, 1970). Occasionally there is a terminal stage of lethargy passing into coma.

PARKINSONISM FOLLOWING ENCEPHALITIS LETHARGICA

PATHOLOGY AND AETIOLOGY

See pages 485 and 579.

SYMPTOMS

It was common to observe some Parkinsonian symptoms in the acute attack of encephalitis and in many cases Parkinsonism developed insidiously during the subsequent 12 months. The interval, however, was sometimes as long as 20 years; or no history of an acute attack was obtainable. Since the greatest incidence of the disease was in early adult life, for 20 years after the epidemic of the 1920s most cases of encephalitic Parkinsonism occurred before the age of 40. Subsequently many cases beginning as late as 60 years of age appeared. With the virtual disappearance of encephalitis lethargica it now seems that this form of the disease is gradually disappearing.

Stiffness, slowness of movement, and weakness usually precede tremor. These symptoms are usually more marked upon, and may be confined to, one side of the body. Sometimes they are even more restricted and involve only one upper limb, or one upper limb and the same side of the face. In the early stages the upper limb is usually more affected than the lower. Rigidity is usually more conspicuous than tremor throughout the course of the illness. The pupillary reactions to accommodation or to light or to both may be impaired, and apathy, depression, or dementia may be conspicuous. There is often an excess of sebaceous secretion over the face, and of saliva which characteristically drips from the open mouth.

Oculogyral Spasm

Spasm of conjugate ocular muscles was a not infrequent complication of Parkinsonism following encephalitis lethargica, but is now comparatively rare. The attacks last from a few seconds to hours. The eyes are usually deviated upwards, with lids retracted, less often laterally, and rarely downwards or obliquely. There may be an associated spasmodic deviation of the head in the same direction and occasionally the patient may fall over backwards. Sometimes the eyes become fixed when the gaze is directed forwards, or in a position of convergence. During the attack the patient's attempts to move the eyes in other directions result in only a very feeble, jerky displacement from the position of spasmodic deviation.

Other Symptoms

Other symptoms occasionally occur, especially torticollis or other dystonic attitudes of the trunk and limbs. Bizarre contractures of the extremities are not infrequently seen in severe post-encephalitic cases but are rare in paralysis agitans.

PROGNOSIS

In most cases Parkinsonism following soon after encephalitis was a progressive condition running a much shorter course than paralysis agitans. In a few cases the disorder seemed to become arrested and this happened most often when the symptoms were predominantly unilateral. In severe cases the patient became quite incapacitated within a year of the onset of symptoms, but at present milder chronic cases are the rule and the disorder often reaches a stationary condition. Progressive amyotrophy resembling motor neurone disease is an occasional late sequel (Greenfield and Matthews, 1954). Death is due to pneumonia, vascular disease, or a general cachexia terminating in coma.

ARTERIOSCLEROTIC 'PARKINSONISM'

Clinical features resembling those of Parkinsonism may develop in the course of cerebral arteriosclerosis, but the resulting clinical picture is not only very variable in itself but is also frequently complicated by the presence of other symptoms of vascular disease. Thus there are usually accompanying signs of pseudobulbar palsy, corticospinal lesions, dementia, or of a lesion of the midbrain.

Some cases are due to arteriosclerosis with low or normal blood pressure, and are, therefore, found in late middle and old age. However, a number of patients with severe hypertension and with consequent multiple small softenings in the cerebral hemispheres and brain stem may develop a slow shuffling gait, facial immobility, emotional lability (pathological over-emotionalism) with rigidity of the limbs, hyperreflexia and extensor plantar responses. These patients often develop other signs of pseudobulbar palsy. The age-incidence is generally later than that of paralysis agitans, though in severely hypertensive patients it may occur earlier in life. The onset is usually insidious, but in some cases follows a 'stroke'; and a series of mild 'strokes' may each be followed by an increase in the severity of the symptoms.

Of symptoms resembling those of Parkinsonism, the bodily attitude, slowness of movement, and the festinating gait are the commonest, and lack of facial expression and tremor are rare. The rigidity is often atypical, being variable in degree and predominating in the flexors of the elbows and in the extensors of the knees. Catatonia is not uncommon. It seems probable that the symptoms are in part due to lesions at a higher level than the corpus striatum, interrupting corticostriate fibres.

The course of the disorder is more rapid than that of paralysis agitans. The condition shows little or no response to treatment with levodopa and other remedies (Godwin-Austen et al., 1971; Parkes et al., 1974). When the blood pressure is high, a fatal cerebral haemorrhage may occur. Progressive dementia, dysphagia, and eventual incontinence render nursing difficult, and the patient succumbs in a few years.

THE DIAGNOSIS OF PARKINSONISM

It is necessary to distinguish the Parkinsonian syndrome from other conditions which may simulate it. Since the most striking Parkinsonian symptoms are tremor and muscular rigidity, Parkinsonism is most likely to be confused with conditions causing one or other of these symptoms.

Other Causes of Tremor

Senile Tremor. Tremor is not uncommon in old age. It differs from Parkinsonian tremor in being finer and more rapid. At first it is absent when the limbs are at rest and occurs only on voluntary movement ('action' tremor). Later it may be present during rest also. It is most marked in the upper limbs, but is more frequently present in the head than Parkinsonian tremor. The rhythmical to-and-fro 'titubating' movements of the head are characteristic. It is not associated with muscular weakness or rigidity.

Benign or 'Essential' Familial Tremor. This is a form of tremor which may occur in several members of the same family, sometimes in successive generations (Critchley, 1949; Larsson and Sjögren, 1960; Critchley, 1972).

It may begin in childhood and usually develops during the first twenty-five years of life. It may be fine and rapid or slower and coarser, is usually absent at rest in the early stages and tends to be increased by voluntary movement and emotion. It is thus classified as an action tremor; senile tremor may be regarded as a similar disorder of sporadic occurrence in late life. It may be generalized or involve especially the hands, lips, and tongue. As a rule it persists and worsens slightly throughout life and no other nervous abnormality occurs. In rare instances paralysis agitans has been observed in a member of a family afflicted with familial tremor. A curious feature of benign familial tremor is that it is almost specifically, though temporarily, relieved by ethyl alcohol (Growdon *et al.*, 1975). Propranolol (Morgan *et al.*, 1973; Sweet *et al.*, 1974; Rajput *et al.*, 1975) and/or diazepam may reduce the tremor slightly; in severe cases stereotaxic surgery is occasionally necessary.

Hysterical Tremor. Two forms of hysterical tremor are encountered: a fine tremor, localized to one limb or generalized, and resembling the shaking of extreme fear, of which it is probably a perpetuation; and a coarse, irregular shaking, intensified by voluntary movement. In common with other hysterical symptoms, hysterical tremor is characterized by its irregularity, variability from time to time, and by a tendency to diminish when the patient's attention is distracted and to increase when it is directed to the affected part of the body. The tremor of acute anxiety states is similar but less florid and variable.

Tremor in Hyperthyroidism. This is a fine, rapid tremor usually confined to the outstretched arms and sometimes more marked on one side than the other. The associated exophthalmos, thyroid enlargement, tachycardia, and flushed and sweating skin usually render diagnosis easy.

Toxic Tremor. Tremor may be a symptom of intoxication with various poisons, especially mercury, cocaine, and alcohol. The tremor of cocaine addiction and chronic alcoholism is fine and is unlikely to be confused with Parkinsonian tremor. The tremor of chronic mercurial poisoning and delirium tremens and that due to withdrawal of barbiturates or other drugs is somewhat coarser, but has not the rhythmical character of Parkinsonian tremor. The 'flapping' or 'wing-beating' tremor (asterixis) of chronic liver disease is also distinctive. In all these cases the cause is usually easily discoverable, and in delirium tremens the acute onset and characteristic mental symptoms are distinctive.

Multiple Sclerosis. In multiple sclerosis intention tremor is common as it is in some other conditions causing cerebellar ataxia. It is absent when the limb is at rest and develops only during voluntary movement, increasing as the limb approaches its objective. In this respect it is the opposite of Parkinsonian tremor, which is present at rest and diminishes on movement. Static tremor is rare in multiple sclerosis, and is most often seen in the head. It disappears when the patient is lying with the neck muscles relaxed. In this disease there are usually nystagmus and signs of corticospinal lesions, which, apart from the character of the tremor, distinguish it from Parkinsonism.

Hereditary Ataxia

Intention tremor similar to that observed in multiple sclerosis is a common feature of several types of inherited cerebellar degeneration. Static tremor, showing certain resemblances to that of Parkinsonism is, however, seen in patients with olivo-ponto-cerebellar degeneration in which, however, the associated features of dementia, cerebellar ataxia and corticospinal tract degeneration are distinctive.

General Paresis. Tremor affecting especially the face, tongue, and hands is an early symptom of general paresis. This is a fine tremor, increased on voluntary movement. The mental changes, Argyll Robertson pupils, signs of corticospinal tract lesions, and positive V.D.R.L. reaction in the blood and spinal fluid will distinguish the condition from Parkinsonism.

The Parkinsonism–Dementia Complex

This is a degenerative disease of unknown aetiology, thought by some to be genetically determined, though this is still uncertain, which occurs only in the Chamorro people of Guam and the Mariana islands. Most affected patients develop bradykinesia, rigidity, and tremor but progressive dementia also occurs and few patients survive for more than a few years. Some patients also develop signs of amyotrophic lateral sclerosis (motor neurone disease) (Hirano et al., 1961, 1966; Brody and Chen, 1969). The pathological changes differ from those of paralysis agitans; the rigidity and tremor may improve with levodopa (Schnur et al., 1971) but the dementia does not.

Corticostriatonigral Degeneration

This familial and progressive disorder [p. 697] is indistinguishable from paralysis agitans in its early stages except that it usually produces severe akinesia and rigidity but little if any tremor; dementia is common and pathological changes in the putamen and globus pallidus are much more severe than in idiopathic Parkinsonism (Adams et al., 1964; Takei and Mirra, 1973). Similar clinical and pathological features may develop in advanced cases of so-called progressive multi-system degeneration (the Shy–Drager syndrome, see page 321), in which, however, severe orthostatic hypotension is usually the presenting feature.

Progressive Supranuclear Palsy

This rare condition (Steele et al., 1964; Behrman et al., 1969; Kurihara et al., 1974) is characterized by progressive paralysis of upward vertical gaze [FIG. 107], paroxysmal dysequilibrium, progressive Parkinsonian features, and often increasing dementia. The neck muscles become rigid and retrocollis is sometimes seen as is corticospinal tract involvement.

Other States of Rigidity

Hysterical Rigidity. This is characterized by the fact that the degree of the rigidity is proportional to the observer's efforts to move the limb. In Parkinsonism the rigidity is, by contrast, a definite quantum which always yields to the exercise of slightly greater force.

Spasticity due to Corticospinal Tract Lesions. This is distinguished by the selective distribution of the rigidity to certain muscle groups, usually the flexors in the upper and the extensors in the lower limbs. Moreover, it tends to be maximal at the beginning of a passive movement and to diminish as the movement proceeds. Parkinsonian rigidity is uniform both in its distribution and throughout the angle of joint movement. In paraplegia-in-flexion hypertonia occurs in the flexors of the lower limbs, but in this condition, as in paraplegia-in-extension, the plantar reflexes are extensor, whereas they are flexor in uncomplicated Parkinsonism.

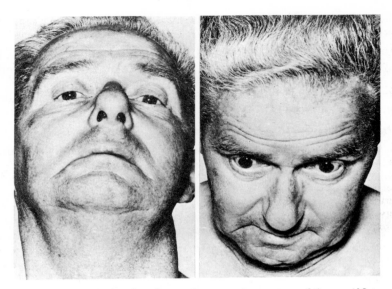

A. Even on head flexion there is no reflex upward movement of the eyes. Note the Parkinsonian features

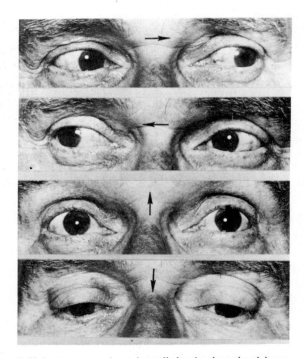

B. Voluntary upward gaze is totally lost but lateral and downward gaze is retained

FIG. 107. Progressive supranuclear palsy.

(Kindly provided by Dr. J. D. Spillane)

Arthritis. Rigidity due to joint disease occasionally simulates Parkinsonism, especially when the vertebral joints are affected as in ankylosing spondylitis. The flexion of the spine and immobility of the head may at first glance be deceptive. Pain in such cases, however, is usually severe at some stage of the disease, and it is easy to demonstrate that the rigidity is bony and not muscular in origin.

TREATMENT

Though the treatment of Parkinsonism is palliative rather than curative, much can be done to relieve the patient's discomfort.

The sufferer from Parkinsonism should be encouraged to lead an active life as long as possible but should avoid fatigue. A 'zip' fastener on the trousers is a convenience. Passive movements are valuable for their temporary effect in diminishing the rigidity, but more as a means of postponing the development of contractures. Re-educational walking exercises under the supervision of a skilled physiotherapist are often valuable. A walking-stick is an invaluable aid in many cases and in patients with severe akinesia a frame walking aid which encourages the patient to lean forwards and to initiate those walking reflexes which are impaired by the disease process may be very helpful. Chairs with seats which can be electrically or mechanically elevated and many other appliances are sometimes useful. For many years the only drugs available to diminish the rigidity were those of the belladonna group, and these also reduce salivation and sweating. Traditional remedies such as hyoscine hydrobromide, belladonna, and stramonium, which undoubtedly reduce rigidity and salivation, have now been supplanted by synthetic antispasmodic drugs. On the whole the most useful are benzhexol (*Artane*), beginning with 2 mg three times a day, and ethopropazine (*Lysivane*), beginning with 50–200 mg a day and increasing the dose in accordance with the patient's tolerance, or orphenadrine hydrochloride (*Disipal*), 50–100 mg up to three times a day. It is often necessary to try several preparations, since the drug which suits one patient may not suit another. Benztropine (*Cogentin*), 1–2 mg at night, and methixene (*Tremonil*), 5–10 mg three times a day, may be a little more successful than other remedies in controlling tremor but no drug is really effective in this respect; in Tennyson's words, 'What drugs can make a wither'd palsy cease to shake?'. All of the drugs mentioned may produce dryness of the mouth, constipation, and blurring of vision. The latter may be helped by adding pilocarpine, 10 mg three times daily. Confusion is an even more important side-effect, particularly in elderly patients and may be accompanied by disturbing visual and auditory hallucinations. Retention of urine may also occur. Such side-effects may even necessitate withdrawal of all drugs in a few cases. Most patients are best treated by a combination of up to two drugs (e.g. *Artane* and *Cogentin*; or *Disipal* and *Tremonil*). The improvement produced by anticholinergic remedies is limited; not more than 80 per cent of patients show up to 30 per cent improvement (Duvoisin, 1965; Esplin, 1965; Calne, 1970). Amphetamine was once widely used for oculogyric crises and depression and may indeed produce limited improvement in Parkinsonism (Parkes *et al.*, 1974) but has been supplanted in the treatment of depression by tricyclic antidepressant drugs, imipramine and its derivatives (Calne, 1970). Beta-adrenergic blocking remedies such as propranolol have been reported to improve tremor (Owen and Marsden, 1965). When the patient becomes bed-ridden much care will be needed to prevent the development of bed-sores and to maintain adequate nutrition.

U

An important recent addition to the therapeutic armamentarium is amantadine hydrochloride, first introduced as an antiviral agent. The drug is undoubtedly beneficial; the usual dose is 100 mg twice daily and some believe it to be the drug of choice in mild and early Parkinsonism. It is believed to act by blocking the presynaptic uptake of dopamine, thereby prolonging its effective half-life following synaptic release and thus decreasing its inactivation in the brain (Grelak et al., 1970). It improves akinesia and rigidity, and tremor to a lesser extent, but is significantly less effective than levodopa (Hunter et al., 1970) though it seems to have an adjuvant effect when combined with the latter (Godwin-Austen et al., 1970; Parkes et al., 1971; Schwab et al., 1972; Cox et al., 1973; Bauer and McHenry, 1974).

The most major advance of the last fifteen years has been the introduction into treatment of levodopa and a vast literature upon the use of this drug has now accumulated. Its effects may be monitored by estimating the concentration of homovanillic acid and its other metabolites in the CSF (Pullar et al., 1970; Curzon et al., 1970). Examination of brain material at autopsy has confirmed that levodopa significantly increases dopamine (Rinne and Sonninen, 1973). It is usual to begin treatment with 250 mg levodopa daily or twice daily, increasing by 250–500 mg daily every three or four days until the maximum tolerated dosage is reached. Side-effects such as nausea and vomiting may be troublesome but can often be controlled by cyclizine or similar remedies. Metoclopramide is also useful in this respect but may rarely cause dyskinesia; pimozide may reduce levodopa-induced involuntary movements but increases Parkinsonian features (Tarsy et al., 1975). While hypotension may result, there is little risk in treating patients with ischaemic heart disease or cerebrovascular disease (Hunter et al., 1971) provided treatment is introduced under supervision in hospital. The most troublesome side-effect is the development of involuntary movements which may include features of chorea, athetosis, and dystonia as well as bizarre foot-paddling and facial dyskinetic movements which are difficult to classify (Mones et al., 1971). These movements usually cease or lessen when the dose is reduced, and they may be reduced by deanol in a dosage of 100 mg three times daily (Miller, 1974). The dose of levodopa which can be tolerated by individual patients varies from 1 g to 8 g daily. It must not be given with amine oxidase inhibitors or pyridoxine, which inhibits its effects. It is usually wise to combine it with anticholinergic remedies and/or amantadine for maximum therapeutic effect and sudden withdrawal of anticholinergic drugs may produce rapid deterioration (Hughes et al., 1971; Horrocks et al., 1973). The drug is effective in paralysis agitans and in post-encephalitic Parkinsonism (Cotzias et al., 1967; Calne et al., 1969; Yahr et al., 1969; Rinne et al., 1970; Mawdsley, 1970; Duvoisin et al., 1972); it is of some benefit in the Parkinsonism-dementia complex and corticostriatonigral degeneration but not in progressive supranuclear palsy or the Shy–Drager syndrome. In supranuclear palsy it may temporarily modify the Parkinsonian features (Mendell et al., 1970; Klawans and Ringel, 1971) but not other features. It improves akinesia and rigidity most but also improves tremor and oculogyric crises (Klawans and Erlich, 1970) and has a marked alerting effect (Marsh et al., 1971) but does not improve dementia and the disease appears to progress despite partial control of its clinical manifestations (Hunter et al., 1973). Occasional cases show a remarkable lack of response for reasons which are difficult to determine (British Medical Journal, 1973 b) and there is sometimes a progressive deterioration after long-term treatment with episodes of severe akinesia and an 'on–off' effect (Markham,

1972) with marked variation in the patient's condition from one part of the day to another, sometimes related to the timing of the medication, the so-called long-term levodopa syndrome (Barbeau, 1972). This may be due to increasing receptor hypersensitivity. It can be overcome to some extent by reducing the dose of levodopa, by a period of temporary withdrawal of the drug, or by combining levodopa with a decarboxylase inhibitor which reduces the peripheral degradation of dopamine, thus making more available in the brain (Calne *et al.*, 1971; Marsden *et al.*, 1973; Mars, 1973; Yahr, 1973). The usual combination of levodopa with L-alpha-methyldopahydrazine (carbidopa) is 250 mg of the former with 25 mg of the latter in a combined tablet such as *Sinemet*. Before giving this combined preparation, levodopa must be withdrawn but other remedies may be continued; the usual dose is 1 tablet once or twice daily at first, increasing to 3 to 6 tablets a day. Side-effects of levodopa treatment are much reduced by this combined remedy which is now becoming standard. There is some recent evidence that bromocriptine, a new dopaminergic agonist, which may be given with levodopa, in a dosage of 2·5 mg twice daily, gradually increasing up to 30 mg daily, may be another useful remedy (Calne *et al.*, 1974).

Surgery

The operations of pallidectomy and ventrolateral thalamotomy, or both combined, have had an established place in the treatment of Parkinsonism since Cooper (1953) showed that infarction of the globus pallidus resulting from anterior choroidal artery ligation improved contralateral rigidity and tremor. In general, surgery is most suitable for idiopathic Parkinsonism with unilateral symptoms in a patient under the age of 65. Severe akinesia, generalized cerebral atheroma, dementia, and severe hypertension are contra-indications (Cooper, 1961; Gillingham *et al.*, 1960). Various stereotaxic techniques are used by different neurosurgeons; chemopallidectomy (injection of alcohol) has now been largely supplanted by methods involving thermocoagulation or freezing (cryothalamotomy). Increasing experience has indicated that tremor can be greatly reduced or abolished and rigidity reduced by these methods but akinesia, speech disturbance, and salivation are uninfluenced. Bilateral operations carried out simultaneously, or with an interval of a few months between the two procedures, are now practicable, even in patients of 70 years or older who are in good general condition, but confusion and permanent intellectual impairment are more common after bilateral procedures and patients must still be carefully selected for surgical treatment which is only one method of treatment in such cases and does not as a rule supplant the use of appropriate drugs (Hankinson, 1960; Cooper, 1965; Selby, 1967). Indeed, the number of operations being performed has fallen dramatically since the introduction of levodopa, although surgery still has a limited place if tremor is poorly controlled by drugs.

REFERENCES

ADAMS, R. D., BOGAERT, L. VAN, and VANDER EECKEN, H. (1964) Striato-nigral degeneration, *J. Neuropath. exp. Neurol.*, **23**, 584.

AMINOFF, M. J., and WILCOX, C. S. (1972) Control of blood pressure in Parkinsonism, *Proc. roy. Soc. Med.*, **65**, 944.

ANGEL, R. W., ALSTON, W., and HIGGINS, J. R. (1970) Control of movement in Parkinson's disease, *Brain*, **93**, 1.

AYD, F. J., Jun. (1961) A survey of drug-induced extrapyramidal reactions, *J. Amer. med. Ass.*, **175**, 1054.

BARBEAU, A. (1972) Long-term appraisal of levodopa therapy, *Neurology* (*Minneap.*), **22**, 22.

BARBEAU, A., CAMPANELLA, G., BUTTERWORTH, R. F., and YAMADA, K. (1975) Uptake and efflux of ^{14}C-dopamine in platelets : evidence for a generalized defect in Parkinson's disease, *Neurology* (*Minneap.*), **25**, 1.

BAUER, R. B., and MCHENRY, J. T. (1974) Comparison of amantadine, placebo, and levodopa in Parkinson's disease, *Neurology* (*Minneap.*), **24**, 715.

BEHRMAN, S., CARROLL, J. D., JANOTA, I., and MATTHEWS, W. B. (1969) Progressive supranuclear palsy, *Brain*, **92**, 663.

BOGAERT, L. VAN (1930) Contribution clinique et anatomique à l'étude de la paralysie agitante, juvénile primitive, *Rev. neurol.* (*Paris*), **2**, 315.

BREWIS, M., POSKANZER, D. C., ROLLAND, C., and MILLER, H. (1966) Neurological disease in an English city, *Acta neurol. scand.*, **24**, Suppl. 42.

BRITISH MEDICAL JOURNAL (1973 *a*) Mental symptoms and Parkinsonism, *Brit. med. J.*, **2**, 67.

BRITISH MEDICAL JOURNAL (1973 *b*) Failure to respond to levodopa, *Brit. med. J.*, **4**, 314.

BRITISH MEDICAL JOURNAL (1974) Mental changes in Parkinsonism, *Brit. med. J.*, **2**, 1.

BRODY, J. A., and CHEN, K.-M. (1969) Changing epidemiologic patterns of amyotrophic lateral sclerosis and Parkinsonism–dementia on Guam, in *Motor Neuron Diseases*, p. 61, New York.

BROWN, E. L., and KNOX, E. G. (1972) Epidemiological approach to Parkinson's disease, *Lancet*, **i**, 974.

BURTON, J. L., and SHUSTER, S. (1970) Effect of L-dopa on seborrhoea of Parkinsonism, *Lancet*, **ii**, 19.

CALNE, D. B. (1970) *Parkinsonism : Physiology, Pharmacology and Treatment*, London.

CALNE, D. B., REID, J. L., VAKIL, S. D., RAO, S., PETRIE, A., PALLIS, C. A., GAWLER, J., THOMAS, P. K., and HILSON, A. (1971) Idiopathic Parkinsonism treated with an extracerebral decarboxylase inhibitor in combination with levodopa, *Brit. med. J.*, **3**, 729.

CALNE, D. B., SPIERS, A. S. D., STERN, G. M., LAURENCE, D. R., and ARMITAGE, P. (1969) L-dopa in idiopathic Parkinsonism, *Lancet*, **ii**, 973.

CALNE, D. B., TEYCHENNE, P. F., CLAVERIA, L. E., EASTMAN, R., GREENACRE, J. K., and PETRIE, A. (1974) Bromocriptine in Parkinsonism, *Brit. med. J.*, **4**, 442.

COOPER, I. S. (1953) Anterior choroidal artery ligation for involuntary movements, *Science*, **118**, 193.

COOPER, I. S. (1961) *Parkinsonism, Its Medical and Surgical Treatment*, Springfield, Ill.

COOPER, I. S. (1965) The surgical treatment of Parkinsonism, *Ann. Rev. Med.*, **16**, 309.

COTZIAS, G. C., VAN WOERT, M. H., and SCHIFFER, L. M. (1967) Aromatic amino acids and modification of Parkinsonism, *New Engl. J. Med.*, **276**, 374.

COX, B., DANTA, G., SCHNIEDEN, H., and YUILL, G. M. (1973) Interactions of L-dopa and amantadine in patients with Parkinsonism, *J. Neurol. Neurosurg. Psychiat.*, **36**, 354.

CRITCHLEY, E. (1972) Clinical manifestations of essential tremor, *J. Neurol. Neurosurg. Psychiat.*, **35**, 365.

CRITCHLEY, M. (1929) Arteriosclerotic Parkinsonism, *Brain*, **52**, 23.

CRITCHLEY, M. (1949) Observations on essential (heredofamilial) tremor, *Brain*, **72**, 113.

CURZON, G., GODWIN-AUSTEN, R. B., TOMLINSON, E. B., and KANTAMANENI, B. D. (1970) The cerebrospinal fluid homovanillic acid concentration in patients with Parkinsonism treated with L-dopa, *J. Neurol. Neurosurg. Psychiat.*, **33**, 1.

DEN HARTOG JAGER, W. A. (1969) Sphingomyelin in Lewy inclusion bodies in Parkinson's disease, *Arch. Neurol.* (*Chic.*), **21**, 615.

DEN HARTOG JAGER, W. A. (1970) Histochemistry of adrenal bodies in Parkinson's disease, *Arch. Neurol.* (*Chic.*), **23**, 528.

DENNY-BROWN, D. (1962) *The Basal Ganglia and Their Relation to Disorders of Movement*, Oxford.

DUVOISIN, R. C. (1965) A review of drug therapy in Parkinsonism, *Bull. N.Y. Acad. Sci.*, **41**, 898.

DUVOISIN, R. C., LOBO-ANTUNES, J., and YAHR, M. D. (1972) Response of patients with postencephalitic Parkinsonism to levodopa, *J. Neurol. Neurosurg. Psychiat.*, **35**, 487.

EARLE, K. M. (1968) Studies on Parkinson's disease including X-ray fluorescent spectroscopy of formalin fixed brain tissue, *J. Neuropath. exp. Neurol.*, **27**, 1.

ESPLIN, D. W. (1965) in *The Pharmacological Basis of Therapeutics*, ed. Goodman, L. S., and Gilman, A., New York.

GILLINGHAM. F. J., WATSON, W. S., DONALDSON, A. A., and NAUGHTON, J. A. L. (1960) The surgical treatment of Parkinsonism, *Brit. med. J.*, **2**, 1395.

GODWIN-AUSTEN, R. B., BERGMANN, S., and FREARS, C. C. (1971) Effect of age and arteriosclerosis on the response of Parkinsonian patients to levodopa, *Brit. med. J.*, **4**, 522.

GODWIN-AUSTEN, R. B., FREARS, C. C., BERGMANN, S., PARKES, J. D., and KNILL-JONES, R. P. (1970) Combined treatment of Parkinsonism with L-dopa and amantadine, *Lancet*, **ii**, 383.

GREENFIELD, J. G. (1958) in *Neuropathology*, ed. Greenfield, J. G., McMenemey, W. H., Meyer, A., and Norman, R. M., p. 530, London.

GREENFIELD, J. G., and BOSANQUET, F. D. (1953) The brain-stem lesions in Parkinsonism, *J. Neurol. Neurosurg. Psychiat.*, **16**, 213.

GREENFIELD, J. G., and MATTHEWS, W. B. (1954) Post-encephalitic Parkinsonism with amyotrophy, *J. Neurol. Neurosurg. Psychiat.*, **17**, 50.

GRELAK, R. P., CLARK, R., and STUMP, J. M. (1970) Amantadine-dopamine interaction: possible mode of action in Parkinsonism, *Science*, **169**, 203.

GROSS, M., BANNISTER, R., and GODWIN-AUSTEN, R. (1972) Orthostatic hypotension in Parkinson's disease, *Lancet*, **i**, 174.

GROWDON, J. H., SHAHANI, B. T., and YOUNG, R. R. (1975) The effect of alcohol on essential tremor, *Neurology (Minneap.)*, **25**, 259.

HALL, A. J. (1931) Chronic epidemic encephalitis, with special reference to the ocular attacks, *Brit. med. J.*, **2**, 833.

HANKINSON, J. (1960) The surgical treatment of Parkinson's disease, *Postgrad. med. J.*, **36**, 242.

HIRANO, A., MALAMUD, N., and ELIZAN, T. S. (1966) Amyotrophic lateral sclerosis and parkinsonism–dementia complex on Guam, *Arch. Neurol. (Chic.)*, **15**, 35.

HIRANO, A., MALAMUD, N., and KURLAND, L. T. (1961) Parkinsonism–dementia complex—an endemic disease on the island of Guam, II. Pathological features, *Brain*, **84**, 662.

HOEHN, M. M., and YAHR, M. D. (1967) Parkinsonism: onset, progression, and mortality, *Neurology (Minneap.)*, **17**, 427.

HORROCKS, P. M., VICARY, D. J., REES, J. E., PARKES, J. D., and MARSDEN, C. D. (1973) Anticholinergic withdrawal and benzhexol treatment in Parkinson's disease, *J. Neurol. Neurosurg. Psychiat.*, **36**, 936.

HUGHES, R. C., POLGAR, J. G., WEIGHTMAN, D., and WALTON, J. N. (1971) Levodopa in Parkinsonism: the effects of withdrawal of anticholinergic drugs, *Brit. med. J.*, **2**, 487.

HUNT, J. R. (1917) Progressive atrophy of the globus pallidus, *Brain*, **40**, 58.

HUNTER, K. R., HOLLMAN, A., LAURENCE, D. R., and STERN, G. M. (1971) Levodopa in Parkinsonian patients with heart-disease, *Lancet*, **i**, 932.

HUNTER, K. R., LAURENCE, D. R., SHAW, K. M., and STERN, G. M. (1973) Sustained levodopa therapy in Parkinsonism, *Lancet*, **ii**, 929.

HUNTER, K. R., STERN, G. M., LAURENCE, D. R., and ARMITAGE, P. (1970) Amantadine in Parkinsonism, *Lancet*, **i**, 1127.

JAKOB, A. (1925) The anatomy, clinical syndromes and physiology of the extrapyramidal system, *Arch. Neurol. Psychiat. (Chic.)*, **13**, 596.

KESCHNER, M., and SLOANE, P. (1931) Encephalitic, idiopathic and arteriosclerotic Parkinsonism, *Arch. Neurol. Psychiat. (Chic.)*, **25**, 1011.

KIM, R. (1968) The chronic residual respiratory disorder in post-encephalitic Parkinsonism, *J. Neurol. Neurosurg. Psychiat.*, **31**, 393.

KLAWANS, H. L., and ERLICH, M. A. (1970) Observations on the mechanism of Parkinsonian blepharospasm and its treatment with L-dopa, *Europ. Neurol.*, **3**, 365.

KLAWANS, H. L., and GOODWIN, J. A. (1969) Reversal of the glabellar reflex in Parkinsonism by L-dopa, *J. Neurol. Neurosurg. Psychiat.*, **32**, 423.

KLAWANS, H. L., and RINGEL, S. P. (1971) Observations on the efficacy of L-dopa in progressive supranuclear palsy, *Europ. Neurol.*, **5**, 115.

KONDO, K., KURLAND, L. T., and SCHULL, W. J. (1973) Parkinson's disease. Genetic analysis and evidence of a multifactorial etiology, *Mayo Clin. Proc.*, **48**, 465.

KUGELBERG, E. (1952) Facial reflexes, *Brain*, **75**, 385.

KURIHARA, T., LANDAU, W. M., and TORACK, R. M. (1974) Progressive supranuclear palsy with action myoclonus, seizures, *Neurology (Minneap.)*, **24**, 219.

KURLAND, L. T. (1958) in *The Pathology and Treatment of Parkinsonism*, ed. Fields, W. S., p. 5, Springfield, Ill.

LANCE, J. W., and McLEOD, J. G. (1975) *A Physiological Approach to Clinical Neurology*, London.

LARSSON, T., and SJÖGREN, T. (1960) Essential tremor, *Acta psychiat. (Kbh.)*, **36**, Suppl. 144.

LEWIS, P. D. (1971) Parkinsonism—neuropathology, *Brit. med. J.*, **3**, 690.

LORANGER, A. W., GOODELL, H., McDOWELL, F. H., LEE, J. E., and SWEET, R. D. (1972) Intellectual impairment in Parkinson's syndrome, *Brain*, **95**, 405.

MARKHAM, C. H. (1972) Thirty months' trial of levodopa in Parkinson's disease, *Neurology (Minneap.)*, **22**, 17.

MARS, H. (1973) Modification of levodopa effect by systemic decarboxylase inhibition, *Arch. Neurol. (Chic.)*, **28**, 91.

MARSDEN, C. D., BARRY, P. E., PARKES, J. D., and ZILKHA, K. J. (1973) Treatment of Parkinson's disease with levodopa combined with L-alpha-methyldopahydrazine, an inhibitor of extracerebral dopa decarboxylase, *J. Neurol. Neurosurg. Psychiat.*, **36**, 10.

MARSH, G. G., MARKHAM, C. H., and ANSEL, R. (1971) Levodopa's awakening effect on patients with Parkinsonism, *J. Neurol. Neurosurg. Psychiat.*, **34**, 209.

MARTIN, J. P. (1967) *The Basal Ganglia and Posture*, London.

MARTIN, W. E., RESCH, J. A., and BAKER, A. B. (1971) Juvenile Parkinsonism, *Arch. Neurol. (Chic.)*, **25**, 494.

MARTIN, W. E., YOUNG, W. I., and ANDERSON, V. E. (1973) Parkinson's disease: a genetic study, *Brain*, **96**, 495.

MAWDSLEY, C. (1970) Treatment of Parkinsonism with laevo-dopa, *Brit. med. J.*, **1**, 331.

MENDELL, J. R., CHASE, T. N., and ENGEL, W. K. (1970) Modification by L-dopa of a case of progressive supranuclear palsy, *Lancet*, **i**, 593.

MILLER, E. (1974) Deanol in the treatment of levodopa-induced dyskinesias, *Neurology (Minneap.)*, **24**, 116.

MINDHAM, R. H. S. (1970) Psychiatric symptoms in Parkinsonism, *J. Neurol. Neurosurg. Psychiat.*, **33**, 188.

MONES, R. J., ELIZAN, T. S., and SIEGEL, G. J. (1971) Analysis of L-dopa induced dyskinesias in 51 patients with Parkinsonism, *J. Neurol. Neurosurg. Psychiat.*, **34**, 668.

MORGAN, M. H., HEWER, R. L., and COOPER, R. (1973) Effect of the beta adrenergic blocking agent propranolol on essential tremor, *J. Neurol. Neurosurg. Psychiat.*, **36**, 618.

NAKANO, K. K., ZUBICK, H., and TYLER, H. R. (1973) Speech defects of parkinsonian patients. Effects of levodopa therapy on speech intelligibility, *Neurology (Minneap.)*, **23**, 865.

OWEN, D. A. L., and MARSDEN, C. D. (1965) Effect of adrenergic β-blockade on Parkinsonian tremor, *Lancet*, **ii**, 1259.

PARKES, J. D., BAXTER, R. C. H., CURZON, G., KNILL-JONES, R. P., KNOTT, P. J., MARSDEN, C. D., TATTERSALL, R., and VOLLUM, D. (1971) Treatment of Parkinson's disease with amantadine and levodopa: a one-year study, *Lancet*, **i**, 1083.

PARKES, J. D., MARSDEN, C. D., REES, J. E., CURZON, G., KANTAMANENI, B. D., KNILL-JONES, R., AKBAR, A., DAS, S., and KATARIA, M. (1974) Parkinson's disease, cerebral arteriosclerosis, and senile dementia, *Quart. J. Med.*, **43**, 49.

PENDERS, C. A., and DELWAIDE, P. J. (1971) Blink reflex studies in patients with Parkinsonism before and during therapy, *J. Neurol. Neurosurg. Psychiat.*, **34**, 674.

POLLOCK, M., and HORNABROOK, R. W. (1966) The prevalence, natural history and dementia of Parkinson's disease, *Brain*, **89**, 429.

POSKANZER, D. C., SCHWAB, R. S., and FRASER, D. W. (1969) in *Third Symposium on Parkinson's Disease*, ed. Gillingham, F. J., and Donaldson, I. M. L., Edinburgh.

PRATT, R. T. C. (1967) *The Genetics of Neurological Disorders*, London.

PRITCHARD, P. B., and NETSKY, M. G. (1973) Prevalence of neoplasms and causes of death in paralysis agitans: a necropsy study, *Neurology (Minneap.)*, **23**, 215.

PULLAR, I. A., WEDDELL, J. M., AHMED, R., and GILLINGHAM, F. J. (1970) Phenolic acid concentrations in the lumbar cerebrospinal fluid of Parkinsonian patients treated with L-dopa, *J. Neurol. Neurosurg. Psychiat.*, **33**, 851.

RAJPUT, A. H., JAMIESON, H., HIRSH, S., and QURAISHI, A. (1975) Relative efficacy of alcohol and propranolol in action tremor, *Canad. J. neurol. Sci.*, **2**, 31.

RINNE, U. K., and SONNINEN, V. (1973) Brain catecholamines and their metabolites in Parkinsonian patients. Treatment with levodopa alone or combined with a decarboxylase inhibitor, *Arch. Neurol. (Chic.)*, **28**, 107.

RINNE, U. K., SONNINEN, V., and SIIRTOLA, T. (1970) L-dopa treatment in Parkinson's disease, *Europ. Neurol.*, **4**, 348.

RUSHWORTH, G. (1962) Observations on blink reflexes, *J. Neurol. Neurosurg. Psychiat.*, **25**, 93.

RUSHWORTH, G. (1968) Neurophysiologie clinique de quelques réflexes dans le domaine du nerf facial, *Electromyography*, **8**, 349.

SCHNUR, J. A., CHASE, T. N., and BRODY, J. A. (1971) Parkinsonism–dementia of Guam: treatment with L-dopa, *Neurology (Minneap.)*, **21**, 1236.

SCHWAB, R. S., POSKANZER, D. C., ENGLAND, A. C., and YOUNG, R. R. (1972) Amantadine in Parkinson's disease. Review of more than two years' experience, *J. Amer. med. Ass.*, **222**, 792.

SCOTT, R. M., and BRODY, J. A. (1971) Benign early onset of Parkinson's disease: a syndrome distinct from classic postencephalitic parkinsonism, *Neurology (Minneap.)*, **21**, 366.

SCOTT, R. M., BRODY, J. A., SCHWAB, R. S., and COOPER, I. S. (1970) Progression of unilateral tremor and rigidity in Parkinson's disease, *Neurology (Minneap.)*, **20**, 710.

SELBY, G. (1967) Stereotactic surgery for the relief of Parkinson's disease, *J. neurol. Sci.*, **5**, 315, 343.

SELBY, G. (1968) Cerebral atrophy in Parkinsonism, *J. neurol. Sci.*, **6**, 517.

STEELE, J. C., RICHARDSON, J. C., and OLAZEWSKI, J. (1964) Progressive supranuclear palsy, *Arch. Neurol. (Chic.)*, **10**, 333.

STERN, P. H., MCDOWELL, F., MILLER, J. M., and ROBINSON, M. B. (1972) Levodopa therapy effects on natural history of Parkinsonism, *Arch. Neurol. (Chic.)*, **27**, 481.

SWEET, R. D., BLUMBERG, J., LEE, J. E., and MCDOWELL, F. H. (1974) Propranolol treatment of essential tremor, *Neurology (Minneap.)*, **24**, 64.

TAKEI, Y., and MIRRA, S. S. (1973) Striatonigral degeneration: a form of multiple system atrophy with clinical Parkinsonism, in *Progress in Neuropathology*, vol. II, ed. Zimmerman, H. M., p. 217, New York.

TARSY, D., PARKES, J. D., and MARSDEN, C. D. (1975) Metoclopramide and pimoxide in Parkinson's disease and levodopa-induced dyskinesias, *J. Neurol. Neurosurg. Psychiat.*, **38**, 331.

YAHR, M. D. (1967) in *Cecil-Loeb Textbook of Medicine*, ed. Beeson, P. B., and McDermott, W., Philadelphia and London.

YAHR, M. D. (1973) *The Treatment of Parkinsonism—The Role of Dopa Decarboxylase Inhibitors* (Advances in Neurology, vol. 2), New York.

YAHR, M. D., DUVOISIN, R. C., SCHEAR, M. J., BARRETT, R. E., and HOEHN, M. M. (1969) Treatment of Parkinsonism with levodopa, *Arch. Neurol. (Chic.)*, **21**, 343.

YAHR, M. D., WOLF, A., ANTUNES, J.-L., MIYOSHI, K., and DUFFY, P. (1972) Autopsy findings in parkinsonism following treatment with levodopa, *Neurology (Minneap.)*, **22**, 56.

WILSON'S DISEASE

Synonyms. Tetanoid chorea (Gowers); pseudosclerosis (Westphal); progressive lenticular degeneration; hepatolenticular degeneration.

Definition. A progressive disease of early life which is due to an autosomal recessive gene and is characterized by a disorder of copper metabolism leading to degeneration of certain regions of the brain, especially the corpus striatum, and cirrhosis of the liver, and clinically by increasing muscular rigidity, tremor, and progressive dementia. Although pseudosclerosis, which was first investigated by Alzheimer, Westphal, and others between 1883 and 1898, and progressive lenticular degeneration, described by Wilson in 1912, were at one time thought to be different diseases, they are now more usually considered to be identical and are both included under the title Wilson's disease.

PATHOLOGY

The pathological change in the nervous system consists of a degeneration of ganglion cells with neuroglial overgrowth, but without evidence of inflammation or vascular abnormality. Macroscopically the most conspicuous abnormality is found in the lentiform nucleus. In about half the recorded cases visible softening and cavitation of both lentiform nuclei have been observed. In other cases the nucleus has appeared shrunken and occasionally its naked-eye appearance is normal. Microscopically, Alzheimer's type 2 cells are present. This change is most marked in the putamen. The caudate nucleus is usually similarly affected though to a lesser extent, but the globus pallidus is less frequently involved. Pericapillary concretions staining heavily for copper can often be found, especially in the putamen. The so-called Opalski cell (see Greenfield, 1958), a large, rounded cell with a large nucleus and a finely granular or foamy cytoplasm which stains a light rose colour with Nissl stains is thought to be specific for Wilson's disease. It is believed to be of glial origin; these cells are rare in the striatum but are most often seen in thalamus, globus pallidus, and substantia nigra. Similar alterations are often present in other parts of the nervous system; for example, in the cerebral cortex, the thalamus, the red nucleus, and the cerebellum.

In the liver the changes are those of a multilobular cirrhosis which possesses no distinctive characteristics apart from a reddish, brown, or even greenish colour due to the presence of copper, and there is often enlargement of the spleen. The typical Kayser–Fleischer ring around the edge of the cornea has been shown to be due to copper deposition.

AETIOLOGY

There is now convincing evidence that the condition is one of autosomal recessive inheritance with a gene frequency of about 1 in 1,000 of the population (Bearn, 1957). The condition usually becomes clinically manifest between 10 and 25 years of age with a slightly earlier age of onset in female subjects

(Strickland *et al.*, 1973); it appears to be ubiquitous in all races, having been reported from India (Dastur *et al.*, 1968) and Taiwan (Strickland *et al.*, 1973), and many cases have been described in the United Kingdom and in the U.S.A. Glazebrook (1945) and Cumings (1948) showed that the concentration of copper in brain and liver was greatly increased in such cases and it was later shown that caeruloplasmin, the copper-carrying protein of the plasma, is reduced to 10 per cent of normal values; Walshe (1967) suggested that a failure to synthesize this protein is the fundamental genetic abnormality. Ingested copper is deposited in the tissues and excreted in increased quantities in the urine. The whole body turnover of copper[67] has been shown to be prolonged, with a greatly reduced release from liver in affected subjects (O'Reilly *et al.*, 1971 *a* and *b*) and in carriers of the gene (O'Reilly *et al.*, 1970). The plasma iron and transferrin are also low (O'Reilly *et al.*, 1968) and there is an increased urinary output of amino acids (Matthews *et al.*, 1952; Denny-Brown, 1953).

SYMPTOMS

Nervous Symptoms

In many cases choreiform movements of the face and hands or flapping tremor are the first symptoms. These movements may occur when the limbs are apparently at rest and yet be abolished by complete relaxation or support. They are increased by voluntary movement. Athetoid and writhing movements of the trunk and limbs have, however, been observed, and one patient in the terminal stage exhibited violent muscular spasms resembling tetanus. In other cases, dysarthria (see below) is the first manifestation. In general, plastic rigidity followed by tremor or athetoid movements characterize the younger patients while tremor precedes rigidity in those in whom the onset is over the age of 20.

Rigidity in its distribution and general character resembles that of Parkinsonism. The limbs become fixed, usually in a position of flexion, and contractures ultimately develop, but in younger patients the terminal state is a bilateral hemiplegic dystonia.

Voluntary movement is impaired, and articulation and deglutition are early and severely affected. Speech may become unintelligible or the patient may even lose entirely the power of articulation. The facies exhibits, as in Parkinsonism, a vacant, expressionless appearance, or a vacuous smile. Loss of emotional control is usually present, and involuntary laughing and crying may occur. There seems always to be some degree of mental deterioration amounting to a mild dementia. There is no essential change in the tendon-jerks or the abdominal reflexes, though muscular rigidity may render them difficult to elicit. The plantar reflexes are flexor and there is no disturbance of sensibility.

Corneal Pigmentation (The Kayser–Fleischer Ring)

Corneal pigmentation was first observed by Kayser and Fleischer. This is a sign of great diagnostic value. It may be invisible in daylight and is best seen with the slit lamp and corneal microscope. Indeed, slit-lamp examination reveals that it is present in virtually all cases. It consists of a zone of golden-brown granular pigmentation about 2 mm in diameter on the posterior surface of the cornea towards the limbus. It is due to the deposit of copper, and may be present before any nervous symptoms have developed.

Symptoms of Cirrhosis of the Liver

Although these may be inconspicuous, in some cases they prove fatal before the patient develops any nervous symptoms. In the early stages pyrexial attacks, with slight jaundice, may occur; later the liver may be enlarged, and ascites, haematemesis, and other symptoms of portal obstruction may be present.

Renal Lesions

Apart from aminoaciduria (Uzman and Denny-Brown, 1948) patients with Wilson's disease sometimes have glycosuria, increased urinary phosphate excretion, low urate excretion, proteinuria, and a reduced glomerular filtration rate. Spontaneous pseudofractures and osteomalacia and osteochondritis have been described (see Bearn, 1957).

Biochemical Changes

Biochemical tests of value include a low serum copper (normal 86–112 μg per 100 ml) and copper oxidase, a low caeruloplasmin in the blood (normal 27–38 mg per 100 ml), and a high urinary copper (normal 24-hour excretion 0–26 μg) especially if this is increased after treatment with BAL or penicillamine. Both total and alpha amino acids are increased in the urine and figures up to 500–600 mg of alpha amino acids a day may be found. Patients do not incorporate radioactive copper, copper-67, normally with caeruloplasmin (Matthews, 1954) and radiocopper turnover may be abnormal in clinically normal heterozygotes. Measurement of copper levels in liver biopsy specimens using neutron activation analysis may give figures more than five times the normal upper limit in cases of Wilson's disease but the copper content is also substantially increased in samples from patients with long-standing biliary obstruction, as in biliary cirrhosis (Smallwood et al., 1968).

DIAGNOSIS

There are few disorders with which Wilson's disease is likely to be confused. No other disease is characterized by the familial occurrence of tremor and rigidity with liver damage in the second decade of life. Corneal pigmentation and symptoms of cirrhosis of the liver, when present, are pathognomonic. Sporadic cases may simulate other disorders in which the corpus striatum is damaged. Double athetosis, which is characterized by muscular rigidity and choreoathetoid movements, is usually congenital. Symptoms are therefore present from an early age, and some improvement may occur. Neurological manifestations of acquired liver disease [p. 829] usually develop much later in life and are non-familial, but juvenile cirrhosis (Lygren, 1959) occasionally gives diagnostic difficulty.

Other rare familial degenerative disorders of the corpus striatum, without liver damage, cause progressive rigidity, spasmodic laughing, dysarthria, and dementia beginning in childhood, e.g. Hallervorden–Spatz disease and progressive pallidal degeneration.

When Wilson's disease is suspected in one member of a family, all the sibs should be examined for evidence of nervous abnormalities, cirrhosis of the liver, corneal pigmentation, and biochemical change. Any of these symptoms, if present, will not only render it possible to anticipate the development of the disorder in other members of the family but will afford support for the diagnosis in the patient already affected.

PROGNOSIS

The course of the disease may be acute, subacute, or chronic, but it is invariably fatal if not treated. In the shortest illness on record death occurred five weeks after the onset of symptoms. Before effective treatment was available 50 per cent of patients died in from 1 to 6 years though a few survived very much longer (Hall, 1921). The prognosis has been transformed by treatment with D-penicillamine.

TREATMENT

Cumings (1951) and Denny-Brown (1953) showed that substantial improvement could follow the use of dimercaprol (BAL) and another chelating agent, calcium versenate, was subsequently tried with some success. Oral potassium sulphide was also given to reduce the absorption of copper. However, the introduction of D-penicillamine in 1956 by Walshe transformed the prognosis of the condition. The drug is given in a daily dosage of 1·0–2·0 g, with an average dose of 1·5 g (Richmond et al., 1964; Goldstein et al., 1971; Strickland et al., 1973). If the drug is given early enough, the affected subjects grow and develop normally and may remain symptom-free for as long as maintenance treatment is continued. Unfortunately, toxic side-effects of penicillamine have begun to be reported in recent years, of which nephropathy leading to the nephrotic syndrome and thrombocytopenia are the most troublesome (Walshe, 1969). In such cases there may be no alternative to withdrawal of treatment; fortunately the recent introduction of triethyl tetramine (Walshe, 1973) which is given in a dosage of 1·2 g daily, has meant that an effective alternative treatment is available. Rarely, when liver disease is exceptionally severe, liver transplantation may be successful (Starzl et al., 1971).

REFERENCES

BEARN, A. G. (1957) Wilson's disease. An inborn error of metabolism with multiple manifestations, Amer. J. Med., 22, 747.

BICKEL, H., NEALE, F. C., and HALL, G. (1957) A clinical and biochemical study of hepatolenticular degeneration (Wilson's disease), Quart. J. Med., 26, 527.

CUMINGS, J. N. (1948) The copper and iron content in the brain and liver in the normal and in hepatolenticular degeneration, Brain, 71, 410.

CUMINGS, J. N. (1951) The effects of B.A.L. in hepatolenticular degeneration, Brain, 74, 10.

DASTUR, D. K., MANGHANI, D. K., and WADIA, N. H. (1968) Wilson's disease in India. I. Geographic, genetic, and clinical aspects in 16 families, Neurology (Minneap.), 18, 21.

DENNY-BROWN, D. (1953) Abnormal copper metabolism and hepatolenticular degeneration, Res. Publ. Ass. nerv. ment. Dis., 32, 190.

GLAZEBROOK, A. J. (1945) Wilson's disease, Edinburgh med. J., 52, 83.

GOLDSTEIN, N. P., TAUXE, W. N., McCALL, J. T., RANDALL, R. V., and GROSS, J. B. (1971) Wilson's disease (hepatolenticular degeneration). Treatment with penicillamine and changes in hepatic trapping of radioactive copper, Arch. Neurol. (Chic.), 24, 391.

GREENFIELD, J. G. (1958) Hepatolenticular degeneration, in Neuropathology, by Greenfield, J. G., Blackwood, W., McMenemey, W. H., Meyer, A., and Norman, R. M., London.

GREENFIELD, J. G., POYNTON, F. J., and WALSHE, F. M. R. (1923-4) On progressive lenticular degeneration. (Hepato-lenticular degeneration), Quart. J. Med., 17, 385.

HALL, H. C. (1921) La dégénérescence hépato-lenticulaire, Paris.

LYGREN, T. (1959) Hepatolenticular degeneration (Wilson's disease) and juvenile cirrhosis in the same family, *Lancet*, **i**, 275.

MATTHEWS, W. B. (1954) The absorption and excretion of radiocopper in hepatolenticular degeneration (Wilson's disease), *J. Neurol. Neurosurg. Psychiat.*, **17**, 242.

MATTHEWS, W. B., MILNE, M. D., and BELL, M. (1952) The metabolic disorder in hepatolenticular degeneration, *Quart. J. Med.*, **21**, 425.

O'REILLY, S., POLLYCOVE, M., and BANK, W. J. (1968) Iron metabolism in Wilson's disease. Kinetic studies with iron[59], *Neurology (Minneap.)*, **18**, 634.

O'REILLY, S., STRICKLAND, G. T., WEBER, P. M., BECKNER, W. M., and SHIPLEY, L. (1971 a) Abnormalities of the physiology of copper in Wilson's disease. I. The whole-body turnover of copper, *Arch. Neurol. (Chic.)*, **24**, 385.

O'REILLY, S., WEBER, P. M., OSWALD, M., and SHIPLEY, L. (1971 b) Abnormalities of the physiology of copper in Wilson's disease. III. The excretion of copper, *Arch. Neurol. (Chic.)*, **25**, 28.

O'REILLY, S., WEBER, P. M., POLLYCOVE, M., and SHIPLEY, L. (1970) Detection of the carrier of Wilson's disease, *Neurology (Minneap.)*, **20**, 1133.

RICHMOND, J., ROSENOER, V. M., TOMPSETT, S. L., DRAPER, I., and SIMPSON, J. A. (1964) Hepato-lenticular degeneration (Wilson's disease) treated by penicillamine, *Brain*, **87**, 619.

SMALLWOOD, R. A., WILLIAMS, H. A., ROSENOER, V. M., and SHERLOCK, S. (1968) Liver-copper levels in liver disease. Studies using neutron activation analysis, *Lancet*, **ii**, 1310.

STARZL, T. E., GILES, G., LILLY, J. R., TAKAGI, H., MARTINEAU, G., SCHROTER, G., HALGRIMSON, C. G., PENN, I., and PUTNAM, C. W. (1971) Indications for orthotopic liver transplantation: with particular reference to hepatomas, biliary atresia, cirrhosis, Wilson's disease and serum hepatitis, *Transplantation Proceedings*, **3**, 308.

STRICKLAND, G. T., FROMMER, D., LEU, M.-L., POLLARD, R., SHERLOCK, S., and CUMINGS, J. N. (1973) Wilson's disease in the United Kingdom and Taiwan. I. General characteristics of 142 cases and prognosis. II. A genetic analysis of 88 cases, *Quart. J. Med.*, **42**, 619.

UZMAN, L., and DENNY-BROWN, D. (1948) Amino-aciduria in hepatolenticular degeneration (Wilson's disease), *Amer. J. med. Sci.*, **215**, 599.

WALSHE, J. M. (1956) Penicillamine: a new oral therapy for Wilson's disease, *Amer. J. Med.*, **21**, 487.

WALSHE, J. M. (1967) The physiology of copper in man and its relation to Wilson's disease, *Brain*, **90**, 149.

WALSHE, J. M. (1969) Management of penicillamine nephropathy in Wilson's disease: a new chelating agent, *Lancet*, **ii**, 1401.

WALSHE, J. M. (1973) Copper chelation in patients with Wilson's disease. A comparison of penicillamine and triethylene tetramine dihydrochloride, *Quart. J. Med.*, **42**, 441.

WALSHE, J. M., and CUMINGS, J. N., eds. (1961) *Wilson's Disease. Some Current Concepts*, Oxford.

WILSON, S. A. K. (1911–12) Progressive lenticular degeneration: a familial nervous disease associated with cirrhosis of the liver, *Brain*, **34**, 295.

WILSON, S. A. K. (1913–14) An experimental research into the anatomy and physiology of the corpus striatum, *Brain*, **36**, 427.

HALLERVORDEN–SPATZ DISEASE AND INFANTILE NEUROAXONAL DYSTROPHY

The rare familial disorder first described by Hallervorden and Spatz in 1922 presents in childhood or adolescence as a progressive, predominantly extra-pyramidal disorder running a protracted course of several years but usually terminating fatally. Clinically the affected children usually show choreoathetosis and progressive dystonia (Yanagisawa *et al.*, 1966); dementia, fits, and signs of corticospinal tract involvement sometimes but not invariably develop. Pathologically the brains of affected individuals showed degeneration of neurones in the globus pallidus and substantia nigra with many rounded hyaline bodies or spheroids and mineral pigment deposits often containing iron. In 1952 Seitelberger reported a disorder of similar clinical presentation [see p. 660] in which hyaline swelling and eventual breakdown of nerve cells were demonstrated in the cerebellum, basal ganglia, and brain stem; the pallidum showed spheroids, spongy degeneration, discoloration, and deposits of pseudocalcium. Defendini *et al.* (1973) have drawn attention to the presence of Lewy-type inclusions in nerve cells in some such cases and point out that the two disorders are difficult if not impossible to distinguish both clinically and pathologically.

REFERENCES

DEFENDINI, R., MARKESBERY, W. R., MASTRI, A. R., and DUFFY, P. E. (1973) Hallervorden–Spatz disease and infantile neuro-axonal dystrophy. Ultrastructural observations, anatomical pathology and nosology, *J. neurol. Sci.*, **20**, 7.

HALLERVORDEN, J., and SPATZ, H. (1922) Eigenartige Erkrankung im extrapyramidalen System mit besonderer Beteiligung des Globus Pallidus und der Substantia Nigra, *Z. ges. Neurol. Psychiat.*, **79**, 254.

SEITELBERGER, F. (1952) Eine unbekannte Form von infantiler Lipoid-Speicher-Krankheit des Gehirns, in *Proceedings of the 1st International Congress of Neuropathology*, vol. 3, p. 323, Turin.

YANAGISAWA, N., SHIRAKI, H., MINAKAWA, M., and NARABAYASHI, H. (1966) Clinicopathological and histochemical studies of Hallervorden–Spatz disease with torsion dystonia, with special reference to diagnostic criteria of the disease from the clinicopathological viewpoint, *Progress in Brain Research*, **21B**, 373.

TORSION DYSTONIA

Synonym. Dystonia musculorum deformans (Oppenheim).

Definition. A syndrome characterized by involuntary movements producing torsion of the limbs and the vertebral column, which may occur as a symptom of more than one pathological state.

AETIOLOGY AND PATHOLOGY

Torsion dystonia is a rare syndrome which was first described by Schwalbe in 1908 in three siblings. Mendel in 1919 collected 30 cases from the literature. Symptomatic dystonia may occur in many neurological disorders including cerebral palsy, infantile hemiplegia, Wilson's disease, Hallervorden–Spatz disease, and intoxication with phenothiazines and other drugs (Zeman and Whitlock, 1968) and in such cases the pathology is that of the primary disorder. Idiopathic torsion dystonia, however, is inherited as an autosomal recessive trait in Ashkenazic Jews and as an autosomal dominant disorder in non-Jewish populations; many cases are sporadic. In the idiopathic disorder extensive neuropathological studies have failed to demonstrate any consistent abnormalities in the basal ganglia or elsewhere (Zeman and Dyken, 1968; Zeman, 1970). However, Wooten *et al.* (1973) and Ebstein *et al.* (1974) have found elevated serum dopamine-beta-hydroxylase levels in such cases, whether of dominant or recessive inheritance, and it seems likely that the disorder may prove to be due to a biochemical abnormality involving central dopaminergic systems. In a recent review of 42 cases, Marsden and Harrison (1974) point out that an onset in childhood is usually associated with a progressive course leading to severe disability, while the course in cases first developing in adult life is much more benign.

SYMPTOMS

In the severe familial cases the onset usually occurs in childhood or adolescence, and the abnormality is frequently first noticed when the patient walks. In Schwalbe's family the disorder began with spasmodic plantar-flexion of the feet, rendering it impossible to place the heel on the ground. The resultant bizarre gait, when first observed in an otherwise healthy child, is often misconstrued as being hysterical. The involuntary movements in the upper limbs consist of rotation or torsion round the long axes and are associated with similar torsion movements of the vertebral column, especially in the lumbar region [FIG. 108].

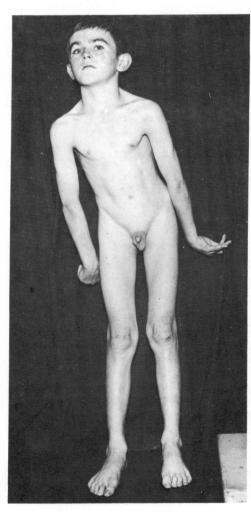

FIG. 108. A case of torsion dystonia; note the abnormal posture of the head, neck, trunk, and upper limbs. (From *An Atlas of Clinical Neurology* 2nd ed., 1975, by J. D. Spillane, reproduced by kind permission of the author

There are frequently lordosis and scoliosis, which are conspicuous when the patient walks, but tend to disappear when he lies down. Other forms of involuntary movement, such as tremor and myoclonic muscular contractions, have been described. Muscular tone is variable, being exaggerated during spasms which may be extremely painful, and sometimes diminished in the intervals between them. Signs of a lesion of the corticospinal tracts are absent. There is no muscular wasting except as a result of cachexia in the terminal stages. The reflexes are normal, and sensibility is unimpaired. Mental changes are absent, and speech and swallowing are usually unaffected until the later stages.

DIAGNOSIS

Torsion dystonia must be distinguished from other forms of involuntary movement, especially from athetosis and from chorea. In athetosis the movements, which are of a slow, writhing character, involve the peripheral parts of the limbs, rather than the proximal as in torsion spasm. Double athetosis, moreover, is usually congenital, and hence the movements develop at an earlier age than torsion spasm. Choreic movements, like athetosis, involve the peripheral parts of the limbs to a greater extent than torsion dystonia. In chorea, however, movements of rotation of the limbs and trunk occur, but they are quicker and briefer than the corresponding movements of torsion spasm. Dystonic movements may develop in the affected limbs after an interval of some years in occasional cases of infantile hemiplegia. Hysteria may cause bizarre involuntary movements resembling torsion dystonia; hysterical involuntary movements, however, rarely involve the trunk and the proximal parts of the limbs, and in hysteria the emotional attitude of the patient to the disorder and the presence of other hysterical symptoms usually settle the diagnosis.

Electromyography may be helpful in diagnosis (Yanagisawa and Goto, 1971), demonstrating tonic non-reciprocal involuntary activity in agonists and antagonists and regular or irregular grouping of action potentials appearing synchronously in many muscles.

PROGNOSIS

In symptomatic dystonia due to Wilson's disease, cerebral palsy, infantile hemiplegia, and other disorders the prognosis is that of the underlying disease. In occasional cases of unknown aetiology spontaneous recovery has been described. In the 'idiopathic' disorder the condition may remain static for many years, especially when the onset is in adult life but in most childhood cases there is slow progressive deterioration and death eventually occurs as a result of the combined effects of cachexia and respiratory or urinary infection.

TREATMENT

Rest and physiotherapy are of little value but diazepam 5 mg three or four times daily or other relaxant drugs are occasionally helpful. Levodopa (Barbeau, 1970; Chase, 1970) alone or with haloperidol (Mandell, 1970) has been recommended but does not seem to be of any long-term benefit. Cooper (1965, 1970) and others have reported substantial improvement following bilateral ventrolateral thalamotomy, a procedure which should certainly be considered in severe cases, although the results of such stereotaxic operations have proved to be variable and unpredictable.

REFERENCES

BARBEAU, A. (1970) Rationale for the use of L-dopa in the torsion dystonias, *Neurology (Minneap.)*, **20**, pt. 2, 96.

CHASE, T. N. (1970) Biochemical and pharmacologic studies of dystonia, *Neurology (Minneap.)*, **20**, pt. 2, 122.

COOPER, I. S. (1965) Clinical and physiologic implications of thalamic surgery for disorders of sensory communication, Part 2 (Intention tremor, dystonia, Wilson's disease and torticollis), *J. neurol. Sci.*, **2**, 520.

COOPER, I. S. (1970) Neurosurgical treatment of dystonia, *Neurology (Minneap.)*, **20**, pt. 2, 133.

EBSTEIN, R. P., FREEDMAN, L. S., LIEBERMAN, A., GOLDSTEIN, M., and PASTERNACK, B. (1974) A familial study of serum dopamine-β-hydroxylase levels in torsion dystonia, *Neurology (Minneap.)*, **24**, 684.

LARSSON, T., and SJÖGREN, T. (1966) Dystonia musculorum deformans. A genetic and population study of 121 cases, *Acta neurol. scand.*, **42**, Suppl. 17.

MANDELL, S. (1970) The treatment of dystonia with L-dopa and haloperidol, *Neurology (Minneap.)*, **20**, pt. 2, 103.

MARSDEN, C. D., and HARRISON, M. J. G. (1974) Idiopathic torsion dystonia (dystonia musculorum deformans). A review of forty-two patients, *Brain*, **97**, 793.

MENDEL, K. (1919) Torsiondystonie, *Mschr. Psychiat. Neurol.*, **46**, 309.

SCHWALBE, M. W. (1908) *Eine eigentümliche tonische Krampfform mit hysterischen Symptomen*, Berlin.

THÉVENARD, A. (1926) *Les dystonies d'attitude*, Thèse, Paris.

WIMMER, A. (1925) Études sur les syndromes extra-pyramidaux, *Rev. neurol. (Paris)*, **2**, 281.

WOOTEN, G. F., ELDRIDGE, R., AXELROD, J., and STERN, R. S. (1973) Elevated plasma dopamine-β-hydroxylase activity in autosomal dominant torsion dystonia, *New Engl. J. Med.*, **288**, 284.

YANAGISAWA, N., and GOTO, A. (1971) Dystonia musculorum deformans. Analysis with electromyography, *J. neurol. Sci.*, **13**, 39.

ZEMAN, W. (1970) Pathology of the torsion dystonias (dystonia musculorum deformans), *Neurology (Minneap.)*, **20**, pt. 2, 79.

ZEMAN, W., and DYKEN, P. (1967) Dystonia musculorum deformans. Clinical, genetic and pathoanatomical studies, *Psychiat. Neurol. Neurochir. (Amst.)*, **70**, 77.

ZEMAN, W., and DYKEN, P. (1968) Dystonia musculorum deformans, in *Handbook of Clinical Neurology*, ed. Vinken, P. J., and Bruyn, G. W., vol. 6, p. 517, Amsterdam.

ZEMAN, W., and WHITLOCK, C. C. (1968) Symptomatic dystonias, in *Handbook of Clinical Neurology*, ed. Vinken, P. J., and Bruyn, G. W., vol. 6, p. 544, Amsterdam.

ZIEHEN (1911) Demonstrat. eines Patienten mit tonischer Torsionsneurose, *Neurol. Zbl.*, **30**, 109.

SPASMODIC TORTICOLLIS

Synonym. Wry neck.

Definition. A rotated attitude of the head, brought about by clonic or tonic contraction of the cervical muscles and occurring as a symptom both of organic disease of the nervous system and of hysteria. Torticollis of organic origin is probably a fragmentary form of torsion spasm. Retrocollis is a similar disorder, in which the neck is extended.

AETIOLOGY AND PATHOLOGY

In the past, confusion as to the nature of torticollis has arisen from a failure to distinguish hysterical torticollis from that occurring as a symptom of organic disease. Since torticollis can be effected voluntarily, it may occur as an hysterical symptom, being then a form of tic. The hysterical nature of the symptoms in such cases is proved by their response to treatment of the primary emotional disorder. There is abundant evidence, however, that torticollis may be due to organic disease of the nervous system, and in such cases there are grounds for regarding it as a limited form of torsion dystonia. It may occur as a sequel to encephalitis lethargica, with or without Parkinsonism, or as a part of other extrapyramidal syndromes. Since torticollis as an isolated symptom is not fatal, pathological investigations are scanty. Cassirer, however, reported a case in which degenerative changes were present in the corpus striatum and were associated with cirrhosis of the liver, and Foerster (1933) one in which bilateral focal lesions of the corpus striatum were present. However, Tarlov (1970) was unable to demonstrate any significant abnormality in extensive pathological studies of the brain of a typical case. Physiologically, torticollis is a disturbance of the normal posture of the head. The rotated posture of the head which follows unilateral labyrinthectomy and lesions of the eighth nerve indicates the import-ance of the labyrinth in the maintenance of the posture of the head, and torticollis is probably due to a disorder of the higher centres concerned in this function, including the corpus striatum. Both sexes are affected, and the onset is usually during adult life. The disorder may be familial.

SYMPTOMS

The development of torticollis is usually insidious but may be sudden, especially when it is hysterical. The rotation of the head is brought about by contraction of the cervical muscles, and though both the superficial and deep muscles of the neck are involved, the muscular contraction is evident to the observer only in the sternomastoid, trapezius, and splenius. The precise posture of the head varies in different cases. Contraction of the sternomastoid alone causes rotation to the opposite side, with flexion of the neck to the side of the contracted muscle. Rotation, however, may occur without lateral flexion, or the head may be flexed to the side to which it is rotated, in such cases con-traction of the sternomastoid on one side being associated with contraction of the splenius and trapezius on the opposite side. The muscles involved become hypertrophied. The disturbance may be predominantly tonic, leading to a sustained posture, or may consist of repeated clonic jerks, as is particularly common in hysterical cases. It may be possible to modify the abnormal posture by altering the position of the patient in relation to gravity, for example, from the erect to the supine, or from the supine to the prone position. There may or may not be resistance to passive movement of the head in the direction opposite to the abnormal position. In a few cases torticollis has been associated with paralysis of rotation to the opposite side. There may be spasm of the facial muscles and platysma on the side to which the head is rotated, or spasmodic torsion move-ments of the upper limb or whole body. The patient not infrequently finds that he can inhibit the torticollis by exerting slight pressure with his finger upon the jaw on the side to which the head is rotated, and the movement ceases during sleep. Pain may occur in the cervical muscles. The reflexes and sensation are normal. Long-continued torticollis may cause cervical spondylosis.

Retrocollis is due to a bilateral contraction of the splenius and trapezius.

DIAGNOSIS

The distinction between hysterical torticollis and torticollis of organic origin may be difficult. Hysteria should be suspected when the symptom develops suddenly in circumstances of mental stress, and also when it can be controlled by relaxation and suggestion, though these measures may also produce transient improvement in the organic disorder which is much more common. Kjellin and Stibler (1974) claim that alkaline end fractions found in isoelectric focusing of samples of cerebrospinal fluid may help to distinguish organic from hysterical cases but this observation remains to be confirmed.

Spasmodic torticollis is distinguished by the age of onset from congenital torticollis, which may be due either to fibrosis of one sternomastoid following a haematoma in the muscle, or to a congenital deficiency of one-half of a cervical vertebra. It is necessary also to exclude as causes of torticollis myositis of the cervical muscles, caries of the cervical spine, and adenitis of the cervical lymph nodes.

PROGNOSIS

Torticollis is almost always intractable, but when it is due to hysteria improvement and even cure may be effected by psychotherapy, abreaction, or hypnosis. Sufficiently radical surgical treatment using radiculectomy and neurectomy has given good results in some cases of organic origin, though the spasm may recur after operation.

TREATMENT

Hysterical torticollis should be treated by psychotherapy or abreaction along the same lines as other hysterical symptoms (Paterson, 1945), and the patient should be taught to practise muscular relaxation. Sedative and tranquillizing drugs such as chlordiazepoxide (*Librium*), 10 mg three or four times daily, or diazepam (*Valium*), 2–5 mg three times a day, may be of some value. Mechanical support to the head may give some relief. Torticollis of organic origin is unlikely to respond to medical measures, though benefit has been claimed to result from treatment with amantadine and haloperidol (Gilbert, 1972). Tetrabenazine, too, is occasionally dramatically successful but its effect is usually only temporary and then at the expense of an unacceptable degree of drug-induced Parkinsonism. Brudny *et al.* (1974) also claim benefit from teaching the patients volitional control with the aid of a feedback display of the electromyogram. Levodopa is of no value (Ansari *et al.*, 1972).

A number of surgical operations have been recommended. Finney and Hughson (1925) divided the accessory nerves and the dorsal divisions of the upper three or four cervical nerves at their points of emergence from the vertebrae. Dandy (1930) combined division of the accessory nerves with interruption of the upper three cervical sensory and motor roots within the spinal canal, and Foerster performed intradural section of both the ventral and dorsal roots of the upper three cervical segments.

Sorensen and Hamby (1966) have reviewed the results obtained in 71 cases treated surgically and found that patients subjected to anterior cervical rhizotomy and subarachnoid section of the spinal accessory nerve did best. In intractable cases simultaneous bilateral lesions produced in ventrolateral thalamic nuclei by stereotaxic methods may be beneficial but the results of this treatment are variable (Cooper, 1965).

REFERENCES

ANSARI, K. A., WEBSTER, D., and MANNING, N. (1972) Spasmodic torticollis and L-dopa. Results of therapeutic trial in six patients, *Neurology (Minneap.)*, **22**, 670.

BRUDNY, J., GRYNBAUM, B. B., and KOREIN, J. (1974) Spasmodic torticollis: treatment by feedback display of the EMG, *Arch. Phys. Med. Rehabil.*, **55**, 403.

COOPER, I. S. (1965) Clinical and physiologic implications of thalamic surgery for disorders of sensory communication, pt. 2 (Intention tremor, dystonia, Wilson's disease and torticollis), *J. neurol. Sci.*, **2**, 520.

DANDY, W. E. (1930) An operation for the treatment of spasmodic torticollis, *Arch. Surg.*, **20**, 1021.

FINNEY, J. M. T., and HUGHSON, W. (1925) Spasmodic torticollis, *Ann. Surg.*, **81**, 255.

FOERSTER, O. (1925) Operative Behandlung des Torticollis spasticus, *Zbl. Chir.*, **53**, 2804.

FOERSTER, O. (1933) Mobile spasm of the neck muscles and its pathological basis, *J. comp. Neurol.*, **58**, 725.

GILBERT, G. J. (1972) The medical treatment of spasmodic torticollis. *Arch. Neurol. (Chic.)*, **27**, 503.

KJELLIN, K. G., and STIBLER, H. (1974) Protein pattern of cerebrospinal fluid in spasmodic torticollis, *J. Neurol. Neurosurg. Psychiat.*, **37**, 1128.

PATERSON, M. (1945) Spasmodic torticollis: results of psychotherapy in 21 cases, *Lancet*, **ii**, 556.

SCHALTENBRAND, G. (1937) Klinik und Behandlung des Torticollis spasticus, *Dtsch. Z. Nervenheilk.*, **145**, 36.

SORENSEN, B. F., and HAMBY, W. B. (1966) Spasmodic torticollis. Results in surgically-treated patients, *Neurology (Minneap.)*, **16**, 867.

TARLOV, E. (1970) On the problem of the pathology of spasmodic torticollis in man, *J. Neurol. Neurosurg. Psychiat.*, **33**, 457.

ATHETOSIS

Definition. Athetosis, or 'mobile spasm', is the term applied to a form of involuntary movement which in some respects resembles chorea, as is recognized by the use of the term 'choreo-athetosis' to describe an intermediate condition. Athetoid movements, however, are slower, coarser, and more writhing than choreic movements. Athetosis is due to a variety of pathological states which damage the basal ganglia.

AETIOLOGY AND PATHOLOGY

The same difficulties are encountered in localizing the lesion responsible for athetosis as in the case of chorea. Nevertheless, there is considerable evidence that it is usually situated in the putamen. Bilateral athetosis is occasionally familial. Athetosis is one of the many involuntary movements which may be induced by the use of drugs such as levodopa or the phenothiazines (Lader, 1970; Singer and Cheng, 1971).

Bilateral Athetosis

Bilateral athetosis may be congenital, when it may be due to the *état marbré* of the corpus striatum described by Oppenheim and Vogt (1911). Rarely bilateral athetosis may develop during adolescence as a progressive disorder terminating in generalized rigidity, as a result of degeneration of the corpus striatum described by C. and O. Vogt (1919) as *état dysmyélinique*. The common pathological factor, according to Denny-Brown (1946), the *état marbré* or status marmoratus, is a disorder of glial formation leading to hypermyelination, involving to a varying extent the cortex, basal ganglia, and other structures, and underlying double athetosis, and some cases of congenital diplegia. Athetosis may rarely occur as a symptom of hepatolenticular degeneration, or may follow kernicterus; cases developing in adult life are usually due to drugs. Paroxysmal kinesigenic choreoathetosis, a disorder in which choreoathetotic, ballistic, and dystonic movements of the extremities occur in brief paroxysmal episodes precipitated by voluntary movement (Kato and Araki, 1969) is probably a form of reflex epilepsy and may respond to treatment with carbamazepine.

Unilateral Athetosis

Unilateral athetosis may also be congenital, being then usually associated with infantile hemiplegia. The brain in such cases may exhibit the Bielschowsky type of cerebral hemiatrophy, in which there is an elective necrosis of the third cortical layer of the precentral gyrus, atrophy of the thalamus, and degeneration and gliosis or false porencephaly of the corpus striatum. Unilateral athetosis may also occur as a result of focal lesions involving the striatum at any age, due, for example, to acute encephalitis or a cerebral vascular lesion complicating the specific fevers in childhood, but senile chorea [see p. 623], which resembles it, is also seen in late middle life and old age, as a result of focal cerebral softening secondary to atheroma.

SYMPTOMS

Congenital athetosis is not usually noticed until the child is several months old, when abnormal postures or movements attract the mother's attention. In the early months of life many such children are hypotonic ('floppy infants') and may be suspected of suffering from the flaccid or hypotonic form of cerebral palsy. Athetosis caused by an acute inflammatory or vascular lesion of the brain may develop rapidly within a few days of the lesion, or insidiously after an interval of several weeks, or even years.

Typical athetosis possesses the following features. One or both halves of the body may be involved. The muscles innervated by the cranial nerves are always much more severely affected when the athetosis is bilateral than when it is unilateral. In bilateral athetosis the patient exhibits frequent grimaces resembling caricatures of normal facial expressions of all kinds. Involuntary laughing and crying are common. The tongue is the site of writhing movements of protrusion and withdrawal, and the patient is often unable to maintain it protruded unless it is held between the teeth. The involuntary movement of the articulatory and pharyngeal muscles leads to dysarthria and dysphagia. The head may be rotated to one or other side, or extended. In unilateral athetosis the facial movements usually consist of little more than an exaggeration of normal expressions. In the upper limbs the peripheral segments exhibit the involuntary movements to a greater extent than the proximal segments. The limb is usually adducted and internally rotated at the shoulder and semiflexed at the elbow. The characteristic posture of the hand is one of marked flexion of the wrist, with flexion at the metacarpophalangeal and extension at the interphalangeal joints, the posture produced by contraction of the interossei, and the thumb is usually adducted, and extended at the two distal joints. This posture is disturbed by slow, writhing movements of flexion and extension at the wrist and at the metacarpophalangeal joints, the fingers remaining extended at the interphalangeal joints, with varying degrees of adduction and abduction. Movements may also occur at the shoulder and elbow, leading sometimes to retraction and internal rotation at the shoulder and extension at the elbow. In severe cases of unilateral athetosis the patient characteristically grasps the affected upper limb with the normal hand, to restrain the movement. He may even sit upon the affected hand or trap it behind his back in a chair in order to restrain the movement. Except in the mildest cases the movements completely interfere with the voluntary use of the limb. The movements of the lower limb are usually less severe than those of the upper, and again are most marked in the distal segments. The foot is usually maintained in the position of talipes equinovarus, often with marked dorsiflexion of the great toe. Athetotic movements are always exaggerated by an attempt to use the limbs in voluntary movement and by nervousness and excitement. They diminish when the patient lies down and disappear during sleep. Though the tone of the muscles is exaggerated during the movements, they are usually found to be hypotonic in the intervals if sufficient relaxation can be obtained. In severe cases, especially of unilateral athetosis, muscular contractures usually develop and the peripheral segments of the limbs become fixed in their characteristic postures.

Double athetosis may be associated with spastic diplegia. Many patients show mild or moderate mental retardation but some with severe athetosis may be normal intellectually.

DIAGNOSIS

The involuntary movements are so distinctive that diagnosis is easy. Choreic movements are more rapid and jerky: those of dystonia slower and to a greater extent around the long axis of the limbs and trunk. Athetosis, in fact, is midway between chorea and dystonia. The age and mode of onset distinguish the cause as either congenital abnormality, progressive degeneration, or acute focal lesion.

PROGNOSIS AND TREATMENT

The medical treatment of athetosis is disappointing. Benzhexol (*Artane*) and sedatives such as phenobarbitone, chlordiazepoxide (*Librium*) and diazepam (*Valium*) may slightly diminish the movements as may dopamine and serotonin antagonists such as tetrabenazine and thiopropazate, but the effect is usually short-lived and disappointing; some improvement may follow re-educational exercises, such as the relaxation exercises advocated by Phelps (1941, 1942), perseveringly carried out over a long period. Surgical measures tried in the past have included section of multiple dorsal roots, excision of a portion of the contralateral precentral gyrus (Bucy and Buchanan, 1932; Bucy, 1951), and anterolateral spinal tractotomy (Putnam, 1933) but none has proved of lasting benefit. Evidence as to the value of stereotaxic thalamotomy is conflicting: Cooper (1955) found it produced alleviation, but Paxton and Dow (1958) found it of no value for congenital athetosis and most authorities now agree that these are the least rewarding cases for stereotaxic surgery.

REFERENCES

Bucy, P. C. (1951) The surgical treatment of extrapyramidal diseases, *J. Neurol. Neurosurg. Psychiat.*, **14**, 108.

Bucy, P. C., and Buchanan, D. N. (1932) Athetosis, *Brain*, **55**, 479.

Carpenter, M. B. (1950) Athetosis and the basal ganglia: Review of the literature and study of forty-two cases, *Arch. Neurol. Psychiat. (Chic.)*, **63**, 875.

COOPER, I. S. (1955) Relief of juvenile involuntary movement disorders by chemo-pallidectomy, *J. Amer. med. Ass.*, **164**, 1297.

DENNY-BROWN, D. (1946) *Diseases of the Basal Ganglia and Subthalamic Nuclei*, New York.

DENNY-BROWN, D. (1962) *The Basal Ganglia and Their Relation to Disorders of Movement*, Oxford.

KATO, M., and ARAKI, S. (1969) Paroxysmal kinesigenic choreoathetosis. Report of a case relieved by carbamazepine, *Arch. Neurol. (Chic.)*, **20**, 508.

LADER, M. H. (1970) Drug-induced extrapyramidal syndromes, *J. Roy. Coll. Phycns Lond.*, **5**, 87.

OPPENHEIM, H., and VOGT, C. (1911) Nature et localisation de la paralysie pseudo-bulbaire congénitale et infantile, *J. Psychol. Neurol. (Lpz.)*, **18**, 293.

PAXTON, H. D., and DOW, R. S. (1958) Two years' experience of chemopallidectomy, *J. Amer. med. Ass.*, **168**, 755.

PHELPS, W. M. (1941) The management of cerebral palsies, *J. Amer. med. Ass.*, **117**, 1621.

PHELPS, W. M. (1942) Evidences of improvement in cases of athetosis treated by re-education, *Res. Publ. Ass. nerv. ment. Dis.*, **21**, 529.

PUTNAM, T. J. (1933) Treatment of athetosis and dystonia by section of extrapyramidal motor tracts, *Arch. Neurol. Psychiat. (Chic.)*, **29**, 504.

SINGER, K., and CHENG, M. N. (1971) Thiopropazate hydrochloride in persistent dyskinesia, *Brit. med. J.*, **4**, 22.

VOGT, C. (1924–5) Sur l'état marbré du striatum, *Jb. Psychiat. Neurol.*, **31**, 256.

VOGT, C., and VOGT, O. (1919) Erster Versuch einer pathologisch-anatomischen Ein-teilungstriärer Motilitätsstörungen nebst Bemerkskungen über seine allgemeine wissenschaftliche Bedeutung, *J. Psychol. Neurol. (Lpz.)*, **24**, 1.

CHOREA

SYDENHAM'S CHOREA

Synonym. St. Vitus' Dance.

Definition. An acute toxi-infective disorder of the nervous system, usually due to acute rheumatism, occurring in childhood and adolescence and characterized by involuntary movements as its most prominent symptom.

PATHOLOGY

Cases of chorea which have come to autopsy have often shown diffuse changes in the brain. Macroscopically, oedema and congestion have been observed. Microscopically, the changes have usually been most marked in the corpus striatum, substantia nigra, and subthalamic nucleus, but cortical abnormalities have also been present. Vasodilatation is conspicuous, but perivascular infiltration with lymphocytes and plasma cells, though sometimes present, is exceptional. There is a diffuse degeneration of ganglion cells, and sometimes perivascular patches of degeneration with compound granular cell infiltration and neuroglial reaction have been described. Encephalitic changes have been described in acute rheumatism (Winkelman and Eckel, 1932; Bruetsch and Bahr, 1939).

AETIOLOGY

Most cases of chorea in childhood are due to acute rheumatism, as is shown by the frequency with which other rheumatic manifestations are present or subsequently develop. Other infections may, however, be the cause, especially scarlet fever and diphtheria; and choreiform movements may be encountered as a symptom of encephalitis lethargica, as a rare complication of chickenpox, in systemic lupus erythematosus (Donaldson and Espiner, 1971; Fermaglich *et al.*, 1973), in patients taking oral contraceptives (Riddoch *et al.*, 1971; Gamboa *et al.*, 1971; Bickerstaff, 1975), and in some individuals with chronic liver disease.

Heredity may play some part in aetiology, since some families appear to be unusually susceptible to acute rheumatism, and there may be a family history either of chorea or of some other rheumatic manifestation. There seems to be a much higher incidence of left-handedness among sufferers from chorea than among the general population.

The white race is more susceptible than the coloured races, and females suffer more than males in the proportion of about three to one. Chorea is rare before the age of 5 and after 20; four-fifths of all cases occur between the ages of 5 and 15.

Mental stress or emotional shock may play a part in precipitating the condition. In a small number of cases chorea occurs during pregnancy—chorea gravidarum. That psychic factors may be in part responsible for this is suggested by the fact that it is relatively commoner in illegitimate pregnancies. There is often, however, a rheumatic history in such cases, and other rheumatic manifestations may be present. Chorea gravidarum usually occurs during the first pregnancy and may recur in subsequent pregnancies. It rarely occurs for the first time in a multipara or after the age of 25. Thyrotoxicosis is a rare association.

SYMPTOMS

Mode of Onset

The onset of chorea is usually insidious, the first complaint being often that the child is clumsy and drops things. When the movements are noticed it is described as restless, fidgety, or unable to keep still. Sometimes the onset is more abrupt and is then often ascribed to a fright.

Involuntary Movements

Involuntary movements are the most prominent symptom of chorea. Choreic movements are best described as quasi-purposive. They are movements of a high order, and although they achieve no purpose, they often resemble fragments of purposive movements following one another in a disorderly fashion. In the face the movements are always bilateral. Frowning, raising the eyebrows, pursing the lips, smiling, and bizarre movements of the mouth and tongue occur. The protruded tongue may be held between the teeth to prevent its sudden withdrawal. The eyes may be rolled from one side to the other, the head turning in the same direction.

In mild cases the speech is not affected; in severe cases there is considerable dysarthria, articulation being slurred and words sometimes being jerked out explosively. In severe cases also mastication and swallowing may be so much disturbed that the patient requires to be artificially fed.

In the upper limb movements occur at all joints. At one moment the elbow may be flexed and the fingers grasping the bedclothes; at the next the arm may be flung out in full extension. Respiration is often jerky and irregular and is frequently impeded by movements involving the abdominal wall and movements of rotation or flexion of the spine. Movements of the lower limbs are usually less conspicuous and are most evident at the periphery. Choreic movements are intensified by voluntary effort and by excitement. They disappear during sleep.

Associated Movements

In chorea the involuntary muscular contractions normally associated with strong voluntary movement are exaggerated, and at the same time incoordinate. When the patient clenches his fist, vigorous associated movements may occur in the face, trunk, and limbs. Yet observation shows that even the synergic extension of the wrist associated with strong flexion of the fingers is not normally carried out. Contraction of the flexors may conflict with, and even overpower, that of the extensors, while the radial and ulnar extensors may not contract synchronously, so that the hand deviates from side to side. This disturbance of associated movement is an early sign of chorea which may precede active involuntary movements, and can be elicited in suspected cases by asking the patient to clench his fists over the observer's fingers, while protruding the tongue.

Voluntary Movement

In mild cases voluntary power is little impaired, though the movements have an abrupt character. For example, if the patient be asked to stretch out the arms, he does so with a sudden movement as though he were flinging his hands away from him. In severe cases the involuntary movements cause considerable incoordination, and voluntary power is thus impaired. Muscular weakness may be marked, as in so-called paralytic chorea, though complete paralysis never develops. Not uncommonly chorea is predominantly unilateral in which case a diagnosis of hemiplegia due to an intracranial lesion may initially be entertained unless the hypotonia and involuntary movements are recognized.

Hypotonia and Posture

Hypotonia is invariably present in chorea, and is best demonstrated by passively extending the wrists and ankles, when a considerable degree of hyperextension can be obtained. The so-called choreic posture of the hand, in which the thumb and fingers are hyperextended at the metacarpophalangeal joints and the wrist is flexed, is merely a manifestation of muscular hypotonia, being an exaggeration of the normal attitude resulting from loss of tone in the antagonistic muscles. The upper limbs are characteristically hyperpronated when outstretched and held above the head.

Reflexes

The cutaneous reflexes in chorea are often exceptionally brisk; the plantar reflexes are flexor. When hypotonia is extreme, the tendon reflexes may be difficult to elicit, but they are usually obtainable and sometimes show a characteristic repetition of the muscular contraction (the 'pendular' reflex).

Sensory changes do not occur, and there is no disturbance of the sphincters.

Mental State

Most choreic children exhibit some emotional lability. In severe cases there may be a persistent state of excitement associated with insomnia—so-called *maniacal chorea*.

The Heart

Since in most cases chorea is due to acute rheumatism it is not surprising that cardiac abnormalities are common. They are not, however, constant. When the heart is involved for the first time during the attack of chorea, the pulse rate is quickened, there is usually slight cardiac dilatation indicated by outward displacement of the apex beat, the apical first sound is somewhat muffled, and there is often a soft systolic murmur in the mitral area. These signs point to myocarditis. When the heart has been affected in previous attacks of rheumatism, signs of valvular damage are more likely to be present. Pericarditis, arthritis, and rheumatic nodules are rarely associated with chorea. Pyrexia is usually absent, unless chorea is complicated by other manifestations of acute rheumatism.

DIAGNOSIS

The diagnosis of chorea is usually simple, since the involuntary movements are distinctive. It is most likely to be confused with habit spasm, in which, however, the same movements are repeated again and again. In athetosis the movements are slower than in chorea and have been well described as mobile spasm. Moreover, in most cases, athetosis in childhood is congenital in origin or is noticed before the age of 5, when chorea is very rare. Hysterical involuntary movements may simulate chorea. These usually occur after the age of 15, and in females, and are an imitation of a case of true chorea. The imitation, however, is never exact. The movements are usually more jerky than those of chorea, and are sometimes rhythmical. There is neither exaggeration nor disorganization of associated movements, and the face usually escapes.

Paralytic chorea may simulate other forms of paralysis in childhood. It is distinguished from hemiplegia by the fact that the upper limb alone is paretic, and by the absence of signs of a corticospinal lesion, especially an extensor plantar reflex. The absence of wasting and of changes in the electrical reaction of the muscles distinguishes it from poliomyelitis. A further diagnostic point is that even in the weak limb slight involuntary movements are present, and they may also be observed elsewhere in the body. Choreiform movements occurring in cerebral palsy are accompanied by other signs of brain damage; however, 'searching' movements superficially resembling those of chorea and sometimes misinterpreted as such, are often seen in 'clumsy children' with minimal cerebral dysfunction due to developmental apraxia (Gubbay, 1975), when the underlying disorder is often difficult to recognize.

In maniacal chorea the mental state may overshadow the physical symptoms, but the history of precedent involuntary movements or the presence of signs of rheumatic endocarditis may enable the correct diagnosis to be made.

Chorea having been diagnosed, the cause can usually be easily ascertained. Many patients show other evidence of the rheumatic infection. Even if these are absent, rheumatism is the most likely cause. Confusion arose in the past from cases of encephalitis lethargica characterized by choreiform movements, though these have not been observed for many years. In such cases the characteristic lethargy was often absent, and the movements were often associated with a reversed sleep rhythm and ocular signs. In adult life, systemic lupus erythematosus, oral contraceptive medication, and chronic liver disease must all be excluded.

Huntington's chorea is distinguished by its onset in later life, usually after the age of 30, by its hereditary character, and its association with progressive dementia.

PROGNOSIS

Death from chorea is rare and occurs in under 2 per cent of cases, usually due to cardiac involvement. It has been suggested that chorea gravidarum carries a less favourable prognosis (Matthews, 1963) but this no longer appears to be the case (Lewis and Parsons, 1966). Most patients recover in from two to three months, rarely in less than six weeks. Recurrences occur in about one-third of all cases: a patient may have two, three, four, or even more attacks (Aron *et al.*, 1965). The average interval between attacks is about one year; it is rarely more than two years. The presence of other rheumatic manifestations, e.g. valvular lesions, does not appear to influence recovery from chorea, but the occurrence of repeated attacks of chorea predisposes to the development of rheumatic carditis and endocarditis. Chorea, as such, leaves no serious sequels, though some mental lability may persist for a while, and slight involuntary movements may be perpetuated as a habit.

TREATMENT

All patients suffering from chorea should be kept in bed for two or three weeks, and should then be allowed to get up only if the movements are considerably diminished in severity. The presence of cardiac complications will probably necessitate longer bed rest, and the condition of the heart must be considered independently. Isolation of the patient is beneficial, and if possible the child should be nursed in a room alone. Excitement is to be avoided, but in all but the most severe cases some quiet occupation should be provided. When the movements are very severe it may be difficult to keep the patient in bed, and more convenient to nurse him upon a mattress placed upon the floor. Special attention must be devoted to the care of the skin and pressure points. If dysphagia is very severe it is rarely necessary to feed the patient by means of a tube. Salicylates and corticosteroid drugs are now known to have no influence upon the disease process. Traditional sedatives such as phenobarbitone, 30 mg three or four times daily, are sufficient in some cases but many patients are dramatically improved with chlorpromazine, 25–50 mg three or four times daily (Lewis and Parsons, 1966) or by diazepam.

During convalescence attention should be paid to re-education of the movements of the limbs. This is best promoted at first by occupations requiring fine manipulation, such as knitting, sewing, bead-threading, drawing, and painting. These, however, are of little value unless carried out under supervision. When the child is up, and if the cardiac condition permits, remedial exercises may be added.

It was once customary to advise removal of infected tonsils but this is no longer recommended and prophylactic penicillin is now preferred in an attempt to prevent recurrence. In chorea gravidarum there is no indication that termination of pregnancy is beneficial.

REFERENCES

ARON, A. M., FREEMAN, J. M., and CARTER, S. (1965) The natural history of Sydenham's chorea, *Amer. J. Med.*, **38**, 83.

BICKERSTAFF, E. R. (1975) *Neurological Complications of Oral Contraceptives*, Oxford.

BRAIN, W. R. (1928) Posture of the hand in chorea and other states of muscular hypotonia, *Lancet*, **i**, 439.

BRUETSCH, W. L., and BAHR, M. A. (1939) Chronic rheumatic brain disease as a factor in the causation of mental illness, *J. Indiana med. Ass.*, **32**, 4.

DONALDSON, I. MacG., and ESPINER, E. A. (1971) Disseminated lupus erythematosus presenting as chorea gravidarum, *Arch. Neurol. (Chic.)*, **25**, 240.

FERMAGLICH, J., STREIB, E., and AUTH, T. (1973) Chorea associated with systemic lupus erythematosus: treatment with haloperidol, *Arch. Neurol. (Chic.)*, **28**, 276.

GAMBOA, E. T., ISAACS, G., and HARTER, D. H. (1971) Chorea associated with oral contraceptive therapy, *Arch. Neurol. (Chic.)*, **25,** 112.

GUBBAY, S. S. (1975) *The Clumsy Child*, London.

LEWIS, B. V., and PARSONS, M. (1966) Chorea gravidarum, *Lancet*, **i,** 284.

LHERMITTE, J., and PAGNIEZ, P. (1930) Anatomie et physiologie pathologiques de la chorée de Sydenham, *Encéphale*, **25,** 24.

MATTHEWS, W. B. (1963) *Practical Neurology*, Oxford.

MEYJES, F. E. P. (1931) Zur Lokalisation und Pathophysiologie der choreatischen Bewegung, *Z. ges. Neurol. Psychiat.*, **133,** 1.

RIDDOCH, D., JEFFERSON, M., and BICKERSTAFF, E. R. (1971) Chorea and the oral contraceptives, *Brit. med. J.*, **4,** 217.

WINKELMAN, N. W., and ECKEL, J. L. (1932) The brain in acute rheumatic fever, *Arch. Neurol. Psychiat. (Chic.)*, **28,** 844.

HUNTINGTON'S CHOREA

Definition. A hereditary disorder characterized pathologically by degeneration of the ganglion cells of the forebrain and corpus striatum, and clinically by choreiform movements and progressive dementia, which usually begin during early middle life.

PATHOLOGY

The brain is small and of diminished weight, the reduction being chiefly, if not entirely, in the forebrain, which shows evidence of marked atrophy affecting the gyri and especially the corpus striatum. The ganglion cells in both the caudate nucleus and in the putamen are reduced in numbers and sometimes almost absent. According to Dunlap (1927), the putamen is more affected than the caudate nucleus and suffers most severely in its second and third fourths. This observer found no loss of cells and no evidence of primary disease in the globus pallidus. Such shrinkage in size as occurred in the latter appeared to be due to destruction of fibres coming from the caudate nucleus and putamen. The degenerative changes are accompanied by an extensive proliferation of neuroglia. However, in four childhood cases Byers *et al.* (1973) found loss of neurones and gliosis in both the globus pallidus and thalamus as well as substantial cerebellar atrophy. On the other hand, Campbell *et al.* (1961) in a patient suffering from the rigid form of the disease found a substantial loss of small nerve cells in the caudate nucleus and putamen with relative sparing of neurones in the shrunken globus pallidus and attributed rigidity to the putaminal lesion, chorea to that in the caudate nucleus. The ganglion cells of the cortex are small and shrunken in appearance, and the white matter of the cerebral hemispheres is reduced in amount, possibly more than the grey.

AETIOLOGY

Huntington's chorea is uncommon in Great Britain but is not uncommon in the United States of America. Though sporadic cases are occasionally encountered, the only known cause is heredity, and the disorder is inherited as a Mendelian dominant. According to Davenport and Muncey (1917) its ancestral source in the United States can be traced to three brothers who migrated there in the seventeenth century. Of a thousand cases in certain districts practically all could be traced to six individuals. Both sexes are affected and transmit the disease with equal frequency. The age of onset of symptoms is usually between 30 and 45, but may be either later or earlier. Exceptionally members of affected sibships have developed the disease in childhood. In an extensive review of the disease in Queensland, Australia, however, Wallace and Hall (1972) found evidence of considerable genetic heterogeneity and suggested that cases of adult and childhood onset may be due to different allelic genes. However, while it is true that cases beginning in childhood or adolescence usually display the rigid form of the disease, many such cases have been described in families in which affected individuals in earlier generations showed the typical onset with choreic movements in middle life and there is no essential difference in the pathological findings in the two varieties (Campbell *et al.*, 1961; Oliver and Dewhurst, 1969); families showing an onset with rigidity in adult life have been described (Bird and Paulson, 1971).

Much attention has been paid recently to the possibility that a specific biochemical abnormality may be present in cases of this disease. Suggestions that it may be due to a disorder of magnesium metabolism have not been confirmed (Fleming *et al.*, 1967) No significant abnormality in lipid composition of white matter has been discovered (Hooghwinkel *et al.*, 1968) and the erythrocyte glycolipids are normal (Wherrett and Brown, 1969), but certain amino acids are reduced in the plasma and CSF of such patients (Perry *et al.*, 1969). There is also evidence of imbalance between central dopamine and acetylcholine activity in such cases (Klawans and Rubovits, 1972), but the administration of L-tryptophan and pyridoxine does not cause any deterioration in motor skill (McLeod and Horne, 1972). However, the enzymes glutamic acid decarboxylase, choline acetylase, and succinate dehydrogenase are all reduced in the corpus striatum of patients with Huntington's chorea (McGeer *et al.*, 1973; Stahl and Swanson, 1974) and there is a loss of GABA-containing neurones (Bird and Iverson, 1974) so that increasing attention is being paid to the metabolism of gamma-aminobutyric acid (GABA) in this disease (Barbeau, 1973, 1975).

SYMPTOMS

The first symptom is usually involuntary movements, which develop insidiously. They are most conspicuous in the face and upper limbs, and are usually more rapid and jerky than the movements of Sydenham's chorea. As the disorder progresses they lead to dysarthria and ataxia of the upper limbs and of the gait. Mental changes gradually develop, usually a few years after the onset of the involuntary movements. They consist of a progressive dementia. Most patients become inert, apathetic, and irritable. Delusions may occur, and outbursts of excitement are not uncommon. Suicide is exceptional.

As Davenport and Muncey showed, the clinical picture does not always exhibit the classical features just described. Dementia may precede involuntary movements or the latter may never appear (Curran, 1930). Alternatively, involuntary movements may not be followed by dementia. Exceptionally Parkinsonian rigidity (the 'rigid' form) takes the place of the involuntary movements (Campbell *et al.*, 1961; Bird and Paulson, 1971). The onset of symptoms in childhood has already been mentioned, and in such cases diffuse extrapyramidal rigidity, fits and pseudobulbar palsy may be the presenting features.

DIAGNOSIS

In typical cases with a family history the diagnosis is easy. In sporadic cases progressive dementia developing in middle life in association with involuntary movements which somewhat resemble tremor may lead to a diagnosis of general paresis. This, however, can easily be excluded by the absence of iridoplegia and by the negative serological reactions. Choreiform involuntary movements are rarely if ever seen in the presenile dementias, in arteriosclerotic dementia, and in Creutzfeld–Jakob disease, but when dementia is the presenting feature in Huntington's disease and when the family history is difficult to obtain, these other conditions may sometimes be considered before involuntary movements appear. The EEG in Huntington's chorea is often of low voltage (Scott *et al.*, 1972) but this finding in an isolated case is of little diagnostic value. In advanced cases air encephalography often shows a characteristic dilatation of the lateral ventricles with absence of the usual indentation due to the body of the caudate nucleus (Gath and Vinje, 1968) but by the time this appearance is present the diagnosis is usually self-evident.

PROGNOSIS

Save in rare cases, the disorder is progressive and terminates fatally, usually in from 10 to 15 years, though it may be much more acute; on the other hand survival for 20 or 30 years is not uncommon.

On account of the dominant heredity, half the children of an affected person may be expected to develop and to be capable of transmitting the disease. Those who remain free from it will not transmit it, but, unfortunately, since symptoms usually do not develop until middle life, it is often impossible in the case of children of an affected parent to decide whether they will transmit the disorder until they have passed the usual age of marriage. When the parent has reached the age of 60 without developing symptoms, it may be assumed that his children are unlikely to develop, and hence to transmit, the disease. Much interest has been aroused recently by the introduction of methods for the detection of the disorder in the preclinical stage. The administration of levodopa 800 mg and carbidopa 200 mg daily for 10 days may evoke choreiform movements in some such cases (Klawans *et al.*, 1970; *British Medical Journal*, 1972) but it is still uncertain as to how early in life and how often this test can be regarded as having predictive reliability. It is possible that measurement of the uptake by platelets of dopamine and 5-hydroxytryptamine (Aminoff *et al.*, 1974) could prove useful as a screening test and without doubt others will be introduced in the next few years (Barbeau *et al.*, 1972).

TREATMENT

The onset of the mental deterioration frequently necessitates institutional care. No form of treatment is known to arrest the progress of the dementia.✓ Chlorpromazine or thiopropazate (*Dartalan*) may help to control the involuntary movements. Lithium carbonate (Aminoff and Marshall, 1974) and methysergide (Klawans *et al.*, 1972) are among the many drugs which have been shown to be of no value. Tetrabenazine 25 mg three times daily is probably the most effective treatment (McLellan *et al.*, 1974). Stereotaxic surgery has been tried in some cases but may accelerate the development of dementia and is therefore contra-indicated as a rule except in rare cases in which there is no trace of intellectual impairment and no evidence of ventricular dilatation on air encephalography.

REFERENCES

AMINOFF, M. J., and MARSHALL, J. (1974) Treatment of Huntington's chorea with lithium carbonate: a double-blind trial, *Lancet*, **i**, 107.

AMINOFF, M. J., TRENCHARD, A., TURNER, P., WOOD, W. G., and HILLS, M. (1974) Platelet uptake of dopamine and 5-hydroxytryptamine and plasma-catecholamine levels in patients with Huntington's chorea, *Lancet*, **ii**, 1115.

BARBEAU, A. (1973) G.A.B.A. and Huntington's chorea, *Lancet*, **ii**, 1499.

BARBEAU, A. (1975) Progress in understanding Huntington's chorea, *Canad. J. neurol. Sci.*, **2**, 81.

BARBEAU, A., CHASE, T. N., and PAULSON, G. W. (1972) *Huntington's Chorea, 1872–1972* (Advances in Neurology, vol. 1), New York.

BELL, J. (1934) Huntington's chorea, *Treasury of Human Inheritance*, vol. iv, pt. 1, London.

BIRD, E. D., and IVERSON, L. L. (1974) Huntington's chorea—post-mortem measurement of glutamic acid decarboxylase, choline acetyltransferase and dopamine in basal ganglia, *Brain*, **97**, 457.

BIRD, M. T., and PAULSON, G. W. (1971) The rigid form of Huntington's chorea, *Neurology (Minneap.)*, **21**, 271.

BRITISH MEDICAL JOURNAL (1972) Presymptomatic detection of Huntington's chorea, *Brit. med. J.*, **3**, 540.

BYERS, R. K., GILLES, F. H., and FUNG, C. (1973) Huntington's disease in children. Neuropathologic study of four cases, *Neurology (Minneap.)*, **23**, 561.

CAMPBELL, A. M. G., CORNER, B., NORMAN, R. M., and URICH, H. (1961) The rigid form of Huntington's disease, *J. Neurol. Neurosurg. Psychiat.*, **24**, 71.

CURRAN, D. (1929–30) Huntington's chorea without choreiform movements, *J. Neurol. Psychopath.*, **10**, 305.

DAVENPORT, C. B., and MUNCEY, E. B. (1916–17) Huntington's chorea in relation to heredity and eugenics, *Amer. J. Insan.*, **73**, 195 (also *Proc. nat. Acad. Sci. (Wash.)*, 1915, **1**, 283).

DAVISON, C., GOODHART, S. P., and SHLIONSKY, H. (1932) Chronic progressive chorea, *Arch. Neurol. Psychiat. (Chic.)*, **27**, 906.

DUNLAP, C. B. (1927) Pathologic changes in Huntington's chorea, *Arch. Neurol. Psychiat. (Chic.)*, **18**, 867.

FLEMING, L. W., BARKER, M. G., and STEWART, W. K. (1967) Plasma and erythrocyte magnesium in Huntington's chorea, *J. Neurol. Neurosurg. Psychiat.*, **30**, 374.

GATH, I., and VINJE, B. (1968) Pneumoencephalographic findings in Huntington's chorea, *Neurology (Minneap.)*, **18**, 991.

HOOGHWINKEL, G. J. M., BRUYN, G. W., and DE ROOY, R. E. (1968) Biochemical studies in Huntington's chorea. VII. The lipid composition of the cerebral white and gray matter, *Neurology (Minneap.)*, **18**, 408.

KLAWANS, H. L., PAULSON, G. W., and BARBEAU, A. (1970) Predictive test for Huntington's chorea, *Lancet*, **ii**, 1185.

KLAWANS, H. L., and RUBOVITS, R. (1972) Central cholinergic–anticholinergic antagonism in Huntington's chorea, *Neurology (Minneap.)*, **22**, 107.

KLAWANS, H. L., RUBOVITS, R., RINGEL, S. P., and WEINER, W. J. (1972) Observations on the use of methysergide in Huntington's chorea, *Neurology (Minneap.)*, **22**, 929.

MCGEER, P. L., MCGEER, E. G., and FIBIGER, H. C. (1973) Choline acetylase and glutamic acid decarboxylase in Huntington's chorea: a preliminary study, *Neurology (Minneap.)*, **23**, 912.

MCLELLAN, D. L., CHALMERS, R. J., and JOHNSON, R. H. (1974) A double-blind trial of tetrabenazine, thiopropazate, and placebo in patients with chorea, *Lancet*, **i**, 104.

MCLEOD, W. R., and HORNE, D. J. DE L. (1972) Huntington's chorea and tryptophan, *J. Neurol. Neurosurg. Psychiat.*, **35**, 510.

OLIVER, J., and DEWHURST, K. (1969) Childhood and adolescent forms of Huntington's disease, *J. Neurol. Neurosurg. Psychiat.*, **32**, 455.

PERRY, T. L., HANSEN, S., DIAMOND, S., and STEDMAN, D. (1969) Plasma-aminoacid levels in Huntington's chorea, *Lancet*, **i**, 806.

SCOTT, D. F., HEATHFIELD, K. W. G., TOONE, B., and MARGERISON, J. H. (1972) The EEG in Huntington's chorea: a clinical and neuropathological study, *J. Neurol. Neurosurg. Psychiat.*, **35**, 97.

STAHL, W. L., and SWANSON, P. D. (1974) Biochemical abnormalities in Huntington's chorea brains, *Neurology (Minneap.)*, **24**, 813.

WALLACE, D. C., and HALL, A. C. (1972) Evidence of genetic heterogeneity in Huntington's chorea, *J. Neurol. Neurosurg. Psychiat.*, **35**, 789.

WHERRETT, J. R., and BROWN, B. L. (1969) Erythrocyte glycolipids in Huntington's chorea, *Neurology (Minneap.)*, **19**, 489.

SENILE CHOREA

Choreiform movements may follow vascular lesions of the brain in middle life and old age. Their onset is usually sudden, and they are generally unilateral. When this is the case they differ only in degree from hemiballismus. Chronic progressive chorea occasionally occurs in the absence of hereditary predisposition. The large and small cells of the caudate nucleus and putamen degenerate but the cerebral cortex is spared (Alcock, 1936). It is difficult to distinguish this from the sporadic occurrence of Huntington's chorea, though it has been stated that the age of onset of senile chorea is usually later than that of Huntington's variety, and that mental symptoms are less likely to occur. The movements are usually less florid and widespread than those of Huntington's chorea. Chlorpromazine is a useful drug in the management of these sporadic cases.

HEMIBALLISMUS

Hemiballismus is the term applied to involuntary movements which affect the limbs unilaterally, though the face may rarely be involved on both sides. Hemiballismus differs from chorea in that the movements affect the proximal parts of the limbs to a greater extent, and hence lead to wide excursions, and they are practically continuous except during sleep. The movements are often so violent [FIG. 109] that the skin of the limbs may be excoriated. The lesion responsible is usually situated in the subthalamic nucleus (corpus Luysii) of the opposite side, but lesions have been observed elsewhere, especially in the corpus striatum and in the pathways connecting it to the subthalamic nucleus (see Whittier, 1947; Meyers *et al.*, 1950; Martin, 1957).

Spontaneous cessation of the movements is rare, and many patients die from exhaustion. Surgical measures which have been found to give relief include extirpation of the precentral cortex, linear cortico-subcortical section, and midbrain pyramidotomy (Meyers *et al.*, 1950) but these operations have now been replaced by stereotaxic thalamotomy (Martin and McCaul, 1959) which is often dramatically successful.

FACIAL DYSKINESIA

A Parkinsonian syndrome and choreiform movements may develop in patients receiving long-term treatment with phenothiazine drugs for psychiatric conditions but usually improve when these drugs are withdrawn. However, distressing facial dyskinetic movements with grimacing, chewing, and intermittent protrusion of the tongue are more disturbing complications of such treatment

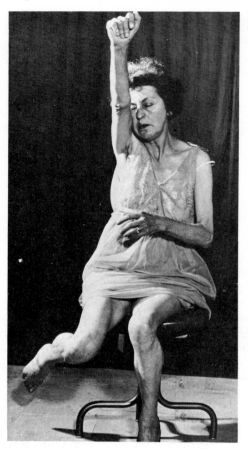

FIG. 109. Hemiballismus (photograph kindly supplied by Dr. J. D. Spillane)

and are unfortunately irreversible (Hunter *et al.*, 1964; Evans, 1965). Sometimes similar movements arise spontaneously in patients not known to be taking drugs (Altrocchi, 1972) and in such cases the aetiology is unknown. Similar orofacial dyskinetic movements also develop in patients receiving levodopa for the treatment of Parkinsonism, but unlike those due to phenothiazines they often disappear when the dose of levodopa is reduced. Tetrabenazine 25 mg four times daily (Godwin-Austen and Clark, 1971) and thiopropazate (Singer and Cheng, 1971) are among the remedies which have been shown to be helpful in reducing these distressing movements.

PALATAL MYOCLONUS

Palatal myoclonus is a condition in which rhythmical movements of the soft palate, occurring 60–180 times a minute develop insidiously. They interfere with speech, swallowing, and respiration and usually persist during sleep. Often pathological examination reveals hypertrophy of the olivary nuclei; the condition appears to be due to a disorder within the olivocerebellar modulatory projection on to the rostral brain stem; the aetiology is unknown (Herrmann and Brown, 1967). Ocular bobbing is a rare accompaniment (Yap *et al.*, 1968).

GILLES DE LA TOURETTE SYNDROME

This bizarre syndrome was first described in 1885 by Gilles de la Tourette who reported 9 cases beginning in childhood with persistent multiple tics and coprolalia, a form of recurrent verbal utterance consisting of the expostulation of obscenities and swear-words. The disease is of unknown aetiology, has no known neuropathology and has been regarded by some as a manifestation of schizophrenia. The vocal tics sometimes are associated with barks or grunts and some patients show echolalia and compulsive imitation of movements or gestures. In a recent report of 22 cases, Sweet *et al.* (1973) found non-specific EEG abnormalities in many but were unable to elucidate any neurological substrate of the disorder, though there was a high incidence of left-handedness. The condition may well prove to be of psychiatric rather than organic origin; haloperidol may be of some value in treatment (*British Medical Journal*, 1973).

REFERENCES

ALCOCK, N. S. (1936) A note on the pathology of senile chorea (non-hereditary), *Brain*, **59**, 376.

ALTROCCHI, P. H. (1972) Spontaneous oral-facial dyskinesia, *Arch. Neurol. (Chic.)*, **26**, 506.

BRITISH MEDICAL JOURNAL (1973) Syndrome of Gilles de la Tourette, *Brit. med. J.*, **2**, 568.

EVANS, J. H. (1965) Persistent oral dyskinesia in treatment with phenothiazine derivatives, *Lancet*, **i**, 458.

GILLES DE LA TOURETTE, G. (1885) Étude sur une affection nerveuse caractérisée par l'incoordination motrice accompagnée d'écholalie et de coprolalie (jumping, latah, myriachit), *Arch. Neurol. (Paris)*, **9**, 19, 158.

GODWIN-AUSTEN, R. B., and CLARK, T. (1971) Persistent phenothiazine dyskinesia treated with tetrabenazine, *Brit. med. J.*, **4**, 25.

HERRMANN, C., Jun., and BROWN, J. W. (1967) Palatal myoclonus; a reappraisal, *J. neurol. Sci.*, **5**, 473.

HUNTER, R., EARL, C. J., and JANZ, D. (1964) A syndrome of abnormal movements and dementia in leucotomized patients treated with phenothiazines, *J. Neurol. Psychiat.*, **27**, 219.

MARTIN, J. P. (1927) Hemichorea resulting from a local lesion of the brain (the syndrome of the body of Luys), *Brain*, **50**, 637.

MARTIN, J. P. (1928) A contribution to the study of chorea. The symptoms which result from injury of the corpus Luysii, *Lancet*, **ii**, 315.

MARTIN, J. P. (1957) Hemichorea (hemiballismus) without lesions in the corpus Luysii, *Brain*, **80**, 1.

MARTIN, J. P., and McCAUL, I. R. (1959) Acute hemiballismus treated by ventrolateral thalamotomy, *Brain*, **82**, 104.

MEYERS, R., SWEENEY, D. B., and SCHWIDDE, J. T. (1950) Hemiballismus. Aetiology and surgical treatment, *J. Neurol. Neurosurg. Psychiat.*, **13**, 115.

SINGER, K., and CHENG, M. N. (1971) Thiopropazate hydrochloride in persistent dyskinesia, *Brit. med. J.*, **4**, 22.

SWEET, R. D., SOLOMON, G. E., WAYNE, H., SHAPIRO, E., and SHAPIRO, A. K. (1973) Neurological features of Gilles de la Tourette's syndrome, *J. Neurol. Neurosurg. Psychiat.*, **36**, 1.

WHITTIER, J. R. (1947) Ballism and the subthalamic nucleus, *Arch. Neurol. Psychiat. (Chic.)*, **58**, 672.

YAP, C.-B., MAYO, C., and BARRON, K. (1968) 'Ocular bobbing' in palatal myoclonus, *Arch. Neurol. (Chic.)*, **18**, 304.

X

13

CONGENITAL AND DEGENERATIVE DISORDERS

CEREBRAL PALSY

The inclusive term 'cerebral palsy' was used by Ingram (1964) to identify a group of chronic non-progressive disorders occurring in young children in which disease of the brain causes impairment of motor function. The impairment of motor function may be the result of paresis, including movement or incoordination, but motor disorders which are transient or are the result of progressive disease of the brain or attributable to abnormalities of the spinal cord are excluded.

The classification of conditions which fall into this group remains a matter of dispute but, modified from Ingram (1964), the following is suggested as being reasonably satisfactory in the present state of knowledge:

Quadriplegia or tetraplegia
Diplegia (including hypotonic, dystonic, and rigid or spastic forms)
Hemiplegia
Bilateral hemiplegia
Ataxia (cerebellar diplegia)
Dyskinesia (dystonic, choreoid, athetoid forms)

To these groups may be added the disputed category of so-called 'minimal cerebral palsy' or 'minimal cerebral dysfunction' (Bax and MacKeith, 1963). The dyskinetic forms of cerebral palsy have been considered in CHAPTER 12.

REFERENCES

BAX, M., and MACKEITH, R. (1963) Minimal cerebral dysfunction, *Little Club Clinics in Developmental Medicine*, No. 10, London.
HOLT, K. S. (1965) *Assessment of Cerebral Palsy*, London.
INGRAM, T. T. S. (1964) *Paediatric Aspects of Cerebral Palsy*, Edinburgh.

CONGENITAL DIPLEGIA

Synonyms. Congenital spastic paralysis; Little's disease.

Definition. The term 'congenital diplegia' is now used to include a group of cases characterized by bilateral and symmetrical disturbances of motility, which are present from birth and which subsequently remain stationary or show a tendency towards improvement. Though commonly the lesion involves chiefly the corticospinal tracts, causing weakness and spasticity which are most conspicuous in the lower limbs, mental defect, involuntary movements, and ataxia may be present either in association with spastic weakness or as the sole manifestations of the cerebral or cerebellar lesion. Diplegia is the term traditionally used when all four limbs are affected but weakness and spasticity are more severe in the lower limbs, while quadriplegia or tetraplegia is the term employed when all four limbs are affected to an equal extent.

AETIOLOGY AND PATHOLOGY

Cerebral palsy is found in between 1 and 2 per 1,000 live births (Courville, 1954; Department of Health, 1970). Of seven affected infants, one is likely to die, one will be grossly crippled physically, two severely mentally retarded, and one will be mildly affected with minor incapacity; the remaining two are likely to require special treatment (Menkes, 1974).

There has been much dispute about the aetiology and pathology of this condition. Plainly it is a disorder of multiple aetiology. Rarely it may be a consequence of gross cerebral maldevelopment, and traumatic intracranial haemorrhage resulting from precipitate, difficult, or instrumental delivery, whether due to tearing of dural venous sinuses or of cerebral veins and whether it is subarachnoid, subdural, or intracerebral is also a rare cause, though it was once thought to be common. Traumatic damage to the brain stem or upper spinal cord is also uncommon (Towbin, 1970). However, abnormal pregnancy, labour, or delivery (Ingram, 1964) or prematurity (Polani, 1958; Prechtl, 1968) are clearly important factors leading to the birth of many diplegic infants. There is growing evidence to indicate that prenatal or perinatal anoxia is a major aetiological factor but that complex neonatal metabolic abnormalities, especially including hypoglycaemia, as well as disorders of cerebral perfusion resulting from brain swelling, increased vascular resistance, and hypotension all play a part in varying degree (Courville, 1971; Menkes, 1974).

Severe anoxia alone may result in massive cystic degeneration of the central cerebral white matter, as Little (1862) originally showed, but this type of pathological change is rare in cases of cerebral palsy. A more common finding, especially in premature infants, is periventricular encephalomalacia (Banker and Larroche, 1962; DeReuck et al., 1972), a disorder in which diminished arterial perfusion gives bilateral areas of necrosis and gliosis, sometimes but not invariably symmetrically distributed in the white and grey matter surrounding the lateral ventricles. In full-term infants it is commoner to find multiple areas of cortical damage varying in distribution and severity and giving lobar or nodular cortical sclerosis (ulegyria), sometimes associated with cystic change (porencephaly) in the subjacent white matter. It is often difficult to distinguish between large intracerebral cysts (porencephaly) which may sometimes be developmental (Kramer, 1956) and multilocular cystic encephalopathy (Crome, 1958) which is usually secondary to vascular damage. In the basal ganglia there may be spongiform degeneration (status marmoratus) or symmetrical demyelination with an appearance like the veining of marble (status dysmyelinatus). The cortical changes are probably a consequence of infarction due to damage to small arteries or veins, but there is still dispute about the pathogenesis of the changes in the basal ganglia, although these, too, have been attributed to the effects of venous haemorrhage resulting from obstruction of the galenic venous system (Schwartz, 1961). Lesions limited to the cerebellum with diffuse damage to the dentate nuclei and cerebellar cortex are seen in cases of ataxic cerebral palsy but are much less common; in such children, clinical diagnosis from cerebellar agenesis, which, however, is often familial (Joubert et al., 1969), may be very difficult. Perinatal damage to the brain stem due to compression of the vertebral arteries during delivery is even more rare (Yates, 1959).

As already mentioned, gross abnormalities of cerebral development, including anencephaly, schizencephaly, lissencephaly, macrogyria, micropolygyria, agenesis of the corpus callosum, and primary microcephaly may all produce some clinical features corresponding to those of cerebral palsy; infants with anencephaly do not survive, but the other disorders listed may all give mental retardation, seizures, and variable degrees of spastic paresis, sometimes compatible with long survival (see Menkes, 1974). Many syndromes of mental retardation due to chromosomal anomalies, specific metabolic defects, and others which are of unknown cause may also be associated with variable neurological abnormalities.

SYMPTOMS

The symptoms depend upon the distribution of the degenerative changes in the brain. These may predominate in the prefrontal region which is concerned especially with psychical functions, in the precentral gyri, or in the subordinate centres concerned in motility and its co-ordination. Thus one function may be affected almost alone, with the production of types of congenital diplegia characterized by the predominance of (1) mental retardation, (2) spastic weakness, (3) involuntary movements, and (4) cerebellar deficiency. Mixed varieties, however, are common. Atonic cerebral palsy is the term which has been applied to cases in which there is hypotonia of the limbs in early infancy and childhood but often with brisk tendon reflexes and extensor plantar responses. In some such patients spasticity develops later; others go on to develop ataxia or athetosis.

Frequently nothing abnormal is noticed about the child at birth and for some time afterwards, though diplegic infants are often difficult to feed. However, the increasing use of the Apgar scoring system in the assessment of the newborn (Drage and Berendes, 1966) and the examination of postural and other reflexes in young infants (Donovan et al., 1962; Paine and Oppé, 1966) often assists in early identification, especially when primitive reflexes which normally disappear with maturation fail to do so. In some cases microcephaly and muscular rigidity are so marked that attention is drawn to them early. Often the child is only regarded as abnormal when it fails to reach one of the landmarks of normal development at the expected time. Thus it may be observed that it fails to take notice of its surroundings, that it does not begin to raise its head when 3 months old, sit up at 6 months, and begin to walk and talk at the end of the first year of life. Diplegic children, too, are usually late in acquiring control of the sphincters.

Mental Retardation

Mental retardation may be the predominant symptom and then may occur in the absence of any gross disturbance of motility, except such clumsiness as results from an inability to learn to control the limbs. In other cases retardation is associated with diplegia. It ranges through all the degrees arbitrarily characterized as severe, moderate, and mild retardation. Frequently the diplegic child appears to be more backward mentally than is actually the case, since his slowness in learning to walk, and his clumsiness in using his hands retard his mental development. Some children, though developing late, ultimately achieve a high degree of intelligence in spite of severe motor disabilities.

Weakness and Spasticity

These symptoms, which are mainly attributable to defective development of, or damage to, the corticospinal and extrapyramidal tracts, are usually remarkably symmetrical on the two sides. Rarely one side is more affected than the other. The lower limbs are usually more severely affected than the upper. The severity of the symptoms of corticospinal defect varies greatly in different cases. When at its slightest, power and tone may be almost normal, the sole indications of the lesion being exaggerated knee- and ankle-jerks, extensor plantar responses, and slight contractures of the calf muscles, leading to a moderate degree of talipes equinovarus. A somewhat more severe lesion causes a spastic paraplegia of the type originally described by Little in 1862, in which weakness and spasticity are confined to the lower limbs and the muscles of the lower trunk. The lower limbs are rigid in a position of plantar flexion of the ankle, extension at the knee, and adduction and internal rotation at the hip, and contractures develop in the spastic muscles. Voluntary power is often fairly strong, though much hampered by the spasticity. The gait is characteristic, since the plantar flexion of the feet causes the child to walk on the toes, while owing to adduction of the hips the knees may rub together, or may be actually crossed, the so-called 'scissors gait'. The tendon reflexes in the lower limbs are much exaggerated, and the plantar reflexes are extensor. The abdominal reflexes are frequently brisk in spite of the severity of the corticospinal lesion. Spinal deformities, such as lordosis and scoliosis, are common.

In the most severe cases (quadriplegia) the upper limbs and bulbar muscles suffer from spastic weakness as well as the lower limbs and the posture may be decerebrate or decorticate, sometimes with preservation of the tonic neck reflexes. In Ingram's (1964) series, no child with quadriplegia was found to be educable. In the upper limbs the rigidity is usually most marked in the flexor muscles, and the involvement of the bulbar muscles leads to spastic dysarthria and in severe cases to dysphagia. Dribbling of saliva is common.

Involuntary Movements

Involuntary movements may be athetotic or choreiform, or may present some of the features of both, being then described as choreo-athetoid. The characteristics of these involuntary movements are described on pages 572 and 611. In double athetosis athetotic or choreiform movements are present on both sides of the body and are increased by voluntary and emotional movements. The involuntary movements are most evident in the slighter cases, being replaced by hypertonia in the most severe examples of the disorder. The face is expressionless in repose, but involuntary laughing and crying frequently occur. There are gross disturbances of articulation, phonation, mastication, and deglutition, and voluntary movement of the limbs is slow and clumsy. In typical double athetosis there is no clinical evidence of damage to the corticospinal tracts and the plantar reflexes are flexor, but it is not uncommon to find athetotic or choreiform movements associated with spastic diplegia of the type described in the previous section.

Cerebellar Diplegia

In this rare form of diplegia the symptoms are those of cerebellar deficiency, especially nystagmus, hypotonia, and ataxia (see Walsh, 1963). In many such cases in early infancy hypotonia dominates the clinical picture; cerebellar diplegia is thus one cause of flaccid or atonic diplegia in infancy although in some other cases demonstrating hypotonia and flaccidity the typical involuntary movements of chorea and/or athetosis make their appearance in the second year of life.

Other Symptoms

Optic atrophy, field defects, and cranial nerve involvement are very rare but squint and nystagmus are common in diplegic children, and epilepsy occurs in about 27 per cent of cases (Ingram, 1964). A moderate degree of skeletal infantilism is usually present, and puberty is not uncommonly delayed.

DIAGNOSIS

In most cases diagnosis is easy, since the symptoms have clearly been present since birth. The presence of muscular rigidity readily distinguishes spastic diplegia from benign congenital hypotonia and progressive spinal muscular atrophy of infants, in both of which conditions the muscles are flaccid. Difficulty may, however, be experienced in distinguishing these conditions from flaccid diplegia (due to cerebellar diplegia or incipient choreo-athetosis) during the first 12 to 18 months of life. It is important to distinguish congenital diplegia from progressive degenerative disorders of the brain developing in early life, such as cerebromacular degeneration and diffuse sclerosis, both of which lead to bilateral spastic weakness. The distinction is based upon the fact that in these two disorders the child is normal at birth and develops normally during the early months of its life, and symptoms, when they develop, become progressively worse, whereas in congenital diplegia the child is abnormal from the beginning and its condition remains stationary or slowly improves. This aspect of differential diagnosis has important genetic implications as cerebral palsy is rarely familial while the degenerative disorders are usually inherited and may affect other sibs.

PROGNOSIS

The prognosis of congenital diplegia depends upon its severity and especially upon the degree of mental retardation. In the most severe cases the child rarely survives more than a year or two, usually succumbing to pneumonia. Even when the disability is only moderately severe, many affected individuals fail to survive beyond the early years of adult life. Although the condition sometimes remains stationary, there is usually a very slow improvement in the motor symptoms, both in those with spastic weakness and in those with involuntary movements, but this depends chiefly upon the mental state of the patient, and little improvement can be expected when severe mental retardation is present. In favourable cases it may be expected that a child will learn to walk, even though he may not do so until he is 5 or 6 years old.

TREATMENT

Treatment consists essentially in the education of movement, combined with the removal as far as possible of the obstacles which result from contractures and deformities. Much, therefore, depends upon the patience and care which are available for the education of the patient. Every effort must be made to help the child to learn to walk, and by means of simple games and occupations involving manipulative skill it must gradually be taught control over the movements of the upper limbs. Intensive physiotherapy is undoubtedly of value in many cases but certain specialized programmes of treatment in centres for the treatment of the cerebral palsied are based upon false concepts of neuromuscular function (Menkes, 1974) and care must be taken that excessive physiotherapeutic effort is not lavished on the hopeless case (Wilson, 1969). In the United Kingdom, assessment and treatment centres established by the National Spastics Society play an invaluable role. Treatment must be tailored to the needs of the individual case. Contractures may be dealt with by tenotomy, and in addition severe abductor spasm may be relieved by dividing the obturator nerve. Drugs such as chlordiazepoxide (*Librium*) and diazepam (*Valium*) have some value in reducing spasticity and in occasional cases intrathecal phenol injections are indicated for the relief of severe spasticity with flexor spasms. Levodopa has been thought to be beneficial in some cases of athetoid cerebral palsy (Rosenthal *et al.*, 1972) but its effects are marginal and other drugs such as tetrabenazine have been tried with little benefit. Stereotaxic surgery has proved to have a very limited role in the treatment of athetosis but may be more helpful in cases with dystonia. Other surgical procedures directed towards the relief of spasticity and deformity have been utilized in selected cases (Samilson, 1975). These operations, however, should only be carried out in children whose mental capacity and voluntary power will enable them to profit by them. Epilepsy must be treated in the usual way.

REFERENCES

BAKER, R. C., and GRAVES, G. O. (1931) Cerebellar agenesis, *Arch. Neurol. Psychiat. (Chic.)*, **25**, 548.

BANKER, B. Q., and LARROCHE, J. C. (1962) Periventricular leukomalacia of infancy: a form of neonatal anoxic encephalopathy, *Arch. Neurol. (Chic.)*, **7**, 386.

COLLIER, J. (1924) Pathogenesis of cerebral diplegia, *Brain*, **47**, 1.

COURVILLE, C. B. (1954) *Cerebral Palsy*, Los Angeles.

COURVILLE, C. B. (1971) *Birth and Brain Damage*, Pasadena.

CROME, L. (1958) Multilocular cystic encephalopathy of infants, *J. Neurol. Neurosurg. Psychiat.*, **21**, 146.

DEPARTMENT OF HEALTH (1970) *Cerebral Palsy*, London.

DEREUCK, J., CHATTHA, A. S., and RICHARDSON, E. P. (1972) Pathogenesis and evolution of periventricular leukomalacia in infancy, *Arch. Neurol. (Chic.)*, **27**, 229.

DONOVAN, D. E., COUES, P., and PAINE, R. S. (1962) The prognostic implications of neurologic abnormalities in the neonatal period, *Neurology (Minneap.)*, **12**, 910.

DRAGE, J. S., and BERENDES, H. (1966) Apgar scores and outcome of the newborn, *Pediat. Clin. N. Amer.*, **13**, 636.

FORD, F. R., CROTHERS, B., and PUTNAM, M. C. (1927) *Birth Injuries of the Central Nervous System*, London.

FREUD, S. (1897) Die infantile Cerebrallähmung, *Spec. Path. Ther. Nothnagel*, **9**, Th. II, Abt. 2, Wien.

HOLT, K. S. (1965) *Assessment of Cerebral Palsy*, London.

INGRAM, T. T. S. (1964) *Paediatric Aspects of Cerebral Palsy*, Edinburgh.

JOUBERT, M., EISENRING, J.-J., ROBB, J. P., and ANDERMAN, F. (1969) Familial agenesis of the cerebellar vermis: a syndrome of episodic hyperpnea, abnormal eye movements, ataxia, and retardation, *Neurology (Minneap.)*, **19**, 813.

KRAMER, W. (1956) Multilocular encephalomalacia, *J. Neurol. Neurosurg. Psychiat.*, **19**, 209.

LITTLE, W. J. (1862) On the influence of abnormal parturition, difficult labor, premature birth, and asphyxia neonatorum on the mental and physical conditions of the child, especially in relation to deformities, *Trans. obstet. Soc. Lond.*, **3**, 293.

MENKES, J. H. (1974) *Textbook of Child Neurology*, Philadelphia.

PAINE, R. S., and OPPÉ, T. E. (1966) Neurological examination of children, *Clin. Dev. Med.*, **20/21**, 1.

POLANI, P. E. (1958) Prematurity and 'cerebral palsy', *Brit. med. J.*, **2**, 1497.
PRECHTL, H. F. R. (1968) Neurological findings in newborn infants after pre- and paranatal complications, in *Aspects of Praematurity and Dysmaturity*, ed. Jonxis, J. H. P., Visser, H. K. A., and Troelstra, J. A., Leiden.
ROSENTHAL, R. K., McDOWELL, F. H., and COOPER, W. (1972) Levodopa therapy in athetoid cerebral palsy, *Neurology (Minneap.)*, **22**, 1.
SAMILSON, R. L. (1975) *Orthopaedic Aspects of Cerebral Palsy*, London, Philadelphia.
SCHWARTZ, P. (1961) *Birth Injuries of the Newborn*, New York.
TOWBIN, A. (1970) Central nervous system damage in the human fetus and newborn infant, *Amer. J. Dis. Child.*, **119**, 529.
WALSH, E. G. (1963) Cerebellum, posture and cerebral palsy, *Little Club Clinics in Developmental Medicine*, No. 8, London.
WILSON, J. (1969) Chronic paediatric neurological disorders, *Brit. med. J.*, **4**, 152, 211.
YATES, P. O. (1959) Birth trauma to vertebral arteries, *Arch. Dis. Child.*, **34**, 436.

CONGENITAL AND INFANTILE HEMIPLEGIA

Definition. 'Congenital hemiplegia' is self-explanatory; 'infantile hemiplegia' is the term applied to hemiplegia which develops during the first few years of life. Like hemiplegia in adult life, it is a symptom of many pathological states; the distinction between congenital and infantile varieties is largely artificial.

AETIOLOGY

The causation of hemiplegia in childhood is often obscure, and there have been comparatively few pathological investigations of acute examples. The most convenient classification is, therefore, one based upon the clinical features and associations of the hemiplegia, and we may recognize the following varieties: (1) congenital hemiplegia; (2) hemiplegia complicating known infections; (3) hemiplegia of acute onset in the absence of any evident predisposing cause; (4) hemiplegia of slow onset.

1. Congenital hemiplegia is rare. There is a history of difficult labour in many such cases, and the commonest cause is probably a vascular lesion occurring during birth. Norman *et al.* (1957) discussed the aetiological factors, viz. a fall in systemic blood pressure, arterial compression owing to displacement of the cranial contents, and obstruction of the great cerebral vein. Ulegyria in the affected hemisphere is common (Benda, 1952); thus the pathogenesis is similar to that in many cases of cerebral diplegia. Less often the condition may be due to a congenital cerebral deformity, such as true porencephaly, aplasia of the cerebral hemisphere, intracranial angioma, or a cerebral vascular lesion or encephalitis occurring during fetal life. Congenital double hemiplegia is distinguished from congenital diplegia by the more severe affection of the upper limbs.

2. Hemiplegia may occur as a complication of many acute infective disorders of childhood, but is much commoner in some than in others. Whooping cough is one of the commonest causes. Less frequently it occurs in association with measles, scarlet fever, diphtheria, chickenpox, smallpox, vaccinia, pneumonia, otitis media, septicaemia due to pyogenic organisms, typhoid fever, typhus, dysentery, mumps, chorea, encephalitis lethargica. The relationship of the hemiplegia to the infection which it complicates is often obscure. In many cases the cerebral lesion is a vascular one. Thus meningeal and intracerebral haemorrhage have frequently been described in whooping cough, and arterial thrombosis and embolism have been observed in diphtheria. Cerebral thrombosis, too,

appears to be the commonest cause of hemiplegia in typhoid and typhus fevers and either cerebral venous thrombosis or cerebral abscess or meningitis may cause hemiplegia in cases of otitis media. In scarlet fever so-called 'acute haemorrhagic encephalitis' has been reported, while in smallpox, chickenpox, vaccinia, and measles the lesion is often a demyelinating encephalitis, which is regarded by some as due to the infecting organism and by others as due to hypersensitivity. Acute poliomyelitis, congenital syphilis, and tuberculous meningitis are very rare causes.

3. Cases of hemiplegia occurring in early childhood without any obvious predisposing cause are slightly more frequent than those which fall within the preceding group. In some cases the hemiplegia is probably a manifestation of an encephalitis or toxic encephalopathy of unknown origin. In the majority, how-ever, it is probably due to a vascular lesion, including haemorrhage from an angioma or aneurysm, or subdural haematoma; infarction is, however, com-moner. Bickerstaff (1964) suggested that in many cases the condition is due to internal carotid artery thrombosis, perhaps as a result of carotid arteritis, result-ing, for instance, from infected lymph nodes in the neck.

Infantile hemiplegia usually develops during the first three years of life and rarely after the age of 6.

4. Hemiplegia of slow onset is very rare in childhood. The causes include intracranial tumour, arising either in one cerebral hemisphere or in the pons, cerebral tuberculoma, and diffuse sclerosis. ·

PATHOLOGY

The pathological changes, as might be expected, are varied. Cases which are examined shortly after the onset of the hemiplegia frequently show focal vascular lesions, including meningeal and intracerebral haemorrhage and infarction. Ischaemic lesions within the fields of individual arteries or in the boundary zones between two arteries have been described. In some cases the pathological picture has been one of so-called 'acute haemorrhagic encephalitis', and the changes of post-infectious encephalomyelitis have been found in small-pox, chickenpox, vaccinia, and measles. In brains examined long after the onset of the hemiplegia the changes commonly found are meningeal thickening, localized atrophic sclerosis, cysts, and pseudoporencephaly. The Sturge-Weber syndrome [see p. 243] is one rare cause of infantile hemiplegia but the associated facial naevus and the characteristic intracranial calcification are distinctive.

SYMPTOMS

Congenital hemiplegia is usually detected at an early age, because it is observed that the child does not move the affected arm and leg normally, or because these limbs feel rigid.

Infantile hemiplegia usually develops suddenly. When it occurs as a complica-tion of an existing infective disease hemiplegia does not usually develop until some days after the onset of the infection, usually during the second week and sometimes not until the patient is convalescent. Convulsions occur at the onset in many cases. Consciousness is lost and the convulsive movements frequently predominate upon and may be confined to the side which subsequently be-comes paralysed. Usually a series of attacks occurs during 24 hours and the patient remains comatose for a variable period, sometimes for several days after the convulsions stop. Headache, vomiting, delirium, and pyrexia frequently usher in the attacks. During the stage of coma the limbs on the affected side are found to be completely flaccid and the plantar reflex is extensor. When the patient recovers consciousness he is hemiplegic, and when the right side of the body is paralysed, usually aphasic also, and sometimes there is intellectual impairment. In less severe cases hemiplegia may develop without convulsions and without loss of consciousness. The cerebrospinal fluid may be normal or may show an increase in protein, red blood cells, or a leucocytosis, depending upon the nature of the cerebral lesion. In a patient with an intracranial angioma there may be a systolic bruit over the cranium or the carotid artery in the neck.

In favourable cases improvement occurs, and in a few weeks or months recovery may be complete. When the hemiplegia does not recover, flaccidity gives place to spasticity in the course of a few weeks and the condition of the limbs on the paralysed side comes to resemble that found in congenital hemiplegia. The upper limb is severely affected as well as the lower and usually becomes spastic in an attitude of flexion, less often in extension. The signs of hemiplegia are described elsewhere [see p. 20]. Disorders of sensation in the affected limbs are found on careful examination in about two-thirds of all patients (Tizard et al., 1954). Owing to the early age of onset the development of the paralysed limbs is retarded and they remain smaller than those of the normal side; muscle fibres on the affected side are atrophic (Erbslöh et al., 1970). Contractures readily develop in both upper and lower limbs. When the paralysis is incomplete, involuntary movements of an athetoid or choreic character may develop on the affected side and dystonic features are seen to develop in occasional cases many years after the onset. Homonymous hemianopia is present on the affected side in 17–27 per cent of cases (Menkes, 1974). Facial weakness is common but involvement of cranial nerves is relatively rare. Epilepsy is much commoner in infantile hemiplegia than in cerebral diplegia and occurs in over 50 per cent of cases. The convulsions usually begin with tonic spasm or clonic movements of the paralysed side, but later they usually become generalized (Ford, 1926) and are attended by loss of consciousness.

DIAGNOSIS

Congenital hemiplegia is readily recognized: hemiplegia acquired in childhood must be distinguished from paralytic chorea, which is preceded by involuntary movements, and acute poliomyelitis which is rarely limited to one upper and lower limb and which is characterized by loss of tendon reflexes and muscular wasting. When the child is seen during the acute stage of a cerebral disturbance the subsequent development of hemiplegia cannot always be anticipated, but the occurrence of repeated convulsions, especially if these are predominantly unilateral, should suggest this possibility.

Hemiplegia of gradual onset is rare in childhood and is usually due to intracranial tumour. Angiography, the EMI scan, air encephalography, or ventriculography may be needed in difficult cases.

PROGNOSIS

Little improvement is likely to occur in congenital hemiplegia, but in mild cases careful education may enable the child to make some use of the paralysed limbs. It is exceptional for the lesion responsible for acquired infantile hemiplegia to prove fatal, but, if the child shows no signs of returning consciousness 48 hours after the onset of the convulsions, the outlook for recovery is poor. The more severe the symptoms of the acute stage, the more likely are mental

defect, aphasia, and hemiplegia to be persistent. Nevertheless, there are exceptions to this rule, and for several weeks after the acute stage there is no sure
method of deciding to what extent recovery of function will occur. Some patients
recover completely, but a considerable proportion remain intellectually impaired
and hemiplegic, and of these more than half become epileptic. Less than a third
become capable of an independent existence (Tizard, 1953). The hope of
considerable improvement should not be abandoned until at least a year has
elapsed after the onset of the illness. Even after this lapse of time some increase
of power and co-ordination may occur in the paralysed limbs in response to
treatment. Almost invariably the affected children eventually walk and in general
lower limb function improves considerably but often little effective movement
returns in the arm and hand.

TREATMENT

When the patient is unconscious the usual measures will be called for [see
p. 1170]. Otherwise treatment in the acute stage depends upon the cause. Cerebral
oedema may require treatment with steroid drugs, and hyperpyrexia with
hypothermia. The after-treatment of hemiplegia, both of the congenital and of
the acquired forms, includes active and passive movements to diminish the
risk of contractures, and the correction of the latter by tenotomy when they
develop. When any voluntary power remains, re-educational exercises should
be instituted. Small doses of anticonvulsants should be given daily over a period
of several years in the hope of preventing the development of epilepsy. Aphasia,
when present, must be treated by attempting to re-educate the child's powers
of speech. In some cases with severe hemiplegia, intractable epilepsy and
behaviour disorder, the operation of hemispherectomy has been advocated and
has resulted in marked reduction in the fits, improved behaviour and intellectual
performance and no significant increase in weakness of the affected limbs
(Krynauw, 1950; McKissock, 1953; Wilson, 1970). Unfortunately, follow-up
studies of such cases have suggested that, except in cases of the Sturge-Weber
syndrome [see p. 243], improvement after the operation is sometimes only
temporary and there is a high morbidity in subsequent years in over a third of
cases, usually due to persistent subdural haemorrhage, obstructive hydrocephalus, and haemosiderosis of the central nervous system due to chronic
bleeding (Falconer and Wilson, 1969). However, these long-term complications
are often remediable so that the operation should still be considered in appropriate cases.

REFERENCES

BENDA, C. E. (1952) *Developmental Disorders of Mentation and Cerebral Palsies*, New York.
BICKERSTAFF, E. R. (1964) Aetiology of acute hemiplegia in childhood, *Brit. med. J.*, **2**, 82.
ERBSLÖH, F., REH, H. E., and ZIEGLER, W. J. (1970) Kontrolaterale Hypotrophie der
    Skeletmuskulatur bei infantiler hemispastischer Cerebralparese, *Arch. Psychiat.
    Nervenkr.*, **213**, 282.
FALCONER, M. A., and WILSON, P. J. E. (1969) Complications related to delayed hemorrhage
    after hemispherectomy, *J. Neurosurg.*, **30**, 413.
FORD, F. R. (1926) Cerebral birth injuries and their results, *Medicine (Baltimore)*, **5**, 122.
FORD, F. R., CROTHERS, B., and PUTNAM, M. C. (1927) *Birth Injuries of the Central Nervous
    System*, London.

FORD, F. R., and SCHAFFER, A. J. (1927) The etiology of infantile acquired hemiplegia, *Arch. Neurol. Psychiat.* (*Chic.*), **18**, 323.

KRYNAUW, R. W. (1950) Infantile hemiplegia treated by removing one cerebral hemisphere, *J. Neurol. Psychiat.*, **12**, 243.

LeCOUNT, E. R., and SEMERAK, C. B. (1925) Porencephaly, *Arch. Neurol. Psychiat.* (*Chic.*), **14**, 365.

McKISSOCK, W. (1953) Infantile hemiplegia, *Proc. roy. Soc. Med.*, **46**, 431.

MENKES, J. H. (1974) *Textbook of Child Neurology*, Philadelphia.

NORMAN, R. M., URICH, H., and McMENEMEY, W. H. (1957) Vascular mechanisms of birth injury, *Brain*, **80**, 49.

TIZARD, J. P. M. (1953) The future of infantile hemiplegics, *Proc. roy. Soc. Med.*, **46**, 637.

TIZARD, J. P. M., PAINE, R. S., and CROTHERS, B. (1954) Disturbances of sensation in children with hemiplegia, *J. Amer. Med. Ass.*, **155**, 628.

WILSON, P. J. E. (1970) Cerebral hemispherectomy for infantile hemiplegia: a report of 50 cases, *Brain*, **93**, 147.

MINIMAL CEREBRAL DYSFUNCTION

It has been suggested that this is a condition of cerebral abnormality which, though not sufficient to cause easily identifiable syndromes of cerebral palsy, is severe enough to cause minor motor dysfunctions, epilepsy, learning difficulties, or abnormalities of behaviour (Bax and MacKeith, 1963). The concept of minimal cerebral dysfunction has been criticized as being 'an escape from making a diagnosis' (Ingram, 1973; *The Lancet*, 1973), and it is true that many cases so diagnosed have proved on careful scrutiny to be suffering from minor degrees of cerebral palsy in all its myriad forms. The hyperkinetic syndrome of infancy and early childhood (*British Medical Journal*, 1975) has sometimes been considered erroneously under this heading. However, the term may still be usefully employed to identify those visuomotor disorders, abnormalities of cognition and execution, which may be found in minor degree in otherwise normal school children (Clements and Peters, 1962; Brenner and Gillman, 1966) and which may result in educational difficulties. Certainly there are some children who show no evidence of a lesion in the primary motor or sensory pathways but who have disorders of skilled movement (praxis), of the recognition and interpretation of sensory information (gnosis), or of speech and related faculties, Some such are the so-called 'clumsy children' described by Gubbay *et al.* (1965) who showed marked clumsiness of movement without paralysis, incoordination, or sensory loss. Improvement with increasing maturity was the rule but educational difficulties were striking initially in the more severely affected cases. It is still uncertain as to whether this syndrome of developmental apraxic or agnosic ataxia (Gubbay, 1975), including the developmental Gerstmann syndrome (Benson and Geschwind, 1970), is due to identifiable pathological changes in the brain, to a disorder of the physiological establishment of cerebral dominance, or sometimes to one cause or the other in different cases.

REFERENCES

BAX, M., and MacKEITH, R. (1963) Minimal cerebral dysfunction, *Little Club Clinics in Developmental Medicine*, No. 10, London.

BENSON, D. F., and GESCHWIND, N. (1970) Developmental Gerstmann syndrome, *Neurology* (*Minneap.*), **20**, 293.

BRENNER, M. W., and GILLMAN, S. (1966) Visuomotor ability in schoolchildren—a survey, *Develop. Med. Child Neurol.*, **8**, 686.
BRITISH MEDICAL JOURNAL (1975) Hyperactivity in children, *Brit. med. J.*, **4**, 123.
CLEMENTS, S. D., and PETERS, J. E. (1962) Minimal brain dysfunctions in the school-age child, *Arch. Gen. Psychiat.*, **6**, 185.
GUBBAY, S. S. (1975) *The Clumsy Child*, London.
GUBBAY, S. S., ELLIS, E., WALTON, J. N., and COURT, S. D. M. (1965) Clumsy children, *Brain*, **88**, 295.
INGRAM, T. T. S. (1973) Soft signs, *Develop. Med. Child Neurol.*, **15**, 527.
THE LANCET (1973) Minimal brain dysfunction, *Lancet*, **2**, 487.

KERNICTERUS

This term has been applied to a disorder of infancy in which pathological examination of the affected brains reveals canary-yellow staining of the meninges, choroid plexus, basal ganglia (especially the globus pallidus), the dentate nuclei, the vermis, the hippocampus, and the medullary nuclei. In the affected areas there is widespread degeneration of neurones and secondary astrocytosis.

The condition is associated with an elevated blood level of indirect bilirubin to 20 mg per 100 ml or more in the neonatal period. Many reported cases have been due to icterus gravis neonatorum (erythroblastosis fetalis or haemolytic disease of the newborn) due to Rh or other rarer forms of blood-group incompatibility in which, for instance, an Rh-positive infant with an Rh-positive father is affected by the passage of antibodies across the placenta from a previously sensitized but Rh-negative mother (Gerrard, 1952). However, with the increasing use of early induction of labour, exchange transfusion, and other methods of treatment and prevention, the incidence of kernicterus due to this cause has declined. However, cases of kernicterus related to other factors, including prematurity, other forms of haemolytic anaemia, sepsis, acidosis, and the many causes of neonatal jaundice continue to be seen occasionally (Brown, 1964). Experimental studies have shown, however, that a high bilirubin alone will not damage the developing brain (Vogel, 1953) and it seems that only vulnerable nerve cells, perhaps abnormal as a result of various metabolic disturbances, will be affected (Lathe, 1955).

The affected infants are usually deeply jaundiced at birth, with bile in the stools and urine, and often show the haematological characteristics of haemolytic anaemia. Many untreated cases are fatal but few cases of neonatal haemolytic anaemia treated with early exchange transfusion now develop kernicterus. The development of the latter is usually heralded by coma, convulsions, and a decerebrate or decorticate posture with extensor spasms alternating with hypotonia. The survivors typically demonstrate nerve deafness, variable degrees of mental retardation, defects of vertical conjugate gaze, and neurological manifestations resembling those of bilateral choreoathetosis and/or dystonia (Evans and Polani, 1950; Byers *et al.*, 1955; Schaffer and Avery, 1971; Menkes, 1974).

REFERENCES

BROWN, A. K. (1964) Management of neonatal hyperbilirubinemia, *Obstet. Gynec.*, **7**, 985.
BYERS, R. K., PAINE, R. S., and CROTHERS, B. (1955) Extra-pyramidal cerebral palsy with hearing loss following erythroblastosis, *Pediatrics*, **15**, 248.

EVANS, P. R., and POLANI, P. E. (1950) The neurological sequelae of Rh sensitisation, *Quart. J. Med.*, **19**, 129.

GERRARD, J. (1952) Kernicterus, *Brain*, **75**, 526.

LATHE, G. H. (1955) Exchange transfusion as a means of removing bilirubin in haemolytic disease of the newborn, *Brit. med. J.*, **1**, 192.

MENKES, J. H. (1974) *Textbook of Child Neurology*, Philadelphia.

PARSONS, L. G. (1947) Haemolytic disease of the new-born, *Lancet*, **i**, 534.

ROBERTS, G. F. (1947) *The Rhesus Factor*, London.

SCHAFFER, A. J., and AVERY, M. E. (1971) *Diseases of the Newborn*, 3rd ed., Philadelphia.

VOGEL, F. S. (1953) Studies on the pathogenesis of kernicterus. With special reference to the nature of kernicteric pigment and its deposition under natural and experimental conditions, *J. exp. Med.*, **98**, 509.

ZIMMERMAN, H. M., and YANNET, H. (1933) Kernikterus: jaundice of the nuclear masses of the brain, *Amer. J. Dis. Child.*, **45**, 740.

ZIMMERMAN, H. M., and YANNET, H. (1935) Cerebral sequelae of icterus gravis neonatorum and their relation to kernikterus, *Amer. J. Dis. Child.*, **49**, 418.

INBORN ERRORS OF METABOLISM INCLUDING THE NEURONAL STORAGE DISORDERS

It may perhaps seem more logical to consider the disorders which fall into this group in CHAPTER 15 which deals with intoxications and metabolic disorders; however, in many of the conditions concerned, the nature of the primary metabolic defect responsible for what has long been considered to be a degenerative disorder has been elucidated only recently; developments in this field are occurring so quickly that no classification will satisfy everyone. Solely for this reason some of these rare diseases are considered here, others in CHAPTER 15; so many new conditions of this type are being discovered almost annually that only the most important disorders can be dealt with; for more comprehensive coverage of the topic see Menkes (1974). The following is a useful working classification of these diseases according to present knowledge.

A. Disorders of amino acid metabolism [see CHAPTER 15].
B. Disorders of lipid metabolism [see TABLE 13.1].
C. Disorders of serum lipoproteins.
D. Disorders of purine metabolism.
E. Disorders of carbohydrate metabolism.
F. Disorders of mucopolysaccharide metabolism.
G. Miscellaneous disorders of unknown aetiology.

THE LIPIDOSES

There are a number of inherited diseases which cause the deposition of abnormal lipid in the central and/or peripheral nervous system and sometimes in other tissues or organs. Within the last few years we have moved away from a clinical classification of these disorders, towards one based upon the nature of the material which is stored in abnormal amount and/or upon the nature of the enzymatic defect which is responsible. Unfortunately the phenotypical presentation of many different metabolic defects may be very similar and yet, on the other hand, apparently identical biochemical defects may occasionally produce very different clinical manifestations so that no single classification is uniformly satisfactory. All, however, are characterized by a progressive course of cerebral and often visual deterioration but varying considerably in tempo in the different varieties. Many of these disorders are now known as the gangliosidoses because various gangliosides are stored in the neurones of the central nervous system. A simplified classification of the lipidoses and of the metabolic defects responsible for them is given in Table 13.1.

TABLE 13.1

CLASSIFICATION OF THE LIPIDOSES

(modified from Cumings (1970), White (1973), Menkes (1974))

Disease	Lipid accumulated	Enzyme defect
Infantile amaurotic idiocy		
Tay–Sachs disease	Ganglioside GM_2	Hexosaminidase A
Sandhoff's disease	Ganglioside GM_2 plus globoside	Hexosaminidase A and B
Late infantile amaurotic idiocy (Batten–Bielschowsky group)		
Generalized GM_1 gangliosidosis	GM_1 ganglioside	beta-galactosidase
Juvenile GM_2 gangliosidosis	GM_2 ganglioside	Hexosaminidase A (partial)
Late infantile form with curvilinear bodies	Ceroid and lipofuscin	Unknown
Juvenile amaurotic idiocy (Spielmeyer–Vogt)	Often ceroid and lipofuscin (in occasional cases GM_2 ganglioside)	Usually unknown (in occasional cases hexosaminidase A—partial)
Neuronal ceroid-lipofuscinosis	Ceroid and lipofuscin	Unknown
Late onset lipidosis (Kufs)	Lipofuscin	Unknown
Niemann–Pick disease	Sphingomyelin	Sphingomyelinase
Gaucher's disease	Glucocerebroside	Glucocerebrosidase
Krabbe's disease	Galactocerebroside	beta-galactosidase
Metachromatic leuco-dystrophy (sulphatide lipidosis)	Sulphatide	Arylsulphatase A
Xanthomatoses		
Hand–Schuller–Christian disease	Cholesterol	Unknown
Farber's disease	Ceramide and gangliosides	Ceramidase
Wolman's disease	Triglyceride and esterified cholesterol	Unknown
Fabry's disease	Trihexosyl ceramide	alpha-galactosidase
Refsum's disease	Phytanic acid	Phytanic acid alpha-hydroxylase
Pelizaeus–Merzbacher disease	Unknown	Unknown
Alexander's disease	Unknown	Unknown
Canavan–van Bogaert–Bertrand disease	Unknown	Unknown

INFANTILE AMAUROTIC FAMILY IDIOCY

Synonyms. Cerebromacular degeneration; Tay–Sachs disease; Sandhoff's disease.

Definition. A disease of early life, frequently occurring in several members of the same family, characterized pathologically by widespread deposit of lipids, mainly gangliosides, in the ganglion cells of the brain and retina, and clinically by progressive mental failure, blindness, and paralysis.

PATHOLOGY

The pathological changes in Tay–Sachs disease (Tay, 1881; Sachs, 1887) and in Sandhoff's disease (Sandhoff *et al.*, 1968) are identical although in the former ganglioside GM_2 alone accumulates in the neurones and in the latter there is also accumulation of globoside. The neurones of the cerebral cortex, the Purkinje cells of the cerebellum, the retinal ganglion cells, and, to a lesser extent, the neurones of the brain stem and spinal cord become ballooned due to the accumulation of lipid, usually with peripheral displacement of the nucleus. Macroscopically the brain is often atrophic with ventricular dilatation and secondary demyelination, sometimes with cavitation of the white matter, but paradoxically in the late stages megalencephaly has been described (Crome and Stern, 1972). Electron microscopic examination of affected nerves, dendrites, and some glial cells shows 'membranous cytoplasmic bodies' (Terry and Weiss, 1963), sometimes called 'zebra bodies' because of the typical concentric laminations which they show due to the accumulation of gangliosides in the presence of phospholipids and cholesterol.

AETIOLOGY

Tay–Sachs disease is largely confined to infants of Ashkenazic Jewish ancestry, but Sandhoff's disease occurs in non-Jewish children. Both disorders are of autosomal recessive inheritance; the former is due to hexosaminidase A deficiency, while in the latter hexosaminidase B is also deficient (Suzuki *et al.*, 1971).

SYMPTOMS

The child is usually normal at birth but between three and six months of age listlessness and apathy develop with failure to reach normal developmental milestones. Convulsions subsequently develop in many cases, often with myoclonic jerking in response to 'startle'. Progressive flaccid paralysis of all four limbs usually develops but in the later stages may be replaced by spasticity and opisthotonus. There is a cherry-red spot at the macula and in early infancy this is virtually pathognomonic; atrophy of the optic disc and retina progress rapidly and eventually there is total blindness, but the pupil reactions are often preserved until relatively late. Progressive enlargement of the head occasionally occurs as a late manifestation; the disease is unresponsive to any form of treatment and invariably terminates fatally in the second or third year of life.

DIAGNOSIS

This is generally easy as no other disease causes such a progressive cerebral degeneration in early infancy in the absence of hepatosplenomegaly and with a cherry-red spot at the macula. A similar cherry-red spot may be seen in some cases of Niemann–Pick disease and in Gaucher's disease but in these cases it usually appears later and is accompanied by enlargement of the liver and spleen; it is also occasionally found in generalized GM_1 gangliosidosis (see below) in which there are also systemic manifestations. Schilder's disease may also cause progressive blindness, dementia, and paralysis in infancy but is of later onset, of variable clinical course, and does not as a rule cause optic atrophy or myoclonus. The EEG in Tay–Sachs disease often shows irregular, generalized spike and wave discharges (Cobb et al., 1952) while in Schilder's disease the changes are non-specific.

An assay of hexosaminidase in the serum will confirm the diagnosis and may also be used to detect heterozygous carriers (Okada and O'Brien, 1969). Antenatal diagnosis is now possible by measuring the hexosaminidase activity of amniotic cells obtained by amniocentesis (O'Brien et al., 1970).

REFERENCES

Cobb, W., Martin, F., and Pampiglione, G. (1952) Cerebral lipidosis: an electroencephalographic study, Brain, **75**, 343.

Crome, L., and Stern, J. (1972) Pathology of Mental Retardation, 2nd ed., Edinburgh and London.

Cumings, J. N. (1970) The lipidoses, in Handbook of Clinical Neurology, ed. Vinken, P. J., and Bruyn, G. W., vol. 10, chap. 15, Amsterdam.

Greenfield, J. G., and Holmes, G. (1925) The histology of juvenile amaurotic idiocy, Brain, **48**, 183.

Hassin, G. B. (1924) A study of the histopathology of amaurotic family idiocy, Arch. Neurol. Psychiat. (Chic.), **12**, 640.

Menkes, J. H. (1974) Textbook of Child Neurology, Philadelphia.

O'Brien, J. S., Okada, S., Chen, A., and Fillerup, D. L. (1970) Tay–Sachs disease: detection of heterozygotes and homozygotes by serum hexosaminidase assay, New Engl. J. Med., **283**, 15.

Okada, S., and O'Brien, J. S. (1969) Tay–Sachs disease: generalized absence of a beta-D-N-acetylhexosaminidase component, Science, **165**, 698.

Sachs, B. (1887) On arrested cerebral development, with special reference to its cortical pathology, J. nerv. ment. Dis., **15**, 541.

Sandhoff, K., Andreae, V., and Jatzkewitz, H. (1968) Deficient hexosaminidase activity in an exceptional case of Tay–Sachs disease with additional storage of kidney globoside in visceral organs, Life Sci., **7**, 283.

Suzuki, Y., Jacob, J. C., Suzuki, K., Kutty, K. M., and Suzuki, K. (1971) GM_2-gangliosidosis with total hexosaminidase deficiency, Neurology (Minneap.), **21**, 313.

Tay, W. (1881) Symmetrical changes in the region of the yellow spot in each eye of an infant, Trans. ophthal. Soc. U.K., **1**, 55.

Terry, R. D., and Weiss, M. (1963) Studies in Tay–Sachs disease: ultrastructure of cerebrum, J. Neuropath. exp. Neurol., **22**, 18.

White, H. H. (1973) Diseases due to inborn metabolic defects, in A Textbook of Neurology, ed. Merritt, H. H., pp. 652–6, Philadelphia.

LATE INFANTILE, JUVENILE, AND LATE ONSET AMAUROTIC IDIOCY

This group of disorders, previously classified under the inclusive title of the cerebromacular or cerebroretinal degenerations, and originally described by Vogt (1905), Spielmeyer (1906), Jansky (1909), Bielschowsky (1914), Batten (1914), and Kufs (1925), among others, is now known to embrace a large number of different degenerative disorders, all characterized by a progressive course, all familial and due as a rule to autosomal recessive inheritance, but resulting from a variety of different metabolic abnormalities, some identified comparatively recently and some as yet unknown. As Menkes (1974) points out, some have been identified as independent disease entities solely as a result of ultrastructural studies. Zeman and Dyken (1969) point out that age of onset alone is an unsafe guide to classification.

Generalized GM₁ Gangliosidosis

This condition, which is also called familial neurovisceral lipidosis, occurs in two main forms. Type I (Norman *et al.*, 1959), also known as pseudo-Hurler's disease, resembles Hurler's disease clinically in that the affected infants are hypotonic at birth, show severe developmental delay, and usually have large frontal bosses, depressed nasal bones, macroglossia, low-set ears, and generalized skeletal deformities. Hepatosplenomegaly is usually found at about 6 months of age and a cherry-red spot is present in about 50 per cent of cases. In type II, progressive mental deterioration, often with convulsions, begins at about 8 to 16 months of age and a cherry-red spot is usually present but bony abnormalities are absent and there is no enlargement of the liver or spleen.

In both varieties the neurones are distended with lipid as in Tay–Sachs disease and membranous cytoplasmic bodies as well as abnormal lysosomal accumulation are usually found ultrastructurally (Suzuki *et al.*, 1968; Derry *et al.*, 1968). As in Hurler's disease, beta-galactosidase is absent in leukocytes and fibroblasts but unlike the latter condition there is no abnormality of mucopolysaccharides.

Other Late Infantile, Juvenile, and Adult Forms

The principal problem in attempting to classify this group of disorders upon any rational basis is that if one excludes the relatively few cases in which an accumulation of GM₂ ganglioside has been found with a partial deficiency of hexosaminidase A (Suzuki and Suzuki, 1970; Menkes *et al.*, 1971), the nature of the accumulated lipid in the remaining cases and of the causal enzymatic defect is still unknown.

In the late infantile cases (Batten–Bielschowsky) there is no racial pre-dominance, a cherry-red spot at the macula is not usually found, and the affected children are usually normal until two to four years of age. The condition usually begins with myoclonic jerking, sometimes with generalized convulsions, and there is progressive ataxia, paralysis, and retinal degeneration with optic atrophy. Parkinsonian features occasionally appear; in most cases there is eventual spastic paralysis, but progression is slow with death usually occurring in late childhood.

By contrast, the juvenile cases (Spielmeyer–Vogt) usually present with pro-gressive impairment of vision and intellect between six and 14 years of age with retinal pigmentation and optic atrophy and slowly developing spastic paralysis without fits or ataxia. A presentation with progressive dystonia (juvenile dystonic lipidosis) has been described (Elfenbein, 1968).

The adult variety (Kufs's disease) which is rare (Kornfeld, 1972) does not usually cause blindness but generally presents with progressive spastic weakness and with epilepsy and/or dementia.

In many of the disorders within this group, vacuolated lymphocytes or cells sometimes resembling the 'sea-blue histiocytes' of Niemann–Pick disease may be found in the peripheral blood. The cerebrospinal fluid protein may be slightly raised. In contrast to the usual finding in Tay–Sachs disease, the electro-retinogram (ERG) is grossly abnormal or absent and the occipital visual evoked response (VER) is greatly increased in amplitude (Harden *et al.*, 1973). The EEG usually shows the typical irregular spike and wave discharge previously thought typical of 'cerebral lipidosis' (Cobb *et al.*, 1952) with an abnormal response to photic stimulation and is indeed much more abnormal in these cases as a rule than in Tay–Sachs disease (Pampiglione and Harden, 1973).

Pathological examination of brain material obtained from such cases shows neuronal swelling less marked than in the gangliosidoses and the material stored is PAS-positive but is not dissolved by the usual lipid solvents. In some such cases Zeman and Donahue (1963) described curvilinear cytoplasmic bodies showing a granular or multiloculated appearance on electron microscopy (Andrews *et al.*, 1971). Subsequently it was shown by histochemical studies (Zeman and Dyken, 1969) that much of the abnormal material was ceroid and lipofuscin and now many of these cases are classified under the inclusive title of **neuronal ceroid-lipofuscinosis** (Pellissier *et al.*, 1974). Indeed Zeman (1969) suggested that if one excludes the gangliosidoses, all of the conditions in this group represent varying manifestations of this primary pathological change, but this view is not universally accepted. However, others have shown that the characteristic cytoplasmic bodies may be found in skeletal muscle, peripheral nerve, and skin examined ultrastructurally (Carpenter *et al.*, 1972) and in the appendix (Rapola and Haltia, 1973). Certainly this type of patho-logical change is now being discovered frequently in cases of late infantile amaurotic idiocy (Santavuori *et al.*, 1973; Haltia *et al.*, 1973). Similar neuronal cytoplasmic bodies have been found in the brains of patients with Morquio's syndrome, which is now believed to belong to the mucopolysaccharidoses (Gilles and Deuel, 1971).

REFERENCES

ANDREWS, J. M., SORENSON, V., CANCILLA, P. A., PRICE, H. M., and MENKES, J. H. (1971) Late infantile neurovisceral storage disease with curvilinear bodies, *Neurology (Minneap.)*, **21**, 207.

BATTEN, F. E. (1914) Family cerebral degeneration with macular change (so-called juvenile form of family amaurotic idiocy), *Quart. J. Med.*, **7**, 444.

BIELSCHOWSKY, M. (1914) Uber spatinfantile familiare amaurotische Idiotie mit Klein-hirnsymptomen, *Deutsch. Z. Nervenheilk.*, **50**, 7.

CARPENTER, S., KARPATI, G., and ANDERMANN, F. (1972) Specific involvement of muscle, nerve, and skin in late infantile and juvenile amaurotic idiocy, *Neurology (Minneap.)*, **22**, 170.

COBB, W., MARTIN, F., and PAMPIGLIONE, G. (1952) Cerebral lipidosis: an electro-encephalographic study, *Brain*, **75**, 343.

DERRY, D. M., FAWCETT, J. S., ANDERMANN, F., and WOLFE, L. S. (1968) Late infantile systemic lipidosis. Major monosialogangliosidosis: delineation of two types, *Neurology (Minneap.)*, **18**, 340.

ELFENBEIN, I. B. (1968) Dystonic juvenile idiocy without amaurosis, a new syndrome: light and electron microscopic observations of cerebrum, *Johns Hopk. Med. J.*, **123**, 205.

GILLES, F. H., and DEUEL, R. K. (1971) Neuronal cytoplasmic globules in the brain in Morquio's syndrome, *Arch. Neurol. (Chic.)*, **25**, 393.

HALTIA, M., RAPOLA, J., SANTAVUORI, P., and KERÄNEN, A. (1973) Infantile type of so-called neuronal ceroid-lipofuscinosis. Part 2. Morphological and biochemical studies, *J. neurol. Sci.*, **18**, 269.

HARDEN, A., PAMPIGLIONE, G., and PICTON-ROBINSON, N. (1973) Electroretinogram and visual evoked response in a form of 'neuronal lipidosis' with diagnostic EEG features, *J. Neurol. Neurosurg. Psychiat.*, **36**, 61.

JANSKY, J. (1909) Uber einen noch nicht beschriebenen Fall der familiaren amaurotischen Idiotie mit Hypoplasie des Kleinhirns, *Z. Erforsch. Behandl. Jugendlich. Schwachsinns*, **3**, 86.

KORNFELD, M. (1972) Generalized lipofuscinosis (generalized Kufs' disease), *J. Neuropath. exp. Neurol.*, **31**, 668.

KUFS, M. (1925) Uber eine Spatform der amaurotischen Idiotie und ihre heredofamiliaren Grundlagen, *Z. Ges. Neurol. Psychiat.*, **95**, 169.

MENKES, J. H. (1974) *Textbook of Child Neurology*, Philadelphia.

MENKES, J. H., O'BRIEN, J. S., OKADA, S., GRIPPO, J., ANDREWS, J. M., and CANCILLA, P. A. (1971) Juvenile GM₂ gangliosidosis, *Arch. Neurol. (Chic.)*, **25**, 14.

NORMAN, R. M., URICH, H., TINGEY, A. H., and GOODBODY, R. A. (1959) Tay–Sachs disease with visceral involvement and its relationship to Niemann–Pick disease, *J. Path. Bact.*, **78**, 409.

PAMPIGLIONE, G., and HARDEN, A. (1973) Neurophysiological identification of a late infantile form of 'neuronal lipidosis', *J. Neurol. Neurosurg. Psychiat.*, **36**, 68.

PELLISSIER, J. F., HASSOUN, J., GAMBARELLI, D., TRIPIER, M. F., ROGER, J., and TOGA, M. (1974) Céroide-lipofuscinose neuronale. Etude ultrastructurale de deux biopsies cérébrales, *Acta Neuropath. (Berl.)*, **28**, 353.

RAPOLA, J., and HALTIA, M. (1973) Cytoplasmic inclusions in the vermiform appendix and skeletal muscle in two types of so-called neuronal ceroid-lipofuscinosis, *Brain*, **96**, 833.

SANTAVUORI, P., HALTIA, M., RAPOLA, J., and RAITTA, C. (1973) Infantile type of so-called neuronal ceroid-lipofuscinosis. Part 1. A clinical study of 15 patients, *J. neurol. Sci.*, **18**, 257.

SPIELMEYER, W. (1906) Ueber eine besondere Form von familiaerer amaurotischer Idiotie, *Neurol. Zbl.*, **25**, 51.

SUZUKI, K., SUZUKI, K., and CHEN, G. C. (1968) Morphological, histochemical and biochemical studies on a case of systemic late infantile lipidosis (generalized gangliosidosis), *J. Neuropath. exp. Neurol.*, **27**, 15.

SUZUKI, Y., and SUZUKI, K. (1970) Partial deficiency of hexosaminidase component A in juvenile GM₂-gangliosidosis, *Neurology (Minneap.)*, **20**, 848.

VOGT, H. (1905) Ueber familiaere amaurotische Idiotie und verwandte Krankheitsbilder, *Mschr. Psychiat. Neurol.*, **18**, 161, 310.

ZEMAN, W. (1969) What is amaurotic idiocy?, *Lipids*, **4**, 76.

ZEMAN, W., and DONAHUE, S. (1963) Fine structure of the lipid bodies in juvenile amaurotic idiocy, *Acta Neuropath.*, **3**, 144.

ZEMAN, W., and DYKEN, P. (1969) Neuronal ceroid-lipofuscinosis (Batten's disease): relationship to amaurotic family idiocy?, *Pediatrics*, **44**, 570.

NIEMANN-PICK DISEASE

Described by Niemann in 1914, this disorder, which is characterized by storage of sphingomyelin in the cells of the reticuloendothelial system and sometimes in the brain, is now known to occur in four distinct forms, all of autosomal recessive inheritance, which have been called types A to D (see Menkes, 1974). The classical form of the disease (type A), which is the commonest, usually affects Jewish children. Many show a cherry-red spot in the retina, and they develop hepatosplenomegaly and intellectual deterioration, usually in the first year of life, accompanied often by jaundice, anaemia, enlargement of the abdomen, and poor physical development. Myoclonus or generalized seizures are common and progressive spastic paralysis usually develops with death occurring before the age of five years (Fredrickson and Sloan, 1972). In some such cases, supranuclear ophthalmoplegia has been reported (Neville *et al.*, 1973). In type B, the viscera are involved but the nervous system is spared, while in type C neurological symptoms do not usually appear until two to four years of age and the clinical course is much slower; in type D the symptoms of nervous system involvement do not appear until even later in childhood and the course is slower still.

Pathologically the brain and retina show ballooned ganglion cells which have a characteristic vacuolated foamy appearance and contain large quantities of sphingomyelin (Crocker, 1961; Lynn and Terry, 1964). Diagnosis can be made by bone marrow examination, which sometimes reveals 'sea-blue histiocytes' (Neville *et al.*, 1973), by rectal biopsy, or by the assay of sphingomyelinase in leucocytes, in skin or bone marrow cultures (Kampine *et al.*, 1967; Sloan *et al.*, 1969), and prenatally in amniotic cell cultures in types A and B, but not in types C and D.

REFERENCES

CROCKER, A. C. (1961) The cerebral defect in Tay–Sachs disease and Niemann–Pick disease, *J. Neurochem.*, **7,** 69.

FREDRICKSON, D. S., and SLOAN, H. R. (1972) Sphingomyelin lipidoses: Niemann–Pick disease, in *The Metabolic Basis of Inherited Disease*, 3rd ed., ed. Stanbury, J. B., Wyngaarden, J. B., and Fredrickson, D. S., p. 783, New York.

KAMPINE, J., BRADY, R., and KANFER, J. (1967) Diagnosis of Gaucher's disease and Niemann–Pick disease with small samples of venous blood, *Science*, **155,** 86.

LYNN, R., and TERRY, R. D. (1964) Lipid histochemistry and electron microscopy in adult Niemann–Pick disease, *Amer. J. Med.*, **37,** 987.

MENKES, J. H. (1974) *Textbook of Child Neurology*, Philadelphia.

NEVILLE, B. G. R., LAKE, B. D., STEPHENS, R., and SANDERS, M. D. (1973) A neuro-visceral storage disease with vertical supranuclear ophthalmoplegia and its relationship to Niemann–Pick disease—a report of nine patients, *Brain*, **96,** 97.

NIEMANN, A. (1914) Ein unbekanntes Krankheitsbild, *Jahrb. Kinderheilk.*, **79,** 1.

SLOAN, H. R., UHLENDORF, B. W., and KANFER, J. N. (1969) Deficiency of sphingomyelin-cleaving enzyme activity in tissue cultures derived from patients with Niemann–Pick disease, *Biochem. Biophys. Res. Commun.*, **34,** 582.

GAUCHER'S DISEASE

This rare disease, first described by Gaucher in 1882, is usually due to an autosomal recessive gene but occasional families showing dominant inheritance have been described (Pratt, 1967). It is due to the storage of cerebroside in the cells of the reticuloendothelial system and sometimes in the brain, resulting from a deficiency of glucocerebrosidase, but so-called juvenile Gaucher's disease is probably now to be regarded as GM_3 gangliosidosis (Menkes, 1974). In the commonest chronic form of the disease there is marked progressive enlargement of the liver and spleen but the nervous system is not involved. In the less common infantile cases (Barlow, 1957; van Bogaert, 1957) there is severe involvement of the brain with progressive apathy, sometimes strabismus, and signs of pseudobulbar palsy with progressive spastic paralysis of the limbs and decerebrate rigidity. Convulsions sometimes occur and the disease is usually fatal before the end of the first year of life. Sometimes radiography of long bones shows areas of rarefaction, particularly in the lower ends of the femora.

Pathologically the characteristic feature in the cells of the spleen, bone marrow, or brain is the presence of large spherical or oval Gaucher cells which show a lacy, striated appearance of the cytoplasm. In the infantile cases the defective enzyme is probably glucosyl ceramide beta-glucosidase (Brady *et al.*, 1966). The diagnosis may also be made by estimation of this enzyme in cultures of leucocytes or skin fibroblasts.

Splenectomy is sometimes performed simply because of the massive splenic enlargement and the risk of rupture in chronic cases but has no influence upon the course of the disease.

REFERENCES

BARLOW, C. (1957) Neuropathological findings in a case of Gaucher's disease, *J. Neuropath. exp. Neurol.*, **16**, 239.

BOGAERT, L. VAN (1957) *Cerebral Lipidoses*, Springfield, Ill.

BRADY, R. O., KANFER, J. N., BRADLEY, R. M., and SHAPIRO, D. (1966) Demonstration of a deficiency of glucocerebroside-cleaving enzyme in Gaucher's disease, *J. clin. Invest.*, **45**, 1112.

GAUCHER, P. (1882) *De l'Epithelioma Primitif de la Rate*, Thèse, Paris.

MENKES, J. H. (1974) *Textbook of Child Neurology*, Philadelphia.

PRATT, R. T. C. (1967) *The Genetics of Neurological Disorders*, London.

KRABBE'S DISEASE

This condition, which is also called globoid cell leucodystrophy, was first delineated by Krabbe in 1916. Galactocerebroside accumulates in the brain and peripheral nerves and sulphatide is reduced. It usually begins at four to six months of age and gives rise to convulsions, restlessness, and irritability followed by progressive rigidity and ultimately bulbar paralysis. Tonic spasms induced by noise or other forms of sensory stimulation are common. Optic atrophy is sometimes seen. Despite the generalized rigidity the tendon reflexes are usually depressed. The disease is uninfluenced by treatment and is invariably fatal within a few months or years, though rare cases with survival into adult life have been described. The cerebrospinal fluid protein is invariably raised and motor and sensory conduction in the peripheral nerves is delayed (Bischoff and Ulrich, 1969; Dunn *et al.*, 1969). A similar disorder has been reported in dogs (Roszel *et al.*, 1972).

The characteristic pathological feature of this disorder is one of widespread demyelination of the white matter of the cerebrum, cerebellum, and spinal cord; the brain shows minimal sparing of the subcortical arcuate fibres. Thus the pathological changes are those of a demyelinating disease [see CHAPTER 11] rather than of a neuronal storage disorder. In the areas of demyelination epithelioid cells and large multinuclear globoid cells, 20–50 μm in diameter, are seen and may also be found in the peripheral nerves (Hogan *et al.*, 1969). Ultrastructurally these cells show cytoplasmic inclusions which are tubular in longitudinal section but irregularly crystalloid in transverse section (Suzuki and Grover, 1970; Liu, 1970; Andrews *et al.*, 1971). The condition appears to be due to an inherited deficiency of galactocerebroside beta-galactosidase (Austin *et al.*, 1970).

REFERENCES

ANDREWS, J. M., CANCILLA, P. A., GRIPPO, J., and MENKES, J. H. (1971) Globoid cell leukodystrophy (Krabbe's disease): morphological and biochemical studies, *Neurology (Minneap.)*, **21**, 337.
AUSTIN, J., SUZUKI, K., ARMSTRONG, D., BRADY, R., BACHHAWAT, B. K., SCHLENKER, J., and STUMPF, D. (1970) Studies in globoid (Krabbe) leukodystrophy (GLD). V. Controlled enzymic studies in ten human cases, *Arch. Neurol. (Chic.)*, **23**, 502.
BISCHOFF, A., and ULRICH, J. (1969) Peripheral neuropathy in globoid cell leukodystrophy (Krabbe's disease). Ultrastructural and histochemical findings, *Brain*, **92**, 861.
DUNN, H. G., LAKE, B. D., DOLMAN, C. L., and WILSON, J. (1969) The neuropathy of Krabbe's infantile cerebral sclerosis (globoid cell leukodystrophy), *Brain*, **92**, 329.
HOGAN, G. R., GUTMANN, L., and CHOU, S. M. (1969) The peripheral neuropathy of Krabbe's (globoid) leukodystrophy, *Neurology (Minneap.)*, **19**, 1094.
KRABBE, K. (1916) A new familial, infantile form of diffuse brain sclerosis, *Brain*, **39**, 74.
LIU, H. M. (1970) Ultrastructure of globoid leukodystrophy (Krabbe's disease) with reference to the origin of globoid cells, *J. Neuropath. exp. Neurol.*, **29**, 441.
ROSZEL, J. F., STEINBERG, S. A., and McGRATH, J. T. (1972) Periodic acid–Schiff-positive cells in cerebrospinal fluid of dogs with globoid cell leukodystrophy, *Neurology (Minneap.)*, **22**, 738.
SUZUKI, K., and GROVER, W. D. (1970) Krabbe's leukodystrophy (globoid cell leukodystrophy): an ultrastructural study, *Arch. Neurol. (Chic.)*, **22**, 385.

METACHROMATIC LEUCODYSTROPHY
(SULPHATIDE LIPIDOSIS)

This disorder was first described by Greenfield in 1933 and in 1950 Brain and Greenfield suggested that it was a form of diffuse cerebral sclerosis which they identified as 'late infantile metachromatic leucoencephalopathy with primary degeneration of the interfascicular oligodendroglia'. However, in 1960 Austin showed that the condition was due to the accumulation of sulphatide (cerebroside sulphate) in neurones but more particularly in myelin and glial cells in the cerebral white matter and also in peripheral nerve; hence the condition is now classified with the lipidoses. Subsequently he demonstrated a primary deficiency of arylsulphatase A (Austin *et al.*, 1965).

The commonest variety of this autosomal recessive condition is the late infantile, which usually develops in the second or third year of life with progressive difficulty in walking, clumsiness in the upper limbs, occasional strabismus, and subsequently progressive spastic (or flaccid) paralysis, dementia, and bulbar paralysis. Death is usual within six months to four years. Convulsions are uncommon, occurring late if at all, but optic atrophy is not infrequent. The tendon reflexes are often lost due to peripheral nerve involvement, motor and sensory nerve conduction velocity is usually slowed (Fullerton, 1964), and the cerebrospinal fluid protein is usually increased.

A juvenile form of the condition has been described (Austin, 1965; Menkes, 1966) beginning between five and seven years of age and progressing slowly. An adult variety is also relatively common (Austin *et al.*, 1968; Betts *et al.*, 1968; Hirose and Bass, 1972) and usually presents with progressive facile euphoric dementia, occasionally with psychotic features, and ultimately with slowly developing signs of corticospinal tract dysfunction and with variable evidence of subclinical polyneuropathy.

Pathologically there is diffuse demyelination of the white matter of the brain, spinal cord, and peripheral nerves with loss of oligodendroglia and with the accumulation of metachromatic granules due to the accumulation of sulphatide in neurones and glial cells but more particularly in the areas of demyelination. These granules stain brown rather than blue with stains such as cresyl violet or thionine. Similar metachromatic granules may be found in the renal tubules and may thus be isolated from centrifuged specimens of urine, and they may also be found in saliva. At autopsy they are also present in gall bladder, pancreas, and liver. Ultrastructurally they are seen as compact 'myelin bodies' in brain or as torpedo-like structures in peripheral nerve (Liu, 1968). Diagnosis has been made in the past by examination of the urine, by brain, peripheral nerve, or rectal biopsy (Julius et al., 1971) or by measurement of urinary arylsulphatase A (Austin et al., 1966; Stumpf and Austin, 1971) but the simplest and most reliable test is by estimating the enzyme in leucocytes obtained from venous blood (Percy and Brady, 1968). The enzyme deficiency is the same in infantile, juvenile, and adult cases, a fact which remains unexplained. This test is also successful in identifying heterozygous carriers (Bass et al., 1970) but treatment of the condition with purified arylsulphatase does not produce clinical benefit (Greene et al., 1969).

REFERENCES

AUSTIN, J. (1960) Metachromatic form of diffuse sclerosis: III. Significance of sulfatide and other lipid abnormalities in white matter and kidney, *Neurology (Minneap.)*, **10,** 470.

AUSTIN, J. (1965) Mental retardation. Metachromatic leucodystrophy, in *Medical Aspects of Mental Retardation*, ed. Carter, C. H., p. 768, Springfield, Ill.

AUSTIN, J., ARMSTRONG, D., FOUCH, S., MITCHELL, C., STUMPF, D., SHEARER, I., and BRINER, O. (1968) Metachromatic leukodystrophy (MLD). VIII. MLD in adults: diagnosis and pathogenesis, *Arch. Neurol. (Chic.)*, **18,** 225.

AUSTIN, J., ARMSTRONG, D., and SHEARER, L. (1965) Metachromatic form of diffuse cerebral sclerosis. V. The nature and significance of low sulfatase activity: a controlled study of brain, liver and kidney in four patients with metachromatic leukodystrophy (MLD), *Arch. Neurol. (Chic.)*, **13,** 593.

AUSTIN, J., ARMSTRONG, D., SHEARER, L., and MCAFEE, D. (1966) Metachromatic form of diffuse cerebral sclerosis. VI. A rapid test for the sulfatase A deficiency in meta-chromatic leukodystrophy (MLD) urine, *Arch. Neurol. (Chic.)*, **14,** 259.

BASS, N. H., WITMER, E. J., and DREIFUSS, F. E. (1970) A pedigree study of metachromatic leukodystrophy. Biochemical identification of the carrier state, *Neurology (Minneap.)*, **20,** 52.

BETTS, T. A., SMITH, W. T., and KELLY, R. E. (1968) Adult metachromatic leukodystrophy (sulphatide lipidosis) simulating acute schizophrenia: report of a case, *Neurology (Minneap.)*, **18,** 1140.

BRAIN, W. R., and GREENFIELD, J. G. (1950) Late infantile metachromatic leucoencephalo-pathy with primary degeneration of the interfascicular oligodendroglia, *Brain*, **73,** 291.

FULLERTON, P. M. (1964) Peripheral nerve conduction in metachromatic leucoencephalo-pathy (sulphatide lipidosis), *J. Neurol. Psychiat.*, **27,** 100.

GREENE, H. L., HUG, G., and SCHUBERT, W. K. (1969) Metachromatic leukodystrophy. Treatment with arylsulfatase-A, *Arch. Neurol. (Chic.)*, **20,** 147.

GREENFIELD, J. G. (1933) A form of progressive cerebral sclerosis in infants associated with primary degeneration of the interfascicular glia, *J. Neurol. Psychopath.*, **13,** 289.

HIROSE, G., and BASS, N. H. (1972) Metachromatic leukodystrophy in the adult. A bio-chemical study, *Neurology (Minneap.)*, **22**, 312.

JULIUS, R., BUEHLER, B., AYLSWORTH, A., PETERY, L. S., RENNERT, O., and GREER, M. (1971) Diagnostic techniques in metachromatic leukodystrophy, *Neurology (Minneap.)*, **21**, 15.

LIU, H. M. (1968) Ultrastructure of central nervous system lesions in metachromatic leukodystrophy with special reference to morphogenesis, *J. Neuropath. exp. Neurol.*, **27**, 624.

MENKES, J. H. (1966) Chemical studies of two cerebral biopsies in juvenile metachromatic leukodystrophy: the molecular composition of cerebrosides and sulfatides, *J. Pediat.*, **69**, 422.

PERCY, A. K., and BRADY, R. O. (1968) Metachromatic leukodystrophy: diagnosis with samples of venous blood, *Science*, **161**, 594.

STUMPF, D., and AUSTIN, J. (1971) Metachromatic leukodystrophy (MLD). IX. Qualitative and quantitative differences in urinary arylsulfatase A in different forms of MLD, *Arch. Neurol. (Chic.)*, **24**, 117.

XANTHOMATOSES

Hand–Schüller–Christian Disease. In this rare disease described by Hand (1893), Schüller (1915), and Christian (1919) there is a massive accumulation of cholesterol in the cells of the reticuloendothelial system and in the bones of the skull. The cholesterol-containing cells show a typical foamy appearance histologically; the liver and spleen are often enlarged and the lymph nodes, lungs, and pleura may be involved. X-rays of the skull and pelvis commonly show extensive areas of rarefaction in membranous bones.

The usual neurological manifestations are diabetes insipidus due to invasion of the pituitary and tuber cinereum by xanthomatous deposits and exophthalmos due to involvement of the orbital tissues. However, plaques of demyelination with foam cells in the brain have been described by Davison (1933) and Feigin (1956), and Elian *et al.* (1969) reported an adult male in whom a large dural xanthoma produced signs of an intracranial space-occupying lesion. Diabetes insipidus usually responds to treatment with pitressin but retardation of growth and mental development are common and the disease is ultimately fatal.

Farber's Disease. This rare disorder, also called lipogranulomatosis (Farber *et al.*, 1957) produces irritability and hoarseness of the cry within the first few weeks of life. Subcutaneous nodules and erythematous swellings develop, usually in relationship to joints, mental and motor retardation are both severe, and the condition is usually fatal before the age of two years. Ceramides and gangliosides accumulate in neurones and glial cells in the central nervous system and in mesenchymal cells in the subcutaneous tissue due to a deficiency of ceramidase (Sugita *et al.*, 1972).

Wolman's Disease. In 1956 Abramov *et al.* described this rare syndrome which resembles clinically Niemann–Pick disease type A and is also charac-terized by failure to gain weight, malabsorption, and adrenal insufficiency. There is massive hepatosplenomegaly and calcification of the adrenals (Wolman *et al.*, 1961; Guazzi *et al.*, 1968). Mental retardation is usual but other neuro-logical manifestations are usually absent. Sudanophilic lipid (triglyceride and free and esterified cholesterol) is stored in the leptomeninges and in liver, spleen, intestine, adrenals, and lymph nodes. Acanthocytosis of red blood cells is common. A defect of acid lipase is responsible.

Cerebrotendinous Xanthomatosis. This rare disease (van Bogaert *et al.*, 1937; Menkes *et al.*, 1968), due to cholestanol (dihydrocholesterol) deposition in the nervous system, gives rise to cataracts, cerebellar ataxia, and dementia, associated with xanthomas of tendons and in the lungs. It is very slowly progressive, uninfluenced by treatment, and can be diagnosed by estimation of cholestanol in the serum and red cells.

REFERENCES

ABRAMOV, A., SCHORR, S., and WOLMAN, M. (1956) Generalized xanthomatosis with calcified adrenals, *Amer. J. Dis. Child.*, **91**, 282.

BOGAERT, L. VAN, SCHERER, H. J., and EPSTEIN, E. (1937) *Une Forme Cerebrale de la Cholesterinose Generalisée*, Paris.

CHRISTIAN, H. A. (1919) Defects in membranous bones, exophthalmos, and diabetes insipidus, *Contr. Med. Biol. Res.*, **1**, 390, New York.

DAVISON, C. (1933) Xanthomatosis and the central nervous system, *Arch. Neurol. Psychiat. (Chic.)*, **30**, 75.

ELIAN, M., BORNSTEIN, B., MATZ, S., ASKENASY, H. M., and SANDBANK, U. (1969) Neurological manifestations of general xanthomatosis. Hand–Schüller–Christian disease, *Arch. Neurol. (Chic.)*, **21**, 115.

FARBER, S., COHEN, J., and UZMAN, L. L. (1957) Lipogranulomatosis: a new lipoglycoprotein 'storage' disease, *J. Mount Sinai Hosp. N.Y.*, **24**, 816.

FEIGIN, I. (1956) Xanthomatosis of nervous system, *J. Neuropath. exp. Neurol.*, **15**, 400.

GUAZZI, G. C., MARTIN, J. J., PHILIPPART, M., ROELS, H., VAN DER EECKEN, H., VRINTS, L., DELBEKE, M. J., and HOOFT, C. (1968) Wolman's disease, *Europ. Neurol.*, **1**, 334.

HEATH, P. (1931) Xanthomatosis or lipoid histiocytosis; report of ocular observations in 2 cases of Christian's syndrome: correlation with other ocular syndromes, *Arch. Ophthal. (Chic.)*, **5**, 29.

MENKES, J. H., SCHIMSCHOCK, J. R., and SWANSON, P. D. (1968) Cerebrotendinous xanthomatosis: the storage of cholesterol within the nervous system, *Arch. Neurol. (Chic.)*, **19**, 47.

MORISON, J. M. W. (1934) Schüller's disease, *Brit. J. Radiol.*, **7**, 213.

SCHÜLLER, A. (1915) Uber eigenartige Schädeldefekte im Jugendalter, *Fortschr. Röntgenstr.*, **23**, 12.

SUGITA, M., DULANEY, J. T., and MOSER, H. W. (1972) Ceramidase deficiency in Farber's disease (lipogranulomatosis), *Science*, **178**, 1100.

WOLMAN, M., STERK, V. V., GATT, S., and FRENKEL, M. (1961) Primary familial xanthomatosis with involvement and calcification of the adrenals, *Pediatrics*, **28**, 742.

FABRY'S DISEASE

This rare disorder (angiokeratoma corporis diffusum) is inherited as an X-linked recessive trait and rarely produces symptoms in heterozygous females (Wise *et al.*, 1962). It is due to the deposition of ceramide tri- and di-hexosides in vacuolated foamy cells in smooth, cardiac, and striated muscle, in the bone marrow, in reticuloendothelial cells, and in the renal glomeruli, resulting from a deficiency of alpha-galactosidase. In the central nervous system the storage of the abnormal lipid is usually confined to the walls of the blood vessels, sometimes resulting in thrombosis, but autonomic neurones are sometimes directly involved (Christensen-Lou and Reske-Nielsen, 1971).

In childhood the presenting feature is usually a punctate rash on the face, buttocks, and genitalia, and fever, abdominal and joint pain as well as weight loss are common. Painful paraesthesiae in the extremities are also common as well as excruciating episodes of abdominal, chest, and muscle pain which may be relieved by diphenylhydantoin (Lockman *et al.*, 1973); the pain may well be due to involvement of dorsal root ganglion cells (Kahn, 1973) or peripheral nerves (Kocen and Thomas, 1970). Corneal opacities may be found on slit-lamp examination. Hypertension and episodes of cerebral infarction or haemorrhage are not uncommon when the condition presents first in adult life. The disease is progressive and is uninfluenced by treatment including intravenous infusion of purified alpha-galactosidase (Mapes *et al.*, 1970). Death is usually due to renal failure.

The diagnosis can be made by renal biopsy or by the demonstration of specific crystalline inclusions on electron microscopy of skin fibroblasts grown in tissue culture (McLean and Stewart, 1974).

REFERENCES

CHRISTENSEN-LOU, H. O., and RESKE-NIELSEN, E. (1971) The central nervous system in Fabry's disease. A clinical, pathological and biochemical investigation, *Arch. Neurol. (Chic.)*, **25**, 351.

KAHN, P. (1973) Anderson–Fabry disease: a histopathological study of three cases with observations on the mechanism of production of pain, *J. Neurol. Neurosurg. Psychiat.*, **36**, 1053.

KOCEN, R. S., and THOMAS, P. K. (1970) Peripheral nerve involvement in Fabry's disease, *Arch. Neurol. (Chic.)*, **22**, 81.

LOCKMAN, L. A., HUNNINGHAKE, D. B., KRIVIT, W., and DESNICK, R. J. (1973) Relief of pain of Fabry's disease by diphenylhydantoin, *Neurology (Minneap.)*, **23**, 871.

MAPES, C. A., ANDERSON, R. L., and SWEELEY, C. C. (1970) Enzyme replacement in Fabry's disease: an inborn error of metabolism, *Science*, **169**, 987.

MCLEAN, J., and STEWART, G. (1974) Fabry's disease: specific inclusions found on electron microscopy of fibroblast cultures, *J. med. Genet.*, **11**, 133.

WISE, D., WALLACE, H. J., and JELLINEK, E. H. (1962) Angiokeratoma corporis diffusum, *Quart. J. Med.*, **31**, 177.

REFSUM'S DISEASE
(HEREDOPATHIA ATACTICA POLYNEURITIFORMIS)

This progressive degenerative disorder of the nervous system was described in 1946 by Refsum in two families in which the affected individuals showed retinal pigmentation, nerve deafness, ataxia, muscular atrophy, and other evidence of peripheral neuropathy. Cammermeyer in 1956 showed that lipid was deposited in the neurones and in macrophages in areas of central and peripheral demyelination in this disease, and in 1965 Richterich *et al.* showed that the lipid which accumulated was 3,7,11,15-tetramethyl hexadecanoic acid (phytanic acid) due to a block in the alpha-oxidation of phytanic to pristanic acid. The condition is due to an autosomal recessive gene; it usually begins between the ages of four and seven years with symptoms and signs of a poly-neuropathy followed by visual deterioration and ataxia. The eyes show optic atrophy and retinal pigmentation without the vascular changes of true retinitis pigmentosa. Less constant features are fixed pupils, nerve deafness, ichthyosis, cataracts, bony abnormalities, and a cardiomyopathy with prolongation of the

QT segment and QRS complex in the electrocardiogram. The peripheral nerves often become hypertrophied and show 'onion-bulb' formation.

The cerebrospinal fluid protein is usually raised to between 100 and 600 mg/100 ml and the serum phytanic acid (normal 0·2 mg/100 ml) is raised to 10–50 mg/100 ml. Motor and sensory nerve conduction in peripheral nerves is markedly slowed. Nerve biopsy is sometimes used to confirm the diagnosis.

The condition runs an indolent course with slow deterioration occurring over many years. A diet devoid of phytol (a derivative of chlorophyll which is a phytanic acid precursor) has been shown to produce striking improvement (Eldjarn et al., 1966; Steinberg et al., 1970; Lundberg et al., 1972).

REFERENCES

CAMMERMEYER, J. (1956) Neuropathologic changes in hereditary neuropathies: manifestation of the syndrome heredopathia atactica polyneuritiformis in the presence of interstitial hypertrophic polyneuropathy, J. Neuropath. exp. Neurol., 15, 340.

ELDJARN, L., TRY, K., STOKKE, O., MUNTHE-KAAS, A. W., REFSUM, S., STEINBERG, D., AUIGUN, J., and MIZE, C. (1966) Dietary effects on serum-phytanic acid levels and on clinical manifestations in heredopathia atactica polyneuritiformis, Lancet, i, 691.

LUNDBERG, A., LILJA, L. G., LUNDBERG, P. O., and TRY, K. (1972) Heredopathia atactica polyneuritiformis (Refsum's disease): experiences of dietary treatment and plasmapheresis, Europ. Neurol., 8, 309.

REFSUM, S. (1946) Heredopathia atactica polyneuritiformis, Acta psychiat. (Kbh.), Suppl. 38.

RICHTERICH, R., VAN MECHELEN, D., and ROSSI, E. (1965) Refsum's disease. An inborn error of lipid metabolism with storage of 3,7,11,15-tetramethyl hexadecanoic acid, Amer. J. Med., 39, 230.

STEINBERG, D., MIZE, C. E., HERNDON, J. H., FALES, H. M., ENGEL, W. K., and VROOM, F. Q. (1970) Phytanic acid in patients with Refsum's syndrome and response to dietary treatment, Arch. Intern. Med., 125, 75.

PELIZAEUS–MERZBACHER DISEASE

This rare demyelinating disorder first described by Pelizaeus (1885) and Merzbacher (1910) most commonly presents as an X-linked recessive disorder beginning before three months of age with jerky head movements, disorganized eye movements, and irregular nystagmus followed by the gradual development of cerebellar ataxia, involuntary movements, and ultimately spasticity in all four limbs (Tyler, 1958). The CSF is normal and the diagnosis is rarely made during life. There is a less common form of the disease of later onset and dominant inheritance (Camp and Lowenberg, 1941; Zeman et al., 1964), and an atypical family with late onset and probable autosomal recessive inheritance has been described (Fahmy et al., 1969). Pathologically there is patchy demyelination of the cerebral white matter, often in perivascular distribution, with accumulation of sphingomyelin but not of cholesterol esters. Seitelberger (1963) postulated a disorder of glycerophosphatide metabolism but the pathogenesis and biochemical basis of the condition are both unknown.

REFERENCES

CAMP, C. D., and LOWENBERG, K. (1941) An American family with Pelizaeus–Merzbacher disease, Arch. Neurol. Psychiat. (Chic.), 45, 261.

FAHMY, A., CARTER, T., PAULSON, G., and NANCE, W. E. (1969) A 'new' form of hereditary cerebral sclerosis, *Arch. Neurol. (Chic.)*, **20**, 468.

MERZBACHER, L. (1910) Eine eigenartige familiär-hereditäre Erkrankungsform, *Z. Ges. Neurol. Psychiat.*, **3**, 1.

PELIZAEUS, F. (1885) Ueber eine eigentümliche Form spastischer Lähmung mit Cerebralerscheinungen auf hereditärer Grundlage, *Arch. Psychiat. Nervenkr.*, **16**, 698.

SEITELBERGER, F. (1963) Contribution to Pelizaeus–Merzbacher's disease, in *Brain Lipids and Lipoproteins and the Leucodystrophies*, ed. Folch-pi, J., and Bauer, H., New York.

TYLER, H. R. (1958) Pelizaeus–Merzbacher disease, *Arch. Neurol. Psychiat. (Chic.)*, **80**, 162.

ZEMAN, W., DEMYER, W., and FALLS, H. F. (1964) Pelizaeus–Merzbacher's disease: a study in nosology, *J. Neuropath. exp. Neurol.*, **23**, 334.

ALEXANDER'S DISEASE

In 1949, Alexander reported a degenerative neurological disorder in an infant characterized by mental retardation and progressive enlargement of the head. Pathologically the condition is characterized by eosinophilic hyaline bodies (Rosenthal fibres) deposited in subpial and perivascular bands distributed randomly throughout the cerebral white matter (Schochet *et al.*, 1968). On electron microscopy these bodies consist of granular osmophilic masses resulting from the conglutination of altered glial filaments. An onset in adult life has been described (Seil *et al.*, 1968) though the condition usually begins in infancy or early childhood. It has also been called hyaline panneuropathy or dysmyelinogenic leucodystrophy.

REFERENCES

ALEXANDER, W. S. (1949) Progressive fibrinoid degeneration of fibrillary astrocytes associated with mental retardation in a hydrocephalic infant, *Brain*, **72**, 373.

SCHOCHET, S. S., LAMPERT, P. W., and EARLE, K. M. (1968) Alexander's disease: a case report with electron microscopic observations, *Neurology (Minneap.)*, **18**, 543.

SEIL, F. J., SCHOCHET, S. S., and EARLE, K. M. (1968) Alexander's disease in an adult: report of a case, *Arch. Neurol. (Chic.)*, **19**, 494.

CANAVAN'S DIFFUSE SCLEROSIS
(VAN BOGAERT–BERTRAND)

Canavan in 1931 described a rare degenerative disorder of early infancy, probably of autosomal recessive inheritance, characterized by progressive mental deterioration and megalocephaly. Van Bogaert and Bertrand (1949) noted the occurrence of the disorder in Jewish families and pointed out that many cases also showed progressive loss of vision and bilateral spastic weakness. Pathologically the condition is characterized by spongy degeneration of the brain with vacuolation in the deeper layers of the cerebral cortex and subjacent white matter; there is also total myelin loss in the white matter of the cerebral and cerebellar hemispheres with relative preservation of neurones and axons and ballooning of the astrocytes (Kamoshita *et al.*, 1967; 1968). Most affected children die before the age of two years. The pathogenesis is unknown although lysosomal enzyme activity is increased in skin fibroblasts cultured from such cases (Milunsky *et al.*, 1972). Menkes (1974) suggests that mitochondrial dysfunction may lead to chronic cerebral oedema which is a feature of such cases; the condition should probably be classified as a dysmyelinating disorder but its pathogenesis is still unknown.

REFERENCES

BOGAERT, L. VAN, and BERTRAND, L. (1949) Sur une idiotie familiale avec dégénérescence spongieuse du nervaxe, *Acta Neurol. Belg.*, **49**, 572.
CANAVAN, M. M. (1931) Schilder's encephalitis periaxalis diffusa, *Acta Neurol. Psychiat. (Chic.)*, **25**, 299.
KAMOSHITA, S., RAPIN, I., SUZUKI, K., and SUZUKI, K. (1968) Spongy degeneration of the brain: a chemical study of two cases including isolation and characterization of myelin, *Neurology (Minneap.)*, **18**, 975.
KAMOSHITA, S., REED, G. B., and AGUILAR, M. J. (1967) Axonal dystrophy in a case of Canavan's spongy degeneration, *Neurology (Minneap.)*, **17**, 895.
MENKES, J. H. (1974) *Textbook of Child Neurology*, Philadelphia.
MILUNSKY, A., KANFER, J. N., SPIELVOGEL, C., and SHAHOOD, J. M. (1972) Elevated lysosomal enzyme activities in Canavan's disease, *Pediat. Res.*, **6**, 425.

COCKAYNE'S SYNDROME

This rare disorder (Cockayne, 1936, 1946; Rowlatt, 1969) of recessive inheritance but unknown aetiology gives mental and physical retardation beginning usually after the first year of life. Clinically it causes microcephaly, dwarfism, a so-called 'bird facies', retinal pigmentation, deafness, large hands and feet, and a thick skull vault and small pituitary fossa as well as mental retardation. Pathologically there is extensive demyelination and atrophy of cerebral, cerebellar, brain stem, and spinal cord white matter with calcification of the cortex and basal ganglia. Peripheral neuropathy is an occasional manifestation (Moosa and Dubowitz, 1970).

REFERENCES

COCKAYNE, E. A. (1936) Dwarfism with retinal atrophy and deafness, *Arch. Dis. Child.*, **11**, 1.
COCKAYNE, E. A. (1946) Dwarfism with retinal atrophy and deafness, *Arch. Dis. Child.*, **21**, 52.
MOOSA, A., and DUBOWITZ, V. (1970) Peripheral neuropathy in Cockayne's syndrome, *Arch. Dis. Child.*, **45**, 674.
ROWLATT, U. (1969) Cockayne's syndrome: report of a case with necropsy findings, *Acta Neuropath. (Berl.)*, **14**, 52.

CHEDIAK–HEGASHI SYNDROME

Chediak (1952) described this syndrome characterized by partial albinism, hepatosplenomegaly, lymphadenopathy, mental retardation, and cerebellar degeneration with nystagmus. Peripheral neuropathy is sometimes present (Donohue and Bain, 1957; Sheramata *et al.*, 1971); the polymorphonuclear leucocytes show peroxidase-positive granules and cytoplasmic inclusions are found in neurones as well as perivascular cellular infiltration in pons, cerebellum, and peripheral nerves.

REFERENCES

CHEDIAK, M. (1952) Nouvelle anomalie leucocytaire de caractère constitutionnel et familial, *Rev. Hemat.*, **7**, 362.
DONOHUE, W. L., and BAIN, H. W. (1957) Chediak–Higashi syndrome, *Pediatrics*, **20**, 416.
SHERAMATA, W., KOTT, S., and CYR, D. P. (1971) The Chediak–Higashi–Steinbrinck syndrome, *Arch. Neurol. (Chic.)*, **25**, 289.

DISORDERS OF SERUM LIPOPROTEINS

A-Beta-Lipoproteinaemia (the Bassen-Kornzweig Syndrome)

This autosomal recessive condition, first described by Bassen and Kornzweig in 1950, presents in childhood, usually between the ages of two and 16 years, with atypical retinitis pigmentosa, progressive cerebellar ataxia, mental retardation, peripheral neuropathy, and steatorrhoea. The red blood cells show a typical 'thorny' malformation (acanthocytosis) and the serum levels of cholesterol, carotenoids, vitamin A, and phospholipids are invariably depressed, with absence of the beta-lipoprotein moiety. Acanthocytosis is not, however, absolutely specific for this syndrome, having been reported in patients with normal serum lipoproteins, including some with anaemia and cirrhosis (Menkes, 1974) and others with various neurological manifestations including Hallervorden–Spatz disease, and adults with mental retardation, extrapyramidal manifestations, and areflexia (Critchley *et al.*, 1968). Pathologically there is demyelination of the spinocerebellar tracts and posterior columns and neuronal loss in the cerebral cortex and anterior horns of the spinal cord (Sobrevilla *et al.*, 1964). The steatorrhoea may improve on a low fat diet but the neurological disorder is progressive and ultimately fatal.

Hypo-Alpha-Lipoproteinaemia (Tangier Disease)

This rare autosomal recessive disorder usually gives rise to peripheral neuropathy and retinitis pigmentosa (Engel *et al.*, 1967). There is almost total absence of high-density plasma lipoproteins; the liver, spleen, lymph nodes, and tonsils are usually enlarged and demonstrate storage of cholesterol esters.

REFERENCES

BASSEN, F. A., and KORNZWEIG, A. L. (1950) Malformation of erythrocytes in a case of atypical retinitis pigmentosa, *Blood*, **5**, 381.
CRITCHLEY, E. M. R., CLARK, D. B., and WIKLER, A. (1968) Acanthocytosis and neurological disorder without beta-lipoproteinemia, *Arch. Neurol. (Chic.)*, **18**, 134.
ENGEL, W. K., DORMAN, J. D., LEVY, R. I., and FREDERICKSON, D. S. (1967) Neuropathy in Tangier disease, *Arch. Neurol. (Chic.)*, **17**, 1.
MENKES, J. H. (1974) *Textbook of Child Neurology*, Philadelphia.
SOBREVILLA, L. A., GOODMAN, M. L., and KANE, C. A. (1964) Demyelinating central nervous system disease, muscular atrophy, and acanthocytosis (Bassen–Kornzweig syndrome), *Amer. J. Med.*, **37**, 821.

DISORDERS OF PURINE METABOLISM

Hyperuricaemia (the Lesch-Nyhan Syndrome)

Catel and Schmidt (1959) first described severe choreoathetosis and spasticity in children with hyperuricaemia, and in 1964 Lesch and Nyhan defined the usual neurological characteristics of this rare X-linked disorder which is thus confined to males. The affected boys usually show mild to moderate mental retardation and choreoathetosis which usually begins in the second year of life but is followed by the development of spasticity in all four limbs. A typical but unexplained feature is self-mutilation with biting of the tongue, lips, and fingers leading to progressive destruction unless the fingers, in particular, are protected. Renal calculi and haematuria ultimately develop and most patients die from renal failure.

The serum uric acid is usually raised and the urinary uric acid:creatine ratio is greater than two (Berman et al., 1968). The condition is due to a deficiency of hypoxanthine-guanine phosphoribosyl transferase (Seegmiller et al., 1967), a defect which can be identified in fibroblasts in culture. Identification of this enzymatic abnormality can be used for the identification of heterozygous female carriers (Migeon et al., 1968) and for antenatal diagnosis in amniotic cell cultures. Allopurinol may reduce the serum uric acid and may delay the development of renal failure but has little or no effect upon the neurological manifestations which have not been explained neuropathologically (Sass et al., 1965; Berman et al., 1969; Menkes, 1974).

REFERENCES

BERMAN, P. H., BALIS, M. E., and DANCIS, J. (1968) Diagnostic test for congenital hyperuricemia with central nervous system dysfunction, *J. Lab. clin. Med.*, **71**, 247.

BERMAN, P. H., BALIS, M. E., and DANCIS, J. (1969) Congenital hyperuricemia, *Arch. Neurol. (Chic.)*, **20**, 44.

CATEL, W., and SCHMIDT, J. (1959) Uber familiare gichtische Diathese in Verbindung mit zerebalen und renalen Symptomen bei einen Kleinkind, *Deutsch Med. Wschr.*, **84**, 2145.

LESCH, M., and NYHAN, W. L. (1964) A familial disorder of uric acid metabolism and central nervous system function, *Amer. J. Med.*, **36**, 561.

MENKES, J. H. (1974) *Textbook of Child Neurology*, Philadelphia.

MIGEON, B. R., DER KALOUSTIAN, V. M., and NYHAN, W. L. (1968) X-linked hypoxanthine-guanine phosphoribosyl transferase deficiency: heterozygote has two clonal populations, *Science*, **160**, 425.

SASS, J. K., ITABASHI, H. H., and DEXTER, R. A. (1965) Juvenile gout with brain involvement, *Arch. Neurol. (Chic.)*, **13**, 639.

SEEGMILLER, J. E., ROSENBLOOM, F. M., and KELLEY, W. N. (1967) Enzyme defect associated with a sex-linked human neurological disorder and excessive purine synthesis, *Science*, **155**, 1682.

DISORDERS OF CARBOHYDRATE METABOLISM

Glycogen Storage Disease. Of all the many disorders of glycogen storage which have been described, only one, namely Pompe's glycogenosis (Cori type II—Cori, 1952-3), a disorder of autosomal recessive inheritance due to amylo-1,4-glucosidase (acid maltase) deficiency, is known to affect the central nervous system. Usually the condition presents shortly after birth with generalized muscular weakness, hypotonia, and cardiomegaly. At autopsy there is evidence of diffuse glycogen storage in the neurones of the cerebral cortex and spinal cord (Crome *et al.*, 1963) but the muscular and cardiac involvement predominate and the condition is usually fatal within the first few months of life. However, it is now apparent that an identical enzymatic defect may give rise to the signs of an acquired myopathy first developing in late childhood, adolescence, or even adult life [see p. 1033].

Galactosaemia and Fructosuria. These rare disorders are considered on page 835.

Glycoprotein Storage. Progressive myoclonic epilepsy in which there is abnormal storage of glycoprotein in the so-called Lafora bodies is considered on page 1135.

REFERENCES

CORI, G. T. (1952–3) Glycogen structure and enzyme deficiencies in glycogen storage disease, *Harvey Lect.*, **48**, 145.

CROME, L., CUMINGS, J. N., and DUCKETT, S. (1963) Neuropathological and neurochemical aspects of generalized glycogen storage disease, *J. Neurol. Neurosurg. Psychiat.*, **26**, 422.

DISORDERS OF MUCOPOLYSACCHARIDE METABOLISM

Gargoylism (Hurler's Disease)

This syndrome, which is characterized by mental and physical retardation, hepatosplenomegaly, clouding of the cornea, a characteristic facial appearance, and multiple skeletal deformities, is now known to embrace at least six (White, 1973) and more probably seven (Menkes, 1974) different disorders, each characterized by varying degrees of storage of chondroitin sulphate and heparitin sulphate in various tissues and organs of the body including the central nervous system (McKusick, 1969). All save the so-called Hunter syndrome (Hunter, 1917), which is inherited as an X-linked recessive trait, are of autosomal recessive inheritance.

Patients with the typical Hurler syndrome often appear normal at birth but towards the end of the first year of life show evidence of mental retardation, clouding of the cornea, widely spaced eyes, flattening of the nasal bridge, thickening of the lips, and an open mouth. The skin is often coarse, an umbilical hernia is common with a protuberant abdomen, the hands are large with short and stubby fingers, and there is often hepatosplenomegaly. Radiological changes are particularly common in the humerus with thickening of the cortex and enlargement of the medulla but many long bones may be abnormal (Caffey, 1952). Progressive spasticity and dementia, sometimes with deafness and optic atrophy, develop and death usually results from bronchopneumonia in childhood. Skin fibroblasts contain excess mucopolysaccharides and typical inclusions seen ultrastructurally (Lyon *et al.*, 1973) and the latter may also be increased in the urine (Renuart, 1966). The lymphocytes often contain metachromatically staining cytoplasmic inclusions (Reilly granules) (Belcher, 1972).

Y

The Hunter type usually spares the cornea and runs a milder course, the Sanfilippo variety affects the nervous system severely but often produces only mild somatic manifestations, the Morquio variety (Gilles and Deuel, 1971) in which keratosulphate is stored in abnormal amounts, causes severe skeletal abnormalities and often less severe nervous system involvement, and the Scheie and Maroteaux–Lamy variants usually spare the nervous system and the intellect (see Menkes, 1974). Antenatal diagnosis through amniotic cell culture is now possible in many of these disorders. No treatment is of any value.

As already noted [p. 642], GM$_1$ gangliosidosis (pseudo-Hurler's disease) gives similar clinical features (mental retardation, hepatosplenomegaly, abnormal facies, and bony abnormalities) but the urinary mucopolysaccharide excretion is normal.

REFERENCES

BELCHER, R. W. (1972) Ultrastructure and cytochemistry of lymphocytes in the genetic mucopolysaccharidoses, *Arch. Path.*, **93**, 1.

CAFFEY, J. (1952) Gargoylism: prenatal and postnatal bone lesions and their early post-natal evolution, *Amer. J. Roentgen.*, **67**, 715.

GILLES, F. H., and DEUEL, R. K. (1971) Neuronal cytoplasmic globules in the brain in Morquio's syndrome, *Arch. Neurol. (Chic.)*, **25**, 393.

HUNTER, C. (1917) A rare disease in two brothers, *Proc. roy. Soc. Med.*, **10**, 104.

LYON, G., HORS-CAYLA, M. C., JONSSON, V., and MAROTEAUX, P. (1973) Aspects ultra-structuraux et signification biochimique des granulations metachromatiques et autres inclusions dans les fibroblastes en culture provenant de lipidoses et de muco-polysaccharidoses, *J. neurol. Sci.*, **19**, 235.

MCKUSICK, V. A. (1969) The nosology of the mucopolysaccharidoses, *Amer. J. Med.*, **47**, 730.

MENKES, J. H. (1974) *Textbook of Child Neurology*, Philadelphia.

RENUART, A. W. (1966) Screening for inborn errors of metabolism associated with mental deficiency or neurologic disorders or both, *New Engl. J. Med.*, **274**, 384.

WHITE, H. H. (1973) Diseases due to inborn metabolic defects, in *A Textbook of Neurology*, ed. Merritt, H. H., p. 652, Philadelphia.

MISCELLANEOUS DISORDERS OF UNKNOWN AETIOLOGY

Menkes' Kinky Hair Disease (Trichopoliodystrophy)

In 1962 Menkes *et al.* described an X-linked recessive disorder characterized by early and severe retardation of growth, peculiar white and 'kinky' hair, frequent epileptic seizures, and focal cerebral and cerebellar degeneration involving particularly the grey matter. The condition is usually fatal in early childhood; French *et al.* (1972) and Ghatak *et al.* (1972) have suggested that it should be entitled 'trichopoliodystrophy' and identified pathological changes in skeletal muscle as well as in the central nervous system. Danks *et al.* (1972) suggest that the condition is due to diminished copper absorption as they found low serum copper and caeruloplasmin levels in such cases.

Alpers' Disease (Progressive Cerebral Poliodystrophy)

This condition, described by Alpers in 1931, is still a poorly defined entity, thought by some to be a heredodegenerative disorder but attributed by others to anoxia (Norman, 1958) or an inflammatory process (Dreifuss and Netsky, 1964). On the whole current evidence suggests that some cases at least which are classified under this title represent an inherited process of autosomal recessive inheritance and unknown aetiology; the disorder has been described in three sibs (Sandbank and Lerman, 1972). It may begin in early infancy or in the first few years of life and leads to progressive dementia, seizures, spasticity, and opisthotonus. It can be diagnosed in life only by brain biopsy which shows almost total neuronal loss in the grey matter of the cerebral cortex with astrogliosis and microgliosis; large disorganized mitochondria may be found (Sandbank and Lerman, 1972).

Cerebral Gigantism

In 1964 Sotos *et al.* described five mentally retarded patients with large faces, large dolicocephalic skulls, widely spaced eyes, high arched palates, and large hands and feet. They showed excessive growth up to about the fifth year of life and subsequently their height, weight, and bone age were two to four years in advance of normal (Gardner-Medwin, 1969). Precocious puberty has been described in the many cases subsequently reported but this syndrome has no known aetiology, and no specific endocrinological or neuropathological features have been identified.

Urbach-Wiethe's Disease (Lipoid Proteinosis)

This rare disorder, probably of autosomal recessive inheritance, is characterized by hoarseness of the voice, cutaneous and mucosal lesions, intracranial calcification, alopecia, ocular and dental abnormalities, photosensitivity, and short stature. In two sibs reported by Newton *et al.* (1971) rage attacks, epilepsy, and severe loss of recent memory were prominent clinical features. The chemical composition of the abnormal material stored in the brain is unknown. The disease may present in childhood, but the course is usually prolonged well into adult life.

REFERENCES

ALPERS, B. J. (1931) Diffuse progressive degeneration of the gray matter of the cerebrum, *Arch. Neurol. Psychiat. (Chic.),* **25,** 469.

DANKS, D. M., CAMPBELL, P. E., STEVENS, B. J., MAYNE, V., and CARTWRIGHT, E. (1972) Menkes' kinky hair syndrome: defect in copper absorption, *Pediatrics,* **50,** 188.

DREIFUSS, F. E., and NETSKY, M. G. (1964) Progressive poliodystrophy, *Amer. J. Dis. Child.,* **107,** 649.

FRENCH, J. H., SHERARD, E. S., LUBELL, H., BROTZ, M., and MOORE, C. L. (1972) Trichopoliodystrophy. I. Report of a case and biochemical studies, *Arch. Neurol. (Chic.),* **26,** 229.

GARDNER-MEDWIN, D. (1969) Cerebral gigantism?, *Develop. Med. Child Neurol.,* **11,** 796.

GHATAK, N. R., HIRANO, A., POON, T. P., and FRENCH, J. H. (1972) Trichopoliodystrophy. II. Pathological changes in skeletal muscle and nervous system, *Arch. Neurol. (Chic.),* **26,** 60.

MENKES, J. H., ALTER, M., and STEIGLEDER, G. K. (1962) A sex-linked recessive disorder with growth retardation, peculiar hair, and focal cerebral and cerebellar degeneration, *Pediatrics,* **29,** 764.

NEWTON, F. H., ROSENBERG, R. N., LAMPERT, P. W., and O'BRIEN, J. S. (1971) Neurologic involvement in Urbach-Wiethe's disease (lipoid proteinosis), *Neurology (Minneap.),* **21,** 1205.

NORMAN, R. M. (1958) Alpers' disease, in *Neuropathology*, ed. Greenfield, J. G., Blackwood, W., McMenemey, W. H., Meyer, A., and Norman, R. M., p. 378, London.

SANDBANK, U., and LERMAN, P. (1972) Progressive cerebral poliodystrophy—Alpers' disease, *J. Neurol. Neurosurg. Psychiat.*, **35**, 749.

SOTOS, J. F., DODGE, P. R., MUIRHEAD, D., CRAWFORD, J. D., and TALBOT, N. B. (1964) Cerebral gigantism in childhood, *New Engl. J. Med.*, **271**, 109.

Infantile Neuroaxonal Dystrophy. This rare disorder, which seems to be due to an autosomal recessive gene, was first described by Seitelberger in 1952. Pathologically it is characterized by the accumulation of large axonal swellings in the grey matter of the brain and spinal cord and by degeneration of the globus pallidus, cerebellum, and long spinal tracts. Optic atrophy and partial denervation of skeletal muscles may also occur. Ultrastructural studies of sections of frontal cortex have shown that the axonal spheroids contain a sponge-like network of tubular structures and that presynaptic terminals are particularly involved (Hedley-Whyte *et al.*, 1968; Herman *et al.*, 1969; Coster *et al.*, 1971). Similar changes are found in muscle biopsy sections involving extra- and intrafusal axons and motor end-plates (Martin and Martin, 1972).

The condition usually begins between the ages of one and three years with arrest of development and motor weakness progressing to paralysis due to a combination of pyramidal tract and lower motor neurone dysfunction; there may be loss of pain sensation in the legs. Convulsions are rare but progressive optic atrophy leads to blindness and most patients die before the end of the first decade.

The EEG usually shows diffuse fast activity, the EMG confirms the presence of denervation and the serum and CSF lactate dehydrogenase activity may be raised. Certain features of the condition resemble those of experimental tocopherol deficiency in animals but no specific biochemical abnormality has yet been detected in these cases, while no effective treatment has yet been introduced. Some authorities believe that the condition is identical with, or closely related to, Hallervorden–Spatz disease [see p. 604] but others are confident that it is an independent entity (Indravasu and Dexter, 1968; Martin and Martin, 1972).

REFERENCES

COSTER, W. DE, ROELS, H., and VANDER EECKEN, H. (1971) Electron microscopical study of neuroaxonal dystrophy, *Europ. Neurol.*, **5**, 65.

COWEN, D., and OLMSTEAD, E. V. (1963) Infantile neuroaxonal dystrophy, *J. Neuropath.*, **22**, 175.

HEDLEY-WHYTE, E. T., GILLES, F. H., and UZMAN, B. G. (1968) Infantile neuroaxonal dystrophy: a disease characterized by altered terminal axons and synaptic endings, *Neurology (Minneap.)*, **18**, 891.

HERMAN, M. M., HUTTENLOCHER, P. R., and BENSCH, K. G. (1969) Electron microscopic observations in infantile neuroaxonal dystrophy: report of a cortical biopsy and review of the recent literature, *Arch. Neurol. (Chic.)*, **20**, 19.

HUTTENLOCHER, P. R., and GILLES, F. H. (1967) Infantile neuroaxonal dystrophy. Clinical, pathological and histochemical findings in a family with 3 affected siblings, *Neurology (Minneap.)*, **17**, 1174.

INDRAVASU, S., and DEXTER, R. A. (1968) Infantile neuroaxonal dystrophy and its relationship to Hallervorden–Spatz disease, *Neurology (Minneap.)*, **18**, 693.

MARTIN, J. J., and MARTIN, L. (1972) Infantile neuroaxonal dystrophy. Ultrastructural study of the peripheral nerves and of the motor end plates, *Europ. Neurol.*, **8**, 239.

SEITELBERGER, F. (1952) Eine unbekannte Form von infantiler lipoidopercher Krankheit des Gehirns, *Proceedings of the First International Congress of Neuropathology*, vol. 3, p. 323, Turin.

SUBACUTE NECROTIZING ENCEPHALOMYELOPATHY

This rare condition, first described by Leigh in 1951, is inherited by an autosomal recessive mechanism and its clinical and pathological features strongly suggest that it is due to an inherited enzyme defect. At first the diagnosis was usually made only at post-mortem but recently many cases have been diagnosed during life and have been found to show raised blood pyruvate levels and a metabolic acidosis. Hommes *et al.* (1968) demonstrated in such cases a marked reduction in serum pyruvate carboxylase, the enzyme which converts pyruvate to oxalacetate. Pathologically the brains of affected individuals show widespread cellular necrosis with capillary proliferation in the optic nerves and chiasm, basal ganglia, and brain stem. The appearances are similar to those of Wernicke's encephalopathy, but the distribution of the lesions is somewhat different, the corpora mammillaria usually being spared (Richter, 1968). Faris and Fleckenstein (1970) suggest a possible relationship between this condition and central pontine myelinolysis [p. 564] and Crome (1970) reported a typical case in which the kidneys showed nephrosis and changes in the glomeruli and renal tubules as well as the accumulation of adventitious lipid material in the intima of many arteries and arterioles. Clinically the affected children show failure to thrive, poverty of movement, hypotonia and spasticity, loss of tendon reflexes, nystagmus, and optic atrophy; convulsions sometimes occur and the condition is usually fatal in six to twelve months. Occasional cases have been reported in adolescence (Hardman *et al.*, 1968) and adult life. In some cases there has been apparent temporary arrest of the disease process following treatment with lipoic acid (0·7 mg/kg body weight (Worsley *et al.*, 1965)).

REFERENCES

CROME, L. (1964) Neuropathological changes in diseases caused by inborn errors of metabolism, in *Neurometabolic Disorders in Childhood*, ed. Holt, K. S., and Milner, J., Edinburgh.

CROME, L. (1970) Subacute necrotizing encephalomyelopathy associated with renal and arterial lesions, *Brain*, **93**, 709.

FARIS, A. A., and FLECKENSTEIN, L. D. (1970) Subacute necrotizing encephalomyelopathy: its relationship to central pontine myelinolysis, *J. Neurol. Neurosurg. Psychiat.*, **33**, 667.

GREENHOUSE, A. H., and SCHNECK, S. A. (1968) Subacute necrotizing encephalomyelopathy. A reappraisal of the thiamine deficiency hypothesis, *Neurology (Minneap.)*, **18**, 1.

HARDMAN, J. M., ALLEN, L. W., BAUGHMAN, F. A., and WATERMAN, D. F. (1968) Subacute necrotizing encephalopathy in late adolescence, *Arch. Neurol. (Chic.)*, **18**, 478.

HOMMES, F. A., POLMAN, H. A., and REERINK, J. D. (1968) Leigh's encephalomyelopathy: an inborn error of gluconeogenesis, *Arch. Dis. Child.*, **43**, 423.

LEIGH, D. (1951) Subacute necrotizing encephalomyelopathy in an infant, *J. Neurol. Neurosurg. Psychiat.*, **14**, 216.

RICHTER, R. B. (1968) Infantile subacute necrotizing encephalopathy (Leigh's disease). Its relationship to Wernicke's encephalopathy, *Neurology (Minneap.)*, **18**, 1125.

WORSLEY, H. E., BROOKFIELD, R. W., ELWOOD, J. S., NOBLE, R. L., and TAYLOR, W. H. (1965) Lactic acidosis with necrotizing encephalopathy in two sibs, *Arch. Dis. Childh.*, **40**, 492.

TUBEROUS SCLEROSIS (EPILOIA)

Synonyms. Bourneville's disease; Brushfield–Wyatt disease.

Definition. A rare congenital disorder characterized pathologically by sclerotic masses in the cerebral cortex, adenoma sebaceum, and tumours in various organs, and clinically by mental deficiency and epilepsy.

PATHOLOGY

Macroscopically the brain may show microgyria or macrogyria, and absence of the corpus callosum has been described. The characteristic sclerotic patches to which the disease owes its name were first described by Bourneville and Brissaud in 1880. They are found in the cerebral cortex and are rare in the cerebellum. They are hard to the touch, and white in appearance, ranging in size from 0·5 to 2 cm in diameter. Microscopically they are composed of glial fibres, and contain in addition large cells, some of which are believed to be abnormal ganglion cells, while others are thought to be derived from spongioblasts. Tumour-like masses are also found in the cerebral ventricles, and these appear to be derived from the ependyma. Occasionally a large glioblastoma or astrocytoma is found. Circular laminated bodies resembling corpora amylacea have been found scattered throughout the cerebral cortex, cerebellum, choroid plexus, and the tumours themselves, and there is often cystic degeneration in the cerebral hemispheres and cerebellum, giving small cavities which may be traversed by fine fibrils. The ganglion cells of the cerebral cortex are reduced in number, and are often atypical. The retinal tumours, phakomas, are composed of neuroglia. Adenoma sebaceum described by Balzar in 1885 and Pringle in 1890 consists of a hyperplasia of sebaceous glands embedded in a vascular matrix. Tumours in other situations include rhabdomyoma of the heart, teratoma, and adenosarcoma of the kidney, and tumours have also been described in the thyroid, thymus, breast, and duodenum. Other occasional associated abnormalities include hydromyelia and spina bifida, and congenital malformations of the heart. The bones may show osteoporosis, cyst formation, and periosteal deposits which are visible radiologically (Holt and Dickerson, 1952).

AETIOLOGY

Beyond the fact that tuberous sclerosis is due to a congenital dysplasia probably occurring at an early stage in embryonic life, little is known about its aetiology. In an analysis of 71 cases Bundey and Evans (1969) found evidence favouring simple autosomal dominant inheritance of the disorder; sometimes the parent of an affected individual had adenoma sebaceum but no neurological abnormality, and involvement of more than one sib was relatively common. However, over 80 per cent of cases appeared to be due to new mutations. The condition is thought to be commoner in males than females and in the white races. It appears to be closely related to the syndrome of neurofibroblastomatosis.

SYMPTOMS

There is a wide range of clinical manifestations which have been reviewed by Nevin and Pearce (1968) and by Bundey and Evans (1969). In severe cases becoming manifest in early childhood severe mental retardation and epilepsy are the rule and the fits often begin in the first year of life. Some children present with 'infantile spasms' and with the EEG changes of so-called hypsarrhythmia (Pampiglione, 1968). More often major convulsions occur, sometimes leading to status epilepticus, but minor and Jacksonian attacks may all occur. Focal neurological signs are uncommon except when a large intracranial neoplasm develops. In some mildly affected adults intelligence is normal but in others there is progressive mental retardation with psychotic episodes. Adenoma sebaceum, or epilepsy, or both may occur in patients of normal intelligence.

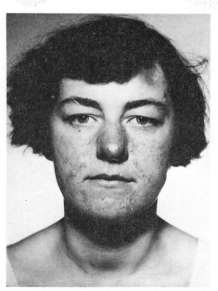

FIG. 110. Adenoma sebaceum in a patient with tuberous sclerosis, from *An Atlas of Clinical Neurology* 2nd ed., 1975, by J. D. Spillane, reproduced by kind permission of the author

Adenoma sebaceum, which is not invariably present, manifests itself at about the fourth or fifth year of life as a pale pink, slightly raised rash, consisting of discrete spots, which fade on pressure, and appear first in the nasolabial folds, spreading over the face in a 'butterfly' pattern, sparing the upper lip [FIG. 110]. A few scattered nodules may also appear on the forehead and neck, but rarely below the clavicles. After the second dentition the adenomas tend to coalesce and darken in colour to a deep red or brown hue. Exceptionally the cutaneous lesion does not make its appearance until puberty or early adult life. Tumours in other situations occasionally grow large enough to cause symptoms. The retinal phakomas, described by van der Hoeve in 1923, are flat, white, round or oval areas about half the size of the optic disc.

DIAGNOSIS

Tuberous sclerosis can be distinguished from other causes of mental deficiency associated with epilepsy only by the presence of adenoma sebaceum or retinal phakomas or of tumours elsewhere. The EEG is usually abnormal but the changes are variable and not diagnostic. Radiographs of the skull may show patchy calcification [FIG. 111] and pneumoencephalography is often diagnostic (Hudolin and Petrovčić, 1957) showing protrusions ('candle-guttering') into the cerebral ventricles [FIG. 112].

PROGNOSIS

Severely affected children often die between the ages of five and 15 years either from intercurrent disease or status epilepticus. Many mildly affected adults have a normal life span, but some die in middle life as a result of a tumour in the brain or in some other organ.

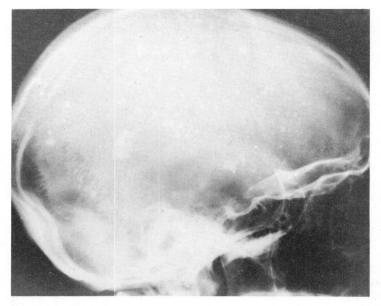

FIG. 111. Patchy intracranial calcification due to tuberous sclerosis in an adult

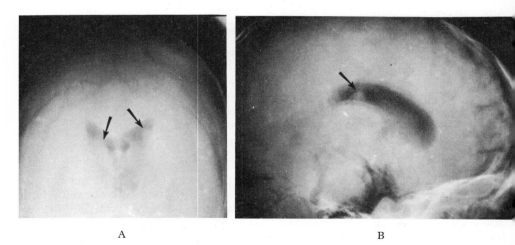

A   B

FIG. 112. Tuberous sclerosis: the pneumoencephalogram shows the characteristic lesions protruding
into the cerebral ventricles. A. Anteroposterior view. B. Lateral view

TREATMENT

Severe mental retardation often necessitates institutional treatment, and the treatment appropriate for epilepsy should be carried out.

REFERENCES

BIELSCHOWSKY, M. (1923-4). Zur Histopathologie und Pathogenese der tuberösen Sklerose, *J. Psychol. Neurol. (Lpz.)*, **30**, 167.

BRUSHFIELD, T., and WYATT, W. (1926) Epiloia, parts I and II. *Brit. J. Child. Dis.*, **23**, 178 and 254.

BUNDEY, S., and EVANS, K. (1969) Tuberous sclerosis: a genetic entity, *J. Neurol. Neurosurg. Psychiat.*, **32**, 591.

CRITCHLEY, M., and EARL, C. J. C. (1932) Tuberose sclerosis and allied conditions, *Brain*, **55**, 311.

FERRARO, A., and DOOLITTLE, G. J. (1936) Tuberous sclerosis, *Psychiat. Quart.*, **10**, 365.

HOLT, J., and DICKERSON, W. (1952) Osseous lesions of tuberous sclerosis. *Radiology*, **58**, 1.

HUDOLIN, V., and PETROVČIĆ, F. (1957) A contribution to the diagnosis of tuberous sclerosis, *J. Neurol. Neurosurg. Psychiat.*, **20**, 125.

KESSEL, F. K. (1949) Some radiologic and neurosurgical aspects of tuberous sclerosis, *Acta psychiat. (Kbh.)*, **24**, 499.

NEVIN, N. C., and PEARCE, W. G. (1968) Diagnostic and genetical aspects of tuberous sclerosis, *J. med. Genet.*, **5**, 273.

PAMPIGLIONE, G. (1968) Some inborn metabolic disorders affecting cerebral electrogenesis, in *Some Recent Advances in Inborn Errors of Metabolism*, ed. Holt, K. S., and Coffey, V. P., Edinburgh.

NEUROFIBROMATOSIS

Synonyms. Neurofibroblastomatosis; von Recklinghausen's disease.

Definition. A disease of congenital origin, characterized by cutaneous pigmentation and the formation of tumours in various tissues. The commonest of these are cutaneous fibromas, mollusca fibrosa, and neurofibromas, but meningiomas and gliomas may also occur. Combinations of these abnormalities have been designated as separate syndromes. Thus Worster-Drought *et al.* (1937) recognized the following:

1. Central type: (*a*) meningeal and perineurial—syndrome of Wishart (1822) which is rare. (*b*) Meningeal only—syndrome of Schultze (1880) which is the rarest. (*c*) Perineurial only—syndrome of Knoblauch (1843) which is the commonest.

2. Peripheral type. The peripheral neurofibromatosis of von Recklinghausen (1882) first described by Tilesius in 1793. The central and peripheral types may also occur in combination. The condition is related to the other phakomatoses, including tuberous sclerosis.

PATHOLOGY

The neurofibromas are tumours usually situated upon peripheral nerves and composed of bundles of long spindle cells. There has been much controversy as to the nature of the cells of which neurofibromas are composed. Russell and Rubinstein (1959) distinguished on histological grounds schwannomas, derived from cells of the neurilemma (sheath of Schwann), and neurofibromas, which they believe to be also of Schwannian origin and not derived from fibroblasts.

Both may be found on the peripheral nerves and also upon the cranial nerves, most frequently upon the vestibulocochlear nerve, but also upon others, especially the vagus, trigeminal, and hypoglossal, and they may occur upon spinal nerve roots, usually the dorsal, or upon the cauda equina. Schwannomas particularly may be solitary. The cutaneous fibromas, or mollusca fibrosa, are formed from the connective tissue elements of the cutaneous nerves. Nerve elements are absent, but there are characteristic whorls of spindle cells. The bone changes associated with neurofibromatosis may consist either of hyperostosis or of rarefaction, with or without cyst formation. According to Thannhauser (1944) the bone lesions in neurofibromatosis and in the osteitis fibrosa cystica of von Recklinghausen are similar. The cause of the 'scalloping' of vertebral bodies seen in some cases [p. 668] is unknown.

Neurofibromas may become sarcomatous. Abnormalities may be present in parts of the nervous system other than the peripheral nerves. Patches of gliosis, neuronal heterotopias and vascular malformations (Pearce, 1967) and ependymal overgrowth may occur in the brain and spinal cord; syringomyelia, and even malignant tumours—glioma and ependymoma—may develop. Glioma of the optic chiasma may be associated with neurofibromatosis, and meningiomas are sometimes present. Pearce (1967), in a study of nine autopsied cases, found a high incidence of intracranial gliomas which were often clinically latent. Rodriguez and Berthrong (1966) reported a patient who had multiple intracranial meningiomas, an acoustic neuroma, multiple ependymomas, and syringomyelia. The condition has been described in association with Cockayne's syndrome [p. 654] (Felgenhauer and Ammann, 1967). Neurofibromatosis is occasionally associated with other congenital abnormalities, such as spina bifida, cerebral meningocele, buphthalmos, syndactyly, and haemangiectatic naevi.

AETIOLOGY

The disease appears to be due to a congenital abnormality of the ectoderm. It is inherited as an autosomal dominant trait. Some members of affected families may show only cutaneous pigmentation, while others exhibit a more extensive clinical picture. Bilateral acoustic neurofibromas sometimes occur in many members of a sibship in successive generations.

SYMPTOMS

Some of the symptoms of neurofibromatosis are always present at birth, for example, cutaneous pigmentation. Others may be absent or may appear later, as a result of slow growth of the neurofibromas or of the reaction of other tissues to these tumours. In some cases, however, the disorder is little, if at all progressive, and may be discovered accidentally. Except in those cases in which gross congenital abnormalities are present, the patient does not usually come under observation on account of symptoms until after the age of 20 years.

Cutaneous Pigmentation

This is almost invariably present. It consists of brownish spots, *café au lait* in colour, varying in size from a pin's head to areas the size of the palm. If five or more of these spots are present on the skin, even in the absence of cutaneous tumours, neurofibromatosis should be suspected. Unlike the *café au lait* spots of Albright's syndrome (polyostotic fibrous dysplasia) the patches of pigmentation in neurofibromatosis usually show a regular outline without deep indenta-tions ('coast of California, rather than coast of Maine'). Occasionally a sheet of diffuse pigmentation may be present on one or both sides of the trunk, corresponding to the cutaneous distribution of several spinal segments. Cutaneous pigmentation is always most evident on the trunk and may be absent from the exposed parts.

Cutaneous Fibromas

Cutaneous fibromas or mollusca fibrosa are soft, pinkish swellings, which may be sessile or pedunculated, and vary in size from a pin's head to an orange. They are frequently present in large num-bers, and are situated chiefly upon the trunk, but some are usually to be found on the face [FIG. 113].

Neurofibromas

Neurofibromas are most readily discovered upon the superficial cutaneous nerves, especially those of the extremities and of the sides of the neck. The tumours are to be felt as movable, bead-like nodules. They may give rise to pain and are occasionally tender on pressure; sometimes they appear to grow within the sheath of a nerve, when pressure may produce pain along the nerve trunk and paraesthesiae in the appropriate dermatome.

Plexiform Neuroma

'Plexiform neuroma' is the term applied to a diffuse neurofibroma-tosis of nerve trunks, which is often associated with an overgrowth of the skin and subcutaneous tissues. In this way large folds of skin may be formed, or there may be a diffuse enlargement of the subcutaneous tissues of a limb, with or without underlying bony abnormality. The commonest sites are the temple, the upper lid, and the back of the neck. The cutaneous hyperplasia has received the names of dermatolysis, pachydermatocele, and elephantiasis

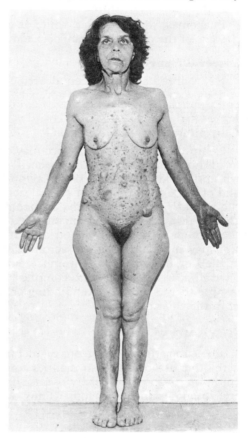

FIG. 113. Neurofibromatosis; note the multiple cutaneous tumours, especially on the trunk, from *An Atlas of Clinical Neurology* 2nd ed., 1975, by J. D. Spillane, reproduced by kind permission of the author

neuromatosa, It is probable that the famous 'Elephant Man' described by Treves was an example of this disorder. A similar hyperplasia may occur in one half of the tongue and in the gums on one side.

Acoustic neuroma is described on pages 241 and 281.

Osseous Manifestations

Kyphoscoliosis is frequently present in neurofibromatosis and may be so severe as to cause compression of the spinal cord. Even in the absence of intrathecal neurofibromas related to the nerve roots a characteristic concave 'scalloping' of the posterior borders of the vertebral bodies may be seen in radiographs of the spine. There may be marked hyperostosis of the bones of the face, with enlargement and rarefaction of the calvarium. These changes may be mainly unilateral. The long bones of the limbs may undergo subperiosteal hyperostosis, and their shafts may be curved.

Retinal Manifestations

Phakomas, which are flat, white or grey, oval or circular masses, about half the size of the optic disc, may occur in the retina (van der Hoeve, 1923).

Visceral Neurofibromas

Neurofibromas have been described on the mucous membranes and in various viscera, including the adrenals. The vagus and sympathetic nerves may also be affected.

Complications

Compression of the spinal cord may occur as a result of severe kyphoscoliosis or of a neurofibroma, or the scoliosis may lead to root pains. Neurofibromas within the skull may give rise to symptoms of increased intracranial pressure, and of focal compression of cranial nerves, especially the eighth [p. 281] or of the brain. Intracranial glioma or meningioma may be present. A sarcomatous change in a neurofibroma manifests itself as a rapid increase in the size of the tumour, with compression and invasion of the neighbouring structures. Epilepsy, mental retardation, acromegaly, adiposogenital dystrophy, infantilism of the Lorain type, phaeochromocytoma of the adrenal, and Addison's disease have all been encountered as complications (Saxena, 1970). Optic atrophy may occur either as an associated finding or as a result of a glioma of an optic nerve or of the chiasm.

DIAGNOSIS

The association of cutaneous pigmentation with neurofibromas and frequently with other associated abnormalities constitutes a unique clinical picture. Difficulties in diagnosis are likely to arise only when some of these clinical features are absent or inconspicuous. Thus a patient may come under observation presenting symptoms of an intracranial tumour, spinal compression, scoliosis with root pains, hyperostosis, or localized elephantiasis. A careful examination of the skin for pigmentation, cutaneous and neural fibromas, will usually enable a correct diagnosis to be made.

PROGNOSIS

The disorder is not always progressive, but the presence of any symptoms in a child or adolescent should lead to a guarded prognosis, as the disorder may later reach its fully developed form. Pregnancy especially may lead to an exacerbation. Frequently the disease does not shorten life nor lead to marked discomfort. In severe cases death may occur from one of the complications described above, from tuberculosis, or after a terminal phase of cachexia.

TREATMENT

Treatment is often palliative. Painful subcutaneous neurofibromas may be treated by excision. Suitable operative treatment may be required for associated intracranial or intraspinal tumours, or when a peripheral neurofibroma compresses a mixed nerve or becomes sarcomatous.

REFERENCES

BIELSCHOWSKY, M., and ROSE, M. (1927) Zur Kenntnis der zentralen Veränderungen bei Recklinghausenscher Krankheit, *J. Psychol. Neurol. (Lpz.)*, **35,** 42.

CROME, L. (1962) Central neurofibromatosis, *Arch. Dis. Child.*, **37,** 640.

FELGENHAUER, W.-R., and AMMANN, F. (1967) Syndrome de Cockayne fruste associé à la neurofibromatose de Recklinghausen, *J. Génét. hum.*, **16,** 6.

FORD, F. R. (1966) *Diseases of the Nervous System in Infancy, Childhood and Adolescence*, 5th ed., p. 995, Springfield, Ill.

HOEVE, J. VAN DER (1923) Augengeschwülste bei der tuberösen Hirnsklerose (Bourneville) und verwandten Krankheiten, *Arch. Ophthal.*, **111,** 1.

KIENBÖCK, R., and RÖSLER, H. (1932) *Neurofibromatose*, Leipzig.

LEHMAN, E. P. (1926) Recklinghausen's neurofibromatosis and the skeleton, *Arch. Derm. Syph. (Chic.)*, **14,** 178.

PEARCE, J. (1967) The central nervous system pathology in multiple neurofibromatosis, *Neurology (Minneap.)*, **17,** 691.

PENFIELD, W., and YOUNG, A. W. (1930) The nature of von Recklinghausen's disease and the tumors associated with it, *Arch. Neurol. Psychiat. (Chic.)*, **23,** 320.

RODRIGUEZ, H. A., and BERTHRONG, M. (1966) Multiple intracranial tumors in von Recklinghausen's neurofibromatosis, *Arch. Neurol. (Chic.)*, **14,** 467.

RUSSELL, W. S., and RUBINSTEIN, L. J. (1959) *Pathology of Tumours of the Nervous System*, pp. 236 et seq., London.

SAXENA, K. M. (1970) Endocrine manifestations of neurofibromatosis in children, *Amer. J. Dis. Child.*, **120,** 265.

THANNHAUSER, S. J. (1944) Neurofibromatosis (von Recklinghausen) and osteitis fibrosa cystica localisata et disseminata (von Recklinghausen), *Medicine (Baltimore)*, **23,** 105.

WEBER, F. P. (1929–30) Periosteal neurofibromatosis, with a short consideration of the whole subject of neurofibromatosis, *Quart. J. Med.*, **23,** 151.

WORSTER-DROUGHT, C., DICKSON, W. E. C., and MCMENEMEY, W. H. (1937) Multiple meningeal and perineural tumours with analogous changes in the glia and ependyma, *Brain*, **60,** 85.

THE HEREDITARY ATAXIAS

Definition. The term 'hereditary ataxia', though by no means completely descriptive, is a convenient one to apply to a group of closely related disorders, all genetically determined, and characterized pathologically by degeneration of some or all of the following parts of the nervous system—the optic nerves, the cerebellum, the olives, and the long ascending and descending tracts of the spinal cord. These localized degenerations occur in various combinations, with corresponding symptoms. Probably these disorders are closely related also to peroneal muscular atrophy, hypertrophic interstitial polyneuropathy, and hereditary sensory neuropathy [see CHAPTER 18] with any of which they may, in occasional families, be combined. The age of onset ranges from childhood to middle life, and the course of these diseases is usually one of slow progression. Many varieties have been described, differing in the distribution of the symptoms. Friedreich's ataxia is relatively common. Some forms of hereditary ataxia are confined to a single family. Each variety tends to breed true, but does not always do so, and more than one form may occur in the same family. In some families there is also a variable association with mental retardation, nerve deafness, and retinitis pigmentosa. By analogy with the storage disorders, including Refsum's disease, already described, and the disorders of amino acid metabolism to be described in CHAPTER 15, it has been postulated that these conditions are likely to be due to a series of enzymatic defects; however, no such defect has yet been identified and it is uncertain as to whether many different genes are involved or whether modification of the effects of only a small number of genes may account for the variable clinical manifestations and the frequency of transitional and hybrid cases. It is impossible to describe in detail all the forms of hereditary ataxia which have been reported. The principal case reports have been reviewed by Pratt (1967). The following are the most important:

1. Hereditary spastic paraplegia.
2. Friedreich's ataxia.
3. The Roussy–Lévy syndrome.
4. The varieties described by Sanger-Brown and Marie.
5. Various forms of progressive cerebellar degeneration.

Brief comment will also be given upon some of the less common syndromes which are difficult to classify.

PATHOLOGY

The pathology of the different varieties of hereditary ataxia will be described in more detail in the appropriate sections. They present the following features in common.

There is a degeneration of the ectodermal elements of the nervous system. The nerve fibres are usually affected more severely than the ganglion cells, but in the later stages these also suffer, though it is difficult to say whether their degeneration is primary or secondary to axonal degeneration. The cerebellum and spinal cord are usually smaller than normal and occasionally show congenital abnormalities. The brunt of the degenerative process usually falls either on the spinal cord or on the cerebellum but both may be involved. In the spinal forms some degenerative changes are usually to be found in all the long ascending and descending tracts, though predominant involvement of certain tracts determines the nature of the clinical picture. Thus the corticospinal tracts are most affected in hereditary spastic paraplegia; the corticospinal tracts, the posterior columns, the posterior spinocerebellar tracts, and the ganglion cells of the dorsal horns of grey matter in Friedreich's ataxia [FIG. 114]; while the changes are most marked in the anterior columns in the cerebellar ataxias. Degeneration is manifest in loss of myelin and destruction of axons, with a reactive gliosis. Recent work has shown that in many varieties there is also axonal degeneration in peripheral nerves (Hughes et al., 1968).

AETIOLOGY

As already stated, the aetiology and pathogenesis of the hereditary ataxias is unknown. All appear to be genetically determined and most affect the sexes equally, but many cases are sporadic and even the individual disease entities vary considerably in their clinical presentation and course and in the mode of inheritance observed in different families (Bell, 1939; Sjögren, 1943; Pratt, 1967). Hereditary spastic paraplegia is sometimes due to an autosomal recessive gene but is more often dominant, while Friedreich's ataxia is usually recessive and less frequently dominant. The Roussy–Lévy syndrome, the Sanger-Brown and Marie varieties and the cerebellar degenerations are often recessive, but numerous families suggestive of dominant inheritance have been reported. Even in these more common varieties and in some of the rarer types there are also reports of X-linked recessive inheritance, so that the position remains confused.

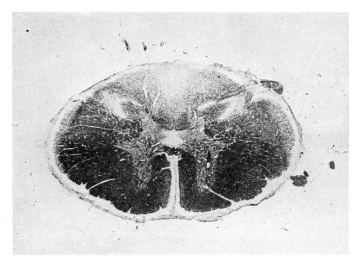

FIG. 114. Friedreich's ataxia. Spinal cord (myelin stain)

CLINICAL VARIETIES

HEREDITARY SPASTIC PARAPLEGIA

Families demonstrating both recessive and dominant inheritance have been described (Schwarz, 1952; Schwarz and Liu, 1956) but there seems to be a greater incidence of the disease in males. The onset of symptoms is usually in childhood, between the ages of 3 and 15 years, rarely in middle age.

PATHOLOGY

The maximal degeneration is found in the corticospinal tracts of the spinal cord, especially from the upper thoracic region downwards. This is associated with slighter degenerative changes in the posterior columns, especially the fasciculus gracilis, and in the large corticospinal cells of the precentral gyrus.

SYMPTOMS

Symptoms are those of a progressive destruction of the corticospinal tracts beginning in the lower limbs. Attention is first attracted to the child on account of its stiff and clumsy gait. The lower limbs are found to be weak and spastic, with exaggerated tendon reflexes and extensor plantar responses. The abdominal reflexes are diminished or lost, and pes cavus is usually present. Later the upper limbs are similarly affected, and finally the muscles innervated from the brain stem, with the production of spastic dysarthria and dysphagia and loss of emotional control. The sphincters are usually slightly affected in the later stages. In spite of degeneration in the posterior columns, no loss of superficial or deep sensibility can usually be detected. Primary optic atrophy and retinal pigmentation have been described. Intelligence is usually normal but mental retardation (Sutherland, 1957), epilepsy (Bruyn and Mechelse, 1962), cardiomyopathy with electrocardiographic abnormalities (Tyrer and Sutherland, 1961), and optic atrophy (Bickerstaff, 1950; van Bogaert, 1952) have been described.

PROGNOSIS

The disease runs a slowly progressive course, weakness and contracture finally confining the patient to bed. However, despite the alarming evidence of spasticity and the clonus and grossly exaggerated lower limb reflexes it is remarkable that patients often manage to walk for 30 years or more after the onset. Death occurs after many years, usually from an intercurrent infection.

FRIEDREICH'S ATAXIA

This disorder is generally recessive but rarely dominant, but sporadic cases occur. The age of onset, interpreted as the age at which symptoms first bring the patient under observation, is usually between 5 and 15 years, though abnormalities such as pes cavus may be discovered in apparently normal members of affected families in early childhood. Exceptionally, symptoms first appear between the ages of 20 and 30, rarely after 30. There is no evidence of linkage between the causal gene and those responsible for any of the blood groups (Powell, 1961).

PATHOLOGY

The spinal cord is unusually small, but the cerebellum is usually normal. Histologically [FIG. 114], the degeneration is most marked in the posterior columns, especially in the fasciculus gracilis. It is most intense in the lower parts of the cord and diminishes towards the medulla. Next to the posterior columns, the lateral columns suffer most, especially the corticospinal tracts and the posterior spinocerebellar tracts, together with the cells of the dorsal nucleus, from which the latter are derived. The anterior spinocerebellar tracts usually escape. There is a reactive gliosis in the degenerated regions. The dorsal root fibres also exhibit degeneration, though their ganglion cells may be little affected. Exceptionally there is some degeneration of the anterior horn cells with resulting muscular weakness and atrophy, often in distal limb muscles.

The heart may show diffuse enlargement due to cardiomyopathy with diffuse fibrosis. Microscopically there is fatty degeneration of the muscle fibres with slight chronic inflammatory infiltration and fibrosis. Even when there is no involvement of lower motor neurones, large diameter myelinated sensory fibres in the peripheral nerves usually show axonal degeneration with secondary demyelination (Hughes et al., 1968; Dyck and Lais, 1972).

SYMPTOMS

As might be deduced from the pathological changes, the cardinal symptoms of Friedreich's ataxia are: ataxia, most marked in the lower limbs, with signs of destruction of the corticospinal tracts, loss of deep reflexes, and, to a variable extent, impairment of sensibility, especially deep sensibility (vibration sense and position and joint sense). In addition, pes cavus and scoliosis are present, and nystagmus and dysarthria indicate a disturbance of cerebellar function at the level of the cranial nerves.

Symptoms appear first in the lower limbs, and it is the ataxic gait which usually first attracts attention. The patient walks on a broad base and tends to reel or stagger. In severe cases he is unable to walk without support on both sides. Standing is similarly affected, and he sways and may be unable to stand without support. The unsteadiness of stance is sometimes intensified by closing the eyes. Ataxia of the lower limbs is usually less evident in movement of the limbs individually when the patient is lying in bed. In the later stages movements of the upper limbs also become ataxic, and intention-tremor is present. Slight involuntary movements, which have sometimes been described as choreiform or myoclonic, are often present in the later stages. These are probably the result of defective co-ordination. Irregular oscillations of the head are common. Nystagmus is present in 70 per cent of cases, and it is usually most marked on lateral ocular deviation. Speech is invariably dysarthric in the later stages, the dysarthria being of the variety associated with cerebellar disease. Speech is usually slow, monotonous, and slurred, and may be explosive or scanning. It is frequently accompanied by vigorous grimaces and associated movements of the facial musculature. Corticospinal tract degeneration leads to weakness, most marked in the lower limbs, with loss of the abdominal reflexes and extensor plantar responses. The tendon reflexes tend to be lost owing to interruption of the reflex arcs on the afferent side. The ankle-jerks are lost before the knee-jerks, and the latter may be exaggerated, owing to the corticospinal lesion, when the former are diminished. The limbs may be either hypotonic or slightly spastic, depending upon the relative severity of loss of afferent impulses from the muscles, which tends to diminish muscle tone, and of the corticospinal tract lesion, which tends to increase it. Sensory changes are inconstant. Shooting pains occasionally occur in the limbs. Postural sense and appreciation of passive movement and of vibration are not infrequently impaired, especially in the lower limbs. In some cases all forms of sensibility are affected. The sphincters are usually unaffected, though incontinence of urine, and more rarely of faeces, may occur in the late stages. Pes cavus and scoliosis are present in almost all cases, the former being usually associated with a slight contracture of the muscles of the calf. Tyrer and Sutherland (1961) suggested that pes cavus is due to unbalanced action of the tibialis posterior muscle but the fact that it may be seen in otherwise unaffected sibs suggests that it and the scoliosis are more probably due to an associated hereditary abnormality of bony development.

Optic atrophy occasionally occurs, and retinal pigmentation has been described. Other rare ocular symptoms include ptosis, abnormalities of the pupillary reflexes, and ophthalmoplegia. Deafness sometimes occurs. Muscular atrophy is a rare complication and is most frequently seen in the hands, leading to claw-hand, which Roth (1948) suggested indicates a relationship to peroneal muscular atrophy. Associated congenital abnormalities include spina bifida occulta and infantilism.

The mental condition of sufferers from Friedreich's ataxia is frequently normal, but schizophrenia has been reported in affected individuals (Shepherd, 1955) and a mild dementia is not uncommon in the later stages, leading to impaired intelligence and irritability. The cerebrospinal fluid is normal. Slight reduction in motor conduction velocity in peripheral nerves, attributed to axonal degeneration in large diameter myelinated fibres, has been described (Salisachs *et al.*, 1975) and abnormalities of sensory conduction and of evoked sensory potentials have also been described (Dyck *et al.*, 1974).

The cardiac changes may lead to heart failure, heart block, and electro-cardiographic abnormalities (Evans and Wright, 1942; Tyrer and Sutherland, 1961). Diabetes mellitus may occur (Tyrer and Sutherland, 1961) with an incidence varying from 8 per cent (Hewer and Robinson, 1968) to 23 per cent (Hewer, 1968) in different reports.

PROGNOSIS

Friedreich's disease is in most cases slowly but steadily progressive. Occasionally, however, it appears to become arrested, and abortive cases are encountered, for example as accidental discoveries in apparently healthy members of affected families, in whom the disorder does not progress. Few patients, however, live for more than 20 years after the onset of symptoms; about three-quarters of all patients show evidence of cardiac dysfunction during life and over half die from heart failure, while diabetic ketosis and intercurrent infection are less common causes of death (Hewer, 1968).

THE ROUSSY-LÉVY SYNDROME

This syndrome (hereditary areflexia with amyotrophy) shows certain affinities with Friedreich's ataxia on the one hand and with peroneal muscular atrophy on the other. The affected patients show mild ataxia, pes cavus, loss of the ankle- and knee-jerks, and peripheral amyotrophy in the upper and lower limbs. The course of the illness is slow with long periods of apparent arrest and the prognosis is therefore much better than that of Friedreich's disease. The finding of multiple 'onion bulbs' in a nerve biopsy obtained from one of the original cases described by Roussy and Lévy (1926) (Lapresle and Salisachs, 1973) suggests that the condition is probably a form of hypertrophic neuropathy [p. 981].

SANGER-BROWN'S AND MARIE'S ATAXIA

Sanger-Brown in 1892 described a variety of hereditary ataxia affecting 24 individuals in five successive generations of the same family. Pathological examination showed degeneration of the cells of the dorsal nucleus, of the posterior columns, and of the posterior spinocerebellar tracts. There was little or no corticospinal tract degeneration, and changes in the cerebellum were slight or absent.

The age of onset lay between 16 and 35 years, the first symptom being ataxia of the lower limbs. The condition differed from Friedreich's ataxia in the presence of optic atrophy, ptosis, diplopia, and, occasionally, of complete internal and external ophthalmoplegia, and exaggerated tendon reflexes and ankle clonus, whereas nystagmus and pes cavus were absent.

A very similar disorder was reported by Neff (1895) in four generations of a single family, 13 individuals being affected. This disorder differed from the ataxia of Sanger-Brown in that the onset of symptoms was delayed until between the ages of 50 and 65, and in some cases even later. Four affected members of Neff's family developed dementia.

Marie, in 1893, under the title of 'hereditary cerebellar ataxia', described a group of patients suffering from signs of cerebellar deficiency and corticospinal tract degeneration with, in some cases, optic atrophy. The onset of symptoms occurred during adolescence, and multiple cases were observed in the same family. Pathological examination of cases exhibiting the clinical features described by Marie has usually shown a slight degree of atrophy of the cerebellum, while in the spinal cord degeneration was most marked in the ascending cerebellar tracts and the anterolateral columns, the corticospinal tracts and posterior columns being little affected. It is doubtful, however, whether this form of cerebellar ataxia can be considered either a clinical or a pathological entity. It is probably a mixed group containing some cases of Friedreich's ataxia together with cases allied to the Sanger-Brown variety. Greenfield (1954) considers that 'hereditary spastic ataxia' covers many families in these groups.

PROGRESSIVE CEREBELLAR DEGENERATION

Although the many forms of progressive cerebellar degeneration have been shown to be very variable in clinical presentation and course, they exhibit a sufficient clinical and pathological similarity to justify their consideration together. The following are the more important varieties that have been described:

Primary parenchymatous degeneration of the cerebellum (Holmes).
Olivopontocerebellar atrophy (Dejerine and Thomas).
Olivorubrocerebellar atrophy (Lhermitte and Lejonne).
Delayed cortical cerebellar atrophy (Rossi, Marie, Foix, and Alajouanine).

As their names imply, these forms of cerebellar degeneration differ in the precise localization of the degenerative process and its incidence upon the brain stem. Their relationship was discussed by Critchley and Greenfield (1948).

Primary Parenchymatous Degeneration of the Cerebellum

Under this title Holmes described four cases occurring in a single family. One case was investigated pathologically. The cerebellum, pons, and medulla were abnormally small, especially the cerebellum, which on microscopical examination showed atrophy of all three cortical layers. This was associated with atrophy and gliosis of the olive and of the olivocerebellar fibres in the medulla and inferior cerebellar peduncle. The midbrain, pons, and spinal cord were normal. The symptoms, the onset of which occurred in early middle life, between the ages of 33 and 40, were those of progressive cerebellar deficiency. Speech became explosive, and nystagmus and ataxia of the upper and lower limbs were present. Vision and the optic nerves were normal; the tendon reflexes were brisk and there was no sensory disturbance.

Olivopontocerebellar Atrophy

This form of cerebellar atrophy was described by Dejerine and Thomas in 1900. Many cases are sporadic but several families showing dominant inheritance have been reported.

The pathological changes consist of atrophy of the ganglion cells of the olives, and of the grey matter of the pons, with degeneration of the middle cerebellar peduncles and to a lesser extent of the inferior cerebellar peduncles. The cerebellum suffers mainly as a result of atrophy of its afferent fibres by these routes. The Purkinje and other ganglion cells of the cerebellar cortex are affected secondarily. It is the olive and the neocerebellum which undergo degeneration.

The central nuclei of the cerebellum are relatively unaffected, but in **olivoru-brocerebellar atrophy** these degenerate, together with the superior peduncles, and degeneration can be traced as far as the red nuclei. A detailed review of olivopontocerebellar degeneration and related disorders has been given by Konigsmark and Weiner (1970). In a family containing many affected members, Landis *et al.* (1974) found in cerebellar biopsies from two patients severe degeneration of Purkinje cells, degeneration of cortical afferent fibres, and variable loss of granule cells. Tubular structures and crystalline inclusions were found on electron microscopy.

The onset of symptoms occurs in late middle life up to the age of 60. The symptoms are those of a slowly progressive cerebellar deficiency, namely, dysarthria, ataxia and tremor of the limbs, ataxic gait, and muscular hypotonia. Nystagmus is usually absent. Voluntary power is well preserved and the reflexes are usually normal, except that the ankle-jerks may be lost. Parkinsonian features may develop, and mental deterioration (dementia) may occur in the later stages. In some cases, spasticity, exaggerated reflexes, and extensor plantar responses rather than hypotonia occur and there is a static tremor superficially resembling that of Parkinson's disease. In some families there is also evidence of posterior column dysfunction (Landis *et al.*, 1974).

Dominant Spino-Pontine Atrophy

This condition, described by Boller and Segarra (1969) and Taniguchi and Konigsmark (1971), gives rise to severe progressive ataxia, nystagmus, dysarthria, hypotonia, hyperreflexia, and extensor plantar responses, beginning usually in adult life with preservation of the intellect and loss of vibration and tactile sensation occurring late. Affected individuals usually die between 30 and 57 years of age. Neuropathological examination shows marked degeneration of the nuclei of the basis pontis and of the cerebellar peduncles, spinocerebellar tracts and posterior columns but the inferior olives are normal and the cerebellar cortex is preserved apart from minimal Purkinje cell loss.

Delayed Cortical Cerebellar Atrophy

This disorder occurs sporadically. Greenfield (1954) and Becker *et al.* (1971) consider that it is indistinguishable from the Holmes type of cerebellar degeneration (above). The condition is normally of late onset and dominant inheritance, presenting with truncal ataxia and dysarthria followed by ataxia of the upper limbs. Pathologically there is atrophy of the vermis and cerebellar hemispheres with loss of Purkinje and granular cells and secondary degeneration of the olivary nuclei (Hoffman *et al.*, 1971). The occurrence of tremor, brisk reflexes, posterior column involvement, and extrapyramidal manifestations in some patients showing a similar clinical presentation (Currier *et al.*, 1972) makes clinical differentiation from olivopontocerebellar atrophy (see above) difficult.

Other Forms of Cerebellar Ataxia

A very large number of other hereditary variants of cerebellar ataxia have been described and the relationship of many of these to the varieties described above is unclear. Thus cerebellar ataxia was one feature of the form described by Ferguson and Critchley (1928) in which corticospinal tract involvement, posterior column type sensory loss, and external ophthalmoplegia were also seen; had it not been for the family history any single case of this disorder would have been impossible to distinguish from multiple sclerosis.

In *dyssynergia cerebellaris myoclonica* (the Ramsay–Hunt syndrome) progressive cerebellar ataxia with nystagmus and dysarthria is accompanied by repeated myoclonus and sometimes mental retardation, but the progressive dementia seen in progressive myoclonic epilepsy [p. 1135] does not occur and no Lafora bodies are found in the brain at post-mortem examination, but there is severe degeneration of the dentate nuclei (Hunt, 1921). Myoclonus may be precipitated by photic stimulation (Kreindler *et al.*, 1959); a similar syndrome associated with nerve deafness has been described (May and White, 1968).

Other rare combinations include ataxia, nerve deafness, mental retardation, and signs of upper and lower motor neurone lesions beginning in infancy (Berman *et al.*, 1973), familial agenesis of the vermis with episodic hyperpnoea, abnormal eye movements, and mental retardation (Joubert *et al.*, 1969) and dominantly inherited cerebellar ataxia of late onset with defective optokinetic nystagmus and absent or abnormal oculovestibular reflexes but with preservation of cochlear function (Philcox *et al.*, 1975). Similar abnormalities of eye movement and of vestibulo-ocular reflexes, with unstable fixation and dysmetria of voluntary saccades may, however, be found in many variants of hereditary ataxia, including Friedreich's ataxia (Baloh *et al.*, 1975).

In the rare autosomal recessive syndrome often called the *Marinesco–Sjögren syndrome* (Marinesco *et al.*, 1931; Sjögren, 1950; Garland and Moorhouse, 1953; Ron and Pearce, 1971), somatic and mental retardation are accompanied by cerebellar ataxia, cataracts, and sometimes by epilepsy, microcephaly, and corticospinal tract dysfunction.

The *Sjögren–Larsson syndrome*, which is also an autosomal recessive disorder (Sjögren and Larsson, 1957), is characterized by congenital ichthyosis, mental retardation, spasticity, epilepsy, macular degeneration, abnormalities of the teeth, and hypertelorism (Guilleminault *et al.*, 1973). Amino acid excretion may be abnormal (Ionasescu *et al.*, 1973) and the condition may be due to an as yet unidentified disorder of lipid metabolism which may possibly be influenced favourably by giving a diet with medium chain triglycerides.

Fahr's disease (familial calcification of the basal ganglia), a condition of autosomal dominant inheritance, usually begins early in life with progressive dementia, convulsions, and rigidity. Calcification in the walls of the vessels of the lenticular and dentate nuclei may be seen on radiographs of the skull (Foley, 1951). Cerebellar ataxia and pigmentary macular degeneration occasionally occur (Strobos *et al.*, 1957).

Other Rare Disorders Tentatively Classified with the Hereditary Ataxias

Other rare combinations of neurological features include neurofibromatosis, peroneal muscular atrophy, congenital deafness, partial albinism, and Axenfeld's defect of the iridocorneal angle occurring in several members of two generations of a family (Bradley *et al.*, 1974), optic atrophy, nerve deafness, and distal neurogenic atrophy (Iwashita *et al.*, 1970), and distal muscular atrophy, ataxia, retinitis pigmentosa, and diabetes mellitus of dominant inheritance without the biochemical features of Refsum's disease (Furukawa *et al.*, 1968).

Usher's syndrome is the name which has been given to the combination of congenital deafness and retinitis pigmentosa giving progressive blindness (Usher, 1914; Vernon, 1969); there is still dispute as to whether this condition is identical with or different from *Hallgren's syndrome*, in which the same two salient clinical features are sometimes associated with vestibulo-cerebellar ataxia and mental retardation in certain members of affected families (Hall-gren, 1959; Merin *et al.*, 1974). Both disorders are usually of autosomal recessive inheritance. Certainly, similar tapeto-retinal degeneration is sometimes seen in association with many of the disorders of the hereditary ataxia group described above (François, 1974).

Xeroderma pigmentosum is a rare autosomal recessive disease characterized by abnormal sensitivity to sunlight with pigmentary changes in the skin, telangiectases, keratoses, and eventually cutaneous carcinomata. Neurological complications include progressive dementia, chorea, nerve deafness, cortico-spinal tract degeneration, peripheral neuropathy, and skeletal abnormalities (Waltimo *et al.*, 1967; Thrush *et al.*, 1974).

Ataxia Telangiectasia

This rare disorder, which is probably of autosomal recessive inheritance and which has been called the Louis–Bar syndrome, is characterized by cerebellar ataxia with onset in infancy and with inability to walk by the age of 10 years. Telangiectasiae are seen in the bulbar conjunctivae and, later, on the skin. Most patients show a deficiency in serum gamma-globulin resulting in a diminished resistance to respiratory infections, one of which eventually proves fatal. Patho-logically the Purkinje and granular cells of the cerebellum are selectively involved. Boder and Sedgwick (1963) reviewed 101 cases, Strich (1966) described the pathological findings in 3 cases, and McFarlin *et al.* (1972) have reviewed the clinical features and immunology of the disorder. The serum alpha-fetoprotein is raised to above 30 mg per ml in all cases, a finding suggesting widespread failure of tissue differentiation, especially in the liver, in such cases (Waldmann and McIntire, 1972).

DIAGNOSIS

The diagnosis of the hereditary ataxias rests upon the onset, in most cases before the age of 20, of progressive symptoms, of which ataxia is usually the most conspicuous, and which frequently include symptoms of bilateral corticospinal tract degeneration, sensory loss, pes cavus and scoliosis, and sometimes optic atrophy. When the disorder is familial and the history of its incidence can be obtained it is usually easy to make a correct diagnosis. Sporadic cases, however, may give rise to difficulty. Hereditary spastic paraplegia must be distinguished from congenital diplegia by the fact that the patient is normal at birth, and the disorder is progressive, whereas in diplegia the symptoms are congenital, and tend to improve, and are not uncommonly associated with mental deficiency and with epilepsy. Friedreich's ataxia must be distinguished from multiple sclerosis and from tabes. It frequently begins before the age of 15, when the onset of multiple sclerosis is rare. Both disorders are characterized by nystagmus, ataxia, and extensor plantar responses, but scoliosis, pes cavus, and loss of the knee- and ankle-jerks are peculiar to Friedreich's disease. The distinction of Friedreich's disease from tabes is based upon the absence in the latter of pes cavus, scoliosis, dysarthria, and extensor plantar responses, and the presence of Argyll Robertson pupils and, in most cases, of positive serological reactions in the blood and cerebrospinal fluid. The diagnosis of a sporadic case of the ataxia described by Ferguson and Critchley (1929) from multiple sclerosis may be extremely difficult, if not impossible.

The progressive hereditary cerebellar degenerations of late middle life are to be distinguished from sporadic spinocerebellar degeneration arising as a complication of carcinoma in the lung or elsewhere; from tumours, by the absence of increased intracranial pressure; from tabes, by the usual preservation of the tendon reflexes, and the absence of sensory loss and of pupillary abnormalities; and from subacute combined degeneration, by the absence of paraesthesiae, sensory loss, and gastric achylia.

From the bewildering variety of combinations of neurological symptoms and signs described above, it is apparent that until specific enzymatic or other biochemical defects underlying various manifestations of these syndromes are identified, classification will always be difficult. Many cases continue to occur which cannot readily be identified as belonging to any of the varieties listed above. As knowledge extends, more and more of these disorders may eventually be considered more appropriately to be due to inborn errors of metabolism. For the present, however unsatisfactory it may be, ignorance of aetiology demands that they can only be classified by 'pattern recognition' of various combinations of signs of neurological dysfunction.

TREATMENT

No treatment which can influence the course of most of these disorders is known. Although the patient will ultimately become bedridden, this should be postponed as long as possible but often a wheelchair or other appropriate aids are required. Re-educational exercises may help to keep the ataxia under control. In Friedreich's ataxia the pes cavus may require surgical treatment or appropriate boots and a spinal support may be needed to control scoliosis. In the later stages care must be taken to avoid as far as possible exposing the patient to the risk of respiratory infections.

REFERENCES

BALOH, R. W., KONRAD, H. R., and HONRUBIA, V. (1975) Vestibulo-ocular function in patients with cerebellar atrophy, *Neurology (Minneap.)*, **25**, 160.

BECKER, P. E., SABUNCU, N., and HOPF, H. C. (1971) Dominant erblicher Typ von 'cerebellarer Ataxie', *Z. Neurol.*, **199**, 116.

BELL, J. (1939) Hereditary ataxia and spastic paraplegia, *Treasury of Human Inheritance*, vol. iv, pt. 3, London.

BERMAN, W., HASLAM, R. H. A., KONIGSMARK, B. W., CAPUTE, A. J., and MIGEON, C. J. (1973) A new familial syndrome with ataxia, hearing loss and mental retardation, *Arch. Neurol. (Chic.)*, **29**, 258.

BICKERSTAFF, E. R. (1950) Hereditary spastic paraplegia, *J. Neurol. Neurosurg. Psychiat.*, **13**, 134.

BODER, E., and SEDGWICK, R. P. (1963) Ataxia-telangiectasia: a review of 101 cases, *Little Club Clinics in Developmental Medicine*, **8**, 110.

BOGAERT, L. VAN (1952) Études sur la paraplégie spasmodique familiale. V. Forme classique pure avec atrophie optique massive chez certains de ses membres. Considérations génétiques sur la paraplégie spasmodique familiale en général, *Acta neurol. belg.*, **52**, 795.

BOLLER, F., and SEGARRA, J. M. (1969) Spino-pontine degeneration, *Europ. Neurol.*, **2**, 356.

BRADLEY, W. G., RICHARDSON, J., and FREW, I. J. C. (1974) The familial association of neurofibromatosis, peroneal muscular atrophy, congenital deafness, partial albinism, and Axenfeld's defect, *Brain*, **97**, 521.

BRUGSCH, H. G., and HAUPTMANN, A. (1944) Familial occurrence of Friedreich's ataxia with Charcot–Marie–Tooth's neural muscular atrophy, *Bull. New Engl. med. Cent.*, **6**, 42.

BRUYN, G. W., and MECHELSE, K. (1962) The association of familial spastic paraplegia and epilepsy in one family, *Psychiat. Neurol. Neurochir.*, **65**, 280.

COURVILLE, C. B., and FRIEDMAN, A. P. (1940) Chronic progressive degeneration of the superior cerebellar cortex (parenchymatous cortical cerebellar atrophy), *Bull. Los Angeles neurol. Soc.*, **5**, 171.

CRITCHLEY, M., and GREENFIELD, J. G. (1948) Olivo-ponto-cerebellar atrophy, *Brain*, **71**, 343.

CURRIER, R. D., GLOVER, G., JACKSON, J. F., and TIPTON, A. C. (1972) Spinocerebellar ataxia: study of a large kindred. I. General information and genetics, *Neurology (Minneap.)*, **22**, 1040.

DEJERINE, J., and THOMAS, A. (1900) L'atrophie olivo-ponto-cérébelleuse, *N. Iconogr. Salpêt.*, **13**, 330.

DYCK, P. J., and LAIS, A. C. (1972) Evidence for segmental demyelination secondary to axonal degeneration in Friedreich's ataxia, in *Clinical Studies in Myology* (International Congress Series No. 295), p. 253, Amsterdam.

DYCK, P. J., LAMBERT, E. H., and NICHOLS, P. C. (1974) Quantitative measurement of sensation related to compound action potential and number and sizes of myelinated and unmyelinated fibers of sural nerve in health, Friedreich's ataxia, hereditary sensory neuropathy, and tabes dorsalis, in *Handbook of Electroencephalography and Clinical Neurophysiology*, vol. 9, p. 83, Amsterdam.

EVANS, W., and WRIGHT, G. (1942) The electrocardiogram in Friedreich's disease, *Brit. Heart J.*, **4**, 91.

FERGUSON, F. R., and CRITCHLEY, M. (1928) Leber's optic atrophy and its relationship with the heredo-familial ataxias, *J. Neurol. Psychopath.*, **9**, 120.

FERGUSON, F. R., and CRITCHLEY, M. (1929) A clinical study of an heredofamilial disease resembling disseminated sclerosis, *Brain*, **52**, 203.

FOLEY, J. (1951) Calcification of the corpus striatum and dentate nuclei occurring in a family, *J. Neurol. Neurosurg. Psychiat.*, **14**, 253.

FRANÇOIS, J. (1974) Tapetoretinal degenerations in spinocerebellar degenerations (heredo-ataxias), Proceedings of the Fourth International Congress of Neurogenetics and Neuroophthalmology, *Acta Genet. med. (Roma)*, **23**, 3.

FRIEDREICH, N. (1863) Ueber degenerative Atrophie der spinalen Hinterstrange, *Virchows Arch. path. Anat.*, **26**, 391.

FRIEDREICH, N. (1876) Ueber Ataxie mit besonderer Berücksichtigung der hereditären Formen, *Virchows Arch. path. Anat.*, **68**, 145.

FURUKAWA, T., TAKAGI, A., NAKAO, K., SUGITA, H., TSUKAGOSHI, H., and TSUBAKI, T. (1968) Hereditary muscular atrophy with ataxia, retinitis pigmentosa, and diabetes mellitus: a clinical report of a family, *Neurology (Minneap.)*, **18**, 942.

GARLAND, H., and MOORHOUSE, D. (1953) An extremely rare recessive hereditary syndrome including cerebellar ataxia, oligophrenia, cataract, and other features, *J. Neurol. Neurosurg. Psychiat.*, **16**, 110.

GREENFIELD, J. G. (1954) *The Spinocerebellar Degenerations*, Oxford.

GUILLEMINAULT, C., HARPEY, J. P., and LAFOURCADE, J. (1973) Sjögren-Larsson syndrome. Report of two cases in twins, *Neurology (Minneap.)*, **23**, 367.

HALDANE, J. B. S. (1941) Partial sex-linkage of recessive spastic paraplegia, *J. Genet.*, **41**, 141.

HALL, G. W., and MACKAY, R. P. (1937) Forms of familial ataxia resembling multiple sclerosis, *Arch. Neurol. Psychiat. (Chic.)*, **38**, 19.

HALLGREN, B. (1959) Retinitis pigmentosa combined with congenital deafness; with vestibulo-cerebellar ataxia and mental abnormality in a proportion of cases, *Acta psychiat. scand.*, **34**, Suppl. 138.

HEWER, R. L. (1968) Study of fatal cases of Friedreich's ataxia, *Brit. med. J.*, **3**, 649.

HEWER, R. L., and ROBINSON, N. (1968) Diabetes mellitus in Friedreich's ataxia, *J. Neurol. Neurosurg. Psychiat.*, **31**, 226.

HOFFMAN, P. M., STUART, W. H., EARLE, K. M., and BRODY, J. A. (1971) Hereditary late-onset cerebellar degeneration, *Neurology (Minneap.)*, **21**, 771.

HOLMES, G. (1907 a) A form of familial degeneration of the cerebellum, *Brain*, **30**, 466.

HOLMES, G. (1907 b) An attempt to classify cerebellar disease, with a note on Marie's hereditary cerebellar ataxia, *Brain*, **30**, 455.

HUGHES, J. T., BROWNELL, B., and HEWER, R. L. (1968) The peripheral sensory pathway in Friedreich's ataxia: an examination by light and electron microscopy of the posterior nerve roots, posterior root ganglia, and peripheral sensory nerves in cases of Friedreich's ataxia, *Brain*, **91**, 803.

HUNT, J. R. (1921) Dyssynergia cerebellaris myoclonica—primary atrophy of the dentate system: a contribution to the pathology and symptomatology of the cerebellum, *Brain*, **44**, 490.

IONASESCU, V., STEGINK, L., MUELLER, S., and WEINSTEIN, M. (1973) Amino acid abnormality in Sjögren–Larsson syndrome, *Arch. Neurol. (Chic.)*, **28**, 197.

IWASHITA, H., INOUE, N., ARAKI, S., and KUROIWA, Y. (1970) Optic atrophy, neural deafness and distal neurogenic amyotrophy, *Arch. Neurol. (Chic.)*, **22**, 357.

JOUBERT, M., EISENRING, J.-J., and ROBB, J. P. (1969) Familial agenesis of the cerebellar vermis. A syndrome of episodic hyperpnea, abnormal eye movements, ataxia and retardation, *Neurology (Minneap.)*, **19**, 813.

KONIGSMARK, G., and WEINER, L. (1970) The olivopontocerebellar atrophies: a review, *Medicine (Baltimore)*, **49**, 227.

KREINDLER, A., CRIGHEL, E., and POILICI, I. (1959) Clinical and electroencephalographic investigations in myoclonic cerebellar dyssynergia, *J. Neurol. Neurosurg. Psychiat.*, **22**, 232.

LANDIS, D. M. D., ROSENBERG, R. N., LANDIS, S. C., SCHUT, L., and NYHAN, W. L. (1974) Olivopontocerebellar degeneration. Clinical and ultrastructural abnormalities, *Arch. Neurol. (Chic.)*, **31**, 295.

LAPRESLE, J., and SALISACHS, P. (1973) Onion bulbs in a nerve biopsy specimen from an original case of Roussy–Lévy disease, *Arch. Neurol. (Chic.)*, **29**, 346.

LEJONNE, P., and LHERMITTE, J. (1909 a) Atrophie olivo-rubro-cérébelleuse, *N. Iconogr. Salpêt.*, **22**, 605.

LEJONNE, P., and LHERMITTE, J. (1909 b) Atrophie olivo-et rubro-cérébelleuse, *Rev. neurol. (Paris)*, **17**, 109.

McFARLIN, D. E., STROBER, W., and WALDMANN, T. A. (1972) Ataxia–telangiectasia, *Medicine*, **51**, 281.

MARIE, P., FOIX, C., and ALAJOUANINE, T. (1922) De l'atrophie cérébelleuse tardive à prédominance corticale, *Rev. neurol. (Paris)*, **29**, 849, 1082.

MARINESCO, G., DRAGANESCO, S., and VASILIU, D. (1931) Nouvelle maladie familiale, caractérisée par une cataracte congénitale et un arrêt du développement somatoneuropsychique, *Encéphale*, **26**, 97.

MARINESCO, G., and TRETIAKOFF, C. (1920) Étude histo-pathologique des centres nerveux dans trois cas de maladie de Friedreich, *Rev. neurol. (Paris)*, **27**, 113.

MATHIEU, P., and BERTRAND, I. (1929) Études anatomo-cliniques sur les atrophies cérébelleuses, *Rev. neurol. (Paris)*, **36**, 721.

MAY, D. L., and WHITE, H. H. (1968) Familial myoclonus, cerebellar ataxia, and deafness: specific genetically-determined disease, *Arch. Neurol. (Chic.)*, **19**, 331.

MERIN, S., ABRAHAM, F. A., and AUERBACH, E. (1974) Usher's and Hallgren's syndromes, Proceedings of the Fourth International Congress of Neurogenetics and Neuroophthalmology, *Acta Genet. med. (Roma)*, **23**, 49.

NEFF, I. H. (1895) A report of thirteen cases of ataxia in adults with hereditary history, *Amer. J. Insan.*, **51**, 365.

PHILCOX, D. V., SELLARS, S. L., PAMPLETT, R., and BEIGHTON, P. (1975) Vestibular dysfunction in hereditary ataxia, *Brain*, **98**, 309.

POWELL, E. D. U. (1961) Blood-group studies in Friedreich's ataxia, *Brit. med. J.*, **1**, 868.

PRATT, R. T. C. (1967) *The Genetics of Neurological Disorders*, London.

RON, M. A., and PEARCE, J. (1971) Marinesco–Sjögren–Garland syndrome with unusual features, *J. neurol. Sci.*, **13**, 175.

ROSSI, I. (1907) Atrophie parenchymateuse primitive du cervelet à localisation corticale, *N. Iconogr. Salpêt.*, **20**, 66.

ROTH, M. (1948) On a possible relationship between hereditary ataxia and peroneal muscular atrophy, *Brain*, **71**, 416.

ROUSSY, G., and LÉVY, G. (1926) Sept cas d'une maladie familiale particulière, *Rev. neurol. (Paris)*, **1**, 427.

SALISACHS, P., CODINA, M., and PRADAS, J. (1975) Motor conduction velocity in patients with Friedreich's ataxia: report of 12 cases, *J. neurol. Sci.*, **24**, 331.

SCHAFFER, K. (1922) Zur Pathologie und pathologischen Histologie der spastischen Heredodegeneration (hereditäre spastische Spinalparalyse), *Dtsch. Z. Nervenheilk.*, **73**, 101.

SCHWARZ, G. A. (1952) Hereditary (familial) spastic paraplegia, *Arch. Neurol. Psychiat. (Chic.)*, **68**, 655.

SCHWARZ, G. A., and LIU, C.-N. (1956) Hereditary (familial) spastic paraplegia: further clinical and pathologic observations, *Arch. Neurol. Psychiat. (Chic.)*, **75**, 144.

SHEPHERD, M. (1955) Report of a family suffering from Friedreich's disease, peroneal muscular atrophy, and schizophrenia, *J. Neurol. Neurosurg. Psychiat.*, **18**, 297.

SJÖGREN, T. (1943) Klinische und erbbiologische Untersuchungen uber die Heredo-ataxien, *Acta psychiat. (Kbh.)*, Suppl. xxvii.

SJÖGREN, T. (1950) Hereditary congenital spinocerebellar ataxia accompanied by congenital cataract and oligophrenia, *Confin. neurol. (Basel)*, **10**, 293.

SJÖGREN, T., and LARSSON, T. (1957) Oligophrenia in combination with congenital ichthyosis and spastic disorders. A clinical and genetic study, *Acta psychiat. scand.*, Suppl. 113, 1.

STRICH, S. J. (1966) Pathological findings in three cases of ataxia-telangiectasia, *J. Neurol. Neurosurg. Psychiat.*, **29**, 487.

STROBOS, R. R. J., DE LA TORRE, E., and MARTIN, J. F. (1957) Symmetrical calcification of the basal ganglia with familial ataxia and pigmentary macular degeneration, *Brain*, **80**, 313.

SUTHERLAND, J. M. (1957) Familial spastic paraplegia: its relation to mental and cardiac abnormalities, *Lancet*, **ii**, 169.

TANIGUCHI, R., and KONIGSMARK, B. W. (1971) Dominant spino-pontine atrophy: report of a family through three generations, *Brain*, **94**, 349.

THRUSH, D. C., HOLTI, G., BRADLEY, W. G., CAMPBELL, M. J., and WALTON, J. N. (1974) Neurological manifestations of xeroderma pigmentosum in two siblings, *J. neurol. Sci.*, **22**, 91.

TYRER, J. H., and SUTHERLAND, J. M. (1961) The primary spinocerebellar atrophies and their associated defects with a study of the foot deformity, *Brain*, **84**, 289.

USHER, C. H. (1914) On the inheritance of retinitis pigmentosa, with notes of cases, *Royal London Ophth. Hosp. Rept.*, **9**, 130.

VERNON, M. (1969) Usher's syndrome—deafness and progressive blindness, *J. chron. Dis.*, **22**, 133.

WALDMANN, T. A., and MCINTIRE, K. R. (1972) Serum-alpha-fetoprotein levels in patients with ataxia-telangiectasia, *Lancet*, **ii**, 1112.

WALTIMO, O., IIVANAINEN, M., and HOKKANEN, E. (1967) Xeroderma pigmentosum with neurological manifestations, *Acta neurol. scand.*, **43**, Suppl. 31, 66.

MOTOR NEURONE DISEASE

Synonyms. Amyotrophic lateral sclerosis; progressive muscular atrophy; progressive bulbar palsy; motor system disease.

Definition. A disease characterized pathologically by degenerative changes, which are most marked in the anterior horn cells of the spinal cord, the motor nuclei of the medulla, and the corticospinal tracts, and clinically by progressive wasting of the muscles, especially those of the upper limbs and those innervated from the medulla, combined with symptoms of corticospinal tract degeneration. The term 'progressive muscular atrophy' is associated especially with the names of Aran (1850) and Duchenne (1847). Charcot (1869) distinguished two varieties —progressive muscular atrophy of Aran and Duchenne, characterized only by lower motor neurone lesions, and a form in which these were associated with symptoms of corticospinal tract lesions and which he called 'amyotrophic lateral sclerosis'. These two varieties are now usually regarded as nosologically similar. When the lower motor neurone lesions predominate, or, as more rarely happens, occur alone, the term 'progressive muscular atrophy' is still generally applied to the disease, and when the muscles innervated from the medulla are predominantly involved it has been termed 'progressive bulbar palsy'. Some authors then use the term 'amyotrophic lateral sclerosis' for those cases in which signs of corticospinal tract disease predominate in the early stages and in which it may initially be difficult or impossible to find evidence of lower motor neurone involvement. In most cases, however, the symptoms of upper and lower motor neurone lesions are mixed, except in the lower limbs, where the latter are frequently absent until the terminal stages. Greenfield (1958) preferred the term amyotrophic lateral sclerosis to motor neurone disease on the grounds that the pathological changes in the spinal cord are not limited to the motor neurones and many American authors use this term as an inclusive one, embracing all varieties of the disease. Motor neurone disease, however, is a better inclusive term.

PATHOLOGY
The Spinal Cord

Naked-eye changes in the spinal cord are slight, but on section the grey matter of the anterior horns appears smaller than normal, and the ventral roots are wasted. Microscopically there is severe degeneration of the ganglion cells of the anterior horns. This change is usually most marked in the cervical enlargement of the cord, but is always widespread, and its severity is not invariably proportional to the clinical condition. The ganglion cells exhibit chromatolysis, which is at first perinuclear. There is frequently a granular deposit of lipochrome. The total number of ganglion cells is much reduced. As a rule all groups within the anterior horn suffer equally. There are exceptions to this, however, but there is no general agreement as to whether some are more susceptible than others. The degeneration is associated with a slight secondary gliosis, and rarely slight perivascular infiltration with round cells has been observed. Large axonal swellings containing large numbers of neurofilaments (spheroids) have been found in the anterior horns and in the brain stem nuclei (Carpenter, 1968). In the variety of familial amyotrophic lateral sclerosis which is common in the Mariana islands and which is often associated with the Parkinsonism–dementia complex [p. 591], Alzheimer's neurofibrillary change is common in cortical neurones and granulovacuolar change in the cells of Ammon's horn of the hippocampus (Hirano et al., 1967), and neurofibrillary tangles have also been observed along with hyaline acidophilic bodies, superficially resembling Lewy bodies, in the anterior horn cells. Similar changes have now been reported in hereditary cases of motor neurone disease occurring in racial groups other than the Chamorro people of the Mariana islands (Metcalf and Hirano, 1971; Takahashi et al., 1972) and even in occasional cases of the commoner sporadic form of the disease in adults (Schochet *et al.*, 1969; Meyers *et al.*, 1974) as well as in juvenile cases (Nelson and Prensky, 1972).

The Weigert-Pal stain or other suitable myelin stains reveal degeneration of the white matter of the spinal cord, which is most marked in, and often confined to, the anterolateral columns [FIG. 115]. The corticospinal fibres suffer most, both the direct and the crossed corticospinal tracts being affected. Corticospinal tract degeneration is never equally severe at all levels. It is not uncommon to find severe changes in the lower thoracic and lumbosacral regions, while the upper thoracic region is but slightly affected, and severe changes are found again in the cervical enlargement, extending up to the medulla. The spinocerebellar tracts usually show degeneration, especially the anterior, and the severity of

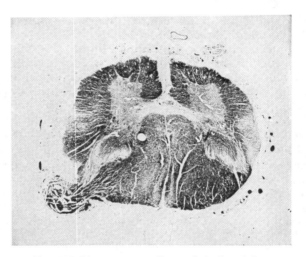

FIG. 115. Motor neurone disease. Spinal cord, L.1

this change varies in different segments. The rubrospinal, vestibulospinal, and tectospinal tracts are also degenerated to a variable extent, and despite the well-known fact that sensory symptoms and signs are absent, slight degeneration is occasionally present in the posterior columns, especially in some familial cases (Engel *et al.*, 1959). The endogenous fibres of the spinal cord which lie close to the grey matter are degenerated in the anterolateral columns, but not in the posterior columns (Smith, 1960).

The Brain Stem

The ganglion cells of the medullary motor nuclei show degenerative changes similar to those in the anterior horn cells of the spinal cord. These alterations are most marked in the hypoglossal nucleus, the dorsal nucleus of the vagus, the nucleus ambiguus, and the trigeminal motor nucleus. The facial nucleus is usually less severely affected. Similar changes have been observed in the sensory nuclei. There is a marked degeneration in the pyramids. Bertrand and van Bogaert (1925) described a case in which corticospinal tract degeneration was severe in the medulla and negligible in the pons and cerebral peduncles. Degeneration has also been described in the inferior cerebellar peduncle, the medial longitudinal fasciculus, the medial and lateral lemnisci, and the reticular formation. The third and fourth nerve nuclei in the midbrain almost invariably escape.

The Cerebral Hemispheres

Naked-eye changes are usually inconspicuous, but slight atrophy of the ascending frontal gyri has been described. Microscopic changes are most marked in the cerebral cortex anterior to the central sulcus. The typical lesion in subacute cases is a lipochrome degeneration of the ganglion cells in the frontal and precentral regions. This change is most marked in the third and fifth cortical layers, the latter of which contains the large corticospinal motor cells of Betz. Degeneration has also been observed in the tangential fibres of the cortex. Some glial overgrowth is usually present in the regions which are the site of atrophy. Degenerative changes are also found in the middle-third of the corpus callosum and in the corticospinal fibres in the posterior limb of the internal capsule (Brownell et al., 1970).

Peripheral Nerves and Muscles

The ventral roots and peripheral nerves exhibit axonal degeneration, with secondary demyelination. Collateral sprouting of surviving motor axons occurs with reinnervation of groups of denervated muscle fibres which may subsequently become denervated again when the reinnervating neurone is involved in the disease process (Wohlfart, 1957). The muscles show characteristic changes of denervation atrophy in that large (or sometimes small and scattered) groups of uniformly atrophic but otherwise normal-appearing muscle fibres are seen lying alongside other groups which are normal or even larger than normal. In long-standing cases there may be so-called 'secondary myopathic change' (Drachman et al., 1967) with some random variation in fibre size, central nuclei, and degeneration or necrosis of individual fibres similar to that seen in myopathic disorders; this change appears to be due to the interplay of denervation and re-innervation and to the trauma to which a weakened muscle is regularly subjected.

AETIOLOGY

Motor neurone disease is a disease of late middle life, usually beginning between the ages of 50 and 70, occasionally as early as the third decade or as late as the eighth. Cases occurring in childhood and early adult life may be difficult or impossible to distinguish clinically from chronic spinal muscular atrophy of the Kugelberg–Welander type [p. 706] unless signs of corticospinal tract dysfunction are prominent. The sporadic disorder occurs world-wide and in all races (Edgar et al., 1973) and has an incidence of about 1 new case in 100,000 of the population per year with a prevalence variably reported as between 2·5–7 per 100,000 (Kurland and Mulder, 1954; Kurtzke, 1969). It is generally more common in males than in females, but not in Finland where geographical isolates of increased incidence have been reported (Jokelainen, 1976); it may be less common in Mexicans (Olivares et al., 1972), but is relatively common in Filipinos (Matsumoto et al., 1972) and in Nigerians, in whom it tends to run an unusually benign course (Osuntokun et al., 1974). Clinically atypical varieties of the disease have been described in certain parts of India (Valmikinathan et al., 1973). The sporadic variety is much the commonest, but many families showing dominant, recessive, or, rarely, X-linked recessive inheritance (Kennedy et al., 1968) have been described in many parts of the world (Pratt, 1967; Liversedge and Campbell, 1974). In such familial cases many atypical variants have been reported including an onset in childhood or adolescence with chronic bulbar palsy (Fazio, 1892; Londe, 1893; Markand and Daly, 1971) or benign proximal forms of the disease.

Amyotrophic lateral sclerosis is endemic in the Chamorro people on the island of Guam and shows there a high familial incidence; it is still uncertain whether this condition, with which the so-called Parkinsonism–dementia complex is often associated (Eldridge et al., 1969), is a genetically determined disorder of dominant inheritance or whether it could be the result of combined genetic and environmental (such as a slow virus) factors (Kurland, 1957; Hirano et al., 1967; Kurland, 1972; Reed et al., 1975). This disorder is probably different from the sporadic form of motor neurone disease which is commonly observed in Europe and in America though it may be clinically indistinguishable. However, dementia has been reported in familial juvenile amyotrophic lateral sclerosis in Holland (Staal and Went, 1968; Bots and Staal, 1973) and, as mentioned above, pathological changes once thought to be confined to the Guam variety are now being discovered in sporadic cases in other parts of the world, so that the nosological position remains uncertain.

The condition has been regarded by some workers, especially in France, as a form of 'chronic poliomyelitis', but this hypothesis is not borne out by the histological appearances or by virological studies. Inflammatory infiltration is rare and scanty, and when it occurs probably should be regarded as a reaction to degeneration. Exceptionally, however, the disease may develop in an individual who suffered many years earlier from acute anterior poliomyelitis and progressive atrophy may then begin in the limb or limbs most severely affected by the acute illness. Hallen et al. (1969) suggest that in such cases the process may indeed be one of chronic poliomyelitis, and that they should be distinguished from sporadic cases, but this view is disputed by others. The condition has also been reported to follow encephalitis lethargica (Milhorat, 1946). Evidence to indicate that the causal virus is responsible for these sequelae is, however, lacking. It is, however, conceivable that injury to anterior horn cells caused by a virus may shorten the active life of some of these cells and the postulate that motor neurone disease is due to a premature ageing process in such cells, perhaps precipitated by unknown environmental factors, has received some support (McComas et al., 1973). Suggestions that the condition may be due to lead intoxication (Campbell et al., 1970), associated with a diffuse angiopathy (Störtebecker et al., 1970; Urbánek and Jansa, 1974), with disorders of lipid and carbohydrate metabolism (Ionasescu and Luca, 1964; Gustafson and Störtebecker, 1972) or with high concentrations of manganese and calcium in the central nervous system (Yase, 1972) are either unsubstantiated as yet or have given no definite clues to the aetiology of the disease. Exocrine pancreatic dysfunction, found in certain cases, is probably an epiphenomenon. The neuronal effects of lead poisoning may certainly simulate this condition (Boothby et al., 1974). Attempts to isolate a causal virus have been uniformly unsuccessful (Cremer et al., 1973; Liversedge and Campbell, 1974). It has been suggested that there is an association between this disorder and malignant disease (Brain et al., 1965; Norris and Engel, 1965; Vejjajiva et al., 1967) and an identical clinical syndrome has been reported in association with macroglobulinaemia with improvement following treatment of the latter condition (Peters and Clatanoff, 1968), but recent work suggests that the association with carcinoma is no more than could be accounted for by chance (Jokelainen, 1976). The CSF homovallinic acid (HVA) is lower in such cases than in control subjects but levodopa is therapeutically ineffective (Mendell *et al.*, 1971). The significance of CSF changes in such cases identified by isoelectric focusing and indicating a 'barrier-damage pattern' (Kjellin and Stibler, 1976) has yet to be determined. There is some evidence of disordered protein metabolism in neurones but not in myelin in such cases (Savolainen and Palo, 1973) and of DNA-directed mRNA synthesis (Mann and Yates, 1974), but whether these abnormalities indicate a fundamental aetiopathogenic mechanism is still uncertain. There is no conclusive evidence that trauma plays any part in aetiology, but it is an old observation that weakness and wasting may first appear in the muscles which are most used by the patient in his occupation, or have been the site of an injury: the significance of this relationship is as yet undetermined.

SYMPTOMS

Mode of Onset

The disease is usually chronic, but may run a subacute course. Correspondingly the onset is generally insidious, but may be more rapid. The nature of the earliest symptoms depends upon which region of the nervous system is first affected. Commonly the first abnormality is observed in the hands, where the patient may be conscious of weakness, stiffness, or clumsiness of movements of the fingers, or his attention may be drawn to the wasting, or he may perceive fascicular twitching. When the shoulder girdle and upper arm muscles are first affected the first symptom is weakness of movements of the shoulder. When degeneration begins in the bulbar motor nuclei the first symptom to be noticed is usually dysarthria or dysphagia. Less frequently the disease begins with spastic paraplegia, or wasting of one or both lower limbs. Cramp-like pains in the limbs are often an early symptom.

Symptoms and Signs of Lower Motor Neurone Degeneration

Degeneration of the anterior horn cells, and of the motor cells of the medulla, leads to weakness and wasting of the muscles which they innervate. Fasciculation is also a conspicuous sign, and occurs in those muscles which are supplied by ganglion cells undergoing active degeneration. It may be limited to a few groups of muscles, or be much more widespread, and its extent is an indication of the diffuseness of the degenerative process. Very rarely, widespread weakness and wasting may occur in the absence of fasciculation. When fasciculation is not immediately evident it can often be evoked by sharply tapping the muscle. Contractures are usually slight. As a rule muscular wasting begins in the hands, the muscles of the thenar eminences being first affected. Not uncommonly one hand may begin to waste some months or even a year before the other. In other cases the onset is symmetrical. The wasting tends to spread to the muscles innervated by the segment of the spinal cord adjacent to that first affected. Hence, after the hands, the forearm muscles are involved, the flexors usually suffering before the extensors. The weakness and atrophy of the hand muscles lead to clumsiness of the finger movements, and some degree of claw-hand usually develops. This deformity is not, however, as a rule severe, since the long flexors and extensors of the fingers, by which it is maintained, are soon themselves affected.

Next in frequency the muscles of the shoulder girdle and upper arm are first involved, those innervated by the fifth cervical spinal segment, especially the deltoids, being earliest affected [FIG. 116]. Those supplied by the sixth cervical segment, namely, the triceps, latissimus dorsi, the sternal part of the pectoralis major and serratus anterior, are usually involved much later, and the upper part of the trapezius also escapes until a late stage. The muscles innervated by the medulla may be the first to suffer or they may be affected simultaneously with, or shortly after, the upper limbs. The tongue is then usually the first to waste

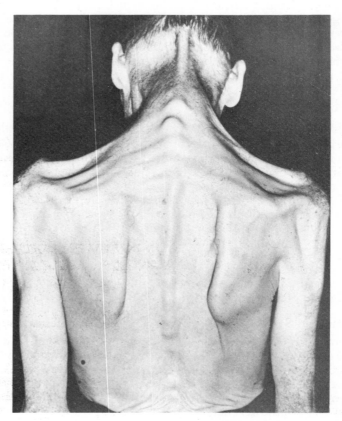

FIG. 116. Widespread wasting of shoulder girdle muscles in advanced motor neurone disease

and becomes shrunken and wrinkled and shows conspicuous fasciculation [FIG. 117]. The orbicularis oris also suffers early, but the orbicularis oculi and other facial muscles are affected later, and less severely. The palate is usually involved shortly after the tongue, together with the extrinsic muscles of the pharynx and larynx. The intrinsic laryngeal muscles usually escape until late. The mandibular muscles usually suffer less severely than the tongue and orbicularis oris. Owing to weakness of the muscles concerned, pursing of the lips and whistling become impossible, and in the later stages saliva runs from the open lips. Protrusion of the tongue is at first weak and later lost. Speech suffers from paresis of the lips, tongue, and palate. The capacity to pronounce labials and dentals is early impaired, and later gutterals. Speech becomes slurred and finally unintelligible. Phonation, however, suffers late, if at all. Swallowing becomes increasingly difficult, and food tends to regurgitate through the nose. Patients usually find semi-solids easier to swallow than either solids or fluids. In progressive bulbar palsy, slurring of speech is often an early symptom and its cause may at first be difficult to identify, especially if there is no fasciculation in the tongue. Later, because of dysphagia, distressing episodes of choking may occur during meals.

Exceptionally the extensor muscles of the cervical spine suffer early [FIG. 116], and when this occurs the head falls forwards. Early involvement of the muscles of the lower limbs is rare. The anterior tibial group and peronei are usually first affected and unilateral or bilateral foot-drop results. This mode of onset may closely simulate polyneuritis, especially when, as occasionally happens, the motor symptoms are associated with muscular pain. It has, therefore, sometimes been called the 'pseudopolyneuritic' form. Exceptionally, weakness begins in the proximal muscles of both the upper and lower limbs and if fasciculation is at first inconspicuous, the condition may simulate a proximal myopathy.

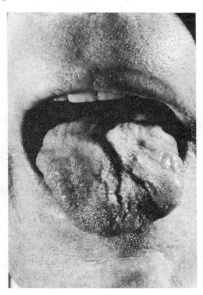

In whatever part of the body muscular wasting begins, in most cases it sooner or later becomes generalized, though progressive bulbar palsy may prove fatal before wasting has had time to develop to a severe extent elsewhere. In the final stages weakness of the trunk muscles renders it impossible for the patient to sit up in bed, and paresis of the respiratory muscles leads to increasing dyspnoea.

Electrodiagnostic Findings

Motor nerve conduction velocity is normal, if the temperature of the limb is controlled, up to a late stage of the disease, as surviving neurones conduct at a normal rate but the amplitude of the compound muscle potential evoked by supramaximal stimulation of its motor nerve may be reduced. In the later stages, demyelination secondary to axonal

FIG. 117. Atrophy of the tongue in motor neurone disease, from *An Atlas of Clinical Neurology* 2nd ed., 1975, by J. D. Spillane, reproduced by kind permission of the author

degeneration may give modest slowing of conduction in surviving motor axons. Methods of estimating electrophysiologically the number of functioning motor units in the extensor digitorum brevis and thenar muscles show a rapid early decline in the number of such units in the early stages of the disease with early functional failure in surviving 'giant' units (Brown and Jaatoul, 1974). Although there is some evidence of abnormal resistance of sensory nerves to ischaemia in such cases (Shahani *et al.*, 1971), sensory nerve function when tested electrophysiologically is normal (Willison, 1962).

Electromyography shows fibrillation potentials on mechanical stimulation by the exploring needle, spontaneous fibrillation and fasciculation potentials when the needle is stationary in the relaxed muscle, and a duration and amplitude of action-potentials greater than normal; even in cases of moderate weakness there may be a marked reduction in the number of spikes on maximal contraction

Z

(Kugelberg, 1949) and synchronization of the activity recorded by two separate electrodes within the same muscle (Buchthal and Pinelli, 1953). 'Giant' motor units of long duration and greatly increased amplitude, presumed to result from the adoption of denervated muscle fibres by axonal sprouts from surviving neurones, are a common finding in this disease (Willison, 1962; Barwick and Richardson, 1974).

Serum Enzymes

It was once thought that neurogenic muscular atrophy occurring in the spinal muscular atrophies, including motor neurone disease, did not cause an increase in serum creatine kinase activity such as that which occurs in the muscular dystrophies and in many other myopathies (Pearce *et al.*, 1964). However, it is now apparent that modest increases in the activity of this enzyme up to 400 I.U./l (normal upper limit 75) in the serum are found in between 50 and 75 per cent of cases of progressive muscular atrophy and amyotrophic lateral sclerosis (Williams and Bruford, 1970; Panitch and Franklin, 1972; Welch and Goldberg, 1972) and have been attributed to secondary myopathic change in the affected muscles (Achari and Anderson, 1974).

Symptoms and Signs of Upper Motor Neurone Degeneration

Save in those cases in which the degeneration is confined to the lower motor neurones the clinical picture is complicated by the symptoms of the upper motor neurone lesions which may be present from the beginning or may develop after muscular wasting. Since weakness and wasting beginning in the lower limbs is relatively uncommon, the legs often present an uncomplicated picture of corticospinal tract degeneration, with weakness and spasticity and extensor plantar responses. In the upper limbs the effect of the addition of an upper to a lower motor neurone lesion is to cause a degree of weakness which is disproportionately great in comparison with the severity and extent of the wasting, and the tendon reflexes are exaggerated in spite of the wasting. It is in the muscles innervated from the medulla that the effects of corticospinal tract degeneration are of the greatest importance. Here we may encounter lower motor neurone degeneration only—progressive bulbar palsy; upper motor neurone degeneration only—'pseudobulbar palsy'; or a combination of the two, which is the most frequent. A lesion of both corticospinal tracts above the medulla, so-called 'pseudobulbar palsy', causes weakness and spasticity of the bulbar muscles and hence leads to dysarthria and dysphagia. The paretic or paralysed muscles are not wasted and hypotonic, as in progressive bulbar palsy, but spastic. The tongue may appear somewhat smaller than normal on account of spasticity, but is not wrinkled and exhibits no fasciculation. The jaw-jerk, palatal, and pharyngeal reflexes are exaggerated, and sneezing and coughing may be excited reflexly. The dysarthria is of the so-called spastic or explosive type. Pseudobulbar palsy, when severe, also leads to an impairment of voluntary control over emotional reactions, as a result of which paroxysmal attacks of involuntary laughing and crying occur. These may take the form of an exaggeration or prolongation of a normal emotional response. Thus a patient laughs because he is amused, but having begun to laugh, is unable to stop. On the other hand, the emotional response may be quite inappropriate, such as uncontrollable laughter on hearing bad news, and then fails to correspond to, or express, the patient's emotional state. When pseudobulbar palsy and progressive bulbar palsy are associated in the same individual, dysarthria and dysphagia are intensified, impairment of emotional control may be present, and an exaggerated jaw-jerk is obtained, in spite of manifest wasting of the bulbar muscles.

The Reflexes

The condition of the reflexes in a given case depends upon the relative preponderance of upper and lower motor neurone degeneration. The palatal and pharyngeal reflexes tend to be lost in the later stages owing to interruption of the reflex arcs concerned. Owing to the presence of corticospinal tract degeneration the abdominal reflexes, which are initially preserved much longer, for instance, than in multiple sclerosis, are eventually diminished or lost, and the plantar reflexes are extensor. The deep reflexes, that is, the jaw-jerk and the tendon reflexes of the limbs, vary between exaggeration and abolition. Degeneration of the lower motor neurones causes impairment, and finally loss, of the reflexes effected by the muscles innervated. Corticospinal degeneration, however, leads to exaggeration of the deep reflexes. Hence it is not uncommon to find exaggerated tendon-jerks in the upper limbs in spite of considerable muscular atrophy. Since in the lower limbs muscular wasting is usually late in developing, the knee- and ankle-jerks are generally exaggerated and the plantar responses become extensor.

Other Symptoms

In the early stages the sphincters are not as a rule severely affected, though slight precipitancy or difficulty of micturition is not uncommon. Later retention or incontinence rarely occurs. Impotence often develops early. There is no sensory impairment. Horner's syndrome is a rare manifestation due to involvement of lateral horn cells in the dorsal cord.

The subcutaneous fat tends to disappear *pari passu* with the muscular wasting, and marked emaciation characterizes the later stages. Mental changes are absent and, although psychosis has occasionally been described, this is probably a coincidence or merely a reaction to a serious and disabling disease. Impairment of emotional control is a disorder of emotional expression and not due to the underlying mental state.

DIAGNOSIS

Motor neurone disease requires to be distinguished from other conditions leading to muscular wasting, especially in the upper limbs, and from other causes of bulbar palsy.

In syringomyelia muscular wasting of the upper limbs is associated with spastic weakness of the lower limbs. Fasciculation, however, is rarely as striking in the wasted muscles as in motor neurone disease, and the characteristic dissociated sensory loss, if not present at the outset, develops at an early stage.

In syphilitic amyotrophy due to meningomyelitis the onset of the weakness and wasting is often accompanied by pain of radicular distribution. Signs of corticospinal tract degeneration are often slight and sensory abnormalities are sometimes found; pupillary abnormalities may be present; the serological reactions are usually positive in either the blood or the cerebrospinal fluid, in which other abnormalities characteristic of syphilis are usually found. Pachymeningitis of the spinal cord secondary to cysticercosis may rarely give a clinical picture indistinguishable from that of motor neurone disease (Kahn, 1972).

Tumour of the spinal cord involving the cervical enlargement is likely to cause muscular wasting in one or both upper limbs, together with spastic paraplegia, but sensory loss is rarely absent, and the changes characteristic of spinal block are usually to be found in the cerebrospinal fluid.

Cervical spondylosis may closely simulate motor neurone disease when it causes muscular wasting and fasciculation in the upper limbs, and spastic weakness in the lower limbs without sensory loss. The course, however, is usually much slower than that of motor neurone disease, and the characteristic X-ray changes are present.

Spinal radiculitis ('neuralgic amyotrophy') causes wasting and weakness of muscles. The fifth cervical nerve is most frequently affected. The onset is usually acute and associated with severe pain in the neck and shoulder. The condition is not progressive, and any change is in the direction of improvement.

Cervical rib may give wasting of the small muscles of one or both hands. Muscular fasciculation, however, is usually absent, and pain along the ulnar border of the hand and forearm is often a prominent symptom, being frequently associated with relative anaesthesia and analgesia in this region, and vascular changes. Moreover, cervical rib can be demonstrated radiographically, though it must be remembered that in the costoclavicular syndrome the same symptoms may be caused by pressure upon a normal first rib or fibrous band. However, digital pressure in the root of the neck will usually reproduce the patient's pain and paraesthesiae.

Lesions of peripheral nerves give rise to little difficulty as a rule, since the distribution of the muscular wasting is at once recognizable as corresponding to the supply of the nerve, and in the case of the median and ulnar nerves is usually associated with sensory abnormalities possessing an equally distinctive distribution. However, a lesion of the deep branch of one ulnar nerve, resulting in wasting of small hand muscles without sensory loss may cause difficulty, but nerve conduction velocity measurements (increased terminal latency) are usually diagnostic.

Polymyositis is usually too acute to give rise to difficulties, and can also be distinguished electromyographically and by muscle biopsy. Various myopathies of late onset, however, may be confused with progressive muscular atrophy. Their diagnosis is discussed on page 1050.

The muscular dystrophies also are unlikely to be confused with amyotrophic lateral sclerosis, since they usually develop at a much earlier age. Dystrophia myotonica, however, is a disorder of adult life, but this condition is readily distinguished on account of the peculiar distribution of the wasting, with its predilection for the sternomastoids, facial muscles and the forearm and leg muscles, the presence of myotonia, the absence of fasciculation, and the association with cataract and other systemic abnormalities.

Peroneal muscular atrophy is distinguished by the peculiar distribution of the wasting, which begins in the periphery of the limbs, but generally in the lower before the upper, and is associated with sensory impairment. This disease, moreover, is usually familial, and the first symptoms often appear in childhood. Scapuloperoneal muscular atrophy [p. 708] may also give rise to difficulty but here again the pattern of weakness and wasting is distinctive.

Arthritis of the hands and fingers generally leads to considerable wasting of the muscles of the hands. The history of pain in the joints and the presence of articular or periarticular swelling, with limitation of joint movement, render the correct diagnosis easy.

It may sometimes be difficult or impossible to distinguish motor neurone disease of unusually early onset from benign spinal muscular atrophy of adolescence or early adult life (*vide infra*) save by the age of onset and benign course of the latter disorder.

Pseudobulbar palsy may be due to vascular lesions involving the corticospinal tracts at any point above the medulla. When these are sudden in onset the condition is unlikely to be confused with amyotrophic lateral sclerosis. When the onset is insidious, the distinction must be based upon the absence of muscular wasting and the presence of arterial degeneration. Myasthenia is distinguished by the characteristic fatigability, the response to edrophonium hydrochloride (*Tensilon*), and the absence of wasting and fasciculation.

In syringobulbia the presence of the characteristic dissociated sensory loss over the face is a distinctive feature.

PROGNOSIS

Motor neurone disease is a progressive disease, but its rate of progress shows considerable variations. In a minority of cases the patient goes rapidly downhill, muscular weakness, wasting, and fasciculation early becoming widespread, and death may occur within a year. In the cases in which the onset is slower the prognosis is influenced by several factors. Those in which the degeneration is for a long time confined to the lower motor neurones do best. Early involvement of the bulbar muscles makes the outlook worse, especially when progressive bulbar palsy is combined with pseudobulbar palsy. In general, patients with progressive bulbar palsy survive about 2–3 years, those with amyotrophic lateral sclerosis 3–5 years, and those with progressive muscular atrophy 3–10 years from the onset of symptoms, but there are many exceptions to this general guide. The prognosis is reviewed by Vejjajiva *et al.* (1967). Temporary arrest may occur, but is uncommon.

TREATMENT

The cause of the disease being in most cases undiscoverable, treatment is limited to dealing with symptoms. Every effort should be made, however, to ascertain whether the patient has been exposed to any form of chronic intoxication. Syphilis may be excluded by the usual serological tests. The patient should avoid fatigue, but should be encouraged to continue at a light occupation as long as possible. Regular moderate exercise to maintain power in innervated muscles is probably beneficial provided the patient does not exhaust himself. Neostigmine, 15 mg orally, two, three, or four times daily with atropine, 0·6 mg, or propantheline, 15 mg twice daily, to overcome its side-effects, may have a temporary beneficial effect upon speech and swallowing in patients with bulbar weakness, and diazepam, 2–5 mg three times daily, may diminish spasticity. Antibiotics may be needed for respiratory and urinary infection. In the late stages tracheostomy may be necessary if dysphagia and choking attacks become severe and the usual attention should be given to the bladder and skin. Temporary but substantial improvement in dysphagia due to pharyngeal paralysis may be achieved by the operation of cricopharyngeal sphincterotomy (Mills, 1973). Tube-feeding or gastrostomy are occasionally required to give appropriate nutriments. Some patients are helped by calipers and toe-springs if foot-drop is troublesome and later a wheel-chair may be necessary. Unfortunately no drug is known which has any influence upon the disease process. In the early stages of the disease, electrophysiological studies may indicate a diminished output of acetylcholine from the affected axon terminals and this may explain transient improvement produced by the administration of neostigmine and its analogues. This finding suggested that guanidine hydrochloride, which increases acetylcholine output, might be of therapeutic benefit in such cases, but controlled trials of treatment have shown no clinical improvement (Norris *et al.*, 1974 *a*) and the drug sometimes causes a striking increase in weakness (Norris *et al.*, 1974 *b*). Antiviral agents have also been shown to be of no benefit (Liversedge and Campbell, 1974).

Opinions vary upon what the affected patient should be told. There is no doubt that a responsible relative should be told the truth, even if one stresses the variability of the clinical course of the condition, emphasizing that some cases are more benign. It has been my custom to tell the affected individual first that the condition is one which is well-recognized, if of unknown cause, and to explain something of research now in progress. In order not to destroy all hope, I believe that it is best to say also that the condition progresses slowly up to a point but then usually becomes arrested, and may even subsequently improve spontaneously, while making it clear that no-one can predict when and if arrest will occur. Comparatively few patients seem to be aware of the deception, even to the end.

REFERENCES

ACHARI, A. N., and ANDERSON, M. S. (1974) Serum creatine phosphokinase in amyotrophic lateral sclerosis, *Neurology (Minneap.)*, **24**, 834.

ARAN, F. A. (1850) Recherches sur une maladie non encore décrite du système musculaire, *Arch. gén. Méd.*, **24**, 5.

BARWICK, D. D., and RICHARDSON, A. T. (1974) Clinical electromyography, in *Disorders of Voluntary Muscle*, 3rd ed., ed. Walton, J. N., p. 1003, Edinburgh and London.

BERTRAND, I., and BOGAERT, L. VAN (1925) Rapport sur la sclérose latérale amyotrophique, *Rev. Neurol. (Paris)*, **32**, 779.

BOOTHBY, J. A., DE JESUS, P. V., and ROWLAND, L. P. (1974) Reversible forms of motor neuron disease: lead 'neuritis', *Arch. Neurol. (Chic.)*, **31**, 18.

BOTS, G. T. A. M., and STAAL, A. (1973) Amyotrophic lateral sclerosis-dementia complex, neuroaxonal dystrophy, and Hallervorden–Spatz disease, *Neurology (Minneap.)*, **23**, 35.

BRAIN, Lord, CROFT, P. B., and WILKINSON, M. (1965) Motor neurone disease as a manifestation of neoplasms (with a note on the course of classical motor neurone disease), *Brain*, **88**, 479.

BROWN, W. F., and JAATOUL, N. (1974) Amyotrophic lateral sclerosis: electrophysiologic study (number of motor units and rate of decay of motor units), *Arch. Neurol. (Chic.)*, **30**, 242.

BROWNELL, B., OPPENHEIMER, D. R., and HUGHES, J. T. (1970) The central nervous system in motor neurone disease, *J. Neurol. Neurosurg. Psychiat.*, **33**, 338.

BUCHTHAL, F., and PINELLI, P. (1953) Action potentials in muscular atrophy of neurogenic origin, *Neurology (Minneap.)*, **3**, 591.

CAMPBELL, A. M. G., WILLIAMS, E. R., and BARLTROP, D. (1970) Motor neurone disease and exposure to lead, *J. Neurol. Neurosurg. Psychiat.*, **33**, 877.

CARPENTER, S. (1968) Proximal axonal enlargement in motor neuron disease, *Neurology (Minneap.)*, **18**, 841.

CHARCOT, J. M., and JOFFROY, A. (1869) Deux cas d'atrophie musculaire progressive avec lésions de la substance grise et des faisceaux antéro-latéraux de la moelle épinière, *Arch. Physiol. norm. Path.*, **2**, 354, 629, 744.

CREMER, N. E., OSHIRO, L. S., NORRIS, F. H., and LENNETTE, E. H. (1973) Cultures of tissues from patients with amyotrophic lateral sclerosis, *Arch. Neurol. (Chic.)*, **29**, 331.

DAVISON, C. (1942) Amyotrophic lateral sclerosis, *Arch. Neurol. Psychiat. (Chic.)*, **46**, 1039.

DRACHMAN, D. B., MURPHY, S. R., NIGAM, M. P., and HILLS, J. R. (1967) 'Myopathic' changes in chronically denervated muscle, *Arch. Neurol. (Chic.)*, **16**, 14.

DUCHENNE, G. B. (1853) Étude comparée des lésions anatomiques dans l'atrophie musculaire progressive et dans la paralysie générale, *Un. méd. Can.*, **7**, 202.

DUCHENNE, G. B. (1860) Paralysis musculaire progressive de la langue, du voile du palais et des lèvres, *Arch. gén. Méd.*, **2**, 283.

EDGAR, A. H., BRODY, J. A., and DETELS, R. (1973) Amyotrophic lateral sclerosis mortality among native-born and migrant residents of California and Washington, *Neurology (Minneap.)*, **23**, 48.

ELDRIDGE, R., RYAN, E., ROSARIO, J., and BRODY, J. A. (1969) Amyotrophic lateral sclerosis and parkinsonism dementia in a migrant population from Guam, *Neurology (Minneap.)*, **19**, 1029.

ENGEL, W. K., KURLAND, L. T., and KLATZO, I. (1959) An inherited disease similar to amyotrophic lateral sclerosis with a pattern of posterior column involvement. An intermediate form?, *Brain*, **82**, 203.

FAZIO, M. (1892) Ereditarieta della parilisi bulbare progressiva, *Riforma. Med.*, **8**, 327.

GREENFIELD, J. G. (1958) in *Neuropathology*, ed. Greenfield, J. G., Blackwood, W., McMenemey, W. H., Meyer, A., and Norman, R. M., p. 545, London.

GUSTAFSON, A., and STÖRTEBECKER, P. (1972) Vascular and metabolic studies of amyotrophic lateral sclerosis. II. Lipid and carbohydrate metabolism, *Neurology (Minneap.)*, **22**, 528.

HALLEN, O., BRUSIS, T., and PFISTERER, H. (1969) Die Myatrophia spinalis postpoliomyelitica chronica. Ein Beitrag zum Problem der sog. Poliomyelitis anterior chronica, *Dtsch. Z. Nervenheilk.*, **195**, 333.

HIRANO, A., KURLAND, L. T., and SAYRE, G. P. (1967) Familial amyotrophic lateral sclerosis, *Arch. Neurol. (Chic.)*, **16**, 232.

IONASESCU, V., and LUCA, N. (1964) Studies on carbohydrate metabolism in amyotrophic lateral sclerosis and hereditary proximal spinal muscular atrophy, *Acta neurol. scand.*, **40**, 47.

JOKELAINEN, M. (1976) The epidemiology of amyotrophic lateral sclerosis in Finland. A study based on the death certificates of 421 patients, *J. neurol. Sci.*, **29**, 55.

KAHN, P. (1972) Cysticercosis of the central nervous system with amyotrophic lateral sclerosis: case report and review of the literature, *J. Neurol. Neurosurg. Psychiat.*, **35**, 81.

KENNEDY, W. R., ALTER, M., and SUNG, J. H. (1968) Progressive proximal spinal and bulbar muscular atrophy of late onset, *Neurology (Minneap.)*, **18**, 671.

KJELLIN, K. G., and STIBLER, H. (1976) Isoelectric focusing and electrophoresis of cerebrospinal fluid proteins in muscular dystrophies and spinal muscular atrophies, *J. neurol. Sci.*, **27**, 45.

KUGELBERG, E. (1949) Electromyography in muscular dystrophies, *J. Neurol. Neurosurg. Psychiat.*, **12**, 129.

KURLAND, L. T. (1957) Epidemiological investigations of amyotrophic lateral sclerosis, *Proc. Mayo Clin.*, **32**, 449.

KURLAND, L. T. (1972) An appraisal of the neurotoxicity of cycad and the etiology of amyotrophic lateral sclerosis on Guam, *Fed. Proc.*, **31**, 1540.

KURLAND, L. T., and MULDER, D. W. (1954) Epidemiologic investigations of amyotrophic lateral sclerosis. I. Preliminary report on geographic distribution, with special reference to the Mariana Islands, including clinical and pathologic observations, *Neurology (Minneap.)*, **4**, 355.

KURTZKE, J. F. (1969) Comments on the epidemiology of amyotrophic lateral sclerosis (ALS), in *Motor Neurone Diseases*, p. 85, New York.

LIVERSEDGE, L. A., and CAMPBELL, M. J. (1974) The central neuronal muscular atrophies and other dysfunctions of the anterior horn cells, in *Disorders of Voluntary Muscle*, 3rd ed., ed. Walton, J. N., p. 775, Edinburgh and London.

LONDE, P. (1893) Paralysie bulbaire progressive infantile et familiale, *Rev. Méd.*, **13**, 1020.

McCOMAS, A. J., UPTON, A. R. M., and SICA, R. E. P. (1973) Motoneurone disease and ageing, *Lancet*, **ii**, 1477.

MANN, D. M. A., and YATES, P. O. (1974) Motor neurone disease: the nature of the pathogenic mechanism, *J. Neurol. Neurosurg. Psychiat.*, **37**, 1036.

MARINESCO, G. (1925) Contribution à l'histo-chimie et à la pathogénie de la maladie de Charcot, *Rev. neurol. (Paris)*, **32**, 513.

MARKAND, O. N., and DALY, D. D. (1971) Juvenile type of slowly progressive bulbar palsy: report of a case, *Neurology (Minneap.)*, **21**, 753.

MATSUMOTO, N., WORTH, R. M., KURLAND, L. T., and OKAZAKI, H. (1972) Epidemiologic study of amyotrophic lateral sclerosis in Hawaii: identification of high incidence among Filipino men, *Neurology (Minneap.)*, **22**, 934.

MENDELL, J. R., CHASE, T. N., and ENGEL, W. K. (1971) Amyotrophic lateral sclerosis. A study of central monoamine metabolism and therapeutic trial of levodopa, *Arch. Neurol. (Chic.)*, **25**, 320.

METCALF, C. W., and HIRANO, A. (1971) Amyotrophic lateral sclerosis. Clinicopathological studies of a family, *Arch. Neurol. (Chic.)*, **24**, 518.

MEYERS, K. R., DORENCAMP, D. G., and SUZUKI, K. (1974) Amyotrophic lateral sclerosis with diffuse neurofibrillary changes, *Arch. Neurol. (Chic.)*, **30**, 84.

MILHORAT, A. T. (1946) Studies in diseases of muscle. XV. Progressive spinal muscular atrophy as a late sequel of acute epidemic encephalitis: report of two cases, *Arch. Neurol. Psychiat. (Chic.)*, **55**, 134.

MILLS, C. P. (1973) Dysphagia in pharyngeal paralysis treated by cricopharyngeal sphincterotomy, *Lancet*, **i**, 455.

NELSON, J. S., and PRENSKY, A. L. (1972) Sporadic juvenile amyotrophic lateral sclerosis. A clinicopathological study of a case with neuronal cytoplasmic inclusions containing RNA, *Arch. Neurol. (Chic.)*, **27**, 300.

NORRIS, F. H., CALANCHINI, P. R., FALLAT, R. J., PANCHARI, S., and JEWETT, B. (1974 *a*) The administration of guanidine in amyotrophic lateral sclerosis, *Neurology (Minneap.)*, **24**, 721.

NORRIS, F. H., FALLAT, R. J., and CALACHINI, P. R. (1974 *b*) Increased paralysis induced by guanidine in motor neuron disease, *Neurology (Minneap.)*, **24**, 135.

NORRIS, F. H., and ENGEL, W. K. (1965) Carcinomatous amyotrophic lateral sclerosis, in *The Remote Effects of Cancer on the Nervous System*, ed. Brain, Lord, and Norris, F. H., p. 24, New York.

OLIVARES, L., SAN ESTEBAN, E., and ALTER, M. (1972) Mexican 'resistance' to amyotrophic lateral sclerosis, *Arch. Neurol. (Chic.)*, **27**, 397.

OSUNTOKUN, B. O., ADEUJA, A. O. G., and BADEMOSI, O. (1974) The prognosis of motor neuron disease in Nigerian Africans—a prospective study of 92 patients, *Brain*, **97**, 385.

PANITCH, H. S., and FRANKLIN, G. M. (1972) Elevation of serum creatine phosphokinase in amyotrophic lateral sclerosis, *Neurology (Minneap.)*, **22**, 964.

PEARCE, J. M. S., PENNINGTON, R. J. T., and WALTON, J. N. (1964) Serum enzyme studies in muscle disease. Part II: Serum creatine kinase activity in muscular dystrophy and in other myopathic and neuropathic disorders, *J. Neurol. Neurosurg. Psychiat.*, **27**, 96.

PETERS, H. A., and CLATANOFF, D. V. (1968) Spinal muscular atrophy secondary to macroglobulinemia. Reversal of symptoms with chlorambucil therapy, *Neurology (Minneap.)*, **18**, 101.

PRATT, R. T. C. (1967) *The Genetics of Neurological Disorders*, London.

REED, D. M., BRODY, J. A., and HOLDEN, E. M. (1975) Predicting the duration of Guam amyotrophic lateral sclerosis, *Neurology (Minneap.)*, **25**, 277.

SAVOLAINEN, H., and PALO, J. (1973) Amyotrophic lateral sclerosis: proteins of neuronal cell membranes, axons and myelin of the precentral gyrus and other cortical areas, *Brain*, **96**, 537.

SCHOCHET, S. S., HARDMAN, J. M., LADEWIG, P. P., and EARLE, K. M. (1969) Intraneuronal conglomerates in sporadic motor neuron disease, *Arch. Neurol. (Chic.)*, **20**, 548.

SHAHANI, B., DAVIES-JONES, G. A. B., and RUSSELL, W. R. (1971) Motor neurone disease.

Further evidence for an abnormality of nerve metabolism, *J. Neurol. Neurosurg. Psychiat.*, **34**, 185.

SMITH, M. A. (1960) Nerve fibre degeneration in the brain in amyotrophic lateral sclerosis, *J. Neurol. Neurosurg. Psychiat.*, **23**, 269.

STAAL, A., and WENT, L. N. (1968) Juvenile amyotrophic lateral sclerosis-dementia complex in a Dutch family, *Neurology (Minneap.)*, **18**, 800.

STÖRTEBECKER, P., NORDSTRÖM, G., PESTÉNY, M. P. DE, SEEMAN, T., and BJÖRKERUD, S. (1970) Vascular and metabolic studies of amyotrophic lateral sclerosis. I. Angiopathy in biopsy specimens of peripheral arteries, *Neurology (Minneap.)*, **20**, 1157.

TAKAHASHI, K., NAKAMURA, H., and OKADA, E. (1972) Hereditary amyotrophic lateral sclerosis. Histochemical and electron microscopic study of hyaline inclusions in motor neurones, *Arch. Neurol. (Chic.)*, **27**, 292.

URBÁNEK, K., and JANSA, P. (1974) Amyotrophic lateral sclerosis. Abnormal cellular inflammatory response, *Arch. Neurol. (Chic.)*, **30**, 186.

VALMIKINATHAN, K., MASCREEN, M., MEENAKSHISUNDARAM, E., and SNEHALATHA, C. (1973) Biochemical aspects of motor neurone disease—Madras pattern, *J. Neurol. Neurosurg. Psychiat.*, **36**, 753.

VEJJAJIVA, A., FOSTER, J. B., and MILLER, H. (1967) Motor neuron disease; a clinical study, *J. neurol. Sci.*, **4**, 299.

WELCH, K. M. A., and GOLDBERG, D. M. (1972) Serum creatine phosphokinase in motor neuron disease, *Neurology (Minneap.)*, **22**, 697.

WILLIAMS, E. R., and BRUFORD, A. (1970) Creatine phosphokinase in motor neurone disease, *Clin. chim. Acta*, **27**, 53.

WILLISON, R. G. (1962) Electrodiagnosis in motor neurone disease, *Proc. roy. Soc. Med.*, **55**, 1024.

WOHLFART, G. (1957) Collateral regeneration from residual motor nerve fibers in amyotrophic lateral sclerosis, *Neurology (Minneap.)*, **7**, 124.

YASE, Y. (1972) The pathogenesis of amyotrophic lateral sclerosis, *Lancet*, **ii**, 292.

CREUTZFELDT-JAKOB DISEASE

In 1920 Creutzfeldt described a case of 'Peculiar focal disease of the central nervous system' and in 1921 and 1923 Jakob added further examples of what he called 'Spastic pseudosclerosis: encephalomyelopathy with disseminated neurogenic lesions'.

Since that time there has been much confusion about the clinical and pathological features of Creutzfeldt–Jakob disease. For some years there was a tendency, particularly in the United Kingdom, to use this diagnostic label to identify groups of cases, sometimes involving more than one member of a family, in which clinical features of Parkinsonism were accompanied by progressive dementia with associated evidence of corticospinal tract dysfunction and sometimes weakness, wasting, and fasciculation of muscles, similar to that seen in motor neurone disease and due to progressive loss of anterior horn cells. These cases, which are rare in Europe and in the United States, show clinical features somewhat similar to those observed in the Parkinsonism–dementia complex, sometimes associated with amyotrophic lateral sclerosis, which is endemic in the island of Guam [pp. 683 and 686]. Some may represent variants of corticostriato-nigral degeneration [p. 591] in which, however, dementia is not usually severe, while others may represent variants of progressive multisystem degeneration [p. 321]. Sometimes these cases are still called spastic pseudosclerosis as Jakob originally suggested. Usually the course is relatively rapid with progressive dementia, dysarthria, spastic weakness of the limbs, Parkinsonian rigidity, tremor, and muscular wasting. In most such cases the pathological changes are different from those recognized now as typical of Creutzfeldt–Jakob disease (see below) and correspond more closely to those of presenile dementia on the one hand and of cortico-striato-nigral degeneration on the other. Diagnostic and nosological difficulty has, however, been compounded by the use of the term cortico-striato-nigral degeneration (Silberman *et al.*, 1961) to identify a case showing the classical pathological changes of Creutzfeldt–Jakob disease (to be described below) and by the fact that clinical features indistinguishable from those of motor neurone disease of rapid progression have been noted in another case with similar pathological findings (Allen *et al.*, 1971).

In 1955, however, Foley and Denny-Brown (1955) described a case corresponding more closely to the clinical picture which Creutzfeldt and Jakob originally reported and others were described by Brownell and Oppenheimer (1965) under the title of subacute presenile polioencephalopathy. The condition which they reported usually began in middle or late life with ataxia, dementia, abnormal movements (often myoclonus), and progressive deterioration leading to stupor with death within a few months. A very similar picture was described by Jones and Nevin (1954) and Nevin *et al.* (1960) under the title of subacute spongiform encephalopathy; they noted in addition visual failure and generalized convulsions in some cases as well as paroxysmal generalized sharp wave complexes in the EEG associated with the myoclonus, with obliteration of normal background activity and widespread slow voltage activity. Pathologically, Brownell and Oppenheimer (1965) noted widespread cell loss and diffuse astrocytic hyperplasia in the cerebral cortex, striatum, and thalamus and granule cell degeneration in the cerebellum, while Nevin *et al.* (1960) stressed the spongiform change with vacuolation and severe loss of nerve cells throughout the cerebral cortex. Subsequently it has become apparent that despite variations in the clinical and pathological picture, Creutzfeldt–Jakob disease and subacute spongiform encephalopathy are virtually identical (Goldhammer *et al.*, 1972; Bubis *et al.*, 1972). Spongiform change is most striking in the more acute cases, which also show the typical EEG findings described by Jones and Nevin (1954) and further documented by Burger *et al.* (1972); in these individuals death has been known to occur within eight to 12 weeks from the onset. When the course extends to several months or even a year or more, diffuse neuronal loss and marked astrocytic hyperplasia is more common (Katzman *et al.*, 1961). No specific biochemical or ultrastructural abnormalities have been described in the brain (Korey *et al.*, 1961; Robinson, 1969; Allen *et al.*, 1971) but transmission experiments have shown that the condition is due to a slow virus [p. 524] and that it can be transmitted to the chimpanzee (Beck *et al.*, 1969). Some authors have suggested that amantidine 100 mg twice daily may produce temporary improvement in such cases (Sanders and Dunn, 1973) but others have found antiviral agents ineffective.

It may thus be concluded that Creutzfeldt–Jakob disease is due to an as yet unidentified slow virus infection and that it may occur in cortical, cortico-striatal, corticospinal, cortico-striato-spinal, and cortico-striato-cerebellar forms. It shows some affinities pathologically with kuru [p. 524]; even if due to an infective agent, it has been reported sometimes to be familial (May *et al.*, 1968).

REFERENCES

ALLEN, I. V., DERMOTT, E., CONNOLLY, J. H., and HURWITZ, L. J. (1971) A study of a patient with the amyotrophic form of Creutzfeld–Jakob disease, *Brain*, **94**, 715.

BECK, E., DANIEL, P. M., MATTHEWS, W. B., STEVENS, D. L., ALPERS, M. P., ASHER, D. M., GAJDUSEK, D. C., and GIBBS, C. J. (1969) Creutzfeld–Jakob disease. The neuropathology of a transmission experiment, *Brain*, **92**, 699.

BROWNELL, B., and OPPENHEIMER, D. R. (1965) An ataxic form of subacute presenile polioencephalopathy (Creutzfeld–Jakob disease), *J. Neurol. Psychiat.*, **28**, 350.

BUBIS, J. J., GOLDHAMMER, Y., and BRAHAM, J. (1972) Subacute spongiform encephalopathy, *J. Neurol. Neurosurg. Psychiat.*, **35**, 881.

BURGER, L. J., ROWAN, A. J., and GOLDENSOHN, E. S. (1972) Creutzfeld–Jakob disease. An electroencephalographic study, *Arch. Neurol. (Chic.)*, **26**, 428.

CREUTZFELDT, H. G. (1920) Über eine eigenartige herdförmige Erkrankung des Zentralnervensystems, *Z. ges. Neurol. Psychiat.*, **57**, 1.

FOLEY, J., and DENNY-BROWN, D. (1955) Subacute progressive encephalopathy with bulbar myoclonus, *J. Neuropath.*, **16**, 133.

GOLDHAMMER, Y., BUBIS, J. J., SAROVAPINHAS, I., and BRAHAM, J. (1972) Subacute spongiform encephalopathy and its relation to Jakob–Creutzfeld disease: report on six cases, *J. Neurol. Neurosurg. Psychiat.*, **35**, 1.

JAKOB, A. (1921) Über eigenartige Erkrankungen des Zentralnervensystems mit bemerkenswerten anatomischen Befunden. Spastische Pseudosklerose-Encephalomyelopathie mit disseminierten Degenerationsherden, *Z. ges. Neurol. Psychiat.*, **64**, 146.

JAKOB, A. (1923) *Spastische Pseudosklerose; die extrapyramidalen Erkrankungen*, p. 215, Berlin.

JONES, D. P., and NEVIN, S. (1954) Rapidly progressive cerebral degeneration (subacute vascular encephalopathy) with mental disorder, focal disturbances and myoclonic epilepsy, *J. Neurol. Neurosurg. Psychiat.*, **7**, 148.

KATZMAN, R., KAGAN, E. H., and ZIMMERMAN, H. M. (1961) A case of Jakob–Creutzfeldt disease. 1. Clinicopathological analysis, *J. Neuropath. exp. Neurol.*, **20**, 78.

KOREY, S. R., KATZMAN, R., and ORLOFF, J. (1961) A case of Jakob–Creutzfeldt disease. 2. Analysis of some constituents of the brain of a patient with Jakob–Creutzfeldt disease, *J. Neuropath. exp. Neurol.*, **20**, 95.

MAY, W. W., ITABASHI, H. H., and DEJONG, R. N. (1968) Creutzfeldt–Jakob disease. II. Clinical, pathologic, and genetic study of a family, *Arch. Neurol. (Chic.)*, **19**, 137.

NEVIN, S., MCMENEMEY, W. H., BEHRMAN, S., and JONES, D. P. (1960) Subacute spongiform encephalopathy—a subacute form of encephalopathy attributable to vascular dysfunction (spongiform cerebral atrophy), *Brain*, **83**, 519.

ROBINSON, N. (1969) Creutzfeldt–Jakob's disease: a histochemical study, *Brain*, **92**, 581.

SANDERS, W. L., and DUNN, T. L. (1973) Creutzfeldt–Jakob disease treated with amantidine, *J. Neurol. Neurosurg. Psychiat.*, **36**, 581.

SILBERMAN, J., CRAVIOTO, H., and FEIGIN, I. (1961) Corticostriatal degeneration of the Creutzfeldt–Jakob type, *J. Neuropath. exp. Neurol.*, **20**, 105.

PERONEAL MUSCULAR ATROPHY

Synonyms. Neural progressive muscular atrophy; Charcot–Marie–Tooth disease.

Definition. A hereditary form of progressive muscular atrophy first described in 1886 by Charcot and Marie and later in the same year by Tooth. Wasting usually begins in the small muscles of the feet and later in those of the hands, and never advances beyond the peripheral parts of the limbs. The condition is closely related to the Roussy–Lévy syndrome [p. 674] and to the Dejerine–Sottas type of familial hypertrophic interstitial polyneuropathy [p. 981].

PATHOLOGY AND AETIOLOGY

Buzzard and Greenfield (1921) described 'interstitial neuritis' in the branches of the peroneal nerve, and Alajouanine *et al.* (1967) found marked proliferation of endoneurial connective tissue with secondary demyelination in lumbar roots. In some cases, changes have also been found in the spinal cord, including degeneration of anterior horn cells and of the cells of the dorsal nuclei, together with posterior column demyelination and inconstant degeneration of the corticospinal tracts, a finding which emphasizes the relationship of the condition, in some families and individuals at least, to the other disorders of the hereditary ataxia group.

It now seems evident that the spinal cord changes are usually secondary to those occurring in the peripheral nerves or else are rarely due to associated inherited degenerative disorder of the central nervous system. New light has been cast upon the classification of the variants of this disorder by the work of Dyck and Lambert (1968 *a* and *b*) and by Thomas *et al.* (1974). It now seems that the commonest (and most benign) form of peroneal muscular atrophy, usually of dominant inheritance, is one in which there is a hypertrophic demyelinating neuropathy of the peripheral nerves, sometimes with palpable nerve enlargement but invariably with Schwann cell proliferation and 'onion-bulb' formation in the affected nerves and gross slowing of motor and sensory nerve conduction velocity. Pathologically the changes in such cases are indistinguishable from those of the Roussy–Lévy syndrome. Dyck and Lambert (1968 *a*) identify as a different disorder the severe Dejerine–Sottas variety of hypertrophic neuropathy, usually of earlier onset and more rapid progression and due to an autosomal recessive trait, but Thomas *et al.* (1974), noting genetic heterogeneity and marked intrafamilial variation in clinical severity and course, doubt whether such a distinction is justified.

Much less common than the hypertrophic variety (Dyck and Lambert, 1968 *a*; Thomas *et al.*, 1974; Bradley, 1974) is the dominant axonal variety, usually of later onset, involving the legs more than the arms, with normal rates of nerve conduction and little sensory involvement. Whether there is a third variety (dominant distal spinal muscular atrophy) with primary involvement of the anterior horn cells rather than of the motor axons of the peripheral nerves is still uncertain. Most authorities believe that this third variant exists and accounts for those cases which present with features of peroneal muscular atrophy but without sensory loss and with subsequent involvement of limb muscles more proximally than is usual in typical peroneal muscular atrophy. The relationship of this third variant to dominantly inherited scapuloperoneal muscular atrophy, a disorder which is usually neuropathic but rarely myopathic (Kaeser, 1965) [see p. 708] is still uncertain.

In the affected skeletal muscles the appearances are those of neurogenic atrophy but 'secondary myopathic change', a frequent sequel of longstanding partial denervation, is often found (Haase and Shy, 1960; Cazzato and Testa, 1969).

The aetiology of the condition is unknown though Dyck *et al.* (1970) found an abnormality of ceramide hexoside metabolism in cases of severe hypertrophic neuropathy. Sporadic cases of all varieties occur; dominant inheritance is usual but autosomal recessive transmission has also been noted in occasional families suffering from each form of the disease and even X-linked recessive inheritance has been described (Herringham, 1889). Members of affected families may show pes cavus and abnormalities of nerve conduction without other clinical symptoms or signs and probably represent a forme fruste of the disorder (Symonds and Shaw, 1926; Dyck *et al.*, 1963; Dyck and Lambert, 1968 *a*).

SYMPTOMS AND SIGNS

The first symptoms are muscular wasting and weakness, which usually begin in the peronei, extensor digitorum longus, or the small muscles of the foot, symmetrically on the two sides. Paralysis of the peronei leads to talipes equino-varus, but when the wasting begins in the intrinsic muscles of the feet pes cavus results. However, there is evidence from cases with the forme fruste of the disease that the pes cavus may be an associated skeletal deformity. Difficulty in walking on the heels is a useful early sign. Not uncommonly it is the deformity of the feet and the resulting laborious 'steppage' gait which bring the patient under observation. Wasting does not usually appear in the hands until a number of years after its onset in the feet. Occasionally, however, both upper and lower extremities are affected simultaneously; exceptionally the hands suffer first. The muscular atrophy, which is occasionally associated with fasciculation, tends to spread very slowly proximally, not involving the muscles longitudinally but transversely. It does not extend above the elbows nor above the junction of the middle and lower thirds of the thigh. This peculiar ascending distribution of the wasting leads to a striking appearance of the limbs. When the lower part of the calf is wasted the 'fat bottle' calf is produced, and wasting of the lower third of the thigh leads to the so-called 'inverted champagne bottle' limb. Ultimately the feet become 'flail', neither dorsiflexion nor plantar flexion being possible. In the cases with a hypertrophic neuropathy which are the majority, motor and sensory nerve conduction are usually greatly slowed in the peroneal nerves and often in the median and ulnar nerves as well, especially if the hands are affected (Dyck *et al.*, 1963; Dyck and Lambert, 1968 *a* and *b*; Nielsen and Pilgaard, 1972). In the cases of presumed axonal degeneration or spinal muscular atrophy, conduction is usually normal (Thomas and Calne, 1974) but in some cases it is nevertheless difficult to be certain whether the primary process is demyelinating and hypertrophic or axonal (Salisachs, 1974). Contractures rarely occur, but are usually slight in proportion to the degree of wasting [FIG. 118].

Electromyography typically shows signs of denervation in the affected muscles and large discrete motor unit action potentials are generally present suggesting that the lesion responsible lies proximally in the motor neurones. Abnormalities of skin temperature control, of orthostatic control of blood pressure, of sweating in the lower extremities, and other features suggesting dysfunction of post-ganglionic sympathetic nerve fibres have been described (Jammes, 1972).

The tendon reflexes are variable. They are usually diminished or lost in the wasted muscles in proportion to the degree of wasting, but loss of the tendon reflexes may precede atrophy. The plantar reflexes are usually lost eventually.

Sensibility may be unaffected, but there is generally loss of vibration sense at the ankles and occasionally some impairment of appreciation of light touch, pain, and temperature over the periphery of the limbs. Deep sensibility is less often affected. Charcot and Marie, in their original paper, described vasomotor changes in the extremities, and perforating ulcers may occur probably due to the presence of an associated hereditary sensory neuropathy (England and Denny-Brown, 1952). Vertebral and other skeletal anomalies and various associated congenital malformations have been reported (Smith, 1958); heart

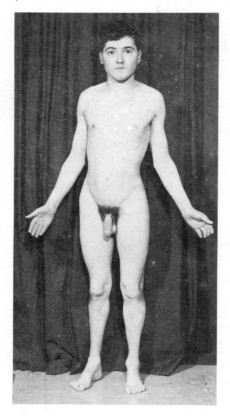

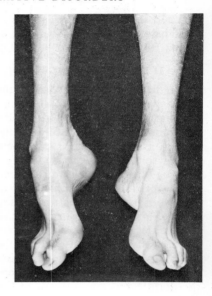

Fig. 118. A case of peroneal muscular atrophy; note the typical atrophy of the distal muscles of the lower limbs with bilateral pes cavus. There was also early wasting of the intrinsic muscles of both hands with complete loss of vibration sense below the knees, from *An Atlas of Clinical Neurology* 2nd ed., 1975, by J. D. Spillane, reproduced by kind permission of the author

block occurred in several members of an affected family (Littler, 1970). The function of the sphincters remains normal.

The cranial nerves are usually normal, but optic atrophy has been described in a few cases (Serratrice *et al.*, 1964) and so, too, has inequality of the pupils, which is possibly due to implication of the ocular sympathetic fibres. Very occasionally the pupils are of the Argyll Robertson type (Alajouanine *et al.*, 1967). Trigeminal neuralgia and anaesthesia rarely occur.

DIAGNOSIS

The onset of the muscular wasting in the lower limbs, and its peculiar ascent from the periphery are distinctive features which usually render the diagnosis easy. In the muscular dystrophies affected muscles waste longitudinally and selectively and the distribution of the wasting is characteristic of the various forms. In Welander's (1951) hereditary distal myopathy the age of onset is later than in peroneal atrophy, and there is no sensory loss. Dystrophia myotonica is distinguished by the presence of myotonia and by the distribution of the wasting, especially its selection of the sternomastoids and the long flexor and extensor muscles of the forearms rather than the small hand muscles. Progressive muscular atrophy usually begins in adult life, and the feet are rarely the site of wasting; fasciculation is usually prominent, weakness and wasting less symmetrical, and the reflexes are often brisk. Friedreich's ataxia, like peroneal atrophy, is an hereditary disorder which gives rise to pes cavus, but nystagmus, ataxia, and extensor plantar responses are peculiar to the former in which, moreover, muscular wasting is less common and overt. Diagnosis from other forms of polyneuropathy may sometimes give rise to difficulty; this is especially true of other varieties of demyelinating polyneuropathy with hypertrophy of peripheral nerves; in such cases, however, the clinical picture is less stereotyped and the course much more rapid, often with relapses and remissions. Whereas an increased protein content in the CSF has been described in the more severe forms of peroneal muscular atrophy with peripheral nerve hypertrophy (Dyck and Lambert, 1968 a), this is rarely as great as in the varieties of steroid-responsive relapsing polyneuropathy which may give similar degrees of peripheral nerve hypertrophy. Other diseases which also give peripheral nerve enlargement, including Refsum's disease, are identified by their other distinctive clinical features.

PROGNOSIS

The disorder runs a very slow course and arrest may occur at any stage. Since the wasting always remains confined to the limbs, the disease does not shorten life and many patients have been reported alive 45 or 50 years after the onset of symptoms. In the case reported by Alajouanine et al. (1967) the patient, whose condition was first diagnosed by Charcot, lived an active life for 60 years and eventually died at the age of 80. In spite of the deformities the degree of disability is often surprisingly slight. Nevertheless, as Thomas et al. (1974) and others have shown, there is sometimes remarkable heterogeneity of clinical presentation and course even within single families, and cases of early onset leading to severe disability with confinement to a wheelchair in late childhood or early adult life do certainly occur but are relatively uncommon.

TREATMENT

No treatment will arrest the course of the disorder. Physiotherapy and various appliances often enable the patient to make the best use of his available resources. Appropriate surgical boots and below-knee calipers with toe-springs or plastic moulded splints worn inside the shoes will usually be required.

REFERENCES

ALAJOUANINE, T., CASTAIGNE, P., CAMBIER, J., and ESCOUROLLE, R. (1967) Maladie de Charcot–Marie. Étude anatomo-clinique, Presse méd., 75, 2745.
BRADLEY, W. G. (1974) The neuropathies, in Disorders of Voluntary Muscle, 3rd ed., ed. Walton, J. N., p. 804, Edinburgh and London.
BUZZARD, E. F., and GREENFIELD, J. G. (1921) Pathology of the Nervous System, London.
CAZZATO, G., and TESTA, G. (1969) Alterazioni miotessutali di tipo 'miopatico' in casi di atrofia muscolare progressiva nevritica di Charcot–Marie–Tooth, Acta Neurol. (Napoli), 24, 171.
CHARCOT, J. M., and MARIE, P. (1886) Sur une forme particulière d'atrophie musculaire progressive souvent familiale, Rev. Médecine, 6, 97.
DYCK, P. J., ELLEFSON, R. D., LAIS, A. C., SMITH, R. C., TAYLOR, W. F., and VAN DYKE, R. A. (1970) Histologic and lipid studies of sural nerves in inherited hypertrophic neuropathy: preliminary report of a lipid abnormality in nerve and liver in Dejerine–Sottas disease, Proc. Mayo Clin., 45, 286.
DYCK, P. J., and LAMBERT, E. H. (1968 a) Lower motor and primary sensory neuron diseases with peroneal muscular atrophy. I. Neurologic, genetic, and electrophysiologic findings in hereditary polyneuropathies, Arch. Neurol. (Chic.), 18, 603.

DYCK, P. J., and LAMBERT, E. H. (1968 b) Lower motor and primary sensory neuron diseases with peroneal muscular atrophy. II. Neurologic, genetic, and electro-physiologic findings in various neuronal degenerations, *Arch. Neurol. (Chic.)*, **18**, 619.

DYCK, P. J., LAMBERT, E. H., and MULDER, D. W. (1963) Charcot–Marie–Tooth disease. Nerve conduction and clinical studies of a large sibship, *Neurology (Minneap.)*, **13**, 1.

ENGLAND, A. C., and DENNY-BROWN, D. (1952) Severe sensory changes, and trophic disorder, in peroneal muscular atrophy (Charcot–Marie–Tooth type), *Arch. Neurol. Psychiat. (Chic.)*, **67**, 1.

HAASE, G. R., and SHY, G. M. (1960) Pathological changes in muscle biopsies from patients with peroneal muscular atrophy, *Brain*, **83**, 631.

HERRINGHAM, W. P. (1889) Muscular atrophy of the peroneal type affecting many members of a family, *Brain*, **11**, 230.

JAMMES, J. L. (1972) The autonomic nervous system in peroneal muscular atrophy, *Arch. Neurol. (Chic.)*, **27**, 213.

KAESER, H. E. (1965) Scapuloperoneal muscular atrophy, *Brain*, **88**, 407.

LITTLER, W. A. (1970) Heart block and peroneal muscular atrophy: a family study, *Quart. J. Med.*, **39**, 431.

NIELSEN, V. K., and PILGAARD, S. (1972) On the pathogenesis of Charcot–Marie–Tooth disease: a study of the sensory and motor conduction velocity in the median nerve, *Acta orthop. scand.*, **43**, 4.

SALISACHS, P. (1974) Wide spectrum of motor conduction velocity in Charcot–Marie–Tooth disease: an anatomico-physiological interpretation, *J. neurol. Sci.*, **23**, 25.

SERRATRICE, G., TATOSSIAN, A., and POINSO, Y. (1964) Amyotrophie de Charcot–Marie associée à une atrophie optique bilatérale, *Presse méd.*, **72**, 2535.

SMITH, C. K. (1958) Vertebral deformities and other anomalies in Charcot–Marie–Tooth disease, *Neurology (Minneap.)*, **8**, 481.

SYMONDS, C. P., and SHAW, M. E. (1926) Familial claw-foot with absent tendon-jerks: a 'forme fruste' of the Charcot–Marie–Tooth disease, *Brain*, **49**, 387.

THOMAS, P. K., and CALNE, D. B. (1974) Motor nerve conduction velocity in peroneal muscular atrophy: evidence for genetic heterogeneity, *J. Neurol. Neurosurg. Psychiat.*, **37**, 68.

THOMAS, P. K., CALNE, D. B., and STEWART, G. (1974) Hereditary motor and sensory polyneuropathy (peroneal muscular atrophy), *Ann. hum. Genet.*, **38**, 111.

TOOTH, H. H. (1886) *The Peroneal Type of Progressive Muscular Atrophy*, Cambridge thesis, London.

WELANDER, L. (1951) Myopathia distalis tarda hereditaria, *Acta med. scand.*, Suppl. 265.

INFANTILE SPINAL MUSCULAR ATROPHY AND RELATED DISORDERS

There has been considerable discussion as to the relationship between two muscular disorders of infancy, namely amyotonia congenita, or myatonia of Oppenheim (1900) on the one hand, and progressive spinal muscular atrophy of infancy on the other; the latter condition was first described by Werdnig (1890) and Hoffmann (1891). Spiller (1913), on clinical grounds, cast doubt upon the distinction of these diseases, and Greenfield and Stern (1927) pointed out that they were pathologically indistinguishable. But it is now believed that in such cases the diagnosis of amyotonia congenita had been wrongly made and that the progressive disorder which terminates fatally is always Werdnig–Hoffmann disease.

Confusion appears to have arisen from the fact that in the past infants showing severe hypotonia and weakness from the moment of birth were usually diagnosed as examples of amyotonia congenita whereas the diagnosis of Werdnig–Hoffmann disease was reserved for the cases in which weakness and hypotonia developed during the first year of life. In fact, as Walton (1956) and Paine (1963) pointed out, the syndrome of diffuse muscular hypotonia and weakness developing early in infancy is one of multiple aetiology and the inclusive term 'amyotonia congenita', which has been utilized to identify the syndrome, is better discarded since in every case an attempt should be made to identify the pathological basis of the disorder. Thus in many such cases with severe weakness and hypotonia, even when present from birth, the condition proves to be one of progressive spinal muscular atrophy; in others the hypotonia is symptomatic, being secondary to mental defect, flaccid cerebral diplegia or to a variety of metabolic or nutritional disorders; there is, however, a small group of cases in which no cause for the hypotonia is discovered and in which slow improvement usually occurs—for the present these cases may be regarded as suffering from 'benign congenital hypotonia', but even this is almost certainly a disorder of multiple aetiology.

PROGRESSIVE SPINAL MUSCULAR ATROPHY OF INFANCY

PATHOLOGY

There is atrophy and chromatolytic degeneration of the ganglion cells of the anterior horns of the spinal cord and, to a variable extent, of the cranial nerve nuclei and of thalamic neurones (Thieffry et al., 1955) but the cortex is usually normal. Rarely there is vacuolation of affected neurones (Kohn, 1971). The ventral roots are small and largely demyelinated. The peripheral nerves exhibit a high proportion of small finely myelinated fibres, and the muscles show simple 'grouped' or neurogenic atrophy with large numbers of very small fibres in groups and rounding and hypertrophy of surviving innervated fibres. The atrophic fibres are of both histochemical types and electron microscopy has shown only the changes associated with denervation though some of the atrophic fibres may have a fetal appearance (Wechsler and Hager, 1962; Shafiq et al., 1967; van Haelst, 1970; Roy et al., 1971). The uptake of uridine by diseased chromatolytic neurones is normal and the nature of the defect in the diseased cells is unknown (Hogenhuis et al., 1967).

AETIOLOGY

The cause of this condition is unknown; it is due to an autosomal recessive gene and thus affects one in four offspring of either sex of two heterozygous carriers. The gene frequency in North-East England has been estimated to be 1 in 80 (Pearn, 1973 a). Unfortunately no method of detecting carriers is available and it is not uncommon to find that two or three successive children of healthy parents may be affected. Although cases have been reported following acute infections it is doubtful if these play a part in aetiology.

SYMPTOMS

Affected children may be normal at birth and often do not begin to exhibit the symptoms of the disorder until they are a few months old. In other cases severe generalized weakness and hypotonia are present from birth, suggesting that the disease process may have begun in fetal life. Reduced fetal movements in the third trimester of pregnancy are often noted by the mothers of affected children (Pearn, 1973 b); when the condition begins in fetal life there may be variable distal contractures of the limbs at birth, so that the condition is one cause of the syndrome of arthrogryposis multiplex congenita (Smith *et al.*, 1963; Tizard, 1974). Muscular weakness usually begins in the muscles of the back, and the pelvic and shoulder girdles, whence it spreads to the proximal, and later to the distal, muscles of the limbs. The affected muscles waste rapidly: though the wasting may be obscured by subcutaneous fat, it may be shown by X-rays. The affected children often adopt a typical posture with abduction and external rotation of the arms at the shoulder and similar abduction and external rotation at the hip joints. Muscular fasciculation is often present and may be seen in the tongue. The intercostal muscles usually become affected and the bulbar muscles may suffer also, but the diaphragm usually escapes until the later stages, so that indrawing of the lower ribs at the diaphragmatic attachment during inspiration is a useful diagnostic sign. The tendon reflexes are lost. Sensibility is unimpaired, and muscle biopsy shows the features of a neurogenic atrophy while electromyography reveals as a rule spontaneous fibrillation and discrete isolated motor unit action potentials of normal or increased size on volition and motor nerve conduction velocity is normal (Buchthal and Zander Olsen, 1970). The CSF is also normal.

DIAGNOSIS

The condition must be distinguished from benign congenital hypotonia which is present at birth, is characterized by generalized muscular hypotonia with less wasting, preservation of the tendon reflexes, absence of complete paralysis, and of involvement of the intercostals, and in which there is a tendency to improvement; and from congenital myopathy, in which also there may be improvement. Muscle biopsy is generally distinctive in each case. Congenital diplegia and other causes of symptomatic hypotonia are usually easily recognized. Infantile polyneuropathy rarely gives a similar picture but is identifiable by a reduced conduction velocity in peripheral nerves and a rise in cerebrospinal fluid protein.

PROGNOSIS

The condition, as its name implies, is generally progressive, and often terminates fatally in a few months, though temporary or even prolonged arrest has been described. In a recent review of 76 cases, Pearn and Wilson (1973) found that in one-third the disease is manifest at or before delivery; all cases showed delayed milestones by five months of age and 95 per cent were dead, usually as a result of respiratory infection or insufficiency, by the age of 18 months.

TREATMENT

No drug treatment of any value is known.

BENIGN SPINAL MUSCULAR ATROPHY OF CHILDHOOD, ADOLESCENCE, AND EARLY ADULT LIFE

In 1956 Kugelberg and Welander described 12 patients occurring in six families, all of whom were suffering from a heredofamilial form of muscular atrophy simulating muscular dystrophy and suggested that this condition, which appeared to be of autosomal recessive inheritance, might prove to be a new syndrome. Many subsequent reports have since appeared indicating that the condition may begin at any age from late infancy, early childhood, or adolescence to early adult life. Proximal muscles of both the upper and lower limbs are usually affected first giving a clinical picture like that of muscular dystrophy, save for the presence of fasciculation in many cases; the electromyogram and muscle biopsy indicate denervation atrophy but the serum creatine kinase activity may be raised and secondary myopathic changes are common in muscle biopsy specimens (Mastaglia and Walton, 1971) while 'myopathic' potentials may also be recorded in the electromyogram from some muscles (Gath et al., 1969). The course of the condition is very variable from case to case but deterioration is usually slow and arrest frequently occurs.

There has been considerable controversy in recent years concerning the relationship of the Kugelberg–Welander syndrome (pseudomyopathic spinal muscular atrophy) to Werdnig–Hoffmann disease. Many authors, having noted the occurrence of severe and much milder cases in the same sibship, as well as apparent arrest, a subsequent benign course, and prolonged survival, even into adult life in some cases, concluded that the two conditions, each of autosomal recessive inheritance, are probably variants of the same disorder (Dubowitz, 1964; Hausmanowa-Petrusewicz et al., 1966; Gardner-Medwin et al., 1967; Hausmanowa-Petrusewicz et al., 1968; Munsat et al., 1969). However, evidence has begun to accumulate to indicate that true Werdnig–Hoffmann disease, beginning at or before birth or, at the latest, before the sixth month of life, is an independent genetic entity (Pearn et al., 1973). Fried and Emery (1971) identify as a second variety, which they call spinal muscular atrophy type II, those cases previously regarded as examples of Werdnig–Hoffmann disease in which the onset is usually between 6 and 15 months of life, in which the disease process often arrests and in which survival, though usually with severe disability, gross skeletal deformity, and multiple contractures, is possible into late childhood, adolescence, or even adult life. In their view this condition differs from spinal muscular atrophy type III (Kugelberg–Welander disease) in which the age of onset is usually later still, in which walking is usually possible, even if beginning late, and the course very much more benign. This view, however, is not universally accepted (Pearn, 1973c) and classification remains controversial (Namba et al., 1970; van Wijngaarden and Bethlem, 1973). It is, however, clear that many patients previously diagnosed as cases of muscular dystrophy (usually of the limb-girdle and facioscapulohumeral varieties) are in fact suffering from chronic spinal muscular atrophy (Walton and Gardner-Medwin, 1974; Tomlinson et al., 1974).

Classification is not made easier by the fact that occasional families demonstrating autosomal dominant (Zellweger et al., 1972) or X-linked recessive (Tsukagoshi et al., 1970) inheritance have been reported. The relationship between this condition and neurogenic scapuloperoneal muscular atrophy (Ricker et al., 1968; Emery et al., 1968; Feigenbaum and Munsat, 1970) which is occasionally X-linked (Thomas et al., 1972) is still uncertain. Inconstant clinical manifestations reported in some cases and families include limb tremor, called minipolymyoclonus by Spiro (1970), oculopharyngeal muscle involvement (Aberfeld and Namba, 1969; Matsunaga et al., 1973), predominantly distal muscular weakness (Meadows et al., 1969; McLeod and Prineas, 1971), extensor plantar responses and other evidence of corticospinal tract dysfunction (Gardner-Medwin et al., 1967), cardiomyopathy (Mawatari and Katayama, 1973; Tomlinson et al., 1974), hyperlipoproteinaemia (Quarfordt et al., 1970), cystinuria and leucinuria (Radu *et al.*, 1974), and chromosomal abnormalities (Ross *et al.*, 1974).

As will be clear from the above comments, the prognosis of the condition is extremely variable and in a sporadic case arising in adult life diagnosis from motor neurone disease can be difficult if not impossible, although in the more benign form of spinal muscular atrophy weakness usually affects proximal muscles rather than distal in the beginning, the course is slow, and bulbar muscle weakness and signs of corticospinal tract dysfunction are rare. The fact that arrest may occur even in severe cases of early onset underlines the necessity of employing measures (attention to posture, appropriate appliances such as spinal supports and splints, vigorous treatment of respiratory infection, etc.) to prevent skeletal deformity and contractures. Physiotherapy (active exercise against resistance when possible) plays a particularly valuable role in this disabling disease as muscle fibres which retain effective innervation may undergo hypertrophy; swimming under supervision may be especially helpful.

SCAPULOPERONEAL MUSCULAR ATROPHY

This uncommon syndrome, previously referred to on pages 692 and 700, shows some resemblance to chronic spinal muscular atrophy on the one hand and to facioscapulohumeral muscular dystrophy on the other. Usually of dominant inheritance, it is sometimes X-linked (Thomas *et al.*, 1972) and sporadic cases are common. It usually begins in early adult life but an onset in adolescence or middle life is sometimes seen. Muscular weakness and wasting in the legs is very similar to that of peroneal muscular atrophy but in the upper limbs the muscular involvement is proximal, usually with winging of the scapulae and variable involvement of other shoulder girdle and upper arm muscles. Early scapular winging and anterior tibial weakness give a picture like that of early facioscapulohumeral dystrophy but the face is spared and the condition is distinguished from peroneal muscular atrophy by the proximal involvement in the upper limbs, the sparing of the small hand muscles and the normal nerve conduction velocity. In most cases the condition appears to be due to a disorder of the anterior horn cells with neurogenic atrophy of muscle (Kaeser, 1965), and there is no evidence of peripheral neuropathy. In some cases and families, however, the same clinical syndrome has been shown to be due to a myopathy (Thomas *et al.*, 1975). The course of the disorder is usually benign and many patients are greatly helped by appliances designed to correct bilateral foot-drop.

BENIGN CONGENITAL HYPOTONIA

SYMPTOMS

This condition, a syndrome of multiple aetiology, is usually present at birth, though frequently it is not observed until the child is old enough to attempt to raise its head. The most striking feature of the disorder is the extreme muscular hypotonia, which makes it possible for the limbs to be placed in bizarre attitudes. The muscles, though somewhat weak, are not paralysed, but the child may be unable to maintain any posture against the force of gravity. It is, therefore, at first unable to raise its head and, later, to sit or to stand, though it is able to move its legs if it is supported beneath the axillae. The tendon reflexes are usually present but may be depressed. The intercostal muscles and diaphragm usually escape. Electromyography may show no abnormality and muscle biopsy often shows no pathological change in muscle fibres though these may be smaller than normal, while rarely they may all be of one histochemical type or else there may be marked disproportion in the number and size of fibres of the two histochemical types (Dubowitz and Brooke, 1974).

DIAGNOSIS

The diagnosis is not easy, as many conditions are characterized by muscular hypotonia in infancy. Congenital laxity of the ligaments (as in families of contortionists) may result in excessive mobility at joints but the muscles are powerful. In Werdnig–Hoffmann disease the weakness and hypotonia are more severe, the tendon reflexes are lost, and there may be indrawing of the lower ribs during inspiration as a result of intercostal weakness. Mental defect and mild flaccid diplegia may be difficult to distinguish in the early stages as may other causes of symptomatic hypotonia. Serum enzyme studies, electromyography, and muscle biopsy are of particular value in excluding spinal muscular atrophy, muscular dystrophy, and other myopathies, while motor nerve conduction velocity measurement and lumbar puncture may be necessary to exclude infantile polyneuropathy. Even so the diagnosis will occasionally remain in doubt and will only be clarified by repeated observation and examination of the child over a period of many months. Many rare and obscure benign congenital myopathies (Turner, 1949; Tizard, 1974) [see p. 1044] may be indistinguishable from benign congenital hypotonia in the early stages. Indeed, as more obscure congenital myopathies are being recognized by modern techniques of investigation, fewer cases of benign infantile hypotonia now remain unexplained than in the past.

PROGNOSIS

The general tendency of the disorder is to improve, and, if the patient survives intercurrent infections, he may ultimately recover completely, though all physical milestones, including walking, are late; some patients have small, weak, and hypotonic muscles throughout life and are then classified as cases of 'benign congenital myopathy'.

TREATMENT

Treatment must be directed to educating voluntary movement.

REFERENCES

ABERFELD, D. C., and NAMBA, T. (1969) Progressive ophthalmoplegia in Kugelberg–Welander disease, *Arch. Neurol. (Chic.)*, **20**, 253.

BATTEN, F. E., and HOLMES, G. (1912–13) Progressive spinal muscular atrophy of infants (Werdnig–Hoffmann type), *Brain*, **35**, 38.

BUCHTHAL, F., and ZANDER OLSEN, P. (1970) Electromyography and muscle biopsy in infantile spinal muscular atrophy, *Brain*, **93**, 15.

DUBOWITZ, V. (1964) Infantile muscular atrophy. A prospective study with particular reference to a slowly progressive variety, *Brain*, **87**, 707.

DUBOWITZ, V., and BROOKE, M. H. (1974) *Muscle Biopsy* (Major Problems in Neurology Series, ed. Walton, J. N.), London.

EMERY, E. S., FENICHEL, G. M., and ENG, G. (1968) A spinal muscular atrophy with scapuloperoneal distribution, *Arch. Neurol. (Chic.)*, **18**, 129.

FEIGENBAUM, J. A., and MUNSAT, T. L. (1970) A neuromuscular syndrome of scapulo-peroneal distribution, *Bull. Los Angeles neurol. Soc.*, **35**, 47.

FRIED, K., and EMERY, A. E. H. (1971) Spinal muscular atrophy type II. A separate genetic and clinical entity from type I (Werdnig–Hoffmann disease) and type III (Kugelberg–Welander disease), *Clin. Genet.*, **2**, 203.

GARDNER-MEDWIN, D., HUDGSON, P., and WALTON, J. N. (1967) Benign spinal muscular atrophy arising in childhood and adolescence, *J. neurol. Sci.*, **5**, 121.

GATH, I., SJAASTAD, O., and LØKEN, A. C. (1969) Myopathic electromyographic changes correlated with histopathology in Wohlfart–Kugelberg–Welander disease, *Neurology (Minneap.)*, **19**, 344.

GREENFIELD, J. G., and STERN, R. O. (1927) The anatomical identity of the Werdnig–Hoffmann and Oppenheim forms of infantile muscular atrophy, *Brain*, **50**, 652.

HAELST, U. VAN (1970) An electron microscopic study of muscle in Werdnig–Hoffmann's disease, *Virchows Arch. Abt. Path. Anat.*, **351**, 291.

HAUSMANOWA-PETRUSEWICZ, I., ASKANAS, W., BADURSKA, B., EMERYK, B., FIDZIANSKA, A., GARBALINSKA, W., HETNARSKA, L., JEDRZEJOWSKA, H., KAMIENIECKA, Z., NIEBROJ-DOBOSZ, I., PROT, J., and SAWICKA, E. (1968) Infantile and juvenile spinal muscular atrophy, *J. neurol. Sci.*, **6**, 269.

HAUSMANOWA-PETRUSEWICZ, I., PROT, J., and SAWICKA, E. (1966) Le problème des formes infantiles et juvéniles de l'atrophie musculaire spinale, *Rev. Neurol.*, **114**, 295.

HOFFMANN, J. (1891) Weiterer Beitrag zur Lehre von der progressiven neurotischen Muskelatrophie, *Dtsch. Z. Nervenheilk.*, **1**, 95.

HOFFMANN, J. (1893) Über chronische spinale Muskelatrophie im Kindesalter, *Dtsch. Z. Nervenheilk.*, **3**, 427.

HOFFMANN, J. (1897) Weiterer Beitrag zur Lehre von der hereditären progressiven spinalen Muskelatrophie im Kindesalter, *Dtsch. Z. Nervenheilk.*, **10**, 292.

HOGENHUIS, L. A. H., SPAULDING, S. W., and ENGEL, W. K. (1967) Neuronal RNA metabolism in infantile spinal muscular atrophy (Werdnig–Hoffmann's disease) studied by radio-autography, *J. Neuropath. exp. Neurol.*, **26**, 335.

KAESER, H. E. (1965) Scapuloperoneal muscular atrophy, *Brain*, **88**, 407.

KOHN, R. (1971) Clinical and pathological findings in an unusual infantile motor neurone disease, *J. Neurol. Neurosurg. Psychiat.*, **34**, 427.

KUGELBERG, E., and WELANDER, L. (1956) Heredo-familial juvenile muscular atrophy simulating muscular dystrophy, *Arch. Neurol. Psychiat. (Chic.)*, **15**, 500.

McLEOD, J. G., and PRINEAS, J. W. (1971) Distal type of chronic spinal muscular atrophy: clinical, electrophysiological and pathological studies, *Brain*, **94**, 703.

MASTAGLIA, F. L., and WALTON, J. N. (1971) Histological and histochemical changes in skeletal muscle from cases of chronic juvenile and early adult spinal muscular atrophy (the Kugelberg–Welander syndrome), *J. neurol. Sci.*, **12**, 15.

MATSUNAGA, M., INOKUCHI, T., OHNISHI, A., and KUROIWA, Y. (1973) Oculopharyngeal involvement in familial neurogenic muscular atrophy, *J. Neurol. Neurosurg. Psychiat.*, **36**, 104.

MAWATARI, S., and KATAYAMA, K. (1973) Scapuloperoneal muscular atrophy with cardio-pathy: an X-linked recessive trait, *Arch. Neurol. (Chic.)*, **28**, 55.

MEADOWS, J. C., MARSDEN, C. D., and HARRIMAN, D. G. F. (1969) Chronic spinal muscular atrophy in adults. I. The Kugelberg–Welander syndrome. II. Other forms, *J. neurol. Sci.*, **9**, 527, 551.

MUNSAT, T. L., WOODS, R., FOWLER, W., and PEARSON, C. M. (1969) Neurogenic muscular atrophy of infancy with prolonged survival. The variable course of Werdnig–Hoffmann disease, *Brain*, **92**, 9.

NAMBA, T., ABERFELD, D. C., and GROB, D. (1970) Chronic proximal spinal muscular atrophy, *J. neurol. Sci.*, **11**, 401.

OPPENHEIM, H. (1900) Über allgemeine und localisierte Atonie der Muskulatur (Myatonie) im frühen Kindesalter, *Mschr. Psychiat. Neurol.*, **8**, 232.

PAINE, R. S. (1963) The future of the 'floppy infant'. A follow-up study of 133 patients, *Develop. med. Child Neurol.*, **5**, 115.

PEARN, J. H. (1973 a) The gene frequency of acute Werdnig–Hoffmann disease (SMA type 1). A total population survey in North-East England, *J. med. Genet.*, **10**, 260.

PEARN, J. H. (1973 b) Fetal movements and Werdnig–Hoffmann disease, *J. neurol. Sci.*, **18**, 373.

PEARN, J. H. (1973 c) *The Spinal Muscular Atrophies of Childhood: a Genetic and Clinical Study*, Ph.D. Thesis, University of London.

PEARN, J. H., CARTER, C. O., and WILSON, J. (1973) The genetic identity of acute infantile spinal muscular atrophy, *Brain*, **96**, 463.

PEARN, J. H., and WILSON, J. (1973) Acute Werdnig–Hoffmann disease. Acute infantile spinal muscular atrophy, *Arch. Dis. Childh.*, **48**, 425.

QUARFORDT, S. H., DeVIVO, D. C., ENGEL, W. K., LEVY, R. I., and FREDRICKSON, D. S. (1970) Familial adult-onset proximal spinal muscular atrophy. Report of a family with type II hyperlipoproteinemia, *Arch. Neurol. (Chic.)*, **22**, 541.

RADU, H., TANASE-MOGOS, I., ROSU, A. M., KILLYEN, I., and IONESCU, V. (1974) A new polygenic disturbance: cystinuria, leucinuria and spinal muscular atrophy, *J. Neurol.*, **207**, 73.

RICKER, K., MERTENS, H.-G., and SCHIMRIGK, K. (1968) The neurogenic scapulo-peroneal syndrome, *Europ. Neurol.*, **1**, 257.

ROSS, R. T., SIMPSON, C. A., and STYLES, S. (1974) Wohlfart Kugelberg Welander syndrome, *Canad. J. neurol. Sci.*, **1**, 130.

ROY, S., DUBOWITZ, V., and WOLMAN, L. (1971) Ultrastructure of muscle in infantile spinal muscular atrophy, *J. neurol. Sci.*, **12**, 219.

SHAFIQ, S. A., MILHORAT, A. T., and GORYCKI, M. A. (1967) Fine structure of human muscle in neurogenic atrophy, *Neurology (Minneap.)*, **17**, 934.

SMITH, E. M., BENDER, L. F., and STOVER, C. N. (1963) Lower motor neuron deficit in arthrogryposis: an EMG study, *Arch. Neurol. (Chic.)*, **8**, 97.

SPILLER, W. G. (1913) The relation of the myopathies, *Brain*, **36**, 75.

SPIRO, A. J. (1970) Minipolymyoclonus: a neglected sign in childhood spinal muscular atrophy, *Neurology (Minneap.)*, **20**, 1124.

THIEFFRY, S., ARTHUIS, M., and BARGETON, E. (1955) Quarante cas de maladie de Werdnig–Hoffmann avec onze examens anatomiques, *Rev. Neurol.*, **93**, 621.

THOMAS, P. K., CALNE, D. B., and ELLIOTT, C. F. (1972) X-linked scapuloperoneal syndrome, *J. Neurol. Neurosurg. Psychiat.*, **35**, 208.

THOMAS, P. K., SCHOTT, G. D., and MORGAN-HUGHES, J. A. (1975) Adult onset scapuloperoneal myopathy, *J. Neurol. Neurosurg. Psychiat.*, **38**, 1008.

TIZARD, J. P. M. (1974) Neuromuscular disorders of infancy, in *Disorders of Voluntary Muscle*, 3rd ed., ed. Walton, J. N., p. 693, Edinburgh and London.

TOMLINSON, B. E., WALTON, J. N., and IRVING, D. (1974) Spinal cord limb motor neurones in muscular dystrophy, *J. neurol. Sci.*, **22**, 305.

TSUKAGOSHI, H., SHOJI, H., and FURUKAWA, T. (1970) Proximal neurogenic muscular atrophy in adolescence and adulthood with X-linked recessive inheritance, *Neurology (Minneap.)*, **20**, 1188.

TURNER, J. W. A. (1949) On amyotonia congenita, *Brain*, **72**, 25.

WALTON, J. N. (1956) Amyotonia congenita: a follow-up study, *Lancet*, **i**, 1023.

WALTON, J. N. (1957) The limp child, *J. Neurol. Psychiat.*, **20**, 144.

WALTON, J. N., and GARDNER-MEDWIN, D. (1974) Progressive muscular dystrophy and the myotonic disorders, in *Disorders of Voluntary Muscle*, 3rd ed., ed. Walton, J. N., p. 561, Edinburgh and London.

WECHSLER, W., and HAGER, H. (1962) Elektronenmikroskopische Befunde an der Skeletmuskulatur bei progressiver spinaler Muskelatrophie, *Arch. Psychiat. Zeitschr. Neurol.*, **203**, 111.

WERDNIG, G. (1890) Über einen Fall von Dystrophia musculorum mit positivem Rückenmarksbefunde, *Wien. med. Wschr.*, **40**, 1796.

WERDNIG, G. (1891) Zwei frühinfantile hereditäre Fälle von progressiver Muskelatrophie unter dem Bilde der Dystrophie, aber auf neurotischer Grundlage, *Arch. Psychiat.*, **22**, 437.

WIJNGAARDEN, G. K. VAN, and BETHLEM, J. (1973) Benign infantile spinal muscular atrophy—a prospective study, *Brain*, **96**, 163.

ZELLWEGER, H., SIMPSON, J., McCORMICK, W. F., and IONASESCU, V. (1972) Spinal muscular atrophy with autosomal dominant inheritance, *Neurology* (*Minneap.*), **22**, 957.

FACIAL HEMIATROPHY

Synonym. Parry–Romberg syndrome.

Definition. A disorder of uncertain aetiology, characterized by progressive wasting of some or all of the tissues of one side of the face and sometimes extending beyond these limits.

PATHOLOGY

Facial hemiatrophy, which was first described by Romberg in 1846, consists essentially of an atrophy which usually involves all the tissues of the face—the skin, the subcutaneous fat and connective tissue, the muscles, cartilage, and bone. The muscular atrophy is due to a disappearance, not of the muscle fibres, but of the fat and connective tissue of the muscle. The tongue and soft palate often suffer in addition. The cartilage of the nose frequently becomes atrophic: that of the ear, larynx, and tarsus is less often affected. The cerebral hemisphere on the affected side may be atrophic. Stief (1933) described vasodilatation in the ipsilateral hemisphere and round cell infiltration of the cervical sympathetic on the affected side.

AETIOLOGY

It is a disorder of early life, usually developing during the second decade, and is sometimes congenital. A number of cases, however, have been observed in which the onset has occurred in middle life or even old age. The cause of the condition is unknown. A relationship to morphoea (localized scleroderma) has been postulated but this could not explain the occasional involvement of other parts of the body on the affected side or the atrophy of the ipsilateral cerebral hemisphere. Various authors have attributed the condition to local trauma or infection, or to lesions of the ipsilateral trigeminal nerve or cervical sympathetic in which indefinite pathological changes have been found (Archambault and Fromm, 1932) but no constant pathological findings have been reported (Ford, 1966) and pathogenesis remains obscure.

SYMPTOMS

Wasting may begin at any point of the face and may either remain limited to one region, so that it has been described as corresponding to one division of the trigeminal nerve, or may spread, either slowly or quickly, to the whole face [FIG. 119], sometimes extending to the side of the neck and even, as in a case of Martin's, involving the breast on the same side. Some authors accept that cases of progressive hemiatrophy of the whole body are closely related. When the disorder is well developed the patient's appearance is striking, the affected half of the face being sunken and wrinkled and presenting the appearance of old age, in marked contrast to the normal side. Very rarely both sides of the face are affected. The atrophy frequently involves the soft palate, tongue, and mucous membrane of the gums on the same side. Muscular weakness is absent.

Falling of the hair of the face and scalp on the affected side is not uncommon. Pigmentary anomalies of the skin, such as vitiligo, frequently occur, and facial naevus has been described. Pains of a neuralgic character may develop and these are frequently associated with tender spots. True tic douloureux may occur. Sensory impairment is rare but cutaneous anaesthesia and analgesia have been encountered. Sweating and lacrimal secretion may be either diminished or increased on the affected side. Ocular sympathetic paralysis—myosis, ptosis, and enophthalmos—has been encountered in a proportion of cases, and Brain saw a case with a unilateral Argyll Robertson pupil. In other cases the pupil on the affected side has been larger than on the normal side.

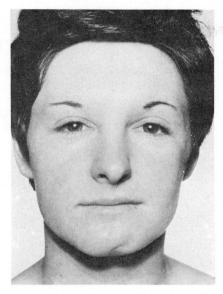

FIG. 119. Early left-sided facial hemiatrophy (kindly supplied by Dr. J. D. Spillane)

Epileptiform convulsions, in some cases Jacksonian and in others generalized, have occurred in a small number of cases. Brain observed one such case in which left facial hemiatrophy was associated with right-sided epilepsy, hemiplegia, hemianaesthesia, hemianopia, and aphasia, and atrophy of the left cerebral hemisphere was demonstrated by encephalography. Migraine is common. Facial hemiatrophy is sometimes associated with syringomyelia, and the presence of scleroderma elsewhere in the body has often been observed.

DIAGNOSIS

The clinical picture is so striking that it can hardly be confused with anything else.

PROGNOSIS

The wasting may become arrested before the whole of the face is involved, but there is no means of determining whether or not this will occur. In mild cases the disorder causes no disability apart from its cosmetic effect.

TREATMENT

No known treatment will arrest the progress of the disease. When trigeminal pain is present, carbamazepine should be tried but constant rather than paroxysmal pain is more likely to respond to standard analgesic remedies.

REFERENCES

ARCHAMBAULT, L., and FROMM, N. K. (1932) Progressive facial hemiatrophy, *Arch. Neurol. Psychiat. (Chic.)*, **27**, 529.

FORD, F. R. (1966) *Diseases of the Nervous System in Infancy, Childhood and Adolescence*, 5th ed., p. 310, Springfield, Ill.

STIEF, A. (1933) Über einen Fall von Hemiatrophie des Gesichtes mit Sektionsbefund, *Z. ges. Neurol. Psychiat.*, **147,** 573.

WARTENBERG, R. (1945) Progressive facial hemiatrophy, *Arch. Neurol. Psychiat. (Chic.)*, **54,** 75.

HEMIHYPERTROPHY

In this rare condition there is hypertrophy of the tissues, including the long bones which are often longer than normal, on one half of the body. Associated anomalies may include congenital heart disease and chromosomal abnormalities (Henry *et al.*, 1973). Focal neurological abnormalities on the affected side are uncommon but focal or generalized epileptic convulsions have been reported as well as congenital indifference to pain on the affected side (Fox and Huott, 1974).

REFERENCES

FOX, J. H., and HUOTT, A. D. (1974) Congenital hemihypertrophy with indifference to pain, *Arch. Neurol. (Chic.)*, **30,** 490.

HENRY, M., LOUIS, J. P., HOEFFEL, J. C., and PERNOT, C. (1973) Congenital hemihypertrophy with aortic, skeletal, and ocular abnormalities, *Brit. med. J.*, **1,** 87.

AGENESIS OF THE CORPUS CALLOSUM

This rare anomaly is often asymptomatic neurologically unless tests designed specifically to test the transfer of information from one cerebral hemisphere to the other can be employed; however, various clinical syndromes resulting from associated developmental abnormalities including hydrocephalus and microgyria have been reported in such cases (Loeser and Alvord, 1968 *a* and *b*). Spontaneous recurrent hypothermia has also been described (Shapiro *et al.*, 1969). Ettlinger *et al.* (1972) have reviewed the behavioural studies which may be useful in establishing the diagnosis.

REFERENCES

ETTLINGER, G., BLAKEMORE, C. B., MILNER, A. D., and WILSON, J. (1972) Agenesis of the corpus callosum: a behavioural investigation, *Brain*, **95,** 327.

LOESER, J. D., and ALVORD, E. C. (1968 *a*) Agenesis of the corpus callosum, *Brain*, **91,** 553.

LOESER, J. D., and ALVORD, E. C. (1968 *b*) Clinicopathological correlations in agenesis of the corpus callosum, *Neurology (Minneap.)*, **18,** 745.

SHAPIRO, W. R., WILLIAMS, G. H., and PLUM, F. (1969) Spontaneous recurrent hypothermia accompanying agenesis of the corpus callosum, *Brain*, **92,** 423.

14

DISORDERS OF THE SPINAL CORD
AND CAUDA EQUINA

ANATOMY OF THE SPINAL CORD
AND CAUDA EQUINA

THE spinal cord lies within the vertebral canal, extending from the foramen magnum, where it is continuous with the medulla oblongata, to the level of the first or second lumbar vertebra. It is oval in shape, being flattened from before backwards, and exhibits two enlargements, in the cervical and lumbar regions, corresponding to the outflow of nerves to the limbs. At its lower end the spinal cord terminates in the conus medullaris, from the end of which a delicate filament, the filum terminale, is prolonged downwards as far as the posterior surface of the coccyx.

The surface of the cord exhibits several longitudinal grooves, the deep anterior median fissure and the shallower posterior median sulcus, while on the lateral aspect are two sulci, the anterolateral and the posterolateral. From the last two a series of root filaments emerge on each side of the cord. At intervals several filaments from the posterolateral sulcus unite to form a dorsal root, upon which is situated a ganglion, the dorsal root ganglion, and similarly those from the anterolateral sulcus unite to form a ventral root. One ventral and the corresponding dorsal root on one side join together just distally to the dorsal root ganglion to form a spinal nerve. Thus from each side there arises a series of spinal nerves, and the spinal cord is regarded as divided into segments, one corresponding to each pair of spinal nerves. There are eight cervical, twelve dorsal or thoracic, five lumbar, five sacral segments, and one coccygeal. Since the spinal cord ends at the first or second lumbar vertebra, all the spinal nerves below the first lumbar descend to their respective foramina in a leash known as the cauda equina.

The spinal cord, like the brain, is surrounded by three meninges. The pia mater is a fibrous membrane, which forms the immediate covering of the cord, and from which fine septa penetrate into its substance. The arachnoid is a delicate, transparent membrane, which lies superficially to the pia mater, from which it is separated by the subarachnoid space; this contains the cerebrospinal fluid, and it is bridged by numerous trabeculae. The arachnoid extends as low as the second sacral vertebra. Outside the arachnoid lies the dura mater, which forms a lining to the vertebral canal, from which it is separated by the epidural space containing fatty tissue, and a thin-walled venous plexus. The dura mater extends a little lower than the arachnoid, to the second or third sacral vertebra. The spinal cord is suspended within its dural sheath by a series of ligamenta denticulata, which extend laterally from the sides of the cord to terminate in tooth-like attachments to the inner aspect of the dura.

On transverse section the substance of the cord is seen to be divided into the central grey and peripheral white matter. The grey matter is composed of ganglion cells and nerve fibres, and the white matter of fibres only. The grey matter forms an H-shaped mass composed of an anterior and a posterior horn on each side, united by the grey commissure, in the centre of which is situated the central canal. The anterior horns of grey matter contain ganglion cells, the axons of which compose the anterior roots and which constitute the lower motor neurones. The cells which innervate the skeletal muscles (alpha motor neurones) measure between 30 μm and 70 μm in diameter (Truex and Carpenter, 1969) and show certain histological characteristics which usually render their differentiation from the gamma motor neurones comparatively easy, as most of the latter are less than 30 μm in diameter (Tomlinson *et al.*, 1973). The large anterior horn cells (motor neurones) are arranged in definite groups (in transverse sections) and columns (in longitudinal sections) and it has been shown by Sharrard (1953, 1955) that specific groups and columns of cells in the cervical and lumbar enlargements consistently innervate various muscle groups and some individual muscles. The total number of limb motor neurones in the lumbosacral cord is remarkably consistent not only on the two sides of the cord but also in different individuals (Tomlinson *et al.*, 1973).

The white matter, which consists of the longitudinal bundles of nerve fibres, is regarded as being divided into three columns. The anterior column lies between the anterior fissure and the anterior horn of grey matter with its emerging roots. The lateral column is situated on the lateral side of the grey matter, between the ventral and dorsal roots, that is, between the anterolateral and posterolateral sulci. The posterior column lies between the posterior median septum and the posterior horn of grey matter and the dorsal root. The paths of the fibres entering the spinal cord by the posterior roots are described elsewhere [see p. 43]. The anatomical situation of the various fibre tracts of the spinal cord is best appreciated by reference to the diagram [FIG. 8, p. 43].

THE BLOOD SUPPLY OF THE SPINAL CORD

Arteries. The spinal cord is richly supplied with blood. There are two posterior spinal arteries, each derived from the corresponding vertebral or posterior inferior cerebellar artery and passing downwards upon the side of the medulla oblongata and throughout the whole length of the spinal cord, where they lie either in front of, or behind, the dorsal nerve roots. The single anterior spinal artery is formed by the union of a branch from each vertebral artery, and descends throughout the whole length of the spinal cord in the anterior median fissure. The spinal arteries are reinforced by segmental arteries, which enter the intervertebral foramina and are derived from the vertebral, intercostal, and lumbar arteries. The two most important of these are one in the lower cervical and one, the artery of Adamkiewicz, in the lower thoracic or upper lumbar region. The spinal cord is thus surrounded by a basocorona or arterial wreath, which unites the spinal arteries and which sends branches horizontally inwards to supply the white matter and the greater part of the posterior horns of grey matter. The anterior horns of grey matter are supplied by branches of the anterior spinal artery, and distributed to the anterior horn on each side alternately.

The direction of blood flow in the anterior spinal artery may not be the same throughout. Bolton (1939) suggested that the direction of blood flow is downwards in the anterior spinal artery, and in the posterior spinal artery down to the lower cervical region; he also suggested that in the dorsal and lumbar regions flow was often upwards. Studies with spinal cord angiography in animals and man (Di Chiro *et al.*, 1970; Di Chiro, 1970; Fortuna *et al.*, 1971; Di Chiro and Fried, 1971) have confirmed that flow is often in a rostral direction even in the lower cervical region but is variable from one individual to another and may be greatly modified by vascular disease. Methods of measuring spinal cord blood flow in animals have been devised (Griffiths, 1973 *a, b,* and *c*) and experimental work has confirmed that motor or sensory activity causes temporary vasodilatation and increased blood flow in the relevant portions of the cord and cauda equina (Blau and Rushworth, 1958). Within the cord the anterior spinal artery supplies all but the posterior part of the posterior columns and posterior horns, which are supplied by the posterior spinal arteries. Descending branches from the spinal arteries also supply the roots of the cauda equina.

Syndromes of spinal cord ischaemia and/or infarction [p. 783] may result from embolism or occlusion of the anterior spinal artery due to atheroma, aortic disease, or a drop in perfusion pressure (Herrick and Mills, 1971; Silver and Buxton, 1974) and may complicate aortography (*The Lancet*, 1973). Posterior spinal artery occlusion due to intrathecal phenol injection has also been described (Hughes, 1970). The motor neurones and the central grey matter in general are more vulnerable to ischaemia than the white matter (Gilles and Nag, 1971; Fried and Aparicio, 1973).

Veins. The spinal veins derived from the substance of the spinal cord terminate in a plexus in the pia mater, in which six longitudinal channels have been described. These pass upwards into the corresponding veins of the medulla oblongata and so drain into the intracranial venous sinuses. Segmental veins pass outwards along the nerve roots to join the internal vertebral venous plexus, in which blood also flows upwards to the intracranial venous sinuses. The posterior half of the cord is drained by the posterior medullary veins; the anterior medullary group can be divided into one lateral and two medial groups (Gillilan, 1970) and the anatomical pattern helps to explain the clinical features of venous infarction of the cord (Hughes, 1971, and see p. 784). Venous drainage through the intervertebral foramina is relatively unimportant, but thrombophlebitis may reach the spinal veins by this route.

REFERENCES

BLAU, J. N., and RUSHWORTH, G. (1958) Observations on the blood vessels of the spinal cord and their responses to motor activity, *Brain*, **81**, 354.

BOLTON, B. (1939) The blood supply of the spinal cord, *J. Neurol. Psychiat.*, **2**, 137.

CORBIN, J. L. (1961) *Anatomie, pathologie artérielle de la moelle*, Paris.

DI CHIRO, G. (1970) Spinal cord angiography, *Proc. roy. Soc. Med.*, **63**, 184.

DI CHIRO, G., and FRIED, L. C. (1971) Blood flow currents in spinal cord arteries, *Neurology* (*Minneap.*), **21**, 1088.

DI CHIRO, G., FRIED, L. C., and DOPPMAN, J. L. (1970) Experimental spinal cord angiography, *Brit. J. Radiol.*, **43**, 19.

FORTUNA, A., LA TORRE, E., and OCCHIPINTI, E. (1971) The direction of blood flow in the cervical cord, *Europ. Neurol.*, **5**, 335.

FRIED, L. C., and APARICIO, O. (1973) Experimental ischemia of the spinal cord: histologic studies after anterior spinal artery occlusion, *Neurology* (*Minneap.*), **23**, 289.

GILLES, F. H., and NAG, D. (1971) Vulnerability of human spinal cord in transient cardiac arrest, *Neurology* (*Minneap.*), **21**, 833.

GILLILAN, L. A. (1970) Veins of the spinal cord: anatomic details; suggested clinical applications, *Neurology* (*Minneap.*), **20**, 860.

GRIFFITHS, I. R. (1973 *a*) Spinal cord blood flow in dogs: 1. The 'normal' flow, *J. Neurol. Neurosurg. Psychiat.*, **36**, 34.

GRIFFITHS, I. R. (1973 b) Spinal cord blood flow in dogs: 2. The effect of the blood gases, *J. Neurol. Neurosurg. Psychiat.*, **36**, 42.

GRIFFITHS, I. R. (1973 c) Spinal cord blood flow in dogs: 3. The effect of blood pressure, *J. Neurol. Neurosurg. Psychiat.*, **36**, 914.

HERRICK, M. K., and MILLS, P. E. (1971) Infarction of spinal cord. Two cases of selective gray matter involvement secondary to asymptomatic aortic disease, *Arch. Neurol. (Chic.)*, **24**, 228.

HUGHES, J. T. (1966) *Pathology of the Spinal Cord*, London.

HUGHES, J. T. (1970) Thrombosis of the posterior spinal arteries: a complication of an intrathecal injection of phenol, *Neurology (Minneap.)*, **20**, 659.

HUGHES, J. T. (1971) Venous infarction of the spinal cord, *Neurology (Minneap.)*, **21**, 794.

THE LANCET (1973) Spinal-cord damage after angiography, *Lancet*, **ii,** 1067.

SHARRARD, W. J. W. (1953) Correlation between changes in the spinal cord and muscle paralysis in poliomyelitis—a preliminary report, *Proc. roy. Soc. Med.*, **46**, 346.

SHARRARD, W. J. W. (1955) The histology of lesions in the lumbo-sacral spinal cord in convalescent and late poliomyelitis, *Proceedings of the Second International Congress of Neuropathology*, p. 437, Amsterdam.

SILVER, J. R., and BUXTON, P. H. (1974) Spinal stroke, *Brain*, **97**, 539.

TOMLINSON, B. E., IRVING, D., and REBEIZ, J. J. (1973) Total numbers of limb motor neurones in the human lumbosacral cord and an analysis of the accuracy of various sampling procedures, *J. neurol. Sci.*, **20**, 313.

TRUEX, R. C., and CARPENTER, M. B. (1969) *Human Neuroanatomy*, 6th ed., p. 247, Baltimore.

PARAPLEGIA

By paraplegia is meant paralysis confined to the lower limbs. This may be caused by a disorder of function at different levels. It may be psychogenic—in hysteria. It may occur as a result of a cerebral lesion, when so placed as to damage the corticospinal fibres from the leg areas of the motor cortex only. Cerebral paraplegia may thus be produced by a meningioma arising in the falx (a parasagittal meningioma), by thrombosis of the superior sagittal sinus, by congenital cerebral lesions (Little's disease), and in rare instances by thrombosis of an unpaired anterior cerebral artery. In such cases the lower limbs are usually spastic in extension. Bilateral brain stem lesions usually cause tetraplegia rather than paraplegia. Paraplegia of flaccid type due to a lesion of the spinal cord is very much commoner and is the form usually encountered. Spinal paraplegia may be associated either with extension or with flexion of the lower limbs, paraplegia-in-extension or paraplegia-in-flexion. Paraplegia may also be caused by a lesion of the anterior horn cells of the lumbosacral region of the spinal cord, e.g. in poliomyelitis or, rarely, motor neurone disease, or by a lesion of the cauda equina, or of the peripheral nerves to the lower limbs, as in polyneuritis, or of the muscles, as in myopathy. We are here concerned mainly with paraplegia due to lesions of the spinal cord.

After a partial lesion of the cord two mutually antagonistic reflex activities emerge, extensor hypertonia and the flexor withdrawal reflex [see p. 56]. The former is recognized as physiologically equivalent to decerebrate rigidity in the animal, which, it will be remembered, is probably dependent upon the connections of the reticular formation nuclei with the spinal cord. The flexor withdrawal reflex, on the other hand, utilizes short spinal reflex arcs. After a lesion which involves the corticospinal tracts only, both sets of reflexes are potentially active, but extensor hypertonia predominates as a persistent tonic activity, giving way only occasionally to the flexor withdrawal reflex when a noxious stimulus excites the latter. If, however, a spinal lesion involves a sufficient transverse extent of the cord to destroy not only the corticospinal fibres but also the descending tracts upon which extensor hypertonia depends, the flexor reflex, freed from its antagonist, manifests greatly heightened activity and dominates the picture. Violent flexor spasms occur in the lower limbs, which in severe cases finally become fixed in an attitude of flexion, with the heels approximated to the buttocks. Paraplegia-in-flexion may be the outcome of a slowly progressive lesion of the cord, in which case it follows paraplegia-in-extension after an intermediate phase in which the balance swings between the two reflex systems. On the other hand, after a traumatic lesion, causing immediate and complete severance of the cord, because the reticulospinal tract is interrupted from the beginning, as soon as the stage of spinal shock has passed, paraplegia-in-flexion tends to develop unless prevented.

PARAPLEGIA-IN-FLEXION

In paraplegia-in-flexion three main reflex activities are demonstrable: (1) the flexor withdrawal reflex, (2) excretory, and (3) sexual reflexes. We must also consider (4) the 'mass reflex', and (5) the tendon reflexes.

1. *The Flexor Withdrawal Reflex* has already been briefly described [see p. 56]. In paraplegia-in-flexion its activity is much enhanced. Its receptive field is enlarged and it may be elicitable by a noxious stimulus applied to any part of the lower limbs and abdominal wall, or even, with a high dorsal lesion, as high as the nipple. The motor response is extremely vigorous, and strong flexion of the lower limb occurs at all joints, with upward movement of the great toe and separation of the other toes. This is usually unilateral, but the opposite lower limb may also become flexed. The activity of the flexor reflex is depressed by spinal shock and by cutaneous or urinary infection. Both its receptive field and its motor response then shrink until it can be obtained only from the outer border of the sole, and yields only a contraction of the inner hamstring muscles.

2. *Excretory Reflexes.* When reflex activity of the divided spinal cord is well established, in traumatic cases about three weeks after transection, reflex evacuation of the bladder and rectum, and reflex sweating occur. The volume of fluid required to evoke reflex contraction of the bladder wall varies in different cases, but is usually about 150–200 ml. Reflex emptying of the bladder can be facilitated by deep breathing or by noxious stimuli applied to the skin of the lower limbs. Reflex evacuation of the rectum occurs in response to a volume of from 100–180 ml. Sweating occurs reflexly in response to cutaneous stimuli from the areas of skin supplied by the fibres of the sympathetic nervous system which leave the spinal cord below the level of the lesion.

3. *Sexual Reflexes.* In paraplegia-in-flexion the cremasteric, dartos, and bulbocavernosus reflexes are present, and reflex erection of the penis and seminal emission can be evoked by handling the organ. Spontaneous priapism may occur. These sexual reflexes may be associated with contractions of the abdominal recti, the leg flexors, and the adductors of the thigh.

4. *The Mass Reflex.* Reflex facilitation is probably responsible for the phenomenon named by Head and Riddoch (1917) the 'mass reflex', in which stimulation of the skin of the lower limbs and, when the lesion is high, of the lower abdominal wall evokes reflex flexion of the lower trunk muscles and the lower limbs, evacuation of the bladder and rectum, and sweating.

5. *The Tendon Reflexes.* The tone of the extensor muscles is minimal in paraplegia-in-flexion, but the tendon reflexes can usually be elicited. Ankle clonus, however, hardly ever occurs.

PARAPLEGIA-IN-EXTENSION

In paraplegia-in-extension tone predominates in the adductors of the hips and the extensors of the hips, knees, and ankles with a resulting posture of extension of the hip and knee and plantar-flexion of the ankles. The knee- and ankle-jerks are exaggerated, and patellar and ankle clonus are frequently present. The elicitation of the knee-jerk may evoke a sharp contraction of the adductors of the opposite hip, the crossed adductor-jerk. Reflex extension of the limb can often be obtained by applying a noxious stimulus, such as a scratch from a pin, to the skin of the upper third of the thigh, and spontaneous extensor spasms may occur.

With this prevalence of extensor tone the flexor withdrawal reflex is relatively inhibited. Its field of elicitation is small compared with that found in paraplegia-in-flexion. After it has been evoked, the limb regains its primary posture of extension by an active return of tone to the extensor muscles. Flexor withdrawal of one limb is usually associated with increased extension of the other, the crossed extensor reflex. The excretory reflexes which accompany paraplegia-in-flexion are absent, and the motor concomitant of erection of the penis is extension instead of flexion of the lower limbs.

SOME RECENT ADVANCES

In occasional cases of paraplegia there is an apparent inconsistency between the degree of spasticity as assessed by flexion or extension of the limb on the one hand and the activity of the tendon reflexes on the other. Marsden *et al.* (1973) have produced evidence to suggest that whereas the tendon jerks depend upon monosynaptic reflexes, the stretch reflex may be due to rapidly conducting long reflex pathways involving the cortex. Swash and Earl (1975) pointed out that in two patients with the Holmes–Adie syndrome and tabes dorsalis, severe transverse cord lesions caused a flaccid paraplegia with absent tendon reflexes; both patients had flexor spasms but there was no spasticity. Measurement of the H-reflex has been used as a method of assessing the excitability of spinal motor neurones in spinal shock and in spasticity and rigidity (Yap, 1967; Diamantopoulos and Zander Olsen, 1967) and experimental work in animals on conduction in demyelinated fibres (McDonald and Robertson, 1972) as well as techniques now being developed of measuring evoked spinal potentials from the skin overlying the spine during peripheral sensory stimulation (Cracco *et al.*, 1975) are likely to make an increasing contribution to our understanding of spinal cord lesions in man. The pathophysiology of paraplegia has recently been reviewed by Lance and McLeod (1975).

REFERENCES

CRACCO, J. B., CRACCO, R. Q., and GRAZIANI, L. J. (1975) The spinal evoked response in infants and children, *Neurology (Minneap.)*, **25**, 31.

DIAMANTOPOULOS, E., and ZANDER OLSEN, P. (1967) Excitability of motor neurones in spinal shock in man, *J. Neurol. Neurosurg. Psychiat.*, **30**, 427.

HEAD, H., and RIDDOCH, G. (1917) The automatic bladder, excessive sweating, and some other reflex conditions, in gross injuries of the spinal cord, *Brain*, **40**, 188.

LANCE, J. W., and McLEOD, J. G. (1975) *A Physiological Approach to Clinical Neurology*, 2nd ed., London.

MARSDEN, C. D., MERTON, P. A., and MORTON, H. B. (1973) Is the human stretch reflex cortical rather than spinal?, *Lancet*, **i**, 759.

McDONALD, W. I., and ROBERTSON, M. A. H. (1972) Changes in conduction during nerve fibre degeneration in the spinal cord, *Brain*, **95**, 151.

MEDICAL RESEARCH COUNCIL (1924) Report of the Committee upon Injuries of the Nervous System, *Spec. Rep. Ser. med. Res. Coun. (Lond.)*, No. 88.

PEDERSEN, E., ed. (1962) Spasticity and neurological bladder disturbances, *Acta neurol. (Kbh.)*, **38**, Suppl. 3.

SCARFF, J. E. (1960) Injuries of the vertebral column and spinal cord, in *Injuries of the Brain and Spinal Cord*, 4th ed., ed. Brock, S., p. 530, New York.

SIMPSON, J. A. (1963) Current neurological concepts of spinal cord injuries, in *Spinal Injuries: a Symposium of the Royal College of Surgeons*, ed. Harris, P., p. 10, Edinburgh.

SWASH, M., and EARL, C. J. (1975) Flaccid paraplegia: a feature of spinal cord lesions in Holmes–Adie syndrome and tabes dorsalis, *J. Neurol. Neurosurg. Psychiat.*, **38**, 317.

WALSHE, F. M. R. (1914–15) The physiological significance of the reflex phenomena in spastic paralysis of the lower limbs, *Brain*, **37**, 269.

WALSHE, F. M. R. (1919) On the genesis and physiological significance of spasticity and other disorders of motor innervation: with a consideration of the functional relationships of the pyramidal system, *Brain*, **42**, 1.

WALSHE, F. M. R. (1923) On variations in the form of reflex movements, notably the Babinski plantar response, under different degrees of spasticity and under the influence of Magnus and de Kleijn's tonic neck reflex, *Brain*, **46**, 281.

WALSHE, F. M. R. (1923) The decerebrate rigidity of Sherrington in man, *Arch. Neurol. Psychiat. (Chic.)*, **10**, 1.

YAP, C.-B. (1967) Spinal segmental and long-loop reflexes and spinal motoneurone excitability in spasticity and rigidity, *Brain*, **90**, 887.

THE INNERVATION OF THE BLADDER AND RECTUM

ANATOMY AND PHYSIOLOGY

The sympathetic fibres to the bladder are derived chiefly from the first and second lumbar ganglia, with contributions from the third and fourth. These fibres ultimately unite to form the presacral nerve or superior hypogastric plexus, which lies in front of the bifurcation of the aorta. From this plexus are derived the two hypogastric nerves, each of which ends in the vesical plexuses on the lateral aspect of the bladder. The parasympathetic nerve supply from the second and third sacral nerves also joins the vesical plexuses. It is doubtful if there is any separately innervated internal sphincter. When the parasympathetic is stimulated the longitudinal fibres of the detrusor pull the neck open and the circular fibres exert pressure on the contents. The physiology of micturition is discussed by Ruch (1960), by Yeates (1973), and by Johnson and Spalding (1974).

In infancy the evacuation of the bladder occurs reflexly, the reflex arc running through the sacral region of the cord. The development of control over bladder evacuation is associated with the growth of inhibition of the evacuation reflex, the path of the inhibitory impulses running in the sympathetic, which maintains closure of the sphincter and inhibition of the detrusor muscles. At the same time it becomes possible voluntarily to overcome this inhibition and so to initiate the act of micturition, which is then completed reflexly. Thus we can recognize three nervous mechanisms controlling bladder function—the sacral reflex arc

A a

for evacuation; the inhibitory influence of the sympathetic; and voluntary control overcoming the last-named and initiating micturition.

Sensation from the bladder concerned with fullness and a desire to micturate travels centrally in the spinothalamic tracts, as does that concerned with urethral pain (Nathan and Smith, 1951), while urethral touch and pressure travel in the posterior columns. The descending motor pathway concerned with voluntary bladder evacuation lies in the lateral columns on an equatorial plane passing through the central canal (Nathan and Smith, 1958). The voluntary initiation of micturition usually occurs in response to an awareness of distension of the bladder. The part of the postcentral gyrus lying at the vertex of the cerebral hemisphere is the cortical centre for sensations derived from the bladder, and the corresponding area of the precentral gyrus is probably the site of origin of motor impulses initiating the act of micturition. It is well recognized that parasagittal lesions which affect this area bilaterally may give rise to retention of urine or sometimes incontinence. Andrew and Nathan (1964) showed that the area concerned is localized in the superior frontal gyrus and that unilateral or, more often, bilateral lesions in this region may give urgency and frequency of micturition and incontinence or sometimes retention; the sensation giving rise to the desire to micturate is diminished or absent.

INVESTIGATION OF BLADDER FUNCTION

In order to diagnose the nature of a bladder disturbance and treat it appropriately it is necessary to test bladder function. *Cystometry* consists in measuring the rise of intravesical pressure induced by increasing volumes of fluid. Either the tidal drainage apparatus is used, or any device by which a funnel and manometer can be attached to the catheter. The intravesical pressure is recorded after the injection of each 50 ml of fluid.

DISTURBANCES OF BLADDER FUNCTION

Lesions involving the Sacral Reflex Arc

Since the sacral reflex arc is concerned in evacuation of the bladder, its interruption usually causes retention of urine, which is produced by the unopposed action of the sympathetic. In tabes dorsalis the reflex is interrupted on its afferent side, owing to degeneration of the afferent neurones. Lesions of the conus medullaris of the spinal cord interrupt the central fibres of the reflex. Lesions of the cauda equina, if they destroy the second and third sacral roots, interrupt both the afferent and the efferent paths of the reflex and hence usually cause retention of urine. Even after severe lesions of the conus or cauda equina, however, 'reflex' evacuation of the bladder may occasionally develop, under the influence of a more peripheral autonomous nervous mechanism, probably the vesical plexus. However, in cauda equina lesions and in tabes the bladder is more usually atonic, that is, it accepts a very large volume of urine without reflexly contracting to raise the intravesical pressure.

Lesions of the Spinal Cord above the Conus Medullaris

Incomplete lesions of the spinal cord may affect principally either the inhibitory fibres destined for the sympathetic outflow or the fibres concerned in the voluntary initiation of micturition. In the former case, the patient complains of difficulty in holding urine, and micturition is precipitate. This is a common symptom in the early stages of multiple sclerosis. Moderately severe but still incomplete lesions of the spinal cord tend to impair voluntary control over micturition, so that retention of urine develops, owing to uninhibited action of the sympathetic. Retention of urine is thus produced by spinal compression in its later stages, by transverse myelitis, and in the more advanced stages of multiple sclerosis.

After complete interruption of conduction in the spinal cord, either by transection or by severe transverse lesions above the conus, there is initially retention during the phase of spinal shock but later there is enhancement of reflex activity in the distal portion, and reflex evacuation of the bladder may then develop through the agency of the sacral reflex arc. It may be facilitated by stimuli applied to the sacral cutaneous areas. But after some massive lesions of the spinal cord the bladder may be atonic, presumably due to concurrent involvement of the cauda equina, perhaps as a result of ischaemia.

Cerebral Lesions

The fibres concerned in the voluntary initiation of micturition may be interrupted at levels of the nervous system above the spinal cord, and retention of urine may then develop, usually in association with severe bilateral corticospinal tract lesions. Lesions involving the vertical region of the precentral cortex on both sides may in the same way cause retention of urine, as Foerster has shown, and impairment of function of this part of the cerebral cortex or of its descending paths is probably responsible for difficulty in micturition and retention of urine, or for urgency and incontinence (Andrew and Nathan, 1964), which are not uncommon symptoms of intracranial tumour, anterior communicating artery aneurysms, and of diffuse cerebral lesions such as presenile dementia or diffuse atherosclerosis.

Nocturnal enuresis in otherwise normal children probably arises in the first place as a result of delay in the development of inhibition of reflex bladder evacuation. Later, for psychological reasons, the child acquires abnormal conditioned reflexes whereby bladder evacuation continues to occur during sleep (Kolvin *et al.*, 1973). Sometimes, however, enuresis in childhood is due to spinal cord or cauda equina lesions associated with spina bifida occulta.

TREATMENT OF BLADDER DISTURBANCES

In the treatment of disturbances of bladder function the underlying physiological principles must be borne in mind. When retention of urine occurs, adequate bladder drainage, usually with the aid of an indwelling catheter, becomes necessary, and steps must be taken to combat the risk of infection of the urinary tract and to treat it, when it develops, with appropriate urinary antiseptics or antibiotics. [See p. 726 for the care of the bladder in paraplegia.]

In view of the fact that retention of urine is usually due to a relative preponderance of sympathetic influence, the action of the parasympathetic may be reinforced by drugs which stimulate its nerve endings. Injection of carbachol, B.P., 1 ml, may be given subcutaneously, or 1 mg of carbachol orally, but if, despite bladder contraction induced by this drug, by bethanechol 10–100 mg, or by distigmine (*Ubretid*), 0·5 mg by injection or 5 mg by mouth, there is no evacuation, catheterization will be required. In chronic cases division of the internal sphincter (bladder neck resection) may help.

Interruption of the sympathetic supply to the bladder by resection of the presacral nerve has been carried out in a small number of cases and good results are claimed for this operation but its effect is rarely lasting. The same operation has been employed to interrupt pain impulses from the bladder in painful conditions such as inoperable carcinoma.

In cases of frequency of micturition or precipitate micturition due to predominant action of the parasympathetic, drugs which paralyse parasympathetic nerve endings are indicated, and propantheline, 15 mg three or four times daily, is useful in such drugs. Emepromium 50 mg two or three times daily is an alternative. These drugs owe what value they possess in the treatment of nocturnal enuresis to their inhibitory effect upon the parasympathetic. Imipramine 50 mg at night (in the adult) or 25 mg (in children) is another remedy which is sometimes of value. Drug treatment alone, however, is rarely successful in this condition and requires to be combined with the education of reflex inhibition produced by suggestion, if necessary in the hypnotic state. Frequently, also, the child requires help to solve his psychological problems at school or in the home. Deconditioning using a pad which, when moistened, causes ringing of a bell, has proved useful in some cases (see Kolvin et al., 1973).

In patients with incontinence after spinal cord lesions every effort must be made to re-establish reflex bladder evacuation at regular intervals. Regular clamping and release of an indwelling catheter every 2–3 hours during the acute stage may help to initiate this process. The atonic bladder of cauda equina lesions can usually be evacuated by manual compression. Satisfactory incontinence apparatuses are available for the male but not, as yet, for the female patient.

THE INNERVATION OF THE RECTUM

The nerve supply of the rectum is identical with that of the bladder and micturition and defaecation are physiologically comparable except that in the rectum voluntary control is exerted over the external sphincter only and the rectum lacks voluntary inhibition.

After destruction of the sacral innervation of the rectum automatic activity, dependent upon a peripheral nervous plexus, develops, the rectum contracting and the sphincter relaxing in response to a rise of tension within the rectum. This reflex activity is rendered more massive and complete when the sacral innervation is intact, e.g. after complete transverse division of the spinal cord above the sacral enlargement. Owing to the small force of the rectal contraction, however, it is at best not very efficient and since the tone of the external sphincter is unaffected by transverse spinal lesions the tendency is for all disturbances of rectal innervation to cause constipation, though after complete transverse division of the spinal cord reflex defaecation may occur and may be facilitated by cutaneous stimuli applied to the sacral cutaneous areas. In most patients with spinal cord or cauda equina lesions, satisfactory control of the bowels is eventually achieved by means of twice-weekly enemas or suppositories or by manual evacuation of the faeces.

REFERENCES

ANDREW, J., and NATHAN, P. W. (1964) Lesions of the anterior frontal lobes and disturbances of micturition and defaecation, Brain, **87,** 233.

DENNY-BROWN, D., and ROBERTSON, E. G. (1933) The state of the bladder and its sphincters in complete transverse lesions of the spinal cord and cauda equina, Brain, **56,** 397.

DENNY-BROWN, D., and ROBERTSON, E. G. (1935) An investigation of the nervous control of defaecation, Brain, **58,** 256.

HOLMES, G. (1933) Observations on the paralysed bladder, *Brain*, **56**, 383.
JOHNSON, R. H., and SPALDING, J. M. K. (1974) *Disorders of the Autonomic Nervous System*, Oxford.
KOLVIN, I., MACKEITH, R. C., and MEADOW, S. R. (1973) *Bladder Control and Enuresis*, London and Philadelphia.
LANGWORTHY, O. R., KOLB, L. C., and LEWIS, L. G. (1940) *The Physiology of Micturition*, Baltimore.
MCLELLAN, F. C. (1939) *The Neurogenic Bladder*, Baltimore.
NATHAN, P. W., and SMITH, M. C. (1951) Centripetal pathway from the bladder and urethra within the spinal cord, *J. Neurol. Neurosurg. Psychiat.*, **14**, 262.
NATHAN, P. W., and SMITH, M. C. (1958) The centrifugal pathway for micturition within the spinal cord, *J. Neurol. Neurosurg. Psychiat.*, **21**, 177.
PEDERSEN, E., ed. (1962) Spasticity and neurological bladder disturbances, *Acta neurol. (Kbh.)*, **38**, Suppl. 3.
RUCH, T. C. (1960) Central control of the bladder, in *Handbook of Physiology*, ed. Field, J., Section I, vol. ii, 1207.
VORIS, H. C., and LANDES, H. E. (1940) Cystometric studies in cases of neurologic disease, *Arch. Neurol. Psychiat. (Chic.)*, **44**, 118.
YEATES, W. K. (1973) Bladder function in normal micturition, in *Bladder Control and Enuresis*, ed. Kolvin, I., MacKeith, R. C., and Meadow, S. R., p. 28, London and Philadelphia.

THE CARE OF THE PARAPLEGIC PATIENT

The general management of a patient suffering from paraplegia requires much care and is as important as the correct treatment of the cause of his disability, for his disorder renders him susceptible to complications which may prove fatal, and, even when less serious, may considerably retard recovery.

DIET

The nutrition of the paraplegic patient is of the utmost importance: the loss of protein through pressure-sores and albuminuria may amount to 50 g daily. The caloric requirements are 3,500, and the diet should include 125 g of protein, a high vitamin intake, and 3,500–4,000 ml of fluid. Milk should be given sparingly as the calcium may increase the risk of urinary calculi. Anaemia may call for iron or even blood transfusion. When protein loss and wasting are severe, courses of treatment with anabolic steroid drugs may be of value.

CARE OF THE SKIN

In paraplegia the skin is extremely liable to injuries which are slow in healing, and readily become infected. The factors which lead to bed-sores are—shock in the early stages after injury, vasomotor paralysis, small traumata, and local ischaemia caused by pressure. Bed-sores are most likely to develop over the bony prominences, especially the heels, the tuber ischii, the sacrum, and the great trochanter.

The paraplegic patient should be nursed if possible on a 'Ripple' bed. Care should be taken that the bed-clothes are warm and dry and free from rucks, and that a hot-water bottle is not placed in contact with the skin. The patient should be bathed daily, the skin being thoroughly cleansed with soap and water, and carefully dried. After this the back is well rubbed with spirit and dusted with a dusting powder. Areas of reddening of the skin or of loss of epidermis may heal quickly if protected by means of a waterproof spray of acrylic resin (*Nobecutane*) or by using a silicone barrier cream or plastic antiseptic spray (*Noxyflex*, *Octaflex*). The posture of the patient should be changed every two hours both by day and night. If he develops an acute infection the liability to bed-sores increases, and he should be moved every hour. The value of pads to protect pressure points is doubtful. The lower limbs should be kept extended and the calves should rest upon small pillows with the heels projecting beyond them. The weight of the bed-clothes is taken from the lower limbs by means of a cradle. If sweating is troublesome, atropine, 0·5 mg, or propantheline, 15 mg, may be given before the patient settles down for the night. As far as possible, contact of the limbs with the bed-clothes should be reduced, and sedatives such as diazepam or nitrazepam may be given if necessary.

THE TREATMENT OF PRESSURE-SORES

If an ulcer has already developed, all necrotic tissue should first be removed to allow free drainage, and cultures should be made weekly. *Trypure Novo* dispersible powder (Evans Medical Ltd.) is helpful in removing sloughs. At first the bed-sores may be cleaned with hydrogen peroxide and a dressing of penicillin (20,000 units in 10 ml of normal saline) applied for a few days. After that eusol or saline dressings or tulle gras should be used. The dressing should be well covered with adhesive plaster attached to skin some distance away from the pressure points and changed every day. Systemic chemotherapy may be required. Occasionally skin-grafting is necessary.

CARE OF THE BLADDER

When retention of urine occurs as a result of a lesion of the nervous system cystitis almost invariably develops, and if untreated leads to ascending pyelonephritis. Retention of urine must therefore be treated by some form of drainage of the bladder. The alternatives available are (1) catheterization every 8 hours, (2) the use of a self-retaining catheter, (3) suprapubic cystostomy. Opinions still differ as to the best way to deal with the paralysed bladder. In general, repeated catheterization or a self-retaining catheter is usually most suitable in the absence of severe urinary infection. Modern fine plastic catheters have reduced the incidence of infection. When urinary infection cannot be otherwise controlled, suprapubic cystostomy may have to be carried out but fortunately it is rarely needed. Manual control of catheter drainage can be obtained by a clip applied to the drainage tube, and operated by the patient. When the catheter has to be removed to be changed, it can be left out for several hours, during which time observations are made on the patient's ability to hold urine, which can be tested by abdominal straining or suprapubic manual pressure. In this way, and by estimations of residual urine, the bladder's recovery of activity can be assessed.

The greatest care must be taken that the catheter and all the vessels and apparatus employed are sterile, and the operator must be scrupulous in his observance of an aseptic technique. Balanitis is a potential source of infection and it may even be advisable that a male patient should be circumcised. If the urinary tract becomes infected the organisms must be cultured and the appropriate chemotherapy or antibiotic used.

Cystoscopy and radiography of the urinary tract, including pyelography, may be necessary to exclude hydronephrosis and renal and vesical calculus; and estimation of renal function may be called for.

The object to be aimed at is an automatic bladder voiding sterile urine. Neither the grossly atonic bladder nor an organ much contracted owing to infection will become automatic. Division of the internal sphincter has been carried out when the detrusor muscle is reflexly active but the sphincter does not relax (Thompson, 1945). Various prostheses utilizing indwelling electrodes have been used in an attempt to stimulate a denervated bladder electrically or alternatively to cause contraction of the external sphincter in order to overcome incontinence, but none has yet entered into common use (see Boyarsky, 1967). For further details of the care of the paralysed bladder see Guttmann (1946), Hardy (1956), Ross et al. (1957), Guttmann (1973), and Johnson and Spalding (1974).

CARE OF THE RECTUM

The constipation which is usually a troublesome complication of paraplegia should be treated by the administration of an aperient at night, two or three times a week, and by washing out the rectum the next day with an enema. In paraplegia the bowel empties itself very slowly after an enema and 'leaking' may occur for an hour or more, a point which is important to bear in mind in order to avoid the bed becoming wet and soiled. If the rectum and large bowel are allowed to become distended, sloughing of the mucous membrane is liable to occur, and in any case abdominal distension causes the patient serious discomfort. Such distension should be treated by the administration of an enema, after which a rectal tube should be left in position. Often regular manual evacuation of faeces by the patient himself (rubber gloves must be supplied to prevent paronychia and other skin sepsis on the hands) is useful.

MUSCULAR SPASMS AND SPASTICITY

Involuntary spasmodic movements of the lower limbs are a troublesome and intractable symptom in many cases of paraplegia. Spasmodic extension may occur when extension is the predominant attitude of the lower limbs. Spasmodic flexion, which is encountered in paraplegia-in-flexion, is much commoner. Flexor movements are reflexly excited by moving contact of the lower limbs with the bed-clothes, a slight movement of the limb being sufficient in many cases to excite a violent flexor spasm. As far as possible, contact of the limbs with the bed-clothes should be reduced. The spasms may be diminished in frequency and severity by the use of sedative drugs, of which the best are diazepam (*Valium*) 5 mg three or four times a day, and baclofen 5 mg three times daily increasing by 5 mg steps every three or four days up to not more than 75 mg daily depending upon tolerance. Dantrolene, 25–50 mg twice daily, increasing up to not more than 800 mg daily, is helpful in some cases; mephenesin carbamate 1–3 g three to five times a day is in general less effective (Calne, 1975).

In patients with no hope of recovery, flexor spasms have been treated by the intrathecal injection of alcohol or preferably of phenol in glycerin, or by anterior rhizotomy. In selected cases of partial paraplegia injection of 1 ml of xylocaine, followed by 1–2 ml of 45 per cent alcohol into the motor points of selected muscles (e.g. hamstrings), after localization of the motor point or motor end-plate zone by electrical stimulation on the skin, is very helpful (Tardieu et al., 1964). Anterior rhizotomy has the disadvantage of leading to muscular wasting and increasing the risk of pressure-sores. In irrecoverable cases division of the obturator nerves and appropriate tenotomies may be helpful. Regular mechanical traction applied to the flexed limbs, combined with appropriate tenotomies have been shown to be valuable by Platt et al. (1958). The use of intrathecal injections is described by Nathan (1959, 1965), by Kelly and Gautier-Smith (1959), and by Calne (1975).

PHYSIOTHERAPY AND COMPENSATORY TRAINING

There are few paraplegic patients who will not be able to get about in a wheel-chair, and many more than was once thought possible can be taught to walk. Physiotherapy therefore aims at obtaining the maximum development of all those muscles in which voluntary power remains, and preventing flexor contractures of the lower limbs. Exercises are carried out with the help of slings as in the Guthrie-Smith apparatus, special attention being paid to the trunk muscles. Passive movements are carried out in the lower limbs once or twice daily. As soon as possible the patient is allowed to sit up in a wheel-chair, the need for frequent changes of posture being still borne in mind. In suitable cases walking is later attempted, and may be achieved even when no voluntary power remains in the lower limbs apart from hip flexion or 'rocking' movements of the pelvis. Appropriate walking instruments or calipers will be necessary, locking at the knee and not carried high enough to exert pressure on the buttocks. A toe-raising spring can be incorporated. When the trunk muscles are paralysed a brace may be necessary. The patient at first must be supported by parallel bars, later he uses elbow-crutches. When the lower limbs are completely paralysed, the pelvis must be rotated and tilted by the abdominal muscles; first one leg, and then the other is swung forward in this way. It may be possible for a patient to learn to 'walk' on crutches by swinging his trunk by means of the pectoralis, latissimus dorsi, serratus anterior, and trapezius muscles if these are over-developed and he has enough strength in his fingers to grasp the crutches, and can move them forward with his pectorals and deltoids. (For details see Deaver and Brown, 1945; Guttmann, 1946; Lowman, 1947; and Guttmann, 1973.)

OTHER MEASURES

In patients with complete transverse cord lesions temperature regulation is impaired due to inability to shiver below the level of the lesion as well as impairment of heat loss mechanisms, so that hypothermia and hyperpyrexia are occasional complications which must be borne in mind (Johnson, 1971). Blood pressure control may also be defective with orthostatic hypotension when the lesion is in the cervical region, but substantial vascular adaptation eventually occurs in most chronic paraplegics (Johnson et al., 1971).

In cases of tetraplegia due to high cervical cord lesions most deaths occur within the first three months; the prognosis has improved greatly with modern methods of care in patients surviving beyond that period. The use of electronic devices which enable the patient to control alarm systems and other electrical equipment with the aid of a mouthpiece, by eye movement, or by a simple manual switch ('POSSUM' or patient-operated selector mechanisms) has been a major advance in improving the level of independence and quality of life (Silver and Gibbon, 1968).

PSYCHOTHERAPY

Not the least important part of the physician's task is to help the patient to adjust himself to a new mode of life—a life not of inactivity but of different activities. At first he will need to be convinced that an active and useful life is still possible. Occupational therapy should be begun early: games play an important part. In most cases the patient must be trained for a new occupation, and the co-operation of an employer sought. Family adjustments have also to be made. Coitus is not always impossible. An erection may be stimulated by handling the penis and, with the co-operation of an instructed wife, success may be achieved. Even when intercourse is impossible, in the case of a wife who is anxious to have a child, ejaculation may follow the intrathecal injection of small doses of neostigmine, following which artificial insemination may be possible (Guttmann, 1973).

INJURIES OF THE SPINAL CORD

AETIOLOGY

The spinal cord may be injured directly by penetrating wounds, for example, stabs or gun-shot wounds, in which case it may be penetrated by a missile or by fragments of bone. More frequently in civil life it suffers indirectly as a result of injuries of the vertebral column, either fractures, dislocations, or fracture-dislocations. The commonest sites of spinal injury in civil life are the lower cervical region and the thoracolumbar junction. The upper cervical region suffers next in frequency (Jefferson, 1928). The epidemiology of spinal cord injury has been fully reviewed by Kurtzke (1975). Though the spinal column may be injured as the result of a blow leading to fracture at the site of the impact, more frequently it is injured by transmitted violence. Forcible extension of the neck may cause fracture of the dens or contusion of the cervical cord, but most spinal injuries are the result of forcible flexion. A blow on the head which does not expend its violence in fracturing the skull may, by forcibly flexing the cervical spine, cause dislocation in the lower cervical region or herniation of an intervertebral disc. Pre-existing cervical spondylosis which narrows the cervical canal greatly increases the risk of damage to the spinal cord by injuries which cause forcible extension of the neck. Blows upon the shoulders, such as are caused by heavy objects falling from a height, result in forcible flexion of the lower part of the spine, which usually yields at the thoracolumbar junction. This type of injury is produced chiefly by industrial accidents. Fracture-dislocation may similarly result from the patient's falling from a height on to the feet or buttocks. Lifting a heavy weight, falls, and strains may precipitate displacement of an intervertebral disc.

The spinal cord may be injured in the infant during birth as a result of violent traction. Such injuries may arise in three ways. Traction on the head may cause dislocation of the upper cervical spine, which is usually immediately fatal. Traction separating the head and shoulders, by exerting tension on the brachial plexus and cervical spinal roots, may injure the spinal cord as well as producing a brachial plexus palsy. In addition, violent traction, especially in a breech presentation, may cause fracture-dislocation in the thoracic or lumbar regions.

Spontaneous fracture-dislocation of the spine may occur when the vertebrae are diseased, for example, in tuberculous caries or in primary or secondary neoplasm of the vertebral column. The blast of a bomb or shell explosion may injure the spinal cord without damaging the spine.

A less common cause of spinal cord injury is decompression sickness (Caisson disease or 'the bends'). Complete or partial paraplegia has been attributed in such cases to arterial infarction secondary to nitrogen bubble emboli, but experimental studies in animals (Hallenbeck et al., 1975) indicate that venous infarction due to obstruction to cord venous drainage into the epidural vertebral venous system may be a more common mechanism.

PATHOLOGY

'*Concussion* of the spinal cord' is a term which has been employed when the cord is injured by transmitted violence without fracture or dislocation of the vertebral column. However, as in the case of head injury [p. 386], it is now doubtful as to whether there is any genuine pathological distinction between concussion and *contusion*, which is defined as bruising of the cord without rupture of the pia mater, resulting from bruising or compression. The contused cord is swollen and may exhibit small haemorrhages. Microscopically, besides oedema and haemorrhages the contused cord exhibits swelling of the axis cylinders and disintegration of their myelin sheaths. In severe cases both completely disappear and the cord may be markedly softened. Ascending and descending degeneration of the long tracts follows the focal lesion. The structural, vascular, physiological, and biochemical changes which follow experimental cord contusion have been reviewed by Dohrmann (1972). *Laceration* of the cord implies an injury of greater severity than contusion, leading to rupture of the pia mater and in the most severe cases the cord is completely transected. Barnett *et al.* (1966) and Nurick *et al.* (1970) have shown that a progressive myelopathy due to ascending cavitation of the cord above the level of the lesion may develop in some cases of traumatic paraplegia some years after the injury. The pathogenesis of this cystic degeneration or traumatic syringomyelia is reviewed by Barnett *et al.* (1973). When a wound penetrates the dura mater, meningitis is liable to occur as a complication of spinal injury. Rupture of the pia in such cases increases the risk of myelitis developing. Injuries of the vertebral column may damage the spinal roots as they pass through the intervertebral foramina.

SYMPTOMS

The symptoms of spinal injury depend upon the severity and situation of the lesion. Injury to the cord does not necessarily follow damage to the vertebral column; for example, dislocation of the cervical spine without injury to the cord is not rare. An injury to the cord in the upper cervical region is usually rapidly, if not immediately, fatal, since it causes paralysis both of the diaphragm and of the intercostal muscles but some such cases now survive with assisted respiration (Silver and Gibbon, 1968).

Complete interruption of the spinal cord leads immediately to flaccid paralysis with loss of all sensation and most reflex activity below the site of the lesion, and paralysis of the bladder and rectum. Muscular paralysis and sensory loss are irrecoverable, but, as after from one to four weeks the stage of spinal shock passes off, reflex activity develops in the divided portion of the cord and the patient presents the picture of paraplegia-in-flexion [see p. 719]. For the motor symptoms of spinal interruption at different levels, see pages 750-2.

Lesions of the cord less severe than complete interruption, such as spinal contusion, may lead to an equally severe immediate disturbance of function, or symptoms may increase in severity for several days *pari passu* with the development of oedema in the cord. Slight spinal injuries cause motor symptoms of incomplete division without complete sensory loss, or, if the injury is limited to one-half of the cord, a partial or complete Brown-Séquard syndrome [see p. 45].

Injuries of the Cauda Equina. Fracture-dislocation of the spine below the first lumbar vertebra damages only the roots of the cauda equina. In civil life unilateral injuries of the cauda are rare, though the severity and extent of the injury may differ on the two sides. Paralysis of the bladder, rectum, and sexual functions immediately follows the injury. The motor, sensory, and reflex disturbances are similar to those more gradually produced by slow compression of the cauda equina and are described on page 751.

DIAGNOSIS

The diagnosis is usually obvious, the only question being the nature and extent of the injury to the cord. Myelography is rarely necessary in such cases. Selective arteriography may help to exclude gross vascular damage (Gargour et al., 1972).

PROGNOSIS

In high cervical cord lesions the immediate danger is due to respiratory paralysis; assisted respiration, when needed, is invariably indicated in such cases as one cannot be certain at the outset as to how much recovery will subsequently take place. With modern methods of management complications such as pneumonia, urinary and cutaneous infection, hypotension, and hypothermia, which were often fatal in the past, are no longer the hazards they once were. It is now clearly possible for a patient with a completely divided cord to retain good general health indefinitely under careful supervision. When the cord has been incompletely divided, the prognosis is better, but, in the absence of infections of the bladder and skin, the limit of functional improvement will be reached when the shock has passed off, usually in two or three months after the injury. After spinal contusion without actual division of the cord substantial recovery often takes place though a variable degree of residual disability is usual. The prognosis of cauda equina injuries is often better than that of injuries of the cord itself, since the roots of the cauda, if not divided, are capable of regeneration.

TREATMENT

Recent evidence derived from experiments upon animals suggests that dexamethasone 5 mg four times daily, if begun within an hour of injury, may reduce the extent of traumatic damage to the spinal cord; dimethyl sulphoxide is also of some value in animals but has yet to be tested in man (de la Torre et al., 1975).

The scope of surgery in the treatment of injuries of the spinal cord has been much discussed, and the modern tendency in this respect is conservative. It has to be recognized that in most cases the maximal injury has been produced at the time of the accident and the condition of the cord is both non-progressive and irreparable. Moreover, for several weeks after the injury spinal shock may render it impossible to decide whether interruption of the cord is complete. When there is reason to believe that the cord has been completely divided, surgery cannot accomplish anything, and open operation may be contra-indicated by the presence of local sepsis, visceral complications, and secondary infective conditions. On the other hand, when there is radiographic evidence of gross bony deformity, disc protrusion or the presence of a foreign body in the spinal canal, and clinical examination indicates that the cord has not been completely divided, and when in such cases recovery of function has begun but has become arrested, surgical intervention offers the hope of relieving compression which may be retarding recovery. In such cases an exploratory laminectomy may be indicated, and may also be required to deal with severe persistent root pains, due to compression of dorsal nerve roots. The most important single measure is immobilization on a flat bed and continuous traction is sometimes indicated in the hope of correcting spinal deformity, but manipulation is rarely if ever indicated because of the risk of increasing damage to the cord. In cases of injury of the cauda equina the most that can be hoped for from operation is the relief of pressure which may be retarding regeneration of the roots. The general management of cases of injury of the spinal cord and cauda equina is described on page 725.

REFERENCES

BARNETT, H. J. M., BOTTERELL, E. H., JOUSSE, A. T., and WYNN-JONES, M. (1966) Progressive myelopathy as a sequel to traumatic paraplegia, *Brain*, **89**, 159.

BARNETT, H. J. M., FOSTER, J. B., and HUDGSON, P. (1973) *Syringomyelia* (Major Problems in Neurology Series, ed. Walton, J. N.), London.

BEDFORD, P. D., COSIN, L. Z., and MCCARTHY, T. F. (1961) Bedsores, *Lancet*, **ii**, 76.

BOYARSKY, S. (1967) *The Neurogenic Bladder*, Baltimore.

BYERS, R. K. (1930) Late effects of obstetrical injuries at various levels of the nervous system, *New Engl. J. Med.*, **203**, 507.

CALNE, D. B. (1975) *Therapeutics in Neurology*, Oxford.

DEAVER, G. G., and BROWN, M. E. (1945) The challenge of crutches, *Arch. phys. Med.*, **26**, 397, 515, 573, 747.

DE LA TORRE, J. C., JOHNSON, C. M., GOODE, D. J., and MULLAN, S. (1975) Pharmacologic treatment and evaluation of permanent experimental spinal cord trauma, *Neurology (Minneap.)*, **25**, 508.

DOHRMANN, G. J. (1972) Experimental spinal cord trauma, *Arch. Neurol. (Chic.)*, **27**, 468.

ELSON, R. A. (1965) Anatomical aspects of pressure sores and their treatment, *Lancet*, **i**, 884.

FEIRING, E. H. (1974) *Brock's Injuries of the Brain and Spinal Cord and Their Coverings*, 5th ed., New York.

FORD, F. R. (1925) Breech delivery in its possible relations to injury of the spinal cord, *Arch. Neurol. Psychiat. (Chic.)*, **14**, 742.

GARGOUR, G. W., WENER, L., and DI CHIRO, G. (1972) Selective arteriography of the spinal cord in posttraumatic paraplegia, *Neurology (Minneap.)*, **22**, 131.

GUTTMANN, L. (1946) Rehabilitation after injuries to the spinal cord and cauda equina, *Brit. J. phys. Med.*, **9**, 162.

GUTTMANN, L. (1973) *Spinal Cord Injuries*, Oxford.

HALLENBECK, J. M., BOVE, A. A., and ELLIOTT, D. H. (1975) Mechanisms underlying spinal cord damage in decompression sickness, *Neurology (Minneap.)*, **25**, 308.

HAMM, F. C. (1945) War wounds of the spinal cord, *J. Amer. med. Ass.*, **129**, 158.

HARDY, A. G. (1956) The care of the bladder in traumatic paraplegia, *Postgrad. med. J.*, **32**, 328.

JEFFERSON, G. (1927-8) Discussion on spinal injuries, *Proc. roy. Soc. Med.*, **21**, 625.

JOELSON, J. J. (1945) War wounds of the spinal cord, *J. Amer. med. Ass.*, **129**, 157.

JOHNSON, R. H. (1971) Temperature regulation in paraplegia, *Paraplegia*, **9**, 137.

JOHNSON, R. H., PARK D., and FRANKEL, H. L. (1971) Orthostatic hypotension and the renin-angiotensin system in paraplegia, *Paraplegia*, **9**, 146.

JOHNSON, R. H., and SPALDING, J. M. K. (1974) *Disorders of the Autonomic Nervous System*, Oxford.

KELLY, R. E., and GAUTIER-SMITH, P. C. (1959) Intrathecal phenol in the treatment of reflex spasms and spasticity, *Lancet*, **ii**, 1102.

KURTZKE, J. F. (1975) Epidemiology of spinal cord injury, *Exp. Neurol.*, **48**, 163.

LOWMAN, E. W. (1947) Rehabilitation of the paraplegic patient, *Arch. Neurol. Psychiat. (Chic.)*, **58**, 610.

NATHAN, P. W. (1959) Intrathecal phenol to relieve spasticity in paraplegia, *Lancet*, **ii,** 1099.

NATHAN, P. W. (1965) Chemical rhizotomy for relief of spasticity in ambulant patients, *Brit. med. J.*, **1,** 1096.

NURICK, S., RUSSELL, J. A., and DECK, M. J. F. (1970) Cystic degeneration of the spinal cord following spinal cord injury, *Brain*, **93,** 211.

PETKOFF, B. P. (1945) War wounds of the spinal cord, *J. Amer. med. Ass.*, **129,** 154.

PLATT, G., RUSSELL, W. R., and WILLISON, R. G. (1958) Flexion spasms and contractures in spinal-cord disease, *Lancet*, **i,** 757.

ROSS, J. C., GIBBON, N. O. K., and DAMANSKI, M. (1957) Recent developments in the treatment of the paraplegic bladder, *Lancet*, **ii,** 520.

SILVER, J. R., and GIBBON, N. O. K. (1968) Prognosis in tetraplegia, *Brit. med. J.*, **4,** 79.

SUTTON, N. G. (1973) *Injuries of the Spinal Cord*, London.

TARDIEU, G., HARIGA, J., TARDIEU, C., GAGNARD, L., and VELIN, J. (1964) Traitement de la spasticité par infiltration d'alcool dilué au point moteur ou par injection épidurale, *Rev. neurol.*, **110,** 563.

THOMPSON, G. S. (1945) Restoration of function by transurethral operation, *Nav. med. Bull. (Wash.)*, **45,** 207.

WALSHE, F. M. R., and ROSS, J. (1936) The clinical picture of minor cord lesions in association with injuries of the cervical spine: with special reference to the diagnostic and localising value of the tendon reflexes of the arm (inversion of the radial reflex), *Brain*, **59,** 277.

War Department. Technical Bulletin, T.B. Med. 162. (1945) Convalescent care and rehabilitation of patients with spinal cord injuries, *War. Med. (Chic.)*, **vii,** 199.

HAEMATOMYELIA AND ACUTE CENTRAL CERVICAL CORD INJURY

Definition. The term 'haematomyelia' implies the occurrence of bleeding within the substance of the spinal cord. Haemorrhages occur within the cord in a variety of pathological states. Petechial haemorrhages are found in acute inflammatory conditions, such as poliomyelitis, in toxic states, in blood diseases, especially those accompanied by purpura, in asphyxia, and as a sequel of severe convulsions. Haemorrhages also occur as a result of injury, in spinal contusion, as well as in laceration of the cord following fracture-dislocation of the spine and the penetration of the spinal canal by missiles. The term 'haematomyelia', however, is usually reserved for a focal extravasation of blood within the spinal cord occurring in the absence of any of the conditions already mentioned.

AETIOLOGY

Haematomyelia in the sense just defined may develop in the absence of any obvious precipitating factor. Not uncommonly, however, it follows an event which may be supposed to have exposed the spinal cord to transmitted violence, though this often seems slight in proportion to the severity of the resulting symptoms. Blows on the spine and falls are sometimes held responsible. There is evidence that a congenital abnormality, for example an intramedullary telangiectasis or angioma, may be one causal factor, and spontaneous haemorrhage into a syringomyelic cavity may occur. The condition has been described as the result of an intramedullary metastasis from a renal carcinoma (Kawakami and Mair, 1973). Haematomyelia usually occurs in early adult life, and males are more frequently affected than females. Recent evidence suggests that, particularly in cases attributable to trauma, a syndrome similar to that produced by haematomyelia is more often due to central softening within the spinal cord rather than haemorrhage, resulting from contusion of the cord such as may occur particularly in the cervical region in patients suffering from previously symptomless cervical spondylosis, frequently after acute flexion or hyper-extension of the neck (Schneider *et al.*, 1958; Cook, 1959).

PATHOLOGY

The cervical enlargement is the commonest site of haemorrhage or central softening. Bleeding occurs primarily in the central grey matter and tends to spread upwards and downwards, assuming a round or oval form, according to its longitudinal extent. It may extend into the white matter, but usually this suffers from compression rather than from direct invasion by the haemorrhage. At first red, the haemorrhage in the later stages becomes brown and may finally be represented by a cystic cavity containing yellow fluid. Surrounding regions of the cord exhibit an infiltration with compound granular cells, and glial reaction. The distribution of central softening without haemorrhage is similar. There is destruction and disappearance of the ganglion cells of both anterior and posterior horns of grey matter at the site of the lesion, and some degree of ascending and descending degeneration is usually found in the tracts of the white matter.

SYMPTOMS

The onset of symptoms in haematomyelia is usually rapidly progressive, though after an injury there may be a sudden impairment of function of the spinal cord, followed later by a progressive increase in symptoms. Sometimes the onset is more gradual, and the symptoms may increase in severity over a period of several days. In cases of central softening after acute flexion or hyper-extension injuries to the neck, neurological disability is usually maximal immediately after the injury and progressive improvement occurs during the subsequent weeks or months (Symonds, 1953). Since the cervical enlargement is the commonest site of haemorrhage, symptoms of a lesion in this situation will alone be described in detail. In some cases the patient complains at the onset of severe pain in the neck radiating down one or both upper limbs. Some-times this pain (hyperpathia) is persistent (Hopkins and Rudge, 1973). In other cases pain is absent, but there may be paraesthesiae, such as numbness and tingling. Muscular weakness rapidly develops. It is often marked in the upper limbs, one of which may suffer more than the other. In the upper limbs the paralysis is due to destruction or compression of the anterior horn cells and hence may be associated with muscular atrophy and diminution or loss of the tendon reflexes. It may be limited to the muscles innervated by the upper segments, cervical 5 and 6, or by the lower segments, cervical 8 and thoracic 1, of the cervical enlargement. Below the level of the lesion the motor symptoms are those of spastic paralysis which may be slight or severe in the lower limbs and may affect the two sides unequally. Sudden and total tetraparesis after relatively minor flexion or extension of the neck, as in a so-called 'whiplash' injury, followed by rapid improvement, is not uncommon in the central cervical syndrome in cases of spondylosis with a narrow cervical canal.

The most prominent sensory changes are due to destruction of the sensory fibres in the grey matter of the cord at the level of the lesion. When this extends into the posterior horns and destroys the ganglion cells, all forms of sensibility will be impaired or lost over the whole or part of the upper limbs. When the destruction is limited to the region of the anterior white commissure there is no disturbance of appreciation of light touch, posture, or passive movement, but analgesia and thermo-anaesthesia occur over several segmental cutaneous areas below the upper level of the haemorrhage, which interrupts the fibres subserving these forms of sensibility at their decussation. The picture is thus similar to that of syringomyelia and a 'cape-like' distribution of the dissociated anaesthesia is frequently seen. It is not uncommon to find also some impairment of appreciation of pain, heat, and cold, over the trunk or lower limbs on one or both sides, owing to compression of the spinothalamic tract. Postural sensibility may be impaired in the lower limbs, but not as a rule to a severe extent, owing to compression of the posterior columns.

The tendon reflexes effected by muscles which are the site of atrophic paralysis are diminished or lost. Those of the lower limbs are usually exaggerated. The abdominal reflexes are diminished or lost and the plantar reflexes are extensor when the corticospinal tracts are damaged. Sphincter disturbances are usually proportional to the severity of the paraplegia.

Dorsal and lumbar haematomyelia are characterized by the rapid development of more or less complete paraplegia and sensory loss below the level of the lesion. Retention of urine is common.

The CSF may be normal or may show an increase in its protein content, with or without xanthochromia.

DIAGNOSIS

Apart from traumatic lesions, there are few conditions in which a lesion of the spinal cord develops so rapidly as in haematomyelia. The onset of transverse myelitis is more often subacute rather than acute, and it is often preceded by pains in the spine. It is often associated with inflammatory changes in the CSF and when, as in some cases, it is syphilitic in origin, the serological reactions in the fluid and probably also in the blood will be positive. Anterior poliomyelitis can be differentiated from haematomyelia by its febrile onset, by the wide but often asymmetrical distribution of the atrophic paralysis, by the absence of sensory loss and of corticospinal lesions, and by the occurrence of a pleocytosis in the CSF. Haemorrhage into a syringomyelic cavity constitutes a form of haematomyelia which it is important to recognize. However, this is a rare complication and haematomyelia is generally distinguishable from the syndrome of syringomyelia by virtue of its acute onset. The pre-existence of syringomyelia may be suggested by a history of painless injuries or trophic lesions of the fingers. The very rare condition of intramedullary abscess of the spinal cord can give a clinical picture very similar to that of haematomyelia but there is usually fever and leucocytosis and evidence of a focus of pyogenic infection elsewhere. The acute central cervical cord syndrome is usually recognized if the significance of the injury, however minor, is appreciated, especially if the radiographs of the cervical spine show spondylosis and a narrow canal.

PROGNOSIS

The mortality rate is low, and most sufferers from haematomyelia survive. Death may rarely occur from upward extension of the haemorrhage leading to paralysis of the diaphragm, through involvement of the spinal origin of the phrenic nerves, or from infection of the urinary tract or other complications of paraplegia. In patients who survive, considerable improvement may be expected and it is often particularly striking in traumatic cases with presumed central cord softening in which it may be concluded that much of the initial disability may have been due to transient disturbance of function due to contusion. Atrophic paralysis and sensory loss due to destruction of the grey matter are permanent, but even these diminish in extent, as recovery occurs in ganglion cells and fibres which have been compressed but not completely destroyed. A steady improvement may be expected in the power of the lower limbs and in many cases this may return to normal, though exaggeration of the tendon reflexes and extensor plantar responses may persist. When haemorrhage has occurred into a syringomyelic cavity, much less improvement in the immediate symptoms can be expected and the prognosis is that of syringomyelia.

TREATMENT

Complete rest is essential with immobilization of the cervical spine; a collar may be helpful. Sedative drugs should be given and analgesics when necessary. When paraplegia is present this will require appropriate treatment. Two weeks after the onset physiotherapy may safely be begun.

REFERENCES

BENDA, C. E. (1929) Zur Klinik der traumatischen Hämatomyelie. Zugleich ein Beitrag zur Differentialdiagnose zwischen Tumor Spinalis und Blutung, *Nervenarzt*, **1**, 28.

CHEVALLIER, P., and DESOILE, H. (1930) L'hématomyélie des jeunes sujets (importance des lésions vasculaires hérédo-syphilitiques), *Rev. Médecine*, **47**, 486.

COOK, J. B. (1959) The relationship of spinal cord damage to cervical spinal injury, *Proc. roy. Soc. Med.*, **52**, 799.

DAVISON, C. (1960) General pathological considerations in injuries of the spinal cord, in *Injuries of the Brain and Spinal Cord*, 4th ed., ed. Brock, S., New York.

DOERR, C. (1906; 1906-7) *Die spontane Rückenmarksblutung (Hämatomyelia)*, Zürich, and *Dtsch. Z. Nervenheilk.*, **32**, 1.

HOPKINS, A., and RUDGE, P. (1973) Hyperpathia in the central cervical cord syndrome, *J. Neurol. Neurosurg. Psychiat.*, **36**, 637.

KAWAKAMI, Y., and MAIR, W. G. P. (1973) Haematomyelia due to secondary renal carcinoma, *Acta Neuropath. (Berl.)*, **26**, 85.

RICHARDSON, J. C. (1938) Spontaneous haematomyelia: a short review and a report of cases illustrating intramedullary angioma and syphilis of the spinal cord as possible causes, *Brain*, **61**, 17.

SCHNEIDER, R. C., THOMPSON, J. M., and BEBIN, J. (1958) The syndrome of acute central cervical spinal cord injury, *J. Neurol. Neurosurg. Psychiat.*, **21**, 216.

SYMONDS, C. P. (1953) The interrelation of trauma and cervical spondylosis in compression of the cervical cord, *Lancet*, **i**, 451.

COMPRESSION OF THE SPINAL CORD

AETIOLOGY AND PATHOLOGY

Compression of the spinal cord may be due to:

Disease of the Vertebral Column. Among the diseases leading to spinal compression are tuberculous osteitis (Pott's disease), secondary carcinoma, and cervical spondylosis with protrusion of intervertebral discs [FIG. 120]. Less frequent causes include primary neoplasms arising from vertebrae, such as sarcoma, myeloma, osteoma, haemangioma, and other forms of osteitis, such as staphylococcal osteitis, syphilitic osteitis, and osteitis deformans of Paget.

Rarely, achondroplasia and severe kyphoscoliosis due to juvenile osteochondritis may have the same effect. The cord may occasionally be compressed by prolapse of an intervertebral disc elsewhere than at the cervical level (e.g. in the dorsal region) or as a result of erosion of vertebrae from without by sarcoma, or by aneurysm of the aorta. Compression due to vertebral injury is described on page 729. High cervical cord compression may result from bony or other anomalies of the craniovertebral junction [p. 1090].

Other Causes of Compression. These include extradural abscess due either to metastatic infection or vertebral osteitis, pachymeningitis due to syphilis, tuberculosis, or exceptionally to pyogenic organisms, infiltration of the meninges with reticulosis or leukaemic deposits, arachnoiditis and arachnoidal cysts, parasitic cysts, such as the hydatid and cysticercus, and extramedullary and intramedullary spinal tumours. Spinal subdural haematoma due to trauma or occurring after lumbar puncture in cases of thrombocytopenia is a rare cause (Edelson *et al.*, 1974).

Vertebral Disease

1. *Separation of the odontoid process* of the axis, occurring either as a congenital abnormality or as the result of trauma or rheumatoid arthritis may, by permitting abnormal movement of the atlas on the axis, lead in time, sometimes after many years, to a delayed myelopathy resulting from compression of the spinal cord (Greenberg, 1968; Stevens *et al.*, 1971).

2. *Intervertebral disc protrusion* is commonest in the cervical region. An acute central prolapse of a disc may give symptoms and signs of acute or subacute cord compression and pain may not be prominent, whereas a lateral protrusion will give pain in the arm due to root compression (brachial neuralgia). Chronic protrusions are the result of degeneration of the discs: they may be single or multiple, and are usually encountered during or after middle age. Such a slow, progressive degenerative process (cervical spondylosis) gives the condition of so-called spondylotic myelopathy. Its effect upon the spinal cord is complex: in addition to directly compressing it, the protruding discs may interfere with its blood supply; while, owing to tethering of the cord by the ligamenta denticulata and of the spinal roots by narrowing of the intervertebral foramina, ordinary neck movements may produce cumulative trauma. The result is a condition of patchy degeneration—cervical myelopathy (Sager, 1969; Wilkinson, 1973).

3. *Neoplasms of the Vertebral Column.* Secondary carcinoma is the commonest vertebral neoplasm. It is rare before the age of 35. The primary growth is more frequently situated within the lung, breast, thyroid, or prostate, less frequently in the uterus, stomach, kidney, or elsewhere. Although the vertebral metastasis may be blood-borne, the spine is not uncommonly involved at the same segmental level as the primary growth, which in such cases probably reaches it via the perineural lymphatics. The carcinomatous deposits erode the spongy portions of the vertebral bodies, which finally collapse. The spinal cord may be compressed as a result of the spinal deformity or by an intravertebral extension of the growth. Usually the spinal roots are compressed earlier than the cord itself so that root pain may be present for some time before vertebral collapse gives acute cord compression.

Sarcoma may arise from a vertebra or invade the spinal column from the neighbouring tissues. Cavernous haemangioma is a rare vertebral tumour but can give rise to spinal cord or nerve root compression and the radiological changes (accentuated vertical striation or a honeycomb pattern) are often, but not invariably, distinctive (McAllister *et al.*, 1975). Myeloma usually arises simultaneously in numerous vertebral bodies and frequently also in other bones, especially the ribs, but solitary myelomas of the spine giving cord compression are not uncommon (Clarke, 1956). Erosion of vertebral bodies leads to collapse. Osteomas are rare tumours which usually arise from the posterior part of a vertebral body and hence compress the cord anteriorly. So-called chondromas are usually intervertebral disc protrusions associated with spondylosis. Deposits of reticulosis and leukaemic metastases usually infiltrate the dura mater extensively on its outer surface but may occasionally invade the cord itself. In such cases pain and symptoms and signs of cord or root compression may occur without any abnormality on plain radiographs and a similar syndrome may result from extradural metastases of carcinoma, but myelography will usually demonstrate the extradural deposits with narrowing of the spinal canal.

4. *Tuberculous spinal osteitis* usually occurs in children and young adults but no age is exempt. It is now much less common in the developed countries than it was 20 or 30 years ago as a result of pasteurization of milk, as most cases of skeletal tuberculosis used to be due to the bovine bacillus. The infective process generally begins in the body of the vertebra, and spreading to adjacent bodies leads to their collapse and so produces an angular deformity of the spine. It is rare for the deformity as such to be an important factor in compression of the spinal cord, which is more frequently due either to an extradural tuberculous abscess or to tuberculous pachymeningitis. In addition to actual compression of the cord, which may, however, be absent, interference with the vascular supply of subjacent segments, either by compression of radicular arteries or endarteritis, is an important factor in the production of paraplegia. Paraplegia occurs in about 11 per cent of patients with Pott's disease, usually within two or three years of the onset, but in some cases after many years of apparent quiescence. The dorsal cord is commonly affected.

5. *Syphilitic spinal osteitis* is now a very rare cause of spinal compression and produces effects similar to those of tuberculous caries. In Paget's *osteitis deformans*, softening and collapse of vertebrae occur without abscess formation. Slowly progressive spastic weakness of the lower limbs due to spinal cord compression may also occur in some *achondroplasic dwarfs* and in patients with severe *kyphoscoliosis* and resultant acute angulation of the vertebral column.

6. *Spinal extradural* or *epidural abscess* is due as a rule to staphylococcal infection, arising either as a result of blood-borne invasion of the extradural space by the infecting organism or, more commonly, resulting from vertebral osteomyelitis. In the early stages the symptoms are those of pain in the back and/or root pains with fever, leucocytosis, and spinal tenderness. If untreated, sensorimotor symptoms in the limbs and sphincter disturbance may herald irreversible paraplegia or tetraplegia due to cord compression and interference with its blood supply. Surgical exploration and decompression of the spinal cord and treatment with the appropriate antibiotics must be carried out before this stage is reached; the condition is a neurosurgical emergency. Spinal subdural abscess has also been described (Hirson, 1965). Very rarely an intramedullary spinal abscess of metastatic origin develops and gives a clinical picture like that of intramedullary tumour of acute onset with pyrexia.

Spinal Tumour

Spinal tumours are conveniently divided into extradural and intradural growths, the latter being further subdivided into those arising outside the spinal cord—extramedullary tumours, and within the cord—intramedullary tumours. Excluding secondary carcinoma of the vertebrae Elsberg (1925) found that 10 per cent of spinal tumours were extradural, 67 per cent were extramedullary, and 14 per cent were intramedullary. More recent experience is variable (Alter, 1975) but Oddsson (1947) found that in a series of 144 spinal tumours, 18 per cent were extradural, 51 per cent extramedullary, 26 per cent intramedullary, and the remainder both extra- and intramedullary. Intramedullary tumours show a higher incidence in childhood (Banna and Gryspeerdt, 1971).

The origin and nature of extradural tumours have been described in the previous section. The commonest extramedullary tumours are meningiomas and neurofibromas. Published figures of relative incidence vary but on balance meningiomas appear to be slightly more common than neurofibromas (Alter, 1975) while the two together are between two and three times as common as spinal gliomas. Neurofibromas usually arise from spinal roots, the posterior more frequently than the anterior. They may be single or multiple and may or may not be associated with generalized neurofibromatosis. Exceptionally, an extramedullary neurofibroma may grow out through an intervertebral foramen, thus adopting a dumb-bell shape. The extraspinal portion may be palpable. Meningiomas may arise either from spinal roots or from the meninges. While neurofibromas may be seen at any level of the spinal canal and occur equally in the two sexes, meningiomas almost always occur in the dorsal region and much more often in females than in males. Sarcomatous changes in spinal meningiomas and primary extramedullary sarcomas are rare. Lipomas occasionally occur but are usually seen in relation to occult spina bifida and spinal dysraphism. Chordomas are rare malignant tumours arising from a remnant of the notochord. Spinal chordomas are almost invariably situated in the sacrococcygeal region (Gessaga et al., 1973). Dermoid cysts and other forms of teratomatous growth may also develop within the spinal canal.

Kernohan et al. (1931), who investigated the histology of intramedullary spinal tumours, claimed to have recognized varieties corresponding to most of the cerebral gliomas. Forty-two per cent of intramedullary tumours, according to these authors, are ependymomas, and the remainder includes spongioblastomas, astroblastomas, medulloblastomas, oligodendrogliomas, ganglioneuromas, very rare intramedullary metastases of carcinoma (Edelson et al., 1972), and haemangioblastomas. Angiomatous malformations are not uncommon and may have a considerable longitudinal extent. They may cause spinal subarachnoid haemorrhage as well as spinal cord compression (Aminoff and Logue, 1974 a) and symptoms of these lesions may first appear in pregnancy (Newman, 1958); spinal subarachnoid bleeding is also occasionally seen in patients with neurofibromas, angioblastic meningiomas, and particularly with ependymomas of the filum terminale (Walton, 1953). Leukaemic deposits may occur within the cord as well as in the extradural space, and gumma and tuberculoma are occasionally found. For some time it was thought that there was an unusually high incidence of spinal cord tumours in patients with syringomyelia; now it seems more probable that secondary ascending or descending cord cavitation as a complication of spinal tumour is a more likely explanation of this association (Barnett et al., 1973). Systemic metastases from primary spinal neoplasms are exceptionally rare but have been described in ependymoma of the filum terminale (Rubinstein and Logan, 1970). By contrast, intra- and extramedullary spinal deposits resulting from intracranial gliomas, especially medulloblastomas, are not uncommon, particularly in children.

Both sexes are equally liable to spinal tumour, which may develop at any age, but in over 80 per cent of cases symptoms first appear between the ages of 20 and 60. There is no significant difference in incidence in different races (Alter, 1975) but meningiomas and neurofibromas are relatively rare in childhood, as indeed are all spinal tumours in comparison to intracranial neoplasms (Ingraham and Matson, 1954; Slooff et al., 1964; Banna and Gryspeerdt, 1971). The thoracic region of the cord is the commonest site of extradural and extramedullary tumours, the lower cervical of intramedullary tumours. Approximately two-thirds of extramedullary tumours are situated on the dorsal or dorsolateral aspects of the cord and approximately one-third on the ventral or ventrolateral aspects (Elsberg, 1925; Alter, 1975).

Meningeal Inflammation

Spinal compression may be due to pachymeningitis. This rare condition is sometimes syphilitic but may be metastatic from a pyogenic infection leading to extradural abscess. Tuberculous pachymeningitis occurs as a result of extension of infection from tuberculous osteitis. The condition known as adhesive spinal arachnoiditis is not completely understood. Adhesions are found between the leptomeninges and may be circumscribed or extensive. Occasionally they enclose encysted collections of CSF. Meningococcal infection, lymphocytic choriomeningitis, syphilis, and spinal trauma may each occasionally play a part in aetiology. Tuberculous meningitis limited to the spinal cord is a cause of adhesive arachnoiditis in some tropical countries (Dastur and Wadia, 1969). Other occasional causes include epidural (Braham and Saia, 1958) and spinal anaesthesia (Payne and Bergentz, 1956), and cryptococcal infection (Davidson, 1968), and very rarely symptomatic arachnoiditis has been described as a sequel to myelography using oily contrast media (Shapiro, 1975). Although adhesive arachnoiditis interferes with the functions of the cord and spinal roots, spinal compression probably plays comparatively little part in its ill effects and it may be that interference with its blood supply is more important.

Papilloedema

Papilloedema is an uncommon complication of spinal tumour (Raynor, 1969; Alter, 1975) and is attributed largely to the effects of the substantial rise in CSF protein which often accompanies these lesions.

Arachnoidal Cysts

These cysts of presumed developmental origin are an occasional cause of spinal cord compression in children, adolescents, and young adults. Commonly they give episodes of radicular pain with signs of spinal cord dysfunction which develop in a step-like manner. Most lie in the dorsal region posterior to the cord and communicate with the subarachnoid space by a narrow orifice which is only easily demonstrable by supine myelography (Nugent et al., 1959; Raja and Hankinson, 1970).

Parasytic Cysts

Hydatid cysts are not uncommon causes of spinal compression in some countries. They are usually extradural. Cysticercus cysts are also occasionally encountered.

Effects of Compression upon the Cord

Spinal compression, however produced, affects the cord in several ways. Direct pressure interferes with conduction in the spinal roots and in the cord itself. Pressure upon the ascending longitudinal spinal veins leads to oedema of the cord below the site of compression. Taylor and Byrnes (1974) suggest that interference with venous drainage may explain symptoms and signs of low cervical cord dysfunction arising in patients with high cervical cord compression. Compression of the longitudinal and radicular spinal arteries also leads to ischaemia of the segments of the cord which they supply. These vascular disturbances cause local oedema of the cord with degeneration of the ganglion cells and of the white matter. Areas of softening may develop—so-called compression myelitis. In general, slow spinal compression affects the pyramidal (corticospinal) tracts first, the posterior columns next, and the spino-thalamic tracts last but there are many exceptions to this rule. It is suggested that this may be due to the fact that the pyramidal tracts are supplied by terminal branches of the anterior spinal artery which are thus most susceptible to compression ischaemia. Alternatively it has been suggested that the pyramidal tract lies closest to the attachments of the ligamentum denticulatum which is subjected to traction when the cord is compressed. Finally, obstruction of the subarachnoid space causes loculation of the CSF below the point of compression and leads to characteristic changes in its composition.

SYMPTOMS

The symptoms of compression of the spinal cord differ to some extent according to whether the source of compression is extradural, extramedullary, or intramedullary and according to its segmental level. The frequency, however, with which it is impossible to determine the relationship of the site of compression to the cord before operation indicates the similarity of the symptoms produced by pressure arising in different situations. It will be convenient, therefore, first to describe the general symptoms of spinal compression, and then to discuss how they may differ according to the site and segmental level of the lesion.

Mode of Onset

The onset of symptoms is usually gradual, especially when they are due to a spinal tumour, but is often rapid in carcinoma of the vertebral column, in spinal extradural abscess, and in acute compression due to other causes. In Pott's disease it is usually gradual but paraplegia may develop acutely. Approximately two-thirds of sufferers from spinal tumour come to operation between the first and second years after the onset of symptoms. Sometimes the interval is considerably longer. The first symptoms are often sensory, the commonest being pain radiating in the distribution of one or more spinal roots. Root pains are usually severe in vertebral collapse from all causes, and in pachymeningitis. In the case of spinal tumours they are most frequently encountered when the tumour is extramedullary (particularly when it is a neurofibroma), and least in intramedullary tumours. The pains may be unilateral or bilateral, and are frequently described as burning or constricting and may be associated with soreness of the skin and tenderness of the deeper structures. They are often intensified by movements of the spine, and by coughing and sneezing, and they may be temporarily relieved by changes in posture. Pain in the back may occur, and is especially frequent in the case of tumours of the cauda equina, and malignant disease of the vertebral column. Compression of the spinothalamic tracts may cause pain of a peculiarly unpleasant character referred to distant parts. Thus pain in a lower limb may be a symptom of compression of the cervical cord. Paraesthesiae may also be produced by compression of the ascending sensory tracts, and take the form of numbness, coldness, or a sense of weight, swelling, or tightness in the limbs. Compression of the posterior columns often gives sensations suggesting that the limb is enclosed in a tight bandage or stocking or that it is being constricted by a tight band or string.

Motor symptoms often develop later than sensory, though the reverse may occur. Weakness, stiffness, and clumsiness of one arm or dragging of one or both legs, especially when tired, are common. When the cervical cord is compressed the order in which the limbs are affected is usually first one upper limb, then the lower limb on the same side, next the opposite lower limb, and finally the opposite upper limb, but cervical spondylosis may present with paraparesis. When the compression is situated below the cervical enlargement motor symptoms are confined to the lower limbs, one usually becoming weak before the other. Exceptionally, paraplegia develops rapidly. This is particularly likely to occur when an acute flexion or hyperextension injury of the neck is experienced by an individual with previously asymptomatic cervical spondylosis. Sphincter disturbances are often late in appearing, even in the case of tumours of the conus medullaris and cauda equina.

The initial symptoms of a spinal angioma are extremely variable and may not appear till middle age. They are rarely those of focal spinal compression, but often indicate an insidiously progressive but rather patchy lesion in the thoracic or lumbar region. Most patients are middle-aged males, disturbances of micturition often appear early and symptoms may be modified by a change in posture (Aminoff and Logue, 1974 a). Exceptional modes of onset are subarachnoid haemorrhage or haematomyelia.

Schäfer (1975) gives a comprehensive review of the differential diagnosis of spinal compression syndromes.

Motor Symptoms

Compression of ventral roots or of the anterior horns of grey matter leads to a progressive lower motor neurone lesion, characterized by weakness, wasting, and fasciculation of the muscles innervated by the affected segments. These symptoms are most conspicuous when the cervical or lumbosacral regions are compressed. Wasting of the intercostal muscles is similarly produced by a lesion of the thoracic cord but may be very difficult to detect.

Compression of the corticospinal tracts causes spastic weakness of the muscles below the level of the lesion. One side of the body is frequently involved before the other, but later spastic paraplegia-in-extension develops and as interruption of conduction in the cord becomes complete this may give place to paraplegia-in-flexion.

Objective Sensory Changes

Compression of dorsal spinal roots at the level of the lesion may cause apparent hyperaesthesia and hyperalgesia (hyperpathia) or 'girdle pain' in the corresponding cutaneous areas. Anaesthesia and analgesia may follow. Compression of the long ascending sensory tracts leads to impairment of sensibility in distant parts of the body. Several forms of dissociated sensory loss are encountered. Compression of the spinothalamic tract causes impairment of appreciation of pain, heat, and cold on the opposite side of the body, but owing to a lamination of the fibres of the tract there may be a slow progressive ascent of the sensory 'level' and certain cutaneous areas may escape. Thus it is common to find sensibility unimpaired over the areas supplied by the sacral segments of the cord ('sacral sparing'). Less frequently the sacral segments are affected early, but an area of normal cutaneous sensibility intervenes between them and an area of sensory loss at a higher level. The final upper limit of the area of analgesia and thermo-anaesthesia is frequently several segments below the level of the lesion. This discrepancy occurs when the uppermost sensory fibres compressed in the cord are those which have decussated several segments below. It is exceptional to find that appreciation of pain, heat, and cold is affected to an equal extent. Not uncommonly cold is still felt over an area which is anaesthetic to heat, and sometimes a cold object, though not recognized as cold, evokes an unpleasant painful sensation. Cutaneous anaesthesia to light touch is frequently absent until the late stages, probably on account of the bilateral path of fibres subserving this form of sensibility. Appreciation of posture, passive movement, and vibration is impaired to a variable extent, and frequently more upon one side than upon the other. Although these forms of sensibility, which depend upon the integrity of the posterior columns, are likely to be affected early when the source of compression is posteriorly situated, they frequently also suffer when the cord is compressed from in front, probably due to pressure against the infolded ligamentum subflavum.

Tenderness of the spine on pressure or percussion may arise in two ways. When vertebrae are diseased, inflamed or subjected to erosion by a tumour, their spinous processes are likely to be tender. When the vertebrae are normal, however, compression of the spinal cord or dorsal roots may lead to tenderness in the region of the spines of the vertebrae innervated by the segments affected. In the latter case the tender vertebra is not necessarily the one overlying the lesion, but is often situated at a lower level, since the segments of the spinal cord do not correspond with the vertebrae in which they are situated (see below). When the cervical cord is compressed, flexing or extending the cervical spine frequently causes pain, numbness, or tingling, radiating into the regions innervated by the affected part of the cord. This symptom (so-called 'electric shock-like' sensations or Lhermitte's sign) may occur with both extramedullary and intramedullary tumours, in cervical myelopathy due to spondylosis and in multiple sclerosis.

The Reflexes

Compression of the spinal cord at a given segmental level leads to diminution or loss of reflexes when the central portion of the reflex arc passes through the segment affected. When the corticospinal tract is simultaneously compressed, reflexes below the level of the lesion show the changes associated with corticospinal lesions, that is, the tendon reflexes are exaggerated, the cremasteric and abdominal reflexes are diminished or lost, and the plantar reflexes are extensor. The reflexes are, therefore, often of value in the localization of a spinal lesion, especially when a reflex mediated by one spinal segment is diminished and one transmitted by a slightly lower segment is exaggerated. For example, a lesion extending down to the fifth or even the sixth cervical segment but not involving the seventh cervical is likely to lead to diminution or loss of the biceps- and supinator-jerks, which depend upon the integrity of the former segments, while the triceps-jerk, of which the reflex arc passes through the seventh cervical segment, may be exaggerated. Thus a tap on the biceps tendon may fail to evoke a biceps jerk but instead there is contraction of triceps due to exaggeration of the triceps jerk which can be obtained by stimulation over a wide field (inversion of the biceps jerk). Similarly, inversion of the radial jerk (finger flexion, occurring in the absence of a radial jerk, on tapping the tendon of the brachioradialis) is a useful clinical indication of a lesion at C5–6. The segmental levels of the various spinal reflexes are given on page 54.

The Sphincters

The sphincters are not as a rule affected in the earliest stages of spinal compression, but later precipitancy or difficulty of micturition usually develops, and later still retention of urine is common, or the bladder may be emptied automatically. Constipation usually occurs, but when there is severe paraplegia there may be incontinence of faeces. Sphincter changes may occur at an earlier stage in the case of tumours involving the cauda equina and conus medullaris than when the compression is situated at a higher level.

Autonomic Symptoms

Autonomic symptoms may be of limited value in the localization of a spinal lesion. When there is considerable interruption of conduction in the spinal cord the control of higher centres over autonomic functions below the level of the lesion is impaired. In such cases excessive sweating frequently occurs over the parts of the body thus isolated from higher control and the regulation of body temperature and blood pressure may be impaired [p. 1070]. Since the sympathetic outflow from the spinal cord is limited to the region between the first thoracic and the second lumbar segments, the upper level of the cutaneous distribution of autonomic disturbances does not as a rule correspond to that of the sensory symptoms of a lesion at a given level of the spinal cord [see p. 750]. Oedema of the lower limbs is often seen in cases of severe spinal compression, as in paraplegia from other causes.

The Spine

The spine may exhibit angular deformity, local tenderness, and pain on movement when the vertebrae are diseased. In cervical spondylosis, however, both pain and limitation of movement are often very slight. A spinal bruit may be present when there is an angioma (Matthews, 1959).

The Cerebrospinal Fluid

Examination of the CSF is of considerable diagnostic importance, since obstruction of the spinal subarachnoid space produces characteristic changes in its chemical composition, and its pressure below the block. Care is, however, necessary in cases of suspected extradural abscess and lumbar puncture should not be performed at or near the site of spinal pain or tenderness in view of the risk of introducing organisms into the subarachnoid space. Furthermore, it must be noted that the removal of CSF by lumbar puncture below a spinal block may render subsequent lumbar myelography impracticable, at least for several days, because of shrinkage of the lumbar subarachnoid space. When there is strong clinical suspicion that the spinal cord is being compressed, therefore, it is often preferable to proceed direct to myelography, examining a specimen of fluid removed at the time, without carrying out a preliminary diagnostic lumbar puncture.

The presence of a tumour of the cauda equina may lead to a failure to obtain CSF by lumbar puncture at the site of election below the fourth lumbar vertebra, if it completely fills the spinal canal at this point. Cisternal myelography will then be indicated.

Chemical Changes. The essential chemical abnormality is a rise in the protein content of the fluid, which usually lies between 0·1 and 0·5 g per 100 ml but may be even higher if the block is complete. In addition the fluid is yellow in colour—xanthochromia—in about 40 per cent of cases, and may coagulate spontaneously. An excess of mononuclear cells in the fluid may be present when the source of compression is inflammatory (e.g. spinal extradural abscess), and exceptionally in cases of tumour. A rise in the protein content of the fluid is most marked in cases of extramedullary spinal compression, and may be slight when the source of pressure is extradural or intramedullary. It is important to note that the protein may be normal or only slightly raised when the cord is compressed in the cervical region, whatever the cause of compression. A rise of the protein content is not uncommon in the fluid removed *above* a tumour of the cauda equina.

Queckenstedt's Test and Manometry. Before myelography became a widely used and relatively innocuous procedure in appropriate cases, Queckenstedt's test, as described on page 128, was widely utilized as a valuable guide to the presence or absence of spinal cord compression. However, experience has indicated that the test gives so many false negative results in cases of cord compression without complete block that it has been largely discarded since, when it is likely to be useful, myelography will almost always be essential. Similarly, manometry, which may indicate subnormal pressure below an obstruction in the spinal subarachnoid space and the absence of normal variations in pressure corresponding to the pulse and respiration, is of very limited diagnostic value. Nevertheless, Queckenstedt's test carried out in various head positions is still sometimes used in the diagnosis of cervical cord compression due to spondylosis; various precise techniques of electromanometry have also been shown to be of some diagnostic value and are reviewed by Lakke (1975). But none of these techniques can supplant myelography as a means of diagnosis and localization of spinal lesions.

Exacerbation of Symptoms following Lumbar Puncture. In cases of spinal subarachnoid block, especially when this is due to a spinal tumour, the withdrawal of CSF below the level of the block by lumbar puncture may lead to a shift in the position of the tumour and a temporary or even permanent intensification of the symptoms, especially root pains, weakness, and retention of urine. Thus hasty lumbar puncture is unwise in cases of suspected spinal tumour. On suspicion of such a diagnosis it is wiser to seek a neurosurgical opinion and to arrange myelography at a time when the neurosurgeon will be able to operate immediately, particularly if clinical deterioration follows the procedure.

Radiography

Radiography of the spine should be carried out in all cases of spinal compression. When this is due to disease of the vertebral column only X-ray examination may enable the cause of the compression to be discovered. It renders visible the vertebral destruction due to tuberculous caries, and other forms of osteitis, secondary carcinoma, primary vertebral neoplasm, and the changes associated with traumatic lesions. It should, however, be noted that a spinal extradural abscess due to acute vertebral osteitis may be present without visible radiological abnormalities in the early stages. Chronic disc protrusion is likely to be associated with narrowing of the corresponding disc space [FIG. 120], and bony spurs from the bodies of adjacent vertebrae: its presence can be confirmed by myelography [FIG. 121]. Many patients, particularly manual workers, have severe degenerative changes in the discs of the cervical spine without symptoms (Irvine *et al.*, 1965; Wilkinson, 1973) so that when radiological findings of spondylosis are present in a patient with signs of spinal cord compression it cannot necessarily be assumed that spondylosis is the cause so that myelography will usually be necessary. A tumour arising within the vertebral canal may by erosion lead to its diffuse enlargement, in which case the distance between the pedicles will be increased, or it may pass outwards through the intervertebral foramen with local destruction of bone. Oblique views will then demonstrate enlargement of the intervertebral foramen and a soft-tissue shadow of a 'dumb-bell' tumour may also be seen.

Myelography

While some workers prefer to use air or oxygen injected intrathecally by lumbar puncture for the demonstration of lesions causing spinal cord compression, most radiologists prefer the use of an opaque oily contrast medium made up of ethyl esters of isomeric iodophenidecyclic acids (*Myodil, Pantopaque*) of which 5–6 ml is usually injected by lumbar puncture with the patient in the sitting position. This preparation is generally non-irritant and few complications are known to result from its use (Bull and McKissock, 1962) although iodine sensitivity should be excluded before it is used. Occasionally low back pain and root pains in the legs and even retention of urine may follow myelography but these complications are as a rule transient; untoward long-lasting sequelae (due to adhesive arachnoiditis—Davies, 1956) are so rare that in Great Britain no attempt is made to remove the injected oil (du Boulay, 1975). In the United States, however, for medicolegal reasons, the lumbar puncture needle is generally left *in situ* and the oil is withdrawn when the radiological examination has been completed. Water-soluble contrast media including methylglucamine iothalamate (*Conray*) and methylglucamate iocarmate (*Dimer-X*) give excellent radiographs but produce acute reactions in an unacceptable proportion of patients (Shapiro, 1975). Following injection the patient is examined on a tilting table under an X-ray screen and anteroposterior and lateral radiographs can be taken at appropriate spinal levels as the flow of contrast medium is observed. Usually the examination is carried out with the patient prone but supine myelography is also essential when a lesion at or near the foramen magnum or an arachnoid cyst lying posterior to the cord is suspected. If the contrast medium is arrested below a compressive lesion or when a lesion in the cauda equina is suspected it may be necessary to inject the medium by cisternal rather than lumbar puncture in order to outline the upper extent of the lesion. In cases of cervical myelopathy radiographs should be taken in several

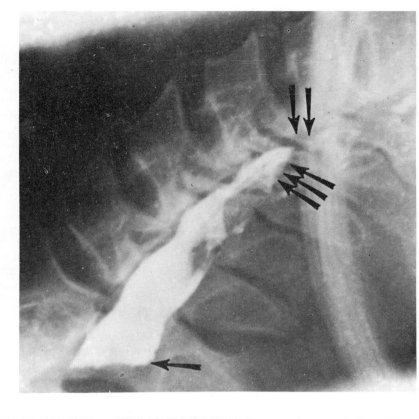

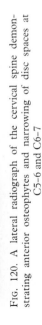

Fig. 121. A myelogram of a patient with cervical myelopathy due to spondylosis. There are a fluid level (the single arrow demonstrates hold-up due to a narrow canal), posterior osteophytes with a disc protrusion (double arrows) and corrugation of the ligamentum subflavum (triple arrows)

Fig. 120. A lateral radiograph of the cervical spine demonstrating anterior osteophytes and narrowing of disc spaces at C5–6 and C6–7

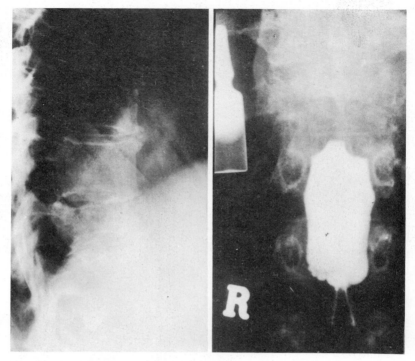

FIG. 122. A radiograph of the spine (on the left) showing collapse of a vertebral body
due to a solitary myeloma with a complete block on myelography (on the right)

positions of the head. When a complete block is present, re-screening after
24 hours may show that some contrast medium has passed the obstruction. The
appearances in the myelogram not only localize the compressive lesion but often
also give an indication as to its nature [FIGS. 122 and 123]. In arachnoiditis there
is usually a patchy hold-up of the medium, while in arteriovenous malformation
of the cord, dilated vessels are often plainly outlined [FIG. 124].

Other Methods of Investigation

Spinal cord angiography, to which reference has already been made, is of
particular value in the diagnosis of spinal vascular malformations but is also
being utilized increasingly as technique improves and complications lessen, to
assist in demonstrating and identifying other spinal lesions (Di Chiro et al.,
1967; Doppman et al., 1969; Vogelsang, 1975). Extradural venography and
lumbar discography (a technique involving the direct injection of contrast
medium into the intervertebral disc) are methods now being used in some centres
especially to demonstrate herniated intervertebral discs but are not yet a part
of routine neuroradiological practice and certainly do not supplant myelography
(Shapiro, 1975). Isotope techniques (myeloscintography) are less valuable in
identifying spinal lesions than gamma-encephalography, but the whole-body
EMI scanner may well make an important contribution in the future.

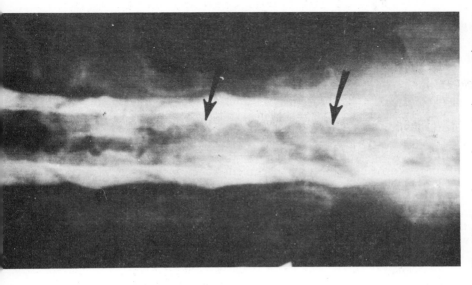

FIG. 124. A myelogram demonstrating an arteriovenous malformation of the dorsal cord; tortuous dilated veins are arrowed

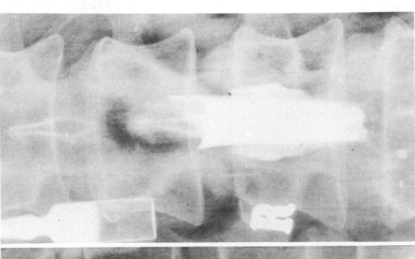

FIG. 123. Lateral and anteroposterior views of a myelogram demonstrating a rounded filling defect due to a neurofibroma of the cauda equina

Symptoms and Signs of Spinal Compression at different Levels

The symptoms of spinal compression at a given level consist of: (1) symptoms of a lower motor neurone lesion, that is, atrophic paralysis with diminution or loss of the tendon reflexes in the muscles innervated by the segments compressed; (2) symptoms of an upper motor neurone lesion, that is, spastic paralysis with exaggeration of the tendon reflexes, diminution or loss of the abdominal and cremasteric reflexes and an extensor plantar reflex on one or both sides below the level of the compression (in advanced cases paraplegia-in-extension in the lower limbs may give place to paraplegia-in-flexion); (3) symptoms of dorsal root irritation, such as girdle pain and hyperpathia, may be present, with a segmental distribution corresponding to the segments compressed; (4) various types of sensory loss already described, with an upper level at or somewhat below the segmental level of the site of compression; (5) autonomic changes, e.g. excessive sweating below the level of the lesion. The following are the principal motor and reflex disturbances resulting from compression of the spinal cord at different levels. The distribution of the sensory changes can best be ascertained from the figures on pages 41 and 42.

The Upper Cervical Region. Spinal compression at this level or at the foramen magnum usually causes considerable pain in the neck and occiput, which is intensified by movements of the cervical spine. Pain, paraesthesiae, and weakness in the upper limbs are early symptoms and loss of proprioceptive sensation in the hands may be particularly prominent. Wasting may occur in both upper limbs although the cervical enlargement is not compressed (Taylor and Byrnes, 1974). Compression of the phrenic nerves or of their nuclei may lead to diminution in the amplitude of the movements of the diaphragm. A tumour in this region may extend upwards through the foramen magnum and cause symptoms through compression of the medulla and of the lowest cranial nerves. Compression of the spinal tract and nucleus of the fifth nerve may cause relative analgesia and thermo-anaesthesia over the face, and the ninth, tenth, and eleventh cranial nerves may also suffer. Signs of corticospinal tract compression are present in both upper and lower limbs with exaggeration of *all* deep tendon reflexes. Postural sense and appreciation of vibration are usually impaired over one or both upper limbs.

The Fifth or Sixth Cervical Segments. Atrophic paralysis is present in the muscles innervated by these segments, namely, the rhomboids, deltoids, spinati, biceps, and brachioradialis. There is spastic paralysis of the remaining muscles of the upper limbs and of the trunk and lower limbs. The biceps- and supinator-jerks are diminished or lost, but are often inverted, as already described [p. 744].

The Eighth Cervical and First Thoracic Segments. Atrophic paralysis involves the flexors of the wrist and fingers and the small muscles of the hands. Paralysis of the ocular sympathetic may be present. The tendon reflexes of the upper limbs are preserved. There is spastic paralysis of the trunk and lower limbs. Compression of the spinal cord at this level is virtually unknown in cervical spondylosis so that wasting of the small hand muscles rarely if ever occurs due to this cause.

Mid-thoracic Region. Atrophic paralysis is confined to the intercostals innervated by the segments involved. Movements of the diaphragm are normal. There is spastic paralysis of the muscles of the abdomen and lower limbs.

Ninth and Tenth Thoracic Segments. The lower halves of the abdominal recti are paralysed; the upper halves are normal. Consequently the umbilicus is drawn upwards when the patient raises his head against resistance. The upper abdominal reflexes are preserved, while those of the lower segments are lost. There is spastic paralysis of the lower limbs.

Twelfth Thoracic and First Lumbar Segments. The abdominal recti are normal, but the lower fibres of obliquus internus and transversus abdominis are paralysed. The abdominal reflexes are preserved, but the cremasteric reflexes are diminished or lost. There is spastic paralysis of the lower limbs.

Third and Fourth Lumbar Segments. Flexion of the hip is preserved. There are atrophic paralysis of quadriceps and the adductors of the hips, with diminution or loss of the knee-jerks, and spastic paralysis of the remaining muscles of the lower limbs, with exaggeration of the ankle-jerks and extensor plantar responses.

First and Second Sacral Segments. Flexion of the hip, adduction of the thigh, extension of the knee, and dorsiflexion of the foot are preserved. There are atrophic paralysis of the intrinsic muscles of the foot and of the calf muscles, and weakness of flexion of the knee and of all muscles moving the hip-joint, except the flexors and adductors. The knee-jerks are preserved; the ankle-jerks and plantar reflexes are lost. The anal and bulbocavernosus reflexes are preserved.

Third and Fourth Sacral Segments. The large bowel and bladder are paralysed and retention of urine and faeces occurs, due to the uninhibited action of the internal sphincters. The external sphincters are paralysed and the anal and bulbocavernosus reflexes are lost. There is usually sensory loss in the perineum and buttocks in 'saddle' distribution. The motility and reflexes of the lower limbs are normal.

Compression of the Cauda Equina

Compression of the cauda equina is most frequently due to a neoplasm, but the nerve roots may be compressed by an associated lipoma in cases of spina bifida occulta, by the constriction of a fibrous band (Léri, 1926), or by chronic arachnoiditis. Perineurial cysts on the posterior sacral roots (Tarlov, 1948) are often asymptomatic but may cause sciatic pain; rarely if ever do they give other manifestations of cauda equina compression. An important source of compression of a single root, or even of multiple roots, occurring sometimes acutely is a displaced intervertebral disc [see p. 924]. Rarely, spondylolisthesis may have the same effect, as may bony stenosis of the lumbar canal (Ehni, 1975) which more often gives the syndrome of recurrent ischaemia or 'claudication' of the cauda equina on effort [see p. 785]. The clinical picture is a variable one, depending upon the site and extent of the source of compression. It may be virtually impossible clinically to distinguish between a neoplasm arising in the cauda equina itself and one arising in the conus medullaris but extending into the cauda. A small tumour may for a long time compress only one or two roots on one side. A large and massive growth may involve the whole of the cauda. For anatomical reasons the lower roots are more likely to be compressed than the upper, since they suffer alone when a growth is situated in the lowest part of the spinal canal, and they are also implicated, together with the upper roots, by tumours at a higher level.

In many cases of compression of the cauda equina by tumour, pain is the earliest symptom. It is usually located in the lumbar or sacral regions of the spine as a dull, aching pain which is liable to be exacerbated by jerky movements, coughing, and sneezing. Less frequently the pain is referred to one or both lower limbs in the distribution of certain of the lower spinal roots, and it may also be referred to the bladder or rectum.

Motor symptoms consist of atrophic paralysis, the distribution of which depends upon the roots affected. Most frequently there is paralysis of the muscles below the knee, though the tibialis anterior may escape, and of the hamstrings and glutei. In such cases the ankle-jerks are diminished or lost, and the plantar reflexes may also be unelicitable; but the knee-jerks are often preserved.

The distribution of the sensory loss also depends upon which spinal dorsal roots are involved. Compression of the lower sacral roots leads to a characteristic saddle-shaped area of anaesthesia and analgesia extending over the perineum, buttocks, and back of the thighs. Compression of the upper sacral and fifth lumbar roots produces an area of sensory loss over the foot and over the posterior and outer aspect of the leg. When the lowest sacral segments are involved, though the external genitals are anaesthetic, and the patient may be unaware of the passage of a catheter through the urethra, some sensibility usually remains in the bladder, so that the patient is aware of its distension, and cystitis may give rise to pain.

Disturbance of function of the bladder and bowel is usual but may be unexpectedly late in developing. Compression of the third and fourth ventral and dorsal sacral roots interrupts the reflex arc upon which evacuation of the bladder and rectum depends. The result is retention of urine and faeces due to the unopposed contraction of the internal sphincters, although the external sphincters are paralysed. Impotence occurs in the male. When the lowest sacral roots are compressed the anal and bulbocavernosus reflexes are lost, but these will be preserved as long as these roots escape.

Trophic symptoms may occur in the lower limbs, which are frequently cold and cyanosed, and tend to become oedematous. Slight injuries over the analgesic areas are apt to lead to sores which are slow to heal.

DIAGNOSIS

The diagnosis of spinal compression involves four stages: (1) Spinal compression must be distinguished from other lesions which may give rise to similar symptoms; (2) when the existence of spinal compression has been established, its segmental level must be determined; (3) an attempt should then be made to decide whether the compression is extradural, extramedullary, or intramedullary; and (4) its pathological nature must be considered.

Diagnosis from other Disorders

When the earliest symptom is pain spinal compression is liable to be confused with visceral disorders of which pain is a prominent symptom, for example, pleurisy, angina pectoris, cholecystitis, gastric and duodenal ulcer, and renal calculus. This error can only be avoided by a thorough examination of the nervous system, which will usually yield some indication of a lesion of the spinal cord, and also by the absence of physical signs of visceral disease. Spinal compression requires to be distinguished from intrinsic cord lesions such as multiple sclerosis, syringomyelia, and motor neurone disease, each of which may be simulated by cervical myelopathy due to spondylosis. On clinical grounds this distinction can usually be made with considerable confidence, but the diagnosis can only be clinched by examination of the CSF and myelography.

Localization of Segmental Level

In the localization of the segmental level of spinal compression segmental symptoms, especially atrophic paralysis and root pains and hyperalgesia, are of the first importance. Next in value is the upper limit of the area of sensory loss, though this is not always easy to define. When it can be accurately determined the segmental level of the upper limit of the area of analgesia may be taken as indicating the lowest segment compressed but it must be remembered that a sensory 'level' for pain sensation may suggest that the lesion is several segments lower than its actual site. Thus a level on the thoracic cage is not infrequently observed in patients with lesions of the cervical cord.

The clinical diagnosis of a tumour of the cauda equina from a tumour of the conus medullaris is often difficult, and may be impossible. If, however, in spite of paralysis of the bladder and rectum, the anal and bulbocavernosus reflexes are preserved and if sensory loss is of the dissociated type, that is, if sensibility to pain, heat, and cold is lost, while that to light touch is preserved, it is likely that the lesion involves the conus rather than the roots. The presence of an extensor plantar response on one or both sides indicates that the spinal cord is compressed at least as high as the fifth lumbar segment.

Relationship of Spinal Segments to Vertebrae. Since the spinal cord terminates at the level of the lower border of the first lumbar vertebra, spinal segments do not correspond numerically with the vertebral arches by which they are enclosed. Having localized a source of compression in terms of spinal segments, and especially in the few cases where the results of myelography are equivocal, the surgeon requires to know beneath which laminal arch he may expect to find it. To ascertain which spinal segment is related to a given vertebra:

For the cervical vertebrae, add 1.
For thoracic 1–6, add 2.
For thoracic 7–9, add 3.
The tenth thoracic arch overlies lumbar 1 and 2 segments.
The eleventh thoracic arch overlies lumbar 3 and 4.
The twelfth thoracic arch overlies lumbar 5.
The first lumbar arch overlies the sacral and coccygeal segments.

It must be remembered that owing to the obliquity of the lower thoracic spinous processes a spinous process in this region is situated at the level of the body of the vertebra below. Despite these valuable clinical guides it is, except in very unusual or urgent circumstances, unwise to operate without confirmation of the level of the lesion by myelography.

The Relationship of the Source of Compression to the Cord

Angular deformity of the spine, and radiographic evidence of vertebral destruction indicate clearly that vertebral disease is responsible for the spinal compression. In the absence of such evidence the differentiation of extradural, extramedullary, and intramedullary sources of spinal compression is often difficult, and may be impossible. In extradural compression root pains not uncommonly occur early, and symptoms of spinal compression are usually bilateral and symmetrical in their development. Motor symptoms usually appear

B b

first, to be followed later by sphincter disturbances, and sensory changes are frequently late. The protein content of the CSF is often not greatly increased and usually lies between 40 and 150 mg per 100 ml. The distinction between extramedullary and intramedullary compression is sometimes impossible before operation but the myelographic findings usually differentiate between the two. The early onset of unilateral root pains and the development of symptoms indicating that compression is mainly exerted upon one-half of the cord favour an extramedullary source of compression. In such cases, moreover, blockage of the spinal subarachnoid space tends to occur early and the protein content of the spinal fluid is usually high. In cases of intramedullary compression root pains are less frequent, motor symptoms are usually bilateral, and sphincter involvement occurs early. An area of dissociated sensory loss extending over a series of segments just below the level of the lesion is suggestive of an intramedullary growth. Subarachnoid blockage occurs later and the protein content of the fluid is usually lower in the case of intramedullary than in the case of extramedullary compression.

Diagnosis of the Cause

1. *Vertebral Disease*. When spinal compression is due to vertebral collapse there is usually considerable pain in, and rigidity of, the spine; angular deformity is common, and radiographic evidence of vertebral destruction will usually be found. *Tuberculous caries* is to be suspected when these symptoms are present in a young patient who shows evidence of infection, such as pyrexia, sweating, and a raised sedimentation rate, with possibly in addition signs of a tuberculous abscess or of a tuberculous focus elsewhere, but it may occur at any age and without general symptoms. *Secondary carcinoma* of the vertebral column is usually seen in middle-aged patients. The onset of the spinal symptoms is often rapid and attended by considerable pain. There may be a history of an operation for carcinoma and, in the absence of this, careful clinical and radiological examination often enable the primary growth to be found. The diagnosis of other forms of vertebral disease, for example, myelomatosis and osteitis deformans of Paget, can usually be established radiographically. When the former is suspected the appropriate tests should be carried out. The presence of *cervical spondylosis* can be demonstrated radiographically, but it must be remembered that this is very common after middle age, and is not always the cause of the patient's symptoms.

2. *Spinal Tumour*. Spinal tumour is to be suspected in cases in which there is a gradual onset and a slowly progressive development of symptoms of spinal compression, in the absence of evident disease of the vertebral column. It is usually impossible to anticipate the nature of the spinal tumour, but a careful search should be made for cutaneous pigmentation and other symptoms of neurofibromatosis, which may be associated with an intrathecal neurofibroma.

3. *Meningitis*. It is often impossible to diagnose either hypertrophic pachymeningitis or arachnoiditis before operation. The occurrence of multiple levels of segmental sensory disturbance, and a patchy or streaky arrest of contrast medium are in favour of arachnoiditis.

Such rare causes of spinal compression as reticulosis, leukaemic deposits, extradural metastases, and parasitic cysts can be suspected only when clinical examination reveals evidence of the disease elsewhere.

PROGNOSIS

General Considerations

The prognosis of compression of the spinal cord depends upon (1) the nature of the source of compression and the extent to which it can be relieved, (2) the severity and duration of the disturbance of function when the patient comes under observation, and (3) the level of the cord compressed. The influence of the nature of the compressing agent upon prognosis is further considered below. The more severe the interruption of conduction in the cord, the less likely is recovery to be complete. Hence the development of paraplegia-in-flexion, which indicates a severe degree of interruption of the cord, is of bad prognostic import, and little functional improvement can be expected in such cases. The longer the history of symptoms of compression, the less complete is recovery likely to be, though even when such symptoms as spastic weakness of the lower limbs have been present for two or more years, a remarkable degree of recovery may occur if the cause can be removed. It cannot be stressed too strongly that rapidly-advancing spinal cord compression demands immediate investigation and treatment so that the latter can be carried out before the circulation to the cord is irreversibly embarrassed. The outlook is best when the site of compression is situated in the middle or lower thoracic regions although it should be remembered that surgical operations in this region, particularly when carried out for the relief of anteriorly-situated lesions, such as the rare dorsal disc protrusions, are hazardous, first because the spinal canal is very narrow in this region, and secondly because the blood supply of the cord is at its most precarious at this point. When the upper cervical cord is compressed the proximity of the spinal centres innervating the diaphragm adds to the risk both of the compression itself and of operations upon this region. Compression of the lumbosacral region and cauda equina is especially liable to lead to disturbance of function of the bladder and bowel, and hence there is a high incidence of infection of the urinary tract in such cases. In all cases of spinal compression the presence of infection of the urinary tract and of severe bed-sores adds to the gravity of the prognosis.

Tuberculous Spinal Osteitis

The mortality rate of tuberculous caries of the spine has been reduced by modern chemotherapy. Spinal compression naturally increases the risk of death, but about 70 per cent of patients with paraparesis recover completely if treated promptly. Others are left with some spastic weakness of the lower limbs. The prognosis both as to life and as to recovery of function is better in children than in adults. The sudden development of paraplegia rapidly becoming complete is usually due to 'concertina' collapse of a vertebral body or to thrombosis of vessels supplying the cord, and in both conditions the outlook is poor. When long-standing paraplegia-in-flexion is present there is no hope of recovery.

Secondary Carcinoma of the Vertebrae

In the past few patients survived more than 12 months after the development of symptoms indicating the presence of metastatic carcinomatous deposits within the vertebral column, death occurring either as a direct result of disturbance of function caused by the primary growth, or from cachexia due to widespread metastases. However, after prompt surgical decompression in appropriate cases followed by radiotherapy and/or chemotherapy, the prognosis is now much better and survival for five years or more is not uncommon in patients with reticulosis, myeloma, and prostatic or testicular tumours (Jameson, 1974).

Spinal Tumour

The prognosis of spinal tumour depends primarily upon the extent to which the growth can be removed. Accordingly, the outlook is much better in the case of extramedullary tumours, a large proportion of which can be removed completely, than when the tumour is intramedullary. Few intramedullary tumours can be successfully removed without considerable damage to the spinal cord although some ependymomas are encapsulated and can be 'shelled out' with subsequent improvement. The mortality rate of operations for spinal tumours is under 5 per cent in the best hands. A considerable functional improvement may be expected to follow the successful removal of a spinal tumour in all but the most advanced cases, even when symptoms of compression have been present for several years. Improvement, however, may be slow and may be expected to continue for a year or more after operation. Angiomas tend to be insidiously progressive in spite of all treatment but some show an unexpectedly benign and remittent course (Aminoff and Logue, 1974 b) and a proportion can be removed successfully (Shephard, 1966; Logue et al., 1974).

Acute Intervertebral Disc Prolapse and Cervical Spondylosis

Acute central protrusion of a cervical intervertebral disc is usually best treated conservatively by means of immobilization of the neck in a plastic collar but if cord compression is severe laminectomy and decompression may be needed and if carried out sufficiently early the prognosis is good. Acute compression of the cauda equina, say by a central disc prolapse, demands immediate operation, especially if the sphincters are involved and here again the prognosis is good. Operative treatment is also indicated as a rule in cord compression due to prolapse of a dorsal intervertebral disc but the operation is risky, recovery is often incomplete, and irreversible paraplegia due to cord infarction is an all-too-frequent complication. In cervical myelopathy due to spondylosis the natural tendency of the disorder is to become arrested, but most patients are left with a varying degree of residual disability.

Arachnoiditis and Arachnoidal Cysts

The response to operation in arachnoiditis is often disappointing and indeed operation is usually contra-indicated when the process is diffuse but the results of surgical removal of arachnoid cysts are usually excellent.

TREATMENT

The treatment of compression of the spinal cord involves (1) the appropriate treatment of the source of the compression, and (2) when paraplegia is present, adequate care of the paralysed limbs, the skin, the urinary tract, and the bowels, along the lines laid down on page 725, for upon the careful treatment of the paraplegia may depend not only the patient's life but also the rate at which recovery of function occurs.

Tuberculous Spinal Osteitis

A patient suffering from tuberculous caries of the spine requires appropriate chemotherapy and orthopaedic treatment, usually immobilization in a plaster bed.

Laminectomy is rarely desirable, since most patients rapidly improve on the treatment described. An exploratory operation, however, may be carried out when paraplegia has continued unimproved after several months of treatment or when a sudden increase in its severity occurs.

Cervical Spondylosis

In some cases immobilization of the neck by means of a plaster or plastic collar has been thought to arrest the progress of cervical myelopathy but the value of this treatment is now recognized to be dubious in contrast to its confirmed beneficial effect in acute cervical intervertebral disc prolapse. In rapidly progressive cases, especially when the patient is relatively young, surgical decompression may be necessary. This is particularly likely to be indicated when myelography indicates that the cord is being compressed by significant disc protrusions at one or two levels and especially if there is infolding of the ligamentum subflavum and a narrow cervical canal (Bradley and Banna, 1968). Surgery is probably contra-indicated if three or more discs are involved. The choice between posterior decompression by laminectomy and anterior removal of the discs with spinal fusion (the Cloward operation) is a matter for decision depending upon clinical and myelographic findings in the individual case.

Lumbar Spondylosis and Spondylolisthesis

Operation in cases of lumbar spondylosis is indicated when chronic sciatic pain due to this cause has resisted conservative treatment or when the cauda equina is compressed by a large acute central disc protrusion. Laminectomy is of dubious value in cases of spondylolisthesis with compression of the cauda equina but spinal fusion may be beneficial, especially in the relief of pain.

Other Spinal Lesions

Surgical decompression is rarely feasible in cases of spinal cord compression due to Paget's disease but is usually indicated in cases of vertebral haemangioma, and sometimes in kyphoscoliosis and achondroplasia.

Secondary Carcinoma of Vertebrae

When multiple vertebrae are involved, treatment can only be palliative as a rule, and morphine should be given in doses adequate for the relief of pain. In many cases of acute compression at a single level emergency laminectomy and decompression is indicated in order to relieve pressure and to obtain a surgical biopsy of the tumour as a preliminary to radiotherapy and chemotherapy. The question as to whether the lesion should be irradiated depends upon the general condition of the patient and the situation and prognosis of the primary lesion being known. Many patients have relief of pain as a result and in some cord compression is relieved so that this treatment is usually indicated if the lesion is radiosensitive and unless the patient is *in extremis* as a result of the primary growth and/or multiple metastases elsewhere. Powerful analgesics and, in selected cases, surgical methods of pain relief (cordotomy, stereotaxic thalamotomy) may be required.

Spinal Tumour

Laminectomy should be performed, and when the tumour is extradural or extramedullary it should be removed as far as possible. Though many intramedullary tumours are inoperable, some, especially ependymomas, are extruded after incision of the cord and after removal of some of these lesions, cord damage is unexpectedly slight. When a spinal tumour for any reason cannot be removed, the operation of laminectomy may lead to a temporary improvement by diminishing the pressure upon the cord. X-ray irradiation may be of value as an accessory method of treatment following operation, especially for intramedullary tumours and sacral chordomas which can rarely be removed. Angiomas show little if any response to radiotherapy; as already mentioned, removal is possible far more often than was thought likely in the past. Considerable benefit has been noted after excision of the superficial fistulous portion of the malformation, intradural ligation of feeding vessels, and excision of draining veins (Logue *et al.*, 1974).

Meningitis and Extradural Abscess

When spinal pachymeningitis is of long standing, it leads to softening of the spinal cord through interference with its vascular supply. In such cases little benefit can be expected to follow operation. At an earlier stage, however, when the symptoms are mainly due to constriction of the cord, improvement may follow laminectomy and removal of granulation tissue. When arachnoiditis is found at operation, an attempt should be made to free the cord from adhesions and to rupture or remove any localized cysts which may be present. Tuberculous spinal meningitis requires the appropriate chemotherapy. Early decompression by laminectomy under antibiotic cover in cases of pyogenic spinal extradural abscess may be followed by complete recovery but if the patient is allowed to become paraplegic before operation is performed, it may be too late.

The rehabilitation of patients suffering from spinal compression who have undergone laminectomy, should include passive movements of the paretic limbs and re-educational exercises, in order to promote functional recovery [see p. 728].

REFERENCES

ABRAHAMSON, L., McCONNELL, A. A., and WILSON, G. R. (1934) Acute epidural spinal abscess, *Brit. med. J.*, **1**, 1114.

ADSON, A. W. (1938) Intraspinal tumors; surgical consideration. Collective review, *Surg. Gynec. Obstet.*, **67**, 225.

ALLEN, I. M. (1930) Tumours involving the cauda equina: a review of their clinical features and differential diagnosis, *J. Neurol. Psychopath.*, **11**, 111.

ALTER, M. (1975) Statistical aspects of spinal cord tumors, in *Handbook of Clinical Neurology*, vol. 19, ed. Vinken, P. J., and Bruyn, G. W., chapter 1, p. 1, Amsterdam.

AMINOFF, M. J., and LOGUE, V. (1974*a*) Clinical features of spinal vascular malformations, *Brain*, **97**, 197.

AMINOFF, M. J., and LOGUE, V. (1974*b*) The prognosis of patients with spinal vascular malformations, *Brain*, **97**, 211.

ANTONI, N. (1962) Spinal vascular malformations (angiomas) and myelomalacia, *Neurology (Minneap.)*, **12**, 795.

BANNA, M., and GRYSPEERDT, G. L. (1971) Intraspinal tumours in children (excluding dysraphism), *Clin. Radiol.*, **22**, 17.

BARNETT, H. J. M., FOSTER, J. B., and HUDGSON, P. (1973) *Syringomyelia* (Major Problems in Neurology Series, ed. Walton, J. N.), London.

BLAKESLEE, G. A. (1928) Compression of the spinal cord in Hodgkin's disease, *Arch. Neurol. Psychiat. (Chic.)*, **20**, 130.

BRADLEY, W. G., and BANNA, M. (1968) The cervical dural canal. A study of the 'tight dural canal' and of syringomyelia by prone and supine myelography, *Br. J. Radiol.*, **41**, 608.

BRAHAM, J., and SAIA, A. (1958) Neurological complications of epidural anaesthesia, *Brit. med. J.*, **2**, 657.

BRAIN, W. R. (1948) Rupture of the intervertebral disk in the cervical region, *Proc. roy. Soc. Med.*, **41**, 509.

BRAIN, W. R., NORTHFIELD, D. W. C., and WILKINSON, M. (1952) The neurological manifestations of cervical spondylosis, *Brain*, **75**, 187.

BRICE, J., and McKISSOCK, W. (1965) Surgical treatment of malignant extradural spinal tumours, *Brit. med. J.*, **1**, 1341.

BUCY, P. C., and OBERHILL, H. R. (1950) Intradural spinal granulomas, *J. Neurosurg.*, **7**, 1.

BULL, J. W. D. (1948) Rupture of the intervertebral disk in the cervical region, *Proc. roy. Soc. Med.*, **41**, 513.

BULL, J. W. D., and McKISSOCK, W. (1962) *An Atlas of Positive Contrast Myelography*, New York.

BUTLER, R. W. (1934–5) Paraplegia in Pott's disease, with special reference to the pathology and aetiology, *Brit. J. Surg.*, **22**, 738.

CAIRNS, H., and RUSSELL, D. S. (1931) Intracranial and spinal metastases in gliomas of the brain, *Brain*, **54**, 377.

CAMPBELL, A. M. G., and PHILLIPS, D. G. (1960) Cervical disk lesions with neurological disorder, *Brit. med. J.*, **2**, 481.

CLARKE, E. (1956) Spinal cord involvement in multiple myelomatosis, *Brain*, **79**, 332.

CRITCHLEY, M., and GREENFIELD, J. G. (1930) Spinal symptoms in chloroma and leukaemia, *Brain*, **53**, 11.

DASTUR, D. K., and WADIA, N. H. (1969) Spinal meningitides with radiculo-myelopathy. Part 2—Pathology and pathogenesis, *J. neurol. Sci.*, **8**, 261.

DAVIDSON, S. (1968) Cryptococcal spinal arachnoiditis, *J. Neurol. Neurosurg. Psychiat.*, **31**, 76.

DAVIES, F. C. (1956) Effect of unabsorbed radiographic contrast media on the central nervous system, *Lancet*, **ii**, 747.

DI CHIRO, G., DOPPMAN, J., and OMMAYA, A. K. (1967) Selective arteriography of arteriovenous aneurysms of spinal cord, *Radiology*, **88**, 1065.

DOPPMAN, J. L., DI CHIRO, G., and OMMAYA, A. K. (1969) *Selective Arteriography of the Spinal Cord*, St. Louis.

DU BOULAY, G. (1975) Myelography, in *Handbook of Clinical Neurology*, vol. 19, ed. Vinken, P. J., and Bruyn, G. W., chapter 8, p. 179, Amsterdam.

EDELSON, R. N., CHERNIK, N. L., and POSNER, J. B. (1974) Spinal subdural hematomas complicating lumbar puncture: occurrence in thrombocytopenic patients, *Arch. Neurol. (Chic.)*, **31**, 134.

EDELSON, R. N., DECK, M. D. F., and POSNER, J. B. (1972) Intramedullary spinal cord metastases, *Neurology (Minneap.)*, **22**, 1222.

EHNI, G. (1975) Effects of certain degenerative diseases of the spine, especially spondylosis and disk protrusion, on the neural contents, particularly in the lumbar region, *Mayo Clin. Proc.*, **50**, 327.

ELKINGTON, J. ST. C. (1936) Meningitis serosa circumscripta spinalis, *Brain*, **59**, 181.

ELSBERG, C. A. (1925) *Tumors of the Spinal Cord*, New York.

ELSBERG, C. A., and CONSTABLE, K. (1930) Tumors of the cauda equina, *Arch. Neurol. Psychiat. (Chic.)*, **23**, 79.

GESSAGA, E. C., MAIR, W. G. P., and GRANT, D. N. (1973) Ultrastructure of a sacro-coccygeal chordoma, *Acta neuropath. (Berl.)*, **25**, 27.

GLOBUS, J. H., and DOSHAY, L. J. (1929) Venous dilatations and other intraspinal vessel alterations, including true angiomata, with signs and symptoms of cord compression, *Surg. Gynec. Obstet.*, **48**, 345.

GREENBERG, A. D. (1968) Atlanto-axial dislocations, *Brain*, **91**, 655.

HASSIN, G. B. (1928) Circumscribed suppurative nontuberculous peripachy-meningitis, *Arch. Neurol. Psychiat. (Chic.)*, **20**, 110.

HIRSON, C. (1965) Spinal subdural abscess, *Lancet*, **ii**, 1215.

HOWELL, C. M. H. (1936-7) Arachnoiditis, *Proc. roy. Soc. Med.*, **30,** 33.

INGRAHAM, F. D., and MATSON, D. D. (1954) Intraspinal tumours, in *Neurosurgery of Infancy and Childhood*, p. 345, Springfield, Ill.

IRVINE, D. H., FOSTER, J. B., NEWELL, D. J., and KLUKVIN, B. N. (1965) Prevalence of cervical spondylosis in a general practice, *Lancet*, **i,** 1089.

JAMESON, R. M. (1974) Prolonged survival in paraplegia due to metastatic spinal tumours, *Lancet*, **i,** 1209.

KERNOHAN, J. W., WOLTMAN, H. W., and ADSON, A. W. (1931) Intramedullary tumors of the spinal cord, *Arch. Neurol. Psychiat. (Chic.)*, **25,** 679.

LAKKE, J. P. W. F. (1975) Detection of obstruction of the spinal canal by CSF manometry, in *Handbook of Clinical Neurology*, vol. 19, ed. Vinken, P. J., and Bruyn, G. W., chapter 5, p. 91, Amsterdam.

LÉRI, A. (1926) *Études sur les affections de la colonne vertébrale*, Paris.

LOGUE, V., AMINOFF, M. J., and KENDALL, B. E. (1974) Results of surgical treatment for patients with a spinal angioma, *J. Neurol. Neurosurg. Psychiat.*, **37,** 1074.

MATTHEWS, W. B. (1959) The spinal bruit, *Lancet*, **ii,** 1117.

MCALLISTER, V. L., KENDALL, B. E., and BULL, J. W. D. (1975) Symptomatic vertebral haemangiomas, *Brain*, **98,** 71.

MONIZ, E. (1925) La pachyméningite spinale hypertrophique et les cavités médullaires, *Rev. neurol. (Paris)*, **32,** 433.

NASSAR, S. I., and CORRELL, J. W. (1968) Subarachnoid hemorrhage due to spinal cord tumors, *Neurology (Minneap.)*, **18,** 87.

NEWMAN, M. J. D. (1958) Spinal angioma with symptoms in pregnancy, *J. Neurol. Neurosurg. Psychiat.*, **21,** 38.

NUGENT, G. R., ODOM, G. L., and WOODHALL, B. (1959) Spinal extradural cysts, *Neurology (Minneap.)*, **9,** 397.

ODDSSON, B. (1947) *Spinal Meningioma*, Copenhagen.

PAYNE, J. P., and BERGENTZ, S. E. (1956) Paraplegia following spinal anaesthesia, *Lancet*, **i,** 666.

PENNING, L. (1961) Atlanto-axial instability and functional X-ray examination, *Medicamundi*, **7,** 113.

RAJA, I. A., and HANKINSON, J. (1970) Congenital spinal arachnoid cysts, *J. Neurol. Neurosurg. Psychiat.*, **33,** 105.

RAYNOR, R. B. (1969) Papilledema associated with tumors of the spinal cord, *Neurology (Minneap.)*, **19,** 700.

ROSS, J. C., GIBBON, N. O. K., and DAMANSKI, M. (1964) Bladder dysfunction in non-traumatic paraplegia, *Lancet*, **i,** 779.

RUBINSTEIN, L. J., and LOGAN, W. J. (1970) Extraneural metastases in ependymoma of the cauda equina, *J. Neurol. Neurosurg. Psychiat.*, **33,** 763.

SAGER, P. (1969) *Spondylosis Cervicalis*, Copenhagen.

SCHÄFER, E.-R. (1975) The spinal compression syndrome, in *Handbook of Clinical Neurology*, vol. 19, ed. Vinken, P. J., and Bruyn, G. W., chap. 17, p. 347, Amsterdam.

SEDDON, H. J. (1934-5) Pott's paraplegia: prognosis and treatment, *Brit. J. Surg.*, **22,** 769.

SHAPIRO, R. (1975) *Myelography*, 3rd ed., Chicago.

SHEPHARD, R. H. (1966) A reappraisal of spinal intradural angiomas with particular emphasis on treatment by excision, *Proc. roy. Soc. Med.* (film), **59,** 796.

SLOOFF, J. L., KERNOHAN, J. W., and MACCARTY, C. S. (1964) *Primary Intramedullary Tumors of the Spinal Cord and Filum Terminale*, Philadelphia, London.

STEVENS, J. C., CARTLIDGE, N. E. F., SAUNDERS, M., APPLEBY, A., HALL, M., and SHAW, D. A. (1971) Atlanto-axial subluxation and cervical myelopathy in rheumatoid arthritis, *Quart. J. Med.*, **40,** 391.

STOOKEY, B. (1924) A study of extradural spinal tumors, *Arch. Neurol. Psychiat. (Chic.)*, **12,** 663.

STOOKEY, B. (1927) Adhesive spinal arachnoiditis simulating spinal cord tumor, *Arch. Neurol. Psychiat. (Chic.)*, **17,** 151.

SYMONDS, C. P., and MEADOWS, S. P. (1937) Compression of the spinal cord in the neighbourhood of the foramen magnum, *Brain*, **60,** 52.

TARLOV, I. M. (1948) Cysts (perineurial) of sacral roots. Another cause (nemovabre) of sciatic pain, *J. Amer. med. Ass.*, **138,** 740.

TAYLOR, A. R., and BYRNES, D. P. (1974) Foramen magnum and high cervical cord compression, *Brain*, **97,** 473.

TILNEY, F., and ELSBERG, C. A. (1926) Sensory disturbances in tumors of the cervical spinal cord, *Arch. Neurol. Psychiat. (Chic.)*, **15,** 444.

VOGELSANG, H. (1975) Angiography, in *Handbook of Clinical Neurology*, vol. 19, ed. Vinken, P. J., and Bruyn, G. W., chapter 10, p. 229, Amsterdam.

WALTON, J. N. (1953) Subarachnoid haemorrhage of unusual aetiology, *Neurology (Minneap.)*, **3,** 517.

WEIL, A. (1931) Spinal cord changes in lymphogranulomatosis, *Arch. Neurol. Psychiat. (Chic.)*, **26,** 1009.

WILKINSON, M. (1973) *Cervical Spondylosis*, 2nd ed., London.

WOLTMAN, H. W., KERNOHAN, J. W., ADSON, A. W., and CRAIG, W. McK. (1951) Intramedullary tumors of spinal cord and gliomas of intradural portion of filum terminale; fate of patients who have these tumors, *Arch. Neurol. Psychiat. (Chic.)*, **65,** 378.

WYBURN-MASON, R. (1943) *Vascular Abnormalities and Tumours of the Spinal Cord*, London.

SYRINGOMYELIA

Definition. A chronic disorder characterized pathologically by the presence of long cavities, surrounded by gliosis, which are situated in the central part of the spinal cord and frequently extend up into the medulla (syringobulbia). The principal clinical features are areas of cutaneous analgesia and thermoanaesthesia, often with preservation of appreciation of light touch and postural sensibility, but with muscular wasting and trophic changes, especially in the upper limbs, and symptoms of corticospinal tract degeneration in the lower limbs. The term 'syringomyelia' was first used by Ollivier in 1824.

PATHOLOGY

The pathological changes characteristic of syringomyelia are most frequently situated in the lower cervical and upper thoracic regions of the spinal cord. Extension to the medulla is common, and the process may reach the pons or even as high as the internal capsule. A thoracolumbar and lumbosacral incidence is rare and is usually due to a true hydromyelia associated with congenital anomalies of the lower spine, although ascending cavitation occurring after traumatic transverse lesions of the cord, or in association with cord tumours, has been reported.

The affected region of the cord is enlarged, mainly in the transverse plane [FIG. 125]. In some cases the enlargement is sufficient to cause erosion of the bones of the spinal canal or at least widening of its anteroposterior diameter (Wells *et al.*, 1959). Transverse section of the cord reveals a cavity surrounded by a zone of translucent gelatinous material. Microscopically, the gelatinous material lining the cavity contains glial cells and fibres. The protein content of the fluid in the cavity is high. In a recent detailed review, Barnett *et al.* (1973) distinguish between 'communicating' and non-communicating syringomyelia; the pathogenesis of these two varieties will be discussed below. There is little difference, however, in the pathological characteristics of the actual cord cavities in the two varieties in most cases; the differences lie in the nature of the associated lesions.

The expansion of the cavity and surrounding gliosis, affecting more severely the less resistant grey matter rather than the more dense white matter, at least in the first instance, lead to compression of the anterior horns of the grey matter, thus causing atrophy of the anterior horn cells, and degeneration of their axons in the ventral roots and peripheral nerves. Extension to the brain stem (syringobulbia) usually occurs first in the posterolateral part of the medulla in the region of the spinal nucleus of the trigeminal nerve and the nucleus ambiguus, so that the earliest signs of brain stem dysfunction are usually due

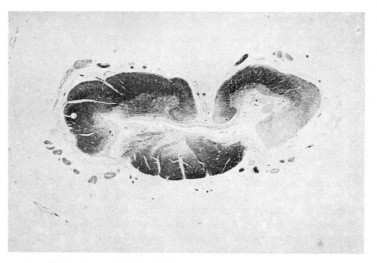

FIG. 125. Syringomyelia: spinal cord. Cavitation surrounded by gliosis

to the involvement of nuclei. Compression of the long ascending and descending tracts of the cord or brain stem occurs somewhat later, and leads to secondary degeneration, which is most marked first in the corticospinal tracts, later in the spinothalamic tracts, and later still the posterior columns. Haemorrhage into a syringomyelic cavity constitutes one uncommon form of haematomyelia.

AETIOLOGY AND PATHOGENESIS

For many years it was thought that syringomyelia was due to a congenital abnormality, perhaps causing abnormal closure of the central canal of the spinal cord in the embryo. Others took the view that the condition was a degenerative disorder of unknown cause. It is now apparent that so-called 'communicating syringomyelia' is the commoner variety (Barnett et al., 1973) and Gardner (Gardner and Angel, 1958; Gardner, 1965) was among the first to stress the relationship of the condition to congenital anomalies and other lesions in the neighbourhood of the foramen magnum, including the Chiari type I anomaly (congenital extension of the cerebellar tonsils below the foramen magnum), craniovertebral developmental abnormalities with or without occult hydrocephalus (Foster et al., 1969), and basal arachnoiditis. Gardner suggested that in such cases abnormalities of this type, as well as the Dandy–Walker syndrome of closure of the foramina of Magendie and Luschka prevented, perhaps intermittently, the egress of cerebrospinal fluid from the fourth ventricle into the subarachnoid space with the result that pressure waves of fluid were forced down into the central canal of the cord which thus became dilated (hydro-myelia). This view is now generally accepted, though opinions differ about the exact nature of the hydrodynamic mechanisms involved (Williams, 1969). The fact that a syringomyelic cavity is sometimes found to lie alongside an apparently normal spinal canal can be accounted for by the fact that with dilatation of the canal, its ependymal lining quickly disappears and diverticula may form which dissect downwards (or sometimes upwards) alongside the canal in the central grey matter. In several large series of cases recently described (Appleby et al., 1968; Barnett et al., 1973) the Chiari type I anomaly has been found to be the commonest congenital anomaly present in such cases but basal arachnoiditis, either developing as a sequel to previous trauma, subarachnoid haemorrhage, or meningitis, or without evident cause, accounts for about a quarter of these cases.

In 'non-communicating syringomyelia', by contrast (Barnett et al., 1973), the condition is more often due to or associated with spinal injury, with or without paraplegia, spinal arachnoiditis, or spinal tumour. In these cases the cavity may develop in the dorsal or lumbar cord first; indeed, except in cases of spina bifida (with which hydromyelia may be associated) the discovery of a lumbar syrinx in a patient without a history of injury should always raise the possibility of a spinal glioma or ependymoma, though intramedullary metastases (Weitzner, 1969) or extramedullary tumours are less often associated with such a lesion. In cases of traumatic paraplegia or arachnoiditis, the cavities usually ascend from the site of the lesion, but in upper cervical lesions downward cavitation is sometimes found. The cavitation has been attributed to a combination of factors including venous obstruction, exudation of protein, and ischaemia (Barnett et al., 1973), while oedema (Feigin et al., 1971) may be another factor.

Brewis et al. (1966) found the prevalence of syringomyelia over all to be 8·4 per 100,000 in an English city. The condition has been described in more than one member of a family (Bentley et al., 1975) and other congenital malformations, including spina bifida, have been found in families containing affected members. It is commoner in males than females and symptoms can appear at any age between 10 and 60 years but usually between 25 and 40.

SYMPTOMS

The symptoms of syringomyelia are readily interpreted as the outcome of the progressive lesion in the central region of the spinal cord.

Mode of onset

The onset is usually insidious but rarely develops rapidly over the course of a few weeks. Wasting and weakness of the small muscles of the hands are common early symptoms, but the patient may notice loss of feeling in the hands or the resulting injuries. Less often pain or trophic lesions first attract attention.

Sensory Symptoms and Signs

At the earliest stage there is an elongated cavity, situated in the central grey matter, and extending longitudinally through several segments, usually in the lower cervical and upper thoracic segments of the cord. The lesion is often predominantly unilateral at first and its effect is to interrupt on one side the decussating sensory fibres derived from several consecutive dorsal roots. Since the fibres which decussate shortly after entering the cord are those which conduct impulses concerned in the appreciation of pain, heat, and cold, these forms of sensibility are impaired while other forms are preserved. This is the dissociated sensory loss described by Charcot, and is usually first observed along the ulnar border of the hand, forearm, and arm, and upper part of the chest and back on one side in a 'half-cape' distribution with a horizontal lower border across the chest wall and ending sharply at the midline. Sometimes, however, the impaired sensibility occupies the 'glove' area. When the lesion is centrally situated from the first, or has extended from one side of the cord to the other, the area of dissociated sensory loss is bilateral. As the lesion extends upwards and downwards in the cord, the area of sensory impairment extends to the radial sides of the upper limbs and the neck, and downwards over the thorax, exhibiting at this stage a distribution *en cuirasse*. The areas over which appreciation of pain, heat, and cold are first impaired, and later lost, are not always, nor even usually, co-terminous, but any one may be more extensive than the others. When the lesion reaches the upper cervical segments, it begins to involve the spinal tract and nucleus of the trigeminal nerve, which receives fibres conducting impulses concerned in the appreciation of pain, heat, and cold from the face. Progressive destruction of these fibres causes extension of the area of dissociated sensory loss in a concentric manner from behind forwards on the face, sensibility on the tip of the nose and upper lip sometimes being last affected. Exceptionally the disorder begins in the medulla, in which case sensibility is first impaired on the face.

The progressive extension of the spinal lesion later causes compression of the lateral spinothalamic tracts on one or both sides, leading to loss of appreciation of pain, heat, and cold over the lower parts of the body. There is sometimes an area of normal sensibility over the abdomen intervening between the area of thoracic anaesthesia due to interruption of the decussating fibres and the area of sensory loss on one or both lower limbs due to compression of the spino-thalamic tracts. Sensation over the posterior aspects of the lower limbs is usually affected last. When the spinothalamic tract is compressed at the level of the medulla, appreciation of pain, heat, and cold is impaired or lost over the whole of the opposite half of the body. The posterior columns are usually the last of the sensory pathways to suffer, but in the late stages appreciation of posture, passive movement, and vibration is likely to be impaired, especially in the lower limbs, and there may be extensive anaesthesia to light touch.

Thermo-anaesthesia may be detected by the patient, owing to the fact that hot water no longer feels hot over the affected parts of the body, and his analgesia exposes him to injuries, especially burns of the fingers, which he does not notice at the time, because they are painless. Spontaneous pains, though usually absent, are sometimes troublesome, and the patient may describe burning, aching, or shooting pains which may in some respects resemble the lightning pains of tabes but more often the pain is continuous and may then cause considerable distress. Such pains in one side of the face or in the upper limb may be the first symptom. When the lesion begins in the thoracicolumbar or lumbosacral regions of the cord the dissociated loss has a corresponding distribution. In non-communicating cases secondary to spinal cord trauma or other lesions, an ascending sensory 'level' after months or years during which the neurological condition had been static usually gives a clue to the presence of this lesion.

Optic atrophy is exceptional, but has occasionally been described, presumably due to associated occult hydrocephalus.

Motor Symptoms and Signs

The earliest motor symptoms are usually muscular weakness and wasting, due to atrophy of the anterior horn cells produced by compression. Since the lesion usually begins in the cervicothoracic region of the cord, muscular wasting usually first appears in the small muscles of the hands. It may be bilateral from the beginning, or one hand may suffer before the other. As the lesion extends, the muscular wasting spreads to involve the forearms, and later the arms, shoulder girdles, and upper intercostals. It is often slight, and is never as severe as is seen in advanced cases of motor neurone disease. Fasciculation is uncommon. Contractures may develop, especially in the muscles of the hand and forearm. Extension of the lesion to the posterolateral part of the medulla often involves the nucleus ambiguus, causing paresis of the soft palate, pharynx, and vocal cord, occasionally causing laryngeal stridor (Alcala and Dodson, 1975). The other motor functions in which the cranial nerves are concerned are less frequently affected, though Brain observed paralysis of the mandibular muscles, lateral rectus, facial muscles, and soft palate on one side as a result of haemorrhage into a syringomyelic cavity in the pons and medulla. The tongue is occasionally involved. Nystagmus is commonly present in syringomyelia. It is variable in character, sometimes being phasic and present on lateral gaze, but may be dissociated in type, while vertical nystagmus on upward gaze is not uncommon (Thrush and Foster, 1973); it has been ascribed to involvement of the vestibular and cerebellar connections within the brain stem. Paralysis of the ocular sympathetic on one or both sides may be present, and leads to small and often irregular pupils, with ptosis and slight enophthalmos. The reaction to light is preserved.

Compression of the corticospinal tracts in the spinal cord causes weakness, with slight spasticity and extensor plantar responses in the majority of cases in the later stages. The loss of power, however, is rarely severe. The tendon reflexes are exaggerated in the lower limbs, and usually diminished or lost in the upper limbs particularly on the side of the dissociated anaesthesia, presumably due to interruption of the reflex arc; only rarely are they exaggerated in the arms, depending upon the predominance of the upper motor neurone lesion. The sphincters are usually little affected. As with the sensory findings, ascending weakness of lower or upper motor neurone type, or both, is an important feature of non-communicating syringomyelia, extending upwards from a spinal lesion.

Trophic Symptoms and Signs

Trophic symptoms are conspicuous. True hypertrophy involving all the tissues may be present in one limb or one-half of the body or even of the tongue. Loss of sweating or excessive sweating may occur, usually over the face and upper limbs. Excessive sweating may be spontaneous or may be excited reflexly when the patient takes hot or highly-seasoned food. Twenty per cent of patients exhibit osteo-arthropathy—Charcot's joints. The shoulders, elbows, and cervical spine are most frequently affected, less often the joints of the hands, the temporomandibular joint, the sternoclavicular and acromioclavicular joints, and the joints of the lower limbs. Atrophy and decalcification of the bones in the region of the joints with erosion of joint surfaces and subsequent bony destruction are the usual radiographic findings [FIG. 126]. The development of the joint changes is not usually associated with pain. The affected joint is often enlarged, and movement evokes loud crepitus but is generally painless. The long bones are

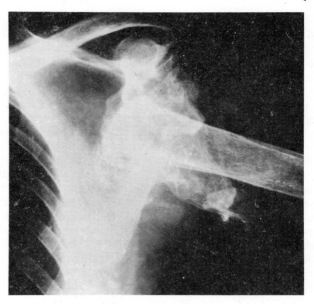

FIG. 126. A Charcot's shoulder joint in syringomyelia

frequently brittle. Trophic changes in the skin include cyanosis, hyperkeratosis, and thickening of the subcutaneous tissues, leading to a swelling of the fingers described as 'la main succulente'. The analgesia, as already described, renders the patient exceptionally liable to minor injuries, and the poor nutrition of the hands delays healing. Ulceration, whitlows, and necrosis of bone are not uncommon. Gangrene rarely occurs. The scars of former injuries are usually evident upon the palmar surface of the fingers [FIG. 127].

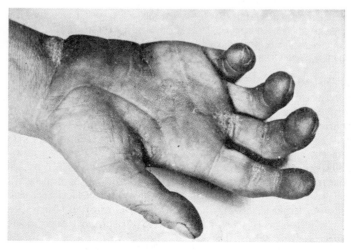

FIG. 127. Hand in syringomyelia, showing muscular wasting and fleshy fingers with scars of burns

Syringobulbia

The medulla may be involved by upward extension from the spinal cord, or may be the initial site of the disorder. In the latter case the onset of symptoms may be sudden or gradual. Trigeminal pain, vertigo, facial, palatal, or laryngeal palsy, or wasting of the tongue may be the presenting symptom. The physical signs of syringobulbia have been described above.

Morvan's Syndrome

Morvan in 1883 described patients with painless whitlows on the fingers of both hands. Subsequently this title has been applied to cases in which there is progressive loss of pain sensation, ulceration, loss of soft tissue, and resorption of the phalanges with muscular atrophy, not only in the hands but sometimes also in the feet, with perforating ulcers. While it is now clear that such changes in the hands may rarely occur in syringomyelia (Barnett et al., 1973), a similar syndrome may occur in some cases of leprosy and in most cases in which all four extremities are involved, the underlying pathology is usually one of hereditary sensory neuropathy or so-called acrodystrophic neuropathy (Spillane and Wells, 1969; Bradley, 1974).

Associated Abnormalities

A large number of abnormalities have been described in association with syringomyelia, occurring either in affected individuals or in members of their families. Bremer (1926) drew attention to the following anomalies: deformities of the sternum, kyphoscoliosis, a difference in the size of the breasts, increase in the ratio between arm and body length, acrocyanosis of the hands, curved fingers, enuresis, and anomalies of the hair and ears. Common abnormalities which may be added to Bremer's list include cervical rib, spina bifida, basilar impression of the skull, fusion of cervical vertebrae (the Klippel–Feil syndrome) with shortening of the neck, and other craniovertebral anomalies, hydrocephalus, and pes cavus (Barnett et al., 1973). Light brown pigmentation either in spots or diffuse sheets, often with a segmental distribution, is occasionally seen, especially on the shoulders.

The Cerebrospinal Fluid

The CSF usually shows no abnormality unless the cavity has been large enough to cause a block when the protein content of the fluid may be raised.

Radiology

Straight radiographs of the cervical spine may show in some cases congenital anomalies (e.g. fusion of vertebral bodies) or may demonstrate that the antero-posterior diameter of the spinal canal is greater than normal. Prone myelography will usually confirm that the spinal cord itself is enlarged and is usually helpful in identifying the cause of non-communicating syringomyelia (such as a spinal tumour or arachnoiditis) but supine examination of the region of the foramen magnum using injected air or contrast medium is necessary to show the descent of the cerebellar tonsils (Chiari type I anomaly) with which many 'communicating' cases are now known to be associated [FIG. 128] (Appleby et al., 1968; Barnett et al., 1973). When no such abnormality is demonstrated air encephalography or even ventriculography with air or contrast medium may be needed to show the closure of the exit foramina of the fourth ventricle or the basal arachnoiditis which is present in some other cases.

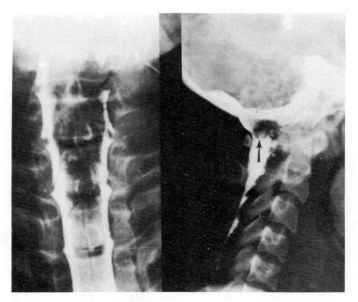

FIG. 128. The myelographic appearances of communicating syringo-myelia in association with a Chiari type I anomaly. The anteroposterior view (on the left) shows marked widening of the upper cervical cord, while the lateral supine view demonstrates the ectopic cerebellar tonsils (arrow)

DIAGNOSIS

There is little difficulty in making a diagnosis of syringomyelia when the disorder is advanced, since the association of wasting and trophic lesions of the hands with extensive dissociated sensory loss, and with symptoms of cortico-spinal tract lesions in the lower limbs is distinctive. The diagnosis is much more difficult in the early stages and this is particularly important if treatment is to be effective. Intramedullary tumour of the spinal cord (especially ependy-moma) may closely simulate syringomyelia. As a rule, however, it progresses more rapidly and blockage of the spinal subarachnoid space, with resulting changes in the CSF, is likely to occur. The same is true of extramedullary spinal tumours with the addition that pain is usually a more prominent symptom of this lesion than of syringomyelia. Haematomyelia, though it may produce similar symptoms to syringomyelia, develops acutely. It must be remembered that haemorrhage into a syringomyelic cavity constitutes one form of haemato-myelia. Cervical spondylosis, though it may cause wasting of proximal upper limb muscles and paraesthesiae in the hands as well as spastic weakness of the lower limbs, does not cause dissociated sensory loss over the upper limbs. Motor neurone disease may simulate syringomyelia when it begins with wasting of the small muscles of the hands, especially when the corticospinal fibres to the lower limbs are simultaneously involved. Sensory loss, however, is absent, and muscular wasting develops much more rapidly. In motor neurone disease muscular fasciculation is almost constantly present and is frequently widespread, whereas in syringomyelia it is less common. Cervical rib may cause symptoms which resemble those of the early stage of syringomyelia, and the distinction between the two is rendered difficult by the fact that they may coexist. Pain along the ulnar border of the hand and forearm is a common result of cervical rib, but rare in syringomyelia, and it is usual for the latter condition to come under observation at a stage at which sensory loss possesses an extent larger than can be attributed to a cervical rib. Peroneal muscular atrophy is distinguished from syringomyelia by the fact that muscular wasting of the lower limbs usually precedes that of the upper. The trophic symptoms of Raynaud's disease may simulate syringomyelia, but the dissociated sensory loss is absent in the former, while in the latter the attacks of blanching of the fingers observed in Raynaud's disease do not occur. Hereditary sensory neuropathy is distinguished by its early onset and by the distal loss of pain sensation in all four limbs.

Syringobulbia presents little difficulty in diagnosis when the medullary lesion is an upward extension of cervical syringomyelia. When it occurs alone, however, it must be distinguished from other lesions of the medulla. Thrombosis of the posterior inferior cerebellar artery, which usually leads to sensory loss similar to that found in syringobulbia, is distinguished by its acute onset. Tumours of the medulla may closely simulate syringobulbia, especially as symptoms of increased intracranial pressure may be slight or absent, but the onset is more rapid, and extension to the pons, leading to paralysis of the lateral rectus or of conjugate ocular deviation and to facial paresis, is common in the case of medullary tumours and rare in syringobulbia. Progressive bulbar palsy is distinguished by the absence of sensory loss. The diagnosis of basilar impression, which may closely simulate or be associated with syringomyelia, can be established only radiographically [see p. 1090].

PROGNOSIS

The course of syringomyelia, if untreated, is progressive, though progress is frequently slow and arrest may occur, so that the patient's condition may remain unchanged for many years. A sudden intensification of symptoms may follow minor trauma (Barnett et al., 1973) or be produced by haemorrhage into a syringomyelic cavity, and occasionally distension of the spinal cord may become so marked as to produce a complete transverse lesion leading to paraplegia. Both of these events, however, are exceptional, and sufferers from syringomyelia frequently live many years, death occurring either from bulbar paralysis, leading to bronchopneumonia, or from some independent disease.

TREATMENT

In the past, apart from physiotherapeutic measures designed to reduce spasticity, delay contractures and improve movement in weakened limbs, treatment of this condition was largely symptomatic. The protection of analgesic areas and early treatment of cutaneous lesions in order to promote healing were also regarded as essential and remain obligatory today. In some cases continuous pain has required powerful analgesics and occasionally surgical methods for its relief, if intractable (medullary tractotomy or stereotaxic thalamotomy), have been required. Some surgeons have recommended laminectomy for decompression of the swollen spinal cord with aspiration or incision and drainage of the cavity but the results of the procedure have usually been disappointing. However, in non-communicating cases secondary to spinal tumour or arachnoiditis, laminectomy with partial or complete removal of the causal tumour, decompression, the drainage of arachnoidal cysts, or the division of fibrous bands tethering the cord may all be of benefit. When ascending cavitation follows a complete traumatic transverse lesion of the cord, the process may be arrested by total excision of a segment of the spinal cord at and just above the level of the injury (Barnett *et al.*, 1973). For many years radiotherapy, introduced first in 1905, had a considerable vogue and was believed to be particularly successful in relieving pain, while some have suggested that sensory loss and muscular weakness and trophic changes were often reduced by this method. In recent years, however, its use has declined progressively.

The recent discovery that in many communicating cases the condition is secondary to hydromyelia resulting from a developmental anomaly (Chiari malformation) in the region of the foramen magnum (Gardner, 1965; Appleby *et al.*, 1968) has prompted many surgeons to recommend that the upper cervical cord and lower medulla should be decompressed at the foramen magnum and that if the exit foramina of the fourth ventricle are occluded they should be opened up and the upper end of the central canal should then be occluded with muscle; aspiration of the central cavity may also be necessary (Hankinson, 1970). If carried out sufficiently early in the course of the disease, the results of these procedures seem encouraging in that dissociated sensory loss may gradually disappear and reflex changes may be reversed; occasionally there is complete recovery. Surgical treatment should thus be seriously considered in all such cases seen within a few years of the onset but is less likely to be helpful if the condition is long-established. When the condition is secondary to basal arachnoiditis or when a Chiari malformation is accompanied by arachnoiditis, the results of this operation are much less satisfactory. Some surgeons now recommend ventriculo-atrial drainage with a Spitz–Holter or other appropriate valve in this type of case, but the results of this procedure are variable and its value has yet to be determined.

REFERENCES

ALCALA, H., and DODSON, W. E. (1975) Syringobulbia as a cause of laryngeal stridor in childhood, *Neurology (Minneap.)*, **25**, 875.

APPLEBY, A., FOSTER, J. B., HANKINSON, J., and HUDGSON, P. (1968) The diagnosis and management of the Chiari anomalies in adult life, *Brain*, **91**, 131.

BARNETT, H. J. M., FOSTER, J. B., and HUDGSON, P. (1973) *Syringomyelia* (Major Problems in Neurology series, ed. Walton, J. N.), London.

BENTLEY, S. J., CAMPBELL, M. J., and KAUFMANN, P. (1975) Familial syringomyelia, *J. Neurol. Neurosurg. Psychiat.*, **38**, 346.

BRADLEY, W. G. (1974) *Disorders of Peripheral Nerves*, Oxford.

BREMER, F. W. (1926) Klinische Untersuchungen zur Ätiologie der Syringomyelie, der 'Status dysraphicus', *Dtsch. Z. Nervenheilk.*, **95**, 1.

BREWIS, M., POSKANZER, D. C., ROLLAND, C., and MILLER, H. G. (1966) Neurological disease in an English city, *Acta neurol. scand.*, **42**, Suppl. 24.

CRUCHET, R., and DELMAS-MARSALET, P. (1939) Sur la maladie de Morvan, *Confin. neurol. (Basel)*, **2**, 32.

CURTIUS, F., and LORENZ, I. (1933) Über den Status dysraphicus, klinischerbiologische und rassenhygienische Untersuchungen an 35 Fällen von Status dysraphicus und 17 Fällen von Syringomyelie, *Z. ges. Neurol. Psychiat.*, **149**, 1.

CZERNY, L. J., and HEINISMANN, J. I. (1930) Beiträge zur Pathologie und Röntgentherapie der Syringomyelie, *Z. ges. Neurol. Psychiat.*, **125**, 573.

FEIGIN, I., OGATA, J., and BUDZILOVICH, G. (1971) Syringomyelia: the role of edema in its pathogenesis, *J. Neuropath. exp. Neurol.*, **30**, 216.

FOSTER, J. B., HUDGSON, P., and PEARCE, G. W. (1969) The association of syringomyelia and congenital cervicomedullary anomalies: pathological evidence, *Brain*, **92**, 25.

GARDNER, W. J. (1965) Hydrodynamic mechanism of syringomyelia; its relationship to myelocele, *J. Neurol. Psychiat.*, **28**, 247.

GARDNER, W. J., and ANGEL, J. (1958) The cause of syringomyelia and its surgical treatment, *Cleveland Clinic Quarterly*, **25**, 4.

HANKINSON, J. (1970) Syringomyelia and the surgeon, in *Modern Trends in Neurology*, ed. Williams, D., p. 127, London.

JONESCO-SISESTI, N. (1929) *Tumeurs médullaires associées à un processus syringomyélique*, Paris.

JONESCO-SISESTI, N. (1932) *La Syringobulbie*, Paris.

LASSMAN, L. P., JAMES, C. C. M., and FOSTER, J. B. (1968) Hydromyelia, *J. neurol. Sci.*, **7**, 149.

MORVAN, A. M. (1883) De la parésie analgésique à panaris des extrémitiés supérieures ou paréso-analgésie des extrémitiés supérieures, *Gazette Hebdomadaire Medecine et de Chirurgie*, **35**, 580.

PETRÉN, K., and LAURIN, E. (1925) Diagnosis of spinal tumors, with especial consideration of Rontgen-ray treatment of tumors and of syringomyelia, *Arch. Neurol. Psychiat. (Chic.)*, **14**, 1.

SCHLESINGER, H. (1902) *Die Syringomyelia*, Leipzig.

SPILLANE, J. D., and WELLS, C. E. C. (1969) *Acrodystrophic Neuropathy*, London.

THRUSH, D. C., and FOSTER, J. B. (1973) An analysis of nystagmus in 100 consecutive patients with communicating syringomyelia, *J. neurol. Sci.*, **20**, 381.

WEITZNER, S. (1969) Coexistent intramedullary metastasis and syringomyelia of cervical spinal cord, *Neurology (Minneap.)*, **19**, 674.

WELLS, C. E. C., SPILLANE, J. D., and BLIGH, A. S. (1959) The cervical spinal canal in syringomyelia, *Brain*, **82**, 23.

WILLIAMS, B. (1969) Hypothesis: the distending force in the production of 'communicating syringomyelia', *Lancet*, **ii**, 189.

MYELODYSPLASIA

Myelodysplasia was the term employed by Fuchs (1909) to describe a condition which he believed to be due to incomplete closure of the neural tube in the embryo. It is frequently familial and sometimes hereditary, and in some respects superficially resembles lumbar syringomyelia. Unlike the latter condition, however, it is non-progressive. The symptoms usually indicate a disturbance of function of the lumbosacral region of the spinal cord, though other parts may be affected. Myelodysplasia is closely related to spina bifida, with which it is almost invariably associated.

Lumbosacral myelodysplasia has been held responsible for a variety of disturbances which are occasionally familial. The following are the principal symptoms: impairment of sphincter control, leading especially to enuresis; deformities of the feet, for example, pes cavus and syndactylism of the toes; wasting of the muscles below the knees, with impairment of the ankle-jerks; dissociated sensory loss of a syringomyelic character over one or both legs; and trophic disturbances of the feet, such as delayed healing of wounds, chronic ulceration, and gangrene. Symptoms usually become apparent in childhood but in less severe lesions the condition first becomes manifest in young or even middle-aged adults. Spina bifida may only be apparent radiologically.

The commonest anatomical abnormality of the spinal cord is *diastematomyelia* (a bifid state of the lower cord). In many cases the two spinal cords are contained within a single dural tube but in others each of the two cords has its own dural sheath and the two are separated by a bony or fibrocartilaginous septum [FIG. 129] which may prevent the normal ascent of the cord as the vertebral column grows or else it may compress one or other spinal cord (James and Lassman, 1964). Either this anomaly itself or other associated lesions within the spinal canal such as lipomas (Lassman and James, 1967), which are commonly present in cases of 'spinal dysraphism' may demand surgical treatment which often produces considerable improvement. Other associated lesions found in some cases include intramedullary dermoids, adhesions in the cauda equina, and ectopic dorsal nerve roots (James and Lassman, 1967), while a low conus medullaris, tethered by a fibrous band to the dura in the region of an

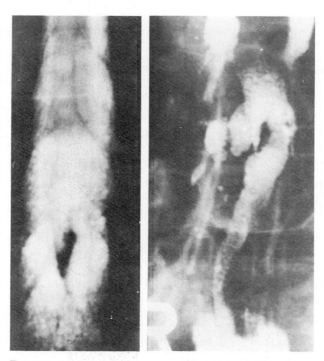

FIG. 129. A myelogram in a case of diastematomyelia; a prone anteroposterior view (on the left) shows diastematomyelia with a midline septum; the supine view (on the right) shows an intrathecal lipoma in the same case

occult spina bifida may give a similar clinical picture (James and Lassman, 1972). Rarely a similar anatomical anomaly in the cervical region may give a clinical picture resembling that of syringomyelia. Myelography is invaluable in differential diagnosis but must usually be performed by the cisternal route under general anaesthesia in children (Gryspeerdt, 1963).

Myelodysplasia is distinguished from syringomyelia by the fact that it is occasionally familial, by its non-progressive character, and by its predominant incidence upon the lower limbs. Other causes of muscular wasting and of trophic lesions of the feet must be excluded, especially peroneal muscular atrophy, hereditary sensory neuropathy, tabes, and gangrene of vascular origin.

The spinal defect upon which the symptoms depend is non-progressive, but there is a tendency for trophic lesions to occur and the patient may be progressively crippled by these.

It seems that in selected cases, particularly when the lesion is in the lumbar region, laminectomy with removal of lipomas or of bands which constrict or tether the spinal cord or its roots is often beneficial.

REFERENCES

BIJE, L. (1956) *Status Dysrhaphicus*, Baarn.
BRUNS, F. (1903) Familiare symmetrischer Gangran und Arthropathie, *Neurol. Zbl.*, **22**, 599.
CURTIUS, F., and LORENZ, I. (1933) Über den Status dysraphicus, klinischerbiologische und rassenhygienische Untersuchungen an 35 Fällen von Status dysraphicus und 17 Fällen von Syringomyelie, *Z. ges. Neurol. Psychiat.*, **149**, 1.
FUCHS, A. (1909) Über den klinischen Nachweis kongenitaler Defektbildungen in den unteren Rückenmarksabschnitten (Myelodysplasia), *Wien. med. Wschr.*, **59**, 2142, 2262.
GRYSPEERDT, G. L. (1963) Myelographic assessment of occult forms of spinal dysraphism, *Acta Radiol.*, **1**, 702.
JAMES, C. C. M., and LASSMAN, L. P. (1964) Diastematomyelia, *Arch. Dis. Childh.*, **39**, 125.
JAMES, C. C. M., and LASSMAN, L. P. (1967) Results of treatment of progressive lesions in spina bifida occulta five to ten years after laminectomy, *Lancet*, **ii**, 1277.
JAMES, C. C. M., and LASSMAN, L. P. (1972) *Spinal Dysraphism (Spina Bifida Occulta)*, London.
LASSMAN, L. P., and JAMES, C. C. M. (1967) Lumbosacral lipomas: critical survey of 26 cases submitted to laminectomy, *J. Neurol. Neurosurg. Psychiat.*, **30**, 174.
LICHTENSTEIN, B. W. (1940) Spinal dysraphism. Spina bifida and myelodysplasia, *Arch. Neurol. Psychiat. (Chic.)*, **44**, 792.
RILEY, H. A. (1930) Syringomyelia or myelodysplasia, *J. nerv. ment. Dis.*, **72**, 1.
THÉVENARD, A. (1942) L'arthropathie ulcéro-mutilante familiale, *Rev. neurol. (Paris)*, **74**, 193.

CAUDAL DYSPLASIA

This rare developmental anomaly, sometimes called the caudal regression syndrome, is characterized by clinical and radiographic evidence of agenesis of the sacrococcygeal segments of the vertebral column and spinal cord; there is associated severe atrophy of the related spinal roots and nerves with grossly impaired innervation of the lower limb musculature (Price *et al.*, 1970). Patients so affected have neurological abnormalities ranging in severity from mild impairment of bladder control to total motor and sensory paralysis below the level of the lesion.

REFERENCE

PRICE, D. L., DOOLING, E. C., and RICHARDSON, E. P. (1970) Caudal dysplasia (caudal regression syndrome), *Arch. Neurol. (Chic.)*, **23**, 212.

SPINA BIFIDA

Synonym. Rachischisis.

Definition. Incomplete closure of the vertebral canal, which is usually associated with a similar anomaly of the spinal cord, or, when less severe, with other less striking intraspinal abnormalities.

AETIOLOGY AND PATHOLOGY

In the early embryo the nervous system is represented by the neural groove, the lateral folds of which unite dorsally to form the neural tube. An arrest in this process of development leads to defective closure of the neural tube, associated with a similar defect in the closure of the bony vertebral canal—spina bifida. A number of varieties of spina bifida are described, differing in respect of the nature and severity of the spinal defect. In the severe form a sac protrudes through the vertebral opening, which yields an impulse on crying and coughing, and compression of which in the infant increases the tension of the fontanelle. The sac may contain meninges only—meningocele; in more severe cases it contains both meninges and the flattened, opened, or bifid spinal cord—myelocele or meningomyelocele. In such cases, when the cutaneous covering is incomplete, there may be a discharge of cerebrospinal fluid. Very rarely the central canal of the cord is closed but dilated—syringomyelocele. Talwalker and Dastur (1970) distinguish six anatomical varieties of meningocele depending upon the association of such additional defects as fistulae, aberrant neural tissue, and tethering of the cord or roots, and three varieties of meningomyelocele which they prefer to call 'ectopic spinal cord'. In the least severe cases there is no protrusion, but a defect in the laminae may be palpable as a depression, which is sometimes covered by a dimple or a tuft of hair (spina bifida occulta). There may, however, be no visible or palpable abnormality and the laminal defect may then be detected radiologically.

The commonest site of spina bifida is the lumbosacral region. Occasionally it is found in the thoracic region, very rarely in the cervical. In lumbosacral spina bifida the spinal cord frequently retains its fetal length and extends as low as the sacrum. James and Lassman (1967, 1972) have found in many cases of spina bifida occulta a variety of lesions including diastematomyelia, intramedullary dermoid, hydromyelia, cauda equina compression due to a fibrous band or to adhesions, ectopic dorsal nerve roots and subcutaneous lumbosacral lipoma communicating with a similar intraspinal lipoma. Spina bifida may be associated with other congenital abnormalities such as hydrocephalus due to atresia of the cerebral aqueduct or the Chiari type I (ectopia of the cerebellar tonsils) or type II (tonsillar ectopia with malformation of the medulla and cervical cord) (Spillane and Rogers, 1959; Emery and MacKenzie, 1973), occipital meningocele, cervical hydromyelia or syringomyelia, hare lip, and cleft palate. There may be general physical hypoplasia, with some degree of mental defect. Severe degrees of spina bifida may be incompatible with survival, the victim being stillborn or surviving birth only a short time. Paralysis of the lower limbs and of the sphincters is usually present in the latter type of case.

Renwick (1972) suggested that spina bifida and anencephaly might be related to the consumption of potatoes affected by 'blight', but this hypothesis has not been supported by subsequent epidemiological studies which did, however, suggest a slightly increased incidence in females and a significant increase in incidence in Rochester, Minnesota in 1944 corresponding to a rubeola epidemic (Haynes et al., 1974). A possible relationship to hardness of water supplies is also unconfirmed to date (Lowe et al., 1971). MacMahon and Yen (1971) noted a threefold increase in the incidence of these malformations in Boston, Massachusetts, in the years 1929–32, corresponding with the years of the great depression. Carter and Evans (1973) have estimated that the risk that a parent with spina bifida may transmit the condition to his or her offspring of either sex is about 3 per cent.

SYMPTOMS AND SIGNS

Spina bifida occulta may give rise to no symptoms and may be an accidental discovery in the course of a routine examination. It is present in 17 per cent of all spines X-rayed (Curtius and Lorenz, 1933). It is of considerable clinical importance, however, since intradural lesions associated with it sometimes give rise to symptoms, the cause of which is not immediately evident. In such cases a careful investigation of the history often shows that symptoms were present at an early age, though improvement may have occurred, to be followed by a relapse in early adult life. However, in occasional cases, symptoms, say due to an intradural lipoma, may not appear until middle or late life. Such a relapse may be due to the effect of growth in causing tension upon the lower end of the cord and cauda equina, which are anchored at an abnormally low level, or to the compression of these structures by a lipoma, dermoid, or constricting band. The symptoms are those of a chronic lesion of the cauda equina, though frequently one function is more conspicuously affected than others.

Frequently it has been noted that the patient was slow in learning to walk and walked clumsily at first. Muscular wasting and weakness may be present in the muscles below the knees, with impairment or loss of the ankle-jerks and contracture of the calf muscles, leading to pes cavus. James and Lassman (1967, 1972) have drawn particular attention to a milder syndrome of progressive muscular imbalance and neurological deficit resulting in deformity of one or both feet in childhood with, in some cases, trophic ulceration and incontinence, and point out that this syndrome resulting from minimal spinal dysraphism always demands investigation as early treatment may prevent progressive deformity. Sensation may be impaired over the cutaneous areas innervated by the lowest sacral segments, leading to the characteristic saddle-shaped area of analgesia over the buttocks and posterior surface of the thighs. Pain is usually inconspicuous. Sphincter disturbances are often prominent. Enuresis may be present, either constantly or intermittently, from infancy. The patient may have been late in gaining control over the bladder as a child, and this may never have become complete. Frequently nocturnal enuresis is associated with precipitate micturition by day. Less often retention of urine develops with secondary hydro-ureter and hydronephrosis and resulting impairment of renal function. Jancke (1916) described a sibship in which enuresis occurred in several generations and was associated with spina bifida in those members who were examined radiographically. The rectal sphincter is less often affected, though constipation or, less frequently, incontinence of faeces may occur. Impotence may be present in the male, either from the beginning of sexual life or after a period of normal potency. Trophic changes are conspicuous in some cases, and are rarely altogether lacking. In milder cases the feet are usually cold and cyanosed, and cutaneous injuries are slow in healing and tend to lead to ulceration, not only of the feet but also of the analgesic skin of the buttocks and thighs. Gangrene of the toes may occur and arthropathies have been described in the feet. These more severe neurological and associated abnormalities, of all degrees of severity up to complete flaccid paraparesis with sphincter paralysis, are more often associated with overt spina bifida than with the occult form. Less common associated abnormalities include global atrophy or oedema of one lower limb, melanoleucoderma, and cutaneous naevi.

Cervical spina bifida occulta may be associated with hydromyelia or diastematomyelia causing symptoms resembling those of syringomyelia in the upper limbs, with wasting and trophic disturbances in the hands, and dissociated sensory loss.

The cerebrospinal fluid as a rule shows no abnormality, though lumbar puncture may be difficult or impossible at the usual level. Radiography shows defective fusion of the laminae in the affected region, usually the first sacral and fifth lumbar. Myelography is usually best performed by the cisternal route in such cases and is often successful in demonstrating diastematomyelia, an unusually low position of the conus medullaris, a typical filling defect due to a lipoma, or even a fibrous band constricting the cauda equina (Gryspeerdt, 1963).

DIAGNOSIS

The diagnosis of severe forms of spina bifida with a protruding sac is easy. Spina bifida occulta, however, may be missed, if it is not borne in mind as a possible cause of the symptoms of which the patient complains. All cases of enuresis for which no cause can be found, especially when precipitate micturition occurs by day, should be carefully examined for the presence of minor neurological signs in the lower limbs, and radiographs of the lumbosacral spine should be taken. The more severe symptoms of spina bifida require to be differentiated from those of a tumour of the cauda equina, while, when trophic lesions are prominent, it is necessary to exclude Raynaud's disease and thrombo-angiitis obliterans. The fact that in spina bifida symptoms have often been present since birth is an important diagnostic point, and the rarity of pain and the non-progressive character of the symptoms will help to exclude a tumour. The cerebrospinal fluid protein content is much more often raised when a tumour is present than in cases of dysraphism. The ischaemia of the fingers characteristic of Raynaud's disease is absent in spina bifida and the arterial pulse is not reduced in volume, as is the case in arterial disease. X-ray examination of the spine and myelography afford confirmatory evidence.

Antenatal Diagnosis. An important recent development has been the discovery that estimation of alpha-fetoprotein in the amniotic fluid (Brock and Sutcliffe, 1972; Allan et al., 1973; Seller et al., 1973) or in the maternal serum (Brock et al., 1974; Wald et al., 1974) may successfully identify a fetus with a severe CNS malformation such as spina bifida cystica or anencephaly. Ultrasonic examination may be a useful but less accurate adjuvant (Campbell et al., 1975). Screening of pregnant women by means of serum alpha-fetoprotein estimation is therefore possible followed by ultrasonic examination and/or amniocentesis (British Medical Journal, 1975), leading in appropriate cases to therapeutic abortion.

PROGNOSIS

In the past, sufferers from the more severe degrees of spina bifida did not long survive. However, in recent years, early surgical treatment carried out in the first few days of life (see below) has resulted in there being many more survivors. Laurence (1974) showed that without operation, in 100 patients with myelocele and meningocele, only 17 will survive into the teens without operation with eight minimally handicapped and five dependent on wheelchairs. With aggressive early operative treatment 50 per cent will survive, 15 being minimally handicapped and 27 dependent on wheelchairs. There was a significantly higher incidence of mental handicap, usually due to hydrocephalus, in the survivors following operation.

In patients suffering complications of occult spina bifida the prognosis is generally very much better, especially now that ascending urinary infection and other renal complications can usually be treated effectively.

TREATMENT

Sharrard (1963) and others showed that the survival rate of sufferers from meningomyelocele may be greatly increased and subsequent disability greatly reduced by operative closure of the sac within the first 48 hours of life. Subsequently neurosurgical treatment may be required for associated hydrocephalus and a variety of orthopaedic procedures may also be needed. Even if the lower limbs appear totally paralysed and anaesthetic, walking may eventually be possible with the aid of appropriate appliances if training is begun sufficiently early, usually towards the end of the second year of life. Incontinence of urine may be controlled in some cases by propantheline given in doses graded according to age, 15 mg three times daily in the adult, while retention of urine may initially require catheterization followed later by bladder neck resection. Urinary infection will require appropriate antibiotics and incontinence of faeces is usually controlled eventually by the use of suppositories, regular enemas or even, in some cases, manual evacuation as the child grows older. The selection of cases for early operation, depending upon the potential quality of life in the survivors and the prospect of independent existence, has been a fertile source of controversy and raises serious ethical problems. Lorber (1973, 1975) has argued against a policy of operating upon all cases; in 37 newborn infants he advised against operation in 25 because of the severity of the malformation and all died within 9 months. Hunt et al. (1973) found the definition of predictive factors difficult but stressed the importance of defining the level of sensory impairment. Smith and Smith (1973) favour operating early upon most infants with low lesions and a low sensory level, but postponing consideration of surgery for at least a month in more severe cases.

There is now good evidence that in cases of spina bifida occulta, operation carried out soon after symptoms first become apparent, to divide a constricting band, remove or decompress a lipoma or a dermoid cyst, may produce considerable improvement and prevent progressive deformity. This is particularly important in childhood so that growth of an affected limb will not be impaired but operation may be equally successful if symptoms first develop in adult life.

REFERENCES

ALLAN, L. D., FERGUSON-SMITH, M. A., DONALD, I., SWEET, E. M., and GIBSON, A. A. M. (1973) Amniotic-fluid alpha-fetoprotein in the antenatal diagnosis of spina bifida, *Lancet*, **ii**, 522.

BRITISH MEDICAL JOURNAL (1975) Antenatal diagnosis of spina bifida, *Brit. med. J.*, **1**, 414.

BROCK, D. J. H., BOLTON, A. E., and SCRIMGEOUR, J. B. (1974) Prenatal diagnosis of spina bifida and anencephaly through maternal plasma-alpha-fetoprotein measurement, *Lancet*, **i**, 767.

BROCK, D. J. H., and SUTCLIFFE, R. G. (1972) Alpha-fetoprotein in the antenatal diagnosis of anencephaly and spina bifida, *Lancet*, **ii**, 197.

CAMPBELL, S., PRYSE-DAVIES, J., COLTART, T. M., SELLER, M. J., and SINGER, J. D. (1975) Ultrasound in the diagnosis of spina bifida, *Lancet*, **i**, 1065.

CARTER, C. O., and EVANS, K. (1973) Children of adult survivors with spina bifida cystica, *Lancet*, **ii**, 924.

CURTIUS, F., and LORENZ, I. (1933) Über den Status dysraphicus, klinischerbäiologische und rassenhygienische Untersuchungen an 35 Fällen von Status dysraphicus und 17 Fällen von Syringomyelie, *Z. ges. Neurol. Psychiat.*, **149,** 1.

EMERY, J. L., and MACKENZIE, N. (1973) Medullo-cervical dislocation deformity (Chiari II deformity) related to neurospinal dysraphism (meningomyelocele), *Brain*, **96,** 155.

GRYSPEERDT, G. L. (1963) Myelographic assessment of occult forms of spinal dysraphism, *Acta radiol. (Stockh.)*, **1,** 702.

HASSIN, G. B. (1925) Spina bifida occulta cervicalis, *Arch. Neurol. Psychiat. (Chic.)*, **14,** 813.

HAYNES, S. G., GIBSON, J. B., and KURLAND, L. T. (1974) Epidemiology of neural-tube defects and Down's syndrome in Rochester, Minnesota, 1935–1971, *Neurology (Minneap.)*, **24,** 691.

HUNT, G., LEWIN, W., GLEAVE, J., and GAIRDNER, D. (1973) Predictive factors in open myelomeningocele with special reference to sensory level, *Brit. med. J.*, **4,** 197.

JAMES, C. C. M., and LASSMAN, L. P. (1967) Results of treatment of progressive lesions in spina bifida occulta five to ten years after laminectomy, *Lancet*, **ii,** 1277.

JAMES, C. C. M., and LASSMAN, L. P. (1972) *Spinal Dysraphism (Spina Bifida Occulta)*, London.

JANCKE (1915–16) Über eine Bettnässerfamilie, zugleich ein Beitrag zur Erblichkeit der Spina bifida, *Dtsch Z. Nervenheilk.*, **54,** 255; also Röntgenbefunde bei Betnässern, *Dtsch Z. Nervenheilk.*, **55,** 334.

LASSMAN, L. P., and JAMES, C. C. M. (1967) Lumbosacral lipomas: critical survey of 26 cases admitted to laminectomy, *J. Neurol. Psychiat.*, **30,** 174.

LAURENCE, K. M. (1974) Effect of early surgery for spina bifida cystica on survival and quality of life, *Lancet*, **i,** 301.

LORBER, J. (1973) Early results of selective treatment of spina bifida cystica, *Brit. med. J.*, **3,** 201.

LORBER, J. (1975) Ethical problems in the management of myelomeningocele and hydrocephalus, *J. roy. Coll. Phycns Lond.*, **10,** 47.

LOWE, C. R., ROBERTS, C. J., and LLOYD, S. (1971) Malformations of central nervous system and softness of local water supplies, *Brit. med. J.*, **2,** 357.

MACMAHON, B., and YEN, S. (1971) Unrecognized epidemic of anencephaly and spina bifida, *Lancet*, **i,** 31.

RENWICK, J. H. (1972) Hypothesis: Anencephaly and spina bifida are usually preventable by avoidance of a specific but unidentified substance present in certain potato tubers, *Br. J. prev. soc. Med.*, **26,** 67.

ROBERTS, J. B. M. (1962) Spina bifida and the urinary tract, *Ann. roy. Coll. Surg. Engl.*, **31,** 69.

SELLER, M. J., CAMPBELL, S., COLTART, T. M., and SINGER, J. D. (1973) Early termination of anencephalic pregnancy after detection by raised alpha-fetoprotein levels, *Lancet*, **ii,** 73.

SHARRARD, W. J. W. (1963) Meningomyelocele: prognosis of immediate operative closure of the sac, *Proc. roy. Soc. Med.*, **56,** 510.

SMITH, G. K., and SMITH, E. D. (1973) Selection for treatment in spina bifida cystica, *Brit. med. J.*, **4,** 189.

SPILLANE, J. D., and ROGERS, L. (1959) Lumbosacral spina bifida cystica with craniovertebral anomalies: report of two cases presenting with neurological disorder in adult life, *J. Neurol. Neurosurg. Psychiat.*, **22,** 44.

TALWALKER, V. C., and DASTUR, D. K. (1970) 'Meningoceles' and 'meningomyeloceles' (ectopic spinal cord). Clinicopathological basis of a new classification, *J. Neurol. Neurosurg. Psychiat.*, **33,** 251.

WALD, N. J., BROCK, D. J. H., and BONNAR, J. (1974) Prenatal diagnosis of spina bifida and anencephaly by maternal serum-alpha-fetoprotein measurement, *Lancet*, **i,** 765.

MYELITIS

Definition. Inflammation of the spinal cord, usually involving both the grey and the white matter, in a considerable part of its transverse extent. When the lesion is limited longitudinally to a few segments, it is described as transverse myelitis; when it spreads progressively upwards, as ascending myelitis.

AETIOLOGY

Myelitis may be a manifestation of meningovascular syphilis [see pp. 461–4]. It may be due to participation of the cord in acute or subacute encephalomyelitis due to a neurotropic virus or in acute disseminated encephalomyelitis, disseminated myelitis and optic neuritis, and acute disseminated encephalomyelitis complicating vaccination, smallpox, measles, chickenpox, or other specific fevers [p. 529]. Thus it has been described as a complication of varicella (White, 1962) and antirabies vaccination (Prussin and Katabi, 1964), to name only two causes, and it may complicate infective mononucleosis [p. 446]. In herpes zoster myelitis, the causal virus has been isolated from the spinal cord (Hogan and Krigman, 1973). An episode indistinguishable from an attack of transverse myelitis may be one presentation of multiple sclerosis.

Myelitis may be due to infections of the cord with pyogenic organisms, which may reach it through a penetrating wound, by extension from osteomyelitis of an adjacent vertebra, by inward spread from pyogenic meningitis, or through the blood stream from a focus of infection in any part of the body, the latter being the route of infection when myelitis rarely complicates typhoid fever or brucellosis. Tuberculous myelitis may follow tuberculous caries of the spine.

PATHOLOGY

To the naked eye the spinal cord at the site of inflammation, which is usually the lower thoracic region, exhibits oedema and hyperaemia, and in severe cases actual softening—myelomalacia. Microscopically, the leptomeninges are congested and infiltrated with inflammatory cells. The substance of the cord exhibits congestion or thrombosis of the vessels with perivascular inflammatory infiltration, and oedema. There is degeneration of the ganglion cells of the grey matter, the myelin sheaths and axis cylinders of the white. The cord is diffusely infiltrated with inflammatory cells and with compound granular corpuscles. There is a hyperplasia of neuroglia. Ascending and descending degeneration can be traced in the long tracts. Abscess of the spinal cord is a very rare form of localized myelitis. The pus is to a variable extent encapsulated and, as it tends to spread longitudinally, the abscess usually assumes a spindle shape [p. 738]. When myelitis is due to pyogenic organisms, these may be demonstrable in films or on culture, and spirochaetes may be present in the syphilitic form, but in myelitis forming part of acute disseminated encephalomyelitis and in the form which occurs sporadically no virus or other infecting organism can often be demonstrated and it seems likely that this is often an acute demyelinating process due to hypersensitivity rather than infection.

SYMPTOMS

The onset of symptoms is acute or subacute, and there is often some pyrexia. There is usually considerable pain in the back at the level of the lesion. Flaccid paralysis, partial or complete, then develops more or less rapidly, being confined to part of the trunk and the lower limbs when the thoracic region of the cord is the part involved. Sensory loss, which may be complete or incomplete, is present and usually exhibits an upper level corresponding to the segmental site of the lesion. There may be a zone of hyperpathia intervening between the area of sensory loss and that of normal sensibility above, and the spine may be tender in this region. There is an impairment of sphincter control, often amounting to complete paralysis of the bladder and rectum. The tendon reflexes are usually at first diminished or lost, and the abdominal reflexes are lost below the level of the lesion. The plantar reflexes may be absent for a few days after the onset and later become extensor. In the ascending form of myelitis there is a more or less rapid upward progression of the level of paralysis and sensory loss.

The cerebrospinal fluid usually contains a considerably increased protein content and an excess of cells, which are polymorphonuclear in cases of pyogenic myelitis, but usually exclusively or predominantly mononuclear in other forms. The V.D.R.L. and other serological reactions are negative, except in syphilitic cases. The gamma-globulin in the fluid is often raised, especially when an episode of 'transverse myelitis' is the first manifestation of multiple sclerosis.

DIAGNOSIS

The rapid onset of the symptoms of a transverse or ascending lesion of the spinal cord usually renders the diagnosis easy. Myelitis is distinguished from acute infective or post-infective polyneuritis (the Guillain-Barré syndrome) by the presence of extensor plantar reflexes, and of partial or complete sensory loss with a segmental upper level. Haematomyelia usually develops after injury; it usually involves the cervical enlargement and causes greater damage to the grey than to the white matter of the cord. Syphilitic myelitis is distinguished by the history of infection and signs of cerebral syphilis, when these are present, and by positive serological reactions in the blood and cerebrospinal fluid. When myelitis forms part of an attack of acute disseminated encephalomyelitis, symptoms of cerebral lesions may be present, and in the cases following vaccination and the specific fevers the causal condition is usually readily discovered from the history. In disseminated myelitis and optic neuritis the diagnosis is clear when the latter precedes the former. Otherwise it must remain in doubt until optic neuritis develops. When myelitis complicates poliomyelitis, the patient exhibits in addition the typical atrophic paralysis. In zoster myelitis the diagnosis is established by the characteristic eruption. Though multiple sclerosis may be suspected as the cause of a transverse lesion of the spinal cord, especially in a young adult, this diagnosis can only be established if there is a history of previous and characteristic lesions of the nervous system, or if signs of this—for example, pallor of the optic discs or nystagmus—are present. Myelitis can be attributed to infection with pyogenic organisms only when a focus of such infection can be found or the organism grown.

PROGNOSIS

The prognosis depends upon the aetiology of the condition and its severity. Pyogenic myelitis is usually fatal, and so is the ascending form but occasional cases of intramedullary abscess have been treated successfully by means of antibiotics and surgical drainage and methods of mechanically-aided respiration have saved many patients who would previously have died of ascending myelitis. Any form of myelitis which is sufficiently severe to lead to a complete functional interruption of the cord is a very grave condition owing to the risk of death from urinary or cutaneous infection. However, even in such cases if complications are treated effectively, recovery is possible. In myelitis forming part of one of the various forms of acute disseminated encephalomyelitis the prognosis is often good, and if the patient survives the acute attack considerable functional recovery is the rule. In sporadic cases of myelitis a guarded prognosis should be given in view of the possibility that the cord lesion may be the first symptom of multiple sclerosis. For the prognosis of syphilitic myelitis see page 463, and for that of acute disseminated myelitis with optic neuritis see page 543.

TREATMENT

The general treatment of the patient must be carried out on the lines indicated for the treatment of paraplegia [see p. 725]. Any specific cause must receive appropriate treatment. For the treatment of syphilitic myelitis see page 463, and for that of acute disseminated myelitis with optic neuritis see page 544.

In those cases in which no cause for the condition can be demonstrated (these are the majority) there is now good evidence that treatment with ACTH, 80 Units intramuscularly daily, when given in the acute phase and continued for several weeks or months in diminishing dosage improves the outcome.

REFERENCES

BUZZARD, E. F., and GREENFIELD, J. G. (1921) *Pathology of the Nervous System*, London.
DAVISON, C., and KESCHNER, M. (1933) Myelitic and myelopathic lesions (a clinico-pathologic study). 1. Myelitis, *Arch. Neurol. Psychiat. (Chic.)*, **29**, 332.
HOGAN, E. L., and KRIGMAN, M. L. (1973) Herpes zoster myelitis, *Arch. Neurol. (Chic.)*, **29**, 309.
HUGHES, J. T. (1966) *Pathology of the Spinal Cord*, London.
PRUSSIN, G., and KATABI, G. (1964) Dorsolumbar myelitis following antirabies vaccination with duck embryo vaccine, *Ann. int. Med.*, **60**, 114.
WHITE, W. H. (1962) Varicella myelopathy, *New Engl. J. Med.*, **266**, 772.

RADIATION MYELOPATHY

A syndrome of slowly progressive paraparesis, due to radiation injury to the spinal cord, may develop one to four years after a course of ionizing radiation given usually to the neck or mediastinum for the treatment of post-cricoid carcinoma or bronchial carcinoma with mediastinal spread. Weakness, spasticity, and sensory loss usually develop gradually, often with impairment of sphincter control (Palmer, 1972) and the condition often becomes arrested. The cerebrospinal fluid is usually normal and so, too, is myelography. However, occasionally cord swelling may result from radiation necrosis giving a myelographic appearance simulating an intramedullary tumour (Marty and Minckler, 1973). The dose of radiation given has almost always exceeded 4,000 r and is usually of the order of 6,000–8,000 r (Pallis *et al.*, 1961). Pathologically, vacuolation and degeneration of the neurones and white-matter degeneration are seen while the spinal arterioles and capillaries are usually greatly thickened and show narrowing of their lumina. Coagulative necrosis of the grey matter at the site of maximal exposure to radiation is sometimes seen (Burns *et al.*, 1972) but vascular occlusion is usually prominent in addition (Palmer, 1972). Similar pathological changes occur in the brain in late radiation encephalopathy (de Reuck and vander Eecken, 1975).

REFERENCES

BURNS, R. J., JONES, A. N., and ROBERTSON, J. S. (1972) Pathology of radiation myelopathy, *J. Neurol. Neurosurg. Psychiat.*, **35**, 888.
DE REUCK, J., and VANDER EECKEN, H. (1975) The anatomy of the late radiation encephalopathy, *Europ. Neurol.*, **13**, 481.
HUGHES, J. T. (1966) *Pathology of the Spinal Cord*, London.
MARTY, R., and MINCKLER, D. S. (1973) Radiation myelitis simulating tumor, *Arch. Neurol. (Chic.)*, **29**, 352.
PALLIS, C. A., LOUIS, S., and MORGAN, R. L. (1961) Radiation myelopathy, *Brain*, **84**, 460.
PALMER, J. J. (1972) Radiation myelopathy, *Brain*, **95**, 109.

SUBACUTE NECROTIC MYELITIS

This condition, first described by Foix and Alajouanine (1926) and subsequently by Greenfield and Turner (1939) and by Mair and Folkerts (1953) is commoner in men than in women and in the older age group, particularly in patients with chronic cor pulmonale. Clinically it is characterized by a slowly progressive and ascending weakness of the lower extremities with variable sensory loss and sphincter disturbance; there are signs of combined upper and lower motor neurone lesions and the clinical picture indicates a slowly progressive disorder of the cauda equina and lower spinal cord extending over several years. The protein content of the cerebrospinal fluid is usually raised and myelography, which is necessary to exclude a spinal tumour, is either negative or may demonstrate dilated blood vessels on the surface of the cord. Pathologically the cord is shown to be necrotic and there is widespread distension and often thrombosis of veins on the surface and within its substance. Some authors believe that the condition is due to a spinal thrombophlebitis (Blackwood, 1963), others that there is true venous angioma formation. No treatment is available though the condition is so rarely diagnosed in life that anticoagulants have not been given an adequate trial.

A disorder of similar clinical presentation, but quite different in its pathological characteristics and entitled 'subacute necrotic myelopathy', has been described as a complication of carcinoma [p. 872].

REFERENCES

BLACKWOOD, W. (1963) in *Greenfield's Neuropathology*, 2nd ed., ed. Blackwood, W., McMenemey, W. H., Meyer, A., Norman, R. M., and Russell, D. S., London.
FOIX, C., and ALAJOUANINE, T. (1926) La myélite nécrotique subaiguë, *Rev. neurol.*, **2**, 1.
GREENFIELD, J. G., and TURNER, J. W. A. (1939) Acute and subacute necrotic myelitis, *Brain*, **62**, 227.
MAIR, W. G. P., and FOLKERTS, J. F. (1953) Necrosis of the spinal cord due to thrombophlebitis (subacute necrotic myelitis), *Brain*, **76**, 563.

LANDRY'S PARALYSIS

In 1859 Landry first described a condition of acute ascending paralysis and subsequently the name 'Landry's paralysis' was commonly given to cases showing such a clinical presentation. It is now well recognized that this is a syndrome and not a single disease entity and the use of the term as a definitive diagnosis can no longer be justified. In very acute cases which present with sensory disturbance in the limbs followed by the rapid development of flaccid areflexic paralysis and a fatal outcome, usually within a few days, the condition can usually be classified pathologically as one of *acute necrotic myelopathy* (Hughes, 1966). *Transverse* or *ascending myelitis* as described above may also give rise to a clinical picture of ascending paralysis of variable severity, while *post-infective polyneuritis* or *polyradiculopathy* (the Guillain-Barré syndrome) is yet another cause. The episodes of ascending paralysis which may follow acute exanthemata or inoculation, particularly with rabies vaccine, are plainly due to acute disseminated or ascending myelitis, while during epidemics, occasional cases of poliomyelitis may present in this way, as may the acute polyneuropathy which complicates some cases of porphyria. A toxin produced by the bite of the Rocky Mountain wood tick has been known to produce similar symptoms which resolve when the tick is removed (Gibbes, 1938) while Symonds (1949) described such a syndrome associated with a high serum potassium due to renal failure. Thus the prognosis and management of cases so-called 'Landry's paralysis' are dependent upon the elucidation of the cause of the syndrome in every case.

REFERENCES

GIBBES, J. H. (1938) Tick paralysis in South Carolina, *J. Amer. med. Ass.*, **111**, 1008.
HUGHES, J. T. (1966) *Pathology of the Spinal Cord*, London.
LANDRY, O. (1859) Note sur la paralysie ascendante aiguë, *Gaz. hebd. Méd.*, **6**, 472.
SYMONDS, C. P. (1949) Reorientation in neurology, *Lancet*, **i**, 677.

SOME OTHER SPINAL CORD LESIONS

Nutritional and metabolic disorders of the spinal cord including syndromes due to B_{12} deficiency, tropical spastic paraplegia, and subacute myelo-opticoneuropathy are described in CHAPTER 15, as are the effects of chemical and electrical injury. Myoclonus as a symptom of spinal cord disease is considered on page 1134.

INFARCTION AND ISCHAEMIA OF THE SPINAL CORD AND CAUDA EQUINA

The Blood Supply of the Spinal Cord and Cauda Equina

In the cervical and upper thoracic regions the major blood supply of the spinal cord is derived from the anterior spinal artery, which is formed by the union of the two anterior spinal branches which arise from the vertebral arteries within the cranial cavity. It runs in the anterior median fissure of the cord and receives small tributaries at different levels from the inferior thyroid arteries and from the costocervical trunk, each of which is derived from the corresponding subclavian artery. The anterior spinal artery supplies the anterior and lateral columns of the cord and the greater part of the spinal grey matter. The two small posterior spinal arteries also arise from the vertebrals intracranially and receive numerous small radicular tributaries entering the spinal cord along the posterior nerve roots; they supply the posterior columns of the cord. There are scanty circumferential vessels on the surface of the cord which form anastomoses between the anterior and posterior spinal vessels.

In the lower thoracic and lumbar regions the anterior and posterior spinal arteries receive large tributaries from the intercostal and lumbar branches of the aorta which contribute the major blood supply of the lower cord. One such vessel, the great anterior radicular artery of Adamkewicz (1882) which usually enters the spinal cord at about the T8 segment but may do so at any level from T8 to L4, appears to be of particular importance. The vessels in the lowest segments of the cord and the roots of the cauda equina receive tributaries from the iliolumbar and lateral sacral branches of the internal iliac arteries. Published work on the anatomy of the spinal cord arterial tree and upon its variable and inconstant but profuse venous drainage has been reviewed by Hughes (1966), by Garland et al. (1966), by Henson and Parsons (1967) by Gillilan (1970), and by Di Chiro and Fried (1971). The contribution made by spinal cord angiography to our understanding of spinal cord blood supply and drainage is mentioned on page 716.

Infarction of the Spinal Cord and Cauda Equina

Occlusion of the *anterior spinal artery* in the cervical region was shown by Spiller (1909) to produce infarction of the anterior and lateral columns of the cord from the fourth cervical to the third thoracic segments. Clinically the onset is abrupt, often with pain in the neck and back and paraesthesiae in the upper limbs followed by flaccid paralysis of both arms with loss of pain and temperature sensation below a variable level in the cervical region but with preservation of light touch and position and joint sense. Initially there is usually also flaccid paralysis of the lower limbs (spinal shock) but if the patient survives spastic weakness of the lower limbs develops with increased reflexes and extensor plantar responses. There is usually retention of urine and of faeces in the early stages but automatic bladder and bowel control may eventually be achieved. In severe cases paralysis remains complete and the prognosis is grave, but when infarction is less extensive the lower limbs may show a remarkable degree of recovery.

Anterior spinal artery occlusion ('spinal stroke') in the dorsal region is commonly a complication of dissecting aneurysm of the aorta, though it may result from embolism as a result of disintegration of an atheromatous plaque in the aorta (Wolman and Bradshaw, 1967) or from a drop in perfusion pressure (Silver and Buxton, 1974), from transient cardiac arrest (Gilles and Nag, 1971), or as a rare complication of spinal angiography (*The Lancet*, 1973). The central grey matter of the cord seems to be especially vulnerable to the effects of ischaemia (Herrick and Mills, 1971). When dissecting aneurysm is the cause, and occasionally in other cases, there is severe pain in the back followed by total and permanent flaccid paralysis of the lower limbs, sphincter paralysis and loss of pain and temperature sensation up to a sensory 'level' at about the umbilicus (corresponding to the T10 segment of the cord), but with preservation of some light touch sensation and of position and joint sense. Thrombosis of posterior spinal arteries complicating intrathecal phenol injection has been described (Hughes, 1970) as has venous infarction of the cord (Hughes, 1971), while infarction of the upper cervical cord, presumed to be due to spasm of spinal arteries, has been described as a sequel of minor spinal trauma in childhood (Ahmann et al., 1975).

While the clinical picture of anterior spinal artery occlusion has been recognized for many years, increasing attention has been paid more recently to the fact that infarction of the cord may sometimes be much more restricted, possibly due to occlusion of one posterior spinal artery or of one or more feeding or radicular arteries. In such cases weakness and sensory impairment may be restricted to one limb or may be asymmetrical in the two lower limbs and considerable or even complete recovery may take place after such a localized infarct. While rare by comparison with intermittent cerebral ischaemia, it also seems probable that transient episodes of weakness and of paraesthesiae in the lower extremities may well be due in many cases to *transient ischaemia of the spinal cord* or *cauda equina* (Wells, 1966; Garland et al., 1966; Henson and Parsons, 1967). Furthermore, there is now pathological evidence to suggest that repeated episodes of ischaemia or focal infarction may give rise to a slowly progressive spastic weakness of the lower limbs with variable sensory loss and signs of mixed upper and lower motor neurone involvement. In such cases of *atherosclerotic myelopathy*, a step-wise clinical course with episodes of deterioration alternating with periods of apparent arrest may suggest the nature of the disease, as may associated clinical evidence of atherosclerosis, but inflammatory, demyelinating, and neoplastic disorders must be excluded by means of radiology, cerebrospinal fluid examination, serological tests to exclude syphilis, and myelography. Rarely, collagen disease such as polyarteritis nodosa or systemic lupus erythematosus (Garcin, 1955) may give rise to episodes of spinal cord infarction.

Spinal cord embolism (Wolman and Bradshaw, 1967) due to the breakdown of an atheromatous plaque in the aorta so that fragments of cholesterol-containing debris are swept into the arteries of the cord, may give episodes of major infarction or chronic ischaemic myelopathy as described above. Similar episodes have been described in cases of subacute bacterial endocarditis; air and fat embolism of the cord appear to be very rare but decompression sickness (Caisson disease, p. 813) occurring during decompression in divers and compressed-air workers, in which bubbles of nitrogen appear in the circulating blood, commonly gives rise to transient episodes of spinal cord dysfunction and occasionally to incomplete or irreversible paraplegia (Haymaker, 1957).

Treatment, other than the usual nursing care of patients with paraplegia, is of little value in cases of spinal cord infarction. Vasodilator drugs may reasonably be given, but seem to be of little value and in cases of intermittent ischaemia or progressive myelopathy there are theoretical reasons for suggesting that anticoagulant drugs may be worthy of a trial. Surgical treatment of an aortic dissecting aneurysm is of no value once cord infarction has occurred.

Intermittent Claudication or Ischaemia of the Spinal Cord or Cauda Equina

In 1906 Dejerine first suggested that transient weakness or numbness of one or both lower limbs occurring during exercise might be due to ischaemia of the spinal cord. It is now well recognized that in some patients the lower spinal cord or the roots of the cauda equina may suffer a degree of compression which is sufficient to restrict their arterial blood supply but is not sufficient to give rise to any symptoms or abnormal physical signs at rest. However, when the patient begins to walk he often develops first aching pain in one or both calves similar to that of true intermittent claudication, but the peripheral pulses in the legs and feet are found to be normal. If he continues to walk, paraesthesiae in one or both feet may then supervene and it is not uncommon for foot-drop to follow (in ischaemia of the cauda equina) or spastic weakness of one or both legs (in

C C

ischaemia of the cord). In suspected cases the symptoms may be precipitated by appropriate exercise under supervision; when the cauda equina is principally affected one or both ankle jerks may disappear, while if the lower cord is being compressed the plantar responses may become extensor.

The condition can usually be shown by radiography and myelography, which are obligatory investigations in such cases, to be due to either a central inter-vertebral disc protrusion (Blau and Logue, 1961) or, in cases involving the cauda equina, a bony stenosis of the lumbar canal resulting from an overgrowth (of unknown aetiology) of the bony laminae (Verbiest, 1954; Joffe *et al.*, 1966). In either event, laminectomy and decompression of the spinal canal usually produces complete relief of symptoms.

REFERENCES

AHMANN, P. A., SMITH, S. A., SCHWARTZ, J. F., and CLARK, D. B. (1975) Spinal cord infarction due to minor trauma in children, *Neurology (Minneap.)*, **25**, 301.

BLAU, J. N., and LOGUE, V. (1961) Intermittent claudication of the cauda equina, *Lancet*, **i**, 1081.

DEJERINE, J. (1906) Sur la claudication intermittente de la moelle épinière, *Rev. neurol.*, **33**, 1.

DI CHIRO, G., and FRIED, L. C. (1971) Blood flow currents in spinal cord arteries, *Neurology (Minneap.)*, **21**, 1088.

GARCIN, R. (1955) Aspects neurologiques du lupus érythémateux disséminé, *Rev. Neurol.*, **92**, 511.

GARLAND, H., GREENBERG, J., and HARRIMAN, D. G. F. (1966) Infarction of the spinal cord, *Brain*, **89**, 645.

GILLES, F. H., and NAG, D. (1971) Vulnerability of human spinal cord in transient cardiac arrest, *Neurology (Minneap.)*, **21**, 833.

GILLILAN, L. A. (1970) Veins of the spinal cord. Anatomic details: suggested clinical applications, *Neurology (Minneap.)*, **20**, 860.

HAYMAKER, W. (1957) Decompression sickness, in *Handbuch der Speziellen Pathologischen Anatomie und Histologie*, vol. 13, ed. Scholz, W., p. 1600, Berlin.

HENSON, R. A., and PARSONS, M. (1967) Ischaemic lesions of the spinal cord: an illustrated review, *Quart. J. Med.*, **36**, 205.

HERRICK, M. K., and MILLS, P. E. (1971) Infarction of spinal cord. Two cases of selective gray matter involvement secondary to asymptomatic aortic disease, *Arch. Neurol. (Chic.)*, **24**, 228.

HUGHES, J. T. (1966) *Pathology of the Spinal Cord*, London.

HUGHES, J. T. (1970) Thrombosis of the posterior spinal arteries. A complication of an intrathecal injection of phenol, *Neurology (Minneap.)*, **20**, 659.

HUGHES, J. T. (1971) Venous infarction of the spinal cord, *Neurology (Minneap.)*, **21**, 794.

JOFFE, R., APPLEBY, A., and ARJONA, V. (1966) 'Intermittent ischaemia' of the cauda equina due to stenosis of the lumbar canal, *J. Neurol. Neurosurg. Psychiat.*, **29**, 315.

LANCET (1973) Spinal-cord damage after angiography, *Lancet*, **ii**, 1067.

SILVER, J. R., and BUXTON, P. H. (1974) Spinal stroke, *Brain*, **97**, 539.

SPILLER, W. G. (1909) Thrombosis of the cervical anterior median spinal artery: syphilitic acute anterior poliomyelitis, *J. nerv. ment. Dis.*, **36**, 601.

VERBIEST, H. (1954) A radicular syndrome from developmental narrowing of the lumbar vertebral canal, *J. Bone Jt. Surg.*, **36B**, 230.

WELLS, C. E. C. (1966) Clinical aspects of spinovascular disease, *Proc. roy. Soc. Med.*, **59**, 790.

WOLMAN, L., and BRADSHAW, P. (1967) Spinal cord embolism, *J. Neurol. Neurosurg. Psychiat.*, **30**, 446.

15

INTOXICATIONS AND METABOLIC DISORDERS

ALCOHOL ADDICTION

AETIOLOGY

ALCOHOL addiction is a symptom of many different mental disorders and every case requires careful psychological investigation. It is more common in males than in females, is rare before the age of 20, and most frequently occurs in middle life. A parental history of alcoholism is frequently present. Alcoholism may be a symptom of loss of self-control associated with the early stages of dementia, due, for example, to general paresis or cerebral arteriosclerosis. It may occur in schizophrenia or in manic-depressive psychosis. Though alcoholism is less common in females than males there appears to be a higher incidence of psychopathic personality in female than in male alcoholics and its incidence in females and in young people is increasing. In some cases the periodicity of the outbreaks of alcoholism is due to a periodically recurrent depression in an individual with cyclothymia. Alcohol addicts who are not frankly psychotic are usually neurotic, and take alcohol as a means of escape from the difficulties of life. Business worries and domestic unhappiness are common secondary causes. The alcohol is often taken in the form of spirits; and the alcohol addict may also be a drug addict. Indeed there is some evidence that there are personality traits common to many of those who become addicted to any drug, of which alcohol is one.

The WHO definition of an alcoholic is: 'Alcoholics are those excessive drinkers whose dependence upon alcohol has attained such a degree that they show a noticeable mental disturbance or an interference with bodily and mental health, their interpersonal relations and their smooth economic and social functioning; or who show the prodromal signs of such development. They therefore need treatment' (D.H.S.S., 1973).

INCIDENCE

It has been estimated that there are 4,390 alcoholics per 100,000 in the U.S.A. and at least 1,100 per 100,000 in Britain (Sim, 1975). The Department of Health and Social Security (D.H.S.S., 1973) estimate that there are about 400,000 alcoholics in England and Wales. There are important and complex differences in the incidence observed in various racial and ethnic groups (Jellinek, 1951; Williams and Glatt, 1965) but almost every country appears to have its 'skidrow' where down-and-out intractable drinkers and those who consume methyl alcohol tend to congregate (Bourne et al., 1966; Edwards et al., 1966; Olin, 1966).

PATHOLOGY

The prolonged consumption of alcohol produces degenerative changes in the central nervous system and in the peripheral nerves, which in their general features are similar to the effects of a large variety of other toxic agents. The brain is atrophied, and microscopically there is degeneration of the ganglion cells of the cerebral cortex. Degeneration of the middle layers of the corpus callosum is said to be characteristic (Marchiafava, 1933; Ironside *et al.*, 1961). In Wernicke's encephalopathy there are proliferation of capillaries, gliosis, and often patchy small haemorrhages in the corpora mammillaria and midbrain (Victor and Adams, 1953). In cases of polyneuritis the peripheral nerves exhibit degeneration of both myelin sheaths and of axis cylinders. There is evidence that the neuropathy, both central and peripheral, is not directly due to the alcohol, but is caused by deficiency of Vitamin B$_1$ [see p. 955]. This is also the cause of Wernicke's encephalopathy, which may complicate chronic alcoholism. Similarly alcoholic pellagra occurs. Victor and Adams (1961) conclude that whereas delirium tremens, alcoholic epilepsy, and alcoholic hallucinosis are due to habituation and alcohol withdrawal, and while Wernicke's disease, Korsakow's syndrome, polyneuropathy, retrobulbar neuropathy, and pellagra are due to nutritional deficiencies which are associated with alcoholism, the pathogenesis of alcoholic cerebellar degeneration, central pontine myelinolysis [see p. 564], of Marchiafava-Bignami disease and of alcoholic dementia is not yet fully understood and some of these disorders could prove to be due to a direct toxic effect of the long-continued ingestion of large quantities of alcohol. Cardiomyopathy and acute and chronic myopathic syndromes involving skeletal muscle have also been described in alcoholic patients (Ekbom *et al.*, 1964; Perkoff *et al.*, 1966).

Chronic malnutrition is common in alcoholic subjects who substitute alcoholic beverages for food; breakfast is often discarded first and later other meals are regularly missed.

SYMPTOMS

Acute Alcoholic Intoxication

The action of alcohol upon the nervous system is paralytic, the highest functions being first affected. The earliest symptoms of intoxication, therefore, are those of altered behaviour, and the social value of alcohol in moderate doses rests upon its power of paralysing those inhibitions which manifest themselves as shyness, and of reducing, in the individual who takes it, his capacity for criticizing his own utterances, and those of others. In larger doses it produces irregularities in conduct, the nature of which depends upon the temperament of the individual, who may be excited, voluble, combative, depressed, or maudlin. There is impairment of memory, especially for recent events. The ability to carry out co-ordinated and complex motor acts is progressively impaired (Drew *et al.*, 1958) and since October 1967 in Great Britain it has been an offence in law to drive a motor vehicle when the blood alcohol exceeds 80 mg/100 ml. In the Scandinavian countries the legal limit is very much lower. Eventually articulation becomes impaired; the conjunctivae are congested; the pupils are usually dilated, but may be contracted, and there may be some impairment of the pupillary reaction to light; nystagmus is invariable and diplopia may occur. In still larger doses alcohol produces unconsciousness, and finally death, through extension of the paralysis to vital centres.

The relationship between the alcoholic content of the blood and the state of the nervous system is variable. A great deal depends upon the body weight of the drinker, upon whether the simultaneous or previous ingestion of food delays the absorption of the alcohol, and upon whether or not the individual in question is accustomed to taking alcoholic drinks. In general there are few if any signs of intoxication with a blood level of below 100 mg/100 ml, although between 50 and 100 mg/100 ml some lack of inhibition and impairment of motor skills, with a slowing of reaction time, are generally apparent. Intoxication is usually clearly apparent in conversation with or on examining the individual with a blood level of 150 mg/100 ml but he is usually still in reasonable control of his behaviour and faculties at about this level, whereas at 200 mg/100 ml the signs of drunkenness are usually evident, and consciousness is generally lost, except in habitual heavy drinkers or alcoholic subjects, at a level between 250 and 300 mg/100 ml. As a very rough guide, up to three single 'tots' of spirit or three half-pints of British beer will, in the average individual, give a blood level within an hour of between 50 and 75 mg/100 ml.

Methyl Alcohol

The consumption of methyl alcohol in the form of methylated spirits, industrial alcohol, anti-freeze, and filtered metal polish is mainly seen in the poor in countries where alcoholic drinks are expensive, or in exceptionally degenerate alcoholics. It may cause severe toxic confusional states, irreversible optic atrophy with bilateral central scotomata or even total blindness and sometimes rapid death.

Pathological Drunkenness

In certain individuals, especially those who have suffered from head injury or organic lesions of the brain, a comparatively small dose of alcohol may rapidly produce the symptoms of acute intoxication and this may also occur in individuals taking barbiturate drugs regularly, in whom alcohol has an additive effect. It must of course be remembered that personal injury is common in alcoholic subjects so that one must be careful not to attribute to intoxication the effects of closed head injuries occurring in such subjects.

Delirium Tremens

The precise cause of delirium tremens is still uncertain. It is most frequently seen as the result of a prolonged debauch in the chronic alcoholic, but may be precipitated in such an individual by acute infection, or operation, or an accident. The sudden deprivation of alcohol is undoubtedly the most important factor.

The onset may be acute, but there is often a prodromal period of nervousness, anorexia, and insomnia. The characteristic symptoms are tremor, and acute confusion, accompanied by hallucinations, which are principally visual. The tremor is coarse and generalized, and is most evident in the face, tongue, and hands. The patient is completely disorientated, and experiences visual hallucinations, which often assume terrifying forms, especially of animals. Auditory hallucinations may also be present, and cutaneous sensations may be interpreted as insects crawling under the skin. The emotional mood is usually one of terror, and the patient may attempt to escape from his surroundings, and attack with violence those around him. Convulsions may occur. In addition to these nervous disturbances, symptoms of a severe toxaemia are present. Hyperpyrexia is not uncommon, and there may be albuminuria. The tongue is furred, the pulse rapid, and cardiac dilatation may occur. Delirium tremens runs an acute course, and in most cases recovery occurs in three or four days. In cases which end fatally, death is due to heart failure in which dehydration plays an important part, or to intercurrent lobar pneumonia to which such individuals are peculiarly subject.

Acute Alcoholic Hallucinosis

This condition occurs in chronic alcoholics, either developing gradually or coming on suddenly after unusual excess. It is characterized by hallucinations which, unlike those in delirium tremens, are predominantly auditory and are often associated with delusions of persecution; signs of delirium are absent.

Dipsomania

This outmoded term has sometimes been used to identify alcoholic subjects who embark upon recurrent drinking-bouts ('the lost week-end'), the craving for alcohol suddenly developing after a period of abstinence.

Korsakow's Psychosis

Korsakow's psychosis, though most frequently the result of chronic alcoholism with polyneuritis, may be due to other causes [see p. 1175]. It is often associated with Wernicke's encephalopathy [see p. 846]. The characteristic feature of Korsakow's psychosis is a disturbance of attention and memory, which leads to disorientation of the patient in space and time. His memory for recent events and his ability to retain new impressions are lost, and he fills the gap by confabulation, that is, the invention of a purely imaginary past. For example, one who has been bedridden for weeks describes with a wealth of detail a walk which he took on the previous day. Many clinical varieties of Korsakow's psychosis have been described, chiefly in terms of variations of the emotional mood, which is usually euphoric.

Alcoholic Cerebellar Degeneration

Victor et al. (1959) described 50 cases of this condition which is characterized by ataxia of stance and gait and of leg movements with little or no involvement of the arms (apart from action tremor which is seen in a few cases); nystagmus and dysarthria are absent in most cases. The condition appeared to progress over a period of a few weeks or months and then to become arrested in most cases. Pathological observations in 11 cases revealed a degeneration of all neurocellular elements of the cerebellar cortex, particularly of the Purkinje cells and also degeneration of the olivary nuclei. In the cerebellum changes were most striking in the anterior and superior aspects of the vermis and of the hemispheres.

Marchiafava-Bignami Disease

This rare condition, originally described in Italian drinkers of crude red wine is now known to occur in other alcoholic patients. It is characterized clinically by disorders of emotional control and cognitive function followed by variable delirium, fits, tremor, rigidity, and paralysis and most patients eventually become comatose and die within a few months. Symmetrical demyelination with subsequent cavitation and destruction of axis cylinders is found in the corpus callosum and often, in varying degree, in the central white matter of the cerebral hemispheres, in the optic chiasm, and in the middle cerebellar peduncles (Victor and Adams, 1961).

Alcoholic Dementia

Prolonged addiction to alcohol leads in many cases to progressive mental deterioration. There is nothing distinctive in the nature of the resulting dementia, which is characterized, like other dementias, by impairment of memory and intellectual capacity, emotional instability, moral deterioration, and carelessness with regard to dress and person. Delusions may be present, a delusion of marital infidelity being particularly common.

Alcoholic dementia may be associated with dysarthria, tremor, sluggish pupillary reactions to light, nystagmus, and muscular weakness.

The full clinical picture of alcoholic polyneuropathy may be present, but even in the absence of this the tendon reflexes are likely to be lost in the lower limbs.

Epilepsy

Epileptic attacks are not uncommon in chronic alcoholism, and are indistinguishable from the convulsions of idiopathic epilepsy. The convulsions of absinthe drinkers are due to the presence in the drink of the convulsant drug thujone. How other forms of alcohol cause epilepsy is not clearly understood. It would appear that fits may occur either at the height of a debauch, or much more often soon after withdrawal of alcohol ('rum fits') when they may be compared with the attacks which occur on the withdrawal of other drugs such as barbiturates.

Polyneuropathy

The symptoms of polyneuropathy which may complicate any form of chronic alcoholism are described on page 955 and pellagra is described on page 849.

Central Pontine Myelinolysis

This rare complication of alcoholism is considered on page 564.

Tobacco-Alcohol Amblyopia

This condition is considered on page 161. In Great Britain it is generally attributed to the effects of pipe tobacco, but American authors consider that heavy alcohol consumption is also a factor.

Alcoholic Myopathy

In 1962 Hed *et al.* described an acute muscular syndrome occurring in alcoholic patients after a debauch. Occasionally, muscle pain, tenderness and oedema were curiously localized in these cases but in others many skeletal muscles were involved. In severely affected individuals widespread muscle fibre necrosis, myoglobinuria, renal damage, and hyperkalaemia were found. Perkoff *et al.* (1966) described a similar reversible acute muscular syndrome occurring in chronic alcoholic patients; painful cramps and muscular tenderness were usually found, the serum creatine kinase activity was often raised and in most cases the serum lactate failed to rise after ischaemic work suggesting that glycogen utilization in the muscles was impaired. A subacute painless myopathy resolving after the withdrawal of alcohol has also been described by Ekbom *et al.* (1964). In a series of 44 cases, Oh (1972) found that 26 suffered from the acute syndrome while 18 had a subacute or chronic myopathy. Konttinen *et al.* (1970) found increased serum creatine kinase activity in 43 of 100 chronic alcoholic subjects.

Hepatic Encephalopathy

This syndrome which may complicate cirrhosis of the liver is not infrequently seen in alcoholic patients and is described on page 829. Increases in serum ornithine carbamoyl transferase and glutamate dehydrogenase activity, indicating liver cell and mitochondrial damage respectively, were found in many alcoholic patients by Konttinen *et al.* (1970), sometimes in the absence of other evidence of cirrhosis.

Other Metabolic Abnormalities

Severe hyponatraemia due to water intoxication and giving rise to disordered consciousness, sometimes with epileptic attacks and/or signs of corticospinal tract dysfunction, associated with alcoholic encephalopathy has been reported in heavy beer drinkers by Demanet *et al.* (1971).

Merry and Marks (1972) have drawn attention to disorders of hypothalamic, pituitary, and adrenal function in alcoholic subjects in whom morning plasma cortisol levels were above normal but fell after the ingestion of moderate amounts of alcohol, in contrast to the findings in control subjects.

Various haematological abnormalities, including disorders of haemopoiesis (Hillman, 1975) and of platelet function (Cowan, 1975) have also been described.

DIAGNOSIS

The diagnosis of both acute and chronic alcoholic poisoning presents little difficulty if a reliable history is available. The early stages of acute alcoholic intoxication must be distinguished from the effects of acute lesions of the nervous system, especially those following head injury, and a smell of alcohol in the breath is not proof that the symptoms are due to intoxication. The diagnosis of alcoholic coma is described on page 1166. The clinical picture in delirium tremens is highly distinctive, though a similar picture follows withdrawal of barbiturates or amphetamines. The history, however, and careful examination of the nervous system will settle the matter. Korsakow's psychosis may be associated with focal cerebral lesions as well as with non-alcoholic forms of polyneuropathy, and these must be distinguished from alcoholism by the history and clinical features. Alcoholic dementia must be distinguished from general paralysis. A history of alcoholic excess does not necessarily mean that this is the cause of the dementia, as alcoholism may complicate general paresis. In doubtful cases the cerebrospinal fluid and the blood serological reactions should be examined. In general paresis characteristic abnormalities are present in the fluid, and the serological reactions both in this and in the blood are positive. In arteriosclerotic dementia there is frequently evidence of focal cerebral vascular lesions; diagnosis from presenile dementia is usually dependent upon the history of alcoholism.

Alcoholic cerebellar degeneration must be distinguished from familial cerebellar ataxia and cerebellar degeneration secondary to carcinoma, while the Marchiafava-Bignami syndrome may simulate a tumour of the corpus callosum and central pontine myelinolysis can produce symptoms and signs similar to those which occur in brain stem tumour, demyelination due to other causes or basilar artery thrombosis. Alcoholic myopathy must be distinguished from McArdle's syndrome of myophosphorylase deficiency and from other forms of endocrine and metabolic myopathy. In all of these conditions the history of excessive alcoholic intake is crucial and it must be remembered that some alcoholics are very adept at concealing the evidence of their heavy and often secret drinking so that even a spouse may be unaware of the true state of affairs at least for a time. Concealment of empty bottles and of evidence of excessive spending on drink are common.

PROGNOSIS

The prognosis of alcohol addiction depends upon the underlying cause, and the stage at which treatment is begun. When the habit is the expression of a psychotic or a seriously unbalanced personality, or when there is a strong hereditary tendency to alcoholism, the outlook is bad. A history of previous 'cures' and relapses also makes the outlook unsatisfactory. Voegtlin and his collaborators (1942) claimed that many patients treated by 'conditional reflex therapy' remained abstainers four years later. In a series of cases of delirium tremens reported by Tavel *et al.* (1961) the mortality rate was 11·8 per cent. The mortality rate of patients with Korsakow's psychosis is also high. In mild cases recovery may be complete. In more severe cases, and cases of long standing, there is likely to be some permanent mental impairment.

The prognosis of chronic alcoholism and the results of treatment are reviewed by McKinley and Moorhead (1967) and by Victor and Adams (1974). Detailed reviews of the many medical consequences of alcoholism may also be found in Seixas *et al.* (1975).

Alcoholic dementia runs a slow course in most cases, lasting for years. In the early stages withdrawal of alcohol leads to marked improvement, sometimes to complete recovery. In long-standing cases the brain has been permanently damaged, and recovery is incomplete. Exceptionally the course is much more rapid, and in a few weeks or months a rapidly progressive dementia terminates in coma and death, often preceded by a terminal hyperpyrexia. Central pontine myelinolysis and the Marchiafava-Bignami disease appear to be universally fatal within a few months of the onset. Alcoholic cerebellar degeneration usually becomes arrested after a period of deterioration and the various forms of myopathy slowly resolve when the alcohol is withdrawn.

TREATMENT

Alcohol Addiction

The successful treatment of alcohol addiction requires thorough supervision, so that the amount of alcohol taken can be completely controlled. If the patient is to be treated in his own home, reliable nurses may be required. Often treatment can only be carried out successfully in an appropriate institution. Even so, many patients display remarkable cunning in obtaining access to supplies of alcohol and experience teaches that most alcoholics are accomplished and plausible liars. Complete and permanent abstinence from alcohol is the aim, but alcohol should never be suddenly withdrawn. The daily dose should be tapered, and in most cases the withdrawal can be accomplished within a week. Delirium tremens or other acute confusional states may follow sudden withdrawal. Diazepam or other appropriate tranquillizers are generally necessary during the withdrawal period; drugs for the treatment of depression (amitriptyline, imipramine) are often necessary in addition. During the period of treatment a careful psychological investigation must be carried out to ascertain the presence of any underlying psychosis or neurosis, and in suitable cases the patient should receive psychotherapeutic treatment and/or appropriate drugs. The necessity for complete and permanent abstinence must be impressed upon the patient, as the slightest lapse in this respect may be followed by relapse. Psychological help may be given by Alcoholics Anonymous (address in England, BM/AAL, London, W.C.1). It is a truism that chronic alcoholism is an incurable disease unless the patient really wishes to be cured when the association with others in a similar plight through A.A. may be invaluable. Unfortunately some patients may forswear alcohol and then become addicted to other drugs.

Voegtlin (1940) treated alcohol addiction by giving an injection of emetine and making the patient drink during the period of nausea, thus endeavouring to establish a conditioned reflex of aversion and aversion therapy has been used successfully by others. Apomorphine may similarly be used. The drug disulfiram (*Antabuse*) acts by sensitizing the patient to even a small dose of alcohol (Hald and Jacobsen, 1948; Martensen-Larsen, 1948). The usual dose is 0·5 g daily; whenever a patient receiving this drug takes alcohol an unpleasant reaction with headache, intense flushing, and vomiting follows due to the release of acetaldehyde into the circulation. Unfortunately, some fatal reactions have been described and it is all too easy for the patient to discontinue the drug on leaving hospital unless very carefully supervised. This drug should only be given in the first instance in hospital; side-effects due to long-term administration include depression, confusion, impotence, peripheral neuropathy, and a metallic taste. Calcium carbimide (*Abstem*), 50 mg twice daily, is similar but less violent in its effects and also less toxic in long-term administration. Victor and Adams (1974) and Sim (1975) review the literature of these and other modes of treatment.

Delirium Tremens

The sufferer from delirium tremens should be treated as a patient with a severe toxaemia involving not only the nervous but also the cardiovascular system. Every effort must be made, therefore, to keep him in bed, and careful nursing supervision is indispensable. It is unnecessary to give alcohol, but a high fluid intake is most important: Tavel *et al.* (1961) say that some severely ill patients may need up to 6 litres a day. Full doses of sedative will be required: those most often used in the past were barbiturates but recent evidence suggests that chlordiazepoxide (*Librium*), 50 mg, may be marginally more effective (Sereny and Kalant, 1965). Phenothiazine derivatives are also valuable but are not without risk of inducing hypotension (Browne *et al.*, 1959). Merry and Marks (1972) recommended diazepam in doses up to 30 mg as required; this drug has less effect in suppressing cortisol activity than the barbiturates. Large doses of the B and C vitamins should be given by injection, say in the form of *Parentrovite*. Smith (1949) recommended ACTH and this drug is now generally given in a dosage of 20–40 units 8-hourly for at least 48 hours. Antibiotic cover to prevent pneumonia and other infections is also necessary for four or five days.

Acute Alcoholic Hallucinosis

Hallucinosis should be treated on the same lines as delirium tremens.

Other Disorders

Korsakow's syndrome, Wernicke's encephalopathy, and alcoholic polyneuropathy should be treated by maintaining adequate nutrition and by the administration of large doses of thiamine and other vitamins. These measures are also appropriate in cases of alcoholic dementia and the other complications listed but have little if any effect in conditions such as cerebellar degeneration or Marchiafava–Bignami disease.

REFERENCES

BOURNE, P. G., ALFORD, J. A., and BOWCOCK, J. Z. (1966) Treatment of skid-row alcoholics, *Quart. J. Stud. Alcohol*, **27**, 242.

BROWNE, I. W., RYAN, J. P. A., and McGRATH, S. D. (1959) The management of the acute withdrawal phase in alcoholism, *Lancet*, **i**, 959.

CARMICHAEL, E. A., and STERN, R. O. (1931) Korsakoff's syndrome: its histopathology, *Brain*, **54**, 189.

COWAN, D. H. (1975) The platelet defect in alcoholism, in *Medical Consequences of Alcoholism*, ed. Seixas, F. A., Williams, K., and Eggleston, S., *Ann. N.Y. Acad. Sci.*, **252**, 328.

DEMANET, J. C., BONNYNS, M., BLEIBERG, H., and STEVENS-ROCMANS, C. (1971) Coma due to water intoxication in beer drinkers, *Lancet*, **ii**, 1115.

DEPARTMENT OF HEALTH AND SOCIAL SECURITY (1973) *Alcoholism*, Medical Memorandum, London.

DREW, G. C., COLQUHOUN, W. P., and LONG, H. A. (1958) Effect of small doses of alcohol on a skill resembling driving, *Brit. med. J.*, **2**, 993.

EDWARDS, G., HAWKER, A., WILLIAMSON, V., and HENSMAN, C. (1966) London's skid row, *Lancet*, **i**, 249.

EKBOM, K., HED, R., KIRSTEIN, L., and ASTROM, K. (1964) Muscular affections in chronic alcoholism, *Arch. Neurol. (Chic.)*, **10**, 449.

HALD, J., and JACOBSEN, E. (1948) A drug sensitizing the organism to ethyl alcohol, *Lancet*, **ii**, 1001.

HED, R., LUNDMARK, C., FAHLGREN, H., and ORELL, S. (1962) Acute muscular syndrome in chronic alcoholism, *New Engl. J. Med.*, **274**, 1277.

HILLMAN, R. S. (1975) Alcohol and hematopoiesis, in *Medical Consequences of Alcoholism*, ed. Seixas, F. A., Williams, K., and Eggleston, S., *Ann. N.Y. Acad. Sci.*, **252**, 297.

IRONSIDE, R., BOSANQUET, F. D., and McMENEMEY, W. H. (1961) Central demyelination of the corpus callosum (Marchiafava-Bignami disease), *Brain*, **84**, 212.

JELLINEK, E. M. (1951) W.H.O. Expert Committee on Mental Health. Subcommittee on Alcoholism. Report, *Wld Hlth Org., techn. Rep. Ser.* **42**, 20.

KONTTINEN, A., HÄRTEL, G., and LOUHIJA, A. (1970) Multiple serum enzyme analyses in chronic alcoholics, *Acta med. scand.*, **188**, 257.

McKINLEY, R. A., and MOORHEAD, H. H. (1967) Alcoholism, in *Progress in Neurology and Psychiatry*, ed. Spiegel, E. A., chap. 26, New York.

MARCHIAFAVA, E. (1932-3) The degeneration of the brain in chronic alcoholism, *Proc. roy. Soc. Med.*, **26**, 1151.

MARTENSEN-LARSEN, O. (1948) Treatment of alcoholism with a sensitizing drug, *Lancet*, **ii**, 1004.

MERRY, J., and MARKS, V. (1972) The effect of alcohol, barbiturate, and diazepam on hypothalamic/pituitary/adrenal function in chronic alcoholics, *Lancet*, **ii**, 990.

OH, S. J. (1972) Alcoholic myopathy: initial review, *Alabama J. med. Sci.*, **9**, 79.

OLIN, J. W. (1966) 'Skid-row' syndrome: a medical profile of the chronic drunkenness offender, *Canad. med. Ass. J.*, **95**, 205.

PERKOFF, G. T., HARDY, P., and VELEZ-GARCIA, E. (1966) Reversible acute muscular syndrome in chronic alcoholism, *New Engl. J. Med.*, **274**, 1277.

ROSENBAUM, M., and MERRITT, H. H. (1939) Korsakoff's syndrome. Clinical study of the alcoholic form, with special regard to prognosis, *Arch. Neurol. Psychiat. (Chic.)*, **41**, 978.

SEIXAS, F. A., WILLIAMS, K., and EGGLESTON, S. (1975) Medical Consequences of Alcoholism, *Ann. N.Y. Acad. Sci.*, **252.**

SERENY, G., and KALANT, H. (1965) Comparative clinical evaluation of chlordiazepoxide and promazine in treatment of alcohol-withdrawal syndrome, *Brit. med. J.*, **1**, 92.

SIM, M. (1975) *Guide to Psychiatry*, 3rd ed., Edinburgh.

SMITH, J. J. (1949) The treatment of acute alcoholic states with A.C.T.H. (adrenocortico-trophic) and A.C.E. (adrenocortical) hormones, *Quart. J. Stud. Alcohol*, **11**, 190.

TAVEL, M. E., DAVIDSON, W., and BATTERTON, T. D. (1961) A critical analysis of mortality associated with delirium tremens, *Amer. J. med. Sci.*, **242**, 18.

VICTOR, M., and ADAMS, R. D. (1953) The effect of alcohol on the nervous system, in *Metabolic and Toxic Diseases of the Nervous System*, p. 526, Baltimore.

VICTOR, M., and ADAMS, R. D. (1961) On the etiology of the alcoholic neurologic diseases, *Amer. J. clin. Nutr.*, **9**, 379.

VICTOR, M., and ADAMS, R. D. (1974) Alcohol, *Harrison's Principles of Internal Medicine*, 7th ed., chap. 111, New York.

VICTOR, M., ADAMS, R. D., and MANCALL, E. L. (1959) A restricted form of cerebellar cortical degeneration occurring in alcoholic patients, *Arch. Neurol. (Chic.)*, **1**, 579.

VOEGTLIN, W. L. (1940) The treatment of alcoholism by establishing a conditioned reflex, *Amer. J. med. Sci.*, **199**, 802.

VOEGTLIN, W. L., LEMERE, F., BROZ, W. R., and O'HOLLAREN, P. (1942) Conditioned reflex therapy of alcoholic addiction: follow-up report of 1042 cases, *Amer. J. med. Sci.*, **203**, 525.

WILLIAMS, G. P., and GLATT, M. M. (1965) Unrecognized drinking, *Lancet*, **ii**, 1294.

DRUG ADDICTION

GENERAL CONSIDERATIONS

Drug addiction may be defined as the habitual use of a drug in order to modify the personality and diminish the strain of life. It is characterized by tolerance (increased doses are required to produce the desired effect), craving, and the development of severe symptoms on deprivation of the drug. Drugs of addiction include opium and its derivatives, morphine, heroin, eucodal, dilaudid, pethidine, and various synthetic drugs; and cocaine. Within recent years addiction to barbiturates, amphetamine and its derivatives and to lysergic acid diethylamide (LSD) and other hallucinogens has been recognized increasingly and, more rarely, addiction to anaesthetic agents has been reported.

Drug habituation is a condition resulting from the repeated consumption of a drug in which there is a desire to continue taking the drug, but little or no tendency to increase the dose. The dependence is psychological and not physical, hence there are no physical symptoms of deprivation. Bromides, nicotine, and marihuana (cannabis) are drugs which may lead to habituation.

ADDICTION TO OPIATES AND OTHER SYNTHETIC ANALGESIC DRUGS

AETIOLOGY

The addict to morphine and to other analgesics often acquires his habit as a result of the legitimate administration of the drug for the relief of physical pain. As tolerance develops, increasing doses are required for this purpose. After a time he finds that he is unable to relinquish the drug without developing the symptoms of deprivation described below. Moreover, to avoid this, he requires increasing doses. Morphine gives the addict no pleasurable sensations. As De Quincey wrote: 'Opium had long ceased to found its empire upon spells of pleasure; it was solely by the tortures connected with the attempt to abjure it that it kept its hold.' Very few, however, who receive narcotics for the relief of pain become addicts. The drug, besides relieving pain, blunts the edge of reality: to the psychologically unstable, therefore, it affords a way of escape from life's difficulties. Having experienced the sedative effects of morphine, they continue to take it for the relief of mental pain or distress, and are thus fettered to their habit by a double bond, psychological and physiological. Adams (1937) classified addicts into four groups:

1. Stabilized addicts who may lead useful lives on a fixed dose.
2. Accidental addicts, not necessarily psychopathic, who have often acquired addiction through treatment of a painful disease.
3. Natural addicts, essentially psychopathic.
4. Criminal addicts, who take to drugs for vicious purposes.

Within recent years, addiction to many synthetic analgesic drugs has been reported and most of the remedies involved are listed by Victor and Adams (1974). They include diacetylmorphine (heroin), dihydromorphinone, codeine and its derivatives, pethidine (meperidine or *Demerol*), methadone, levorphan, *d*-propoxyphene, and phenazocine; these remedies resemble the opiates pharmacologically, but vary in their patterns of abuse and addictive properties. Pentazocine, another synthetic remedy, has a low addictive tendency, but occasional cases of physical dependency have been described (Wood *et al.*, 1974).

Doctors and nurses form a considerable proportion of addicts, since they have ready access to the drugs. Residence in a country where they are readily obtainable may also facilitate the acquisition of the habit. The number of drug addicts in the United States was officially said in 1955 to be 44,905, in Canada 3,295, and in Great Britain about 470, but numbers have greatly increased within the last 20 years and Victor and Adams (1974) estimate that there are now over 400,000 addicts in New York city alone; the incidence in Great Britain and Europe is much less but has nevertheless increased alarmingly.

SYMPTOMS OF ADDICTION

The psychopathic addict undergoes a progressive mental deterioration, with loss of interest in his environment, intellectual efficiency, and self-respect. He becomes quite untrustworthy, and will commit almost any crime to obtain a supply of his drug, if he is faced by the prospect of deprivation. Physically he represents a picture of chronic toxaemia, including the specific symptoms attributable to the pharmacological action of the drug. He is wasted and shows trophic changes in the hair and nails. The pupils are usually contracted, and react sluggishly to light. The alimentary tract suffers severely; the appetite is poor and constipation is always present. There is severe fatigability, and muscular weakness, frequently with some ataxia. The pulse is of small volume, and the extremities are cold. Slight albuminuria may be present. Carelessness leads to infection of the skin at the site of the injections, and the resulting scars are usually to be found, while in some cases abscesses or ulcers may be present when the patient comes under observation.

SYMPTOMS OF DEPRIVATION

The addict who is suddenly deprived of his drug exhibits a highly characteristic train of symptoms. As the time for his usual injection passes he becomes restless and apprehensive, and yawning and sneezing develop, followed by the symptoms of an acute coryza. He feels cold, and contraction of the smooth muscles of the skin produces the appearance described as 'goose-flesh'. Later he complains of cramps in the abdomen, back, or lower limbs. His face is contracted in his distress; perspiration is excessive, and muscular spasms and twitching occur, most violently in the lower extremities. There is often a general tremor and the patient may be violent in his demands for the drug. Later, vomiting and diarrhoea occur, and lead to a stage of circulatory collapse, which may even terminate in death.

The pharmacology of drug addiction is fully discussed by Isbell and Fraser (1950) and by Sim (1975). Many explanations of the symptoms of deprivation have been proposed. The most plausible is a modification of Dixon's 'release' theory. Since morphine depresses many autonomic functions, tolerance must involve the balancing of increasing doses by a progressively higher 'gearing' of autonomic activity. When the morphine is suddenly withdrawn the autonomic nervous system 'races' like a motor-car engine when the clutch is suddenly thrown out. Nevertheless, psychological factors must also play some part, since it is said that in prisons, where abrupt withdrawal without medication has been common, abstinence symptoms are often less severe.

TREATMENT

Not every drug addict requires treatment. Stabilized addicts leading useful lives on a fixed dose, especially when past middle age, are often best left un-treated. In Great Britain, the right of every doctor to prescribe opiates for addicts has now been proscribed by law and all addicts must now obtain their drugs from licensed doctors, usually working in psychiatric units or in centres for the treatment of drug addiction which have been established.

Treatment which should be carried out in an institution has been reviewed by Wolff (1945–6), by Isbell and Fraser (1950), by the British Inter-departmental Committee (1961), by Clemmesen (1963) and by Victor and Adams (1974). Abrupt withdrawal and very slow withdrawal are both now regarded as un-satisfactory. Generally the drug is reduced over a period of 7 to 10 days. It is now regarded as unnecessary to cover the withdrawal by large doses of drugs of the atropine group. Circulatory collapse and pulmonary oedema may require fluid restriction, diuretics, the use of pressor amines, and assisted respiration (Clemmesen and Lassen, 1963). Adjuvant therapy includes the judicious use of sedatives and hypnotics, maintenance of fluid balance, and simple psycho-therapy. Methadone and chlorpromazine in doses up to 100 mg three times daily may be used to suppress the abstinence symptoms, and are then withdrawn. The use of opiate antagonists such as cyclazocine is now being tested (Victor and Adams, 1974).

The after-treatment of the morphine addict is important, if a relapse is to be prevented. Convalescence under medical supervision should last for three months. Any painful condition which has necessitated morphine in the past should as far as possible be remedied. Psychotherapy may be required. It is desirable that the patient should abstain from alcohol, which may predispose to a relapse.

COCAINE ADDICTION

Coca leaves are chewed in South America for their sedative effects and their power of abolishing fatigue. Cocaine as a drug of addiction may be injected sub-cutaneously, drunk as coca wine, smoked, or taken as snuff. It acts to some extent as a sexual stimulant, and is stated to produce a sense of internal peace. Addicts suffer from mental deterioration, and, in severe cases, from confusional insanity. Hallucinations, especially of insects crawling under the skin, are common, and epilepsy may occur. Cocaine sniffing may lead to ulceration of the nasal septum. Addicts who are suddenly deprived of cocaine do not suffer, like morphine addicts, from severe deprivation symptoms. Treatment, therefore, is not required to counteract these, but is similar to the after-treatment of the morphine addict. Cocainism, however, is much more difficult to cure than morphine addiction.

REFERENCES

ADAMS, E. W. (1937) *Drug Addiction*, London.
BALL, J. C., and CHAMBERS, C. K. (1970) *The Epidemiology of Opiate Addiction in the United States*, Springfield, Ill.
CLEMMESEN, C. (1963) Treatment of narcotic intoxication, *Dan. med. Bull.*, **10**, 97.
CLEMMESEN, C., and LASSEN, N. A. (1963) Treatment of circulatory shock in narcotic poisoning, *Dan. med. Bull.*, **10**, 100.
DOLE, V. P., and NYSWANDER, M. E. (1968) Methadone maintenance and its implication for theories of narcotic addiction, *Res. Publ. Ass. nerv. ment. Dis.*, **46**, 359.
ISBELL, H., and FRASER, H. F. (1950) Addiction to analgesics and barbiturates, *Pharmacol. Rev.*, **2**, 355.
MAIER, H. W. (1928) *La cocaïne*, Paris.
SIM, M. (1975) *Guide to Psychiatry*, 3rd ed., Edinburgh.
VAILLANT, G. E. (1966) A 12-year follow-up of New York narcotic addicts, *Arch. gen. Psychiat.*, **15**, 599.
VICTOR, M., and ADAMS, R. D. (1974) Opiates and other analgesic drugs, in *Harrison's Principles of Internal Medicine*, 7th ed., chap. 112, New York.
WOLFF, P. O. (1945-6) The treatment of drug addicts, *Bull. Wld. Hlth. Org.*, No. 12.
WOOD, A. J., MOIR, D. C., CAMPBELL, C., DAVIDSON, J. F., GALLON, S. C., HENNEY, E., and McALLION, S. (1974) Medicines evaluation and monitoring group: central nervous system effects of pentazocine, *Brit. med. J.*, **1**, 305.
Report of the Interdepartmental Committee on Drug Addiction (1961), London, H.M.S.O.

SEDATIVES AND HYPNOTICS

Barbiturates, chloral, sulphonal, and allied drugs may be taken as drugs of habituation, either alone or with morphine, and addicts may become tolerant of enormous doses. All these drugs produce similar symptoms, both in cases of acute poisoning and in addicts, though some have in addition individual peculiarities.

Habituation to Synthetic Hypnotics

When taken habitually (Glatt, 1966) these drugs lead to mental deterioration, dysarthria, nystagmus, muscular weakness, tremor, and incoordination. There is usually considerable emaciation. Veronal and sulphonal may lead to haemato-porphyrinuria and polyneuropathy. Chloral has a markedly toxic effect on the heart and on the skin, causing reddening of the face and a papular eruption. Treatment is carried out by means of gradual withdrawal: sudden withdrawal may cause convulsions. The general management is the same as that for morphine addiction.

The introduction within recent years of many new sedative and tranquillizing remedies has been followed by reports of habituation to many of these including meprobamate, glutethimide, chlordiazepoxide, diazepam, and many more. When taken to excess, these drugs give symptoms like those of acute or chronic barbiturate intoxication (see below) and long-term habituation followed by withdrawal can result in withdrawal symptoms including hallucinations and delirium.

The phenothiazines, by contrast, and related remedies such as reserpine and the butyrophenones (e.g. haloperidol) may cause cholestatic jaundice, agranulocytosis, epileptiform attacks, orthostatic hypotension, skin sensitivity reactions, and extrapyramidal manifestations including drug-induced Parkinsonism and orofacial dyskinesia [see pp. 581 and 623].

Barbiturate Poisoning

In Great Britain the increasing use of barbiturates and of other sedative drugs for suicidal attempts has meant that this group of drugs now exceed coal-gas poisoning as a method of attempted suicide (Cumming, 1961) and there are probably over 3,000 hospital admissions annually due to this cause. Because of the frequency with which these drugs are used for suicidal attempts, efforts are being made in Great Britain to proscribe their use as so many more satisfactory sedatives and hypnotics are now available, though even the modern tranquillizing remedies such as diazepam and nitrazepam are not without risk as mentioned above.

In mild cases slurred speech, drowsiness, ataxia, and nystagmus are apparent but when the dose ingested is large the patients are stuporose or comatose and there is eventually total areflexia with hypotension and oliguria. Small blisters filled with serum may appear on the limbs in severe cases. Hypothermia and cardiac arrest may occur (Fell *et al.*, 1968).

Management consists first in aspirating stomach contents, in identifying when possible the causative agent in stomach contents, blood or urine (or by searching the patient's belongings or questioning the relatives or family doctor concerning drugs which were in the patient's possession). Maintenance of an adequate airway, often by intubation, of the blood pressure by the use of appropriate drugs (e.g. methedrine), of the fluid and electrolyte intake by intravenous therapy and the administration of appropriate antibiotics with intensive nursing care to prevent pulmonary collapse and bed-sores are all essential. The use of analeptic drugs such as bemegride and amiphenazole has now been generally discarded in favour of the elimination of the offending drug by dialysis with the artificial kidney in severe cases. Catheterization is usually necessary and assisted respiration may be required for several days. With such measures recovery from very severe poisoning is now possible (Kennedy *et al.*, 1969).

Chronic barbiturate intoxication has also become much more common in recent years (see Victor and Adams, 1974). The clinical picture resembles that of alcoholic intoxication; as in alcoholism, delirium and withdrawal convulsions may follow withdrawal and treatment is similar to that of delirium tremens.

REFERENCES

CUMMING, G. (1961) *The Medical Management of Acute Poisoning*, London.
ESSIG, C. F. (1966) Non-narcotic addiction, *J. Amer. med. Ass.*, **196,** 714.
ESSIG, C. F. (1972) Chronic abuse of sedative–hypnotic drugs, in *Drug Abuse*, ed. Zarafonetis, C. J. D., Philadelphia.
FELL, R. H., GUNNING, A. J., BARDHAN, K. D., and TRIGER, D. R. (1968) Severe hypothermia as a result of barbiturate overdose complicated by cardiac arrest, *Lancet*, **i,** 392.
FLANDIN, C., BERNARD, J., and JOLY, F. (1934) *L'intoxication par les somnifères (intoxication barbiturique)*, Paris.

GLATT, M. M. (1966) Controlled trials of non-barbiturate hypnotics and tranquillisers, *Psychiat. Neurol.*, **152,** 28.

KENNEDY, A. C., LINDSAY, R. M., BRIGGS, J. D., LUKE, R. G., YOUNG, N., and CAMPBELL, D. (1969) Successful treatment of three cases of very severe barbiturate poisoning, *Lancet*, **i,** 995.

VICTOR, M., and ADAMS, R. D. (1974) Barbiturates (Chapter 113), Depressants, stimulants and psychotogenic drugs (chap. 114) in *Harrison's Principles of Internal Medicine*, 7th ed., New York.

WRIGHT, J. T. (1955) The value of barbiturate estimations in the diagnosis and treatment of barbiturate intoxication, *Quart. J. Med.*, N.S. **24,** 95.

CHRONIC BROMIDE INTOXICATION

Chronic bromide intoxication is now rare but may still result from the prolonged administration of bromide for therapeutic purposes. It used to be most often encountered in patients suffering from neurosis, hyperthyroidism, or epilepsy. Since the bromides are now much less frequently used, commoner sources of bromide intoxication are compounds of bromide with urea, such as carbromal and bromvaletone.

Bromide tends to replace the chlorides in the body, and a greater amount of bromide will be absorbed by a person with a low chloride intake than by one who is taking larger amounts of chloride. The blood bromide level is a rough index of the degree of intoxication, though individual susceptibility varies greatly. The normal level of bromide in the blood is under 3 mg per 100 ml. According to Barbour *et al.* (1936), levels of under 100 mg per 100 ml can usually be ignored; those between 100 and 200 mg per 100 ml are likely to be associated with symptoms of intoxication in elderly patients or in those with impaired cardiovascular or renal efficiency, and levels of over 200 mg per 100 ml produce symptoms in most cases. There is evidence that bromide, like chloride, is excreted into the stomach and so may be reabsorbed.

In mild cases the symptoms are largely subjective, and consist of depression, fatigability, inability to concentrate, loss of memory, lack of appetite, and poor sleep. In more severe cases the mental state is usually one of confusion with some disorientation. The occurrence of terrifying hallucinations, especially at night, is rather characteristic. Physical symptoms are variable: when severe they consist of slurred speech, tremor and ataxia of the upper limbs, a staggering gait, and diminution or loss of the tendon reflexes. In more severe cases still the patient becomes stuporose. The rash usually regarded as characteristic of bromide intoxication is frequently absent.

The bromide must be immediately discontinued and the patient given increased sodium chloride and fluid by the mouth. Washing out the stomach helps to eliminate the drug. In severe cases the artificial kidney may be used. Restlessness is controlled if necessary by chlorpromazine or diazepam.

REFERENCES

BARBOUR, R. F., PILKINGTON, F., and SARGANT, W. (1936) Bromide intoxication, *Brit. med. J.*, **2,** 957.

MINSKI, L., and GILLEN, J. B. (1937) Blood bromide investigations in psychotic epileptics, *Brit. med. J.*, **2,** 850.

MARIHUANA (HASHISH, CANNABIS INDICA)

This drug which has been used by certain races in the Orient and in South America has recently been used more widely in Western countries, being often smoked in cigarettes. Its use is still illegal; it is a drug of habituation and not of addiction and in itself it is a minor nuisance rather than a serious social evil. It produces a transient sense of well-being and sometimes reversible hallucinations. Its major danger is that for social reasons it may introduce its habituees to narcotics.

There has been considerable pressure in the United States and in Europe by certain groups who wish the social use of the drug to be legalized, partly on the grounds that its use is so widespread in many countries that existing laws are being continuously flouted, partly because it is believed by some that its very illegality encourages many young people to use it, and partly because there are many who believe it to be less of a social evil than alcohol. Clearly its occasional or intermittent use in low dosage does no lasting harm, but personality changes, loss of drive and purpose, academic failure, and various emotional symptoms have been reported in habitual users who may also show reversal of sleep rhythm and impairment of recent memory (Kolansky and Moore, 1971). Campbell *et al.* (1971) suggest that heavy and prolonged smoking may lead to cerebral atrophy demonstrable by pneumoencephalography, but this view has been challenged by others.

AMPHETAMINE ADDICTION

Amphetamines and their derivatives are commonly taken by young people in order to obtain temporary uplift or mental alertness, or to reduce desire for sleep. Addiction may also occur in young and middle-aged women who have received these drugs in therapeutic doses for the treatment of depression or fatigue or obesity. Connell (1958) has described acute psychotic states of a paranoid or hallucinatory nature while psychopathic and irresponsible behaviour is also common. Fits may occur as a result of intoxication or withdrawal. A common sign of addicts is continuous chewing, grinding of the teeth or licking of the lips, sometimes resulting in ulceration.

OTHER STIMULANTS

Caffeine (a cup of tea or coffee contains 100–150 mg, and this drug is also a constituent of cola drinks) is a mild stimulant which, when taken to excess may cause insomnia, tachycardia, mild cardiac arrhythmias, and diuresis, but serious side-effects are rare. Cigarette smoking with consequent absorption of nicotine has a mild stimulant effect and may affect reaction time (Ashton *et al.*, 1972) and the 'contingent negative variation' in the EEG of human subjects (Ashton *et al.*, 1974), but there are no known long-term neurological ill-effects of smoking.

Monoamine oxidase inhibitors (e.g. phenelzine and tranylcypromine) have been widely used in the treatment of neurotic depression; in excess they have been known to cause insomnia, agitation, orthostatic hypotension, limb oedema, and even mania and convulsions. The principal danger of these remedies is that if they are taken along with tyramine-containing foods or beverages (cheese, 'Marmite', beer, and red wine), severe hypertensive reactions may occur, sometimes causing intense headache, cardiac arrhythmias, cerebral vascular accidents, and even death. Similar cross-reactions may occur with pheno-thiazines and narcotic remedies.

Tricyclic antidepressive remedies and dibenzazepine derivatives such as imipramine or amitryptiline and their derivatives have proved invaluable in the treatment of depressive illness but may on occasion cause not only dryness of the mouth, constipation, blurring of vision, and other parasympathetomimetic effects, but on occasion orthostatic hypotension, agitation, restlessness and even ataxia, blood dyscrasia, and, rarely, convulsions (especially in epileptics or individuals with a low convulsive threshold).

HALLUCINOGENIC AGENTS

The use of hallucinogenic drugs such as LSD and mescaline is increasing and in some universities and other circles has developed almost into a cult. The danger of these drugs is that the induced hallucinations are sometimes terrifying and rarely pleasurable and the view that they produce increased perception is a dangerous delusion. Irreversible psychosis may result and addiction is increasing.

REFERENCES

ASHTON, H., MILLMAN, J. E., TELFORD, R., and THOMPSON, J. W. (1974) The effect of caffeine, nitrazepam and cigarette smoking on the contingent negative variation in man, *Electroenceph. clin. Neurophysiol.*, **37**, 59.
ASHTON, H., SAVAGE, R. D., TELFORD, R., THOMPSON, J. W., and WATSON, D. W. (1972) The effects of cigarette smoking on the response to stress in a driving simulator, *Brit. J. Pharmacol.*, **45**, 546.
CAMPBELL, A. M. G., EVANS, M., THOMSON, J. L. G., and WILLIAMS, M. J. (1971) Cerebral atrophy in young cannabis smokers, *Lancet*, **ii**, 1219.
CONNELL, P. H. (1958) *Amphetamine Psychosis*, Maudsley Monographs, No. 5, London.
GOODMAN, L. S., and GILMAN, A. (1970) *Pharmacological Basis of Therapeutics*, 4th ed., New York.
KOLANSKY, H., and MOORE, W. T. (1971) Effects of marihuana on adolescents and young adults, *J. Amer. med. Ass.*, 216, 486.
SIM, M. (1975) *Guide to Psychiatry*, 3rd ed., Edinburgh.
VICTOR, M., and ADAMS, R. D. (1974) Depressants, stimulants and psychotogenic drugs, in *Harrison's Principles of Internal Medicine*, 7th ed., chap. 114, New York.

ANTICONVULSANT DRUGS

Anticonvulsants such as phenobarbitone, phenytoin, and primidone are occasionally used, especially by epileptic patients, for suicidal attempts. The symptoms and signs of acute poisoning and its management are similar to those described for barbiturate intoxication. During prolonged administration in the management of epilepsy the appearance of side effects such as drowsiness, dysarthria, nystagmus, and ataxia may be due to variable absorption and utilization rates in different subjects or to changes in the excipient used in the preparation given (Tyrer *et al.*, 1970) and can often be prevented by the estima-tion of blood levels (Kutt and Penry, 1974). More troublesome side effects include depression of folate metabolism with megaloblastic anaemia (Reynolds, 1973), chronic lymphadenopathy, choreoathetosis and encephalopathy (McLellan and Swash, 1974), and irreversible cerebellar degeneration (Dam, 1970) which is fortunately rare. The possibility that phenytoin may rarely be carcinogenic (*The Lancet*, 1971) and that it and other anticonvulsants may have a teratogenic effect when taken during pregnancy (Annegers *et al.*, 1974) has also been raised but remains unproven.

REFERENCES

ANNEGERS, J. F., ELVEBACK, L. R., HAUSER, W. A., and KURLAND, L. T. (1974) Do anticonvulsants have a teratogenic effect?, *Arch. Neurol. (Chic.)*, **31**, 364.
DAM, M. (1970) Number of Purkinje cells in patients with grand mal epilepsy treated with diphenylhydantoin, *Epilepsia*, **11**, 313.
KUTT, H., and PENRY, J. K. (1974) Usefulness of blood levels of antiepileptic drugs, *Arch. Neurol. (Chic.)*, **31**, 283.
THE LANCET (1971) Is phenytoin carcinogenic?, *Lancet*, **ii**, 1071.
MCLELLAN, D. L., and SWASH, M. (1974) Choreo-athetosis and encephalopathy induced by phenytoin, *Brit. med. J.*, **2**, 204.
REYNOLDS, E. H. (1973) Anticonvulsants, folic acid, and epilepsy, *Lancet*, **i**, 1376.
TYRER, J. H., EADIE, M. J., SUTHERLAND, J. M., and HOOPER, W. D. (1970) Outbreak of anticonvulsant intoxication in an Australian city, *Brit. med. J.*, **4**, 271.

LEAD POISONING

AETIOLOGY

The nervous symptoms of plumbism are usually due to chronic poisoning with lead. Industrial lead poisoning was at one time common, but has now been reduced by legislative restrictions. Lead poisoning still occurs, however, especially among plumbers and painters. In such cases the principal route of absorption of the lead is probably the digestive tract, though some may enter the body through the lungs. Water which passed through lead pipes was an occasional source of poisoning in the past, and beer and cider were sometimes similarly contaminated. The first glass of these beverages, which had stayed in a lead pipe all night, was particularly poisonous. Sucking lead paint or pica are still the commonest causes of poisoning in children (Barltrop, 1968). Cosmetics containing lead are an occasional source of poisoning, which may also follow the use of lead obtained from diachylon plaster as a home-made abortifacient. Lead tetra-ethyl is a highly poisonous substance which has caused encephalopathy in the United States. It is used in small quantities in some forms of petrol. Because of its potential environmental effect due to inhalation of vehicle exhaust fumes, many countries are now introducing legislation to reduce the lead content of motor fuel.

At least 90 per cent of ingested lead is not absorbed and adults excrete about 0·3 mg daily in the faeces, while the usual amount in infants is 0·13 mg daily with an upper limit of 0·18 mg (Barltrop and Killala, 1967). That which is absorbed from the gut first enters the erythrocytes and then is stored in liver, kidney, and bone; very little if any is laid down in the brain or skeletal muscle; later that stored in liver and kidney is gradually transferred to bone (Barltrop, 1968, 1969). In chronic lead poisoning, as Aub and his fellow workers showed, 95 per cent of the lead is stored in the bones as insoluble phosphate. This lead storage is facilitated by a diet rich in calcium. In states of acidosis the stored lead is released into the blood stream, and its excretion in the faeces and urine is much increased. Hunter and Aub (1926–7) showed that mobilization and excretion of lead can be similarly effected by parathyroid extract (parathormone). The undue mobilization of lead may precipitate an attack of encephalopathy.

It has long been known that in lead neuropathy the muscles paralysed are usually those most used in the patient's occupation. Fullerton (1966) has shown that this heavy metal produces both axonal degeneration and demyelination in the peripheral nerves of guinea-pigs, but Hopkins (1970) was unable to produce lead neuropathy in the baboon.

PATHOLOGY

Lead exerts its toxic action by combining with essential SH-groups of certain enzymes involved in porphyrin synthesis and carbohydrate metabolism; in particular it depresses delta-aminolaevulinic acid dehydratase activity, and a possible correlation between infantile ingestion of lead and mental retardation has been postulated (Millar *et al.*, 1970; Beattie *et al.*, 1975). Enzymes concerned with haem synthesis are also suppressed, thus accounting for the high incidence of anaemia, and renal tubular function is also impaired. In the central nervous system, early neuropathological studies suggested that the metal produced widespread degeneration of cerebral and spinal cord neurones but this now appears much less certain and the oedema of lead encephalopathy is associated with relatively little deposition of lead in the brain when compared with other tissues (Kehoe, 1961 *a* and *b*; Goldstein and Diamond, 1974). In acute lead encephalopathy the brain is pale and oedematous, with an excess of fluid in the subarachnoid space. Meningeal irritation may also occur (Smith *et al.*, 1960). In guinea-pigs in which lead produced combined axonal degeneration and demyelination in peripheral nerves, epileptic seizures were also common and could be provoked by noise or movement (Fullerton, 1966). Similar seizures, in the absence of any recognizable pathological changes in the brain other than oedema, were seen in the baboon (Hopkins, 1970).

SYMPTOMS

Acute Encephalopathy

This is an acute cerebral disturbance which is rare in adults but is commonly seen in children aged 1 or 2, and characterized by convulsions, delirium, and coma, often associated with papilloedema, and sometimes with cervical rigidity. The cerebrospinal fluid frequently shows abnormality; its pressure is increased, and there is an excess of globulin and of cells, which in adults are usually lymphocytes, though in children polymorphonuclear cells may be present. An increase in the sugar content of the fluid has also been described, and the presence of lead in it has been demonstrated. Between 20 and 30 per cent of children who suffer from this condition suffer from recurring fits as a sequel (Coffin *et al.*, 1966).

Chronic Encephalopathy

Mental changes and epileptiform convulsions have been observed as chronic manifestations of lead poisoning. Primary optic atrophy occasionally occurs. Laryngeal palsy is a rare symptom which was described by Gowers and by Harris, who saw a case of bilateral abductor paralysis.

Lead Neuropathy

This condition usually affects the extensor muscles of the wrist and fingers, as a rule bilaterally, though the right side may suffer alone, especially in right-handed individuals. Wrist- and finger-drop occur, and the loss of synergic extension of the wrist causes weakness of flexion of the fingers. The brachioradialis muscle escapes and so, as a rule, does the abductor pollicis longus. In the upper-arm type of palsy the spinati, deltoid, biceps, brachialis, and brachioradialis muscles are affected. These are the abductors and external rotators of the shoulder and flexors of the forearm, and this distribution of paralysis may occur in workers employing these muscles chiefly, for example, in men making batteries. The lower limbs are occasionally affected, the muscles paralysed being those supplied by the common peroneal nerve, with the exception of the tibialis anterior, which usually escapes. It is characteristic of lead neuropathy that it is predominantly motor, and sensory symptoms and signs are usually slight or absent. Occasionally the muscular weakness and wasting is so widespread that it simulates progressive muscular atrophy but there is no evidence that lead intoxication plays any part in the pathogenesis of motor neurone disease.

The paralysed muscles waste and demonstrate electrophysiological evidence of denervation with mild slowing of motor nerve conduction velocity, but fasciculation and sensory changes are absent.

Other Symptoms

Other symptoms of lead poisoning are of diagnostic importance. The blue line should be sought on the gums. There may be a history of colic and indeed lead colic is often the most prominent symptom in adults. There is often a secondary anaemia, with stippling of the red cells—punctate basophilia. Cardiovascular hypertrophy with high blood pressure may be present, or symptoms of renal tubular dysfunction. Gout is a rare complication today. In chronic lead poisoning in children X-rays may show a 'lead line', a band of increased density, at the diaphysial end of the growing bones. The normal content of lead in the blood is 10–60 μg per litre. In lead encephalopathy there may be 100–200 μg per ml in the blood, and 100–1,000 μg or more per litre of urine.

DIAGNOSIS

Acute lead encephalopathy must be distinguished from uraemia, in which there is always a high blood-urea content, and from hypertensive encephalopathy in which the blood pressure is usually higher. Meningitis may be simulated. Lead neuropathy is distinguished from a lesion of the radial nerve by the escape of the brachioradialis and by its gradual onset and by the involvement of muscles, perhaps on the opposite side or others not supplied by the radial nerve. In various other forms of polyneuropathy, foot-drop is usually associated with wrist-drop; pain in the limbs is often a prominent symptom; and there is usually sensory loss with a 'glove and stocking' distribution. Moreover, the blue line on the gums and other symptoms of lead poisoning are absent. In all doubtful cases the blood should be examined for evidence of anaemia and punctate basophilia, and lead should be sought in the urine and faeces.

Patients with lead poisoning excrete increased quantities of coproporphyrin III and of delta-amino-laevulinic acid in the urine so that a urinary screening test for porphyrin should be performed when the diagnosis is suspected.

PROGNOSIS

The outlook in acute encephalopathy is always serious, especially when convulsions occur, but with modern methods of treatment the prognosis has improved, and recovery, when it occurs, is often complete, but the patient may be left mentally retarded, blind, or epileptic. Little improvement is to be expected in chronic encephalopathy. In lead neuropathy the prognosis is good, provided the patient abstains from contact with lead. Recovery, however, is usually slow, and may take one to two years.

TREATMENT

The patient with lead poisoning must be removed from contact with lead, and must never return to an occupation which exposes him to it. If he does so, relapse is certain. The first question to be settled is whether the patient requires active elimination of the lead or not. The treatment of lead poisoning has been revolutionized by the introduction of chelating agents. Disodium calcium ethylene-diamine-tetra-acetate (CaEDTA, *Versene*) forms with lead a chelate, which is a stable, water-soluble, and virtually non-ionized complex, which is excreted by the kidneys. Its successful use has been reported by Browne (1955) and Sidbury (1955), who treated nine patients. The drug can be given both orally and intravenously. The oral dose used by Sidbury was 30 mg per kg of body weight given before breakfast and supper with liberal amounts of water. Two methods have been used for the intravenous route: slow infusion of 1 g on the first day and 2 g a day thereafter for a total of five days in divided doses, twice daily in 250 ml of 5 per cent glucose in water; or 400 mg was given once or twice a day in 5 or 10 ml of saline. For children the dose is 60–75 mg per kg of body weight, given in the same ways. Both seemed equally satisfactory. There was marked improvement or complete disappearance of symptoms in all cases, including those of lead encephalopathy, on the third day of treatment, when blood and urine analyses showed that most of the readily available lead had been excreted. An alternative method of treatment is BAL in doses of 2–4 mg per kg of body weight given every 4 hours for up to 10 days. Indeed some authorities suggest combined therapy with calcium versenate and BAL; in mild cases, penicillamine 1·0–1·5 g daily for three to five days may be sufficient (Poskanzer and Bennett, 1974). Since lead is deposited in the bones, patients who have been exposed to lead for long periods cannot eliminate the metal in a short time. They may therefore relapse and require further courses of treatment. Wrist-drop and finger-drop may require to be treated by a splint. Lumbar puncture or the use of dexamethasone, 5 mg three or four times daily to reduce cerebral oedema, may be helpful in the immediate treatment of encephalopathy and if convulsions occur, anticonvulsants may be required.

REFERENCES

BARLTROP, D. (1968) Lead poisoning in childhood, *Postgrad. med. J.*, **44**, 537.
BARLTROP, D. (1969) Environmental lead and its paediatric significance, *Postgrad. med. J.*, **45**, 129.
BARLTROP, D., and KILLALA, N. J. P. (1967) Faecal excretion of lead by children, *Lancet*, **ii**, 1017.
BEATTIE, A. D., MOORE, M. R., GOLDBERG, A., FINLAYSON, M. J. W., GRAHAM, J. F., MACKIE, E. M., MAIN, J. C., McLAREN, D. A., MURDOCH, R. M., and STEWART, G. T. (1975) Role of chronic low-level lead exposure in the aetiology of mental retardation, *Lancet*, **i**, 589.
BROWNE, R. C. (1955) Metallic poisons and the nervous system, *Lancet*, **i**, 775.
COFFIN, R., PHILLIPS, J. L., STADLES, W. I., and SPECTOR, S. (1966) Treatment of lead encephalopathy in children, *J. Pediat.*, **69**, 198.
CUMINGS, J. N. (1959) *Heavy Metals and the Brain*, Oxford.
FULLERTON, P. M. (1966) Chronic peripheral neuropathy produced by lead-poisoning in the guinea-pig, *J. Neuropath. exp. Neurol.*, **25**, 214.

GOLDSTEIN, G. W., and DIAMOND, I. (1974) Metabolic basis of lead encephalopathy, in *Brain Dysfunction in Metabolic Disorders*, ed. Plum, F., A.R.N.M.D., vol. 53, New York.

HOPKINS, A. (1970) Experimental lead poisoning in the baboon, *Brit. J. industr. Med.*, **27**, 130.

HUNTER, D. (1930) Goulstonian lectures. The significance to clinical medicine of studies in calcium and phosphorus metabolism, *Lancet*, **i**, 897, 947, 999.

HUNTER, D., and AUB, J. C. (1926–7) Lead studies. XV. The effect of the parathyroid hormone on the excretion of lead and of calcium in patients suffering from lead poisoning, *Quart. J. Med.*, **20**, 123.

KEHOE, R. A. (1961 *a*) The metabolism of lead in man in health and disease. 2. Metabolism under abnormal conditions, *J. roy. Inst. publ. Hlth*, **24**, 101.

KEHOE, R. A. (1961 *b*) Present hygienic problems relating to the absorption of lead, *J. roy. Inst. publ. Hlth*, **24**, 177.

THE LANCET (1955) Chelating agents, *Lancet*, **i**, 754.

McKHANN, C. F. (1932) Lead poisoning in children: the cerebral manifestations, *Arch. Neurol. Psychiat. (Chic.)*, **27**, 294.

MILLAR, J. A., BATTISTINI, V., CUMMING, R. L. C., CARSWELL, F., and GOLDBERG, A. (1970) Lead and delta-aminolaevulinic acid dehydratase levels in mentally retarded children and in lead-poisoned suckling rats, *Lancet*, **ii**, 695.

MORRIS, C. E., HEYMAN, A., and POZEFSKY, T. (1964) Lead encephalopathy from whiskey, *Neurology (Minneap.)*, **14**, 493.

POSKANZER, D. C., and BENNETT, I. L., Jr. (1974) Heavy metals, in *Harrison's Principles of Internal Medicine*, 7th ed., chap. 110, New York.

SIDBURY, J. B., Jr. (1955) Lead poisoning, *Amer. J. Med.*, **17**, 932.

SMITH, J. F., McLAURIN, R. L., NICHOLS, J. B., and ASBURY, A. (1960) Studies in cerebral oedema and cerebral swelling, *Brain*, **83**, 411.

MANGANESE POISONING

This is an industrial disease due to the inhalation of manganese dust and occurs particularly in manganese miners in Chile and in some parts of central Europe. The clinical features, which often appear within 6–9 months of exposure, are those of an extrapyramidal syndrome like Parkinsonism with slurred, monotonous speech, slowness and clumsiness of movement, facial masking and anteropulsion or retropulsion. Personality change in the form of irritability and variable euphoria may be succeeded by intense fatigue, lethargy, and somnolence. Little improvement usually follows removal of the patient from exposure to the dust but chelating agents or BAL may be of some value and levodopa relieves the Parkinsonian features.

MERCURY POISONING

Acute mercurial poisoning may produce neurological symptoms and signs, but gastro-intestinal and renal damage usually dominate the clinical picture. Chronic mercurial poisoning in children may give 'pink disease' [p. 974] and one form in adults is Minamata disease. Chronic exposure to this metal in industry and even in police officers exposed to mercurial finger-print powder (which is no longer used) may give rise to a syndrome of tremor, variable limb weakness and ataxia and personality change often characterized by fatigability, insomnia, irritability, and erethism (childish over-emotionalism). In the central nervous system there is often selective damage to the granular cell layer of the cerebellum. The condition may result either from organic or inorganic mercurial poisoning as in the inhalation of mercury vapour in thermometer workers (Vroom and Greer, 1972), the excessive use of mercurous chloride laxatives (Davis *et al.*, 1974), or through eating bread made from wheat treated with methyl mercury as in a recent epidemic in Iraq (Rustam and Hamdi, 1974). BAL or chelating agents should be given in such cases and penicillamine may also be effective.

Minamata Disease

Between 1953 and 1956 a disorder characterized by symptoms and signs of peripheral neuropathy, cerebellar ataxia, visual and hearing loss and inconstant pyramidal tract involvement, and sometimes by the development of a progressive encephalopathy, was noted in villagers living near Minamata Bay in Kyushu Island, Japan. In fatal cases widespread neuronal damage was found in the granular layer of the cerebellum and in the cerebral cortex. The condition usually followed the ingestion of fish and circumstantial evidence suggested that it was due to the toxic action of a mercurial compound contained in the effluent which flowed into Minamata Bay from a fertilizer factory.

REFERENCES

COHEN, M. M. (1955) Cerebral intoxication, in *Clinical Neurology*, ed. Baker, A. B., Chapter 15, pp. 866–943, London.
DAVIS, L. E., WANDS, J. R., WEISS, S. A., PRICE, D. L., and GIRLING, E. F. (1974) Central nervous system intoxication from mercurous chloride laxatives, *Arch. Neurol. (Chic.)*, **30**, 428.
HUNTER, D. (1975) *The Diseases of Occupations*, 5th ed., London.
MCALPINE, D., and ARAKI, S. (1958) Minamata disease, *Lancet*, **ii**, 629.
POSKANZER, D. C., and BENNETT, I. L., Jun. (1974) Heavy metals, in *Harrison's Principles of Internal Medicine*, 7th ed., chap. 110, New York.
RUSTAM, H., and HAMDI, T. (1974) Methyl mercury poisoning in Iraq—a neurological study, *Brain*, **97**, 499.
VROOM, F. Q., and GREER, M. (1972) Mercury vapour intoxication, *Brain*, **95**, 305.

SOME OTHER POISONS WITH NEUROLOGICAL EFFECTS

The other heavy metals including arsenic and lead, as well as a variety of organic and inorganic chemicals, are known to produce polyneuropathy, sometimes associated with other neurological manifestations; they are considered in CHAPTER 17, while the effects of cyanide intoxication are described in CHAPTER 16 along with the nutritional disorders.

Thallium poisoning produces symptoms varying from mild polyneuropathy with alopecia to irreversible coma and death (Bank *et al.*, 1972; Kennedy and Cavanagh, 1976). In such cases there are demyelination of peripheral nerves, degeneration of posterior root ganglia, and less distinctive changes in the central nervous system. Podophyllum taken as an abortifacient can cause disordered consciousness and polyneuropathy (Clark and Parsonage, 1957) and hexachlorophene bathing of infants may cause a brain stem vacuolar encephalopathy (Shuman *et al.*, 1975). Skeletal fluorosis due to the excessive dietary ingestion of fluoride may produce spastic paraplegia due to spinal cord compression (Singh *et al.*, 1961).

REFERENCES

BANK, W. J., PLEASURE, D. E., SUZUKI, K., NIGRO, M., and KATZ, R. (1972) Thallium poisoning, *Arch. Neurol. (Chic.)*, **26**, 456.

CLARK, A. N. G., and PARSONAGE, M. J. (1957) A case of podophyllum poisoning with involvement of the nervous system, *Brit. med. J.*, **2**, 1155.

KENNEDY, P., and CAVANAGH, J. B. (1976) Spinal changes in the neuropathy of thallium poisoning, *J. neurol. Sci.*, **29**, 295.

SHUMAN, R. M., LEECH, R. W., and ALVORD, E. C. (1975) Neurotoxicity of hexachlorophene in humans. II. A clinicopathological study of 46 premature infants, *Arch. Neurol. (Chic.)*, **32**, 320.

SINGH, A., JOLLY, S. S., and BANSAL, B. C. (1961) Skeletal fluorosis and its neurological complications, *Lancet*, **i**, 197.

ORAL CONTRACEPTIVES

Neurological side-effects of oral contraceptives include cerebral vascular accidents (Altshuler *et al.*, 1968; and see p. 328) and choreiform movements which usually resolve when the drug is withdrawn (Lewis and Harrison, 1969). An increased frequency and severity of attacks of migraine and epilepsy has also been described (Bickerstaff, 1975).

REFERENCES

ALTSHULER, J. H., McLAUGHLIN, R. A., and NEUBUERGER, K. T. (1968) Neurological catastrophe related to oral contraceptives, *Arch. Neurol. (Chic.)*, **19**, 264.

BICKERSTAFF, E. R. (1975) *Neurological Complications of Oral Contraceptives*, Oxford.

LEWIS, P. D., and HARRISON, M. J. G. (1969) Involuntary movements in patients taking oral contraceptives, *Brit. med. J.*, **4**, 404.

CARBON MONOXIDE POISONING

AETIOLOGY

Carbon monoxide poisoning may occur as the result of the accidental or suicidal inhalation of coal-gas or of gas from a motor-car exhaust. Carbon monoxide may also be present in dangerous quantities in the air of coal-mines, especially after explosions. By combining with the haemoglobin of the blood to form carboxyhaemoglobin, carbon monoxide reduces the capacity of the blood to take up oxygen, and so leads to anoxaemia.

Absorption of the gas is cumulative, so that a concentration of 0·1 per cent will saturate the blood up to 50 per cent. Effort increases absorption.

PATHOLOGY

In fatal cases the blood is cherry-red in colour and coagulates slowly. All the tissues are reddened. There is oedema of the lungs, and haemorrhages are found in the pleura and intestinal mucosa. Changes in the nervous system are of special importance and exhibit a predilection for the cerebral cortex, the hippocampus, cerebellum, and the corpus striatum. The changes are those of anoxia (see p. 15) and similar appearances may be found to follow cardiac arrest or may complicate open-heart surgery. However, there are significant differences between the effects of hypoxic anoxia and those of carbon monoxide poisoning in relation to oxygen availability and utilization (Astrup and Pauli, 1968), though the neurological effects are similar. There is focal or laminar necrosis of the second and third cortical layers and often of the superficial white matter with striking degeneration in the Purkinje cells of the cerebellum and in Sommer's sector of Ammon's horn of the hippocampus. There may also be variable degrees of degeneration of the basal ganglia and occasional demyelination of the central white matter. When the patient survives for several days there is likely to be extensive ischaemic necrosis of the cerebral cortex and the lesions of the globus pallidus may progress to softening. Chronic exposure to minimal concentrations of carbon monoxide is believed to play a role in atherogenesis in cigarette smokers (Wanstrup et al., 1969).

SYMPTOMS

McNally (1931) stated that the severity of the symptoms can be correlated with the degree of saturation of the blood with the gas. When this is less than 10 per cent there are no symptoms. At between 10 and 20 per cent the patient complains of slight headache and a tight sensation in the forehead, and there is a dilatation of the cutaneous vessels. At between 30 and 50 per cent there is severe headache, weakness, giddiness, dimness of vision, nausea, vomiting, and collapse. At between 50 and 60 per cent the patient becomes comatose and may convulse. Paralysis of the heart and respiration occurs, with tachycardia, tachypnoea, cyanosis, and, in some cases, glycosuria. Only a small proportion, even of patients who become comatose, end with permanent symptoms. Garland and Pearce (1967) have drawn particular attention to the striking variation in the clinical picture which may occur in such cases, including such features as major seizures, cortical blindness, dysphasia, apraxia and various forms of agnosia with mental changes ranging from retardation to frank psychotic behaviour. Some patients leave hospital apparently recovered only to relapse into coma in from one to three weeks, or into a state of akinetic stupor, or confusion and visual agnosia with catatonic postures. Polyneuropathy is a rare complication (Snyder, 1970).

No explanation has yet been advanced for this syndrome of so-called postanoxic encephalopathy but there is some evidence that its incidence is reduced if activity is greatly limited in the early stages after poisoning (Plum et al., 1962). A mild Parkinsonian syndrome may make its appearance within six weeks of recovery from the initial coma.

PROGNOSIS

In mild cases there is usually complete recovery, but in severe cases the patient may remain comatose for days or even for weeks, and on recovery may exhibit symptoms of permanent damage to the brain, including dementia, aphasia, apraxia, choreo-athetoid movements, Parkinsonian features and polyneuropathy. However, even a confusional state lasting for as long as two months does not necessarily mean that the patient may not recover completely (Garland and Pearce, 1967).

TREATMENT

The patient should at once be moved from exposure to the gas, preferably to the open air, care being taken to protect the body from loss of heat. Inhalations of oxygen should be given and these may with advantage contain 5 per cent of carbon dioxide to increase the pulmonary ventilation, the object being as rapidly as possible to replace carboxyhaemoglobin by oxyhaemoglobin. If the patient is unconscious, artificial respiration should be carried out by administering the mixture of oxygen and carbon dioxide with a respirator. Smith *et al.* (1962) recommend treatment with oxygen at two atmospheres pressure and exposure to hyperbaric oxygen in a pressure chamber is being used increasingly in severe cases; this is especially valuable when carbon monoxide poisoning is complicated by barbiturate poisoning or a cerebrovascular accident. Suitable treatment for heart failure may be required. In the later stages treatment is symptomatic.

REFERENCES

ASTRUP, P., and PAULI, H. G. (1968) A comparison of prolonged exposure to carbon monoxide and hypoxia in man, *Scand. J. clin. Lab. Invest.*, **22**, Suppl. 103.

DENNY-BROWN, D. (1960) Diseases of the basal ganglia, *Lancet*, **ii**, 1104.

DRINKER, C. K. (1938) *Carbon Monoxide Asphyxia*, New York.

GARLAND, H., and PEARCE, J. (1967) Neurological complications of carbon monoxide poisoning, *Quart. J. Med.*, **36**, 445.

MCNALLY, W. D. (1931) Carbon monoxide poisoning, *Illinois med. J.*, **59**, 383.

MEYER, A. (1958) in *Neuropathology*, by Greenfield, J. G., Blackwood, W., McMenemey, W. H., Meyer, A., and Norman, R. M., p. 234, London.

MEDICAL RESEARCH COUNCIL. Carbon monoxide poisoning. Use of carbon dioxide–oxygen mixture, *Brit. med. J.* (1958), **2**, 1408.

PLUM, F., POSNER, J. B., and HAIN, R. F. (1962) Post-anoxic encephalopathy, *Arch. intern. Med.*, **110**, 18.

SMITH, G., LEDINGHAM, I. McA., SHARP, G. R., NORMAN, J. N., and BATES, E. H. (1962) Treatment of coal-gas poisoning with oxygen at 2 atmospheres pressure, *Lancet*, **i**, 816.

SNYDER, R. D. (1970) Carbon monoxide intoxication with peripheral neuropathy, *Neurology (Minneap.)*, **20**, 177.

STRECKER, E. A., TAFT, A. E., and WILLEY, G. F. (1927) Mental sequelae of carbon monoxide poisoning, with reports of autopsy in two cases, *Arch. Neurol. Psychiat. (Chic.)*, **17**, 552.

WANSTRUP, J., KJELDSEN, K., and ASTRUP, P. (1969) Acceleration of spontaneous intimal-subintimal changes in rabbit aorta by a prolonged moderate carbon monoxide exposure, *Acta path. microbiol. scand.*, **75**, 353.

WILSON, G., and WINKLEMAN, N. W. (1924) Multiple neuritis following carbon monoxide poisoning: a clinicopathologic study, *J. Amer. med. Ass.*, **82**, 1407.

CAISSON DISEASE

AETIOLOGY AND PATHOLOGY

Caisson disease, also known as compressed-air sickness, diver's paralysis, and 'the bends', first made its appearance with the introduction of high-pressure caissons for submarine work. It also occurs in tunnel workers and others who work in compressed air. Divers may work in caissons which are open at the bottom and in which the air must be maintained at a high pressure, usually 30 to 35 lb/in², to balance the pressure of the water, which increases in proportion to the depth. As a result of the increased air pressure in the caisson, the tissues of those working in it absorb the gases of the air. If such individuals are suddenly transferred to normal atmospheric pressure, these gases, especially the nitrogen, are liberated in the tissues in the form of small bubbles, in a manner exactly comparable to the liberation of bubbles of carbon dioxide in a bottle of soda water when the cork is removed. The nitrogen is especially soluble in the body fats, and is thus liberated in large amounts in the nervous system. For this reason also fat men are more liable to caisson disease than those of spare build. The liberation of bubbles of gas causes not only disruption of the nerve tissue but also interference with its blood supply through blockage of small vessels.

SYMPTOMS

The first symptom is usually pain situated in the limbs, trunk, and epigastrium, and sometimes associated with vomiting. The pain usually begins in the knees and hips and aseptic necrosis of one or both femoral heads is an important sequel. Headache and vertigo may occur and in severe cases the patient may rapidly become comatose. Scintillating scotomata and paraesthesiae in the extremities are important premonitory symptoms (Behnke, 1974). Hemiplegia or paraplegia with sensory loss may occur.

PROGNOSIS

In severe cases the condition is fatal. In less severe cases recovery usually occurs, sometimes in a few hours, but disability may persist for days, weeks, or months. In some cases, symptoms and signs of paraparesis may persist indefinitely [p. 785].

TREATMENT

Prophylaxis consists in the slow decompression of workers exposed to high pressures. When symptoms have developed, immediate recompression is necessary, the patient being placed in an air lock for this purpose, and restoration to normal pressure must be extremely slow. Otherwise treatment is symptomatic.

MOUNTAIN SICKNESS

Fatigue, dyspnoea, clubbing of the fingers, cyanosis, and somnolence with polycythaemia and a haematocrit often exceeding 70 per cent are the usual manifestations of this disorder (Monge's disease) and are readily relieved by a return to lower altitudes. Pulmonary oedema is a less common manifestation.

REFERENCES

BEHNKE, A. R. (1974) Disorders due to alterations in barometric pressure, in *Harrison's Principles of Internal Medicine*, 7th ed., chap. 117, New York.
BENNETT, P. B., and ELLIOTT, D. H. (1969) *The Physiology and Medicine of Diving*, London.
DU BOIS, E. F. (1929) Physiology of respiration in relationship to the problems of naval medicine: part vi, Deep diving, *Nav. med. Bull. (Wash.)*, **27**, 311.
HILL, L. E. (1912) *Caisson Sickness and the Physiology of Work in Compressed Air*, London.
HULTGREN, H. N., and GROVER, R. F. (1968) Circulatory adaptation to high altitude, *Ann. rev. Med.*, **19**, 119.
PATON, W. D. M., and WALDER, D. N. (1954) Compressed air illness, M.R.C. Special Report Series, No. 281, London, H.M.S.O.

ELECTRIC SHOCK

PATHOLOGY

The pathological changes produced in the nervous system by electric shock are highly characteristic. They consist of chromatolysis of the ganglion cells, dilatation of the perivascular spaces, vascular lesions ranging from focal petechial haemorrhages to actual disruption of large vessels, changes in the peripheral nerves such as fragmentation of the axons and neurilemma, and a peculiar spiral-like appearance of the muscle fibres. These changes may be associated with electrical burns of the skin.

AETIOLOGY AND PATHOGENESIS

There has been much discussion as to the precise way in which electric shock injures the nervous system. The heating effect of the current may sometimes be sufficient to cause severe damage, as in legal electrocution or lightning stroke. Bodily tissues vary considerably in their resistance to the flow of electrical current, whether due to electrocution or lightning. Bone and skin are relatively resistant, whereas blood, muscle, and nervous tissue are good conductors (Wallace and Petersdorf, 1974). The point of contact with earth is important, as is the pathway of current through the body; thus contact with the leg or foot is likely to be less harmful than if the electrical shock enters via the head or hand and is then conducted to one or both feet; the duration of contact is also important. Cardiac arrhythmia and arrest and tetanic muscular contraction followed sometimes by muscle necrosis and consequent myoglobinuria are important complications of severe shock.

Changes in the central nervous system are most likely to occur when the current has been applied directly to the skull. The extreme variability of conditions is no doubt responsible for the unpredictability of the results of exposure to electric currents. Eleven thousand volts may cause only slight injury (Critchley, 1934). On the other hand, forty volts has been known to prove fatal. Death from electric shock, however, is rare, especially considering the risks of exposure in civilized life.

SYMPTOMS

A severe electric shock causes immediate loss of consciousness. If the patient does not lose consciousness there is usually severe pain associated with bizarre sensory disturbances, especially visual hallucinations. A typical immediate sequel of the shock is a transitory flaccid paraplegia with objective sensory disturbance, both disappearing after about 12 hours. Critchley classified the neurological sequelae of electric shock as follows: (1) cerebral, (2) spinal, (3) mixed cerebrospinal affection, (4) peripheral nerve lesions, isolated or multiple, and (5) psychological disorders, hysteria being particularly common. Symptoms of an isolated cerebral lesion are rare, but spinal atrophic paralyses leading to a clinical picture not unlike motor neurone disease are not uncommon. Both immediate spastic tetraplegia (So and Lee, 1973) and delayed myelopathy (Holbrook et al., 1970) giving wasting of muscles in the upper limbs and paraparesis have been described. Brachial neuropathy may follow a shock to the upper limbs and Critchley described a lasting polyneuropathic syndrome following lightning stroke.

PROGNOSIS

Generalizations about prognosis are impossible on account of the varied character of the clinical picture.

TREATMENT

The first essential is immediate artificial respiration and, if necessary, external cardiac massage since by these methods it may be possible to revive a victim even though the heart has apparently ceased to beat. It is difficult to know how long artificial respiration should be carried on in the absence of any response, but there is some evidence that resuscitation has been effective even after a period of several hours. During artificial respiration the general treatment of shock should be carried out, and the after-treatment will depend upon the nature of the sequelae.

REFERENCES

CRITCHLEY, M. (1934) Neurological effects of lightning and of electricity, *Lancet*, **i**, 68.
HOLBROOK, L. A., BEACH, F. X. M., and SILVER, J. R. (1970) Delayed myelopathy: a rare complication of severe electrical burns, *Brit. med. J.*, **4**, 659.
JELLINEK, S. (1932) *Elektrische Verletzungen*, Leipzig.
MORRISON, L. R., WEEKS, A., and COBB, S. (1930) Histopathology of different types of electric shock on mammalian brains, *J. industr. Hyg.*, **12**, 324.
PRITCHARD, E. A. B. (1934) Changes in the central nervous system due to electrocution, *Lancet*, **i**, 1163.
SO, S. C., and LEE, M. L. K. (1973) Spastic quadriplegia due to electric shock, *Brit. med. J.*, **2**, 590.
WALLACE, J. F., and PETERSDORF, R. G. (1974) Electrical injuries, in *Harrison's Principles of Internal Medicine*, 7th ed., chap. 120, New York.

HEAT STROKE

Heat stroke is characterized by partial or complete loss of consciousness, hyperpyrexia, convulsions, and delirium following excessive exposure to sun or heat. The body temperature usually exceeds 41·1 °C, there is lack of sweating and circulatory collapse (Climatic Physiology Committee, 1958). Occasional cases have been described with permanent neurological sequelae after recovery, including cerebellar ataxia, dysarthria, mild dementia, and polyneuropathy (Mehta and Baker, 1970).

REFERENCES

CLIMATIC PHYSIOLOGY COMMITTEE (1958) A classification of heat illness, *Brit. med. J.*, **1**, 1533.
MEHTA, A. C., and BAKER, R. N. (1970) Persistent neurological deficits in heat stroke, *Neurology* (*Minneap.*), **20**, 336.

POISONING WITH ORGANOPHOSPHORUS INSECTICIDES

Many organophosphorus insecticides in common use are powerful inhibitors of both cholinesterase and pseudocholinesterase and the compounds in this group most toxic to man are the so-called 'nerve gases'. The clinical features of mild poisoning include miosis and widespread muscular weakness and fasciculation. In more severe poisoning, respiratory distress, cardiac arrhythmia, widespread paralysis, and cardiac arrest may occur (Namba *et al.*, 1970, 1971). The different preparations differ in their relative toxicity, but in many instances early treatment with pralidoxine 1 g intravenously followed by 0·5 g/hour by intravenous infusion with atropine sulphate 5 mg intravenously every 20–30 minutes is effective (Ladell, 1958; Namba *et al.*, 1971).

REFERENCES

LADELL, W. S. S. (1958) Treatment of anticholinesterase poisoning, *Brit. med. J.*, **2**, 141.
NAMBA, T., GREENFIELD, M., and GROB, D. (1970) Malathion poisoning. A fatal case with cardiac manifestations, *Arch. environm. Hlth (Chic.)*, **21**, 533.
NAMBA, T., NOLTE, C. T., JACKREL, J., and GROB, D. (1971) Poisoning due to organophosphate insecticides, *Amer. J. Med.*, **50**, 475.

SNAKE BITE

Snake venom neurotoxins comprise a heterogeneous group of proteins, their neurotoxic fractions being closely associated with, but distinct from, the cholinesterase, ribonuclease, and deoxyribonuclease fractions of the venom (Porges, 1953; Pearn 1971). The bites of many venomous snakes may be followed by widespread muscular weakness and above all by respiratory paralysis, though sea-snake bites may be followed by widespread necrosis of skeletal muscle and hepatic and renal damage (Marsden and Reid, 1961). Treatment is based upon the use of assisted respiration and intravenous injections of polyvalent antivenene (Pearn, 1971).

REFERENCES

MARSDEN, A. T. H., and REID, H. A. (1961) Pathology of sea-snake poisoning, *Brit. med. J.*, **1**, 1290.
PEARN, J. H. (1971) Survival after snake-bite with prolonged neurotoxic envenomation, *Med. J. Aust.*, **2**, 259.
PORGES, N. (1953) Snake venoms, their biochemistry and mode of action, *Science*, **117**, 47.

TETANUS

Definition. Tetanus is an intoxication of the nervous system with the exotoxin of the tetanus bacillus. It is characterized by the progressive development of muscular rigidity which is subject to paroxysmal exacerbations.

AETIOLOGY

Tetanus is due to infection with the *Clostridium tetani*, a Gram-positive, anaerobic organism which bears spores. The spore is oval or rounded, and develops at one end of the bacillus, which then presents the appearance of a drumstick. The *Cl. tetani* is actively motile, its movement being due to flagella. Fildes (1929) showed by immunological methods that a number of types exist, not all of which are toxic.

The *Cl. tetani* is widely distributed in the soil, and is found in the faeces of many animals, especially horses, and of a small proportion of normal human beings. The disease arises in man through contamination of wounds with the spores of the organism, especially as a result of accidents in which road dust or soil is introduced into the wound. Other, less common, sources of tetanus infection include vaccination, infection of wounds by contaminated dressings or catgut, and the injection of infected drugs, especially in narcotic addicts. Tetanus neonatorum, due to infection of the stump of the umbilical cord in newly born infants, and puerperal tetanus are common in some tropical countries.

The mere introduction of tetanus spores into a wound is not sufficient to cause the disease. It usually appears to be necessary that other organisms should also be present. There is frequently a foreign body, such as a splinter. The *Cl. tetani* do not spread beyond the wound, but they produce an exotoxin, by which the nervous system is poisoned. Animal experiments have suggested that the toxin reaches the nervous system by ascending the axis cylinders of the peripheral nerves. It has been shown that the dorsal root ganglia act as a filter which prevents the toxin entering the spinal cord by the dorsal roots. Its portal of entry is thus confined to the ventral roots. There is, however, some recent evidence to suggest that the toxin may also spread by the blood stream; thus Zacks and Sheff (1966) have found that the toxin could be isolated from brain, spinal cord, skeletal muscle, and spleen after injecting it into mice. Zacks *et al.* (1966) have also shown vesicles and dense intra-mitochondrial inclusions in the skeletal muscle of such animals. Tetanic muscular spasms are probably due to the fact that the toxin blocks the inhibitory interneurones in the spinal cord and in human subjects there is widespread myopathic change in the affected skeletal muscles with a concomitant rise in serum creatine kinase activity, and electron microscopy shows evidence of post-synaptic damage to the motor end-plates (Eyrich *et al.*, 1967). In experimental tetanus, chromatolysis of anterior horn cells with hyperaemia and spinal cord haemorrhages are seen, but spinal synaptic endings are morphologically normal (Tarlov *et al.*, 1973). Having reached the brain stem and spinal cord, the toxin produces its characteristic effects by disturbing the normal regulation of the reflex arc. Afferent stimuli not only produce an exaggerated effect, but also reciprocal innervation is abolished and both prime movers and antagonists contract. Hence arises the characteristic muscular spasm.

When a small amount of toxin is slowly absorbed it reaches the anterior horn cells by the route already described. In such cases the first symptom is local spasm of the muscles in the neighbourhood of the wound. When a slightly larger amount of toxin is produced it enters the circulation by way of the lymphatics and reaches the nervous system diffusely by ascending all the peripheral motor nerves. The larger the volume of toxin, the more remains unabsorbed by the anterior horn cells and available to poison distant synapses and ultimately the vital centres. There is then no local tetanus; trismus is usually the first symptom and the spasm subsequently spreads rapidly, to involve the arms, trunk, and legs.

PATHOLOGY

Tetanus is essentially a disorder of function of the nervous system and no constant structural changes have been observed, though hyperaemia may occur in the spinal cord and brain, especially in the anterior horns of grey matter and there may be rupture of fibres and haemorrhages and consequent myopathic change (Eyrick *et al.*, 1967) in the muscles which have been subjected to violent spasms.

SYMPTOMS
Incubation Period

The incubation period varies, but is usually 7 or 8 days. In patients who have had a prophylactic inoculation of antitoxin it may extend to several weeks. Exceptionally it is as short as one or two days or, conversely, it may seem, on occasion, to be as long as two or three weeks, when the clinical syndrome may be

D d

milder than in the average case, or the spasms may even be curiously localized in one or more limbs (local tetanus). Such a prolonged incubation period is commonest in those who have previously been immunized.

Descending Form

A prodromal phase of restlessness and irritability has been described. The first motor symptom is usually trismus, which is rapidly followed, or may be preceded, by stiffness of the neck. At this stage the patient is likely to attribute his symptoms to a chill. Within a few hours, however, the spasm extends to other muscles and dysphagia is often an early complaint. Spasm of the facial muscles may lead either to pursing of the lips or to retraction of the angles of the mouth—the risus sardonicus. The eyes may be partly closed through contraction of the orbicularis oculi, or the eyebrows may be elevated by spasm of the frontalis. Examination reveals the presence of rigidity of the musculature of the limbs and trunk. There may be slight opisthotonus. The muscles of the abdominal wall are rigid, and the lower limbs, which are usually affected more than the upper, are fixed in a position of extension. As the disease progresses, this persisting general rigidity undergoes paroxysmal exacerbations which are attended by severe cramp-like pains. Opisthotonic spasm usually occurs in these attacks, but in some cases the spine is bent in other directions, for example, forwards or laterally. Spasm of the larynx and respiratory muscles leads to dyspnoea, and profuse sweating occurs. These convulsive paroxysms may be excited by external stimuli, for example, by attempting to feed the patient. Between the paroxysms the general muscular rigidity persists. The tendon reflexes are exaggerated, but, with the exceptions described below, there are no signs of organic lesions of the nervous system. Consciousness is retained to the end.

Death may occur in a convulsive attack from asphyxia, or, when severe spasms recur frequently, from heart failure. The disease may be apyrexial, but some fever is not uncommon, and hyperpyrexia is an important and serious complication in severe cases, the temperature even continuing to rise after death. Other risks include a negative nitrogen balance leading to uraemia, hypotension, and gastric dilatation, all most liable to occur between the 7th and 14th days, and motor paresis. Laryngeal spasm, apnoea, and pneumonia are also risks. In favourable cases the severity and frequency of the spasms gradually diminish, but the general rigidity frequently persists for several weeks, trismus often being the last abnormality to disappear.

Ascending or Local Form

In this form of tetanus the first symptom is local spasm of the muscles in the neighbourhood of the wound, whence persistent or intermittent spasm spreads to neighbouring muscles and in severe cases to the other limbs, head, and trunk. After recovery from this form of the disease the original local spasm may persist for days or weeks. In one reported case due to injury by a porcupine quill, severe rigidity was present in one upper limb only (though trismus was also present in the early stages) for over five months, and in the first two or three months any attempt to use the affected limb produced severe spasms localized to it—'recruitment spasm' (Struppler et al., 1963).

Cephalic Tetanus

Cephalic tetanus is a rare variety of the ascending form and follows wounds of the head, face, and neck. Muscular paralysis is frequently present, usually

involving the facial muscles on one side (Vakil *et al.*, 1973) and may be associated with facial spasm on the opposite side. Trismus and pharyngeal spasm
usually develop. When the wound has involved the orbit, ptosis, external
ophthalmoplegia, and iridoplegia have been observed on one or both sides.
Cephalic tetanus may remain localized or become generalized. It is rarely
fatal, but, when recovery occurs, facial paralysis and spasm may persist for
weeks.

Splanchnic Tetanus

This term has been applied to a form of tetanus which follows abdominal
wounds and in which the bulbar and respiratory muscles are early and severely
affected.

Autonomic Manifestations

Common autonomic manifestations in tetanus include tachycardia, irregularities of cardiac rhythm, peripheral vasoconstriction, profuse sweating,
hyperpyrexia, increased carbon dioxide output, and increased urinary catecholamine excretion, presumed to be due to involvement of the sympathetic
nervous system (Kerr *et al.*, 1968), while episodes of profound arterial hypotension, responsive to carbon dioxide inhalation, have also been recorded
(Corbett *et al.*, 1973).

Modified Tetanus

The symptoms of tetanus may be considerably modified by a previous immunization or prophylactic inoculation of antitoxin. The incubation period in
such cases is usually longer than normal. There is a tendency for the spasm to
remain localized to the muscles in the neighbourhood of the wound, and often,
when generalized tetanus ensues, convulsions are absent, and if they occur are
likely to be slight.

DIAGNOSIS

Conditions causing trismus may be confused with tetanus. Trismus is sometimes produced by painful lesions in the neighbourhood of the jaw such as
dental abscess, or it may follow mandibular block with local anaesthetics. The
presence of the causative lesion and the localized character of the spasm enable
these cases to be distinguished from tetanus. Trismus may also occur in encephalitis, and in some cases, post-vaccinal encephalitis in which trismus was a prominent symptom was at first regarded as tetanus. Symptoms of organic lesions of
the brain and spinal cord are always present in such cases and distinguish them
from tetanus. The convulsions of strychnine poisoning superficially resemble
those of tetanus, but develop more rapidly. Moreover, the fact that they follow
reflex excitation is apparent from the beginning, whereas this is a late feature in
tetanus. Strychnine poisoning also differs from tetanus in that muscular relaxation is complete between the paroxysms, and the upper limbs are more severely
affected. A history of poisoning can usually be obtained. Rabies may also be confused with tetanus, but in this condition trismus is absent and dysphagia is the
most conspicuous symptom. Further, muscular relaxation occurs between the
paroxysms and there is almost always a history of a bite by a rabid animal. Tetany
is distinguished from tetanus by the fact that the muscular spasm always begins
in the periphery of the limbs and leads to the characteristic attitude of the hands.
Trismus occurs only in the most severe attacks. Hysteria may cause either trismus

or generalized rigidity associated with opisthotonos. Hysterical trismus, however, is not always associated with rigidity elsewhere, while hysterical opisthotonus usually forms part of a hysterial convulsion which develops suddenly without pre-existing rigidity, is attended by apparent impairment of consciousness, and is frequently associated with other signs of hysteria. Nevertheless, hysterical trismus with associated spasms is sufficiently common, often after minor injury, to give diagnostic difficulty in some cases; electromyography may be useful in such cases.

PROGNOSIS

The prognosis of tetanus unmodified by immunization or prophylactic inoculation of antitoxin is always extremely grave, though the outlook was somewhat improved by treatment with antitoxic serum. In one series of cases the mortality before the introduction of treatment with serum was 79 per cent and afterwards 57·7 per cent. Corresponding figures for the London Hospital quoted by Fildes (1929) were 81·7 per cent and 71·8 per cent. In general, the shorter the incubation period the worse is the prognosis, and few patients with an incubation period of less than six days used to recover. Cole (1937–8) stressed the prognostic importance of the interval between the first symptom and the first generalized reflex spasms, which he called 'the period of onset'. Nevertheless, the new methods of treatment recently introduced offer the hope of saving life even when the incubation period is short, and the mortality rate is now 30 per cent or less. There may be some persistent motor weakness for many months after recovery. Illis and Taylor (1971), in a follow-up study, found that many patients suffered from irritability, sleep disorders, fits, myoclonus, decreased libido, or postural hypotension, and many showed electroencephalographic abnormalities.

TREATMENT

The patient should be nursed in isolation, if possible in an intensive care unit, and should be kept as quiet as possible. The curative value of antitoxin is limited by the fact that the nervous system is largely impenetrable by immune bodies. Nevertheless, antitoxin can neutralize circulating toxin and so reduce the dose, perhaps to one the tissues can neutralize. A massive dose (100,000 units) should be given intravenously. In fact, some authors nowadays doubt whether antitoxin is necessary, but many still recommend surgical toilet of the wound, if identified, in an attempt to remove the tetanus bacilli and spores.

The modern treatment of severe tetanus is based upon the elimination of muscle spasm by tubocurarine chloride in doses of 15 mg repeated as necessary up to a daily total of 150–650 mg, while artificial respiration is carried out with intermittent positive-pressure equipment through a tracheostomy tube, and naso-oesophageal feeding is employed.

Chlorpromazine is effective in the control of spasms and can be given either in a dosage of 100–150 mg four- or six-hourly intramuscularly or, in neonates, 25 mg four- or six-hourly. Cole and Youngman (1969) recommended paraldehyde, but more recently diazepam given intravenously is preferred to this drug and to chlorpromazine by many authors. Antibiotics are given to prevent pulmonary infection. The continuous supervision of an anaesthetist and laryngologist is required. Nutrition and fluid and electrolyte balance must be watched, and many nursing difficulties need to be overcome (Shackleton, 1954; Forbes and Auld, 1955; Adams, 1958; Smith, 1958; Adams et al., 1959).

REFERENCES

ABEL, J. J., and others. Researches on tetanus, *Bull. Johns Hopk. Hosp.*, II, 1935, **56,** 84; III, 1935, **56,** 317; IV, 1935, **57,** 343; V, 1936, **59,** 307; VI, 1938, **62,** 91; VII, 1938, **62,** 522; VIII, 1938, **62,** 610.

ADAMS, E. B. (1958) Clinical trials in tetanus, *Proc. roy. Soc. Med.*, **51,** 1002.

ADAMS, E. B., WRIGHT, R., BERMAN, E., and LAURENCE, D. R. (1959) Treatment of tetanus with chlorpromazine and barbiturates, *Lancet*, **i,** 755.

COLE, L. (1937–8) The treatment and prognosis of tetanus, *Proc. roy. Soc. Med.*, **31,** 1205.

COLE, L., and YOUNGMAN, H. (1969) Treatment of tetanus, *Lancet*, **i,** 1017.

CORBETT, J. L., SPALDING, J. M. K., and HARRIS, P. J. (1973) Hypotension in tetanus, *Brit. med. J.*, **3,** 423.

EYRICH, K., AGOSTINI, B., SCHULZ, A., MÜLLER, E., NOETZEL, H., REICHENMILLER, H. E., and WIEMERS, K. (1967) Clinical and morphological studies of skeletal muscle changes in tetanus, *Germ. med. Mth.*, **12,** 469.

FILDES, P. (1929) Bacillus tetani, in *A System of Bacteriology*, vol. 3, p. 298, London.

FORBES, G. R., and AULD, M. (1955) Management of tetanus, *Amer. J. Med.*, **18,** 947.

ILLIS, L. S., and TAYLOR, F. M. (1971) Neurological and electroencephalographic sequelae of tetanus, *Lancet*, **i,** 826.

KERR, J. H., CORBETT, J. L., PRYS-ROBERTS, C., SMITH, A. C., and SPALDING, J. M. K. (1968) Involvement of the sympathetic nervous system in tetanus, *Lancet*, **ii,** 236.

SHACKLETON, P. (1954) The treatment of tetanus, *Lancet*, **ii,** 155.

SHERRINGTON, C. S. (1917) Observations with antitetanus serum in the monkey, *Lancet*, **ii,** 964.

SMITH, A. C. (1958) The treatment of severe tetanus by paralysing drugs and intermittent pressure respiration, *Proc. roy. Soc. Med.*, **51,** 1006.

STRUPPLER, A., STRUPPLER, E., and ADAMS, R. D. (1963) Local tetanus in man, *Arch. Neurol. (Chic.)*, **8,** 162.

TARLOV, I. M., LING, H., and YAMADA, H. (1973) Neuronal pathology in experimental local tetanus, *Neurology (Minneap.)*, **23,** 580.

VAKIL, B. J., SINGHAL, B. S., PANDYA, S. S., and IRANI, P. F. (1973) Cephalic tetanus, *Neurology (Minneap.)*, **23,** 1091.

ZACKS, S. I., HALL, J. A. S., and SHEFF, M. F. (1966) Studies in tetanus. IV. Intramitochondrial dense granules in skeletal muscles from human cases of tetanus intoxication, *Amer. J. Path.*, **48,** 811.

ZACKS, S. I., and SHEFF, M. F. (1966) Studies on tetanus. V. *In vivo* localization of purified tetanus neurotoxin in mice with fluorescein-labelled tetanus antitoxin, *J. Neuropath. exp. Neurol.*, **25,** 422.

BOTULISM

Definition. A form of food poisoning due to intoxication with the exotoxin of the *Clostridium botulinum* derived from infected foodstuffs, especially those preserved in tins, and characterized by extreme weakness and fatigability of both striated and unstriated muscle.

AETIOLOGY

The *Cl. botulinum* is a large, Gram-positive, anaerobic, spore-bearing organism, which is an inhabitant of the soil in certain regions and may contaminate food. It finds a most congenial environment in food preserved in tins, especially vegetables and fruit, and both bought and home-preserved foodstuffs may be contaminated with it. The commonest type is so-called Type E, and Type E spores have been shown to be plentiful in North American soil and littoral waters (Meyers, 1956). It produces a powerful exotoxin, to which the toxic effects are due. Tinned food infected with the bacillus may often be detected as tainted. Production of gas in the tin may abolish the normal vacuum, and the food often has a peculiar rancid odour and taste. This, however, may be disguised by sauces and dressings. There are many examples of severe and fatal poisoning occurring in a person who had only tasted the food to see if it was tainted. Cooking at boiling temperature for a few minutes destroys the toxin, but boiling at high altitudes may be less effective (Cherington, 1974). There have been outbreaks of botulism in many countries, especially in Germany, where it was first attributed to eating infected sausages—hence the name, derived from 'botulus', a sausage—and in the United States. An outbreak leading to a number of deaths occurred at Loch Maree in Scotland in 1922. Botulism has frequently been observed in domestic animals which have eaten the remains of tainted food, and fowls which have been thus intoxicated may die before symptoms appear in human beings, who have eaten the same food. Contamination of fish by Type E may occur before they are caught and Whittaker et al. (1964) reported eight simultaneous cases due to eating white chubb fish from the Great Lakes area, fish which was contaminated with Type E spores.

Botulinus toxin acts presynaptically, by abolishing the release of acetylcholine at cholinergic nerve endings (Burgen et al., 1949; Zacks, 1964).

PATHOLOGY

The changes in the nervous system consist of severe congestion of both the brain and meninges, leading to oedema and perivascular haemorrhages.

SYMPTOMS

In man, symptoms usually develop between 18 and 36 hours after the ingestion of the tainted food, less frequently as early as 12 hours or as late as 48 hours or longer afterwards. In about one-third of all cases an acute gastro-intestinal disturbance, characterized by nausea, vomiting, and diarrhoea, occurs, but in most cases this is absent, constipation, probably due to paresis of the smooth muscle of the intestines, occurring early and persisting throughout the illness.

The earliest symptoms of muscular weakness are usually visual. Dimness of vision occurs as a result of paresis of accommodation; the pupils sometimes become dilated, and lose their reaction to light, and ptosis usually develops early. Paresis of the external ocular muscles leads to diplopia, and nystagmus may be present. In some cases complete ocular immobility occurs. Vertigo is not uncommon. Owing to weakness of the muscles concerned, swallowing and talking become difficult; attempts to swallow lead to choking and regurgitation of food through the nose; and there may be complete aphonia. Weakness of the jaw muscles renders mastication difficult or impossible, the muscles of the trunk and limbs also become extremely weak, and respiratory insufficiency or paralysis may follow. The muscular disturbance appears to be an extreme degree of fatigability, rather than an actual paralysis, since the patient may be able to carry out a movement moderately well on one occasion but be then unable to repeat it. The tendon reflexes are preserved and the plantar reflexes are flexor. There is usually no sensory disturbance. In most cases consciousness remains unimpaired up to the end, though occasionally there is a terminal coma, and terminal convulsions have been described.

The cerebrospinal fluid is usually normal. The temperature remains normal, unless a complicating infection, such as bronchopneumonia, develops. The pulse is usually rapid. Death occurs either from respiratory paralysis or bronchopneumonia.

DIAGNOSIS

The most useful diagnostic features are: (1) a previously healthy patient; (2) absence of fever; (3) abdominal symptoms; (4) weakness, malaise, and fatigability; (5) cranial nerve signs; and (6) a likely food source.

In cases in which an acute gastro-intestinal disturbance occurs the diagnosis from other forms of acute gastro-enteritis cannot usually be made before the onset of muscular weakness, unless domestic animals have already shown signs of poisoning. The dilated pupils may suggest belladonna poisoning, but the unclouded mental condition enables this to be excluded. When the diagnosis is doubtful it may be confirmed by the demonstration of the *Cl. botulinum* or of its toxins in the remains of food which has been consumed.

Supramaximal stimulation of a peripheral nerve with recording of the evoked muscle action potential may give a decremental response at low rates of stimulation but an increase in amplitude during stimulation at 50 Hz, as in the Eaton–Lambert syndrome [p. 1025] (Cherington, 1974).

PROGNOSIS

The mortality varies in different outbreaks; in the past it often ranged between 16 and 65 per cent but the outlook is much better with modern treatment. Death usually occurs between the fourth and eighth day. Convalescence is very slow but eventual recovery is usually complete.

TREATMENT

Prophylaxis consists in the careful scrutiny of all tinned foods, and the rejection, without tasting it, of any which appears to be tainted. The cooking of tinned products for ten minutes before use abolishes all risk of botulism. Antitoxin appears to possess greater prophylactic than curative value, but it can seldom be used before the onset of muscular symptoms. Fifty thousand units of a polyvalent serum should be employed. The stomach should be washed out and a purge administered to remove as far as possible any toxin which may not have yet been absorbed. Antibiotics should also be given orally and parenterally, penicillin being the drug of choice in order to destroy surviving organisms in the gastro-intestinal tract which may still be producing exotoxin. Complete rest is of great importance to protect the muscles from all avoidable fatigue, and sedatives should be given if necessary. Nasal feeding and artificial respiration may be required.

Temporary improvement may follow an injection of edrophonium or neostigmine, but sustained improvement usually results from guanidine hydrochloride given in a dosage of 250 mg every four hours for several days (Cherington, 1974).

REFERENCES

Burgen, A. S. V., Dickens, F., and Zatman, L. J. (1949) Action of botulinum toxin on the neuro-muscular junction, *J. Physiol. (Lond.)*, **109**, 10.
Cherington, M. (1974) Botulism: ten-year experience, *Arch. Neurol. (Chic.)*, **30**, 432.
Meyer, K. F. (1956) The status of botulism as a world health problem, *Bull. Wld Hlth Org.*, **15**, 28.

Monro, T. K., and Knox, W. W. N. (1923) Remarks on botulism as seen in Scotland in 1922, *Brit. med. J.*, **1**, 279.

Petty, C. J. (1965) Botulism; the disease and the toxin, *Amer. J. med. Sci.*, **249**, 345.

Whittaker, R. L., Gilbertson, R. B., and Garrett, A. S. (1964) Botulism, Type E. Report of 8 simultaneous cases, *Ann. intern. Med.*, **61**, 448.

Zacks, S. I. (1964) *The Motor End-plate*, Philadelphia.

SAXITOXIN POISONING

Saxitoxin, a powerful neurotoxic agent, may produce symptoms in human subjects eating mussels or other shellfish which have been contaminated by dinoflagellates of the genus *Gonyaulax* which only occur in the sea at certain times of the year and in certain weather conditions. Epidemics have been reported from the Pacific Coast of the U.S.A. and from many places in Europe. An outbreak in Northumberland affecting 78 individuals was described by McCollum *et al.* (1968); while the condition has been fatal all patients in this series recovered. Symptoms, which usually developed within 30 minutes to 12 hours after eating mussels, included paraesthesiae in the limbs and circumoral distribution, muscular weakness, ataxia, headache, vomiting, and choking sensations. Recovery was usually complete within 24–72 hours.

REFERENCE

McCollum, J. P. K., Pearson, R. C. M., Ingham, H. R., Wood, P. C., and Dewar, H. A. (1968) An epidemic of mussel poisoning in North-East England, *Lancet*, **ii**, 767.

ERGOTISM

'Ergotism' is the term applied to poisoning with the toxins produced by the fungus *Claviceps purpurea* of rye. Two forms occur, one characterized by gangrene—the gangrenous form—the other by muscular spasms and generalized convulsions—the convulsive form, which is now very rare.

Poisoning with ergot was usually due in the past to the consumption of bread made from contaminated flour. The gangrenous form is occasionally produced by the administration of ergot as an abortifacient. Very rarely it may result from the excessive use of ergotamine tartrate given as a treatment for migraine (Hudgson and Hart, 1964) or of the closely-related drug dimethysergide (*Deseril*) given as a prophylactic in this condition, though retroperitoneal fibrosis is a more important complication of treatment with the latter remedy. Many patients who take abnormally large amounts of these drugs may complain of pains in the limbs and of paraesthesiae, blanching of digits and coldness in the extremities but the fully-developed syndrome of ergotism is rare. Ergotism was rare in Britain, but commoner on the continent of Europe, where it was especially prevalent during the Middle Ages. Epidemics occurred in France, Germany, Sweden, Norway, Finland, Russia, and elsewhere, and in the last-named country it is apparently still endemic. The gangrenous and convulsive forms differed in their geographical distribution, the former occurring to the west, and the latter to the east, of the Rhine, though mixed epidemics were sometimes observed where these regions meet. There is reason to believe that the gangrenous form was due to poisoning with ergotoxin or ergotamine, but the convulsive form appeared to depend upon the coexistence of two factors, namely consumption of an unknown constituent of ergot, not the alkaloid, together with a deficiency of vitamin A in the diet (Mellanby, 1931; Barger, 1931).

Convulsive ergotism was associated with degeneration of the spinal cord, especially of the dorsal columns, and also of the peripheral nerves. Thickening of the media and hyaline degeneration of the intima of the arteries, sometimes associated with thrombosis, are the changes found in the gangrenous form.

The onset of gangrenous ergotism may be insidious or rapid. Gangrene is usually preceded by severe burning pains, hence the name St. Anthony's fire. Gangrene may involve only the nails, or the fingers or toes or whole limbs, the gangrenous part separating spontaneously without pain or the loss of blood. Convulsive ergotism began with muscular fasciculation, followed by clonic and tonic muscular spasms, leading to abnormal postures and finally, in severe cases, generalized convulsions. Anaesthesia of the limbs, hemiplegia, and paraplegia sometimes occurred.

REFERENCES

BARGER, G. (1931) Ergot and Ergotism, London.
HUDGSON, P., and HART, J. A. L. (1964) Acute ergotism: report of a case and a review of the literature, Med. J. Aust., 2, 589.
MELLANBY, E. (1931) The experimental production and prevention of degeneration in the spinal cord, Brain, 54, 247.
VON STORCH, T. J. C. (1938) Complications following the use of ergotamine tartrate. Their relation to the treatment of migraine headache, J. Amer. med. Ass., 111, 293.

THE NEUROLOGICAL MANIFESTATIONS OF ACUTE PORPHYRIA

The porphyrias are disorders involving the metabolism of porphyrins and porphyrin precursors (Dean, 1969). They may be symptomless, may cause cutaneous lesions, or may be responsible for an acute illness (acute porphyria) which gives psychological, neurological, and abdominal symptoms. Dean divides this group of conditions first into the three varieties of hepatic porphyria, namely porphyria variegata (protocoproporphyria, the South African type), acute intermittent porphyria (pyrroloporphyria, the Swedish type) and coproporphyria (Goldberg et al., 1967). In addition there are other rare varieties of non-hepatic porphyria including the erythropoietic type (congenital porphyria) in which there are anaemia, splenomegaly, and pink staining of the teeth and of bones without neurological manifestations, and symptomatic porphyria which presents largely with cutaneous manifestations precipitated often by alcoholism but not by barbiturates, or else by eating bread made from wheat treated with hexachlorophene.

Macalpine et al. (1968) have suggested that King George III of England suffered from a psychotic illness due to porphyria and gave reasons for suggesting that the disorder was present in many members of the Royal Houses of Stuart, Hanover, and Prussia.

AETIOLOGY AND PATHOLOGY

The South African and Swedish types of porphyria and coproporphyria are all inherited as autosomal dominant traits. The Swedish type is commonest in Europe (Waldenstrom, 1957) and is seen most often in females between 16 and 50 years. Acute attacks are often precipitated by drugs, especially barbiturates, light sensitivity does not occur, and there is a high excretion of porphobilinogen G and of delta-amino-laevulinic acid during the acute attacks and for a long time afterwards. In the South African type (Dean and Barnes, 1958) the age and sex incidence is similar, acute attacks are always precipitated by drugs and are often fatal; light sensitivity (porphyria variegata) is found in many affected individuals, particularly males, and there is a high excretion of porphobilinogen in the acute attack but this returns to normal as soon as the patient recovers. Faecal excretion of protoporphyrin is normal in acute intermittent porphyria but is raised in the South African variety. Coproporphyria is less common than the other two types; there is excessive excretion of coproporphyrin in the stools, acute attacks of neurological dysfunction may be precipitated by barbiturates but there are no skin changes, and both urinary coproporphyrin and uroporphyrin are increased in the attacks. In acute attacks, especially in the Swedish type, there is a greatly increased activity of delta-amino-laevulinic acid synthetase, the rate-limiting enzyme of haem biosynthesis, in liver biopsy specimens, along with excessive urinary excretion of certain porphyrogenic steroids (Goldberg et al., 1969; Sweeney et al., 1970; The Lancet, 1972). In many cases uroporphyrinogen-I synthetase activity is reduced in the red blood cells.

The pathological changes in the nervous system were studied by Hierons (1957) who found evidence of demyelination in peripheral nerves and abnormalities of the anterior horn cells. There were no specific abnormalities in the brain and it seemed likely that the mental disturbances observed in acute attacks are of metabolic origin. Dagg et al. (1965) drew attention to the similarity of lead poisoning to acute porphyria. In both conditions there is a considerable increase in the excretion of delta-amino-laevulinic acid. They suggest that the abdominal, cardiovascular, and neurological manifestations may be explained on a neurogenic basis with focal demyelination of peripheral and autonomic nerves and in the central nervous system. However, Cavanagh and Mellick (1965) found no evidence of demyelination in the peripheral nerves of four fatal cases and suggested that the lesion lay distally in the axon. Mustajoki and Seppäläinen (1975) found slowing of sensory and to a lesser extent of motor conduction in the peripheral nerves in 20 patients with the Swedish and 5 with the South African variety of porphyria between attacks. The current view is that the neuropathy of this condition is predominantly axonal but that there is often some secondary demyelination.

SYMPTOMATOLOGY

The syndrome of acute intermittent porphyria may present with the acute clinical picture, or with cutaneous lesions alone, or with a combination of the two. The biochemical lesion may exist without producing any symptoms, particularly in the sibs of affected patients.

The onset of symptoms usually occurs in adolescence or early adult life, and the acute manifestations are frequently precipitated by the administration of barbiturates, sulphonamides, chloroquine, griseofulvin, the sulphones, and many other drugs (Garcin, 1964), or over-indulgence in alcohol.

Early symptoms of involvement of the nervous system include restlessness, emotional instability and mood disorder, sometimes going on to a confusional state. Epileptic attacks are common, and are sometimes the presenting feature. Severe cerebral involvement may lead to stupor or coma, or status epilepticus.

The other characteristic clinical picture is a polyneuropathy, usually predominantly motor, and leading to muscular weakness, initially chiefly proximal in the limbs, but becoming generalized and sometimes involving the respiratory and bulbar muscles. Though subjective sensory symptoms are common, objective sensory loss is rare.

General symptoms often usher in the attacks, especially acute abdominal pain with nausea, vomiting, and constipation. Hypertension may occur, and there may be impairment of renal function. In the South African type the skin may exhibit scars, erosions, or bullae, and a bronze pigmentation and hirsutism are common.

During the acute attack, the urine contains large amounts of the porphyrin precursors, delta-amino-laevulinic acid and porphobilinogen. In the Swedish type, there is very little increase in urinary and faecal porphyrin excretion except in the acute attack, while in the South African type urinary and faecal porphyrins show a much greater increase, again particularly during an attack. The urine from patients with acute intermittent porphyria is not necessarily abnormally coloured, even during the attack, though in many cases the patient will have noted darkening, and the typical 'port-wine' colour which darkens on standing, at the outset.

DIAGNOSIS

As far as the neurological symptoms are concerned, it is necessary to bear in mind the possibility of porphyria as a cause of otherwise unexplained confusional states, coma, epilepsy, or polyneuropathy occurring particularly in early adult life, and especially if the symptoms have been precipitated by the administration of any of the drugs known to be apt to precipitate acute porphyria. On suspicion of the diagnosis, estimation of urinary porphyrin excretion is indicated. The Watson–Schwarz reaction using Ehrlich's aldehyde reagent is a useful screening test for the Swedish variety even between attacks but is only positive in the other two varieties in the acute attacks (Dean, 1969).

PROGNOSIS

Acute porphyria is always a serious disease but the mortality rate has fallen since intermittent positive pressure respiration was introduced (Dean, 1969). In Berman's (1961) series of 81 cases, there were 22 deaths, only 12 of which were attributed solely to the porphyric illness. In 10 cases the cause of death was cardio-respiratory failure, and in 2 cardiac arrest—a mortality rate of 15·6 per cent. All those patients had severe paralysis. However, even though the patient may be gravely ill, complete recovery may occur.

TREATMENT

Prophylaxis obviously includes the avoidance of the drugs known to precipitate attacks in the case of known sufferers, and the investigation of sibs for evidence of asymptomatic metabolic disorder. Treatment is primarily symptomatic, and the usual treatment of bulbar and respiratory paralysis may be called for. Otherwise, chlorpromazine seems to be of particular value for relief of pain and other symptoms. It may be given in a dose of 25–50 mg three or four times a day, and a single dose of 100 mg is reported to have been followed by a complete remission (Welby et al., 1956). Gajdos and Gajdos-Torok (1961) suggested that the intramuscular injection of adenosine-5-monophosphoric acid may produce prompt improvement, but further experience has not confirmed the value of this treatment.

REFERENCES

BERMAN, S. (1961) Neurologic disorders in porphyria. A brief clinical survey of 81 cases. Reports at the VII International Congress in Neurology, Rome, p. 33.

CAVANAGH, J. B., and MELLICK, R. S. (1965) On the nature of the peripheral nerve lesions associated with acute intermittent porphyria, *J. Neurol. Psychiat.*, **28**, 320.

DAGG, J. H., GOLDBERG, A., LOCHHEAD, A., and SMITH, J. A. (1965) The relationship of lead poisoning to acute intermittent porphyria, *Quart. J. Med.*, **34**, 163.

DEAN, G. (1969) The porphyrias, *Brit. med. Bull.*, **25**, 48.

DEAN, G., and BARNES, H. D. (1955) The inheritance of porphyria acuta, cutanea tarda, and symptomless porphyrinuria, *Brit. med. J.*, **2**, 89.

DEAN, G., and BARNES, H. D. (1958) Porphyria. A South African screening experiment, *Brit. med. J.*, **1**, 298.

DOBRINER, K., and RHOADS, C. P. (1940) The porphyrins in health and disease, *Physiol. Rev.* **20**, 416.

EALES, L. (1960) Cutaneous porphyria, *S. Afr. J. Lab. clin. Med.*, **6**, 63.

EALES, L. (1961) Porphyrins and the porphyrias, in *Annual Reviews of Medicine*, Palo Alto, Calif.

GAJDOS, A., and GAJDOS-TOROK, M. (1961) Adenosine therapy for porphyria, *Lancet*, **ii**, 175.

GARCIN, R. (1964) Porphyries aiguës. Introduction générale, *Soc. Méd. Hôp. Paris*, **115**, 1089.

GOLDBERG, A. (1959) Acute intermittent porphyria, *Quart. J. Med.*, **28**, 183.

GOLDBERG, A., MOORE, M. R., BEATTIE, A. D., HALL, P. E., McCALLUM, J., and GRANT, J. K. (1969) Excessive urinary excretion of certain porphyrinogenic steroids in human acute intermittent porphyria, *Lancet*, **i**, 115.

GOLDBERG, A., RIMINGTON, C., and LOCHHEAD, A. C. (1967) Hereditary coproporphyria, *Lancet*, **i**, 632.

HAEGER, B. (1958) Urinary δ-aminolaevulinic acid and porphobilinogen in different types of porphyria, *Lancet*, **ii**, 606.

HIERONS, R. (1957) Changes in the nervous system in acute porphyria, *Brain*, **80**, 176.

THE LANCET (1972) Enzymes in the hepatic porphyrias, *Lancet*, **ii**, 121.

MACALPINE, I., HUNTER, R., and RIMINGTON, C. (1968) Porphyria in the Royal Houses of Stuart, Hanover and Prussia, *Brit. med. J.*, **1**, 7.

MASON, V. R., COURVILLE, C., and LISKIND, E. (1933) The porphyrins in human disease, *Medicine (Baltimore)*, **12**, 355.

MUSTAJOKI, P., and SEPPÄLÄINEN, A. M. (1975) Neuropathy in latent hereditary hepatic porphyria, *Brit. med. J.*, **2**, 310.

SWEENEY, V. P., PATHAK, M. A., and ASBURY, A. K. (1970) Acute intermittent porphyria. Increased ALA-synthetase activity during an acute attack, *Brain*, **93**, 369.

WALDENSTROM, J. (1957) The porphyrias as inborn errors of metabolism, *Amer. J. Med.*, **22**, 758.

WELBY, J. C., STREET, J. P., and WATSON, C. J. (1956) Chlorpromazine in the treatment of porphyria, *J. Amer. med. Ass.*, **162**, 174.

SUBACUTE MYELO-OPTICO-NEUROPATHY
(S.M.O.N.)

Since 1956 many cases of a neurological syndrome characterized by symptoms and signs of spinal cord and peripheral nerve involvement and optic atrophy, often with abdominal symptoms, have been reported, largely from Japan (Tsubaki *et al.*, 1965; Nakae *et al.*, 1971; Sobue *et al.*, 1972) but also from Australia (Selby, 1972), Singapore (Tay, 1973), and the United Kingdom (Spillane, 1971). A viral cause has been postulated (Nakamura and Inoue, 1972) but ample clinical, biochemical, and epidemiological evidence is now available (*The Lancet*, 1971; Nakae *et al.*, 1973) to indicate that the condition results from self-medication with clioquinol (*Entero-Vioform*) and/or related remedies, usually taken in large doses over a long period of time as a treatment for diarrhoea or other abdominal symptoms. A myeloneuropathy has been produced in dogs by the administration of this drug (Tateishi *et al.*, 1972); a striking fall in the incidence of the syndrome occurred when this drug and related remedies became available only on a doctor's prescription.

REFERENCES

THE LANCET (1971) More on S.M.O.N., *Lancet*, **ii**, 1244.

NAKAE, K., YAMAMOTO, S., and IGATA, A. (1971) Subacute myelo-optico-neuropathy (S.M.O.N.) in Japan, *Lancet*, **ii**, 510.

NAKAE, K., YAMAMOTO, S., SHIGEMATSU, I., and KONO, R. (1973) Relation between sub-acute myelo-optic neuropathy (S.M.O.N.) and clioquinol: nationwide survey, *Lancet*, **i**, 171.

NAKAMURA, Y., and INOUE, Y. K. (1972) Pathogenicity of virus associated with subacute myelo-optico-neuropathy, *Lancet*, **i**, 223.

SELBY, G. (1972) Subacute myelo-optic neuropathy in Australia, *Lancet*, **i**, 123.

SOBUE, I., MUKOYAMA, M., TAKAYANAGI, T., NISHIGAKI, S., MATSUOKA, Y., and ANDO, K. (1972) Myeloneuropathy with abdominal disorders in Japan, *Neurology* (*Minneap.*), **22**, 1034.

SPILLANE, J. D. (1971) S.M.O.N., *Lancet*, **ii**, 1371.

TATEISHI, J., IKEDA, H., SAITO, A., KURODA, S., and OTSUKI, S. (1972) Myeloneuropathy in dogs induced by iodoxyquinoline, *Neurology* (*Minneap.*), **22**, 702.

TAY, C. H. (1973) S.M.O.N. in Singapore, *Lancet*, **i**, 1519.

TSUBAKI, T., TOKOKURA, Y., and TSUKAGOSHI, H. (1965) Subacute myelo-optico-neuropathy following abdominal symptoms, *Jap. J. Med.*, **4**, 181.

THE NEUROLOGICAL SYMPTOMS OF HEPATIC FAILURE

Neurological symptoms may appear as the result of hepatic failure from any cause, e.g. acute virus hepatitis, eclampsia, portal cirrhosis, Wilson's disease, haemochromatosis, acute chemical poisoning, or the terminal stages of biliary cirrhosis. They may arise spontaneously or be precipitated in patients with chronic liver disease by gastro-intestinal haemorrhage, acute alcoholic intoxication, the administration of morphine or barbiturates, paracentesis, diuretics, or surgery. They may also follow the operation of portacaval anastomosis (Sherlock, 1963).

The causes of the disturbances of central nervous function are complex, and are discussed by Summerskill *et al.* (1956), by Sherlock (1963), and by Victor (1974). The essential factor appears to be that as a result of abnormal anastomoses between the portal and systemic arterial systems, either arising naturally or produced by surgery, nitrogenous material intended for the liver enters the systemic circulation. Similar symptoms may be observed after liver transplantation (Parkes *et al.*, 1970 *a*). Measurement of the blood ammonia gives a rough index of the severity of the condition which has more recently been called porto-systemic encephalopathy. Duffy *et al.* (1974) have shown that alpha-ketoglutaramate, a metabolite of glutamine not previously demonstrated in mammalian tissue, is increased four- to tenfold in patients with hepatic encephalopathy and suggest that this substance may exert a toxic effect on the nervous system by competing for glutamic acid receptors in the brain.

One of the most constant pathological features in the brain is the presence in the cortex and in the basal ganglia of Alzheimer type 2 astrocytes which show no cytoplasm with ordinary staining methods (Adams and Foley, 1953). These cells are also present in Wilson's disease. Cavanagh and Kyu (1969) suggest that the astrocytic abnormality may be due to a defect in function of the mitotic spindle and there is also evidence of microtubular dysfunction (*The Lancet*, 1971; Cavanagh, 1974) which may not only give a lead to the nature of the metabolic abnormality but also to new concepts of astrocytic function.

Neurological symptoms in chronic hepatic disease may be intermittent, and sometimes predominantly psychiatric, for long periods. In other cases, and in acute hepatic failure, they develop rapidly and progressively. Psychiatric symptoms consist of changes in the personality, abnormalities of mood and behaviour, and drowsiness deepening into stupor and coma. Speech is likely to be slurred, and there may be dyphasia. A 'flapping' tremor (so-called asterixis) is rather characteristic when the arms are outstretched, but may occur in other toxic states also. Neurological signs suggestive of focal cerebral damage or dysfunction are occasionally seen (Pearce, 1963). Extrapyramidal rigidity and tremor may be present with or without signs of corticospinal lesions or cerebellar deficiency. Muscle twitching may occur. More recently myelopathy with spasticity and increased limb reflexes but with flexor plantar responses has been described (Liversedge and Rawson, 1966) but Pant *et al.* (1968), on the basis of neuropathological studies, suggest that this syndrome is more likely to be due to a restricted form of encephalopathy with descending degeneration of the corticospinal tract rather than to a myelopathy. An increased terminal latency or diminution in the size of the sensory evoked response in electrophysiological studies of peripheral nerve function (Seneviratne and Peiris, 1970) indicates the presence of a subclinical peripheral neuropathy in many cases. In some cases a syndrome of chronic choreo-athetosis has been observed (Toghill *et al.*, 1967).

In severe cases delta waves which may be triphasic will be present in the EEG. In milder cases there is a slowing of the dominant frequency. The EEG can be used as a sensitive indicator of the response to treatment as well as for diagnosis (Laidlaw and Read, 1961; Parkes *et al.*, 1970 b). The cerebrospinal fluid is usually normal.

The clinical and biochemical signs of the causal hepatic disorder will be present. Jaundice may be slight or absent in chronic hepatic failure due to cirrhosis.

Treatment consists first in reducing the absorption of nitrogenous substance from the bowel. Hence a protein intake of less than 20 g daily is necessary and neomycin, 1–2·5 g daily (Dawson *et al.*, 1957), may be given in an attempt to sterilize the bowel and to reduce absorption. *Lactobacillus acidophilus* has been used for the same purpose (Macbeth *et al.*, 1965) while surgical exclusion of the colon has also been successful (Walker *et al.*, 1965). In acute hepatic coma, extracorporeal perfusion of a baboon liver has been shown to relieve the symptoms (Abouna *et al.*, 1972). Levodopa 5 g given by gastric tube in 100 ml water (Parkes *et al.*, 1970 b) has been shown to produce striking temporary improvement in the level of consciousness and in the EEG in hepatic coma, while the cognitive deficits of chronic hepatic encephalopathy are also improved by continuing treatment with this drug in standard dosage (Elithorn *et al.*, 1975).

REFERENCES

ABOUNA, G. M., FISHER, L. McA., STILL, W. J., and HUME, D. M. (1972) Acute hepatic coma successfully treated by extracorporeal baboon liver perfusions, *Brit. med. J.*, **1**, 23.

ADAMS, R. D., and FOLEY, J. M. (1953) The neurological disorder associated with liver disease, in *Metabolic Disorders of the Nervous System*, A.R.N.M.D., Baltimore.

BROWN, I. A. (1957) *Liver–brain Relationships*, Springfield, Ill.

CAVANAGH, J. B. (1974) Liver bypass and the glia, in *Brain Dysfunction in Metabolic Disorders*, ed. Plum, F., A.R.N.M.D., vol. 53, New York.

CAVANAGH, J. B., and KYU, M. H. (1969) Colchicine-like effect on astrocytes after portocaval shunt in rats, *Lancet*, **ii**, 620.

DAWSON, A. M., McLAREN, J., and SHERLOCK, S. (1957) Neomycin in the treatment of hepatic coma, *Lancet*, **ii**, 1263.

DUFFY, T. E., VERGARA, F., and PLUM, F. (1974) α-Ketoglutaramate in hepatic encephalopathy, in *Brain Dysfunction in Metabolic Disorders*, ed. Plum, F., A.R.N.M.D., vol. 53, New York.

ELITHORN, A., LUNZER, M., and WEINMAN, J. (1975) Cognitive deficits associated with chronic hepatic encephalopathy and their response to levodopa, *J. Neurol. Neurosurg. Psychiat.*, **38**, 794.

LAIDLAW, J., and READ, A. E. (1961) The EEG diagnosis of manifest and latent delirium, *J. Neurol. Psychiat.*, **24**, 58.

THE LANCET (1971) The astrocyte in liver disease, *Lancet*, **ii**, 1189.

LIVERSEDGE, L. A., and RAWSON, M. D. (1966) Myelopathy in hepatic disease and portacaval anastomosis, *Lancet*, **i**, 277.

MACBETH, W. A. A. G., KASS, E. H., and McDERMOTT, W. V. (1965) Treatment of hepatic encephalopathy by alteration of intestinal flora with *Lactobacillus acidophilus*, *Lancet*, **i**, 399.

PANT, S. S., REBEIZ, J. J., and RICHARDSON, E. P. (1968) Spastic paraparesis following portacaval shunts, *Neurology (Minneap.)*, **18**, 134.

PARKES, J. D., MURRAY-LYON, I. M., and WILLIAMS, R. (1970 a) Neuropsychiatric and electroencephalographic changes after transplantation of the liver, *Quart. J. Med.*, **39**, 515.

PARKES, J. D., SHARPSTONE, P., and WILLIAMS, R. (1970 b) Levodopa in hepatic coma, *Lancet*, **ii**, 1341.

PEARCE, J. M. S. (1963) Focal neurological syndromes in hepatic failure, *Postgrad. med. J.*, **39**, 653.

READ, A. E., LAIDLAW, J., and SHERLOCK, S. (1961) Neuropsychiatric complications of portacaval anastomosis, *Lancet*, **i**, 961.

SENEVIRATNE, K. N., and PEIRIS, O. A. (1970) Peripheral nerve function in chronic liver disease, *J. Neurol. Neurosurg. Psychiat.*, **33**, 609.

SHERLOCK, S. (1963) *Diseases of the Liver and Biliary System*, 3rd ed., Oxford.

SUMMERSKILL, W. H. J., DAVIDSON, E. A., SHERLOCK, S., and STEINER, R. E. (1956) The neuropsychiatric syndrome associated with hepatic cirrhosis and an extensive portal collateral circulation, *Quart. J. Med.*, **25**, 245.

TOGHILL, P. J., JOHNSTON, A. W., and SMITH, J. F. (1967) Choreoathetosis in porto-systemic encephalopathy, *J. Neurol. Psychiat.*, **30**, 358.

VICTOR, M. (1974) Neurologic changes in liver disease, in *Brain Dysfunction in Metabolic Disorders*, ed. Plum, F., A.R.N.M.D., vol. 53, New York.

WALKER, J. G., EMLYN-WILLIAMS, A., CRAIGIE, A., ROSENOER, V. M., AGNEW, J., and SHERLOCK, S. (1965) Treatment of chronic portal-systemic encephalopathy by surgical exclusion of the colon, *Lancet*, **ii**, 861.

BIOCHEMICAL DISORDERS ASSOCIATED WITH MENTAL RETARDATION

An increasing number of biochemical disorders has been discovered during recent years to be associated with retardation of mental development. Some of these are considered elsewhere in this book, for example, erythroblastosis foetalis [see p. 637], lead poisoning [see p. 804], and the lipidoses and leuco-dystrophies [see p. 638]. Some conditions remain to be considered, which have in common their liability to produce mental subnormality, though it will be noticed that in some cases the same or allied disorders may be detected in adult life. The subject has recently been reviewed by the World Health Organization (1969), by Raine (1972), by Crome and Stern (1972), and by Menkes (1974).

AMINO ACID DISORDERS

Crome and Stern (1972) have tabulated over 100 metabolic disorders, over 30 involving amino acid metabolism, which may be associated with mental retardation. Many of these can only be recognized by means of highly specialized chromatographic techniques applied to the examination of infants' urine. Ideally, were it not for the many difficulties, such screening tests should be carried out in all new-born infants. In addition, prenatal diagnosis through amniocentesis, allowing selective abortion, is being utilized increasingly in the case of those inborn errors of metabolism or chromosomal abnormalities which can be identified in amniotic cells in culture (Harris, 1975). Only some of the commoner and more important conditions will be considered here.

PHENYLKETONURIA

Phenylketonuria, also known as phenylpyruvic oligophrenia, is a hereditary (recessive) metabolic disorder first described by Fölling in 1934. It is characterized by a defect in the hydroxylation of phenylalanine to tyrosine, which leads to the urinary excretion of phenylpyruvic acid. Unless the condition is detected and treated during the first few weeks of life, amentia generally results though it is now clear that occasionally mildly-affected individuals may first be recognized in adult life and may show only minor degrees of subnormality. It has been estimated (Brimblecombe *et al.*, 1961) that there are about 40 new cases in the United Kingdom every year. The importance of recognizing such cases is that they may transmit the disease in its more severe form to their children.

The child usually appears normal at birth, but subsequently fails to develop and may suffer from convulsions. Most such children have blonde hair and a fair complexion, and skin changes have been described, which may be the result of diminished skin pigmentation. The degree of mental deficiency is usually severe, and is associated with a non-specific clumsiness of gait and movement, and often with stereotyped repetitive movements. The EEG shows 'a marked generalized abnormality with poverty of rhythmic activity, excess of large irregular slow waves, and large discharges with variable focal distribution' (Pampiglione, 1961).

The presence of phenylpyruvic acid in the urine is demonstrated by adding to the acidified urine a few drops of fresh 5 per cent ferric chloride solution, which produces a deep bluish-green colour. A simple and more reliable paper-strip test is now available (Brimblecombe *et al.*, 1961). A level of phenylalanine in the serum exceeding 20 mg/100 ml is usually associated with moderate or severe mental retardation, while a figure below that level may be compatible with normal intellectual development, but there are marginal cases in which management presents a difficult problem (*British Medical Journal*, 1971).

Treatment consists in putting the child as early as possible on a diet containing a restricted amount of phenylalanine. This was discussed in detail by Brimblecombe *et al.* (1961). They stated that of all the 10 cases that they had been able to discover in which treatment was begun by the age of 6 weeks, and in which the dietary control of phenylalanine was satisfactory, there was no example of mental deficiency. They also drew attention to the dangers of excessive phenylalanine restriction. Fisch *et al.* (1969), reviewing 12 years of experience, confirmed that affected children treated at an early age had significantly higher developmental and intelligence quotients than those treated later.

HARTNUP DISEASE

Baron *et al.* (1956) first described this hereditary metabolic disorder. Milne *et al.* (1960) collected from the literature 11 patients who were members of 7 unrelated families. The disease appears to be inherited as an autosomal recessive factor. It is characterized by renal amino-aciduria and an excessive excretion of indican and indolic acids. The condition is a disorder of cellular transport of monocarboxylic amino acids in the kidney and intestine.

A curious feature of the disorder is the episodic character of the symptoms. The main clinical features are a photosensitive rash typical of pellagra, mental deterioration, and attacks of cerebellar ataxia. The disease occurs in childhood and tends to improve with increasing age, and in some patients the clinical manifestations have been very mild. The rash may respond to nicotinamide therapy and the attacks of ataxia recover spontaneously. It is suggested that the cerebellar ataxia may be due to intoxication by retained indolic acids, in which case alkalinization of the urine by sodium bicarbonate will increase the excretion of indolic acids and provide an easy method of therapy.

OTHER SYNDROMES ASSOCIATED WITH AMINO ACID DISORDERS

A number of other syndromes, mostly rather rare, have been found to be associated with disorders of the metabolism of amino acids. The term *oculocerebral dystrophy* (Lowe's syndrome or cerebro-oculorenal syndrome) is characterized by eye changes, such as cataract, enophthalmos and corneal opacities, mental retardation, and amino-aciduria. In another syndrome, mental retardation, convulsions, and ataxia are associated with excretion of large quantities of arginin-succinic acid in the urine (argininosuccinicaciduria— Farriaux *et al.*, 1974). Other disorders include carnosinaemia with fits and mental retardation due to carnosinase deficiency (Terplan and Cares, 1972), hyperammonaemia with episodic vomiting, lethargy, ataxia, and mental retardation (Freeman *et al.*, 1970); homocystinuria with mental retardation, epilepsy, ectopia lentis, and a Marfanoid appearance (Carson and Raine, 1971); and many more. There are also two syndromes in which mental retardation is associated with amino acids in the urine which give it a characteristic smell, leading to the terms oast-house syndrome and maple-syrup syndrome. Oast house disease (Hooft *et al.*, 1964) is also characterized by convulsions, hypotonia, oedema, and diarrhoea as well as retardation due to methionine malabsorption; in maple syrup urine disease, convulsions, vomiting, opisthotonus, and severe retardation occur due to leucinosis caused by a defect in the decarboxylation of branched chain fatty acids (Westall, 1964); cases responsive to treatment with thiamine have been described (Scriver *et al.*, 1971). Amino-aciduria is also characteristic of Wilson's disease. Abnormalities of myelin development in the amino-acidurias have been reviewed by Prensky *et al.* (1968), and the neuro-pathological changes in several of these diseases by Martin *et al.* (1968). The disorders now recognized with their clinical and biochemical manifestations are reviewed comprehensively by Crome and Stern (1972) and Menkes (1974).

REFERENCES

BARON, D. N., DENT, C. E., HARRIS, H., HART, E. W., and JEPSON, J. B. (1956) Hereditary pellagra-like skin rash with temporary cerebellar ataxia, constant renal amino-aciduria, and other bizarre biochemical features, *Lancet*, **ii**, 421.

BRIMBLECOMBE, F. S. W., BLAINEY, J. D., STONEMAN, M. E. R., and WOOD, B. S. B. (1961) Dietary and biochemical control of phenylketonuria, *Brit. med. J.*, **2**, 793.

BRITISH MEDICAL JOURNAL (1971) Problems of phenylketonuria, *Brit. med. J.*, **4**, 695.

CARSON, N. A. J., and RAINE, D. N. (1971) *Inherited Disorders of Sulphur Metabolism*, Edinburgh.

CROME, L. C., and STERN, J. (1972) *Pathology of Mental Retardation*, 2nd ed., London.

FARRIAUX, J.-P., CARTIGNY, B., DHONDT, J.-L., KINT, J., LOUIS, J., DELATTRE, P., and FONTAINE, G. (1974) A propos d'une observation d'arginino-succinylurie néo-natale, *Acta paediat. belg.*, **28**, 193.

FISCH, R. O., TORRES, F., GRAVEM, H. J., GREENWOOD, C. S., and ANDERSON, J. A. (1969) Twelve years of clinical experience with phenylketonuria. A statistical evaluation of symptoms, growth, mental development, electroencephalographic records, serum phenylalanine levels, and results of dietary management, *Neurology (Minneap.)*, **19**, 659.

FÖLLING, A. (1934) Über Ausscheidung von Phenylbrenztraubensäure in den Harn als Stoffwechselanomalie in Verbindung mit Imbezillität, *Ztschr. f. physiol. Chem.*, **227**, 169.

FREEMAN, J. M., NICHOLSON, J. F., SCHIMKE, R. T., ROWLAND, L. P., and CARTER, S. (1970) Congenital hyperammonemia: association with hyperglycinemia and decreased levels of carbamyl phosphate synthetase, *Arch. Neurol. (Chic.)*, **23**, 430.

HARRIS, H. (1975) *Prenatal Diagnosis and Selective Abortion*, Cambridge, Mass.

HOOFT, C., TIMMERMANS, J., SNOECK, J., ANTENER, I., OYAERT, W., and VAN DEN HENDE, C. (1964) Methionine malabsorption in a mentally defective child, *Lancet*, **ii**, 20.

MARTIN, J. J., VAN BOGAERT, L., and GUAZZI, G. C. (1968) Déterminations cérébrales des amino-aciduries, *Confin. neurol.*, **30**, 97.

MENKES, J. H. (1974) *Textbook of Child Neurology*, Philadelphia.

MILNE, M. D., CRAWFORD, M. A., GIRAO, C. B., and LOUGHRIDGE, L. W. (1960) The metabolic disorder in Hartnup disease, *Quart. J. Med.*, **29**, 407.

PAMPIGLIONE, G. (1961) EEG in inborn errors of metabolism. Reports at the VII international Congress of Neurology, Rome, p. 15.

PRENSKY, A. L., CARR, S., and MOSER, H. W. (1968) Development of myelin in inherited disorders of amino acid metabolism, *Arch. Neurol. (Chic.)*, **19**, 552.

RAINE, D. N. (1972) Management of inherited metabolic disease, *Brit. med. J.*, **2**, 329.

SCRIVER, C. R., MACKENZIE, S., CLOW, C. L., and DELVIN, E. (1971) Thiamine-responsive maple-syrup-urine disease, *Lancet*, **i**, 310.

TERPLAN, K. L., and CARES, H. L. (1972) Histopathology of the nervous system in carnosinase enzyme deficiency with mental retardation, *Neurology (Minneap.)*, **22**, 644.

WESTALL, R. G. (1964) Dietary treatment of a child with maple syrup urine disease (branched-chain ketoaciduria), in *Neurometabolic Disorders in Childhood*, ed. Holt, K. S., and Milner, J., p. 94, Edinburgh and London.

WORLD HEALTH ORGANIZATION (1969) Biochemistry of mental disorders, *Wld Hlth Org. techn. Rep. Ser.*, No. 427.

DISORDERS OF CARBOHYDRATE METABOLISM

GALACTOSAEMIA

Mental retardation can be associated with an abnormal metabolism of lactose, due to a defect of the enzyme galactose-l-phosphate uridyl transferase, which is inherited as an autosomal recessive factor. The mental defect occurs with varying degrees of severity, and in severe cases enlargement of the liver is associated with jaundice, and the child later develops cataracts. A reducing substance will be found in the urine, and the diagnosis is established by incubating red blood cells obtained from the umbilical cord with galactose. In affected babies an accumulation of galactose-l-phosphate can be demonstrated. In such cases a lactose-free diet appears to give good results (Menkes, 1974).

FRUCTOSURIA

Two metabolic disorders are associated with fructosuria. The first is essential fructosuria, which is symptomless, and may be confused with diabetes mellitus on account of the positive result of testing the urine with Benedict's solution. The other syndrome is known as fructose intolerance, a hereditary disorder in which the absorption of fructose leads to an abnormally high blood fructose associated with hypoglycaemia. There is a deficiency of fructose-l-phosphate aldolase in liver, kidney, and small intestinal mucosa. This condition may be, but is not always, associated with mental retardation, and spastic paraparesis has been described (Rennert and Greer, 1970). Dormandy and Porter (1961) reported a case of familial fructose and galactose intolerance.

HYPOGLYCAEMIA

According to Moncrieff (1960) there are various forms of hypoglycaemia in childhood, and as a result of repeated or prolonged hypoglycaemic attacks severe cerebral damage may occur, with mental deterioration. The pathological changes in such cases are similar to those of anoxia [see p. 810] with widespread neuronal damage (Anderson et al., 1967) but the Purkinje cells of the cerebellum are peculiarly sensitive to hypoglycaemia so that surviving children are often ataxic. Ingram et al. (1967) reviewed 26 children who suffered from hypoglycaemic coma between the ages of 10 weeks and 11 years. Twelve were diabetic, 1 had islet cell adenomatosis, and in 13 the cause of the hypoglycaemia was unknown. Nine of the 23 children seen at follow-up were mentally retarded, 4 were epileptic, and 10 showed signs of ataxia or ataxic diplegia. In addition to the idiopathic type, and hypoglycaemia in diabetes and islet cell adenomatosis, episodes of hypoglycaemia may occur in association with a raised blood fructose, and the same thing may happen in galactosaemia.

REFERENCES

ANDERSON, J. M., MILNER, R. D. G., and STRICH, S. J. (1967) Effects of neonatal hypoglycaemia on the nervous system: a pathological study, J. Neurol. Neurosurg. Psychiat., 30, 295.

DORMANDY, T. L., and PORTER, R. J. (1961) Familial fructose and galactose intolerance, Lancet, i, 1189.

INGRAM, T. T. S., STARK, G. D., and BLACKBURN, I. (1967) Ataxia and other neurological disorders as sequels of severe hypoglycaemia in childhood, Brain, 90, 851.

MENKES, J. H. (1974) *Textbook of Child Neurology*, Philadelphia.
MONCRIEFF, A. (1960) Biochemistry of mental defect, *Lancet*, **ii,** 273.
RENNERT, O. M., and GREER, M. (1970) Hereditary fructosemia, *Neurology (Minneap.),* **20,** 421.

OTHER DISORDERS OF CARBOHYDRATE METABOLISM

Subacute necrotizing encephalomyelopathy (Leigh's disease) has been considered on page 661. Other rare disorders associated with mental retardation which give somewhat similar manifestations include infantile lactic acidosis, isovaleric acidaemia, methylanalonic acidaemia, propionic acidaemia, and several more (Crome and Stern, 1972). Intermittent cerebellar ataxia and choreoathetosis provoked by fever and/or excitement with an absence of neurological abnormality between attacks has now been reported as a consequence of pyruvate decarboxylase deficiency (Blass *et al.*, 1971). Aspartylglucosaminuria, a rare condition causing structural abnormalities, hyperactivity, skin changes, recurrent infection, infantile diarrhoea (in some cases), and moderate or severe retardation may be especially common in Finland (Palo and Mattsson, 1970; Arstila *et al.*, 1972).

REFERENCES

ARSTILA, A. U., PALO, J., HALTIA, M., RIEKKINEN, P., and AUTIO, S. (1972) Aspartylglucosaminuria I: fine structural studies on liver, kidney and brain, *Acta neuropath. (Berl.),* **20,** 207.
BLASS, J. P., KARK, R. A. P., and ENGEL, W. K. (1971) Clinical studies of a patient with pyruvate decarboxylase deficiency, *Arch. Neurol. (Chic.),* **25,** 449.
CROME, L. C., and STERN, J. (1972) *Pathology of Mental Retardation*, 2nd ed., London.
PALO, J., and MATTSSON, K. (1970) Eleven new cases of aspartylglucosaminuria, *J. ment. Defic. Res.*, **14,** 168.

SOME OTHER METABOLIC DISORDERS

Serious infantile protein–calorie malnutrition, as in kwashiorkor, has a profound effect upon brain development and may be associated with slight deficits in intelligence and delayed physical growth (Elliott and Knight, 1972; *The Lancet*, 1972 *a*). Endemic cretinism due to maternal iodine deficiency is another important cause (Pharoah *et al.*, 1971). Hypercalcaemia of infancy due to hyperreactivity to vitamin D or overdosage with this vitamin (Seelig, 1969) may also cause mental retardation.

SOME ENDOCRINE CAUSES OF MENTAL RETARDATION AND OF OTHER NEUROLOGICAL SYMPTOMS

A *diencephalic syndrome* of infancy has been described giving severe emaciation and growth retardation but intellect is usually normal and in most cases hypothalamic gliomas or gliomas of the optic nerve are eventually demonstrated (Pelc and Flament-Durand, 1973).

In *diabetes insipidus* due to lesions of the neurohypophysis or of its afferent neurosecretory cells originating in the supraoptic and paraventricular nuclei of the hypothalamus, thirst and polyuria result from a diminished output of antidiuretic hormone (ADH); the condition may be hereditary or idiopathic and usually responds to treatment with vasopressin (Green *et al.*, 1967); the intellect is well preserved. However, in *nephrogenic diabetes insipidus* the renal tubules are incapable of responding to ADH, the affected infants excrete large quantities of very dilute urine with a specific gravity usually below 1·006, and the polyuria leads to severe hypertonic dehydration which, if untreated, is rapidly fatal. Massive and frequent administration of fluid is necessary to correct the dehydration and associated hypernatraemia; even so, the survivors are often mentally retarded (Ruess and Rosenthal, 1963). The condition, being inherited as an X-linked recessive trait, usually affects only males; it is resistant to vaso-pressin treatment due to a defect in the specific adenyl cyclase of the renal tubules (Thorn, 1970).

Other causes of *hypernatraemia* in infancy, including excessive intake result-ing from the use of certain dried milks in the first six months of life, may cause convulsions, disordered consciousness, and, if severe, permanent brain damage (Morris-Jones *et al.*, 1967). In adults, hypernatraemia, hypodipsia, and hypovo-laemia have been described as an effect of hypothalamic or suprasellar tumours (Vejjajiva *et al.*, 1969; Lascelles and Lewis, 1972). By contrast, *hyperosmolal coma* with *hyponatraemia* and associated hyperglycaemia, often causing cerebral oedema with a raised CSF pressure, is a well-recognized complication of diabetic ketosis (Espinas and Poser, 1969; Clements *et al.*, 1971; *The Lancet*, 1972 *b*) but has also been described as a consequence of severe burns, during peritoneal dialysis, and in steroid therapy, and sometimes causing focal epileptic seizures (Maccario *et al.*, 1965; Boyer, 1967; Boyer *et al.*, 1967). Confusion and mild delirium and even coma with hyponatraemia and hypoglycaemia may also occur in Addison's disease, especially during crises (Plum and Posner, 1972), while psychotic symptoms are common in Cushing's disease (Spillane, 1951) but coma is rare.

Hypopituitarism [p. 276] is usually associated with symptoms and signs of adrenal and/or thyroid insufficiency and with gonadal dysfunction (Fraser, 1970), and the form which may occur in childhood after traumatic infarction of the anterior lobe of the pituitary (Daniel *et al.*, 1959) may cause coma to be unusually prolonged after minor head injury. When it is secondary to tumours of the pituitary region the symptoms of the tumour itself often dominate the clinical picture and the same is true of *acromegaly* in which, however, the endocrine abnormality *per se* is sometimes associated with minor mental changes (Kanis *et al.*, 1974) and with neuromuscular dysfunction [p. 1032].

As stated above, cretinism in infancy is an important cause of mental retarda-tion; in adult life *myxoedema* may be associated with profound mental symptoms ('myxoedematous madness'), with hypothermic coma (Macdonald, 1958; Plum and Posner, 1972), or with cerebellar ataxia (Barnard *et al.*, 1971). Both cretinism and myxoedema may also give symptoms of muscular dysfunction [p. 1031]. *Thyrotoxicosis* is usually associated with anxiety, tremor, and hyper-activity but is a rare cause of stupor and coma in hyperacute cases, while by contrast, apathetic thyrotoxicosis with depression and apathy in elderly subjects has been described (Thomas *et al.*, 1970).

Finally, it should be mentioned that in *idiopathic hypoparathyroidism* (Simp-son, 1952), mental retardation, epilepsy, and incipient tetany are common, and epilepsy and papilloedema have also been reported in true hypoparathyroidism after thyroid surgery (Willison and Whitty, 1957). Mental defect with epilepsy and intracranial calcification is also common in pseudohypoparathyroidism but mental defect alone is more often seen in pseudo-pseudohypoparathyroidism

(Dickson *et al.*, 1960). Spinal cord compression due to ectopic calcification has been reported in pseudohypoparathyroidism (Cullen and Pearce, 1964). The neuromuscular disorders commonly observed in disorders of calcium metabolism are described on page 1033.

REFERENCES

BARNARD, R. O., CAMPBELL, M. J., and MCDONALD, W. I. (1971) Pathological findings in a case of hypothyroidism with ataxia, *J. Neurol. Neurosurg. Psychiat.*, **34**, 755.

BERMAN, P. H., BALIS, M. E., and DANCIS, J. (1969) Congenital hyperuricemia: an inborn error of purine metabolism associated with psychomotor retardation, athetosis and self-mutilation, *Arch. Neurol. (Chic.)*, **20**, 44.

BOYER, J., GILL, G. N., and EPSTEIN, F. H. (1967) Hyperglycemia and hyperosmolarity complicating peritoneal dialysis, *Ann. intern. Med.*, **67**, 568.

BOYER, M. H. (1967) Hyperosmolar anacidotic coma in association with glucocorticoid therapy, *J. Amer. med. Ass.*, **202**, 1007.

CLEMENTS, R. S., BLUMENTHAL, S. A., MORRISON, A. D., and WINEGRAD, A. I. (1971) Increased cerebrospinal-fluid pressure during treatment of diabetic ketosis, *Lancet*, **ii**, 671.

CULLEN, D. R., and PEARCE, J. M. S. (1964) Spinal cord compression in pseudo-hypoparathyroidism, *J. Neurol. Neurosurg. Psychiat.*, **27**, 459.

DANIEL, P. M., PRICHARD, M. M. L., and TREIP, C. S. (1959) Traumatic infarction of the anterior lobe of the pituitary gland, *Lancet*, **ii**, 927.

DICKSON, L. G., MORITA, Y., COWSERT, E. J., GRAVES, J., and MEYER, J. S. (1960) Neurological, electroencephalographic and heredo-familial aspects of pseudohypoparathyroidism and pseudo-pseudohypoparathyroidism, *J. Neurol. Neurosurg. Psychiat.*, **23**, 33.

ELLIOTT, K., and KNIGHT, J. (1972) *Lipids, Malnutrition and the Developing Brain*, Amsterdam, London, New York.

ESPINAS, O. E., and POSER, C. M. (1969) Blood hyperosmolality and neurologic deficit, *Arch. Neurol. (Chic.)*, **20**, 182.

FRASER, R. (1970) Human pituitary disease, *Brit. med. J.*, **4**, 449.

GREEN, J. R., BUCHAN, G. C., ALVORD, E. C., and SWANSON, A. G. (1967) Hereditary and idiopathic types of diabetes insipidus, *Brain*, **90**, 707.

KANIS, J. A., GILLINGHAM, F. J., HARRIS, P., HORN, D. B., HUNTER, W. M., REDPATH, A. T., and STRONG, J. A. (1974) Clinical and laboratory study of acromegaly: assessment before and one year after treatment, *Quart. J. Med.*, **43**, 409.

THE LANCET (1972 *a*) Nutrition and the developing brain, *Lancet*, **ii**, 1349.

THE LANCET (1972 *b*) Hyperosmolal coma, *Lancet*, **ii**, 1071.

LASCELLES, P. T., and LEWIS, P. D. (1972) Hypodipsia and hypernatraemia associated with hypothalamic and suprasellar lesions, *Brain*, **95**, 249.

MACCARIO, M., MESSIS, C. P., and VASTOLA, E. F. (1965) Focal seizures as a manifestation of hyperglycemia, without ketoacidosis, *Neurology (Minneap.)*, **15**, 195.

MACDONALD, D. W. (1958) Hypothermic myxoedema coma, *Brit. med. J.*, **2**, 1144.

MCKERAN, R. O., ANDREWS, T. M., HOWELL, A., GIBBS, D. A., CHINN, S., and WATTS, R. W. E. (1975) The diagnosis of the carrier state for the Lesch–Nyhan syndrome, *Quart. J. Med.*, **44**, 189.

MORRIS-JONES, P. H., HOUSTON, I. B., and EVANS, R. C. (1967) Prognosis of the neurological complications of acute hypernatraemia, *Lancet*, **ii**, 1385.

PELC, S., and FLAMENT-DURAND, J. (1973) Histological evidence of optic chiasma glioma in the 'diencephalic syndrome', *Arch. Neurol. (Chic.)*, **28**, 139.

PHAROAH, P. O. D., BUTTFIELD, I. H., and HETZEL, B. S. (1971) Neurological damage to the fetus resulting from severe iodine deficiency during pregnancy, *Lancet*, **i**, 308.

PLUM, F., and POSNER, J. B. (1972) *The Diagnosis of Stupor and Coma*, 2nd ed., Philadelphia.

RUESS, A. L., and ROSENTHAL, I. M. (1963) Intelligence in nephrogenic diabetes insipidus, *Amer. J. dis. Child.*, **105**, 358.

SEELIG, M. S. (1969) Vitamin D and cardiovascular, renal, and brain damage in infancy and childhood, *Ann. N.Y. Acad. Sci.*, **147**, 537.

SIMPSON, J. A. (1952) The neurological manifestations of idiopathic hypoparathyroidism, *Brain*, **75**, 76.

SPILLANE, J. D. (1951) Nervous and mental disorders in Cushing's syndrome, *Brain*, · **74**, 72.

THOMAS, F. B., MAZZAFERRI, E. L., and SKILLMAN, T. G. (1970) Apathetic thyrotoxicosis, *Ann. intern. Med.*, **72**, 679.

THORN, N. A. (1970) Antidiuretic hormone synthesis, release and action under normal and pathological circumstances, *Advances in Metabolic Disorders*, **4**, 39.

VEJJAJIVA, A., SITPRIJA, V., and SHUANGSHOTI, S. (1969) Chronic sustained hypernatraemia and hypovolaemia in hypothalamic tumour, *Neurology* (*Minneap.*), **19**, 161.

WILLISON, R. G., and WHITTY, C. W. M. (1957) Parathyroid deficiency presenting as epilepsy, *Brit. med. J.*, **1**, 802.

SOME NON-METABOLIC CAUSES OF MENTAL RETARDATION

Microbial causes of mental retardation, including cytomegalovirus infection, rubella, and toxoplasmosis (Stern *et al.*, 1969), are considered on pages 523, 537, and 448.

CHROMOSOMAL ANOMALIES

Crome and Stern (1972) have listed 22 chromosomal anomalies which may be associated with mental retardation. A detailed review of these disorders would be out of place in a textbook of neurology. Among the commoner syndromes are the '*Cri du chat*' syndrome due to partial deletion of the short arm of chromosome S, characterized by low birth weight, microcephaly, cat-like cry, severe retardation, and hypertelorism; Klinefelter's syndrome with hypogenitalism, dwarfism, and a eunuchoid appearance and an XXY or XXXY chromosome constitution; Turner's syndrome or ovarian dysgenesis, with retarded growth, webbed neck, amenorrhoea, deafness in many cases, and an XO chromosomal pattern; and Down's syndrome (mongolism). Severe neuropathological abnormalities have also been reported in the Trisomy E (17–18) syndrome (Michaelson and Gilles, 1972).

Down's Syndrome (Mongolism)

This is the commonest syndrome associated with mental retardation, occurring in about 1 in 650 live births. It is usually due to trisomy of chromosome G, occasionally D/G translocation, G/G translocation, or mosaicism. Accurate diagnosis of the nature of the chromosomal anomaly is important in order to be able to advise the parents upon the risk of involvement of further children.

The principal clinical features are mental and physical retardation (often relatively mild but varying in severity) and a typical mongoloid appearance of the face with abnormalities of the skull, skeleton, hands, and feet and of the palmar creases. Congenital heart lesions and other visceral abnormalities are often present. The patients are usually simple and affectionate, may sometimes be capable of benefiting from limited education, and may also be able to undertake relatively menial tasks. Those patients who survive beyond the age of 40 years usually show clinical and neuropathological evidence of presenile dementia (Ohara, 1972; Ellis *et al.*, 1974).

REFERENCES

CROME, L. C., and STERN, J. (1972) *Pathology of Mental Retardation*, 2nd ed., London.
ELLIS, W. G., McCULLOCH, J. R., and CORLEY, C. L. (1974) Presenile dementia in Down's syndrome, *Neurology (Minneap.)*, **24**, 101.
MICHAELSON, P. S., and GILLES, F. H. (1972) Central nervous system abnormalities in Trisomy E (17–18) syndrome, *J. neurol. Sci.*, **15**, 193.
OHARA, P. T. (1972) Electron microscopical study of the brain in Down's syndrome, *Brain*, **95**, 681.
STERN, H., ELEK, S. D., BOOTH, J. C., and FLECK, D. G. (1969) Microbial causes of mental retardation: the role of prenatal infections with cytomegalovirus, rubella virus, and toxoplasma, *Lancet*, **ii**, 443.

MENTAL RETARDATION SYNDROMES OF UNDETERMINED CAUSE

Many other syndromes of mental retardation accompanied by morphological changes in the nervous system and skeleton have been described in which no specific chromosomal or biochemical anomaly has yet been discovered. Crome and Stern (1972) list over 50 syndromes which have been identified including the de Lange syndrome (retardation, dwarfism, and characteristic facial and cranial appearances), Donohue's syndrome or leprechaunism, the Maroteaux–Lamy syndrome (osteosclerosis, short phalanges, delayed fontanelle closure, clavicular dysplasia, mild retardation), the Treacher Collins syndrome (craniofacial deformity, malar hypoplasia, microgenitalia, deafness), Cockayne's syndrome [p. 654], Menkes kinky hair disease [p. 658], the Prader–Willi syndrome (hypotonia, hypometria, hypogonadism, and mental retardation), the Riley–Day syndrome of dysautonomia [p. 1072], and Sotos' syndrome of cerebral gigantism [p. 659].

Despite the enormous number of syndromes associated with mental retardation which are now recognized, it is still the case that the commonest cause remains that of so-called 'non-specific retardation' (Benton, 1969; Menkes, 1974) which may sometimes be familial (Dekaban and Klein, 1968), a fact which constitutes a major public health problem and a challenge to future research.

REFERENCES

BENTON, A. L. (1969) Neuropsychological aspects of mental retardation, *J. spec. Educ.*, **4**, 3.
CROME, L. C., and STERN, J. (1972) *Pathology of Mental Retardation*, 2nd ed., London.
DEKABAN, A. S., and KLEIN, D. (1968) Familial mental retardation, *Acta genet., Basel*, **18**, 206.
MENKES, J. H. (1974) *Textbook of Child Neurology*, Philadelphia.

CARBON DIOXIDE INTOXICATION

In patients with chronic respiratory disease, especially chronic bronchitis and emphysema, it has become increasingly apparent that neurological manifestations may result from the fact that the respiratory centre appears to become insensitive to carbon dioxide which is retained in the circulation as bicarbonate as a result of chronic alveolar hypoventilation. Chronic alveolar hypoventilation is also being recognized increasingly as a complication of various neuromuscular disorders including myasthenia gravis, muscular dystrophy, and dystrophia myotonica (Buchsbaum *et al.*, 1968); often in such cases severe diaphragmatic weakness can be demonstrated. In some such cases a chronic syndrome characterized by headache, lethargy, drowsiness, and fluctuating confusion persists over a period of many weeks or months. In some cases, however, an acute syndrome characterized by severe headache and vomiting, convulsions, papilloedema, and rapid impairment of consciousness has been described, due to increasing cerebral oedema, and may be precipitated by the administration of oxygen. In many such patients it is necessary to give steroid drugs and diuretics to reduce brain swelling but intermittent positive pressure respiration, monitored by measurements of the blood $p(O_2)$ and $p(CO_2)$ is the most effective treatment, in order to remove the accumulated CO_2 and, in time, to restore the sensitivity of the respiratory centre. In cases of neuromuscular disease with chronic respiratory insufficiency and CO_2 retention it may be difficult to decide whether or not assisted respiration is justified on ethical grounds. In muscular dystrophy of the Duchenne type this treatment is rarely justified in order briefly to prolong life in the presence of severe disability, but in other patients, suffering for instance from limb-girdle dystrophy or spinal muscular atrophy, severe respiratory insufficiency may develop at a time when the patient is still mobile. Intermittent external pulmonary insufflation with a respirator of the Bird type may be very effective in some such cases and may prolong useful life for many years.

REFERENCES

BUCHSBAUM, H. W., MARTIN, W. A., TURINO, G. M., and ROWLAND, L. P. (1968) Chronic alveolar hypoventilation due to muscular dystrophy, *Neurology (Minneap.)*, **18**, 319.

FISHMAN, A. P., TURINO, G. M., and BERGOFOLLY, E. H. (1957) The syndrome of alveolar hypoventilation, *Amer. J. Med.*, **23**, 333.

MANFREDI, F., SIEKER, H. O., SPOTO, A. P., and SALTZMAN, H. A. (1960) Severe carbon dioxide intoxication, *J. Amer. med. Ass.*, **173**, 999.

PLUM, F., and POSNER, J. B. (1972) *The Diagnosis of Stupor and Coma*, 2nd ed., Philadelphia.

STUART-HARRIS, C. H., and HANLEY, T. (1957) *Chronic Bronchitis, Emphysema and Cor Pulmonale*, Bristol.

16

DEFICIENCY DISORDERS

THE isolation of the vitamins and the study of their physiological properties and of the effects of their lack upon animals in experimental conditions led to the hope that vitamin deficiency in man would be recognizable in a similarly clear-cut manner, but greater clinical experience of nutritional disorders during the Second World War produced a more critical approach to a problem which is now seen to be more complex than was thought at first. The sick man suffering from nutritional deficiency has usually been partially starved for a long time. His disorder is often chronic; different vitamins are likely to have been lacking in varying proportions in different circumstances; other dietary elements will probably have been inadequate also; acute and chronic gastrointestinal and other infections are complicating factors acting both by their toxins and also by interfering with the absorption of food. We are thus presented with varying and partially overlapping clinical pictures which we are often unable to correlate with particular forms of deficiency. It seems best, therefore, first to review the physiology of those vitamins whose lack is believed to cause nervous disorders and then to describe the chief syndromes which appear to be caused by nutritional deficiency.

The B Group of Vitamins

Experimental work has led to the isolation of a number of factors in the vitamin B complex, four of which need especially to be considered in relation to nervous disease: these are vitamin B_1 (thiamine or aneurine), nicotinic acid, riboflavine, and pyridoxine. The B group of vitamins are present in greatest amount in brewers' yeast, in the germ and aleurone layer of ripe wheat, and also in egg yolk and mammalian liver, and in smaller amounts in milk, green vegetables, potatoes, and meat.

Vitamin B_1 (Thiamine)

This vitamin plays an important part in the glycolytic and pentose phosphate pathways of glucose metabolism. It forms a compound with pyrophosphoric acid which acts as co-enzyme to the enzyme which breaks down pyruvic acid, one of the intermediate products in the breakdown of glucose. A deficiency of thiamine, by interfering with the breakdown of pyruvic acid, leads to an accumulation of pyruvate in the blood, which can be detected chemically. Experimental workers have described the signs of acute and chronic deficiency in pigeons. Acute deficiency causes opisthotonus, chronic deficiency 'locomotor ataxia', weakness of the legs, and cardiac failure. Histologically there is a degeneration of the peripheral nerves, and haemorrhages are found in the brain. Experimental thiamine deficiency in rats caused 'ragged-red' muscle fibres with abnormal mitochondria and lipid droplets as well as demyelination in peripheral nerves (Kark *et al.*, 1975).

The minimum requirement of thiamine in the day's food is not more than

1·5–2 mg. Thiamine deficiency may be detected by a subnormal blood level (less than 3 μg per 100 ml), diminished urinary excretion after a test dose, or a raised level of pyruvate in the blood.

Nicotinic Acid

Nicotinic acid or niacin acts as a co-enzyme in intracellular oxidation processes. The daily requirements of an adult are probably about 20 mg. A saturation test has been used to detect nicotinic acid deficiency in man. The essential amino acid tryptophan is a niacin precursor. Deficiency of nicotinic acid produces in dogs a condition known as 'black-tongue', which is very similar to human pellagra.

Riboflavine

Riboflavine also acts as a co-enzyme in the breakdown of carbohydrate. It is the precursor of two flavoprotein co-enzymes, namely flavin mononucleotide and flavine adenine dinucleotide, and thus plays a central role in many important metabolic processes (Rivlin, 1970; Van Itallie and Follis, 1974). The daily minimal requirement in man is probably 2–3 mg. Riboflavine deficiency causes angular stomatitis, glossitis, injection of the limbus of the cornea, and in some cases abnormal vascularization of the cornea.

Pyridoxine

Vitamin B_6 is a combination of three naturally occurring pyridines, namely pyridoxine, pyridoxal, and pyridoxinine. The first is found mainly in plant foods, the latter two in animal products; in the average diet, pyridoxine is the main source of vitamin activity. Pyridoxine (vitamin B_6) aids the conversion of tryptophan to N-methyl nicotinamide. In infants reared on a pyridoxine-deficient diet, convulsions and anaemia were noted. In adults living on a diet deficient in this vitamin or in those receiving desoxypyridoxine, or more often, isoniazid given for the treatment of tuberculosis (both of these substances are pyridoxine antagonists), symmetrical polyneuropathy, optic atrophy and/or microcytic anaemia may develop and each can be corrected by administration of this vitamin. Pyridoxine also antagonizes the action of levodopa.

REFERENCES

BEAUPRE, E. M., and GROUNEY, P. M. (1963) Pyridoxine-responsive anaemia with neuropathy, *Ann. intern. Med.*, **59**, 724.

BICKNELL, F., and PRESCOTT, F. (1953) *The Vitamins in Medicine*, 3rd ed., London.

KARK, R. A. P., BROWN, W. J., EDGERTON, V. R., REYNOLDS, S. F., and GIBSON, G. (1975) Experimental thiamine deficiency. Neuropathic and mitochondrial changes induced in rat muscle, *Arch. Neurol. (Chic.)*, **32**, 818.

RIVLIN, R. S. (1970) Riboflavin metabolism, *New Engl. J. Med.*, **283**, 463.

SPILLANE, J. D. (1964) Drug-induced neurological disorders, *Proc. roy. Soc. Med.*, **57**, 135.

STANNUS, H. S. (1944) Some problems in riboflavin and allied deficiencies, *Brit. med. J.*, **2**, 103, 140.

SWANK, R. L. (1940) Avian thiamin deficiency. A correlation of pathology and clinical behaviour, *J. exp. Med.*, **71**, 683.

SWANK, R. L., and PRADOS, M. (1942) Avian thiamine deficiency, *Arch. Neurol. Psychiat. (Chic.)*, **47**, 97.

VAN ITALLIE, T. B., and FOLLIS, R. H. (1974) Thiamine deficiency, ariboflavinosis and vitamin B_6 deficiency, in *Harrison's Principles of Internal Medicine*, 7th ed., chap. 78, New York.

VILTER, R. W., MUELLER, J. E., GLAZER, H. S., JARROLD, A. J., THOMPSON, C., and HAWKINS, V. R. (1963) The effect of vitamin B$_6$ deficiency produced by desoxy-pyridoxine in human beings, *J. Lab. clin. Med.*, **42**, 335.

BERIBERI

AETIOLOGY

The discovery that beriberi was due to dietary deficiency and that one substance lacking in the diet of natives suffering from this disorder was the water-soluble vitamin now known as vitamin B$_1$, or thiamine, which was contained in the germinal layer discarded from polished rice, was of the greatest value in the prevention and treatment of the disease. The designation of this vitamin, the antineuritic vitamin, however, tended to obscure the problems in the aetiology of beriberi which still remain unsolved. It is clear that thiamine is not an antineuritic vitamin in the sense that its absence from the diet necessarily causes neuritis, for this does not occur in animals unless they are given carbohydrates, and in man a fall in the ratio of thiamine to carbohydrate and protein in the diet is also a causal factor, beriberi occurring when the ratio of mg of thiamine per 1,000 non-fat calories falls below 0·3. Since we now know that thiamine is necessary for the normal metabolism of carbohydrates, these observations seem to show that the nervous system and heart suffer in beriberi either from an inability to metabolize carbohydrates normally or because the pentose phosphate pathway is needed not only for carbohydrate metabolism but also for lipid synthesis. Other causal factors are chronic diarrhoea which interferes with the absorption of thiamine, liver disease which probably impairs its storage, and physical exertion which increases the need of the tissues for it. Some believe that a lack of other vitamins of the B group contributes to the causation of beriberi.

Any or all of these factors may combine with dietary deficiency to cause beriberi among prisoners of war or ill-nourished people. There is no doubt that beriberi can occur also in patients whose diet is not deficient in thiamine but who suffer from a disorder of the alimentary canal which renders its absorption defective. Such lesions include pyloric stenosis, gastro-enterostomy, ulcerative colitis, dysentery, and steatorrhoea. In addition to impairing absorption these disorders may lead to the adoption of a deficient diet. Chronic alcoholism may cause beriberi by leading to a defective intake and absorption of thiamine. At the same time the high calorie value of the alcohol increases the need for thiamine and hence the relative deficiency. Pregnancy also increases the demand for the vitamin. Vitamin B deficiency is also seen, even in highly-developed countries, in elderly people living alone on inadequate diets and it may even result from the anorexia which sometimes accompanies chronic endogenous depression.

PATHOLOGY

The changes in the peripheral nervous system are those of axonal neuropathy with secondary demyelination (Prineas, 1970) [see p. 943], involving both the somatic and autonomic nerves. This is the so-called 'dry' form. The affected neurones exhibit degenerative changes, especially at the periphery, and chromatolysis is found in the ganglion cells of the anterior horns and dorsal root ganglia of the spinal cord, and of the motor nuclei of the cranial nerves. The changes in the muscles are those characteristic of degeneration of the lower motor neurones. In the 'wet' form of beriberi there are myocardial degeneration, with enlargement of the right side of the heart, chronic venous congestion of the liver and spleen, effusions in the pleural cavities and pericardium, ascites, and oedema of the skin and subcutaneous tissues. Patients dying in the acute stage of the disease exhibit congestion and haemorrhagic injection of the pyloric end of the stomach and the duodenum.

SYMPTOMS AND SIGNS

The onset in some cases is very rapid, especially in infants—'the acute pernicious' type of Wright, but fulminating beriberi is occasionally seen in the adult (Baron and Oliver, 1958). In others it is more gradual, and mild or larval forms occur. In the most acute cases nervous symptoms typical of polyneuropathy develop within twenty-four or forty-eight hours. These consist of paraesthesiae and tenderness of the limbs, sensory loss, and progressive atrophic paralysis, with loss of reflexes. The paralysis may rapidly spread to involve all the muscles of both upper and lower limbs and finally the laryngeal muscles, intercostals, and diaphragm. Symptoms of cardiac involvement include dyspnoea and palpitations, tachycardia, cardiac dilatation, and signs of heart failure. Oedema may be slight or extreme. Disturbance of function of the alimentary canal leads to flatulence, and constipation or diarrhoea.

In chronic cases the clinical picture is that of a more or less severe polyneuropathy with or without cardiac failure. The presence or absence of oedema is the basis of the distinction between the so-called 'wet' and 'dry' forms of the disease.

DIAGNOSIS

The diagnosis of polyneuropathy in general is discussed on page 945. In the wet form of beriberi the combination of polyneuropathy and cardiac failure is unique. The dry form requires to be distinguished from neuropathy due to other causes. Tenderness of the calves and excessive sensitivity of the skin on the soles of the feet are often more striking in B_1-deficiency neuropathy than in any other. Beriberi should be suspected when the diet has been deficient for any reason or a disorder of the alimentary canal has interfered with absorption. The pyruvic acid in the blood is often raised in beriberi above the normal content of 0·4–1·0 mg per 100 ml, and in doubtful cases a pyruvate tolerance test may be helpful (Joiner et al., 1950) but measurement of urinary thiamine (less than 65 μg per g creatinine is considered abnormal) or of erythrocyte transketolase activity may be more reliable. It should be remembered that many heavy metals produce polyneuropathy by acting as competitive inhibitors of co-enzyme A or by combining with SH groups which are necessary in this reaction so that the possibility of occult heavy metal poisoning should be borne in mind. If such a metal is responsible then an abnormal pyruvate tolerance test may not be corrected by the administration of thiamine.

PROGNOSIS

In untreated fulminating cases death may occur within a few days from heart failure. Patients who survive the acute stage without treatment are likely to be left with the symptoms of a chronic polyneuritis with or without heart failure. Most patients who receive early and thorough treatment during the acute stage make a complete recovery, and remain well as long as they continue to take an adequate diet. Treatment may bring about some improvement in patients who have reached the chronic stage, but they may not recover completely.

TREATMENT

The heart failure must be treated by rest in bed. The diet should consist of frequent small feeds with a minimum of carbohydrates and fluid. Thiamine, 50 mg should be injected intramuscularly at once. There is usually an immediate response, but diuretics and digoxin may also be needed. Oral treatment with 50 mg thiamine three times daily should be continued for some days, the dose later being reduced to a maintenance level of 5–10 mg daily. The usual physio-therapeutic treatment of polyneuropathy should be carried out, a diet rich in thiamine should be given, and the possibility that the patient is also suffering from the lack of other vitamins should be borne in mind. Indeed, it is wise to give nicotinic acid, riboflavine, and pyridoxine as well and to be sure that there is no evidence of associated vitamin B_{12} deficiency. Chronic alcoholics should be treated for alcohol addiction. Patients in whom deficiency is secondary to disease of the stomach, duodenum, or intestine or to endogenous depression will need appropriate treatment.

REFERENCES

BARON, J. H., and OLIVER, L. C. (1958) Fulminating beriberi, Lancet, i, 354.
BICKNELL, F., and PRESCOTT, F. (1953) The Vitamins in Medicine, 3rd ed., London.
GOODHART, R. S., and SINCLAIR, H. M. (1940) Deficiency of vitamin B₁ in man as deter-mined by the blood cocarboxylase, J. biol. Chem., 132, 11.
JOINER, C. L., McARDLE, B., and THOMPSON, R. H. S. (1950) Blood pyruvate estimations in the diagnosis and treatment of polyneuritis, Brain, 73, 431.
PRINEAS, J. (1970) Peripheral nerve changes in thiamine-deficient rats, Arch. Neurol. (Chic.), 23, 541.
SPILLANE, J. D. (1973) Tropical Neurology, London.
VICTOR, M., and ADAMS, R. D. (1961) On the etiology of the alcoholic neurological diseases, Amer. J. clin. Nutr., 9, 379.
WALSHE, F. M. R. (1918–19) On the 'deficiency theory' of the origin of beri-beri in the light of clinical and experimental observations on the disease with an account of a series of 40 cases, Quart. J. Med., 12, 320.
WILLIAMS, R. R. (1961) Toward the Conquest of Beriberi, Cambridge, Mass.
WRIGHT, H. (1903) On the classification and pathology of beri-beri, Stud. Inst. med. Res. Kuala Lumpur, No. 3.

WERNICKE'S ENCEPHALOPATHY

Synonym. Polio-encephalitis haemorrhagica superior.

Definition. An acute or subacute disorder affecting chiefly the midbrain and hypothalamus, caused by vitamin deficiency, chiefly if not exclusively of thiamine, and characterized pathologically by congestion, capillary prolifera-tion, and petechial haemorrhages, and clinically by disorders of memory and consciousness, ophthalmoplegia, and ataxia.

AETIOLOGY

Experimental work shows that a pathological condition which appears to be identical with Wernicke's encephalopathy can be produced in animals by putting them on a diet deficient in thiamine. In man the fasting level of pyruvate in the blood has been found to be invariably elevated, and to return to normal after the administration of thiamine parallel with the clinical improvement of the patient.

It has been suggested, however, that the Wernicke syndrome may not represent a simple thiamine deficiency, being complicated in some cases by lack of other nutritional factors.

The deficiency may be due to various causes. An inadequate diet was the cause of Wernicke's encephalopathy occurring in prisoners of war, and in civil life the causes are the same as those which produce beriberi, namely, inadequate diet, chronic alcoholism (Victor and Adams, 1961), gastro-intestinal disorders, especially carcinoma of the stomach, and persistent vomiting of pregnancy. The condition has also been recorded as occurring after gastrectomy, as a complication of the vomiting due to digitalis poisoning (Richmond, 1959), and of chronic haemodialysis (Lopez and Collins, 1968).

The rare condition of subacute necrotizing encephalopathy or Leigh's disease [p. 661] which occurs in acidotic infants in which raised blood levels of lactate and pyruvate are found is a closely related disorder, resulting, however, from an inborn error of metabolism and not from primary thiamine deficiency (Procopis et al., 1967).

PATHOLOGY

Recent observations have confirmed Wernicke's original description of the pathology of this disorder, the essential lesion consisting of foci of marked congestion with many small petechial haemorrhages affecting particularly the hypothalamus and the grey matter of the upper part of the brain stem. The corpora mammillaria are constantly involved, and frequently there is also a zone of congestion with petechiae in the grey matter immediately surrounding the third ventricle, i.e. throughout the hypothalamus and medial part of the thalamus on each side. Foci are also frequently seen in the posterior colliculi of the midbrain, and less frequently in the grey matter of the floor of the fourth ventricle and other regions. They have also been described in the optic nerves. Histologically the essential lesion appears to be the vascular disorder, namely, great dilatation and proliferation of capillaries with small perivascular haemorrhages. Damage to the nerve cells is usually surprisingly slight. In recent years a number of chronic and atypical cases have been reported with less widespread pathological changes (Grunnet, 1969). '

SYMPTOMS AND SIGNS

The onset is usually insidious. Vomiting and nystagmus are early symptoms. The patient may experience a sense of unreality; he has difficulty in concentrating and sleeps badly. This condition passes into a confusional state which ends in stupor and coma. Hypothermia presumed to be due to posterior hypothalamic involvement has been reported (Philip and Smith, 1973). In less severe and acute cases the mental changes are usually those of Korsakow's syndrome [p. 1175] with defects of recent memory and confabulation. The ophthalmoplegia usually begins with weakness of the lateral recti and horizontal and/or vertical nystagmus with variable defects of conjugate gaze are common (Cogan and Victor, 1954). There is usually some degree of ataxia of the limbs. Retinal haemorrhages may be present. In many cases Wernicke's encephalopathy is accompanied by polyneuropathy, but this is not always so.

DIAGNOSIS

The diagnosis should be suggested by the occurrence of cerebral symptoms in a patient in whom one of the predisposing causes already mentioned is present, and may be confirmed by finding a raised pyruvate level in the blood. Wernicke's encephalopathy is most likely to be confused with acute encephalitis in which, however, fever is likely to be present, and there will probably be a pleocytosis in the cerebrospinal fluid. Associated features of the Korsakow syndrome and polyneuropathy will clinch the diagnosis.

PROGNOSIS

Wernicke's encephalopathy if untreated is often fatal. In prisoner-of-war camps the condition when diagnosed early and treated with the inadequate supplies of thiamine usually available had a mortality rate of 50 per cent. Intensive early treatment, however, usually leads to rapid and complete recovery, except that in some cases the Korsakow syndrome may persist for many months or occasionally for years after recovery from the acute stage. The latter syndrome does not respond to thiamine as completely and promptly as Wernicke's encephalopathy and recovery from it may be incomplete [see p. 1175].

TREATMENT

The treatment is that of beriberi [see p. 846]. In view of the possibility that other deficiencies besides that of thiamine may be present it is advisable to give nicotinic acid as for pellagra and 5 mg of riboflavine daily in addition.

REFERENCES

CAMPBELL, A. C. P., and BIGGART, J. H. (1939) Wernicke's encephalopathy (polio-encephalitis haemorrhagica superior): its alcoholic and non-alcoholic incidence, *J. Path. Bact.*, **48,** 245.

CAMPBELL, A. C. P., and RUSSELL, W. R. (1941) Wernicke's encephalopathy: the clinical features and their probable relationship to vitamin B deficiency, *Quart. J. Med.*, N.S. **10,** 41.

COGAN, D. G., and VICTOR, M. (1954) Ocular signs of Wernicke's disease, *Arch. Ophthal.*, **51,** 204.

GRUNNET, M. L. (1969) Changing incidence, distribution and histopathology of Wernicke's polioencephalopathy, *Neurology (Minneap.)*, **19,** 1135.

JOLLIFFE, N., WORTIS, H., and FEIN, H. D. (1941) The Wernicke syndrome, *Arch. Neurol. Psychiat. (Chic.)*, **46,** 569.

LOPEZ, R. I., and COLLINS, G. H. (1968) Wernicke's encephalopathy, *Arch. Neurol. (Chic.)*, **18,** 248.

MEYER, A. (1944) The Wernicke syndrome, *J. Neurol. Psychiat.*, **7,** 66.

PHILIP, G., and SMITH, J. F. (1973) Hypothermia and Wernicke's encephalopathy, *Lancet*, **ii,** 122.

PRADOS, M., and SWANK, R. L. (1942) Vascular and interstitial cell changes in thiamine-deficient animals, *Arch. Neurol. Psychiat. (Chic.)*, **47,** 626.

PROCOPIS, P. G., TURNER, B., and SELBY, G. (1967) Subacute necrotizing encephalopathy in an acidotic child, *J. Neurol. Neurosurg. Psychiat.*, **30,** 349.

RICHMOND, J. (1959) Wernicke's encephalopathy associated with digitalis poisoning, *Lancet*, **i,** 344.

VICTOR, M., and ADAMS, R. D. (1961) On the etiology of the alcoholic neurological diseases, *Amer. J. clin. Nutr.*, **9,** 379.

WORTIS, H., BUEDING, E., STEIN, M. H., and JOLLIFFE, N. (1942) Pyruvic acid studies in the Wernicke syndrome, *Arch. Neurol. Psychiat. (Chic.)*, **47,** 215.

PELLAGRA

Definition. A disease which appears to be caused chiefly by deficiency of an element in the vitamin B_2 complex, nicotinic acid, though lack of other essential food factors may also be important. It is characterized by cutaneous lesions, mental changes, glossitis, diarrhoea, and degeneration of the brain, spinal cord, and peripheral nerves.

AETIOLOGY

Pellagra is endemic in the poorer strata of the population in many South European countries, in Africa, and especially in the Southern States of the U.S.A. It is rare in Great Britain, where it has been found most often in elderly individuals living alone and in alcoholics. It may occur at any age, and both sexes are affected with equal frequency. It was once commonly, but not exclusively, found among white maize-eaters. It has been shown to be due to a dietary deficiency of nicotinic acid which is also known as the pellagra-preventing (P.P.) factor. It has also been demonstrated that the amino acid, tryptophan, is a nicotinic acid precursor and dietary deficiency of tryptophan or nicotinic acid or both may produce the syndrome. The administration of nicotinic acid produces immediate improvement in patients suffering from pellagra, and will prevent the development of pellagra if added to a diet which otherwise produces it. As in the case of other deficiency diseases, defective absorption of nicotinic acid from the alimentary canal is sometimes the cause of 'secondary' pellagra which may occur even though there is an ample supply of the essential substance in the diet. 'Secondary' pellagra may thus occur after dysentery or long-continued diarrhoea, after operation or cancer involving the stomach or small intestine, and in alcohol addicts. The combination of alcoholism and a deficient diet is an important cause of pellagra in some countries. Pellagra-like skin lesions may be seen in Hartnup disease, due to an inborn error of metabolism in which cerebellar ataxia, amino-aciduria, and an excretion of excess indole-acetic acid in the urine are observed. Rarely, similar skin lesions also appear in patients treated with isoniazid, a vitamin B_6 inhibitor. Finally, in patients with the carcinoid syndrome (malignant argentaffinoma), the circulating serotonin may cause tryptophan deficiency and a pellagra-like syndrome. The disease of dogs, canine black tongue, like human pellagra, can be prevented and cured by nicotinic acid. Maize is said to contain an antivitamin to nicotinic acid.

PATHOLOGY

The meninges are thickened and the brain may be oedematous or atrophic. Chromatolysis and pigmentation are found in the ganglion cells throughout the central nervous system and in the autonomic ganglia. The spinal cord exhibits demyelination of many of the long tracts. This is most marked in the posterior columns in the upper thoracic and cervical regions, but the corticospinal and spinocerebellar tracts also suffer. Changes in the peripheral nerves are less conspicuous, and consist mainly of patchy demyelination. Pigmentation and hyaline degeneration have been described in the cerebral arterioles and capillaries.

The principal lesions outside the nervous system are atrophy of the stomach and intestine, and ulceration of the large bowel.

E E

SYMPTOMS AND SIGNS

In endemic areas the disease may run a protracted course lasting for many years. The first attack and subsequent exacerbations tend to occur in the spring. The early attacks are characterized by gastro-intestinal disturbances, especially diarrhoea, associated with the development of the cutaneous lesions. The latter begin as an erythema involving the parts of the body exposed to light, while later the deeper layers of the skin are involved, leading to desquamation, thickening, and finally atrophy. Exceptionally the cutaneous lesions may be absent. The tongue exhibits glossitis, with loss of the epithelium, and similar changes occur in the pharynx. Gastric achylia is the rule and porphyrinuria is sometimes present. Nervous changes develop later. Many abnormal mental states occur, depending no doubt partly on the psychological constitution of the patient. Mania and melancholia may develop, the latter sometimes leading to suicide. Often the terminal state is a dementia. Visual impairment and diplopia may occur. Dysarthria and dysphagia may develop in the later stages, together with tremor and ataxia, especially in the lower limbs. The tendon jerks may be increased at first, but later tend to be lost. The plantar reflexes may be extensor, but spastic paraparesis is a relatively rare manifestation. Sensory symptoms consist of pain in the limbs with tenderness of the muscles and superficial anaesthesia and analgesia. There may be loss of appreciation of passive movements of the toes.

Nicotinic acid deficiency has also been regarded as the cause of an encephalopathy leading to stupor or coma occurring alone or associated with pellagra, polyneuropathy, ophthalmoplegia, or scurvy. Urinary excretion tests may be of value in diagnosis.

DIAGNOSIS

The clinical picture is unique, and can hardly be confused with anything else, but in the absence of the cutaneous lesions the nervous condition may resemble subacute combined degeneration.

PROGNOSIS

The prognosis in the past was poor, most patients after many years ending their days in mental hospitals. Early treatment on modern lines, however, may be expected to bring about a cure in many cases.

TREATMENT

Treatment is primarily dietetic. However, in acutely ill patients, water and electrolyte disturbances may demand intravenous fluid. Nicotinamide should be given rather than nicotinic acid to avoid the vasomotor side-effects of the latter remedy. In the early stages 100 mg may be given if need be intravenously or intramuscularly; later 200 mg two or three times a day by mouth is sufficient. Frequent small meals should be given at first followed by a high calorie diet; as many vitamin deficiencies are multiple, thiamine and riboflavine should usually be given as well.

REFERENCES

BICKNELL, F., and PRESCOTT, F. (1953) *The Vitamins in Medicine*, 3rd ed., London.
ELLINGER, P., BENESCH, R., and HARDWICK, S. W. (1945) Nicotinamide methochloride elimination tests on normal and nicotinamide-deficient persons, *Lancet*, **ii,** 197.

GRANT, J. M., ZSCHIESCHE, E., and SPIES, T. D. (1938) The effect of nicotinic acid on pellagrins maintained on a pellagra-producing diet, *Lancet*, **i,** 939.

GREENFIELD, J. G., and HOLMES, J. M. (1939) A case of pellagra. The pathological changes in the spinal cord, *Brit. med. J.*, **1,** 815.

JOLLIFFE, N., BOWMAN, K. M., ROSENBLUM, L. A., and FEIN, H. D. (1940) Nicotinic acid and deficiency encephalopathy, *J. Amer. med. Ass.*, **114,** 307.

LANGWORTHY, O. R. (1931) Lesions of the central nervous system characteristic of pellagra, *Brain*, **54,** 291.

MOSER, H., VICTOR, M., and ADAMS, R. D. (1974) Metabolic and nutritional diseases of the nervous system, in *Harrison's Principles of Internal Medicine*, 7th ed., chap. 332, New York.

SEBRELL, W. H. (1938) Vitamins in relation to the prevention and treatment of pellagra, *J. Amer. med. Ass.*, **110,** 1665.

SPIES, T. D. (1938) The response of pellagrins to nicotinic acid, *Lancet*, **i,** 252.

SPILLANE, J. D. (1947) *Nutritional Disorders of the Nervous System*, Edinburgh.

SPILLANE, J. D. (1973) *Tropical Neurology*, London.

SYDENSTRICKER, V. P. (1958) The history of pellagra, its recognition as a disorder of nutrition and its conquest, *Amer. J. clin. Nutr.*, **6,** 409.

SYDENSTRICKER, V. P., and CLECKLEY, H. M. (1941) Effects of nicotinic acid in stupor, lethargy and various other psychiatric disorders, *Amer. J. Psychiat.*, **98,** 83.

NUTRITIONAL NEUROPATHIES OF OBSCURE ORIGIN

For many years doctors practising in the tropics (Spillane, 1969, 1973) have been familiar with clinical pictures which have been found to occur either alone or in association with beriberi, pellagra, or ariboflavinosis. Fresh attention was directed to these syndromes during the Spanish Civil War and the Second World War. They appear to be due to defective nutrition though some may be due to toxic substances in food; various views are held about their causation. Treatment with riboflavine, thiamine, and nicotinic acid has not afforded conclusive evidence that any of these alone is the deficient factor and it seems probable that in many cases there are multiple deficiencies as well as some imbalance between various constituents of the diet.

Painful Feet. There are burning sensations in the soles, especially severe at night and accompanied by hyperalgesia and sweating, and later by a changeable and patchy hyperaesthesia. Other nervous abnormalities are usually absent. This syndrome has been attributed to deficiency of nicotinic acid, but deficiency of pantothenic acid now seems more likely to be the cause.

Spinal Ataxia (Tropical Neuropathy). This begins with dysaesthesiae in the feet, gradually followed by unsteadiness of gait. Sensory loss is prominent. Appreciation of vibration is lost first in the lower limbs, then awareness of passive movement, first in the toes, then more proximally. Cutaneous sensory loss appears later and spreads up to the knees or even the waist. The knee- and ankle-jerks are usually exaggerated but the plantar reflexes are flexor. The condition has been the subject of extensive reports from West Africa (Money, 1961; Monekosso, 1964), from Tanganyika (Haddock *et al.*, 1962), and from Senegal (Collomb *et al.*, 1967). In many cases the clinical picture is purely one of sensory ataxia, often of remarkably sudden onset, but amblyopia and optic atrophy and pyramidal tract involvement have been found to be associated in some cases. Collomb *et al.* (1967) pointed out that in Senegal polyneuropathy occurred in 63 per cent of cases, spastic paraparesis in 21 per cent, and a combination of spasticity and ataxia in 16 per cent. Optic and auditory nerve involvement were present in 32 per cent; they pointed out that most sufferers had severe protein malnutrition and evidence of nicotinic acid and riboflavine deficiency.

Osuntokun (1968) reported 84 cases seen in Western Nigeria and found plasma and urinary thiocyanate levels to be raised in such patients. He gave reasons for suggesting that the condition is due to chronic exposure to dietary cyanide, obtained from culinary derivatives of cassava, the tuber of manioc. Pathological changes found included extensive demyelination in peripheral nerves and similar ultrastructural changes were found in the peripheral nerves of rats treated with cyanide (Williams and Osuntokun, 1969). However, treatment with riboflavine and hydroxocobalamin had no effect upon the course of the illness (Osuntokun *et al.*, 1970). It is still uncertain, however, as to whether this Nigerian ataxic neuropathy is the same condition as that which presents with very similar clinical manifestations in Senegal and other tropical countries (Spillane, 1969, 1973).

Cranial Nerve Disorders. The commonest of these is acute or subacute retrobulbar neuropathy. Nerve-deafness, laryngeal palsy, anosmia, and trigeminal anaesthesia may also occur, with or without spinal ataxia. In Moore's cases (1937) retrobulbar neuritis was associated with soreness of the tongue and mouth and scrotal dermatitis while Monekosso and Ashby (1963) found an association of nutritional amblyopia and spinal ataxia in occasional cases.

In the West Indian amblyopia described by McKenzie and Phillips (1968), optic disc pallor is accompanied by central or paracentral scotomata and the authors consider that cyanide intoxication may be a causal factor. Plainly the condition shows close affinities to tropical ataxic neuropathy as described above, in which optic atrophy, nerve deafness, and sensory spinal ataxia are the commonest three manifestations (Osuntokun *et al.*, 1969).

Strachan's Syndrome

This unexplained disorder, rarely reported in alcoholics in the United States or occurring as a complication of chronic liver disease or non-tropical sprue, is almost certainly of nutritional origin though no single deficiency factor has yet been identified (Moser *et al.*, 1974). Progressive optic atrophy and peripheral paraesthesiae are the predominant symptoms with progressive ataxia and loss of both superficial and deep sensation associated with degeneration of sensory neurones and posterior root ganglia and ascending demyelination of the posterior columns of the cord. Motor involvement is uncommon, vertigo and deafness occur occasionally, and in some cases glossitis, corneal ulceration, and genital dermatitis are seen (the so-called orogenital syndrome). It will be seen that this rare syndrome shows several similarities clinically to tropical ataxic neuropathy.

Spastic Paraplegia. This was the rarest of these disorders among prisoners of war. Mental changes may occur at the onset. Spillane (1947) points out its resemblance to lathyrism. Cruickshank *et al.* (1961) reported cases of paraplegia of gradual or sudden onset in Jamaica associated with loss of posterior column sensibility, retrobulbar neuritis, nerve-deafness, and occasionally distal wasting of the limb muscles. Montgomery *et al.* (1964) analysed the clinical findings in 206 cases and the pathological findings in 10. There were 25 cases with ataxia, optic atrophy, and nerve-deafness resembling the other tropical neuropathies described above, and almost certainly due to malnutrition. In 181 cases, however, the picture was one of a spastic paraparesis; most patients showed positive blood tests for syphilis, but these were negative in the spinal fluid. Pathologically the affected spinal cords often showed evidence of chronic meningo-myelitis. They considered the possibility that toxic food substances (bush tea) or nutritional deficiencies could in some way modify the clinical and pathological picture of neurosyphilis and so produce this syndrome. Mani *et al.* (1969) described 35 cases from Southern India which seemed identical to those observed in Jamaica. They found no evidence of cyanide intoxication in their cases and nothing to indicate that syphilis was responsible. While unidentified dietary toxins may account for the condition they raised the possibility that it could be due to a slow virus infection.

Amblyopia (Behrman, 1962) and spastic paraplegia (Jefferson, 1963) have been reported in West Indian immigrants to the United Kingdom but in these cases, too, the aetiology remains unexplained (Spillane, 1969, 1973). Spastic paraparesis certainly occurs in some cases of Nigerian tropical neuropathy but there the pathological changes in the spinal cord seem different from those found in the West Indies. On the other hand the amblyopic, auditory, and sensory ataxic syndromes observed in many tropical countries show many similarities. Much further work will be required to determine how many different syndromes exist and to identify the causal factors in each of them.

Treatment

The treatment of these tropical neuropathies must include the provision of a full balanced diet with vitamin supplements, particularly of the B group. If given before irreversible pathological changes have occurred there is sometimes, but not always, an encouraging response; in cases of West Indian or South Indian spastic paraplegia the usual treatment for syphilis should also be given but improvement, if any, is usually slight.

Lathyrism

The consumption of lathyrus peas, which are often eaten in India, may produce a slowly-progressive spastic paraplegia, especially when the peas are contaminated with seeds of the weed akta (*vicia sativa*) which contain certain alkaloids and a cyanogenetic glycoside. The toxic principle has been identified as beta-amino-proprionitrile (Sinclair and Jelliffe, 1961).

REFERENCES

BEHRMAN, S. (1962) African race-influenced bilateral amblyopia among West Indian immigrants in the United Kingdom, *Brit. J. Ophthal.*, **46**, 554.

BRAIN, W. R. (1947) Malnutrition of the nervous system, *Brit. med. J.*, **2**, 763.

COLLOMB, H., QUERE, M. A., CROS, J., and GIORDANO, G. (1967) Les neuropathies dites nutritionnelles au Sénégal, *J. neurol. Sci.*, **5**, 159.

CRUICKSHANK, E. K., MONTGOMERY, R. D., and SPILLANE, J. D. (1961) Obscure neuro-logic disorders in Jamaica, *Wld Neurol.*, **2**, 99.

DENNY-BROWN, D. (1947) Neurological conditions resulting from prolonged and severe dietary restriction, *Medicine (Baltimore)*, **26**, 41.

HADDOCK, D. R. W., EBRAHIM, G. J., and KAPUR, B. B. (1962) Ataxic neurological syn-drome found in Tanganyika, *Brit. med. J.*, **2**, 1442.

JEFFERSON, J. M. (1963) Jamaican neuromyelopathy, *Midl. med. Rev.*, **3**, 37.

McKenzie, A. D., and Phillips, C. I. (1968) West Indian amblyopia, *Brain*, **91**, 249.

Mani, K., Mani, A., and Montgomery, R. D. (1969) A spastic paraplegic syndrome in South India, *J. neurol. Sci.*, **9**, 179.

Monekosso, G. L. (1964) Clinical survey of a Yoruba village, *W. Afr. med. J.*, **13**, 47.

Monekosso, G. L., and Ashby, P. H. (1963) The natural history of an amblyopia syndrome in Western Nigeria, *W. Afr. med. J.*, **12**, 226.

Money, G. L. (1961) Etiology of funicular myelopathies in Tropical Africa, *Wld Neurol.*, **2**, 526.

Montgomery, R. D., Cruickshank, E. K., Robertson, W. B., and McMenemey, W. H. (1964) Clinical and pathological observations on Jamaican neuropathies—a report on 206 cases, *Brain*, **87**, 425.

Moore, D. F. (1937) Nutritional retrobulbar neuritis followed by partial optic atrophy, *Lancet*, **i**, 1225.

Moser, H., Victor, M., and Adams, R. D. (1974) Metabolic and nutritional diseases of the nervous system, in *Harrison's Principles of Internal Medicine*, 7th ed., chap. 332, New York.

Osuntokun, B. O. (1968) An ataxic neuropathy in Nigeria. A clinical, biochemical and electrophysiological study, *Brain*, **91**, 215.

Osuntokun, B. O., Langman, M. J. S., Wilson, J., and Aladetoyinbo, A. (1970) Controlled trial of hydroxocobalamin and riboflavine in Nigerian ataxic neuropathy, *J. Neurol. Neurosurg. Psychiat.*, **33**, 663.

Osuntokun, B. O., Monekosso, G. L., and Wilson, J. (1969) Relationship of a degenerative tropical neuropathy to diet: report of a field survey, *Brit. med. J.*, **1**, 547.

Sinclair, H. M., and Jelliffe, D. B. (1961) *Tropical Nutrition and Dietetics*, London.

Spillane, J. D. (1947) *Nutritional Disorders of the Nervous System*, Edinburgh.

Spillane, J. D. (1969) Tropical neurology, *Proc. roy. Soc. Med.*, **62**, 403.

Spillane, J. D. (1973) *Tropical Neurology*, London.

Spillane, J. D., and Scott, G. I. (1945) Obscure neuropathy in the Middle East, *Lancet*, **ii**, 262.

Williams, A. O., and Osuntokun, B. O. (1969) Peripheral neuropathy in tropical (nutritional) ataxia in Nigeria, *Arch. Neurol. (Chic.)*, **21**, 475.

VITAMIN B₁₂ NEUROPATHY (SUBACUTE COMBINED DEGENERATION OF THE SPINAL CORD)

Synonyms. Posterolateral sclerosis; combined system disease.

Definition. A deficiency disease, usually associated with pernicious anaemia, and characterized pathologically by degeneration of the white matter of the spinal cord, which is most evident in the posterior and lateral columns, and of the peripheral nerves and brain, and clinically by paraesthesiae, sensory loss, especially impairment of deep sensibility, ataxia, and paraplegia. Subacute combined degeneration was described as progressive pernicious anaemia in tabetic patients by Leichtenstern in 1884, and the spinal cord changes were associated with the anaemia by Lichtheim in 1887. The first complete clinical and pathological account was given by Russell *et al.* in 1900. The therapeutic value of liver was the discovery of Minot and Murphy in 1926 and led to the recognition of extrinsic and intrinsic factors by Castle and his collaborators. Lester Smith in England and Rickes and his colleagues in America isolated the essential factor, cyanocobalamin, vitamin B₁₂, from the liver in 1948. Richmond and Davidson (1958) for various reasons suggested that vitamin B₁₂ neuropathy is a better name than subacute combined degeneration.

PATHOLOGY

Macroscopic changes in the nervous system are slight. Slight cerebral atrophy has been described, and on section of the cord demyelination is evident in the greyish appearance of the white matter. Microscopically, two types of lesion are found in the spinal cord, necrotic foci and degeneration of the long tracts. It has been suggested that the latter may be secondary to the former. The necrotic foci, which first appear in the lower cervical and upper thoracic regions of the spinal cord, are irregular patches of demyelination situated in the white matter, near the surface, and are possibly related to the entering blood vessels. They are most marked in the posterior columns, and the corticospinal and ascending cerebellar tracts. Degeneration of the long tracts is most evident in the upper part of the cord in the ascending tracts, and in the lower part in the descending tracts. Both types of lesion are characterized by demyelination, and in the most severely affected regions both the myelin sheaths and the axis cylinders disappear, leaving vacuolated spaces separated by a fine glial meshwork [FIG. 130]. Similar focal areas of degeneration have been described in the white

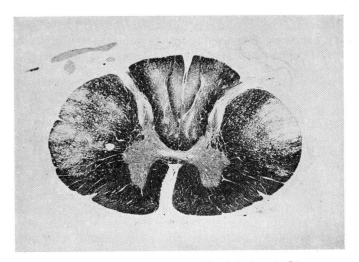

FIG. 130. Vitamin B₁₂ neuropathy. Spinal cord; C3

matter of the brain, together with more diffuse degenerative changes in the cerebral association fibres (Adams and Kubik, 1944). Comparatively recently it has been shown that peripheral nerve lesions are almost invariable with loss of the larger myelinated fibres in distal sensory nerves and evidence of axonal degeneration in teased single fibres (McLeod et al., 1969; Bradley, 1974) although in experimental vitamin B₁₂ deficiency in monkeys, segmental demyelination predominates (Torres et al., 1971).

In most cases the pathological changes of pernicious anaemia are found in patients dying of vitamin B₁₂ neuropathy. These include glossitis, anaemia, hyperplasia of the red marrow in the long bones, slight or moderate enlargement of the spleen, and the presence of iron in the reticulo-endothelial system. Magnus and Ungley (1938) described in pernicious anaemia a profound atrophy of all coats of the stomach wall, localized to the body and sparing the pyloroduodenal region. The sera of about 60 per cent of patients with pernicious anaemia contain antibodies which are capable of interfering with the ability of intrinsic factor to promote normal physiological handling of vitamin B_{12}. Immunofluorescent techniques have revealed that the antigen involved is a constituent of gastric parietal cells (*British Medical Journal*, 1966).

AETIOLOGY

Vitamin B_{12} neuropathy is a disease of middle life, the average age of onset being about 50. It may, however, begin as early as 26 or as late as 70. Both sexes are equally affected. Its familial occurrence is rare, but is well authenticated, and families have been described in which multiple cases of vitamin B_{12} neuropathy and pernicious anaemia have occurred in the same family, sometimes in more than one generation.

In almost all cases vitamin B_{12} neuropathy is associated with megaloblastic anaemia, but the relationship between the two disorders is a complicated one. At first it was believed that the degeneration of the spinal cord was secondary to the anaemia, but that this view is incorrect is shown by the fact that the anaemia may be slight or even, exceptionally, absent, when the spinal degeneration is severe, while only 10 per cent of patients with Addisonian anaemia suffer from vitamin B_{12} neuropathy (see Waters and Mollin, 1961). It must also be noted that psychiatric syndromes of confusion, depression, and dementia have been observed as a result of avitaminosis B_{12} with normal findings in the peripheral blood and marrow (Strachan and Henderson, 1965). There is also evidence to suggest that tobacco amblyopia may be due to traces of cyanide in tobacco smoke which interfere with the utilization of vitamin B_{12} and that the condition may be corrected by the administration of hydroxocobalamin but not by cyanocobalamin (see below) (Chisholm et al., 1967).

It is now known that the importance of gastric achylia lies not in the absence of the gastric acidity but in the lack of an intrinsic factor, secreted by the normal stomach, which facilitates the absorption of an extrinsic factor, contained in the food. This is cyanocobalamin, a cobalt-containing complex isolated in a red crystalline form from the liver by Smith (1948) and Rickes et al. (1948) and called by the latter vitamin B_{12}. Recent work suggests that the only function of the intrinsic factor is to render possible the absorption of extrinsic factor; this occurs in the terminal portion of the ileum; it is necessary for normal haemopoiesis and the maintenance of the nutrition of the nervous system. While failure to secrete intrinsic factor is the usual fault, impaired absorption may cause vitamin B_{12} neuropathy; so, too, may inadequate intake, as in vegans, a sect of strict vegetarians, who refuse to eat any animal products (Smith, 1962).

Although vitamin B_{12} neuropathy is usually associated with pernicious anaemia, the blood count may be normal. Vitamin B_{12} neuropathy may also occur after the operations of partial or total gastrectomy (Williams et al., 1969), intestinal disease, such as idiopathic steatorrhoea, regional ileitis, tropical sprue (Iyer et al., 1973), and resections, diverticulosis and fistulae of the small intestine (Pallis and Lewis, 1974). In such cases a megaloblastic anaemia may be due to either folic acid or vitamin B_{12} deficiency, and folic acid given for the anaemia may aggravate the neurological symptoms of B_{12} deficiency. Another rare cause of B_{12} neuropathy is inherited (autosomal recessive) congenital malabsorption of vitamin B_{12}. Malabsorption due to biologically inert intrinsic factor or to pancreatic disease or the effects of various drugs has also been described but no cases of neurological dysfunction due to these rare causes have been described (Pallis and Lewis, 1974).

SYMPTOMS AND SIGNS

Nervous Symptoms

The clinical picture is usually a mixture of posterior column, corticospinal tract, and peripheral nerve degeneration, but involvement of the optic nerves and brain is not uncommon.

The onset of symptoms is usually gradual, but is sometimes rapid. The first symptoms are generally paraesthesiae, and consist of tingling sensations, first felt in the tips of the toes, and later in the fingers. Less frequently both upper and lower extremities are thus involved simultaneously, or both the hands may be first affected. Other paraesthesiae of which patients complain include sensations of numbness, coldness, and tightness, while sharp stabbing pains occasionally occur and many patients describe sensations as if the extremities were swollen or encased in tight bandages or constricting bands. The paraesthesiae, which usually begin in the periphery of the lower limbs, tend to spread slowly towards and up the trunk, and a sense of constriction around the chest or abdomen is common. Motor symptoms consisting of weakness and ataxia develop at a variable interval after the paraesthesiae, and begin in the lower limbs. The patient may first notice that he easily becomes tired when walking, or that he walks unsteadily and tends to stumble.

Objective sensory changes are almost constantly present, and the forms of sensibility mediated by the posterior columns are always affected. Postural sensibility and appreciation of passive movement and of vibration are impaired first in the lower, and later in the upper limbs. Cutaneous sensibility to light touch, pin-prick, heat, and cold is impaired at first over the periphery of the extremities, leading to the characteristic 'glove and stocking' distribution of superficial sensory loss. The calves may be tender on pressure. The proximal border of the anaesthetic areas moves gradually towards the trunk, and on the trunk itself moves slowly upwards.

In some cases weakness and spasticity, in others sensory ataxia, predominate in the lower limbs, but both weakness and ataxia are usually present in all four limbs, and are more severe in the lower. Inco-ordination in the lower limbs, which is mainly the outcome of defective postural sensibility, is evident in the ataxic gait and the presence of Romberg's sign. Moderate muscular wasting is usually present in the later stages in the extremities, especially in the peripheral muscles.

The reflexes vary considerably. In more than 50 per cent of cases the ankle-jerks are absent when the patient comes under observation; the knee-jerks are lost rather less frequently; in other cases both are exaggerated. The plantar reflexes are flexor at first in about 50 per cent of cases, but later become extensor in all but a small proportion. In a few cases, in which the degeneration is confined to the posterior columns, ataxia is the predominant symptom throughout and signs of corticospinal defect are lacking. Conversely, spastic paraplegia may alone be present.

Sphincter disturbances consist, in the early stages, of difficult or precipitate micturition, and later of retention of urine or incontinence. Impotence occurs early.

Bilateral primary optic atrophy with some visual impairment is observed in about 5 per cent of cases and may even be the presenting feature, when central scotomata may be found (Freeman and Heaton, 1961) [see p. 161]; nystagmus may be present. The pupils may be small, but react normally. Otherwise the cranial nerves are usually normal, though dysarthria may occur rarely.

Mental changes sometimes occur and their importance has been stressed by McAlpine (1929), Holmes (1956), Fraser (1960), Strachan and Henderson (1965), and Pallis and Lewis (1974). They may be present in the absence of anaemia and of signs of spinal cord disease. There may be a mild dementia, with impaired memory and intellectual capacity, or a confusional psychosis with disorientation and paranoid tendencies, or Korsakow's syndrome; or the mental disorder may be predominantly affective, and then manifests itself in irritability or depression with a suicidal tendency. The cerebrospinal fluid is normal. In cases of pernicious anaemia, with or without symptoms and signs of involvement of the brain and spinal cord, the EEG may show diffuse slow activity and returns to normal after appropriate treatment (Samson *et al.*, 1952; Walton *et al.*, 1954).

Associated Symptoms

Gastric achlorhydria is constantly present in Addisonian anaemia, but free acid may be present in the gastric juice when the neuropathy is due to nutritional deficiency or malabsorption. There is usually anaemia, commonly macrocytic, characterized by a high mean cell volume, the presence of megalocytes or even megaloblasts in the circulating blood, poikilocytosis, anisocytosis, poly-chromatophilia, and leucopenia, with a relative lymphocytosis. Even when the blood count is apparently normal it may be possible to demonstrate an excessive number of the large red cells characteristic of pernicious anaemia or an abnormal marrow on sternal puncture. Glossitis is common, but appears to be more closely related to the anaemia than to the neurological symptoms. It may be slight or absent when the anaemia is not severe. Other symptoms may be present if the anaemia is severe. These include dyspnoea, the characteristic lemon tint of the skin, cardiac dilatation, haemic murmurs, and oedema, which is most marked in the lower limbs. The spleen is palpable in only a small proportion of cases. Gastro-intestinal symptoms are common, especially anorexia, flatulence, and diarrhoea, particularly when the neuropathy is secondary to intestinal disease. Bodily nutrition is well maintained at first, but general wasting is marked in the later stages if treatment is delayed.

DIAGNOSIS

The neurological picture must be distinguished from tabes, multiple sclerosis, spinal cord compression, polyneuropathy, and Strachan's syndrome [p. 852]. Tabes is distinguished by the absence of extensor plantar responses, except in taboparesis. Reflex iridoplegia is usually present in tabes, and in most cases the V.D.R.L. reaction is positive in either the blood or the cerebrospinal fluid, if not in both.

In multiple sclerosis there may be evidence of the disseminated character of the lesions, and especially of cerebral involvement, with pallor of the optic discs and nystagmus. The ankle-jerks are usually exaggerated in multiple sclerosis and very rarely diminished. Difficulty in diagnosis is most likely to arise in the form of multiple sclerosis characterized by progressive spastic paraplegia which is not uncommon in middle-aged patients. This, however, usually runs a much more chronic course than subacute combined degeneration, and anaemia and gastric achlorhydria are absent.

Spinal compression may lead to an ataxic paraplegia of gradual onset. Careful investigation of the physical signs, however, often indicates a well-defined level at the upper limit of the motor disability and sensory loss, and characteristic changes will usually be found in the cerebrospinal fluid and on myelography. Cervical spondylosis may cause a myelopathy closely resembling the spinal lesions of vitamin B$_{12}$ neuropathy, but in addition cervical spondylosis and the neuropathy may coexist, in which case the most careful investigation of both will be required to assess their relative importance.

Polyneuropathy may simulate subacute combined degeneration, when paraesthesiae, occurring in the extremities, are associated with ataxia of the lower limbs, loss of the tendon reflexes, and sensory loss of the 'glove and stocking' distribution. It is not surprising that there should be a close resemblance between the two conditions, since it is certain that many symptoms of vitamin B$_{12}$ neuropathy are in fact due to involvement of the peripheral nerves. Furthermore there is evidence from investigations of pyruvate metabolism that vitamin B$_{12}$ and B$_1$ deficiency may coexist (Hornabrook and Marks, 1960). In 'pure' polyneuropathy, however, there is never any evidence of involvement of the corticospinal tracts. Pain and tenderness of the muscles and muscular weakness in the distal segments of the limbs are more severe as a rule than in vitamin B$_{12}$ neuropathy.

When vitamin B$_{12}$ neuropathy is suspected on neurological grounds a blood count should be made and the gastric acidity investigated. The presence of anaemia and of gastric achlorhydria affords strong support for the diagnosis, since, apart from their accidental occurrence, these symptoms are not constantly associated with any condition with which vitamin B$_{12}$ neuropathy is likely to be confused. If there is no anaemia sternal marrow puncture may still show the characteristic abnormality of red cell formation, but this too may be normal. In untreated cases an assay of the serum vitamin B$_{12}$ is diagnostic. The normal range using the *Euglena gracilis* test is from 100 to 960 pg per ml. In vitamin B$_{12}$ neuropathy the serum vitamin B$_{12}$ is usually below 80 pg per ml. It should be noted that chlorpromazine and other drugs may interfere with estimation of the serum B$_{12}$, giving falsely low levels (Herbert *et al.*, 1965). Another useful test is the investigation of vitamin B$_{12}$ absorption using radioactive B$_{12}$ (Berlyne *et al.*, 1957). In pernicious anaemia the absorption is almost nil, but if the intrinsic factor is given as well it becomes normal. When doubt remains as to whether a low serum B$_{12}$ is due to Addisonian pernicious anaemia or to some other cause the Schilling test (measurement of the urinary output of radioactive vitamin B$_{12}$ after oral administration) and a search for gastric parietal-cell antibodies in the serum may be valuable (Wintrobe and Lee, 1974).

PROGNOSIS

The average duration of the illness of pernicious anaemia before the introduction of the modern treatment was about two years. Now it is possible by means of cyanocobalamin or hydroxocobalamin to restore the blood to normal and maintain the patient in good health indefinitely. Such patients need never develop vitamin B$_{12}$ neuropathy. When this has already developed, it can always be arrested, but the degree of recovery depends upon the stage which the disease has reached. The peripheral nerves are capable of regeneration, but this is not possible in the spinal cord, though doubtless here already damaged fibres may be restored to normal. A striking improvement therefore may be expected in the polyneuritic symptoms with disappearance of paraesthesiae and pains in the limbs, sensory loss of the 'glove and stocking' distribution, and muscular wasting if present, and with return of the tendon reflexes and improvement in co-ordination. Extensor plantar reflexes and spastic weakness and gross loss of postural sensibility, however, usually persist unchanged. Even in patients in whom the disease has been arrested by treatment the development of an infection, especially localized suppuration, may lead to an exacerbation.

TREATMENT

The essential factor which is lacking in vitamin B_{12} neuropathy must be administered to the patient intramuscularly in the form of vitamin B_{12}. The intramuscular route is by far the best; oral treatment requires very large doses and work suggesting that oral treatment with vitamin B_{12}-peptide may be equally effective (Mooney and Heathcote, 1963) has not been confirmed. The state of the blood is no guide to the dosage required for the nervous symptoms (Ungley, 1949), which is usually much larger than that needed to combat the anaemia.

Treatment should be begun with 1,000 μg of vitamin B_{12} given every 2 or 3 days for 5 doses to restore the tissue stores. After this 100 μg should be given weekly for 6 months, after which 100 μg a month is usually sufficient but may need to be increased if infection or renal insufficiency develops. Vitamin B_{12} must be given for the rest of the patient's life. Folic acid is not only useless for the treatment of vitamin B_{12} neuropathy but may be deleterious as the administration of a folate load can produce a secondary B_{12} deficiency with exacerbation of neurological symptoms.

The diet should be ample and well supplied with vitamins. If there is any suspicion of B_1 deficiency, thiamine should be given. Re-educational exercises and physiotherapy are of some value. Analgesics and sedatives may be required at first and in advanced cases, which are now fortunately rare, the usual care of the skin, bladder, rectum, and paralysed muscles necessitated by paraplegia will be required.

REFERENCES

ADAMS, R. D., and KUBIK, C. S. (1944) Subacute combined degeneration of the brain, *New Engl. J. Med.*, **231**, 1.

BERK, L., DENNY-BROWN, D., FINDLAND, M., and CASTLE, W. B. (1948) Effectiveness of vitamin B_{12} in combined system disease, *New Engl. J. Med.*, **239**, 328.

BERLYNE, G. M., LIVERSEDGE, L. A., and EMERY, E. W. (1957) Radioactive vitamin B_{12} in the diagnosis of neurological disorders, *Lancet*, **i**, 294.

BRADLEY, W. G. (1974) *Disorders of Peripheral Nerves*, Oxford.

BRITISH MEDICAL JOURNAL (1966) Parietal-cell antibody and gastritis, Leading Article, *Brit. med. J.*, **1**, 643.

CHISHOLM, I. A., BRONTE-STEWART, J., and FOULDS, W. S. (1967) Hydroxocobalamin versus cyanocobalamin in the treatment of tobacco amblyopia, *Lancet*, **ii**, 450.

DAVISON, C. (1931) Changes in the spinal cord in subacute combined degeneration following liver therapy, *Arch. Neurol. Psychiat. (Chic.)*, **25**, 1394.

FRASER, T. N. (1960) Cerebral manifestations of Addisonian pernicious anaemia, *Lancet*, **ii**, 458.

FREEMAN, A. G., and HEATON, J. M. (1961) The aetiology of retrobulbar neuritis in Addisonian pernicious anaemia, *Lancet*, **i**, 908.

GILDEA, E. F., KATTWINKEL, E. E., and CASTLE, W. B. (1930) Experimental combined system disease, *New Engl. J. Med.*, **202**, 523.

GREENFIELD, J. G., and CARMICHAEL, E. A. (1935) The peripheral nerves in cases of subacute combined degeneration of the cord, *Brain*, **58**, 483.

HERBERT, V., GOTTLIEB, C. W., and ALTSCHULE, M. D. (1965) Apparent low serum-vitamin-B_{12} levels associated with chlorpromazine, *Lancet*, **ii**, 1652.

HOLMES, J. M. (1956) Cerebral manifestations of vitamin B$_{12}$ deficiency, *Brit. med. J.*, **2**, 1394.

HORNABROOK, R. W., and MARKS, V. (1960) The effect of vitamin B$_1$ therapy on blood-pyruvate levels in subacute combined degeneration of the cord, *Lancet*, **ii**, 893.

IYER, G. V., TAORI, G. M., KAPADIA, C. R., MATHAN, V. I., and BAKER, S. J. (1973) Neurologic manifestations in tropical sprue, *Neurology (Minneap.)*, **23**, 959.

MCALPINE, D. (1929) Nervous and mental aspects of pernicious anaemia, *Lancet*, **ii**, 643.

MCLEOD, J. G., WALSH, J. C., and LITTLE, J. M. (1969) Sural nerve biopsy, *Med. J. Austral.*, **2**, 1092.

MAGNUS, H. A., and UNGLEY, C. C. (1938) The gastric lesion in pernicious anaemia, *Lancet*, **i**, 420.

MOLLIN, D. L. (1957-8) The megaloblastic anaemias, in *Lectures on the Scientific Basis of Medicine*, vol. 7, p. 94, London.

MOLLIN, D. L. (1959) Radioactive B$_{12}$ in the study of blood diseases, *Brit. med. Bull.*, **15**, 8.

MOONEY, F. S., and HEATHCOTE, J. G. (1963) Oral treatment of subacute combined degeneration of spinal cord, *Brit. med. J.*, **1**, 1585.

PALLIS, C. A., and LEWIS, P. D. (1974) *The Neurology of Gastrointestinal Disease*, London.

RICHMOND, J., and DAVIDSON, S. (1958) Subacute combined degeneration of the spinal cord in non-Addisonian anaemia, *Quart. J. Med.*, **27**, 517.

RICKES, E. L., BRINK, N. G., KONIUSZY, F. R., WOOD, T. R., and FOLKERS, K. (1948) Crystalline vitamin B$_{12}$, *Science*, **107**, 396.

RUSSELL, J. S. R., BATTEN, F. E., and COLLIER, J. (1900) Subacute combined degeneration of the spinal cord, *Brain*, **23**, 39.

SAMSON, D. C., SWISHER, S. N., CHRISTIAN, R. M., and ENGEL, G. L. (1952) Cerebral metabolic disturbance and delirium in pernicious anemia, *Arch. int. Med.*, **90**, 4.

SMITH, A. D. M. (1962) Veganism: a clinical survey with observations on vitamin B$_{12}$ metabolism, *Brit. med. J.*, **1**, 1655.

SMITH, E. L. (1948) Purification of anti-pernicious anaemia factors from liver, *Nature (Lond.)*, **161**, 638.

STRACHAN, R. W., and HENDERSON, J. G. (1965) Psychiatric syndromes due to avitaminosis B$_{12}$ with normal blood and marrow, *Quart. J. Med.*, **34**, 303.

STRAUSS, M. B., and CASTLE, W. B. (1932) The extrinsic (deficiency) factor in pernicious and related anaemias, *Lancet*, **ii**, 111.

TORRES, I., SMITH, W. T., and OXNARD, C. E. (1971) Peripheral neuropathy associated with vitamin B$_{12}$ deficiency in captive monkeys, *J. Path.*, **105**, 125.

UNGLEY, C. C. (1949) Subacute combined degeneration of the cord, *Brain*, **72**, 382.

WALTON, J. N., KILOH, L. G., OSSELTON, J. W., and FARRALL, J. (1954) The electro-encephalogram in pernicious anaemia and subacute combined degeneration of the cord, *Electroenceph. clin. Neurophysiol.*, **6**, 45.

WATERS, A. H., and MOLLIN, D. L. (1961) Studies on the folic acid activity of human serum, *J. clin. Path.*, **14**, 335.

WILLIAMS, J. A., HALL, G. S., THOMPSON, A. G., and COOKE, W. T. (1969) Neurological disease after partial gastrectomy, *Brit. med. J.*, **3**, 210.

WINTROBE, M. M., and LEE, G. R. (1974) Pernicious anaemia and other megaloblastic anaemias, in *Harrison's Principles of Internal Medicine*, 7th ed., chap. 305, New York.

FOLATE DEFICIENCY

Folate deficiency produced by malabsorption (as in steatorrhoea and intestinal 'blind-loop' syndromes) or by the use of anticonvulsant drugs, causes haematological abnormalities identical with those of pernicious anaemia, but until recently was not considered to cause neurological symptoms and signs. However, it has recently been shown that some patients with polyneuropathy and myelopathy (Grant *et al.*, 1965; Reynolds *et al.*, 1973) and others with mental illness, including dementia (Carney, 1967) may be shown to be folate-deficient, with serum values of less than 2 μg/ml. In some such cases improvement follows the administration of folic acid, 5 mg three times daily. In patients with epilepsy who develop folate deficiency and megaloblastic anaemia due to anticonvulsant therapy, it should be noted that the administration of folic acid may lower blood anticonvulsant levels so that the dose may require adjustment if fits are to be controlled (Baylis *et al.*, 1971). While the exact role of folate in the aetiology of these neurological disorders remains to be determined it would appear that estimation of the serum folate should be carried out in cases of unexplained polyneuropathy, myelopathy, and dementia. However, Pallis and Lewis (1974), in a detailed review, find much of the evidence relating neurological symptomatology on the one hand to folate deficiency on the other unconvincing.

REFERENCES

BAYLIS, E. M., CROWLEY, J. M., PREECE, J. M., SYLVESTER, P. E., and MARKS, V. (1971) Influence of folic acid on blood-phenytoin levels, *Lancet*, **i**, 62.
CARNEY, M. W. P. (1967) Serum folate values in 423 psychiatric patients, *Brit. med. J.*, **2**, 512.
GRANT, H. C., HOFFBRAND, A. V., and WELLS, D. G. (1965) Folate deficiency and neurological disease, *Lancet*, **ii**, 763.
HERBERT, V. (1964) Studies of folate deficiency in man, *Proc. roy. Soc. Med.*, **57**, 377.
PALLIS, C. A., and LEWIS, P. D. (1974) *The Neurology of Gastrointestinal Disease*, London.
REYNOLDS, E. H., ROTHFELD, P., and PINCUS, J. H. (1973) Neurological disease associated with folate deficiency, *Brit. med. J.*, **2**, 398.

NEUROLOGICAL COMPLICATIONS OF OTHER HAEMATOLOGICAL DISORDERS

The neurological complications which occasionally occur in a variety of blood diseases are mentioned in many sections of this book. Thus the complications of leukaemia, myeloma, and reticulosis are described in CHAPTER 17. The neurological manifestations of infectious mononucleosis are described on page 446 and have recently been reviewed by Silverstein *et al.* (1972). Polycythaemia vera, which may present with symptoms suggesting cerebral haemorrhage, cerebrovascular insufficiency, or even intracranial neoplasm (Kremer *et al.*, 1972) is mentioned on page 323. Intracerebral, subdural, or subarachnoid haemorrhage may also complicate the bleeding diseases including haemophilia and the various forms of thrombocytopenic purpura [p. 368] and symptoms and signs of cerebral dysfunction are common in thrombotic microangiopathy [p. 378]. These and the neurological effects of other microangiopathies, including vascular involvement in the collagen diseases, in scurvy and vitamin K deficiency, as a consequence of anticoagulant therapy and as a rare complication of hereditary haemorrhagic telangiectasia, as well as the anoxic consequences of profound anaemia are reviewed comprehensively by Lumsden (1970). Relatively little attention has been paid in the literature to the fact that in sickle-cell anaemia, in thalassaemia (Cooley's anaemia), and in other inherited haemoglobinopathies accompanied by haemolytic anaemia of varying severity, neurological manifestations are not uncommon and may even be the presenting clinical features. Complications of *sickle-cell disease* include mental changes, disordered consciousness, convulsions, meningism or frank meningitis (often pneumococcal), and cranial nerve palsies, cerebrovascular accidents, and paraparesis have all been described (Adeloye and Odeku, 1970), while in *thalassaemia*, strokes and/or convulsions occasionally occur as well as recurrent attacks of focal cerebral ischaemia, and proximal myopathy is relatively common (Logothetis *et al.*, 1972). *Acanthocytosis* of the red cells is a well-known accompaniment of α-beta-lipoproteinaemia (the Bassen–Kornzweig syndrome) [p. 655] but has also been described in patients with involuntary movements, evidence of proximal myopathy, areflexia, and bladder dysfunction in whom the serum lipoproteins were normal (Aminoff, 1972).

REFERENCES

ADELOYE, A., and ODEKU, E. L. (1970) The nervous system in sickle cell disease, *Afr. J. med. Sci.*, **1**, 33.

AMINOFF, M. J. (1972) Acanthocytosis and neurological disease, *Brain*, **95**, 749.

KREMER, M., LAMBERT, C. D., and LAWTON, N. (1972) Progressive neurological deficits in primary polycythaemia, *Brit. med. J.*, **3**, 216.

LOGOTHETIS, J., CONSTANTOULAKIS, M., ECONOMIDOU, J., STEFANIS, C., HAKAS, P., AUGOUSTAKI, O., SOFRONIADOU, K., LOEWENSON, R., and BILEK, M. (1972) Thalassemia major (homozygous beta-thalassemia), *Neurology (Minneap.)*, **22**, 294.

LUMSDEN, C. E. (1970) Pathogenetic mechanisms in the leucoencephalopathies in anoxic-ischaemic processes, in disorders of the blood and in intoxications, in *Handbook of Clinical Neurology*, ed. Vinken, P. J., and Bruyn, G. W., vol. 9, chap. 20, Amsterdam.

SILVERSTEIN, A., STEINBERG, G., and NATHANSON, M. (1972) Nervous system involvement in infectious mononucleosis, *Arch. Neurol.*, **26**, 353.

17

THE NEUROLOGICAL MANIFESTATIONS OF NEOPLASMS ARISING OUTSIDE THE NERVOUS SYSTEM

THE presence of a neoplasm in the body may affect the nervous system in a number of different ways. The most familiar is by the spread of metastases to the nervous system itself, or the structures by which it is contained. During recent years, however, a number of other effects, the pathogenesis of many of which is obscure, have been noted.

Cerebral Metastatic Neoplasms

The commonest sites of a primary carcinoma, likely to give rise to cerebral metastases, are the bronchus, breast, kidney, stomach, prostate, and thyroid. It often happens that it is the symptoms of a cerebral metastasis which first bring the patient under medical observation. This is particularly common in the case of carcinoma of the bronchus. Indeed the primary growth may be so small as not to be evident on plain X-rays of the lung. At the other extreme there may be a latent interval of many years between the removal of the primary growth and the development of a cerebral metastasis, e.g. in the case of a breast carcinoma.

The clinical features, diagnosis, and management of secondary carcinoma of the brain are described elsewhere [pp. 247 and 289–91]. Two diagnostic points are of importance: it may be possible to demonstrate the presence of neoplastic cells in the CSF, especially when there is dural infiltration at the base of the brain as commonly occurs in breast cancer (Horton *et al.*, 1973) or in carcinomatosis of the meninges (Jacobs and Richland, 1951; Olson *et al.*, 1974); and electroencephalography or more probably isotope or EMI scanning may show abnormalities suggestive of multiple metastases when only one may be causing clinical symptoms (Strang and Ajmone-Marsan, 1961).

The likelihood that a cerebral metastasis is solitary is of obvious importance in relation to treatment. Russell and Rubinstein (1959) noted that in a series of 117 cases of cerebral metastasis from bronchial carcinoma a solitary secondary was found in the brain in 30 per cent, but in only 2 of these cases were solitary metastases the only secondary growth found in the body, though in 6 others the extracranial deposits were restricted to the hilar glands.

Direct Invasion of the Nervous System by Tumour

The commoner tumours which arise outside the nervous system, but within the skull or spinal canal, are considered in the sections dealing with intracranial and spinal tumours. Other tumours arising from structures in the neighbourhood of the nervous system, and directly invading it, are comparatively rare. They include chordomas, osteomas, chondromas and sarcomas of bone, glomus jugulare tumours, malignant tumours arising in the orbit, nasal sinuses, and nasopharynx. Myeloma is considered below.

Carcinomatous Meningitis

Sometimes metastatic carcinoma of the nervous system may present with the clinical features of subacute meningitis as the result of spread of a metastatic growth to the basal leptomeninges. The identification of tumour cells in the cerebrospinal fluid is a valuable aid to diagnosis [see p. 131 and Olson *et al.*, 1974].

Cranial Metastases

The main clinical importance of metastatic growths in the cranial bones is that such tumours readily spread to the dura and may then lead to a subdural haematoma.

Spinal Metastases

Metastatic carcinoma of the spine is discussed elsewhere [see pp. 737 and 757].

Direct Invasion of Plexuses and Peripheral Nerves

Nerve plexuses or peripheral nerves are sometimes invaded either by a primary tumour or by metastatic growths in neighbouring lymph nodes. This is particularly likely to occur in the case of tumours of the apex of the lung (Pancoast's tumour) but also in carcinoma of the thyroid, breast, uterus, and rectum. Infiltration of the lumbosacral plexus by pelvic cancer, giving lower limb pain, weakness, and sensory loss, is well recognized. Involvement of peripheral nerves by haematogenous metastases is rare except in lymphoma.

Myeloma (Plasmacytoma)

Myelomas may arise within the bones of the skull, or the spine (Clarke, 1954), and may then invade the nervous system secondarily [see p. 248]. Headache, nausea and vomiting, and general malaise are common symptoms in multiple myelomatosis and are sometimes misconstrued as being due to intracranial disease. Compression of the spinal cord, cauda equina, and spinal roots are common and symptomatic herpes zoster, hypercalcaemic encephalopathy, and the carpal tunnel syndrome have all been described (Currie and Henson, 1971).

Polyneuropathy has been described in association with multiple myeloma by Victor *et al.* (1958) and is not the result of compression of nervous structures by tumour tissue. The pathological change in the peripheral nerves is degenerative, and the lower limbs may be affected alone, or with the upper as well. Thickened carpal ligaments may lead to the carpal tunnel syndrome. The condition is unrelated to amyloid disease, and in some cases clinical, radiological, and even biochemical evidence of myeloma may at first be lacking.

NEUROLOGICAL COMPLICATIONS OF THE RETICULOSES

Macroglobulinaemia (Waldenström's Syndrome)

Some 25 per cent of patients with macroglobulinaemia suffer from neurological complications, some of which appear to be due to increased serum viscosity and macroglobulin levels. The subject has been reviewed by Solomon (1965). The principal abnormalities are retinopathy, with papilloedema and haemorrhages in some cases, various manifestations of encephalopathy, including strokes, with headache, auditory symptoms, such as tinnitus, deafness, and vertigo, and postural hypotension. Peripheral neuropathy also occurs but the pathogenesis of this condition is unclear (Gotham *et al.*, 1963). Symptoms due to increased blood viscosity may be relieved by plasmaphoresis but it is now more usual to treat the condition with cyclophosphamide or other cytotoxic agents which may produce some improvement (Bouroncle *et al.*, 1964).

Progressive Multifocal Leuco-encephalopathy

Progressive multifocal leuco-encephalopathy was originally described by Åström *et al.* (1958) and by Cavanagh *et al.* (1959). The subject was reviewed by Richardson (1965) who had access to 44 cases.

It is characterized by foci of demyelination in the white matter of the cerebral hemispheres, sometimes also involving the brain stem and cerebellum and, sparsely, the spinal cord. These areas range in size from some just visible to the naked eye to large confluent areas. Usually the myelin sheaths disappear with preservation of the axis cylinders. Inflammatory infiltration is often absent but there is a characteristic change in most cases in the astrocytes, which are enlarged with bizarre nuclei, often showing mitotic changes, and in all cases, the nuclei of the oligodendrocytes are paler than normal and contain inclusion bodies (Martin and Banker, 1969).

Progressive multifocal leuco-encephalopathy is a rare disorder, usually occurring as a terminal event in patients suffering from disorders of the reticuloendothelial or blood-forming systems, i.e. the reticuloses and myelocytic leukaemias (Davies *et al.*, 1973). It has also been observed in sarcoidosis, tuberculosis, and in a small number of cases of carcinomatosis and other disorders but rarely may arise spontaneously in apparently healthy individuals (Fermaglich *et al.*, 1970). It was speculatively thought to be due to the invasion of the nervous system by a virus in patients who, owing to their primary disorder, had lost the normal immune reactions, and this view has now been confirmed by the observations of Zu Rhein and Chou (1965), Silverman and Rubinstein (1965), and Howatson *et al.* (1965), who, with the electron microscope, identified in the oligodendrocytes particles which appeared to be forms of polyoma virus. The virus may be identified in paraffin-embedded tissues (Morecki and Porro, 1970); it has been isolated and identified in culture as being a member of the polyoma SV_{40} subgroup of papova viruses (Padgett *et al.*, 1971), now generally called the JC type (Weiner *et al.*, 1973). The demyelination is attributed to destruction of the oligodendrocytes by the virus and the changes in the nuclei of the astrocytes to viral invasion.

The disorder usually terminates fatally in three to six months from the onset, but remission and survival for five years have both been reported (Hedley-Whyte *et al.*, 1966). It is characterized by symptoms of massive destruction of the white matter in the cerebral hemispheres and/or cerebellum, i.e. hemiplegia, quadriplegia, aphasia, visual field defects or blindness, dysarthria, and ataxia. Convulsions are uncommon. The patient dies in coma. The cerebrospinal fluid is usually normal.

Subacute 'Poliomyelitis'

Walton *et al.* (1968) reported a patient with Hodgkin's disease who developed subacute muscular weakness and wasting and in whom pathological examination revealed inflammatory changes like those of poliomyelitis in the anterior horns of the spinal cord; no virus was identified.

Leukaemia

In recent years, neurological complications of acute leukaemia in childhood have been reported with increasing frequency and have been attributed to the longer survival achieved with modern treatment; they are seen most often in lymphoblastic leukaemia but also in the other varieties (West *et al.*, 1972). Unilateral or bilateral facial palsy is a well-recognized manifestation. In these cases, cerebral involvement has been attributed to the entry of leukaemic cells into the brain at the sites of intracranial petechial haemorrhage. However, Currie and Henson (1971) have pointed out that focal symptoms and signs indicative of intracranial as well as less-common intraspinal lesions may occur in acute leukaemia in adults as well as in children and in patients with chronic lymphatic and myeloid leukaemia. Leukaemic cells can often be identified in the spinal fluid. Intrathecal methotrexate (8 mg/m² of body surface weekly for five weeks) or cytosine arabinoside (30 mg/m²) (*The Lancet*, 1972) and/or craniospinal irradiation with 2,400 r (*British Medical Journal*, 1973) have been employed in treatment but it should be noted that a necrotizing encephalopathy has been reported as a consequence of intraventricular methotrexate (Shapiro *et al.*, 1973).

The Lymphomas

It has been recognized for many years that intracerebral deposits of Hodgkin's lymphoma, follicular lymphoma, reticulum-cell sarcoma, and lymphosarcoma may give rise to neurological symptoms and signs suggestive of an intracranial space-occupying lesion (John and Nabarro, 1955; Whisnant *et al.*, 1956; Sokal and Glaser, 1956; Hutchinson *et al.*, 1958; Sohn *et al.*, 1967), while spinal cord, cauda equina or root compression, symptomatic herpes zoster, and peripheral nerve or plexus lesions are even more common than intracranial lesions (Currie and Henson, 1971). Intracerebral Burkitt's lymphoma has also been described (Magrath *et al.*, 1974). Multifocal leukoencephalopathy has been described above. Polyneuropathy similar to that which may complicate carcinoma (see below) (Walsh, 1971) and polymyositis (Rose and Walton, 1966) are also well-documented complications, as is hypercalcaemic stupor (Schott, 1975).

NEUROPATHY AND MYOPATHY ASSOCIATED WITH CARCINOMA

During recent years abnormalities in various parts of the nervous system and in the muscles have been noticed to occur with increasing frequency in association with neoplasms of the viscera, but unrelated to the presence of metastases. Denny-Brown (1948) under the heading 'Primary Sensory Neuropathy with Muscular Changes associated with Carcinoma' described 2 cases of bronchial carcinoma in patients whose predominant neurological symptoms were gross loss of sensibility and an associated ataxia. Lennox and Prichard (1950) reported 5 cases of peripheral neuritis among 299 cases of carcinoma of the bronchus. Brain *et al.* (1951) reported 4 cases of subacute cortical cerebellar degeneration associated with carcinoma of the bronchus in 2 and of the ovary in 1.

There have been many additions to the literature and the subject was reviewed by Brain and Norris (1965). Brain and Adams (1965) provided the following classification of these disorders in terms of the anatomical level involved.

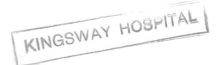

CLASSIFICATION OF NON-METASTATIC CARCINOMATOUS NEUROLOGICAL DISEASES

I. ENCEPHALOPATHY
    1. Multifocal leuco-encephalopathy
    2. Diffuse polio-encephalopathy
       (*a*) With mental symptoms
       (*b*) Subacute cerebellar degeneration
       (*c*) Brain stem lesions
    3. Encephalopathy due to disordered metabolic or endocrine functions or nutritional deficiency, especially
       (*a*) Hypercalcaemia with or without bone metastases
       (*b*) Hyperadrenalism
       (*c*) Hypoglycaemia
       (*d*) Hyponatraemia and water intoxication
       (*e*) Hyperviscosity states especially in macroglobulinaemia

II. MYELOPATHY
    1. Chronic myelopathy
       (*a*) Long tract degeneration
       (*b*) Long tract and neuronal degeneration
       (*c*) including cases simulating motor neurone disease
    2. Subacute necrotic myelopathy
    3. Nutritional myelopathy

III. NEUROPATHY
    1. Sensory neuropathy with dorsal column degeneration
    2. Peripheral sensorimotor neuropathy (polyneuropathy or neuritis)
    3. Metabolic, endocrine, and nutritional neuropathies

IV. MUSCULAR DISORDERS
    1. Polymyopathy
    2. Disorders of neuromuscular transmission
       (*a*) Myasthenic myopathy with paradoxical potentiation
       (*b*) Myasthenia gravis
    3. Polymyositis and dermatomyositis
    4. Metabolic myopathies secondary to disordered endocrine function, especially
       (*a*) Hyperadrenalism
       (*b*) Hypercalcaemia
       (*c*) Hyperthyroidism

THE INCIDENCE OF CARCINOMATOUS NEUROMYOPATHY

Croft and Wilkinson (1965) published a survey of the incidence of carcinomatous neuromyopathy in a large number of men and women with carcinoma at various sites. Their figures showed that in a consecutive series of 1,476 cases of cancer at various sites, there was an over-all incidence of neuromyopathy of 6·6 per cent, the highest figures being 16·4 per cent for carcinoma of the ovary, 14·2 per cent for carcinoma of the lung, and 9 per cent for carcinoma of the stomach, compared with 4·4 per cent for carcinoma of the breast. Table 17.1 shows the incidence of different types of carcinomatous neuromyopathy encountered in the unselected series of 1,476 patients with cancer and in 44 cases specifically referred to them as suffering from neuromyopathy (the selected group).

TABLE 17.1

Type of Neuromyopathy

	Cerebellar degeneration	Motor neurone type	Sensory neuropathy	Mixed peripheral neuropathy	Myasthenic	Neuromuscular	Other	Total
Unselected series	3 (2·9%)	3 (2·9%)	— —	15 (14·6%)	2 (1·9%)	72 (70%)	8 (7·7%)	103
Selected group	6 (13·6%)	3 (6·8%)	6 (13·6%)	14 (31·8%)	— —	10 (22·8%)	5 (11·4%)	44
All patients	9 (6·1%)	6 (4·1%)	6 (4·1%)	29 (19·7%)	2 (1·4%)	82 (55·8%)	13 (8·8%)	147

Croft and Wilkinson used the term 'neuromuscular' here to cover a considerable group of cases of muscular wasting in which it was impossible to be sure on clinical grounds whether the condition was primarily myopathic or neuropathic, or both combined. Thus their figures showed that lung carcinoma is responsible for over 50 per cent of all cases of neuromyopathy associated with carcinoma and that evidence of neuromyopathy is to be found in 14·2 per cent of all patients with lung carcinoma routinely examined, and in 4·4 per cent of all patients with breast carcinoma. The neuromuscular type of disturbance accounted for approximately 50 per cent of the types of neuromyopathy encountered irrespective of the site of the primary growth. Campbell and Paty (1974) also found a high incidence of asymptomatic neuromuscular disease in patients with lung cancer. More than half the patients they studied showed electromyographic evidence of neuromyopathy (i.e. a combination of 'myopathic' motor units with spontaneous and other activity suggesting nerve fibre loss but with normal nerve conduction: an axonal neuropathy was postulated).

PATHOLOGY
Neuropathology

Progressive multifocal leuco-encephalopathy has already been dealt with [p. 866]. Apart from this, when the central nervous system is involved as a remote effect of carcinoma and in the absence of metastases, the pathological picture may be described as a polio-encephalomyelopathy, that is, it is characterized by neuronal destruction and inflammatory infiltration, both diffuse and perivascular, the neuronal degeneration and inflammatory infiltration varying independently of one another. These changes are always to some extent diffuse, but when the damage falls predominantly upon one particular part of the nervous system, this determines the clinical picture, and this relative selectivity in many cases is responsible for the recognizable syndromes. In the brain the inflammatory changes may affect predominantly the limbic lobe, the brain stem, or the cerebellum, when loss of Purkinje cells is always a striking feature, and in some cases none can be found. Vick et al. (1969), in reporting a case of carcinomatous cerebellar degeneration with associated evidence of diffuse encephalomyelitis and radiculitis of sensory neurones, suggested that the degeneration of Purkinje cells might well be of toxic or metabolic origin and that the diffuse inflammatory changes were more probably due to an unidentified infective agent. In the spinal cord the anterior horn cells may be destroyed at varying levels, and there may be ascending and descending tract degeneration.

In some cases the cells of the posterior root ganglia are widely destroyed, and this results in Wallerian degeneration in the posterior columns and peripheral nerves.

The peripheral nerves are often attacked, leading to a peripheral sensorimotor neuropathy, studied by Croft et al. (1967), Croft and Wilkinson (1969), Trojaborg et al. (1969), Campbell and Paty (1974), and others. Croft et al. (1967) found evidence of both axonal loss and demyelination in peripheral nerves, sometimes with sparse lymphocytic infiltration, but it is now generally agreed that the primary lesion is axonal and that any demyelination is secondary.

Many attempts have been made, so far without success, in an effort to show that these neurological manifestations of neoplasia are immunological in origin. Paty et al. (1974) found some evidence of cellular sensitivity to peripheral nerve antigens in patients with carcinomatous neuromyopathy but concluded that this probably resulted from a secondary reaction to previously sequestrated neural antigens. Nevertheless, a carcinomatous myopathy in a patient who showed a marked leukaemoid reaction with medullary plasmocytosis and progressive hypergammaglobulinaemia has been described (Bruyn and Joshua, 1971).

The Pathology of the Muscles

The pathological changes in the muscles may be slight in proportion to the degree of muscular weakness. Shy and Silverstein (1965) reported changes suggestive of a myopathic lesion, i.e. loss of cross-striations, floccular, cloudy and granular changes, and internally placed nuclei with an increase of endomysial connective tissue. Many cases showed basophilic fibres with large vesicular nuclei, and prominent nucleoli characteristic of regeneration of muscle. Inflammatory changes were inconstant and not usually marked. Polymyositis and dermatomyositis developing after middle life are often associated with occult or overt malignant disease (Rose and Walton, 1966; Adams, 1974; Pearson and Currie, 1974), but it now seems evident that the acute necrotizing myopathy without phagocytosis or inflammatory change which is sometimes found in patients with carcinoma (Brownell and Hughes, 1975) is different from polymyositis in the accepted sense of the term and its pathogenesis remains obscure.

CLINICAL FEATURES

Encephalitic Form

When the brain is chiefly involved, symptoms will depend upon the region chiefly affected. The onset of symptoms is often insidious and may cover a wide range of psychiatric disorders, such as dementia, deterioration of memory, or disorder of mood, such as depression, anxiety, or agitation. When the brain stem is chiefly affected, the symptoms will depend upon the distribution of the lesions, ranging from ophthalmoplegia to bulbar palsy, often with nystagmus, ataxia, sometimes involuntary movements, and evidence of bilateral pyramidal tract damage. Severe central hypoventilation has been described in a case in which neuronal intracytoplasmic inclusions were demonstrated in the cerebral cortex but no virus could be isolated (Kaplan and Itabashi, 1974).

Subacute Cerebellar Degeneration

This syndrome has been reviewed by Brain and Wilkinson (1965) and by Vick et al. (1969). The onset is usually subacute with rapidly progressive loss of cerebellar function, leading to ataxia in both upper and lower limbs and dysarthria. Nystagmus, however, is absent in half the cases. The tendon reflexes may be diminished or lost, and the plantar reflexes extensor.

Myelopathy

The symptoms may resemble those of motor neurone disease. The patient may present with symptoms of bulbar palsy, weakness of one or both upper limbs or of the lower limbs, or of generalized weakness and lassitude. Wasting and fasciculation are found in the affected muscles. The tendon reflexes may be exaggerated or diminished and the plantar reflexes may be flexor or extensor. Brain et al. (1965) noted that carcinomatous motor neurone disease often ran a more benign course than the classical disorder. Considerable doubt has been expressed recently as to whether true motor neurone disease is ever truly a manifestation of carcinoma; many authorities believe that either the two disorders may be associated coincidentally or that the clinical manifestations of carcinomatous neuromyopathy may sometimes resemble those of motor neurone disease though the underlying pathological process is different.

Sensory Neuropathy

This is the clinical condition associated with degeneration of the posterior root ganglion cells. The patient develops, usually subacutely, sensory impairment, which tends to involve all forms of sensation in both upper and lower limbs, and is often accompanied by distressing paraesthesiae. There is sensory ataxia, and the tendon reflexes are likely to be diminished or lost. Muscular wasting and weakness may also be present.

Peripheral Sensorimotor Neuropathy (Polyneuropathy)

Croft et al. (1967) divided their patients into three groups. These were: (1) a mild and often terminal peripheral neuropathy occurring in the course of known malignant disease; (2) subacute or acute severe peripheral neuropathy, often occurring before any evidence of malignant disease is present; and (3) patients similar to those in the second group but in whom the neuropathy follows a remitting, or sometimes relapsing, course.

The symptoms are the classical ones of a polyneuropathy with distal weakness and wasting and sensory loss, symmetrical in the upper and lower limbs with diminution or loss of tendon reflexes.

Sometimes the clinical and investigative features give evidence in such cases of an isolated polyneuropathy, but much more often there is also electromyographic evidence of myopathy (Campbell and Paty, 1974). While slowing of motor nerve conduction velocity suggesting demyelination of peripheral nerves has been reported (Croft et al., 1967), in most cases motor and sensory conduction is normal or only slightly reduced (Trojaborg et al., 1969; Campbell and Paty, 1974).

Cerebrospinal Fluid

Both in patients with involvement of the central nervous system and in those with polyneuropathy the CSF is often normal, but a moderate rise in protein and of gamma-globulin is sometimes seen, though a pleocytosis is uncommon.

Symptoms of Neuromyopathy

The carcinomatous neuromyopathies are by far the commonest of the remote effects of malignant disease. Symptoms of muscular weakness may, and often do, ante-date the symptoms of malignancy, sometimes by several years. The predominant complaints of all patients are difficulty in standing, in rising from a sitting position, and in climbing stairs, sometimes with pain in the legs and peripheral paraesthesiae. The muscles most frequently involved are the proximal ones. Involvement of the bulbar muscles may occur, but is relatively uncommon. The tendon reflexes in the affected muscles are diminished or lost and occasionally fasciculation is seen. The symptoms of a neuromyopathy may be associated with those of one of the characteristic central nervous system syndromes.

Electrodiagnostic tests give results characteristic of a myopathy. There is a short mean action potential duration and a marked increase in the number of short polyphasic potentials. Many patients may show electrical evidence of neuropathic involvement as well.

The Myasthenic Syndrome

One of the rarer manifestations of malignancy is the myasthenic syndrome, usually associated with bronchogenic carcinoma (see Lambert and Rooke, 1965 and page 1025). The initial symptom is weakness and easy fatigability of the legs, less frequently the arms; some patients may have blurring of vision or ptosis. There is an appreciable delay in the development of strength and the onset of maximal voluntary contraction, but with prolonged exertion weakness develops more rapidly than in normal persons. The fatigability may not respond at all to edrophonium or neostigmine or to a lesser extent than in myasthenia gravis; it is, however, corrected by guanidine in a dose of 30–45 mg/kg body weight per day in four divided doses. The response of such patients to various muscle relaxant drugs is different from that of patients with myasthenia gravis (Croft, 1958; Simpson, 1974).

There are characteristic electrical reactions. The action potential and the twitch evoked in a muscle by a single supramaximal stimulus are greatly reduced in amplitude even though the strength of voluntary contraction may be normal or nearly so. Repetitive stimulation of the nerve at a slow rate produces a further decrease in amplitude but stimulation at fast rates leads to a progressive increase in the amplitude of the evoked potential (paradoxical potentiation). Electromyography often shows evidence of a myopathy and the diagnosis can easily be missed if studies of neuromuscular transmission are not performed. While this myasthenic–myopathic disorder (now often called the Eaton–Lambert syndrome) is most often seen in patients with bronchogenic carcinoma, it may rarely occur in patients with other forms of malignant disease and even in occasional young patients who show no evidence of neoplasia (Brown and Johns, 1974).

SUBACUTE NECROTIC MYELOPATHY

This rare disorder is characterized clinically by a subacute onset of the symptoms of an ascending lesion of the spinal cord, partial or complete, and usually terminating fatally in days or weeks. The patient develops paraplegia with some impairment of sensibility and loss of sphincter control. The cerebrospinal fluid may be normal but more frequently there is a rise of protein and there may be an excess of cells, either mononuclear or polymorphs. Pathologically there is a massive and symmetrical necrosis which may extend to the whole spinal cord or involve principally the thoracic region. The blood vessels show adventitial thickening and fibrosis, and necrosis.

Mancall and Rosales (1964) found 9 cases in the literature and added 2 more of their own. In 10 out of the 11 cases the myelopathy was associated with a carcinoma. In the 11th case there was a sarcoma, and the condition may be associated with reticulum-cell sarcoma.

NEUROMETABOLIC DISORDERS ASSOCIATED WITH NEOPLASMS

It is now well recognized that tumours of various kinds may disturb metabolism, and so lead to neurological symptoms which may bring the patient under observation. The most important of such symptoms are mental disturbances and muscular weakness. The principal syndromes of this kind were reviewed by Brain and Norris (1965) and summarized by Brain and Adams (1965).

Hypercalcaemia

The production of hypercalcaemia by a tumour of the parathyroid gland has long been recognized. However, there are at least two other ways in which tumours arising elsewhere may produce hypercalcaemia. It is thought that a tumour arising in some organ other than the parathyroid gland may produce a parathormone-like substance which leads to hypercalcaemia. Sarcoidosis may also produce hypercalcaemia in a manner not fully understood. When a tumour metastasizes widely to bones the resulting bone destruction may liberate calcium into the blood stream faster than it can be excreted, and so cause a hypercalcaemia. Myelomatosis may also produce this effect. Hypercalcaemia, however produced, may lead to cerebral symptoms, such as drowsiness, confusion or stupor, or to muscular weakness (Lemann and Donatelli, 1964; Watson, 1963; Dent and Watson, 1964; Currie and Henson, 1971; Schott, 1975).

Adrenal Hypercorticism

Various tumours, including bronchial adenoma, bronchogenic carcinoma, thymoma, or pancreatic carcinoma, may secrete ACTH (Williams *et al.*, 1974) and so lead to adrenal hypercorticism. This may not in the early stages lead to the typical symptoms of Cushing's syndrome, but may give hypokalaemic alkalosis, the symptoms of Cushing's syndrome developing only later. Clinically this syndrome may present with symptoms of a confusional psychosis or dementia, or those of a myopathy (O'Riordan *et al.*, 1966; Friedman *et al.*, 1966).

Hypoglycaemia

Some tumours other than those arising in the pancreas may produce hypoglycaemia. These have usually been of mesenchymal origin. It is thought that in some cases the tumour elaborates a material with insulin-like activity which nevertheless differs in structure from insulin, while in other cases some other explanation is necessary to understand the mode of production of the hypoglycaemia. The presenting symptoms are likely to be those familiar as a result of hypoglycaemia, namely, an encephalopathy characterized by stupor, coma, and convulsions.

Hyponatraemia

Hyponatraemia is most likely to occur in association with a bronchogenic carcinoma or adenoma which secretes a substance like vasopressin with the effects of antidiuretic hormone (inappropriate ADH secretion). The result is hyponatraemia, hypotonicity of extracellular fluid, and a hypertonic urine with sodium loss. The patient usually presents with water intoxication and encephalopathy characterized by coma, convulsions, and a raised pressure of the CSF. Treatment depends upon fluid restriction (see Welt, 1974).

REFERENCES

ADAMS, R. D. (1974) Pathological reactions of the skeletal muscle fibre in man, in *Disorders of Voluntary Muscle*, 3rd ed., ed. Walton, J. N., chap. 6, Edinburgh and London.

ADAMS, R. D., DENNY-BROWN, D., and PEARSON, C. M. (1953) *Diseases of Muscle*, London.

ÅSTRÖM, K.-E., MANCALL, E. L., and RICHARDSON, E. P. (1958) Progressive multifocal leuko-encephalopathy, *Brain*, **81**, 93.

BOURONCLE, B. A., DALTA, P., and FRAJOLA, W. J. (1964) Waldenström's macroglobulin-aemia; report of three patients treated with cyclophosphamide, *J. Amer. med. Ass.*, **189**, 729.

BRAIN, W. R., and ADAMS, R. D. (1965) A guide to the classification and investigation of neurological disorders associated with neoplasms, in *The Remote Effects of Cancer on the Nervous System*, ed. Brain, W. R., and Norris, F., chap. 21, New York.

BRAIN, W. R., CROFT, P. B., and WILKINSON, M. (1965) Motor neurone disease as a manifestation of neoplasm (with a note on the course of classical motor neurone disease), *Brain*, **88**, 479.

BRAIN, W. R., DANIEL, P. M., and GREENFIELD, J. G. (1951) Subacute cerebellar degeneration and its relation to carcinoma, *J. Neurol. Neurosurg. Psychiat.*, **14**, 59.

BRAIN, W. R., and HENSON, R. A. (1958) Neurological syndromes associated with carcinoma, *Lancet*, **ii**, 971.

BRAIN, W. R., and NORRIS, F. (1965) *The Remote Effects of Cancer on the Nervous System*, New York.

BRAIN, W. R., and WILKINSON, M. (1965) Subacute cerebellar degeneration associated with neoplasms, *Brain*, **88**, 465.

BRITISH MEDICAL JOURNAL (1973) Irradiation of C.N.S. in leukaemia, *Brit. med. J.*, **2**, 377.

BROWN, J. C., and JOHNS, R. J. (1974) Diagnostic difficulties encountered in the myasthenic syndrome sometimes associated with carcinoma, *J. Neurol. Neurosurg. Psychiat.*, **37**, 1214.

BROWNELL, B., and HUGHES, J. T. (1975) Degeneration of muscle in association with carcinoma of the bronchus, *J. Neurol. Neurosurg. Psychiat.*, **38**, 363.

BRUYN, G. W., and JOSHUA, D. (1971) Myopathy with leukemoid reaction secondary to alveolar-bronchiolar cell carcinoma, *Neurology (Minneap.)*, **21**, 1114.

CAMPBELL, M. J., and PATY, D. W. (1974) Carcinomatous neuromyopathy: 1. Electro-physiological studies, *J. Neurol. Neurosurg. Psychiat.*, **37**, 131.

CAVANAGH, J. B., GREENBAUM, D., MARSHALL, A. H. E., and RUBINSTEIN, L. J. (1959) Cerebral demyelination associated with disorders of the reticuloendothelial system, *Lancet*, **ii**, 524.

CLARKE, E. (1954) Cranial and intracranial myelomas, *Brain*, **71**, 61.

CROFT, P. B. (1958) Abnormal responses to muscle relaxants in carcinomatous neuropathy, *Brit. med. J.*, **1**, 181.

CROFT, P. B., URICH, H., and WILKINSON, M. (1967) Peripheral neuropathy of sensori-motor type associated with malignant disease, *Brain*, **90**, 31.

CROFT, P. B., and WILKINSON, M. (1965) The incidence of carcinomatous neuromyopathy with special reference to carcinoma of the lung and the breast, in *The Remote Effects of Cancer on the Nervous System*, ed. Brain, W. R., and Norris, F., chap. 6, New York.

CROFT, P. B., and WILKINSON, M. (1969) The course and prognosis in some types of carcinomatous neuromyopathy, *Brain*, **92**, 1.

CURRIE, S., and HENSON, R. A. (1971) Neurological syndromes in the reticuloses, *Brain*, **94**, 307.

DAVIES, J. A., HUGHES, J. T., and OPPENHEIMER, D. R. (1973) Richardson's disease (progressive multifocal leukoencephalopathy), *Quart. J. Med.*, **42**, 481.

DENNY-BROWN, D. (1948) Primary sensory neuropathy with muscular changes associated with carcinoma, *J. Neurol. Neurosurg. Psychiat.*, **11**, 73.

DENT, C. E., and WATSON, L. C. A. (1964) Hyperparathyroidism and cancer, *Brit. med. J.*, **2**, 218.

FERMAGLICH, J., HARDMAN, J. M., and EARLE, K. M. (1970) Spontaneous progressive multifocal leukoencephalopathy, *Neurology (Minneap.)*, **20**, 479.

FRIEDMAN, M., MARSHALL-JONES, P., and ROSS, E. J. (1966) Cushing's syndrome: adrenocortical hyperactivity secondary to neoplasms arising outside the pituitary-adrenal system, *Quart. J. Med.*, **35**, 193.

GOTHAM, J. E., WEIN, H., and MEYER, J. S. (1963) Clinical studies of neuropathy due to macroglobulinaemia (Waldenström's syndrome), *Can. med. Ass. J.*, **89**, 806.

HEATHFIELD, K. W. G., and WILLIAMS, J. R. B. (1954) Peripheral neuropathy and myopathy associated with bronchogenic carcinoma, *Brain*, **77**, 122.

HEDLEY-WHYTE, E. T., SMITH, B. P., TYLER, H. R., and PETERSON, W. P. (1966) Multifocal leukoencephalopathy with remission and five year survival, *J. Neuropath. exp. Neurol.*, **25**, 107.

HENSON, R. A., RUSSELL, D. S., and WILKINSON, M. (1954) Carcinomatous neuropathy and myopathy, *Brain*, **77**, 82.

HORTON, J., MEANS, E. D., CUNNINGHAM, T. J., and OLSON, K. B. (1973) The numb chin in breast cancer, *J. Neurol. Neurosurg. Psychiat.*, **36**, 211.

HOWATSON, A. F., NAGAI, M., and ZU RHEIN, G. (1965) Polyoma-like virions in human demyelinating brain disease, *Canad. Med. Ass. J.*, **93**, 379.

HUTCHINSON, E. C., LEONARD, B. J., MAWDSLEY, C., and YATES, P. O. (1958) Neurological complications of the reticuloses, *Brain*, **81**, 75.

JACOBS, L. L., and RICHLAND, K. J. (1951) Carcinomatosis of the leptomeninges, *Bull. Los Angeles neurol. Soc.*, **16**, 335.

JOHN, H. T., and NABARRO, J. D. N. (1955) Intracranial manifestations of malignant lymphoma, *Brit. J. Cancer*, **9**, 386.

KAPLAN, A. M., and ITABASHI, H. H. (1974) Encephalitis associated with carcinoma, *J. Neurol. Neurosurg. Psychiat.*, **37**, 1166.

LAMBERT, E. H., and ROOKE, E. D. (1965) Myasthenic state and lung cancer, in *The Remote Effects of Cancer on the Nervous System*, ed. Brain, W. R., and Norris, F., chap. 8, New York.

LAMBERT, E. H., ROOKE, E. D., EATON, L. M., and HODGSON, C. H. (1961) Myasthenic syndrome occasionally associated with bronchial neoplasm. Neurophysiologic studies, in *Myasthenia Gravis*, ed. Viets, H. R., p. 362, Springfield, Ill.

THE LANCET (1972) Treating the nervous system in acute leukaemia, *Lancet*, **i**, 297.

LEMANN, J., and DONATELLI, A. A. (1964) Calcium intoxication due to primary hyperparathyroidism: a medical and surgical emergency, *Ann. intern. Med.*, **60**, 447.

LENNOX, B., and PRICHARD, S. (1950) The association of bronchial carcinoma and peripheral neuritis, *Quart. J. Med.*, **19**, 97.

LLOYD, O. C., and URICH, H. (1959) Acute disseminated demyelination of the brain associated with lymphosarcoma, *Lancet*, **ii**, 529.

MAGRATH, I. T., MUGERWA, J., BAILEY, I., OLWENY, C., and KIRYABWIRE, Y. (1974) Intracerebral Burkitt's lymphoma: pathology, clinical features and treatment, *Quart. J. Med.*, **43**, 489.

MANCALL, E. L., and ROSALES, R. K. (1964) Necrotizing myelopathy associated with visceral carcinoma, *Brain*, **87**, 639.

MARTIN, J. B., and BANKER, B. Q. (1969) Subacute multifocal leukoencephalopathy with widespread intranuclear inclusions, *Arch. Neurol. (Chic.)*, **21**, 590.

MORECKI, R., and PORRO, R. S. (1970) Progressive multifocal leukoencephalopathy: identification of virions in paraffin-embedded tissues, *Arch. Neurol. (Chic.)*, **22**, 253.

OLSON, M. E., CHERNIK, N. L., and POSNER, J. B. (1974) Infiltration of the leptomeninges by systemic cancer, *Arch. Neurol. (Chic.)*, **30**, 122.

O'RIORDAN, J. L., BLANSHARD, G. P., MOXHAM, A., and NABARRO, S. (1966) Cortico-trophin-secreting carcinomas, *Quart. J. Med.*, **35**, 137.

PADGETT, B. L., WALKER, D. L., ZU RHEIN, G. M., and ECKROADE, R. J. (1971) Cultivation of papova-like virus from human brain with progressive multifocal leuco-encephalopathy, *Lancet*, **i**, 1257.

PATY, D. W., CAMPBELL, M. J., and HUGHES, D. (1974) Carcinomatous neuromyopathy: immunological studies, *J. Neurol. Neurosurg. Psychiat.*, **37**, 142.

PEARSON, C. M., and CURRIE, S. (1974) Polymyositis and related disorders, in *Disorders of Voluntary Muscle*, 3rd ed., ed. Walton, J. N., chap. 16, Edinburgh and London.

RICHARDSON, E. P. (1965) Progressive multifocal leukoencephalopathy, in *The Remote Effects of Cancer on the Nervous System*, ed. Brain, W. R., and Norris, F., chap. 2, New York.

ROSE, A. L., and WALTON, J. N. (1966) Polymyositis: a survey of 89 cases with particular reference to treatment and prognosis, *Brain*, **89**, 747.

RUSSELL, D. S., and RUBINSTEIN, L. J. (1959) *Pathology of Tumours of the Nervous System*, p. 213, London.

SCHOTT, G. D. (1975) Hypercalcaemic stupor as a presentation of lymphosarcoma, *J. Neurol. Neurosurg. Psychiat.*, **38**, 382.

SHAPIRO, W. R., CHERNIK, N. L., and POSNER, J. B. (1973) Necrotizing encephalo-pathy following intraventricular instillation of methotrexate, *Arch. Neurol (Chic.)*, **28**, 96.

SHY, G. M., and SILVERSTEIN, I. (1965) A study of the effects upon the motor unit by remote malignancy, *Brain*, **88**, 515.

SILVERMAN, L., and RUBINSTEIN, L. J. (1965) Electron microscopic observations on a case of progressive multifocal leukoencephalopathy, *Acta neuropath. (Berl.)*, **5**, 215.

SIMPSON, J. A. (1974) Myasthenia gravis and myasthenic syndromes, in *Disorders of Voluntary Muscle*, 3rd ed., ed. Walton, J. N., chap. 17, Edinburgh and London.

SOHN, D., VALENSI, Q., and MILLER, S. P. (1967) Neurologic manifestations of Hodgkin's disease, *Arch. Neurol. (Chic.)*, **17**, 429.

SOKAL, J. E., and GLASER, G. H. (1956) An unusual neurologic syndrome in Hodgkin's disease, *Ann. intern. Med.*, **44**, 1250.

SOLOMON, A. (1965) Neurological manifestations of macroglobulinemia, in *The Remote Effects of Cancer on the Nervous System*, ed. Brain, W. R., and Norris, F., chap. 12, New York.

STRANG, R., and AJMONE-MARSAN, C. (1961) Brain metastases, *Arch. Neurol. (Chic.)*, **4**, 8.

TROJABORG, W., FRANTZEN, E., and ANDERSEN, I. (1969) Peripheral neuropathy and myopathy associated with carcinoma of the lung, *Brain*, **92**, 71.

VICK, N., SCHULMAN, S., and DAU, P. (1969) Carcinomatous cerebellar degeneration, encephalomyelitis and sensory neuropathy (radiculitis), *Neurology (Minneap.)*, **19**, 425.

VICTOR, M., BANKER, B. Q., and ADAMS, R. D. (1958) The neuropathy of multiple myeloma, *J. Neurol. Neurosurg. Psychiat*, **21**, 73.

WALSH, J. C. (1971) Neuropathy associated with lymphoma, *J. Neurol. Neurosurg. Psychiat.*, **34**, 42.

WALTON, J. N., TOMLINSON, B. E., and PEARCE, G. W. (1968) Subacute 'poliomyelitis' and Hodgkin's disease, *J. neurol. Sci.*, **6**, 435.

WATSON, L. C. A. (1963) Hypercalcaemia and cancer, *Postgrad. med. J.*, **39**, 646.

WEINER, L. P., NARAYAN, O., PENNEY, J. B., HERNDON, R. M., FERINGA, E. R., TOUR-TELLOTTE, W. W., and JOHNSON, R. T. (1973) Papovavirus of JC type in progressive multifocal leukoencephalopathy, *Arch. Neurol. (Chic.)*, **29**, 1.

WELT, L. G. (1974) Disorders of fluids and electrolytes, in *Harrison's Principles of Internal Medicine*, 7th ed., chap. 264, New York.

WEST, R. J., GRAHAM-POLE, J., HARDISTY, R. M., and PIKE, M. C. (1972) Factors in pathogenesis of central-nervous-system leukaemia, *Brit. med. J.*, **3**, 311.

WHISNANT, J. P., SIEKERT, R. G., and SAYRE, G. P. (1956) Neurologic manifestations of the lymphomas, *Medical Clinics of North America*, **40**, 1151.

WILLIAMS, G. H., DLUHY, A. G., and THORN, G. W. (1974) Diseases of the adrenal cortex, in *Harrison's Principles of Internal Medicine*, 7th ed., chap. 86, New York.

ZU RHEIN, G., and CHOU, S. M. (1965) Particles resembling papova viruses in human cerebral demyelinating disease, *Science*, **148**, 1477.

18

DISORDERS OF PERIPHERAL NERVES

TUMOURS OF NERVES

THE connective tissue of a peripheral nerve may be the site of a tumour, either benign—a fibroma, or malignant—a sarcoma. Such tumours do not differ from similar tumours elsewhere. Tumours peculiar to peripheral nerves consist of tumours arising from the nerve elements and those arising from the nerve sheaths. Primary tumours of the nerve elements are extremely rare, but a neuroepithelioma has occasionally been described on a peripheral nerve. The peripheral fibroblastoma, neurinoma, neurofibroma, Schwannoma, or neurilem-moma is a tumour arising from the nerve sheath. Neurofibromas on peripheral nerves may be single but are much more often seen in von Recklinghausen's neurofibromatosis [p. 665]. Peripheral nerves may, of course, be compressed or invaded by primary or secondary tumours arising in other tissues. Tumours involving peripheral nerves are reviewed in detail by Kramer (1970), Seddon (1972), and Dyck *et al.* (1975).

TRAUMATIC AND ALLIED LESIONS OF PERIPHERAL NERVES

Work carried out by Seddon and his collaborators did much to elucidate the nature of the different degrees of nerve injury. Seddon (1944) described three well-defined types of nerve injury. *Neurotmesis* is complete anatomical division. *Axonotmesis* is a 'lesion in continuity' in which more or less of the supporting structure of the nerve is preserved but there is nevertheless such extensive division of axons that true Wallerian degeneration occurs peripherally. *Neurapraxia* is the term applied to a 'transient block', a minimal lesion producing paralysis which is usually incomplete, is unaccompanied by peripheral degeneration, and recovers rapidly and completely. The subject is reviewed in the light of experience gained in the Second World War in *Medical Research Council Special Report Series*, No. 282, 1954 and more recently it has been considered in detail by Sunderland (1968) and Seddon (1972).

Ischaemic Lesions. Ischaemic lesions may involve motor and sensory nerves and also the muscles. They may occur as a result of arterial injury or occlusion, of which tourniquet paralysis is one form; or closed limb fractures, giving arterial injury which may cause Volkmann's ischaemic paralysis. The anterior tibial syndrome is a form of ischaemic paralysis of the muscles in which the anterior tibial muscles after being subjected to unaccustomed effort, swell within their tight fascial compartment and may undergo partial or complete infarction. Richards (1951) reviewed the effects of ischaemia upon peripheral nerves, pointing out as Seddon (1972) has done, that arterial occlusion involves muscle, peripheral nerve, and even bone, to an equal extent; he also stressed the importance of chronic ischaemic neuropathy resulting from more gradual ischaemia resulting from progressive arterial disease. Fullerton (1963) and others have also shown that local ischaemia due to pressure is one of the factors giving rise to symptoms and signs when peripheral nerves or roots are compressed.

Pressure Neuropathy. Repeated or prolonged pressure upon a nerve leads to ischaemia, but also to mechanical deformation of the myelin sheath with local oedema (Rudge *et al.*, 1974; Neary and Eames, 1975). The initial disturbance of function is neurapraxial but this may be followed by axonotmesis, and if the pressure is not relieved perineurial fibrosis develops and prevents recovery. This is the lesion underlying the neuropathy caused by herniated intervertebral disc, narrowed intervertebral foramen, cervical rib, median nerve compression in the carpal tunnel, ulnar nerve compression at the elbow, meralgia paraesthetica, and other so-called entrapment neuropathies.

NEUROTMESIS

Neurotmesis occurs as a result of open wounds, direct blunt injuries, severe traction upon the nerve, and some forms of local chemical poisoning, e.g. by misplaced injections. Retrograde degeneration occurs in the central stump for 2 or 3 cm and the peripheral stump undergoes Wallerian degeneration. The axons of the central end soon sprout, and form a neuroma composed of nerve fibres and scar tissue on the central stump (Sunderland, 1968; Spencer, 1974).

SYMPTOMS AND SIGNS OF COMPLETE DIVISION

Complete division of a mixed peripheral nerve causes motor, sensory, vasomotor, sudomotor, and trophic symptoms corresponding in anatomical distribution to the region in which these functions are supplied by the divided nerve.

Motor Symptoms

Interruption of the motor fibres of the nerve leads to a lower motor neurone paralysis of the muscles which it innervates. The muscles innervated exhibit a flaccid paralysis, and rapidly waste. The reflexes in which they participate are diminished or lost. Investigation of the motor functions of a nerve involves testing the patient's power to contract the muscles both as prime movers and also as synergists (M.R.C., 1976). The observer must be on his guard to detect trick movements, for it is often possible for a movement which is normally effected by a paralysed muscle to be carried out by another muscle when the segment of the limb is first placed in an appropriate position. Electromyography is particularly valuable in identifying the muscles which are paralysed, while if the nerve which has been divided is one in which conduction can be measured electrically, soon after the injury has occurred conduction in the segment distal to the lesion quickly becomes greatly slowed and is later lost.

Sensation

The methods of carrying out tests of sensibility are described elsewhere [see p. 36]. Division of a sensory nerve causes complete loss of cutaneous sensibility only over the area exclusively supplied by the nerve, the *autonomous zone*. This is surrounded by an *intermediate zone*, which is the area of the nerve's territory overlapped by the supply of adjacent nerves. The autonomous and intermediate zones together constitute the *maximal zone* which is the full extent of the nerve's distribution. The cutaneous area over which appreciation of light touch is lost is usually considerably greater than the area characterized by a loss of appreciation of pin-prick. The area over which appreciation of pin-prick is lost is often ill defined and merges gradually into the intermediate zone in which this form of sensibility is present, though impaired. In some cases, even of complete division of a nerve, the completely analgesic area is surrounded by a zone in which, although a stronger stimulus than normal is necessary to evoke pain, the painful sensation is more than usually disagreeable ('hyperpathia'). The term 'deep sensibility' is used to include the appreciation and localization of pressure, and the pain induced by deep pressure, and the recognition of posture and passive movements of the joints. Impairment of deep sensibility, when present as a result of nerve division, is confined to an area which is less extensive than that anaesthetic to light touch.

Vasomotor, Sudomotor, and Trophic Functions

Vasomotor and trophic disturbances which follow destruction of a motor or a mixed nerve are probably due, at least in part, to the interruption of efferent sympathetic fibres concerned in vasoconstriction. These disturbances are most marked after injuries of the median, ulnar, and sciatic nerves. After complete division of a nerve the analgesic area of skin becomes dry and inelastic, and ceases to sweat. The surface becomes scaly owing to retardation of desquamation; the affected area is blue and colder than normal, especially in cold weather; and the limb becomes oedematous when it is allowed to hang down. The analgesic area is exceptionally liable to injury, and when injured heals slowly, so that ulcers may develop. The growth of the nails and hair is retarded (Simpson, 1970). Adhesions between tendons and their sheaths, and fibrous changes in the muscles and joints are to be regarded as complications rather than as direct results of the nerve injury, since they can be prevented by repeated passive movements of the joints.

AXONOTMESIS

This type of lesion is best illustrated by the experimental crushing of a peripheral nerve with forceps, after which all the nerve fibres are broken but the connective tissue of the nerve survives to some extent (Seddon, 1972). It may be associated with open wounds or follow direct blunt injuries, such as fractures and dislocations, traction or compression, as well as local action by physical and chemical agents. Peripheral to the injury degeneration is complete, but in acute cases regeneration always occurs, and functional recovery is always more rapid and more complete than after complete division and suture. At first, however, the symptoms are the same as after neurotmesis.

NEURAPRAXIA

In neurapraxia, although the functions of the nerve are temporarily impaired or even apparently completely lost, recovery occurs so quickly that it is impossible that it could be caused by regeneration. Lesions of this type may be produced by any of the causes of axonotmesis, provided the axons are not actually severed. Pressure is the commonest cause. In neurapraxia according to Seddon (a) the loss of function is predominantly motor; (b) there is little wasting, and the electrical reactions of the muscles persist unchanged; (c) subjective sensory disturbances—numbness, tingling, and burning—are common; (*d*) objective sensory disturbances are generally partial, and often minimal as far as touch, pain, heat, and cold are concerned; (*e*) loss of postural sensibility and vibration sense are common; (*f*) loss of sweating is unusual; and hence conduction distal to the lesion is preserved. The lesion is usually therefore a dissociated one, the motor and proprioceptive fibres suffering most, probably because the largest fibres are the most vulnerable, but in occasional cases all motor and sensory function is temporarily lost. Recovery is fairly rapid, beginning usually after a few days or weeks, and becoming complete within six or eight weeks, though, occasionally, complete restoration of function may be delayed until the fourth month. Recovery progresses irregularly and follows no anatomical order, but is always complete.

DIAGNOSIS OF THE NATURE OF A NERVE LESION

The appropriate treatment of a peripheral nerve lesion depends upon an accurate diagnosis of its nature and severity. The symptoms of neurotmesis and axonotmesis are for a long time indistinguishable. It is possible to wait until sufficient time has elapsed for regeneration to occur and, if it does not, to conclude that the nerve has been completely divided, but if suture is delayed more than five or six months the prospects of recovery are impaired. Moreover, the whole of a nerve may not be equally severely injured and combinations of neurotmesis, axonotmesis, and neurapraxia occur. It is always necessary to take into account the nature of the injury since experience is often a guide to the type of nerve injury to be expected. It is often possible to recognize neurapraxia by the features described above. Electromyography and studies of nerve conduction, to be described below, are of considerable value. However, as Bradley (1974) points out, these tests are of little value in distinguishing between neurotmesis and axonotmesis and when the lesion is proximal or when there is a considerable probability, from the nature of the injury, that actual division of the nerve has taken place, exploration within two or three months of the injury is usually indicated. Particular difficulties may arise in distinguishing between traction injuries of the brachial plexus (in which, after axonotmesis, regeneration and some degree of functional recovery may be anticipated) on the one hand, and avulsion of roots from the spinal cord on the other. Myelography may be useful in making this distinction, as may loss of the axon 'flare' response and of sensory nerve action potentials evoked from the anaesthetic area; if both are lost, the lesion probably lies proximal to the posterior root ganglia so that avulsion is likely and recovery is impossible.

SPECIAL METHODS IN THE DIAGNOSIS OF NERVE LESIONS

In many cases clinical examination and electromyography will suffice to diagnose lesions of peripheral nerves and follow their progress towards recovery but methods of measuring both motor and sensory conduction velocity have greatly increased diagnostic precision. Other methods are occasionally helpful. Gilliatt and Wilson (1954) and Fullerton (1963) have drawn attention to the increase in sensory symptoms produced by temporary ischaemia obtained by applying a pneumatic tourniquet to the limb. *Sweating* responses after exposure

F f

to heat may be used to demarcate a denervated area (Guttmann, 1940) [see p. 1069]. This may be particularly useful in distinguishing between a lesion of a spinal root, plexus and peripheral nerve, e.g. cervical rib and ulnar neuropathy, and in demonstrating a peripheral nerve lesion coexisting with a lesion of the spinal cord, e.g. a lateral popliteal nerve lesion in a patient anaesthetic from a spinal injury. However, Seddon (1972) has found this method of little value in clinical practice. *Procaine nerve-block* (Highet, 1942 *b*) may be applied either to an injured nerve or to neighbouring nerves when the diagnosis is complicated by anomalous muscle movements or when it is uncertain to which nerve a sensory area belongs.

ELECTROPHYSIOLOGICAL TECHNIQUES

The older electrical methods (e.g. Erb's 'reaction of degeneration'—see p. 28) and even the charting of strength duration curves (Wynn-Parry, 1974) which have been used to detect evidence of partial or complete denervation of skeletal muscle, have now been largely supplanted by more sophisticated methods of diagnosis, including electromyography and measurement of motor and sensory nerve conduction velocity. Methods of studying neuromuscular transmission, which are of particular importance in the diagnosis of myasthenia gravis and the myasthenic–myopathic syndrome, are described on pages 1020–22.

Electromyography

This technique normally involves the recording of the electrical activity of muscle at rest, during minimal voluntary contraction, and during full contraction. Surface electrodes may be used in order to identify which muscle or muscle groups are participating in voluntary movement, but for diagnostic work it is necessary to insert a concentric needle electrode into the muscle, to amplify the activity and to display it on a cathode ray oscilloscope, while simultaneously rendering the potentials audible in a loudspeaker (see Norris, 1963; Mayo Clinic, 1971; Licht, 1971; Richardson and Barwick, 1974; Lenman, 1975). Additional sophistications of diagnostic techniques have been used by some workers utilizing such methods as integration of the electromyogram (Lenman, 1959, 1974), automatic frequency analysis (Walton, 1952; Fex and Krakau, 1957; Rose and Willison, 1967; Dowling *et al.*, 1968), single fibre electromyography (Ekstedt, 1964), and intracellular recording (Brooks and Hongdalarom, 1968; McComas and Johns, 1974).

Normal Muscle. When a normal muscle is tested at rest there is no evidence of electrical activity. On slight voluntary contraction motor-unit potentials of 300–2,000 μV in amplitude, and 4–8 ms in duration, are recorded. These are usually monophasic, biphasic, or triphasic in shape, but up to five per cent of potentials recorded from normal muscle may be polyphasic. On vigorous voluntary contraction of the muscle an interference pattern develops. Since the patient recruits as many motor units as possible, and they fire asynchronously, each one interferes with the ones which precede and follow it [FIG. 131].

One method of quantitative electromyography depends upon the measurement of mean action potential duration and amplitude, based upon the accurate measurement of at least 20 single action potentials recorded during voluntary contraction (Kugelberg, 1949; Buchthal *et al.*, 1954; Lenman, 1974); the amplitude and duration of such potentials increases with age.

Additional information can now be obtained by techniques which have been described for estimating the numbers and sizes of motor units in certain limb muscles and especially in the extensor digitorum brevis muscle of the foot (McComas *et al.*, 1971; Campbell *et al.*, 1973; Ballantyne and Hansen, 1974). Information relating to the integrity of the reflex arc, motor neurone excitability, and the activity of the muscle spindles can be obtained by recording the H and F reflexes or by studying the tonic contraction evoked by vibration applied to the muscle (Magladery *et al.*, 1951; Lance *et al.*, 1966; Hagbarth and Eklund, 1966; Marsden *et al.*, 1969; Lenman, 1974; Lance and McLeod, 1975).

NORMAL ELECTROMYOGRAM

Submaximal contraction
individual motor units
visible

1mV

50 ms

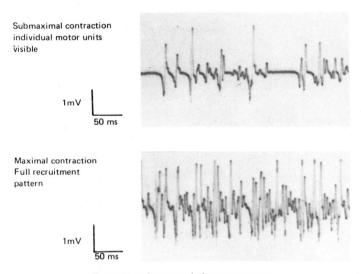

Maximal contraction
Full recruitment
pattern

1mV

50 ms

FIG. 131A, the normal electromyogram

Upper: Submaximal contraction. Note that the individual motor units here vary between 1·5 and 3 mV in amplitude and are of approximately 5–7 ms duration.

Lower: During maximal contraction there is a full 'interference pattern'; the spikes of greater amplitude represent action potentials derived from motor units lying relatively close to the recording electrode, while those of lower amplitude are derived from motor units lying some distance away.

ELECTROMYOGRAM IN MYOPATHY

Submaximal contraction
Full recruitment pattern
Low amplitude polyphasic
units

500μV

50 ms

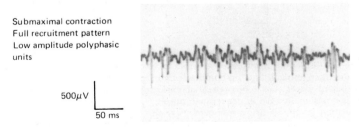

FIG. 131B, the electromyogram in myopathy

The constituent motor units are greatly reduced in amplitude and duration and many are polyphasic.

(FIGURE 131 A, B, and C kindly provided by Dr. R. Weiser.)

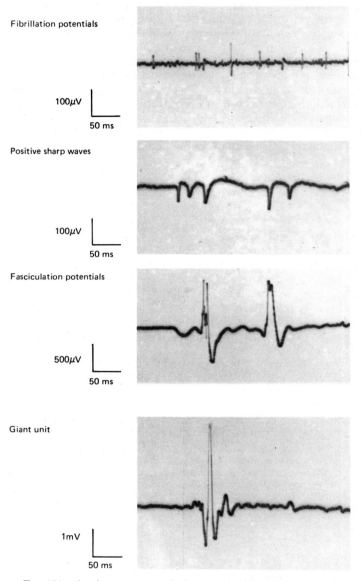

Fibrillation potentials

100μV

50 ms

Positive sharp waves

100μV

50 ms

Fasciculation potentials

500μV

50 ms

Giant unit

1mV

50 ms

FIG. 131c, the electromyogram in denervation. *From top to bottom*:

(i) Spontaneous fibrillation; this is recorded from relaxed resting muscle; the individual potentials measure no more than about 100 μV in amplitude and are of about 1 ms duration.

(ii) Positive sharp waves (saw tooth potentials) also recorded from relaxed resting muscle; this phenomenon is occasionally seen in denervated muscle.

(iii) Fasciculation potentials firing spontaneously, also recorded from relaxed resting muscle in a patient with motor neurone disease; these potentials are morphologically indistinguishable from motor unit action potentials.

(iv) A giant motor unit action potential of approximately 5 mV in amplitude occurring during volitional activity in a patient with motor neurone disease.

Completely Denervated Muscle. After complete transection of a nerve, and when sufficient time—about two weeks—has elapsed to allow the distal segment to degenerate, fibrillation potentials are evident in the resting muscle. A fibrillation potential, which arises from the spontaneous discharge of a single muscle fibre, is usually 50–100 μV in amplitude, 1–2 ms in duration, and monophasic or biphasic in shape. On attempted voluntary contraction no motor unit action potentials are produced. A total absence of such potentials on attempted volition may be found whether the lesion is neurapraxial or due to neurotmesis or axonotmesis; however, in neurapraxia, unlike the other two types of lesion, fibrillation does not occur. Hence if no fibrillation potentials are recorded two or three weeks after apparent total denervation of a muscle, it is likely that the lesion is neurapraxial. On the other hand, when fibrillation potentials are recorded this does not necessarily mean that all motor axons have been divided; it simply indicates that this is true of some. Another type of spontaneous activity sometimes recorded from resting denervated muscle is that of so-called positive sharp waves or so-called 'saw-tooth' potentials.

Partially Denervated Muscle. The electromyogram recorded from partially denervated muscle is what might be expected from a combination of degeneration of some lower motor neurones with preservation of others. If the needle is in the region of muscle fibres denervated due to axonal division, fibrillation potentials will be observed. On slight voluntary contraction intact motor units will fire, and the size, shape, and duration of their motor unit potentials will be normal, but vigorous muscular contraction will not bring into action a sufficient number of additional units to produce a normal interference pattern [FIG. 131]. Thus the interference pattern is reduced.

While the above description applies to acute partial denervation due, for instance, to an incomplete lesion of a motor root or peripheral nerve, there are certain essential differences between this pattern of activity and that more often observed in diseases giving rise to chronic progressive denervation, such as, for instance, motor neurone disease as but one example. If the denervating process is active, fibrillation and positive sharp waves are often found but such activity may be absent or difficult to find if the process is very chronic or has become arrested. However, in such cases, *fasciculation potentials* may be recorded, occurring spontaneously and repetitively when the muscle is at rest; these potentials are morphologically indistinguishable from motor unit action potentials. They usually indicate the presence of a lesion situated proximally in the motor neurone (e.g. in the anterior horn cell) and axon reflexes may play a part in their pathogenesis (Stalberg and Trontelj, 1970). Fasciculation may also be a benign phenomenon (Trojaborg and Buchthal, 1965) and can be exceptionally profuse in one form of myokymia.

It must also be recognized that in chronic denervating processes, surviving axons may produce collateral sprouts which then 'adopt' and reinnervate denervated muscle fibres so that some surviving motor units become much larger than normal in both amplitude and duration (so-called 'giant motor units', which are particularly common in motor neurone disease).

Myopathic Muscle. In myopathy there is a disorder of function which is not based on the pattern of innervation. Fasciculation does not occur and usually there is no spontaneous fibrillation either but in some cases of myopathy (and especially in polymyositis) the disease process may affect intramuscular nerve endings or alternatively focal necrosis of part of a muscle fibre may separate the remainder of the fibre from its motor end-plate so that fibrillation potentials may then be seen. On slight voluntary contraction there may be some normal muscle fibres which respond, but these will be fewer than usual. Consequently the population of muscle fibres within the individual motor units is reduced so that the duration and amplitude of the motor unit potentials is diminished and many are broken-up or polyphasic. On maximal contraction more motor units may fire, but as these will have diseased muscle fibres in them there will be a low-voltage and complex interference pattern made up of many short-duration and polyphasic potentials [FIG. 131].

Myotonia is associated with characteristic chains of oscillations of high frequency which are evoked by movement of the exploring needle within the muscle and which give rise to a characteristic recurring 'dive-bomber' sound in the loud-speaker. Typically myotonic discharges wax and wane, beginning slowly, building up to a crescendo, and then fading gradually. They must be distinguished from other bizarre high-frequency discharges (sometimes called 'pseudomyotonic') which begin and end abruptly and give a sound which is more constant; the pathophysiology of these discharges is poorly understood and they may be recorded as spontaneous activity in many disorders as diverse as motor neurone disease, polyneuropathy, muscular dystrophy, and a variety of metabolic myopathies, so that, unlike true myotonic discharges, they lack diagnostic specificity.

Measurement of Nerve Conduction Velocity

Techniques of measuring motor and sensory nerve conduction velocity have been greatly refined in recent years and have added considerable precision to the diagnosis of peripheral nerve lesions, nerve entrapment syndromes, and diseases of peripheral nerve, especially polyneuropathy (see Kaeser, 1970; Downie, 1974; Bradley, 1974). Motor conduction in the fastest-conducting fibres is usually measured by applying a supramaximal stimulus to a motor nerve at two or more different points through bipolar electrodes applied to the skin over the trunk of the nerve and then recording the evoked muscle action potential from an appropriate muscle supplied by the nerve [FIG. 132A]. The latency from the stimulus to the initial rise of the muscle action potential is measured in milliseconds for each stimulus, as is the distance between the pairs of the stimulating electrodes so that the conduction velocity in m/s in various segments of the trunk of the nerve may readily be calculated. In the case of the median nerve [FIG. 132A] the interval between the stimulus applied at the wrist and the initial rise of the muscle action potential in the abductor pollicis brevis or opponens pollicis is known as the terminal latency. Temperature has a profound effect upon nerve conduction so that the skin temperature of the limb must be carefully maintained at 20–25 °C. Sensory conduction can be measured similarly by applying stimuli to ring electrodes upon a finger [FIG. 132B] and then recording the sensory nerve action potential through cutaneous electrodes applied over the trunk of the nerve (orthodromic conduction) or by stimulating the nerve trunk and recording from the digital ring electrodes (antidromic conduction). The sensory nerve action potential is small so that averaging techniques (Gilliatt *et al.*, 1965; Buchthal and Rosenfalck, 1966) or the use of needle recording electrodes inserted close to the nerve are sometimes required. Well-established methods are now available for studying conduction in the median, ulnar, radial, and digital nerves in the upper limb (Trojaborg, 1970; Casey and Le Quesne, 1972; Downie, 1974; Bradley, 1974) and in the common peroneal, posterior tibial, and sural nerves in the lower (Gilliatt *et al.*, 1961; Behse and Buchthal, 1971). Conduction velocity is normally lower in children than in adults (Wagner and Buchthal, 1972). In the median nerve, maximum motor conduction velocity is normally 49–68 m/s, sensory conduction 60–70 m/s, and the terminal motor latency 2·0–4·5 ms. Conduction velocity in the ulnar nerve is similar, while in the common peroneal nerve maximum motor conduction

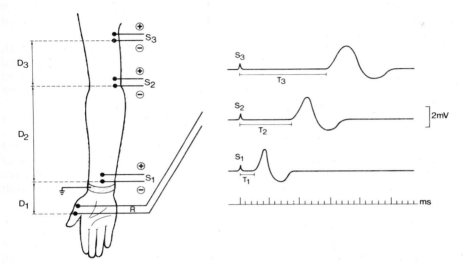

FIG. 132A, diagrammatic representation of the technique of measuring maximum motor conduction velocity in the median nerve

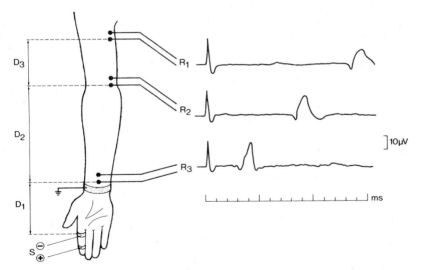

FIG. 132B, diagrammatic representation of the technique for measuring maximum sensory conduction velocity in the median nerve by orthodromic stimulation

(For fuller details see text. FIGURE 132 is reproduced from *Disorders of Peripheral Nerves*, by W. G. Bradley, Blackwell, Oxford 1974, by kind permission of the author and publishers.)

is 45–55 m/s, sensory conduction 45–70 m/s, and terminal motor latency 3·4–6·8 ms.

As previously mentioned, nerve conduction distal to a neurapraxial lesion of a peripheral nerve may remain normal at a time when its function is severely impaired. When a peripheral nerve is compressed as in entrapment neuropathies, motor and sensory conduction across the site of the lesion may be either lost or greatly reduced, while, for instance, in compression of the median nerve in the carpal tunnel, terminal latency is greatly increased. In demyelinating neuropathies, conduction is markedly delayed along affected nerve trunks, while in axonal neuropathies conduction velocity in surviving axons may be normal, but as the number of axons responding to stimulation is reduced, the evoked muscle or sensory action potentials are greatly reduced in amplitude or dispersed, while in 'dying-back' axonal neuropathies, terminal motor and sensory latency may be prolonged.

SYMPTOMS OF RECOVERY

Recovery of function after complete division of a nerve occurs by means of a down-growth of the nerve fibres from the central end, and can therefore take place only when the divided ends lie in apposition or have been brought together by suture. The time required for recovery depends principally upon the distance which the regenerating fibres have to travel from the site of injury to their normal destinations and also upon the integrity of the peripheral sheaths of Schwann cells into which the regenerating axons must grow. Mechanisms of regeneration in myelinated nerves have been studied by Thomas (1966, 1970) and by Orgel et al. (1972) and in unmyelinated nerves by Dyck and Hopkins (1972), Aguayo et al. (1973), and Thomas and King (1974). After complete division and suture many axons are misdirected so that recovery is often incomplete. The average rate of motor nerve regeneration in man is 1·5 mm per day. There has been much theoretical discussion concerning the interpretation of sensory changes which characterize returning function, but there is considerable agreement as to the facts. The first indication that nerve fibres have passed into the distal part of the nerve may be a peculiar sensitivity of the nerve trunk below the site of the union. Mechanical stimulation readily evokes a tingling sensation which is referred by the patient into the cutaneous territory of the nerve (Tinel's sign). Before other objective signs of recovery appear, the patient may say that the part feels more life-like or is less numb. The first objective sign of returning function is a diminution in the area of impairment of deep sensibility. Painful sensibility returns next, but for a long time exhibits characteristics which distinguish it from normal painful feeling. During this stage of recovery, a stronger stimulus than normal may be required to evoke pain, but the response is of a peculiarly unpleasant quality, and is a diffuse and badly localized sensation ('hyperpathia' or the stage of 'protopathic sensation' according to Head). Somewhat later the affected area becomes sensitive to the extremes of heat and cold. The appreciation of light touch, and its accurate localization and tactile discrimination—Head's 'epicritic sensation'—do not recover until many months after the return of painful sensibility, and frequently never recover completely. When recovery of appreciation of light touch occurs it is associated with the disappearance of the uncomfortable and irradiating character of painful sensibility.

With the return of painful sensibility, vasomotor changes become less conspicuous and the skin heals more readily. There is frequently considerable sensory recovery before there is any return of motor power. The response of the paralysed muscles to faradic stimulation may return before voluntary muscular contraction, but this is not always the case. In testing voluntary power the limb should always be placed in such a position that the movement to be carried out is not opposed by the force of gravity. Further, when a muscle can act both as a prime mover and as a synergist it should be tested in both these capacities, as return of power may be demonstrable in one before the other.

The above description of recovery applies only to a nerve which has been completely divided and sutured. After axonotmesis recovery is somewhat more rapid and much more often complete; after neurapraxia, as already stated, it is more rapid still, and always complete.

The following scheme is recommended by the Medical Research Council to assess recovery, which is divided into motor (voluntary power) and sensory:

I. MOTOR RECOVERY

Stage 0. No contraction.

Stage 1. Return of perceptible contraction in the proximal muscles.

Stage 2. Return of perceptible contraction in both proximal and distal muscles.

Stage 3. Return of function in both proximal and distal muscles of such an extent that all *important* muscles are of sufficient power to act against resistance.

Stage 4. Return of function as in stage 3 with the addition that *all* synergic and isolated movements are possible.

Stage 5. Complete recovery.

II. SENSORY RECOVERY

Stage 0. Absence of sensibility in the autonomous zone.

Stage 1. Recovery of deep cutaneous pain sensibility within the autonomous zone.

Stage 2. Return of some degree of superficial cutaneous pain and touch sensibility within the autonomous zone.

Stage 3. Return of superficial cutaneous pain and touch sensibility throughout the autonomous zone with disappearance of any over-response.

Stage 4. Return of sensibility as in stage 3 with the addition that there is recovery of 2-point discrimination within the autonomous zone.

TREATMENT

NON-OPERATIVE TREATMENT

Treatment is directed to avoiding swelling of the paralysed part, to maintaining the nutrition of the paralysed muscles, preventing contractures in their antagonists, and keeping the joints mobile, so that when regeneration of the nerve fibres occurs the limb may be in the best possible condition to profit by the return of nervous function. Even if operation on the nerve should be required, the treatment of the limb is the same before and after operation. In the past, firm splinting was commonly employed in order to keep a paralysed muscle in a relaxed position and to preclude movement which was thought to promote contracture of antagonists. Seddon (1972) has reviewed the objective evidence in detail and has concluded that except in cases of Erb's paralysis, when the arm should be splinted at the shoulder in a position of abduction and external rotation, splinting generally has little to commend it, as immobilized muscles tend to atrophy and become fibrotic more quickly. Hence while over-stretching of paralysed muscles must be avoided, regular passive movement is generally indicated and only those light spring-loaded splinting devices which allow movement against slight resistance in the initially paralysed muscles when they begin to show evidence of voluntary contraction are indicated. There is also some dispute about the value of regular electrical stimulation, but Seddon (1972) concludes that repetitive square wave stimulation of paralysed muscles at a frequency of about 40 stimuli per minute is of some value. As soon as voluntary power begins to return, the patient may be encouraged to assist recovery by active exercises, in which at first the movement is assisted by the physiotherapist. Later re-education in skilled movements forms an important part of the treatment, and the patient must be prevented from carrying out 'trick movements'.

OPERATIVE TREATMENT

The technique of the surgery of the peripheral nerves does not come within the scope of this book, but it is desirable to discuss the indications for surgical treatment, which have been considerably clarified by experience during the Second World War. On the whole, recovery is more complete after secondary suture than after primary suture. In all cases of open wounds, therefore, when there is a risk of infection, primary suture should never be performed. If the nerve is seen, its condition should be noted, and, if it has been divided, steps taken to prevent retraction of the stumps. Secondary suture can then be performed two or three months later. An exception to this rule has been made by some surgeons in the case of small penetrating wounds of warfare and clean glass cuts which almost invariably heal well after suture, but Seddon prefers secondary suture for these injuries also. When the patient presents himself with a healed wound and the past treatment of the nerve injury is unknown, the nerve should be explored, unless the clinical condition and electrophysiological tests suggest that the lesion is neurapraxial. After closed injuries with fractures medical treatment should be carried out for long enough to permit regenerating nerve fibres to reach the most proximal muscle supplied by the nerve, calculating the rate of regeneration at 1 mm a day and allowing a slight margin. If there is then no recovery of function in that muscle, the nerve should be explored. Ballantyne and Campbell (1973), who carried out serial electrophysiological studies after segmental repair of sectioned human peripheral nerves, found that maximum improvement of sensory function was observed at 15 months after suture but improvement in conduction in motor fibres sometimes continued for up to 47 months. Cragg and Thomas (1964) studied experimentally the conduction velocity in regenerated peripheral nerve fibres.

In severe traction injuries of the brachial plexus, when there is evidence [p. 895] of distraction of roots or spinal nerves, surgical treatment is ineffective. For many years nerve grafting has been used to bridge large defects in peripheral nerves. Autografts may be successful but their use is limited by the size of the nerve and the length of the graft required. Allografts have often been unsuccessful in the past because of rejection of the grafted segment of nerve, but Gye et al. (1972), among others, have shown that the use of allografts combined with immunosuppression with drugs such as azathioprine may be much more successful after severe injury or even in diseases such as leprosy (McLeod *et al.*, 1975).

CAUSALGIA

SYMPTOMS

Causalgia is a distressing symptom, usually associated with incomplete lesions of a peripheral nerve. Though it may occur as a result of a lesion of any nerve, it is most frequently met with when the inner cord of the brachial plexus or the median or the sciatic nerve is damaged. It consists of intense and persistent burning pain, which is subject to paroxysmal exacerbations, which may be excited not only by actual contact with the limb but also by any event which excites an emotional reaction in the patient. The pain usually begins a week or two after the injury. The appearance of the affected limb is characteristic. In a case of median nerve causalgia the hand is pink and sweating; the skin is tight and glossy; the nails are curved, grow rapidly, and are tender; the finger pads are wasted, so that the nail-beds protrude; the joints are stiff and swollen, and the bones rarefied and brittle. Tenderness may be evoked either by superficial or by deep stimulation or both, in a small proportion of cases only by the latter. Superficial tenderness usually extends over the whole cutaneous area innervated by the nerve, and thus is more extensive than the area of anaesthesia produced by nerve section, which corresponds to the area exclusively supplied by the nerve. The affected nerve may be tender throughout the whole length of the limb, even as high as the brachial plexus. There may be little or no associated muscular paralysis. Owing to the extreme tenderness of the affected part the patient makes every effort to protect the limb from all forms of external stimulation. Similar symptoms may be referred to the stump following amputation.

Many attempts have been made in the past to explain causalgia; the most plausible explanation has been elaborated on the basis of the 'gate theory' of sensation of Melzack and Wall (1965) [p. 39]. If large diameter sensory fibres are selectively damaged by injury, the 'gate' mechanism is then biased in favour of small fibre influences (*The Lancet*, 1972) so that all somatic input from the affected area of skin produces hyperpathia. It has also been suggested that there may be false synapses (ephapses) between afferent fibres subserving pain in sympathetic nerves with somatic sensory afferents, but this is much less certain and the exact role played by the autonomic nervous system has not yet been established.

TREATMENT

The most effective treatment appears to be sympathetic block with local anaesthetic, followed by sympathectomy if the pain is relieved. Surgical excision of the affected segment of nerve followed by resuturing and/or procaine block of somatic afferents and even cordotomy have been shown as a rule to be ineffective. There is some recent evidence (Meyer and Fields, 1972) to indicate that repetitive selective electrical stimulation of large sensory fibres of peripheral nerves may be remarkably effective, even in some cases in which sympathectomy has failed; this evidence gives some support to the theory of aetiology based upon the 'gate control' hypothesis.

Symptoms superficially resembling those of causalgia sometimes develop in amputation stumps in which painful neuromata on the distal ends of severed nerves develop. In such cases, the severe spontaneous pain may be reproduced by pressure upon the neuroma. Excision of the neuroma or repeated injection of local anaesthetic or phenol may give relief but repeated percussion of the neuroma in the amputation stump with an appropriate instrument may be more effective in the long run.

SYMPTOMS AND TREATMENT OF INDIVIDUAL NERVE LESIONS

THE PHRENIC NERVE

The phrenic nerve is derived from the anterior primary divisions of the third, fourth, and fifth cervical spinal nerves, the main contribution coming from the fourth. It is the motor nerve to the diaphragm. Irritation of the phrenic nerve causes a dry, unproductive, 'barking' cough: rarely it may cause hiccup. Paralysis of the nerve causes loss of movement of the diaphragm on the affected side. The effects of this are most evident when the lesion is bilateral. The diaphragm fails to descend on inspiration and may actually be drawn upwards. There is increased eversion of the costal margins with indrawing of the upper abdominal wall on inspiration. Diaphragmatic paralysis causes no symptoms as long as the patient is at rest, but dyspnoea may occur on exertion. Bilateral paralysis in patients with spinal muscular atrophy or limb-girdle muscular dystrophy may sometimes give severe alveolar hypoventilation with hypercapnia, requiring assisted respiration. The resulting diminution in expansion of the bases of the lungs renders the patient liable to develop a basal bronchopneumonia.

Diaphragmatic paralysis is most frequently produced by lesions involving the anterior horn cells of the spinal cord in the third, fourth, and fifth cervical segments, for example, direct trauma, poliomyelitis, transverse myelitis, and tumours of the spinal cord. The phrenic nerve may be intentionally divided for therapeutic purposes or injured during operations on the neck, and may be compressed by aneurysm of the aorta or by intrathoracic neoplasms or enlargement of the mediastinal glands. It may undergo degeneration in polyneuritis due to alcohol, diphtheria, lead, or other toxins or may be involved in post-infective polyneuropathy (the Guillain–Barré syndrome). In such cases the velocity of conduction in the nerve, which can be measured electrically (Davis, 1967), is usually reduced.

THE NERVES OF THE UPPER LIMB

THE BRACHIAL PLEXUS

The brachial plexus [FIG. 133] is formed from the anterior primary divisions of the fifth, sixth, seventh, and eighth cervical and the first thoracic spinal nerves. It sometimes receives a contribution from the second thoracic nerve. Variations in the position of the brachial plexus are not uncommon. In the so-called 'prefixed' type there is a contribution from the fourth cervical nerve; the fifth cervical branch is large and there may be no branch from the second thoracic. In the 'post-fixed' type there may be no branch from the fourth cervical, and that from the fifth is comparatively small, whereas the second thoracic branch is quite distinct. The spinal segmental representation of muscles may be slightly higher or slightly lower than normal, according to whether the plexus is pre-fixed or post-fixed.

The contributions to the plexus from the anterior primary divisions soon divide into anterior and posterior trunks, and from these are formed the three cords of the plexus. The lateral cord is formed by a union of anterior trunks of the fifth, sixth, and seventh nerves. From it arise the lateral anterior thoracic and musculocutaneous nerves and the lateral head of the median nerve. The medial or inner cord is formed by a combination of the anterior trunk of the eighth cervical with the contribution of the first thoracic nerve to the plexus. It gives origin to the medial head of the median nerve, the ulnar nerve, the medial cutaneous nerves of the arm and forearm, and the medial anterior thoracic

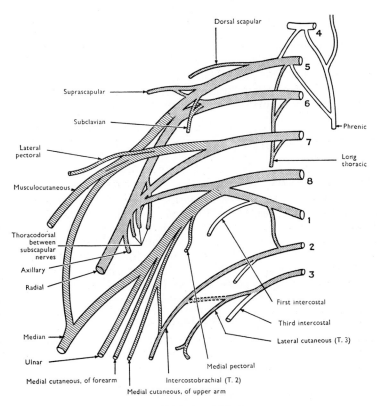

FIG. 133. Right brachial plexus

nerve. The posterior cord is formed by the union of the posterior trunks from the fifth, sixth, seventh, and eighth cervical and sometimes the first thoracic nerves. It gives rise to the axillary and radial nerves, the two subscapular nerves, and the nerve to the teres major.

Certain muscles are innervated by nerves which leave the brachial plexus proximal to the formation of the three cords. The most important of these are: the dorsal scapular nerve, from the fifth cervical, which supplies the levator scapulae and the rhomboid muscles; the long or posterior thoracic nerve, from the fifth, sixth, and seventh cervical nerves, which supplies the serratus anterior; and the suprascapular nerve, from the fifth and sixth cervical nerves, which supplies the supraspinatus and the infraspinatus. For details of methods of examination of individual muscles and their innervation by roots and peripheral nerves, see Medical Research Council (1976).

LESIONS OF THE BRACHIAL PLEXUS

If we consider with the brachial plexus the spinal nerves from which it is derived we find that it is liable to damage at many points and from many causes. One or more of the spinal nerves may be involved by a lesion of the cervical spine, including congenital abnormality such as fusion of vertebrae—Klippel-Feil syndrome—fracture-dislocation, herniated intervertebral disc, spondylosis occurring alone or with any of the foregoing, and, rarely, tuberculous or syphilitic caries or malignant deposits. The plexus itself is liable to be damaged by stabs and gun-shot wounds, by fracture of the clavicle, and by dislocation of the upper end of the humerus. Its component parts may be torn by forcible separation of the head and shoulder or by abduction of the arm, or compressed by abnormalities of the thoracic outlet (the space between the clavicle and first rib). The plexus is occasionally involved in neoplastic deposits in cervical lymph nodes or invaded by apical pulmonary neoplasm, and it may be compressed by a neurofibroma. The character of the motor and sensory disturbances resulting from lesions of the brachial plexus depends upon the situation of the lesion and the part of the plexus involved.

Total Plexus Paralysis

This is a rare occurrence. When the lesion is close to the vertebral column all the muscles supplied by the plexus will be paralysed and the cervical sympathetic may also be involved. When the plexus is involved at the level of the cords, the spinati, rhomboids, serratus anterior, pectorals, and cervical sympathetic may escape. Appreciation of light touch, pain, and temperature is lost over the forearm and hand and over the outer surface of the arm in its lower two-thirds. Postural sensibility and appreciation of passive movement are lost in the fingers. All the tendon reflexes in the upper limb are lost.

Upper Plexus Paralysis (Erb-Duchenne type)

This is due to a lesion of the branch from the fifth cervical nerve to the brachial plexus. Occasionally the sixth cervical contribution may be involved, but this is exceptional. Upper plexus paralysis is usually the result of indirect violence, the nerve being torn by undue separation of the head and shoulder. It is a common form of birth injury resulting from traction on the head when there is difficulty in delivering one shoulder. It may occur in adults as a result of a fall on the shoulder forcing the head to one side as on falling violently from a motor cycle, and occasionally follows an anaesthetic in patients in whom, during the operation, the arm has been held abducted and externally rotated. The muscles paralysed as a result of interruption of the fifth cervical branch are the biceps, deltoid, brachialis, brachioradialis, supraspinatus, infraspinatus, and the rhomboids. When the sixth cervical branch is involved in addition, there may be weakness, but not as a rule complete paralysis, of the serratus anterior, latissimus dorsi, triceps, pectoralis major, and extensor carpi radialis.

The position of the limb resulting from upper plexus paralysis is characteristic. It hangs at the side internally rotated at the shoulder, with the elbow extended and the forearm pronated. There is wasting of the paralysed muscles. Paralysis of the deltoid renders abduction at the shoulder impossible. The elbow cannot be flexed on account of paralysis of the flexors. External rotation at the shoulder is lost owing to paralysis of the spinati. Movements of the wrist and fingers are unaffected. The biceps and supinator jerks are lost. Sensory loss may be absent, but there is sometimes a small area of anaesthesia and analgesia overlying the deltoid.

The results of operative treatment of upper plexus paralysis are disappointing, and surgical intervention is inadvisable, except in those rare instances in which the upper part of the plexus has been divided by a stab or gun-shot wound. It is contra-indicated if tests show the lesion to be proximal to the dorsal root ganglia (Bonney, 1954; Seddon, 1972). The 'flare' response which follows local scratching of the skin is an axon reflex which is lost in lesions occurring distal to the ganglia. Thus if the 'flare' response is present, and particularly if myelography demonstrates a traumatic meningocele (Seddon, 1972) or a pattern of root-sleeve filling which indicates that the fifth root or spinal nerve has been torn from its origin from the spinal cord, the prognosis is very poor. The arm should be put up in an adjustable abduction splint with a movable joint at the elbow, and the usual after-treatment of peripheral nerve lesions should be carried out. When the lesion is distal to the ganglia, however, the prognosis is on the whole better as actual division or tearing of the nerve is much less common, especially when the cause of the paralysis is birth injury. Complete recovery occurs in at least 50 per cent of cases. In infants recovery is often rapid and may be complete in from three to six months. In adults it may take as long as two years. Seddon (1972) gives detailed advice about splints, prostheses, and operations involving muscle transplantation which may be of value in such cases. Holler and Hopf (1968) have drawn attention to aberrant reinnervation after partial recovery due to regeneration which may give rise to synkinetic movements of shoulder girdle muscles and one-half of the diaphragm.

Lower Plexus Paralysis (Dejerine–Klumpke type)

The contribution of the first thoracic nerve to the brachial plexus may be torn as a result of traction on the arm when it is in an abducted position. Lower plexus paralysis is sometimes encountered as a result of birth injury, or may be produced by a fall during which the patient endeavours to save himself by clutching something with the hand. The first thoracic nerve is usually affected alone, but the eighth cervical may also be involved. The resulting paralysis and wasting involves all the small muscles of the hand, a claw-hand resulting from the unopposed action of the long flexors and extensors of the fingers. When the eighth cervical nerve is also involved there may be wasting and weakness of the ulnar flexors of the wrist and fingers. Cutaneous anaesthesia and analgesia are present in a narrow zone along the ulnar border of the hand and for a variable distance up the forearm. There is frequently an associated paralysis of the cervical sympathetic.

LESIONS OF THE CORDS OF THE PLEXUS

The effects of lesions of the cords of the plexus can readily be deduced from a knowledge of their respective contributions to the nerves of the upper limb which have already been described.

The Lateral Cord. The lateral cord is occasionally injured in dislocations of the humerus. Its interruption causes paralysis of the biceps, coracobrachialis, and of all the muscles supplied by the median nerve, except the intrinsic muscles of the hand. Sensation is affected to a variable extent on the radial aspect of the forearm.

The Posterior Cord. This is rarely damaged. A lesion of the posterior cord causes paralysis of the muscles supplied by the axillary and radial nerves, and loss of sensibility over the areas of their cutaneous supply.

Middle Plexus Paralysis. This is also rare and is equivalent to interruption of the posterior cord with the addition of paralysis of the latissimus dorsi as a result of involvement of the thoracodorsal nerve.

The Medial Cord. Injury to the medial cord of the plexus is most commonly produced by subcoracoid dislocation of the humerus. It causes paralysis of the muscles supplied by the ulnar nerve, together with those intrinsic muscles of the hand which are supplied by the median. Sensory loss occurs along the ulnar border of the hand and forearm. Treatment is that appropriate to the individual nerves involved.

Diagnosis of the Site of the Lesion

It is important in relation to both prognosis and treatment to decide the precise site of the lesion. Axon responses to histamine and reflex vasodilatation to cold may decide this, being absent when the lesion is distal to the dorsal root ganglion and present when it is proximal (Bonney, 1954; Seddon, 1972).

COSTOCLAVICULAR SYNDROMES INCLUDING CERVICAL RIB

AETIOLOGY AND PATHOLOGY

The adoption by man of an upright posture and the release of his upper limb as an organ of prehension has imposed certain stresses upon the nervous and vascular supply of the limb, and rendered the bony structure of the upper thoracic outlet liable to congenital abnormalities which may interfere with nerves and blood vessels. There may be a rudimentary rib derived from the seventh cervical vertebra—cervical rib, which may be associated with a prefixed brachial plexus. The first true rib may be congenitally abnormal. The brachial plexus may be post-fixed, and the contribution from the first thoracic nerve may be unusually large with an addition from the second thoracic segment.

The production of symptoms by these factors is complex. The eighth cervical and first thoracic contributions to the plexus may rest upon, and be compressed by, a cervical rib, an enlarged seventh cervical transverse process, a fibrous band uniting this process to the first rib or by the edge of the scalenus anterior muscle. Or it may be compressed by an abnormal or even a normal first rib. The subclavian artery in such cases often arises at a higher level than normal, and may be similarly compressed, or, on abducting the arm, by the clavicle, as it lies between the clavicle and the first rib.

While the scalenus anterior muscle may play a part in the production of symptoms there seems to be no justification for isolating a 'scalenus anterior syndrome'. The mutual relations of the various structures of the upper thoracic outlet are constantly being altered by the respiratory movements and by movements of the upper limb, which contribute a cumulative traumatic factor, which may in time lead to the production of fibrous tissue—an additional element in compression. The third part of the subclavian artery may become the site of aneurysmal dilatation (Naylor, 1958), in which thrombosis may be a source of embolism in the upper limb (Rob and Standeven, 1958) or even in the vertebral artery giving brain stem ischaemia, or the artery itself may become thrombosed. Finally, loss of tone in the shoulder girdle, or the traction due to carrying heavy weights, or dropping of the shoulder-girdle after thoracoplasty, may precipitate symptoms in middle life though the bony abnormalities are congenital, or may cause symptoms even when the bony structures are normal. These factors probably explain why in right-handed persons symptoms usually occur on the right side, though cervical ribs are generally bilateral, and why women are more prone than men to develop symptoms in middle life.

Symptoms may be either nervous or vascular, or both, and the vascular symptoms can be explained as being due to intermittent or persistent vascular occlusion. The occasional coexistence of Horner's syndrome is difficult to explain except as a result of traction upon the cervicothoracic ganglion. It must be remembered that cervical ribs are a fairly common abnormality, and are frequently present without causing symptoms: in fact it has been estimated that symptoms occur in only 5 to 10 per cent of cases. Moreover, they may be associated with other developmental abnormalities, notably syringomyelia.

Symptoms rarely arise in childhood, but occur with increasing frequency between the third and fifth decades of life.

SYMPTOMS AND SIGNS

With Structural Abnormalities. The onset is usually gradual, and the symptoms of which the patient complains may be mainly sensory, motor, or vascular, or a combination of these may be present. The commonest sensory symptom is pain, which is referred to the ulnar border of the hand and distal half of the forearm and may be associated with numbness, tingling, or other paraesthesiae. Typically the pain is relieved by raising the hand above the head, which diminishes the pressure of the nerve upon the rib. Careful sensory investigation frequently reveals either hyperalgesia or relative analgesia in a narrow zone corresponding to the cutaneous distribution of the eighth cervical or first thoracic segment along the ulnar border of the hand and of the distal part of the forearm or occasionally on the medial aspect of the upper arm. Exceptionally, pain in the neck at the site of the rib may be the only symptom of which complaint is made. Motor symptoms consist of weakness and wasting, the distribution of which depends in part upon the position of the plexus. It is usually confined to the small muscles of the hand (Gilliatt et al., 1970), and may begin either in those supplied by the median or in those supplied by the ulnar nerve. Less frequently the muscles of the ulnar side of the forearm are affected, and this is most likely to occur when the plexus is post-fixed. Horner's syndrome may be present.

Vascular symptoms are due to compression of the subclavian artery. Attacks of blanching or cyanosis of the fingers occur, and sometimes even gangrene. The radial pulses are frequently unequal, being of smaller volume upon the affected side, and can sometimes be obliterated when the shoulder is retracted. The course of the subclavian arteries is frequently abnormal when cervical ribs are present, and the artery can be felt passing obliquely across the posterior triangle of the neck from a point 1·5–2·5 cm above the lower border of the sternomastoid to a point behind the middle of the clavicle. Thrombosis or stenosis of the artery may occur, and there is often a systolic bruit or palpable thrill over the vessel. Symonds reported a case in which the thrombus extended from the subclavian artery on the right side into the right common carotid, and caused embolism of the right internal carotid; vertebral artery embolism is probably more common (Gunning *et al.*, 1964). There may also be an aneurysm distal to the point of pressure with embolism of the digital arteries.

The cervical rib may be visible or palpable as a bony swelling in the neck, pressure over which may cause pain or tingling referred to the ulnar border of the hand and forearm, or obliteration of the radial pulse. The presence of cervical ribs can be demonstrated radiographically, but it must be remembered that the symptoms may be due to a fibrous band, which will not be seen in radiograms, or to a normal first rib. The whole cervical and upper thoracic spine should be included in the X-rays.

Without Structural Abnormalities. Though the symptoms may be as severe as in the former group they tend to be less so, and to be sensory rather than motor, and subjective rather than objective. Pain and paraesthesiae are referred along the ulnar border of the forearm and hand. Nocturnal acroparaesthesiae (pain and tingling in the hands, occurring especially at night, and often in middle-aged women) (Heathfield, 1957; Dick and Zadik, 1958) were often attributed in the past to this 'costoclavicular outlet syndrome' but are now known in the great majority of cases to be due to compression of the median nerve in the carpal tunnel.

DIAGNOSIS

A cervical rib is distinguished from motor neurone disease by the presence of pain and analgesia, and by the absence of fasciculation. In syringomyelia, wasting of the small muscles of the hands is associated with analgesia and thermo-anaesthesia, but the sensory loss is usually much more extensive than that associated with a cervical rib, and signs of corticospinal tract degeneration are likely to be present; however, the two conditions may co-exist. The radiographic demonstration of the presence of a rib must not, therefore, be taken as proof that the rib is the cause of the patient's symptoms. Tumour of the apex of the lung will usually be visible radiographically. Lesions of the median or ulnar nerves may be confused with cervical rib, but the diagnosis is established by the characteristic distribution of the motor and sensory symptoms of lesions of these nerves. Clinically, the single most useful diagnostic sign is that of reproducing the patient's pain and paraesthesiae on the affected side by rolling the cords of the brachial plexus under the examiner's fingers in the supraclavicular fossa. Measurement of nerve conduction velocity is invaluable in distinguishing the condition from peripheral nerve lesions; often in compression of the inner cord of the plexus due to cervical rib or a constricting fibrous band, the sensory evoked potential normally produced by stimulating the little finger on the affected side is lost (Gilliatt *et al.*, 1970). For other causes of wasting in the hands see page 909.

TREATMENT

Only surgical treatment affords permanent relief from a structural abnormality, and to obtain the best results it should be undertaken early. The precise operation required depends upon the nature of the abnormality present but the characteristic clinical syndrome described above, even in the absence of any radiological abnormality, demands exploration of the root of the neck. It may be necessary simply to divide a constricting fibrous band or to remove a cervical rib or a large seventh cervical transverse process, or a portion of the first rib, if that is the offender. It may be sufficient to divide the scalenus anterior muscle, thus allowing the first rib to drop. Following operation there is rapid relief of the sensory symptoms, and considerable improvement in muscular power may be expected. If there is severe muscular atrophy before operation, it is unlikely that full recovery will occur: hence the importance of operating early. When symptoms occur without any demonstrable physical abnormality in middle life (this is now known to be rare), in suitable cases exercises designed to strengthen the muscles which lift the shoulder girdle may be helpful.

THE LONG THORACIC NERVE

The long thoracic nerve is derived by three roots from the fifth, sixth, and seventh cervical nerves. The upper two roots pass through the scalenus medius muscle. The nerve, which supplies the serratus anterior, is injured alone most frequently as a result of pressure upon the shoulder, either from a sudden blow or from the prolonged pressure of carrying weights on the shoulder. Occasionally it is involved in shoulder-girdle neuritis ('neuralgic amyotrophy') [see p. 938], and it may be involved in inflammation secondary to apical pleurisy. Isolated lesions of this nerve are comparatively rare but 'winging' of the scapula, presumably due to this cause, is occasionally seen as a sequel of pneumonia or of other infective illnesses or may rarely arise spontaneously for no obvious cause.

The serratus anterior fixes the scapula to the chest wall when forward pressure is exerted with the upper limb. It brings the scapula forward when the upper limb is thrust forward, as in a fencing lunge, and it assists in elevating the limb above the head by rotating the scapula. Paralysis of the serratus anterior causes no deformity of the scapula when the limb is at rest. If, however, the patient is asked to push the limb forward against resistance, the inner border of the scapula becomes winged, especially in its lower two-thirds [FIG. 134]. He is unable to raise the limb above the head in front of him and on abducting the arm the scapula is seen to ride up on the posterior chest wall on the affected side and can be seen to do so when facing the patient. The usual treatment of the paralysed muscle is carried out, but recovery does not always occur.

THE SUPRASCAPULAR NERVE

This nerve supplies the infraspinatus and supraspinatus. Because of its relatively short course following its origin from the brachial plexus, isolated traumatic lesions of this nerve are rare (Sunderland, 1968) though it is occasionally damaged as a sequel of scapular fracture (Seddon, 1972). Kopell and Thompson (1963) suggest that the nerve may suffer entrapment as it passes through the suprascapular foramen and that this is an often unrecognized source of shoulder pain following upper extremity injury. However, they admit that in most such cases there is a 'frozen shoulder' due to pericapsulitis of the joint and that motor paralysis and weakness are rare; it is thus difficult to be certain how much of the patient's pain is due to the joint lesion and how much to nerve entrapment; the concept of an entrapment syndrome of this nerve is not yet completely accepted.

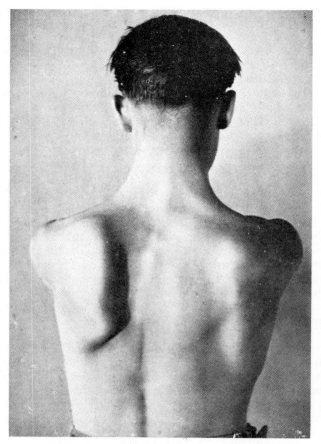

FIG. 134. Winging of the scapula due to paralysis of the left
serratus anterior

THE AXILLARY (CIRCUMFLEX) NERVE

The axillary nerve arises from the posterior cord of the brachial plexus. It innervates the teres minor and deltoid muscles, and supplies cutaneous sensibility to an oval area, the long axis of which extends from the acromion process to half-way down the outer aspect of the arm [FIG. 7, p. 41]. Injury to the axillary nerve, therefore, causes wasting and paralysis of the deltoid muscle, with paralysis of abduction of the arm and anaesthesia and analgesia corresponding to its cutaneous supply, though in clinical practice the actual area of sensory loss is often no more than a small area near the insertion of the deltoid muscle. The axillary nerve may be injured as a result of surgical lesions in the region of the neck of the humerus and is the nerve most often involved in shoulder girdle neuritis ('neuralgic amyotrophy') in which case there is usually severe and persistent pain in the shoulder region for several hours or even for one or two days before the paralysis is noted. The usual treatment for peripheral nerve lesions [p. 889] is given.

THE RADIAL OR MUSCULOSPIRAL NERVE

The radial nerve constitutes the termination of the posterior cord of the brachial plexus and is derived from the fifth, sixth, seventh, and eighth cervical spinal nerves. It innervates the following muscles in the order given: triceps, anconeus, brachioradialis, extensor carpi radialis longus, and, through the pos-. terior interosseous nerve, extensor carpi radialis brevis, supinator, extensor digitorum, extensor digiti minimi, extensor carpi ulnaris, the three extensors of the thumb, and extensor indicis. It supplies sensibility to the lower half of the radial aspect of the arm and the middle of the posterior aspect of the forearm. It also carries sensation from a variable area on the dorsum of the hand extending from the wrist distally as far as the interphalangeal joint of the thumb and the metacarpophalangeal joints of the index and middle fingers, and bounded laterally by the radial border of the thumb, and medially by the axis of the middle metacarpal [FIGS. 7 a and 7 b].

Complete interruption of the radial nerve in or above the axilla causes paralysis and wasting of all the muscles it supplies. Paralysis of the triceps leads to inability to extend the elbow. Paralysis of the brachioradialis is detected through failure of this muscle to contract when the patient flexes the elbow with the forearm midway between pronation and supination, the brachioradialis acting as a flexor of the elbow and not as a supinator. Paralysis of the supinator leads to loss of supination. Paralysis of the extensors of the wrist and fingers causes wrist-drop and finger-drop. Not only is the patient unable to extend the wrist as a primary movement, but synergic extension of the wrist fails to occur in association with flexion of the fingers, with a resulting impairment of the power of this movement. In investigating extension of the thumb special attention must be paid to extension at the carpometacarpal and metacarpophalangeal joints, since extension at the terminal joint may be carried out by some of the intrinsic muscles of the hand. The long extensors of the fingers produce extension only at the metacarpophalangeal joints, extension at the other joints being brought about by the interossei and lumbricals. In a case of radial paralysis, when the patient attempts to extend the fingers, the last-named muscles contract synergically and produce flexion at the metacarpophalangeal and extension at the interphalangeal joints. Following a pressure palsy of the radial nerve sensory loss is variable and may be absent but if present is found usually on the dorsum of the hand between the thumb and index finger. Radial nerve conduction studies may be helpful in determining the site of the lesion [p. 886].

When the nerve is injured, as most frequently happens, in the lower third of the arm, the triceps usually escapes paralysis, and the branch to the brachioradialis, and less frequently that to the extensor carpi radialis longus, may also escape, the distribution of the paralysis coinciding with that following a lesion of the *posterior interosseous nerve*. The radial nerve is frequently injured where it winds round the humerus as a result of fractures of that bone. It is also liable to compression in the axilla through the use of a crutch, and when the arm of an anaesthetized patient is allowed to hang over the edge of the operating table, and during sleep, especially when the patient is intoxicated. In such cases pressure may be due to the arm hanging over the back of a chair ('Saturday-night paralysis'). As Kopell and Thompson (1963) point out, the deep branch of the radial nerve can be compressed by the fibrous edge of the extensor carpi radialis brevis, or as it passes through a slit in the supinator muscle, and this can give signs comparable to those of radial nerve palsy without sensory abnormalities, the picture being effectively that of a posterior interosseous nerve lesion. This may follow trauma and is not infrequently associated with a 'tennis elbow' syndrome. However, there have been many reports of 'idiopathic' posterior interosseous nerve lesions occurring in the absence of trauma and resulting from entrapment in the supinator or compression by a fibrous band (Hustead *et al.*, 1958; Goldman *et al.*, 1969; Spinner, 1972).

In such cases a light splint must be used to maintain extension of the wrist, but although extension at the metacarpophalangeal joints must be ensured, these joints should not be rigidly fixed. A system of spring extension should, therefore, be used for the fingers. The thumb and finger-tips are covered with the fingers of a leather or plastic glove, to which springs are attached. These are carried back over the dorsum of the hand to be attached to a bracelet, which is fixed to the splint beneath the wrist.

The prognosis of lesions of the radial nerve is good as most are due to simple pressure and are thus neurapraxial. Even after complete division and suture, signs of returning muscular function are usually evident in from four to eight months, according to the level of the lesion. When the posterior interosseous nerve is involved and electrical tests indicate a complete lesion the nerve should be explored.

THE MUSCULOCUTANEOUS NERVE

The musculocutaneous nerve is a branch of the lateral cord of the brachial plexus, its fibres being derived from the fifth and sixth cervical spinal nerves. It supplies the biceps and part of the brachialis, the principal flexors of the elbow, and its sensory distribution is to the radial border of the forearm as low as the carpometacarpal joint of the thumb [FIGS. 7 *a* and 7 *b*].

Division of the musculocutaneous nerve, therefore, causes weakness of flexion of the elbow-joint, though some power of flexion can still be carried out by the brachioradialis and the part of the brachialis which is innervated by the radial nerve. Sensation is impaired over the cutaneous distribution of the nerve. The musculocutaneous nerve is rarely injured alone, but may be damaged by dislocation of the head of the humerus or by penetrating wounds. Very rarely it may, like the radial nerve, be affected by simple pressure and transient paralysis of the biceps has been known to occur in a man falling asleep with his wife's head lying across his upper arm.

The forearm should be supported in a sling and the usual treatment of a peripheral nerve lesion carried out.

THE MEDIAN NERVE

The fibres of the median nerve are derived from the sixth, seventh, and eighth cervical and first thoracic spinal segments. It is formed by the union of two heads from the inner and outer cords of the brachial plexus. In the forearm it supplies the following muscles, to which branches are given in the order named: pronator teres, flexor carpi radialis, palmaris longus, flexor digitorum superficialis, flexor pollicis longus, flexor digitorum profundus, pronator quadratus. In the hand it usually supplies the two radial lumbricals, opponens pollicis, abductor pollicis brevis, and the outer head of the flexor pollicis brevis. Sometimes it supplies the first dorsal interosseous. Seddon (1972) describes anomalies in the nerve supply of the muscles of the hand.

Traumatic Lesions. After a complete lesion of the median nerve above its highest muscular branch there is, therefore, paralysis of pronation of the forearm. Occasionally this may result from compression of one or both heads which form the nerve as a result of sclerosis in the wall of the axillary artery to which they are closely related in the axilla. More often the nerve can be trapped or compressed as it passes through the pronator teres muscle at the elbow (the pronator syndrome—Spinner, 1972) or kinked against the fibrous edge of the flexor digitorum superficialis (Kopell and Thompson, 1963). The radial flexor of the wrist is paralysed, so that when the wrist is flexed against resistance the hand deviates to the ulnar side. There is inability to flex the terminal phalanx of the thumb and the phalanges of the index finger. There is weakness of flexion of the phalanges of the remaining fingers, especially the middle finger, but not

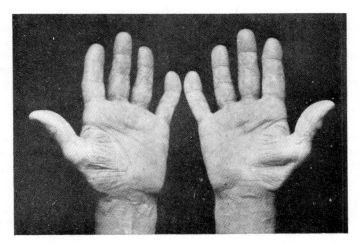

FIG. 135. Partial thenar atrophy due to compression of both median nerves in the carpal tunnel

complete paralysis, since the ulnar half of the flexor digitorum profundus is supplied by the ulnar nerve. Flexion at the metacarpophalangeal joints is carried out by the interossei and lumbricals, of which only the two outer lumbricals are innervated by the median nerve. Paralysis of the muscles of the thenar eminence supplied by the median nerve leads to weakness of abduction of the thumb, a movement which must be tested in a plane at right angles to the palm, and opposition of the thumb is lost. Wasting is present in the paralysed muscles and is especially conspicuous in the lateral half of the thenar eminence, rendering the first metacarpal unduly prominent [FIG. 135]. A lesion of the median nerve or of the anterior interosseous nerve in the middle of the forearm may paralyse the superficial flexors of the thumb and index finger, while allowing those of the other three fingers, the branches to which leave the nerve at a higher level, to escape. When the nerve is injured at the wrist, paralysis is confined to the hand. When investigating muscular power after a median nerve lesion it must be remembered that the abductor pollicis longus may be used in a trick movement as a radial flexor of the wrist, and that opposition of the thumb may be simulated by the combined action of the adductors and the abductor pollicis longus.

Sensory loss following a lesion of the median nerve is somewhat variable, especially in regard to the appreciation of pin-prick [see FIGS. 7a and 7b, pp. 41-2]. Loss of this form of sensibility may be confined to the skin over the terminal phalanges of the index and middle fingers, the affected area being somewhat more extensive on their palmar than on their dorsal aspect. Appreciation of pin-prick is, however, more often lost over a somewhat larger area, including the palmar aspect of the terminal phalanx of the thumb. Loss of appreciation of light touch is more constant in its outline, which runs along the radial border of the thumb to the base of the thenar eminence, thence across the palm to the cleft between the middle and ring fingers, and includes approximately half of the palmar aspect of the ring finger on the radial side. On the dorsum it includes the radial aspect of the terminal two-thirds of the ring finger and the dorsal aspect of the middle and index fingers as far proximally as the middle of the proximal phalanges. From the radial side of the index finger the border passes along the fold of the first interosseous space and up the inner border of the thumb as far as the ulnar edge of the nail. Deep sensibility is usually lost in the terminal phalanges of the index and middle fingers. The median nerve is the commonest site of causalgia, which only occurs, however, when the lesion is incomplete. Nerve conduction velocity measurement [p. 886] is invaluable in localizing accurately the site of the lesion (Buchthal *et al.*, 1974).

The median nerve may be injured at any point of its course by stab or gunshot wounds. It is occasionally damaged in dislocation of the shoulder. The commonest acute traumatic lesion in civil life is a cut at the wrist, usually the result of the hand having been put through a window pane. In such cases the ulnar nerve may also be damaged.

The Anterior Interosseous Nerve

Isolated lesions of this nerve, developing apparently spontaneously, are not uncommon (Kiloh and Nevin, 1952) and usually give rise simply to paralysis of flexion of the terminal phalanges of the thumb and index finger (Smith and Herbst, 1974). The diagnosis can readily be confirmed electrophysiologically (O'Brien and Upton, 1972). While the paresis may recover spontaneously (Gardner-Thorpe, 1974), if there is no recovery in a few months, exploration may be indicated as a fibrous band constricting the nerve or compression by a tendon or aberrant muscle belly may be found (Spinner, 1972).

TREATMENT

To prevent stretching of the paralysed muscles the thumb may be held in a position of palmar abduction and opposition by means of a splint consisting of a leather or plastic cuff at the wrist to which are attached two light springs which run to a moulded cylinder fitted over the metacarpophalangeal joint and perhaps made from a cast of the thumb (Highet, 1942a; Seddon, 1972). The usual treatment for the paralysed muscles is carried out. Causalgia requires special treatment, see page 891. Signs of returning sensibility usually precede motor recovery. After suture of the nerve the latter occurs in from three months to a year, depending upon the situation of the lesion and the distance of individual muscles below it. Voluntary power usually reappears first in pronator teres and in flexor carpi radialis. Sensory recovery is frequently incomplete, especially in respect of appreciation of light touch upon the index finger, but the proportion of useful motor and sensory recoveries is high—88 and 79 per cent respectively (Seddon, 1949).

THE CARPAL TUNNEL SYNDROME

Compression of the median nerve in the carpal tunnel (Brain et al., 1947) occurs spontaneously, chiefly in middle-aged women, and in pregnancy (Wilkinson, 1960). It may also occur after fractures and arthritis involving the wrist-joint, in acromegaly, myxoedema (Murray and Simpson, 1958), the nephrotic syndrome and amyloidosis, and in pyogenic infections of the hand. It results either from lesions which reduce the size of the carpal tunnel, from tenosynovitis with swelling of flexor tendon sheaths due to over-use, or from soft tissue swelling due to fluid retention (as in pregnancy or myxoedema). It is rarely familial, due to an abnormally small size of the carpal tunnel (Danta, 1975), and a similar syndrome has been noted to develop spontaneously in guinea pigs (Fullerton and Gilliatt, 1967). Pain and tingling are felt in the cutaneous distribution of the nerve to the digits, often awakening the patient at night, and constituting the commonest form of acroparaesthesiae. Cutaneous sensory loss over the digits renders the manipulation of small objects difficult, and is some-times accompanied by wasting and weakness of abductor brevis and opponens pollicis, causing conspicuous hollowing of the outer thenar eminence [FIG. 135]. Often, however, pain and paraesthesiae may be the only symptoms for many months and years and are accentuated by using the hand or by warmth. The only abnormal physical signs may be some blunting of sensation in the thumb and fingers supplied by the median nerve and/or tingling in the appropriate distribution produced by a sharp tap over the carpal ligament. The application of a tourniquet to the upper arm above arterial blood pressure may quickly produce ischaemic paraesthesiae in the affected fingers (Gilliatt and Wilson, 1954; Fullerton, 1963). The demonstration of increased terminal latency on stimulation of the median nerve at the wrist is a valuable diagnostic sign (Simpson, 1956; Fullerton, 1963; Preswick, 1963; McLeod, 1966). Studies of antidromic sensory conduction from the fingers supplied by the median nerve when compared with sensory conduction in the ulnar nerve may be even more useful (Kemble, 1968; Buchthal and Rosenfalck, 1971; Loong and Seah, 1971) but some patients with the carpal tunnel syndrome have been found to have a subclinical ulnar neuropathy (Sedal et al., 1973).

The carpal tunnel syndrome in pregnancy may be expected to recover after labour (Wilkinson, 1960). Diuretics, immobilization, and local injections of hydrocortisone (Foster, 1960) may produce temporary improvement, but in most long-standing cases only surgical division of the transverse carpal ligament is likely to be effective.

THE ULNAR NERVE

The ulnar nerve is derived from the eighth cervical and first thoracic spinal nerves. It gives off no branches above the elbow, where it lies behind the medial condyle of the humerus. It supplies branches to the following muscles in the forearm in the order stated: flexor carpi ulnaris, and the inner half of flexor digitorum profundus. In the hand it usually supplies the palmaris brevis, the muscles of the hypothenar eminence, the two medial lumbricals, the palmar and dorsal interossei, the transverse and oblique heads of the adductor pollicis, and the medial head of the flexor pollicis brevis. The first dorsal interosseous muscle is sometimes supplied by the median. Seddon (1954 a) described the anomalies of the nerve supply of the muscles of the hand.

Interruption of the ulnar nerve at or above the level of the elbow causes paralysis of these muscles. As a result of paralysis of the flexor carpi ulnaris the hand deviates to the radial side on flexion of the wrist against resistance. Another method of demonstrating weakness of this muscle is as follows: the patient closes his hand and the examiner adducts it, placing his finger on the tendon of the flexor carpi ulnaris. When the patient extends his fingers this tendon can normally be felt to tighten. Paralysis of the ulnar half of the flexor digitorum profundus abolishes flexion of the little finger at the interphalangeal joints, and weakens flexion of the ring finger at these joints. Paralysis of the muscles of the hypothenar eminence abolishes abduction of the little finger, and impairs flexion of this finger at the metacarpophalangeal joint. Paralysis of the interossei abolishes abduction and adduction of the fingers. In examining this movement it is important that the hand should be kept with the palm pressed against a flat surface, as the long extensors and flexors of the fingers act to some extent as abductors and adductors. Further, the fingers cannot be held with the meta-carpophalangeal joints flexed and the interphalangeal joints extended. Paralysis of the transverse and oblique heads of the adductor pollicis weakens adduction of the thumb, and this is most evident when the patient attempts to press the thumb firmly against the index finger.

Wasting of the paralysed muscles is evident on the ulnar side of the flexor aspect of the forearm, the hypothenar eminence, the interosseous spaces, and the ulnar half of the thenar eminence [FIG. 136]. Paralysis of the small muscles of the hand causes 'claw-hand', this posture being produced by the unopposed action of their antagonists. Since the interossei cause flexion of the fingers at the metacarpophalangeal joints and extension at the interphalangeal joints, when these muscles are paralysed the opposite posture is maintained by the long flexors and extensors, namely, hyperextension at the metacarpophalangeal joints and flexion at the interphalangeal joints. This is usually most marked in the ring and little fingers, since the two radial lumbricals, which are supplied by the median nerve, to some extent compensate for loss of action of the interossei on the index and middle fingers.

After a lesion of the ulnar nerve at or above the elbow loss of deep sensibility is usually limited to the little finger. The area of analgesia to pin-prick is variable, but usually covers the little finger, the ulnar border of the palm, and often the ulnar half of the ring finger. The area of anaesthesia to light touch includes the little finger and the ulnar half of the ring finger, together with the ulnar border of the hand, both on the dorsum and the palmar aspects as far as the wrist, the area being bounded on the radial side by a line continuous with the axis of the ring finger [FIGS. 7 a and 7 b].

When the ulnar nerve is divided at the wrist, the flexor carpi ulnaris and the ulnar half of the flexor digitorum profundus escape paralysis, which is confined to the small muscles of the hand supplied by the nerve. When the lesion is below the point at which the dorsal branch is given off, the area of sensory loss is less than that described above. On the palmar aspect of the hand the area over which sensibility is lost is the same as when the nerve is divided above the wrist, but on the dorsal aspect appreciation of light touch is lost over the terminal two phalanges of the little finger, and the ulnar half of these phalanges of the ring finger, and loss of appreciation of pin-prick is usually confined to the terminal phalanx of the little finger. In such cases all the muscles supplied by the ulnar nerve in the hand are likely to be affected. When the deep palmar branch alone is involved there is no sensory loss and the hypothenar muscles escape.

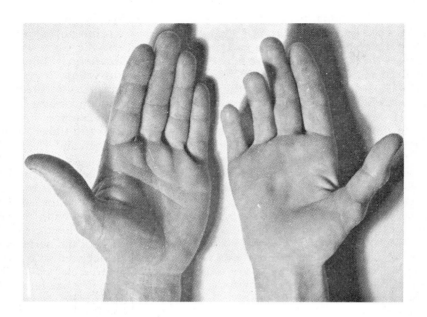

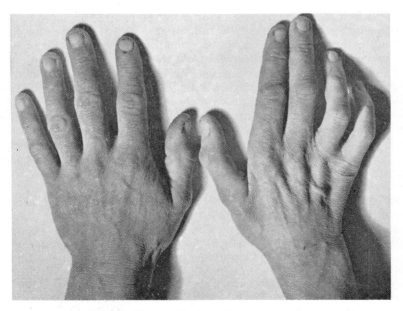

Fig. 136. The hand in right ulnar nerve paralysis

Ulnar Nerve Lesions

Lesions of the ulnar nerve above the elbow are rare, but it may be involved in a penetrating wound. At the elbow it may suffer as a result of fractures and dislocations involving the lower end of the humerus, and the elbow-joint. In such cases the injury to the nerve may be immediate. Occasionally, however, it is involved years after an injury which has led to cubitus valgus ('tardy ulnar palsy'—Gilliatt, 1975). Similarly the nerve may be damaged by osteophytic outgrowths following arthritis of the elbow-joint, by a ganglion, or by a Charcot elbow. However, the commonest site of chronic irritation or compression of the nerve in this situation is as it passes between the humeral and ulnar heads of the flexor carpi ulnaris (the cubital tunnel syndrome) (Kopell and Thompson, 1963; Spinner, 1972; Eisen and Danon, 1974).

In individuals possessing a shallow groove for the nerve behind the internal condyle of the humerus or an unusual degree of physiological cubitus valgus, the nerve may suffer from undue mobility, tending to slip forwards over the internal condyle when the elbow is flexed. Occupations involving repeated flexion of the elbow occasionally cause symptoms through the long-continued minor trauma involved. In all these cases of chronic injury of the nerve at the elbow-joint the lesion is a localized pressure neuropathy associated with fibrous thickening of the nerve at the site of trauma, where a spindle-shaped swelling can often be felt. The earliest symptoms are pain and paraesthesiae referred to the cutaneous distribution of the nerve. These symptoms may at first be apparent only when the patient awakens in the morning after sleeping with the elbow flexed. In long-standing cases there are usually weakness and wasting of the muscles innervated by the nerve in addition. Pressure on the nerve behind the elbow, or where it enters the cubital tunnel, may then reproduce the patient's paraesthesiae. Ulnar paralysis is occasionally met with as a result of pressure on the nerve at the elbow during sleep. At the wrist the ulnar nerve may be injured by cuts, and the median nerve may be simultaneously involved. The entire palmar branch of the nerve, including its superficial sensory component is occasionally compressed or injured on the anterior aspect of the wrist. A pressure neuropathy of the deep palmar branch of the ulnar nerve sometimes occurs in individuals whose occupation involves prolonged or recurrent pressure upon the outer part of the palm and an isolated lesion of this branch has been described in a diabetic subject (Finelli, 1975). In such cases the muscles of the hypothenar eminence usually escape damage and there is no sensory loss. Both at the wrist and in the palm the cause of compression may be a ganglion.

Motor nerve conduction time may be valuable in localizing the lesion, estimating its severity, and assessing recovery (Ebeling et al., 1960; Gilliatt and Thomas, 1960; Payan, 1970). When the lesion is at the elbow, motor conduction is markedly slowed in the segment of the nerve around the elbow, while in lesions of the deep palmar branch of the nerve, conduction in the forearm is normal but terminal latency is increased.

TREATMENT

The treatment of lesions of the ulnar nerve is conducted on the same general lines as for other peripheral nerve lesions. Highet's 'knuckle-duster' splint was designed to maintain the hand in a posture of flexion at the metacarpophalangeal and extension at the interphalangeal joints (Highet, 1942 a). It was modified in order to restore the metacarpal arch (Bowden, 1954 b), and even better spring-loaded splints which do not prevent voluntary contraction in recovering muscles are now available (Seddon, 1972). When the nerve is the site of pressure neuropathy as a result of abnormalities of the elbow-joint or wrist, an appropriate operation will be required to free it from pressure. When the nerve suffers from chronic irritation, it must be brought to lie in front of the internal condyle of the humerus. In such cases operation rapidly relieves sensory symptoms, but recovery of voluntary power is necessarily slower. In a series of 23 cases, good functional recovery took place in 74 per cent but muscle wasting was least likely to improve (Harrison and Nurick, 1970). In lesions of the deep palmar branch of the nerve, exploration is usually indicated, as it may be possible to remove a ganglion which is compressing the nerve. After suture of the nerve, sensibility usually begins to recover before voluntary power. Motor recovery, which occurs to a useful extent in about 80 per cent of cases (Seddon, 1949), usually begins in the flexor carpi ulnaris and flexor digitorum profundus, and is most complete in these muscles and in the abductor digiti minimi. It may take two years after suture at the elbow.

DIGITAL NERVE NEUROPATHY

As Kopell and Thompson (1963) point out, one or more digital nerves in the hand may suffer compression in the intermetacarpal tunnel. This gives rise to burning pain and sensory impairment on the contiguous halves of two adjacent digits. Repeated digital nerve blocks with local anaesthetic agents may relieve the discomfort but not the sensory impairment.

DIAGNOSIS OF WASTING OF THE MUSCLES OF THE HAND

Lesions of the median and ulnar nerves require to be diagnosed from other causes of wasting of muscles of the hand. These muscles are innervated by the anterior horn cells of the first thoracic segment of the spinal cord, with an occasional minimal contribution from the eighth cervical. The causes of wasting, therefore, include lesions of the lower motor neurones at any point between this spinal segment and the muscles, together with certain other conditions in which primary muscular degeneration or reflex muscular wasting occurs.

Lesions of Acute Onset Involving the Anterior Horns

The commonest of such acute lesions is *poliomyelitis*. This is usually easily distinguished by the acute onset, commonly in childhood, the non-progressive character of the wasting, the presence of muscular wasting with a patchy and asymmetrical distribution elsewhere in the body, the cyanosis of the affected extremity, and the absence of sensory loss. Acute post-infective polyradiculopathy (the Guillain–Barré syndrome) usually affects proximal limb muscles more severely than distal, at least at first, and like other forms of polyneuropathy (see below) it usually affects all four limbs. *Vascular lesions of the spinal cord* are a rare cause. Thrombosis of a branch of the anterior spinal artery may cause destruction of the anterior horn cells. In such cases the corticospinal and spinothalamic tracts are usually damaged simultaneously. *Haematomyelia* or cord contusion following acute hyperextension injuries of the neck may also damage anterior horn cells in the cervical enlargement. Wasting is usually not confined to muscles innervated by the first thoracic segment and is usually associated with extensive sensory loss over the upper limbs and often with involvement of the long ascending and descending tracts of the cord.

Lesions of Slow Onset Involving the Anterior Horns

The commonest chronic lesion is *motor neurone disease*, which frequently begins with wasting of the small muscles of one or both hands. This condition is distinguished by its progressive course, the presence of muscular fasciculation and, sooner or later, wasting of other muscle groups, the frequent coexistence of corticospinal tract degeneration, and the absence of sensory loss. In *syringomyelia* wasting of the hand muscles is often an early symptom. Fasciculation is usually slight. The diagnosis depends upon the characteristic associated analgesia and thermo-anaesthesia, trophic lesions, and the frequent involvement of the corticospinal tracts. In *tumour of the spinal cord* the signs of a progressive focal lesion at the cervical enlargement are usually accompanied by pain and evidence of involvement of long ascending and descending tracts.

Lesions of the Ventral Roots

The ventral roots are occasionally involved in the localized *leptomeningitis of syphilitic origin*, or in *arachnoiditis* in which the substance of the cord usually also suffers. The ventral root lesion can be distinguished from a lesion of the anterior horn cells only when the dorsal roots are also involved, leading to root pains, often with some impairment of sensibility over the segmental cutaneous areas.

Lesions of the Spinal Nerve

The spinal nerve consists of a fusion of the ventral and the dorsal root, and a lesion of the first thoracic nerve, therefore, causes root-pain and frequently some sensory loss along the ulnar border of the hand and forearm, in addition to muscular wasting of the small muscles of the hand. The spinal nerve may be the site of neuropathy, though this is rare in the case of the first thoracic nerve and this nerve is rarely affected by intervertebral disc disease or spondylosis, in which conditions, contrary to widespread misconceptions, wasting of small hand muscles is excessively rare. It may, however, be compressed as a result of vertebral body collapse or extradural deposits of carcinoma or reticulosis. A traumatic lesion of the first thoracic spinal nerve is responsible for the *Dejerine-Klumpke type of birth palsy*. Lesions involving the first dorsal segment of the spinal cord, its ventral roots and spinal nerve, usually cause paralysis of the cervical sympathetic, the pre-ganglionic fibres of which leave the cord at this level.

Lesions of the Medial Cord of the Brachial Plexus

Lesions of the medial cord of the plexus, for example the pressure of a *cervical rib*, cause wasting of some or all the muscles supplied by the ulnar nerve, including those in the forearm together with the small muscles of the hand supplied by the median. Often all small hand muscles only are affected first. The distribution of pain and sensory loss involves the eighth cervical and first thoracic segmental areas, that is, roughly, the supply of the ulnar nerve, together with part of the ulnar border of the forearm and arm.

Lesions of the Median and Ulnar Nerves

All lesions situated between the anterior horn cells of the first thoracic segment and the medial cord of the brachial plexus, inclusive, cause wasting of the small muscles of the hand. Distally to the medial cord of the plexus the innervation of these muscles is divided between the ulnar and median nerves. Lesions of these nerves, as already described, are distinguished by the characteristic distribution of the muscular wasting and sensory loss. Apart from localized lesions of these nerves, wasting of the small muscles of the hand may occur in various forms of *polyneuropathy* in which sensory loss of peripheral distribution and tenderness of the muscles are usually present, and the same symptoms usually occur in the lower limbs. In *peroneal muscular atrophy* wasting of the hands usually follows that of the legs and feet. The onset of the wasting in early life, its gradual ascent of the limbs stopping short at the elbows and knees, and the associated peripheral sensory impairment are distinguishing features.

Muscular Dystrophy

Wasting of the small muscles of the hand is found in some forms of *muscular dystrophy*, especially the so-called *distal* type of *myopathy*, and much less frequently in *dystrophia myotonica* in which forearm muscles are wasted but not so much those of the hands. The diagnosis depends upon the age of onset, the symmetrical character, distribution, and progressive course of the wasting, the absence of muscular fasciculation, sensory loss and signs of involvement of the central nervous system, and the familial or hereditary nature of the disorder.

Trophic Disorders

Reflex muscular wasting secondary to *arthritis* of the joints of the hand must not be overlooked. It is easily recognized on account of pain, swelling, and bony changes in the joints. In the so-called *shoulder-hand syndrome*, pericapsulitis of the shoulder-joint is often associated initially with painful swelling of the hand but subsequently there may be atrophy of the small hand muscles and even of the bones (Sudeck's atrophy). *Ischaemia* due to arteriosclerosis or thrombo-angiitis is a rare cause of muscular wasting, more frequently seen in the lower than in the upper limb. *Ischaemic contracture* caused by fractures in the region of the elbow or other major arterial lesions leads to paralysis, wasting, and contracture of the muscles of the forearm and hand, with or without sensory loss, due to compression and degeneration of the nerves.

Electrodiagnosis

Electromyography, measurement of motor and sensory nerve conduction velocity and of distal latency [pp. 882–8] have greatly improved diagnostic precision in lesions causing wasting of the small hand muscles and studies of multisegmental efferent and afferent conduction velocity are particularly valuable (Jušić and Milić, 1972).

THE NERVES OF THE LOWER LIMB
THE LUMBOSACRAL PLEXUS

The lumbar plexus is formed by contributions from the twelfth thoracic and the first, second, third, and fourth lumbar spinal nerves; the sacral plexus, from the fourth and fifth lumbar and the first, second, and third sacral nerves. The principal nerves derived from the lumbar plexus are the femoral and the obturator, and from the sacral plexus the sciatic and the superior and inferior gluteal nerves. The lumbosacral plexus may be compressed by pelvic metastases or one of its roots by a protruded intervertebral disc. It may be injured by the pressure of the fetal head or obstetric forceps during delivery and it is occasionally affected by pelvic deposits of endometriosis; either the obturator or the sciatic nerves may thus be damaged on one or both sides. The lumbosacral cord is most frequently affected, leading to unilateral or bilateral paralysis of the anterior tibial and peroneal muscles. (See also under the sciatic nerve, p. 914.)

THE LATERAL CUTANEOUS NERVE OF THE THIGH

The lateral cutaneous nerve of the thigh is derived from the dorsal parts of the second and third lumbar nerves. Passing through the psoas major muscle it enters the thigh beneath the lateral end of the inguinal ligament, and, piercing the fascia lata of the thigh about 4 inches distal to the anterior superior iliac spine, it divides into an anterior and a posterior branch which supply sensibility to the lateral aspect of the thigh and the lateral part of its anterior aspect from the buttock almost as low as the knee [FIGS. 7 a and 7 b]. Either where the nerve emerges from the pelvis or where it passes through or beneath the inguinal ligament or through the fascia lata it may become constricted by fibrous tissue with the production of pain, numbness, and paraesthesiae referred to the cutaneous distribution of the nerve, especially of its anterior branch. Much less often there is also pain radiating along the groin, due to a connection with the ilio-inguinal nerve (Teng, 1972). This condition, which is known as 'meralgia paraesthetica', usually afflicts middle-aged men but also occurs in women, particularly when overweight. It may follow the application of a plaster jacket or corset and occasionally develops secondarily to tilting of the pelvis in patients suffering from lumbar intervertebral disc prolapse. The pain and numbness are often brought on by walking or standing for long periods. The site of the pain, which is usually associated with relative anaesthesia and analgesia of the skin of the outer aspect of the thigh, is distinctive. The disorder is usually benign, has little more than a nuisance value, and may remit spontaneously. When pain is more troublesome repeated infiltration of local anaesthetic around the lateral half of the inguinal ligament may relieve symptoms, but if this is unsuccessful, operative decompression or division of the nerve may be indicated (Stevens, 1957; Teng, 1972).

THE OBTURATOR NERVE

The obturator nerve is derived from the second, third, and fourth lumbar nerves by roots which are situated anteriorly to those of the femoral nerve. The union of these roots occurs in the psoas muscle and the nerve emerges from the pelvis by the obturator foramen. It gives a branch to the hip-joint and supplies the following muscles: adductor longus and gracilis, adductor brevis usually, and sometimes pectineus, obturator externus, and adductor magnus. Its cutaneous supply is variable and is distributed to the skin of the distal two-thirds of the medial aspect of the thigh [FIGS. 7 a AND 7 b]. It also supplies a branch to the knee-joint.

Injury to the obturator nerve causes paralysis of the adductors of the thigh, except for the flexor fibres of the adductor magnus, which are innervated by the sciatic. Sensory loss is usually absent. The nerve is most frequently injured in the course of a difficult labour, or occasionally as a result of dislocation of the hip. The usual treatment of lower motor neurone paralysis is applied to the paralysed muscles.

The nerve may occasionally be compressed in the obturator canal by an obturator hernia or as a result of osteitis pubis following genito-urinary surgery.

Pain down the medial aspect of the thigh is the most prominent symptom and may demand intrapelvic section of the nerve at the expense of permanent adductor paralysis (Kopell and Thompson, 1963).

THE ILIOINGUINAL NERVE

This nerve, derived from the first and second lumbar roots, innervates a narrow band of skin across the upper thigh, inguinal region, iliac crest, and the base of the scrotum (or labia). It contains motor fibres to the lower portions of the transversalis and internal oblique muscles. It is rarely affected by direct injury or by a misplaced herniorrhaphy incision and may suffer entrapment near to the anterior superior iliac spine, especially in patients with abnormalities of the hip joint, and dysfunction of this nerve may sometimes play a part in the pathogenesis of direct inguinal hernia. Pain in the groin, sometimes causing the patient to adopt a flexed posture, is the usual manifestation and injection of local anaesthetic around the nerve usually affords relief (Kopell and Thompson, 1963).

THE FEMORAL NERVE

The femoral nerve is derived from the lumbar plexus, arising from the dorsal parts of the second, third, and fourth lumbar nerves, posterior to the obturator nerve. The nerve is formed in the psoas major muscle, and after passing through the pelvis enters the thigh beneath the inguinal ligament, lateral to the femoral sheath and femoral vessels. In the abdomen it sends a branch to the iliacus muscle and in the femoral triangle it breaks up into terminal branches which supply the pectineus, sartorius, and quadriceps. It gives articular branches to the hip- and knee-joints. Its intermediate and medial cutaneous branches supply the medial and internal aspects of the thigh in its lower two-thirds, and by the saphenous nerve it supplies sensibility to the inner aspect of the leg and foot as far distally as midway between the medial malleolus and the base of the great toe [FIGS. 7 a and 7 b].

After a lesion of the femoral nerve there may be slight weakness of flexion of the hip owing to paralysis of the iliacus, but the principal motor disturbance is weakness of extension of the knee owing to paralysis of the quadriceps, which is wasted. As a result of this the leg gives way in walking and cannot be used to raise the body on stairs. The knee-jerk is lost, and sensibility is lost over the cutaneous area innervated by the nerve. Causalgia may occur in the distribution of the saphenous nerve after partial lesions of the nerve.

The femoral nerve may be involved in psoas abscess or in new growths within the pelvis, or injured as a result of fractures of the pelvis or of the femur, or by dislocation of the hip. Lesions of this nerve are rarely seen as a result of gun-shot wounds of the thigh, as the proximity of the femoral artery renders the majority of such injuries rapidly fatal. The commonest lesion is a neuropathy which is sometimes secondary to diabetes ('diabetic amyotrophy'), to lumbar spondylosis, or of unknown aetiology. In a series of 23 cases, Thage (1965) found that seven were due to diabetes, two were traumatic, one was due to neurinoma, five to lumbar disc lesions, and eight were idiopathic. Measurement of femoral nerve conduction velocity and terminal latency are invaluable in diagnosis (Thage, 1974).

The usual treatment of lower motor neurone paralysis should be applied to the quadriceps.

G g

THE SCIATIC NERVE

The sciatic nerve is derived from the sacral plexus, which is formed by a fusion of the ventral primary divisions of the fourth and fifth lumbar and of the first, second, and third sacral spinal nerves. The nerve is composed of two divisions which are destined to form the tibial (medial popliteal) and common peroneal (lateral popliteal) nerves. These two divisions, though bound together by connective tissue, are separable up to the sacral plexus from which they are separately derived, the tibial coming from the ventral divisions of the fourth and fifth lumbar and first, second, and third sacral nerves, while the common peroneal comes from the dorsal divisions of the fourth and fifth lumbar and first and second sacral nerves. The sciatic nerve, in addition to its two principal components, contains nerves to the hamstrings and a nerve to the short head of the biceps muscle. It leaves the pelvis by passing through the great sciatic notch below the piriformis muscle into the buttock and then descends in the back of the thigh, lying midway between the great trochanter of the femur and the ischial tuberosity. It terminates at a variable point between the sciatic notch and the proximal part of the popliteal fossa by dividing into the common peroneal and tibial nerves.

In addition to supplying motor nerves to the semitendinosus, semimembranosus, the long and short heads of the biceps, and part of adductor magnus, the sciatic is the motor nerve to all the muscles below the knee. The superficial peroneal branch of the common peroneal nerve supplies the peronei longus and brevis; the deep peroneal nerve supplies the tibialis anterior, extensor digitorum longus, extensor hallucis longus, peroneus tertius, and extensor digitorum brevis. The tibial nerve supplies muscular branches in the following order: gastrocnemius, popliteus, plantaris, and soleus, and by the terminal part innervates the popliteus, the deep part of the soleus, tibialis posterior, flexor digitorum longus, and flexor hallucis longus. The medial and lateral plantar nerves supply the small muscles of the feet.

After complete interruption of the sciatic nerve there is paralysis of flexion of the knee, which is carried out by the hamstrings, and of all the muscles below the knee. Foot-drop occurs as a result of paralysis of the anterior tibial group of muscles and peronei. The patient is able to stand and walk, but drags the toes of the affected foot and is unable to stand on his toes on the paralysed side.

The sensory distribution of the sciatic nerve lies entirely below the knee [FIGS. 7 a and 7 b]. After complete division of the nerve, light touch is the form of sensibility which is lost most extensively. Anaesthesia to cotton wool extends over the whole of the foot, with the exception of a zone about 4 cm wide along the inner aspect, extending about 5 cm distal to the internal malleolus, which is supplied by the saphenous nerve. On the leg the area of anaesthesia to light touch includes the outer aspect, roughly from the midline in front to the midline behind as far up as 5 cm below the upper end of the fibula. Analgesia to pinprick is less extensive than anaesthesia to light touch. Below, the two areas approximately coincide, but above, the area of analgesia is less extensive than that of anaesthesia by about 5–7·5 cm. Appreciation of pressure and of vibration is lost over the whole of the foot, with the exception of the proximal two-thirds of the inner aspect, and position and joint sense are lost in the toes.

The knee-jerk is unaffected, but the ankle-jerk is lost and so also is the plantar reflex. Vasomotor and trophic changes are usually conspicuous after complete division. The leg is congested and swollen, especially when dependent. The skin is dry, and sweating is lost over the foot, except in the saphenous area along the inner border. Perforating ulcers may develop on the sole.

The sciatic nerve may be damaged as a result of fractures of the pelvis or femur, and gunshot wounds of the buttock and thigh. In civil life one of the commonest causes of a sciatic nerve lesion is a misplaced injection given too far medially in the buttock, while there is evidence that rarely the nerve may undergo entrapment or compression as it traverses the sciatic notch. It may be compressed within the pelvis by neoplasms, or by the fetal head during delivery. The common peroneal division is much more susceptible to injury than the tibial. Complete division of the nerve is rare. Differential diagnosis is discussed in the section on sciatica.

THE COMMON PERONEAL (LATERAL POPLITEAL) NERVE

After division of the common peroneal nerve there is paralysis with wasting of the peronei and of the anterior tibial group of muscles. The power of dorsiflexion of the foot and toes and of eversion of the foot is lost, and foot-drop results. Inversion is lost when the foot is dorsiflexed, but a weak movement of inversion is possible in association with plantar flexion. When the nerve is divided above the point of origin of its lateral cutaneous branch, sensation is impaired over the dorsum of the foot, including the first phalanges of the toes, and over the antero-external aspect of the leg in its lower half or two-thirds, the area of anaesthesia to light touch being somewhat more extensive than the area of anaesthesia to pin-prick [FIGS. 7 a and 7 b]. When the lesion is situated below the origin of the lateral cutaneous branch, sensation is impaired over the dorsum of the foot only, and the anaesthetic area is usually bounded by a line passing upwards from the space between the fourth and fifth toes parallel with the outer border of the foot. Deep sensibility is unimpaired.

The common peroneal nerve may be injured as a result of penetrating wounds in the neighbourhood of the knee-joint, and of fractures involving the upper end of the fibula. It is sometimes entrapped or compressed or irritated by fibrous constricting bands as it winds round the neck of the fibula and may suffer from compression by a tight bandage applied to the knee, or by pressure during sleep. In certain occupations, as in slaters working on roofs, the nerve may be compressed if the individual habitually works with one leg flexed and lying under the other with its outer aspect against the roof surface. In such cases of entrapment of the nerve, the muscles which it innervates do not always suffer equally. The peronei are usually more severely affected than the anterior tibial group, and the area of sensory loss is often less than that found after complete division.

A common peroneal nerve palsy, of which the most striking symptom is foot-drop, may result from the causes mentioned and often recovers in two or three months but sometimes surgical exploration of the nerve at the fibular neck is required (Sidey, 1969). The diagnosis can be confirmed by measurements of nerve conduction velocity in the nerve. Slowing of sensory conduction across the segment of the nerve which passes around the neck of the fibula localized the lesion accurately in 64 per cent of a series of 47 patients (Singh et al., 1974).

It is important to recognize that the amplitude of the muscle action potential recorded by surface electrodes over the extensor digitorum brevis muscle and evoked by supramaximal stimulation of the nerve may be larger on stimulation at the knee than at the ankle. This may result from the fact that an anomalous branch of the superficial peroneal nerve (the accessory deep peroneal nerve) which passes alongside the peroneus brevis muscle and behind the lateral malleolus may supply the lateral part of the extensor digitorum brevis (Lambert, 1969; Gutmann, 1970; Infante and Kennedy, 1970).

THE TIBIAL (MEDIAL POPLITEAL) NERVE

After division of the tibial nerve the calf muscles and the muscles of the sole are paralysed and wasted and the foot assumes the position of talipes calcaneo-valgus. The ankle-jerk is lost, and the plantar reflex may also be unelicitable. There is as a rule no loss of deep sensibility. There is anaesthesia to light touch over the skin of the sole, including the plantar aspect of the toes and the dorsal aspect of their terminal phalanges. The area of analgesia is less extensive and does not include the toes [FIGS. 7 a and 7 b].

POSTERIOR TIBIAL NERVE

Rarely the posterior tibial nerve may be compressed behind and below the medial malleolus giving rise to burning pain in the sole of the foot and toes and sensory loss over almost the entire sole of the foot (the tarsal tunnel syndrome). If the condition is due to an abnormal posture of the foot, the use of an appropriate support may be helpful, but if it results from venous engorgement (in patients with varicose veins) or tenosynovitis, surgical decompression is occasionally required unless the causative factors can be relieved by other measures (Kopell and Thompson, 1963).

PLANTAR AND INTERDIGITAL NERVES

Plantar nerves may occasionally be compressed as they enter the medial aspect of the sole of the foot giving a picture of sensory loss slightly less extensive than that of posterior tibial nerve compression (Kopell and Thompson, 1963). Neuropathies of plantar interdigital nerves giving rise to pain and analgesia in the adjacent halves of two contiguous toes have also been described and may rarely be associated with neuroma formation.

TREATMENT

After lesions of the sciatic nerve and of the common peroneal nerve it is important to prevent dropping of the foot. The patient should, therefore, wear a night-splint, and during the day the foot-drop should be overcome by wearing a shoe with a toe-raising spring or by the use of a light moulded plastic splint worn inside the shoe. The usual treatment of peripheral nerve lesions should be carried out, including passive and active movement and electrical stimulation. Recovery is always slow after complete division of the nerve and suture (Seddon, 1972). When the sciatic nerve trunk has been divided return of voluntary power cannot be expected for from a year to eighteen months, and may take much longer. It may be necessary to carry out treatment for three years. In the case of division of the common peroneal nerve return of power may be expected to be demonstrable in from nine moths to a year, but it is likely to be at least two years before the maximum degree of recovery is attained. Useful motor recovery occurs in about 50 per cent of cases after suture. In the case of the tibial nerve motor recovery is better than sensory. In the rare cases of posterior tibial or plantar nerve compression, surgical decompression is indicated in intractable cases, while in certain cases of interdigital neuropathy, excision of a neuroma or division of the affected nerves may be necessary to relieve persistent pain.

REFERENCES

AGUAYO, A. J., PEYRONNARD, J. M., and BRAY, G. M. (1973) A quantitative ultrastructural study of regeneration from isolated proximal stumps of transected unmyelinated nerves, *J. Neuropath. exp. Neurol.*, **32**, 256.

BALLANTYNE, J. P., and CAMPBELL, M. J. (1973) Electrophysiological study after surgical repair of sectioned human peripheral nerves, *J. Neurol. Neurosurg. Psychiat.*, **36**, 797.

BALLANTYNE, J. P., and HANSEN, S. (1974) Computer method for the analysis of evoked motor unit potentials. I. Control subjects and patients with myasthenia gravis, *J. Neurol. Neurosurg. Psychiat.*, **37**, 1187.

BARNES, R. (1954) Peripheral nerve injuries, *Spec. Rep. Ser. med. Res. Coun. (Lond.)*, **282**, 156.

BEHSE, F., and BUCHTHAL, F. (1971) Normal sensory conduction in the nerves of the leg in man, *J. Neurol. Neurosurg. Psychiat.*, **34**, 404.

BONNEY, G. (1954) The value of axon responses in determining the site of lesion in traction injuries of the brachial plexus, *Brain*, **77**, 588.

BOWDEN, R. E. M. (1954 a) Peripheral nerve injuries, *Spec. Rep. Ser. med. Res. Coun. (Lond.)*, **282**, 263.

BOWDEN, R. E. M. (1954 b) Peripheral nerve injuries, *Spec. Rep. Ser. med. Res. Coun. (Lond.)*, **282**, 298.

BRADLEY, W. G. (1974) *Disorders of Peripheral Nerves*, Oxford.

BRAIN, W. R., WRIGHT, A. D., and WILKINSON, M. (1947) Spontaneous compression of both median nerves in the carpal tunnel, *Lancet*, **i,** 277.

BROOKS, J. E., and HONGDALAROM, T. (1968) Intracellular electromyography. Resting and action potentials in normal human muscle, *Arch. Neurol. (Chic.)*, **18**, 291.

BUCHTHAL, F. (1957) *An Introduction to Electromyography*, Copenhagen.

BUCHTHAL, F., PINELLI, P., and ROSENFALCK, P. (1954) Action potential parameters in normal human muscle and their physiological determinants, *Acta physiol. scand.*, **32**, 219.

BUCHTHAL, F., and ROSENFALCK, A. (1966) Evoked action potentials and conduction velocity in human sensory nerves, *Brain Research*, **3**, special issue.

BUCHTHAL, F., and ROSENFALCK, A. (1971) Sensory conduction from digit to palm and from palm to wrist in the carpal tunnel syndrome, *J. Neurol. Neurosurg. Psychiat.*, **34**, 243.

BUCHTHAL, F., ROSENFALCK, A., and TROJABORG, W. (1974) Electrophysiological findings in entrapment of the median nerve at wrist and elbow, *J. Neurol. Neurosurg. Psychiat.*, **37**, 340.

CAMPBELL, M. J., McCOMAS, A. J., and PETITO, F. (1973) Physiological changes in ageing muscles, *J. Neurol. Neurosurg. Psychiat.*, **36**, 174.

CASEY, E. B., and LE QUESNE, P. M. (1972) Digital nerve action potentials in healthy subjects, and in carpal tunnel and diabetic patients, *J. Neurol. Neurosurg. Psychiat.*, **35**, 612.

CRAGG, B. G., and THOMAS, P. K. (1964) The conduction velocity of regenerated peripheral nerve fibres, *J. Physiol.*, **171**, 164.

DANTA, G. (1975) Familial carpal tunnel syndrome with onset in childhood, *J. Neurol. Neurosurg. Psychiat.*, **38**, 350.

DAVIS, D. R. (1949) Some factors affecting the results of treatment of peripheral nerve injuries, *Lancet*, **i,** 877.

DAVIS, J. N. (1967) Phrenic nerve conduction in man, *J. Neurol. Neurosurg. Psychiat.*, **30**, 420.

DICK, T. B. S., and ZADIK, F. R. (1958) Acroparaesthesiae and the carpal tunnel, *Brit. med. J.*, **2**, 288.

DOWLING, M. H., FITCH, P., and WILLISON, R. G. (1968) A special purpose digital computer (Biomac 500) used in the analysis of the human electromyogram, *Electroenceph. clin. Neurophysiol.*, **25**, 570.

DOWNIE, A. W. (1974) Studies in nerve conduction, in *Disorders of Voluntary Muscle*, 3rd ed., ed. Walton, J. N., chap. 27, Edinburgh and London.

DOWNIE, A. W., and SCOTT, T. R. (1967) An improved technique for radial nerve conduction studies, *J. Neurol. Neurosurg. Psychiat.*, **30**, 332.

DYCK, P. J., and HOPKINS, A. P. (1972) Electron microscopic observations on degeneration and regeneration of unmyelinated fibres, *Brain*, **95**, 223.

DYCK, P. J., THOMAS, P. K., and LAMBERT, E. H. (1975) *Peripheral Neuropathy*, Philadelphia.

EBELING, P., GILLIATT, R. W., and THOMAS, P. K. (1960) A clinical and electrical study of ulnar nerve lesions in the hand, *J. Neurol. Neurosurg. Psychiat.*, **23**, 1.

EISEN, A., and DANON, J. (1974) The mild cubital tunnel syndrome, *Neurology (Minneap.)*, **24**, 608.

EKSTEDT, J. (1964) Human single muscle fiber action potentials, *Acta physiol. scand.*, **61**, Suppl. 226.

FEX, J., and KRAKAU, C. E. T. (1957) Some experiences with Walton's frequency analysis of the electromyogram, *J. Neurol. Neurosurg. Psychiat.*, **20**, 178.

FINELLI, P. F. (1975) Mononeuropathy of the deep palmar branch of the ulnar nerve, *Arch. Neurol. (Chic.)*, **32**, 564.

FOERSTER, O. (1929) in LEWANDOWSKY's *Handbuch der Neurologie*, Ergänzungsband, 2. Teil 1. Abschnitt. Spezielle Anatomie und Physiologie der peripheren Nerven, Berlin.

FOERSTER, O. (1929) in LEWANDOWSKY's *Handbuch der Neurologie*, Ergänzungsband, 2. Anschnitt. Die Symptomatologie der Schussverletzungen der peripheren Nerven, Berlin.

FOERSTER, O. (1929) in LEWANDOWSKY's *Handbuch der Neurologie*, Ergänzungsband, 2. Teil 3. Abschnitt. Die Therapie der Schussverletzungen der peripheren Nerven, Berlin.

FOSTER, J. B. (1960) Hydrocortisone and the carpal-tunnel syndrome, *Lancet*, **i**, 454.

FULLERTON, P. M. (1963) The effect of ischaemia on nerve conduction in the carpal tunnel syndrome, *J. Neurol. Neurosurg. Psychiat.*, **26**, 385.

FULLERTON, P. M., and GILLIATT, R. W. (1967) Median and ulnar neuropathy in the guinea-pig, *J. Neurol. Neurosurg. Psychiat.*, **30**, 393.

GARDNER-THORPE, C. (1974) Anterior interosseous nerve palsy: spontaneous recovery in two patients, *J. Neurol. Neurosurg. Psychiat.*, **37**, 1146.

GILLIATT, R. W. (1975) Peripheral nerve compression and entrapment, *Eleventh Symposium on Advanced Medicine*, London.

GILLIATT, R. W., GOODMAN, H. V., and WILLISON, R. G. (1961) The recording of lateral popliteal nerve action potentials in man, *J. Neurol. Neurosurg. Psychiat.*, **24**, 305.

GILLIATT, R. W., LE QUESNE, P. M., LOGUE, V., and SUMNER, A. J. (1970) Wasting of the hand associated with a cervical rib or band, *J. Neurol. Neurosurg. Psychiat.*, **33**, 615.

GILLIATT, R. W., MELVILLE, I. D., VELATE, A. S., and WILLISON, R. G. (1965) A study of normal nerve action potentials using an averaging technique (barrier grid storage tube), *J. Neurol. Neurosurg. Psychiat.*, **28**, 191.

GILLIATT, R. W., and SEARS, T. A. (1958) Sensory nerve action potentials in patients with peripheral nerve lesions, *J. Neurol. Neurosurg. Psychiat.*, **21**, 109.

GILLIATT, R. W., and THOMAS, P. K. (1960) Changes in nerve conduction with ulnar lesions at the elbow, *J. Neurol. Neurosurg. Psychiat.*, **23**, 312.

GILLIATT, R. W., and WILSON, T. G. (1954) Ischaemic sensory loss in patients with peripheral nerve lesions, *J. Neurol. Neurosurg. Psychiat.*, **17**, 104.

GOLDMAN, S., HONET, J. C., SOBEL, R., and GOLDSTEIN, A. S. (1969) Posterior interosseous nerve palsy in the absence of trauma, *Arch. Neurol. (Chic.)*, **21**, 435.

GUNNING, A. J., PICKERING, G. W., ROBB-SMITH, A. H. T., and ROSS RUSSELL, R. (1964) Mural thrombosis of the subclavian artery and subsequent embolism in cervical rib, *Quart. J. Med.*, **33**, 133.

GUTMANN, L. (1940) Topographic studies of disturbances of sweat secretion after complete lesions of peripheral nerves, *J. Neurol. Psychiat.*, **3**, 197.

GUTMANN, L. (1970) Atypical deep peroneal neuropathy, *J. Neurol. Neurosurg. Psychiat.*, **33**, 453.

GYE, R. S., McLEOD, J. G., HARGRAVE, J. C., POLLARD, J. D., LOEWENTHAL, J., and BOOTH, G. C. (1972) Use of immuno-suppressive agents in human nerve grafting, *Lancet*, **i**, 647.

HAGBARTH, K. E., and EKLUND, G. (1966) Motor effects of vibratory muscle stimuli in man, in *Muscle Afferents and Motor Control* (Proceedings of the First Nobel Symposium), ed. Granit, R., p. 177, Stockholm.

HARRISON, M. J. G., and NURICK, S. (1970) Results of anterior transposition of the ulnar nerve for ulnar neuritis, *Brit. med. J.*, **1**, 27.

HEATHFIELD, K. W. G. (1957) Acroparaesthesiae and the carpal-tunnel syndrome, *Lancet*, **ii**, 663.

HIGHET, W. B. (1942 *a*) Splintage of peripheral nerve injuries, *Lancet*, **i**, 555.

HIGHET, W. B. (1942 *b*) Procaine nerve block in the investigation of peripheral nerve injuries, *J. Neurol. Psychiat.*, **5**, 101.

HOLLER, M., and HOPF, H. C. (1968) Posttraumatische Synkinesien zwischen Zwerchfell und Muskeln des Plexus brachialis, *Dtsch. Z. Nervenheilk.*, **193**, 141.

HUSTEAD, A. P., MULDER, D. W., and MACCARTY, C. S. (1958) Non-traumatic, progressive paralysis of the deep radial (posterior interosseous) nerve, *Arch. Neurol. Psychiat. (Chic.)*, **79**, 269.

INFANTE, E., and KENNEDY, W. R. (1970) Anomalous branch of the peroneal nerve detected by electromyography, *Arch. Neurol. (Chic.)*, **22**, 162.

JUŠIĆ, A., and MILIĆ, S. (1972) Nerve potentials and afferent conduction velocities in the differential diagnosis of amyotrophy of the hand, *J. Neurol. Neurosurg. Psychiat.*, **35**, 861.

KAESER, H. E. (1970) Nerve conduction velocity measurements, in *Handbook of Clinical Neurology*, ed. Vinken, P. J., and Bruyn, G. W., vol. 7, chap. 5, Amsterdam.

KEMBLE, F. (1968) Electrodiagnosis of the carpal tunnel syndrome, *J. Neurol. Neurosurg. Psychiat.*, **31**, 23.

KILOH, L. G., and NEVIN, S. (1952) Isolated neuritis of the anterior interosseous nerve, *Brit. med. J.*, **1**, 850.

KOPELL, H. P., and THOMPSON, W. A. L. (1963 and 1975) *Peripheral Entrapment Neuropathies*, Baltimore.

KRAMER, W. (1970) Tumours of nerves, in *Handbook of Clinical Neurology*, ed. Vinken, P. J., and Bruyn, G. W., vol. 8, chap. 23, Amsterdam.

KUGELBERG, E. (1947) Electromyograms in muscular disorders, *J. Neurol. Neurosurg. Psychiat.*, **10**, 122.

KUGELBERG, E. (1949) Electromyography in muscular dystrophies, *J. Neurol. Neurosurg. Psychiat.*, **12**, 129.

LAMBERT, E. H. (1969) The accessory deep peroneal nerve: a common variation in innervation of extensor digitorum brevis, *Neurology (Minneap.)*, **19**, 1169.

LANCE, J. W., DE GAIL, P., and NIELSON, P. D. (1966) Tonic and phasic spinal cord mechanisms in man, *J. Neurol. Neurosurg. Psychiat.*, **29**, 535.

LANCE, J. W., and McLEOD, J. G. (1975) *A Physiological Approach to Clinical Neurology*, 2nd ed., London.

THE LANCET (1972) Causalgia, *Lancet*, **i**, 1170.

LENMAN, J. A. R. (1959) A clinical and experimental study of the effects of exercise on motor weakness in neurological disease, *J. Neurol. Neurosurg. Psychiat.*, **22**, 182.

LENMAN, J. A. R. (1974) Integration and analysis of the electromyogram and related techniques, in *Disorders of Voluntary Muscle*, 3rd ed., ed. Walton, J. N., chap. 29, Edinburgh and London.

SPINAL RADICULOPATHY DUE TO
INTERVERTEBRAL DISC DISEASE

Disorders of the spinal column associated with lesions of the intervertebral discs are by far the commonest cause of painful root compression. Such lesions are situated chiefly in the cervical and lumbar regions of the spine, though they occur occasionally in the thoracic region (Logue, 1952; Carson *et al.*, 1971). The principal cause is undoubtedly the tendency of the intervertebral discs to degenerate with increasing age and this no doubt explains the occurrence of degeneration of both cervical and lumbar intervertebral discs in the same patient. Other factors, especially trauma, may play a part.

The intervertebral disc consists of a central portion, the nucleus pulposus, which obeys the laws of fluids and is surrounded by the annulus fibrosus, a strong but somewhat fibro-cartilaginous and elastic membrane binding the bodies of the vertebrae together. When force is exerted upon the disc it is distributed laterally in all directions, and if the force is too strong for the resistance of the annulus fibrosus the nucleus pulposus will herniate through it. Such protrusions may occur either in the midline or posterolaterally into the spinal canal [see FIG. 121, p. 747], or more laterally into the intervertebral foramen [FIG. 137]. This is described as a nuclear herniation. There is, however, another type of disc protrusion, the annular protrusion, which is produced in

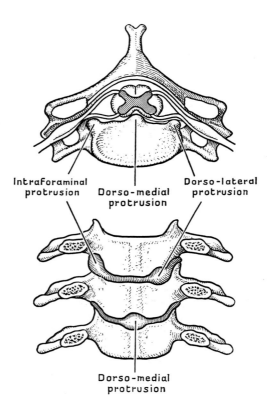

Intraforaminal protrusion   Dorso-medial protrusion   Dorso-lateral protrusion

Dorso-medial protrusion

FIG. 137. Sites of intervertebral disc protrusion

a different way. A degenerated intervertebral disc tends to collapse, in which case the annulus bulges in all directions. The protruded material becomes vascularized and its fibrous elements are increased. A nuclear herniation is originally soft, but in time undergoes a similar transformation into fibrocartilage, so that the end result of both a nuclear and an annular protrusion may be a hard calcified boss. For anatomical reasons the effects of cervical and lumbar protrusions are somewhat different and must be considered separately.

CERVICAL DISC LESIONS AND BRACHIAL RADICULOPATHY

Cervical intervertebral discs are bounded on their lateral margins by an articulation known as the apophyseal joint which lies on the anteromedial side of the intervertebral foramen, the posterior boundary of which is formed by the articulation between the pedicles of the two adjacent vertebrae. The cervical spinal roots may therefore be compressed, either by posterolateral protrusions of the intervertebral disc into the spinal canal or, as the radicular nerve, within the intervertebral foramen, either by an acute disc protrusion or as the result of narrowing of the foramen by osteophytes, especially those arising from apophyseal joints. Such pressure, as Frykholm (1951) showed, leads to fibrosis of the root sheaths.

The pathological changes of the chronic syndrome of cervical spondylosis may involve one pair of intervertebral joints or more than one and are more often related to single or multiple annular protrusions with eventual bony boss formation, though this process may occur in patients who have suffered previous acute protrusions; when the joint lesions are multiple the joints affected may be adjacent to one another or they may not. Since age, manual labour, and recurrent minor trauma are probably the chief factors in causing degeneration of the intervertebral discs, most patients are middle-aged or older, but acute cervical disc protrusion may occur at an earlier age.

Acute Protrusions

Acute protrusions may occur either spontaneously or as the result of trauma. A patient suffering from an acute protrusion usually gives a history of recurrent attacks of pain in the neck often diagnosed as 'fibrositis'. Suddenly a pain more severe and lasting than the previous ones occurs. The neck may feel as though it is fixed, and both active and passive movements cause an intensification of the pain, which may be very severe. Anteroposterior movements of the head (which occur mainly at the atlanto-occipital joints) and rotation (which occurs largely at the atlanto-axial joint) are restricted only by protective muscle spasm. It is lateral movements which are particularly painful, especially towards the side of the lesion (Spurling's sign). The pain is also referred within the distribution of the spinal nerve which is compressed. On examination the neck is usually held rigidly, and sometimes slightly flexed towards the side of the lesion. The muscles innervated by the spinal nerve compressed may be somewhat weak and hypotonic, but severe muscular weakness or wasting are unusual. The tendon reflexes mediated by the affected segment are diminished, and sometimes lost. It may be possible to demonstrate some hyperalgesia and hyperaesthesia within the corresponding dermatome, or some diminution of cutaneous sensibility. Plain X-rays usually show little abnormality, though there may be slight narrowing of the affected intervertebral disc. Myelography may show an indentation of the column of contrast medium or obliteration of the corresponding root sheath. Discography [p. 748] is now often used in the diagnosis of lumbar disc protrusions but the potential risks still outweigh its advantages in the diagnosis of cervical lesions.

The treatment of spontaneous acute protrusion of an intervertebral disc involving one spinal nerve in the neck is a combination of traction on the head, to relieve pressure upon the protruding disc, and/or immobilization. In the acute phase a soft 'Gamgee' tissue collar or one made of newspaper may be helpful and powerful analgesics are usually required. After the acute phase has passed, immobilization may be continued by means of a plastic collar. If these methods fail surgical exploration may be required (Yoss et al., 1957) but this is rarely necessary in acute cervical disc lesions most of which respond quickly to conservative treatment. Acute central protrusions causing spinal cord compression [p. 737] also respond rapidly, as a rule, to immobilization, but laminectomy is occasionally needed if symptoms and signs of cord dysfunction are severe and do not quickly improve.

It is important also to recognize that the prognosis of acute cervical disc protrusions may be very unpredictable after industrial injury where financial compensation may be involved. In such cases pain in the neck and arm, if not responding rapidly to treatment, may breed tension and anxiety which in turn increase pain which may be very persistent, especially if the position is complicated by the motive of possible financial gain. In such cases 'hysterical' weakness and sensory loss may develop in the affected limb and it is difficult to distinguish with confidence between a genuine hysterical overlay (subconscious motivation) and malingering (conscious motivation). 'Collar-dependence' is also common with resultant stiffness of the cervical muscles. While antidepressive and tranquillizing remedies such as diazepam are often helpful in such cases, rehabilitation and persuasion to discard the collar are often very difficult, at least until the compensation claim is settled; the longer settlement is delayed, the worse the prognosis.

CERVICAL SPONDYLOSIS

The duration and the history of symptoms of cervical spondylosis are extremely variable and radicular symptoms may be acute, subacute, or insidious in their onset. To avoid confusion, this term should be reserved for the syndrome resulting from subacute or chronic central and lateral protrusion of cervical intervertebral discs and should not be used in cases of acute protrusion as described above. In fact, radicular symptoms are often absent in cases of cervical cord compression (myelopathy) (Phillips, 1975); this syndrome is described on page 737. Involvement of one spinal nerve leads to symptoms resembling those of a spontaneous acute protrusion of a single intervertebral disc into the intervertebral foramen, as described above. Pain, however, is not always limited to one dermatome, but may extend down the upper limb to involve to a greater or lesser extent all the digits, in which case a clinical picture resembling the classical one of 'brachial neuritis or neuralgia' is produced. An insidious onset is characterized by dysaesthesiae consisting of a burning and tingling sensation, sometimes accompanied by pain, radiating down the upper limb into one or more digits and tending sometimes to be particularly troublesome at night. Motor symptoms are usually slight or absent and only exceptionally is there a complaint of weakness, but occasionally wasting accompanied by fasciculation may be severe enough to simulate motor neurone disease.

On examination of the patient there is commonly some diminution of the appreciation of light touch and pin-prick within the distribution of the dermatomes corresponding to the affected radicular nerves. There may also be localized areas of tenderness in the corresponding muscles. Appreciation of posture and passive movement is usually unimpaired. There is likely to be slight muscular wasting accompanied by hypotonia in the muscles innervated by the affected spinal nerves, but muscular weakness is usually slight. Pseudomyotonia in the affected hand has been reported (Satoyoshi et al., 1972). The tendon reflexes innervated from the affected segments are likely to be diminished or lost and if there is evidence of associated myelopathy, 'inversion' of the biceps or radial reflexes may be observed [p. 744]. Active and passive movements of the neck are somewhat limited in extent, but relatively painless. There may be some local tenderness on pressure.

Plain X-rays usually show narrowing of intervertebral discs with posterior osteophytes, and, in the oblique views, of the intervertebral foramina owing to the projection of osteophytes from the apophyseal joints.

It is uncommon to find evidence of spondylotic radiculopathy without some evidence of associated myelopathy, while by contrast, myelopathy often occurs without evidence of root involvement. Nevertheless, myelography, while demonstrating a central bulge of one or more intervertebral discs, a narrow spinal canal (The Lancet, 1972), or posterior indentation due to infolding of the ligamentum subflavum (Taylor, 1953), may also demonstrate associated lateral protrusions of the affected discs. The effect of cervical movement upon spinal cord and root compression has been reviewed by Adams and Logue (1971 a and b).

TREATMENT

In some cases a simple radiculopathy responds to immobilization in a plaster or plastic collar which is usually required for two or three months. Both traction and manipulation have their advocates, but the latter is probably not free from risk. Surgical decompression of the intervertebral foramina has been carried out, but is rarely required. Laminectomy and posterior decompression continues to be useful in cases with associated myelopathy (Bishara, 1971; Adams and Logue, 1971 c) but there is increasing evidence that in selected cases of myelopathy without substantial root or spinal nerve involvement the anterior operation of removal of the affected disc or discs, followed by spinal fusion (the Cloward operation) gives superior results (Phillips, 1973). Various forms of physiotherapy are useful adjuvants to treatment. In the acute stage analgesic drugs and rest in bed are necessary with the arm supported on a pillow, and when the patient gets up, in a sling, but care must be taken that immobilization does not lead to a 'frozen shoulder'.

LUMBAR DISC LESIONS AND SCIATICA

The term sciatica is applied to a benign syndrome characterized especially by pain beginning in the lumbar region and spreading down the back of one lower limb to the ankle, usually intensified by coughing or sneezing, and associated with little weakness or sensory loss but sometimes with diminution or loss of the ankle-jerk. In most cases spontaneous recovery occurs rather slowly with some liability to recurrence. It has been established that sciatica thus defined is usually due to herniation of one or more of the lumbar intervertebral discs. It seems best, therefore, to discuss sciatica under this heading and to consider other causes of sciatic pain in relation to diagnosis.

AETIOLOGY

Lumbar disc protrusion is often the result of trauma, a history of which is obtainable in at least half of all cases. The commonest type of stress is that produced by lifting a heavy object in a bent-forward position or by a fall in a similar posture. Since 75 per cent of patients are in or beyond the fourth decade it would appear that degenerative changes which begin in the prime of life predispose towards herniation but the syndrome is not uncommon in young adults and may even occur in children. The changes in the lumbar spine associated with pregnancy may also cause it. Thickening of the ligamentum flavum has often been noted in addition.

The age-incidence shows a peak with 35 per cent of cases in the fourth decade, and between 75 and 80 per cent of patients are males. Almost all lumbar herniations occur between the fourth and fifth lumbar or fifth lumbar and first sacral bodies, with a relative frequency of two to three. A disc protrusion compresses the spinal nerve which is running to the foramen one segment below, the fourth lumbar disc the fifth lumbar nerve, and the fifth lumbar disc the first sacral nerve. Sometimes protrusions occur from two or more discs. The compressed nerve becomes swollen and tense. Occasionally an acute lumbar disc protrusion results in the sequestration of a portion of the disc which acts as a major space-occupying lesion in the lumbar canal, involving multiple spinal nerves in the cauda equina.

SYMPTOMS

In most cases the onset is subacute, and sciatica is frequently preceded by lumbar pain, which may have occurred intermittently for years. The pain may immediately follow an injury such as a strain or a fall, or there may be a latent interval of days or even weeks. After two or three days of pain in the lumbar spine the pain radiates down the back of one leg from the buttock to the ankle. It is often possible to distinguish three elements in the pain: (1) pain in the back, aching in character and intensified by spinal movements; (2) pain deep in the buttock and thigh, also aching or gnawing in character and influenced by the posture of the limb; and (3) pain radiating to the leg and foot, momentarily increased by coughing and sneezing. When the first sacral root is compressed the pain radiates to the outer border of the foot. When the pressure is upon the fifth lumbar root it spreads from the outer aspect of the leg to the dorsum or the inner border of the foot. In general the pain is intensified by stooping, sitting, and walking. The patient is usually most comfortable lying in bed on the sound side with the affected leg slightly flexed at the hip and knee. The pain interferes with sleep and when it is very severe he may be able to obtain relief only by getting up and walking about. There is often a feeling of numbness, heaviness, or deadness in the leg, especially along the outer side of the foot.

There may be muscular weakness and slight wasting, not only of the muscles supplied by the sciatic nerve, but sometimes also of other muscles of the lower limb. Compression of the first sacral root causes weakness of the small muscles of the foot and the calf muscles and the ankle-jerk is diminished or lost. Compression of the fifth lumbar root causes weakness of the peronei—occasionally complete foot-drop—and the ankle-jerk is preserved. The knee-jerk may be slightly exaggerated, partly as a reflex result of the pain and partly owing to hypotonia of the hamstrings, the antagonists of the quadriceps, but if the fourth lumbar root is involved it may be diminished. The plantar reflex is flexor. Weakness of extension of the hallux on the affected side is a valuable sign of a fifth lumbar root lesion and examination of the 'great-toe reflex', evoked by a sharp tap with a tendon hammer upon a finger which is so placed upon the dorsum of the proximal phalanx of the toe that it stretches slightly the extensor hallucis longus, is also useful in diagnosis (Taylor and Wienir, 1969). There is tenderness on pressure in the buttock and thigh, straight-leg-raising is limited by pain, and stretching the sciatic nerve by extending the knee with the hip flexed causes severe pain—Lasègue's sign. There is rarely much sensory loss, though often there is some blunting of light touch and pin-prick over the outer half of the foot and three outer toes and lower part of the outer aspect of the leg when the first sacral root is involved. The fourth and fifth lumbar cutaneous areas are shown in FIGURES 7 a and 7 b. Scoliosis is often associated with sciatica, the lumbar spine being laterally flexed, usually towards the affected side, less frequently towards the opposite side. Some rigidity of the lumbar spine is usually present, and there may be a tender spot at the level of the fifth lumbar transverse process. In the case of large central disc protrusions in the lumbar region pain is sometimes bilateral though often more severe on one side, muscular weakness is more widespread, several tendon reflexes may be lost (e.g. one knee-jerk and both ankle-jerks), sensory loss is more extensive, indicating involvement of motor roots, and sphincter control may be impaired. Such a cauda equina syndrome (Shephard, 1959) should be regarded as a neurosurgical emergency. An excess of protein, up to 70 or 80 mg per 100 ml, is present in the CSF in about 80 per cent of cases, but the cell count is normal.

X-ray examination should be carried out in all cases of sciatica, since many causes of sciatic pain are associated with bony changes visible in radiograms. Straight X-rays are not always of value in the diagnosis of herniated disc. The L5–S1 disc space is often normally narrower than that of the other lumbar discs, so that little stress can be laid upon narrowing at this level. Narrowing of the L4–5 space is more likely to be significant especially if associated with sclerosis of adjacent vertebral bodies. Spondylolisthesis at L4–5, but more often at L5–S1, may give not only low back pain but also symptoms and signs of root compression resembling those of intervertebral disc prolapse and is usually readily demonstrable by X-ray. Myelography may demonstrate a filling defect, but is only indicated as a rule if pain is unusually persistent despite adequate rest or immobilization or if there are physical signs of such a degree and extent that surgical treatment is contemplated; a herniated disc may be present in spite of a negative myelogram. Protrusion of the lumbar posterior longitudinal ligament, which is often apparent on myelography, may give symptoms simulating those of disc prolapse (Beatty et al., 1968), as may cysts on sacral nerve roots (Tarlov, 1938; Plewes and Jacobson, 1970) and lumbar canal stenosis [see p. 786]; the latter is often associated with symptoms of cauda equina dysfunction which develop during exertion and are relieved by rest; it, too, is readily demonstrated by this technique.

DIAGNOSIS

Sciatica due to a lumbar disc protrusion must be distinguished from: (1) compression of the nerve roots by a tumour within the spinal canal; (2) root compression resulting from spondylolisthesis, sacral cysts, other developmental anomalies or lumbar canal stenosis; (3) inflammatory or granulomatous processes involving the cauda equina; (4) inflammatory, degenerative, and neoplastic lesions of the spine and pelvis involving the roots; and (5) neoplasms of the pelvic viscera. The principal points of distinction are that in herniated disc the onset of symptoms is fairly rapid, the buttock and posterior aspect of the thigh over the course of the sciatic nerve are usually tender on pressure, muscular wasting is slight, sensory loss is slight, and the course of the disorder during the first months after the onset is stationary or tends towards improvement. In the other lesions mentioned the onset is usually more gradual, the nerve is not tender on pressure, muscular wasting is conspicuous, and sensory loss is more pronounced. Further, these symptoms are progressive.

In such cases the abdomen and pelvis must be thoroughly examined for sources of compression, and the lumbar spine and pelvis should be X-rayed. Attention must also be paid to the general condition of the patient, and inquiry made for symptoms suggestive of a pelvic neoplasm and as to recent loss of weight. Rectal examination should never be omitted; and in women vaginal examination is advisable also. A complete examination of the nervous system is required to exclude tumours within the spinal canal and syphilis as a cause of sciatic pain, and if these are suspected CSF examination and/or myelography are usually indicated.

The distinction of sciatica from femoral neuropathy has been described in the section dealing with the latter.

Herniated disc requires to be distinguished from arthritis of the hip-joint, with which sciatica may be associated. In herniated disc movements of the hip-joint are painless, provided the sciatic nerve is not stretched. The lower limb can be rotated and abducted without pain, whereas these movements are painful and often limited in arthritis of the hip. In the latter condition the ankle-jerk is preserved. X-rays will confirm the diagnosis.

Congenital abnormalities of the lumbosacral junction, such as spondylolisthesis and sacralization of the fifth lumbar vertebra, may cause low back pain but only occasionally true sciatica, unless the fifth lumbar root is compressed. This abnormality will be apparent on the X-ray film. Other causes of low back pain which must be considered in differential diagnosis include contusion due to local injury to the back or one buttock, sometimes associated with transient sciatic pain, osteoarthrosis of apophyseal or neurocentral joints without significant disc protrusion, sacro-iliac strain, and ankylosing spondylitis which will usually be apparent radiologically. Local lumbar pain is not uncommon in some women during menstruation and/or pregnancy and in patients in the para-menopausal age group similar symptoms but without, as a rule, radiation to the legs, may be the result of muscular tension associated with anxiety and/or depression and may respond to treatment with appropriate remedies. As in the case of industrial injuries to the cervical region [see p. 926] symptoms of low back strain with or without intervertebral disc protrusion may be aggravated and perpetuated and the clinical picture clouded by the compensation issue.

Vascular lesions within the distribution of the femoral artery, such as atheroma and thrombo-angiitis obliterans, are occasional causes of pain in the leg in middle age and later in life: intermittent claudication is not always present in these cases. The diagnosis is readily established by diminution in the volume of the femoral, dorsalis pedis, or posterior tibial pulses. The syndrome of intermittent ischaemia of the cauda equina with pain, paraesthesiae or weakness of the leg occurring only on exertion and relieved by rest can usually be distinguished from sciatica, due to a single lateral disc protrusion, by myelography [see p. 746].

The demonstration of defects in motor and/or sensory nerve conduction or of partial denervation of muscles innervated by the affected root by electromyography may also be of considerable value in some cases.

PROGNOSIS

In mild cases the stage of severe pain lasts only two or three weeks and the patient recovers in a month or two, except that he may from time to time experience aching in the course of the nerve and stooping may still excite some pain in the affected leg. In more severe cases there may be slight improvement after several weeks, but the condition then becomes stationary and the patient continues to suffer from considerable pain for a number of months. Recovery, however, ultimately occurs in most cases, except for the residual symptoms just mentioned. In a study of 73 unselected cases treated with bed rest alone, Pearce and Moll (1967) found that 70 per cent recovered satisfactorily but the remaining 30 per cent required other measures. Recovery may occur even though the disc protrusion remains. For this reason, perhaps, relapses are common. In some cases they occur at frequent intervals, so that the patient is hardly free from pain over a period of several years. In other cases the second attack may be delayed until ten or more years after the first. Operation gives good results in 90 per cent of cases operated upon, but even after operation a relapse may occur.

TREATMENT

Most patients with lumbar intervertebral disc protrusion recover completely if treated conservatively. Operation should therefore be reserved for patients with large central disc protrusions involving multiple roots (in whom it is obligatory, especially if the sphincters are involved) and for those with marked motor weakness (e.g. foot-drop) present from the outset. It is probably indicated also in those whose symptoms do not respond to other measures and become chronic, those who relapse, and those with gross and persistent symptoms of root compression, sufficiently severe to cause disability. Probably not more than 10 per cent will require operation, but the percentage will be higher among manual workers, in whom inability to do the necessary physical work may itself constitute an indication for surgery.

Conservative treatment consists of rest in bed and analgesics, to which may be added various measures designed to immobilize the lower part of the spine and the affected lower limb. When rest in bed for two or three weeks has been tried and failed, immediate relief is sometimes given by the application of a plaster jacket which fixes the lumbar spine in slight extension. The patient, who is allowed to walk about, should wear the plaster for three months. Alternatively many patients are relieved by the application of continuous lumbar traction for two or three weeks followed by the provision of a light lumbar support or corset which is worn for three months or longer. Manipulation also has its advocates and is remarkably successful in some patients with intractable pain but the outcome is difficult to predict in advance (Doran and Newell, 1975). An 'overlay' of depression and anxiety commonly occurs in patients with lumbar disc disease and as a result of tension in the lumbar muscles accentuates and perpetuates pain. Antidepressive remedies and tranquillizing drugs such as amitriptyline and diazepam are particularly valuable in some patients. About

70 per cent of patients respond satisfactorily to conservative treatment (Pearce and Moll, 1967) but in those who continue to have pain, provided there is no evidence of a severe 'functional overlay', surgical treatment is probably indicated.

Sacral Epidural Injection

In some cases benefit may be derived from stretching the nerve roots by epidural injection at the sacral hiatus. This can readily be palpated at the lower end of the sacrum, where it is covered by the dorsal sacrococcygeal ligament. The foramen is bounded above by the concave lower border of the sacrum in the midline and at the sides by the two lateral tubercles. The patient either lies on one side or assumes the knee-elbow position. The site of the injection is painted with antiseptic and anaesthetized with procaine, and a fine lumbar-puncture needle is passed through the ligament upwards and slightly forwards. Twenty ml of 1 per cent procaine solution are first injected, and this is followed by an injection of normal saline, of which 80 ml or more can sometimes be injected, the solution being at body temperature. Coomes (1961) used 50 ml of 0·5 per cent procaine alone and found the effects of such an injection to be superior to those of bed rest alone. The object of the injection being to stretch the nerve roots, a sufficient volume of fluid must be injected to raise the tension in the epidural space. It is necessary, therefore, to continue injecting saline until a considerable resistance is encountered, provided always that it does not cause pain. Epidural injection yields relief of pain in about 50 per cent of cases. Sometimes the result is dramatic, the patient being completely and permanently relieved. A second injection may be given after an interval of two or three days if necessary.

Lumbar Extradural Injection

Another form of treatment now enjoying an increasing vogue is that of giving an extradural injection of a corticosteroid preparation; the technique of lumbar injection was described by Barry and Kendall (1962). In a controlled trial Dilke et al. (1973) found that the effects of 80 mg of methylprednisolone injected in 10 ml of normal saline gave excellent relief of pain and other symptoms.

Chemonucleolysis

Chymopapain, a proteolytic enzyme derived from papaya latex, can break down mucopolysaccharide–protein complexes which form an important part of the structure of intervertebral discs. Smith and Brown (1967) carried out discography by injecting contrast medium through a lateral approach directly into the nucleus pulposus of the affected disc or discs and followed this with an injection of 2 mg of chymopapain in 0·5 ml of distilled water. The injection caused severe pain in the back for 12–24 hours but sciatic pain was usually relieved in 24 hours. Potential risks of the method include sensitivity reactions and disc space infection but others have shown that the technique is effective in relieving symptoms rapidly (Nordby and Lucas, 1973; Graham, 1974). The method, which is likely to be used increasingly, seems to give results superior to those of surgery in many cases but no controlled trial has yet been reported (British Medical Journal, 1974).

Physiotherapy

Local heat, diathermy, massage, and other traditional forms of treatment commonly used in cases of sciatica and various forms of low back pain have a useful palliative effect in some cases. Once the phase of acute pain has passed, graduated exercises are of considerable value in improving the mobility of the affected portion of the spine, in relieving muscular spasm or secondary scoliosis, and in improving power in weakened muscles.

RADICULITIS OF THE CAUDA EQUINA

Rarely the cauda equina is the site of a radiculopathy of obscure origin, of subacute or insidious onset. The symptoms and signs are those of a cauda equina lesion [see p. 751], and the inflammatory nature of the process may be suggested by a pleocytosis, usually mononuclear, in the cerebrospinal fluid with some rise of protein. Such a syndrome has been described in ankylosing spondylitis (Matthews, 1968) but in most instances, repeated investigation or eventual pathological observations in such cases has demonstrated that the condition is due either to tumour (e.g. ependymoma of the filum terminale), to mechanical compression of roots, or to ischaemia of roots resulting from atherosclerosis or stenosis of the lumbar canal. Other neurological disorders occasionally associated with ankylosing spondylitis include multiple sclerosis, focal epilepsy, and peripheral nerve lesions, but a cauda equina syndrome is probably the commonest (Thomas *et al.*, 1974).

REFERENCES

ADAMS, C. B. T., and LOGUE, V. (1971 *a*) Studies in cervical spondylotic myelopathy. I. Movement of the cervical roots, dura and cord, and their relation to the course taken by the extrathecal roots, *Brain*, **94**, 557.

ADAMS, C. B. T., and LOGUE, V. (1971 *b*) Studies in cervical spondylotic myelopathy. II. Observations on the movement and contour of the cervical spine in relation to the neural complications of cervical spondylosis, *Brain*, **94**, 569.

ADAMS, C. B. T., and LOGUE, V. (1971 *c*) Studies in cervical spondylotic myelopathy. III. Some functional effects of operations for cervical spondylotic myelopathy, *Brain*, **94**, 587.

BARRY, P. J. C., and KENDALL, P. H. (1962) Corticosteroid infiltration of the extradural space, *Ann. phys. Med.*, **6**, 267.

BEATTY, R. S., SUGAR, O., and FOX, T. A. (1968) Protrusion of the posterior longitudinal ligament simulating herniated lumbar intervertebral disc, *J. Neurol. Neurosurg. Psychiat.*, **31**, 61.

BISHARA, S. N. (1971) The posterior operation in treatment of cervical spondylosis with myelopathy: a long-term follow-up study, *J. Neurol. Neurosurg. Psychiat.*, **34**, 393.

BOSANQUET, F. D., and HENSON, R. A. (1957) Sensory neuropathy in diabetes mellitus, *Folia psychiat. neerl.*, **60**, 107.

BRADFORD, F. K., and SPURLING, R. G. (1941) *The Intervertebral Disk*, Springfield, Ill.

BRITISH MEDICAL JOURNAL (1974) Dissolving discs, *Brit. med. J.*, **2**, 625.

CARSON, J., GUMPERT, J., and JEFFERSON, A. (1971) Diagnosis and treatment of thoracic intervertebral disc protrusions, *J. Neurol. Neurosurg. Psychiat.*, **34**, 68.

COOMES, E. N. (1961) A comparison between epidural anaesthesia and bed rest in sciatica, *Brit. med. J.*, **1**, 20.

DANDY, W. E. (1944) Newer aspects of ruptured intervertebral disks, *Ann. Surg.*, **119**, 481.

DILKE, T. F. W., BURRY, H. C., and GRAHAME, R. (1973) Extradural corticosteroid injection in management of lumbar nerve root compression, *Brit. med. J.*, **2**, 635.

DORAN, D. M. L., and NEWELL, D. J. (1975) Manipulation in the treatment of low back pain: a multi-centre study, *Brit. med. J.*, **2**, 161.

FALCONER, M. A., MCGEORGE, M., and BEGG, A. C. (1948 a) Surgery of lumbar inter-vertebral disk protrusion, *Brit. J. Surg.*, **35**, 225.

FALCONER, M. A., MCGEORGE, M., and BEGG, A. C. (1948 b) Cause and mechanism of symptom-production in sciatic and low-back pain, *J. Neurol. Neurosurg. Psychiat.*, **11**, 13.

FRYKHOLM, R. (1951) Cervical nerve root compression resulting from disc degeneration and root-sleeve fibrosis, *Acta chir. scand.*, Supp. 160.

GRAHAM, C. E. (1974) Backache and sciatica. A report of 90 patients treated by intradiscal injection of chymopapain (discase), *Med. J. Aust.*, **1**, 5.

THE LANCET (1972) Signs and symptoms in cervical spondylosis, *Lancet*, **ii**, 70.

LOGUE, V. (1952) Thoracic intervertebral disc prolapse with spinal cord compression, *J. Neurol. Neurosurg. Psychiat.*, **15**, 227.

LOVE, J. G., and SCHORN, V. G. (1965) Thoracic disk protrusions, *J. Amer. med. Ass.*, **191**, 627.

LOVE, J. G., and WALSH, M. N. (1940) Intraspinal protrusion of intervertebral disks, *Arch. Surg. (Chic.)*, **40**, 454.

MCALPINE, D., and PAGE, F. (1951) Sensory neuropathy due to posterior root ganglion degeneration, *Arch. Mddx Hosp.*, **1**, 250.

MACEY, H. B. (1940) Clinical aspects of protruded intervertebral disks, *Arch. Surg. (Chic.)*, **40**, 433.

MATTHEWS, W. B. (1968) The neurological complications of ankylosing spondylitis, *J. neurol. Sci.*, **6**, 561.

MEDICAL RESEARCH COUNCIL (1976) *Aids to the Examination of the Peripheral Nervous System*, 3rd ed., London.

NORDBY, E. J., and LUCAS, G. L. (1973) A comparative analysis of lumbar disk disease treated by laminectomy or chemonucleolysis, *Clinical Orthopaedics and Related Research*, **90**, 119.

O'CONNELL, J. E. A. (1944) Maternal obstetrical paralysis, *Surg. Gynec. Obstet.*, **29**, 374.

O'CONNELL, J. E. A. (1950) The indications for and results of the excision of lumbar intervertebral disk protrusions, a review of 500 cases, *Ann. roy. Coll. Surg. Engl.*, **6**, 403.

PEARCE, J., and MOLL, J. M. H. (1967) Conservative treatment and natural history of acute lumbar disc lesions, *J. Neurol. Neurosurg. Psychiat.*, **30**, 13.

PENNYBACKER, J. (1940) Sciatica and the intervertebral disk, *Lancet*, **ii**, 532.

PHILLIPS, D. G. (1973) Surgical treatment of myelopathy with cervical spondylosis, *J. Neurol. Neurosurg. Psychiat.*, **36**, 879.

PHILLIPS, D. G. (1975) Upper limb involvement in cervical spondylosis, *J. Neurol. Neurosurg. Psychiat.*, **38**, 386.

PLEWES, J. L., and JACOBSON, I. (1970) Sciatica caused by sacral-nerve-root cysts, *Lancet*, **ii**, 799.

SATOYOSHI, E., DOI, Y., and KINOSHITA, M. (1972) Pseudomyotonia in cervical root lesions with myelopathy, *Arch. Neurol. (Chic.)*, **27**, 307.

SHEPHARD, R. H. (1959) Diagnosis and prognosis of cauda equina syndrome produced by protrusion of lumbar disk, *Brit. med. J.*, **2**, 1434.

SHINNERS, B. M., and HAMBY, W. B. (1949) Protruded lumbar intervertebral discs, *J. Neurosurg.*, **6**, 450.

SMITH, L., and BROWN, J. E. (1967) Treatment of lumbar intervertebral disc lesions by direct injection of chymopapain, *J. Bone Jt Surg.*, **49B**, 502.

SPURLING, R. G., and GRANTHAM, E. G. (1940) Neurologic picture of herniations of the nucleus pulposus in the lower part of the lumbar region, *Arch. Surg. (Chic.)*, **40**, 375.

TARLOV, I. M. (1938) Perineurial cysts of the spinal nerve roots, *Arch. Neurol. Psychiat. (Chic.)*, **40**, 1067.

TAYLOR, A. R. (1953) Mechanism and treatment of spinal-cord disorders associated with cervical spondylosis, *Lancet*, **i**, 717.

TAYLOR, T. K. F., and WIENIR, M. (1969) Great-toe reflexes in the diagnosis of lumbar disc disorder, *Brit. med. J.*, **2**, 487.

THOMAS, D. J., KENDALL, M. J., and WHITFIELD, A. G. W. (1974) Nervous system involvement in ankylosing spondylitis, *Brit. med. J.*, **1**, 148.

WILKINSON, M. (1960) The morbid anatomy of cervical spondylosis and myelopathy, *Brain*, **83**, 589.

YOSS, R. E., CORBIN, K. B., MacCARTY, C. S., and LOVE, J. G. (1957) Significance of symptoms and signs in localization of involved root in cervical disk protrusion, *Neurology (Minneap.)*, **7**, 673.

'INTERSTITIAL NEURITIS'

While 'interstitial neuritis' was a diagnosis commonly made in the past to explain a lesion of a single peripheral nerve for which no obvious cause could be demonstrated, there is growing evidence to indicate that such an inflammatory process does not exist as a specific pathological entity. In most cases so diagnosed in the past it is now well recognized that the condition almost certainly resulted from mechanical compression of the nerve in question or of its component roots, or from ischaemia, due either to peripheral vascular disease (Richards, 1951; Gairns *et al.*, 1960) or to a diffuse inflammatory disorder of arteries such as polyarteritis nodosa (Lovshin and Kernohan, 1948) in which an arteritis of the vasa nervorum may occur resulting in a 'mononeuritis multiplex'. It is also well recognized that some individuals have a peculiar liability to develop peripheral nerve lesions (of the lateral popliteal, ulnar, or median nerves and less frequently of other mixed nerves) as a result of transient and minimal trauma; these patients may develop recurrent palsies of the affected nerve or nerves and this liability often appears to be inherited (Earl *et al.*, 1964). The pathogenesis of this form of '*hereditary neuropathy with liability to pressure palsy*', in which there is evidence of some loss of myelinated fibres and extensive segmental demyelination with marked slowing of conduction in many peripheral nerves at a time when symptoms may be absent (Davies, 1954; Behse *et al.*, 1972), is unknown. Manifestations of multiple peripheral nerve entrapment are also seen occasionally in rare inherited metabolic disorders including amyloidosis and mucopolysaccharidosis (Karpati *et al.*, 1974).

REFERENCES

BEHSE, F., BUCHTHAL, F., CARLSEN, F., and KNAPPEIS, G. G. (1972) Hereditary neuropathy with liability to pressure palsies: electrophysiological and histopathological aspects, *Brain*, **95**, 777.

DAVIES, D. M. (1954) Recurrent peripheral-nerve palsies in a family, *Lancet*, **ii**, 266.

EARL, C. J., FULLERTON, P. M., WAKEFIELD, G. S., and SCHUTTA, H. S. (1964) Hereditary neuropathy with liability to pressure palsies, *Quart. J. Med.*, **33**, 481.

GAIRNS, F. W., GARVEN, H. S. D., and SMITH, G. (1960) The digital nerves and the nerve endings in progressive obliterative vascular disease, *Scot. med. J.*, **5**, 382.

KARPATI, G., CARPENTER, S., EISEN, A. A., WOLFE, L. S., and FEINDEL, W. (1974) Multiple peripheral nerve entrapments, *Arch. Neurol. (Chic.)*, **31**, 418.

LOVSHIN, L. L., and KERNOHAN, J. W. (1948) Peripheral neuritis in periarteritis nodosa, *Arch. intern. Med.*, **82**, 321.

RICHARDS, R. L. (1951) Ischaemic lesions of peripheral nerves: a review, *J. Neurol. Psychiat.*, **14**, 76.

'NEURITIS' OF THE FACE AND SCALP

Pain is commonly experienced in the distribution of one or more of the cutaneous nerves of the face and scalp and has been attributed to 'neuritis', but the nature of the pathological process in such cases is speculative. In some cases there may well be mechanical compression or irritation of the affected nerve, in others emotional tension is almost certainly a factor. The term 'neuritis' may reasonably be used to identify cases in which the aetiology cannot be identified with certainty provided it is not taken to imply the presence of a specific pathological process. Occasionally all the branches of one trigeminal nerve are involved. More frequently the affection is limited to one branch, usually the supra-orbital or auriculotemporal, less often the infra-orbital. The cutaneous distribution of the great occipital nerve is also a common site of pain.

SYMPTOMS

The onset is often acute, and pain in the face and scalp may follow a cold, tonsillitis, or an attack of influenza. The patient complains of pain situated within the distribution of the affected nerve. The pain usually occurs in paroxysms lasting for several hours, most frequently towards the close of the day, when he is fatigued. An attack of pain is also readily precipitated by exposure to cold. When the pain is severe it interferes with sleep. It is of a dull, aching character, intensified by exacerbations in which it is described as shooting along the course of the nerve. There is often hyperpathia in the area of skin supplied by the nerve, and when this includes the scalp it is noticed on combing and brushing the hair. The nerve trunk is tender on pressure, which causes irradiation of pain throughout the nerve. The cutaneous hypersensitivity is readily demonstrated by pricking with a pin.

DIAGNOSIS

There are numerous causes of paroxysmal pain in the face and scalp, and careful investigation is required to exclude other conditions before falling back on a diagnosis of 'neuritis'.

Infection of the nasal air sinuses is a common cause of such pain, frontal sinusitis being associated with supra-orbital pain, and infection of the maxillary antrum with pain in approximately the distribution of the infra-orbital nerve. In ethmoiditis the pain is chiefly at the root of the nose, and in infection of the sphenoidal sinus is usually referred to the forehead or occiput. In acute cases of sinus infection there is usually a history of influenza or a cold in the head with or without a purulent nasal discharge. There may be visible oedema over the frontal sinus or antrum. Transillumination and examination of the nose will usually reveal the site of infection, and in doubtful cases the sinuses should be X-rayed.

The tympanic membranes should always be examined to exclude a latent otitis media.

The teeth are a common cause of facial pain. Search should be made for carious teeth, and the possibility that there is an unerupted tooth must always be considered. This may be present, as may also a buried root, in an apparently edentulous patient, and can be detected only by X-ray examination. Pain of dental origin is often accentuated by chewing or by the ingestion of hot or cold foods. Pain on chewing, and radiating into the temple or down over the mandible, is also a feature of some cases of temporomandibular arthrosis due to dental malocclusion (Costen's syndrome). The pharynx should also be examined for the presence of a growth, which may occasionally cause pain referred to the ear and neck.

The eye is occasionally the source of referred neuralgic pain, the commonest ocular cause being glaucoma, which may be missed unless this possibility is borne in mind. Pain may also be referred to the face in disease of the heart and lungs as in the case of pain in the lower jaw developing on exertion in angina pectoris.

Intractable neuralgia may follow herpes zoster involving the first division of the trigeminal nerve. The history of the eruption and the residual scars render the diagnosis easy. Trigeminal neuralgia, by contrast, is distinguished by the brevity of the attacks of pain and the characteristic precipitating factors. Trigeminal neuropathy, usually giving numbness, but occasionally pain, is a rare manifestation of connective tissue disease, such as systemic lupus (Ashworth and Tait, 1971).

In migraine the headache occurs in attacks or paroxysms which are often associated with vomiting and preceded by the characteristic aura. There is usually a long history. Periodic migrainous neuralgia ('cluster headache') gives attacks of severe pain in and around the eye, lasting for up to two hours and occurring daily or twice daily in bouts lasting for several weeks or months.

Temporal or cranial arteritis occurs in the elderly and often gives rise to pain and tenderness in the scalp, particularly in the temporal and occipital regions; the temporal arteries are usually tortuous and tender and the erythrocyte sedimentation rate is raised.

Tabes is an occasional cause of paroxysmal pain in the face or scalp, but is readily recognized by its other clinical features.

The various intracranial causes of pain in the face and head must also be borne in mind, especially lesions of the trigeminal fibres in the brain stem such as syringobulbia, and thrombosis of the posterior inferior cerebellar artery, in both of which pain is usually associated with analgesia and thermo-anaesthesia.

Occipital pain may be due to lesions of the cervical region of the spinal cord or of the vertebral column at this level, especially cervical spondylosis. Pain and stiffness in the neck and occipital muscles ('stiff neck') is often a banal, self-limiting disorder of undetermined cause, but has been noted occasionally to occur in epidemic forms ('epidemic cervical myalgia'—Davies, 1960); a viral aetiology has been postulated but remains unproven.

Psychogenic pain is distinguished by its lack of relation to a nerve trunk, its failure, often, to respond to analgesic drugs, and by the patient's exaggerated emotional reaction to the pain. However, it must be stressed that chronic tension of the muscles attached to the scalp, occurring in association with anxiety and/or depression, may give rise to pain of exactly the type described, and this is not infrequently unilateral. This is particularly true of the so-called 'atypical facial pain' which usually occurs in the upper jaw in young or middle-aged women and which is often attributed erroneously to 'neuritis' but which in the great majority of cases is of purely psychogenic origin. Other aspects of the differential diagnosis of facial pain are also considered on page 176.

PROGNOSIS

In most cases the prognosis in patients with acute episodes of pain in the face and scalp is good and there is a rapid response to treatment. Occasionally, however, especially in individuals of a neurotic temperament, the pain proves intractable.

TREATMENT

The first essential is to exclude the organic causes of facial pain referred to above by means of appropriate investigations. Simple analgesic drugs are often effective but the fact that many cases respond even more satisfactorily to a combination of antidepressive and tranquillizing remedies is sufficient to indicate that in a high proportion of such cases there is no organic cause for the pain.

If a pain persists despite the measures outlined it is occasionally necessary to inject the nerve trunk with 2 per cent procaine solution, the supra-orbital nerve being injected at the supra-orbital notch, the infra-orbital at its foramen, by the methods described in the section on trigeminal neuralgia. The great occipital nerve can be similarly injected, and when occipital pain is due to cervical myalgia relief may sometimes be obtained from procaine injection of any tender spots in the muscles. Posterior cervical and/or occipital pain in spondylosis will sometimes require temporary immobilization in a cervical collar.

BRACHIAL NEURITIS

The term 'brachial neuritis' was formerly used to describe the symptoms which are now known usually to be caused by radiculopathy due to cervical spondylosis. No distinctive clinical picture of true brachial neuritis exists and like 'sciatic neuritis' the term has ceased to serve a useful purpose.

SHOULDER-GIRDLE NEURITIS (NEURALGIC AMYOTROPHY)

Localized neuritis of one or more nerves innervating the shoulder-girdle muscles was well recognized before the Second World War and was also observed during the war, especially in the Near East (Spillane, 1943; Parsonage and Turner, 1948). The patients were often in hospital for an operation or acute infection. Pain is usually the initial symptom; it may be intense for several days and is followed by muscular wasting and weakness. The muscles most often affected are the serratus anterior, spinati, deltoid, and trapezius in that order. When the deltoid is involved there may be sensory loss over the distribution of the axillary (circumflex) nerve. More recent experience has shown that in more than a third of cases there is no history of antecedent illness, infection, or trauma, that other muscles including biceps and forearm muscles are less commonly involved, that clinical and/or electrophysiological evidence (slowing of nerve conduction with electromyographic evidence of denervation) gives evidence of bilateral brachial plexus involvement in about one-quarter of all cases, and that very rarely there is a mild lymphocytic pleocytosis or rise in protein in the cerebrospinal fluid (Weikers and Mattson, 1969; Tsairis et al., 1972). Despite the severity of the initial pain and/or paralysis, recovery of muscle power is usually excellent, beginning within one or two months, but complete functional recovery may take up to three years or longer (Tsairis et al., 1972); only occasionally is paralysis permanent, especially in deltoid or serratus anterior. The cause is unknown but an identical syndrome may follow 7–10 days after the injection of foreign serum ('serum neuropathy'). Treatment is symptomatic; in the first few days pain of an intense burning character in the shoulder and arm may be so severe that powerful analgesics are required. When the acute phase is over, active exercises should be encouraged as soon as possible.

INTERCOSTAL NEUROPATHY

Intercostal neuropathy is a rare disorder which is diagnosed much more frequently than it occurs. It is characterized by paroxysmal pain throughout the distribution of an intercostal nerve, associated frequently with cutaneous tenderness in the area supplied by the nerve, especially at the point of emergence of its lateral cutaneous branch. Before diagnosing this condition the utmost care must be taken to exclude the many other disorders which may be associated with similar pain which may be due to inflammation of spinal dorsal roots, especially in syphilis or arachnoiditis, or their compression by a neoplasm of the spinal cord. It may precede or follow an attack of herpes zoster. The spinal nerve may be compressed as a result of localized collapse of the vertebral column, most commonly due to tuberculous caries, secondary carcinoma, or traumatic lesions. Spondylosis is often associated with root pains, and these may also be produced by scoliosis. Pleurisy, both tuberculous and neoplastic, is sometimes mistakenly diagnosed as intercostal neuralgia, and the thorax is a common site of referred pain in visceral disease, especially diseases of the upper abdominal viscera including cholecystitis and carcinoma of the body or tail of the pancreas. Pain in the distribution of an intercostal nerve is also seen in some patients after thoracotomy and may be intractable. Another important, if uncommon, cause of this syndrome is the so-called 'rib-tip' syndrome due to increased mobility of the anterior ends of the lower ribs (*British Medical Journal*, 1976).

TREATMENT

Intercostal neuropathy should be treated with analgesics. Local anaesthetic injections may give temporary relief and if all else fails the nerve may be injected with alcohol or phenol, care being taken that the needle does not penetrate the pleura. In occasional cases, surgical division of two or three intercostal nerves close to the spine may be needed but even after this operation pain may recur after a few months. Even posterior rhizotomy at the appropriate levels does not always afford permanent relief.

FEMORAL 'NEURITIS'

The term femoral 'neuritis' dates from the time when sciatica was attributed to sciatic neuritis and a similar clinical picture within the distribution of the femoral nerve was thought to be due to an inflammation of its roots. It is now recognized, however, that this syndrome is often due to an intervertebral disc protrusion in the upper lumbar spine, pain being referred into the third or fourth lumbar dermatome and accompanied by wasting and weakness of the quadriceps and diminution or loss of the knee-jerk. It may also be due to diabetes ('diabetic amyotrophy'), to ischaemia as in 'mononeuritis multiplex' due to polyarteritis nodosa and other disorders, or to involvement of the nerve in inflammatory or neoplastic processes in the pelvis. Treatment depends upon the nature of the lesion. Thage (1974) gives a detailed review of the causes of weakness and wasting of the quadriceps muscle, including femoral neuropathy.

SCIATIC 'NEURITIS'

As in the case of brachial and femoral 'neuritis' it is now doubtful whether true sciatic 'neuritis' ever occurs except as part of a more diffuse inflammatory or toxic process involving many nerves. Isolated sciatic nerve lesions almost invariably prove to be due to trauma or to compression of the nerve or of its component roots.

REFERENCES

ASHWORTH, B., and TAIT, G. B. W. (1971) Trigeminal neuropathy in connective tissue disease, *Neurology* (*Minneap.*), **21,** 609.
BRADLEY, W. G. (1974) *Disorders of Peripheral Nerves*, Oxford.
BRITISH MEDICAL JOURNAL (1976) Rib pain, *Brit. med. J.*, **1,** 358.
DAVIES, D. M. (1960) Epidemic cervical myalgia, *Lancet*, **i,** 1275.
HARRIS, W. (1926) *Neuritis and Neuralgia*, London.
PARSONAGE, M. J., and TURNER, J. W. A. (1948) Neuralgic amyotrophy. The shoulder-girdle syndrome, *Lancet*, **i,** 973.
SPILLANE, J. D. (1943) Localized neuritis of the shoulder girdle, *Lancet*, **ii,** 532.
SUNDERLAND, S. (1968) *Nerves and Nerve Injuries*, Edinburgh and London.
TAYLOR, R. A. (1960) Heredofamilial mononeuritis multiplex with brachial predilection, *Brain*, **83,** 113.
THAGE, O. (1974) *Quadriceps Weakness and Wasting. A Neurological, Electrophysiological and Histological Study*, Copenhagen.
TSAIRIS, P., DYCK, P. J., and MULDER, D. W. (1972) Natural history of brachial plexus neuropathy, *Arch. Neurol.* (*Chic.*), **27,** 109.
WEIKERS, N. J., and MATTSON, R. H. (1969) Acute paralytic brachial neuritis, *Neurology* (*Minneap.*), **19,** 1153.

POLYNEURITIS (POLYNEUROPATHY)

Synonyms. Multiple symmetrical peripheral neuritis; multiple neuritis.

Definition. Polyneuritis is a clinical picture, the essential feature of which is an impairment of function of many peripheral nerves simultaneously, resulting in a symmetrical distribution of flaccid muscular weakness, and usually also of sensory disturbances, affecting as a rule the distal more than the proximal segments of the limbs, and sometimes also involving the cranial nerves. A simultaneous disorder of cerebral function, leading to mental disturbances, is sometimes associated. Polyneuritis thus defined may be caused by a very large number of agencies, which may operate in many different ways and even at different points of the peripheral nerves. Among such agencies are numerous endogenous and exogenous toxins, acute inflammatory processes which directly attack the nerves, ischaemia, and numerous metabolic disorders including vitamin deficiency.

Peripheral neuritis was recorded by Lettsom in 1789 and an epidemic in Paris was described by Robert Graves in 1828. Todd first conceived that the terminal branches of the peripheral nerves might undergo degeneration, and this was demonstrated pathologically by Dumenil in 1864. Joffroy in 1879 contributed to the classification of polyneuritis and Grainger Stewart gave it the name multiple symmetrical peripheral neuritis in 1881. Korsakow described the mental changes sometimes associated with alcoholic polyneuritis in 1889.

As Simpson (1962) pointed out, except in the case of leprosy, true inflammation in peripheral nerves is relatively uncommon and most such disorders are more correctly termed 'neuropathy'. Recent pathological studies have demonstrated that many polyneuropathies are demyelinating (the myelin sheath and/or Schwann cell are attacked by the disease) but some are due to axonal degeneration, often with secondary demyelination. In demyelinating neuropathies nerve conduction is usually markedly delayed, while in axonal degenerations there may be no conduction at all, or, if denervation is partial, the surviving axons conduct at a normal rate.

While many forms of polyneuropathy affect both sensory and motor fibres, some appear to involve motor fibres selectively and others sensory fibres, while there is now good evidence to indicate that sometimes heavily myelinated, rapidly conducting fibres are predominantly involved, while in other cases finely myelinated or even unmyelinated fibres are attacked. Some processes which involve the axon primarily appear to involve its entire length, others begin distally ('dying-back' neuropathies). The factors which determine such selective involvement of Schwann cells, myelin, axons, and different classes of fibres are still poorly understood (Bradley, 1974; Dyck *et al.*, 1975).

AETIOLOGY

The following classification includes the most important causes (see also *Classification of the Neuromuscular Diseases—Research Group on Neuromuscular Diseases of the World Federation of Neurology*, 1968 and as revised by Gardner-Medwin and Walton, 1974):

1. TOXIC SUBSTANCES

(a) *Metals*: Antimony, arsenic, bismuth, copper, lead, mercury (pink disease, Minimata disease), phosphorus, thallium.

(b) *Drugs, organic chemicals, and other toxic substances*: Acrylamide, aniline, 'bush tea', carbon monoxide, carbon bisulphide, carbon tetrachloride, chloral, chloretone, chloroquine, clioquinol, cyanogenetic glycosides, cytotoxic agents including vincristine sulphate, DDT, dinitrobenzol, disulfiram, emetine, ethionamide, glutethimide, immune sera, isoniazid, n-hexane, nitrofurantoin, pentachlorphenol, phenytoin, stilbamidine, streptomycin, sulphanilamide and its compounds, sulphonal, tetrachlorethane, thalidomide, trichlorethylene, triorthocresylphosphate (ginger paralysis and apiol paralysis).

2. DEFICIENCY, METABOLIC, AND HAEMATOLOGICAL DISORDERS

Beriberi, chronic alcoholism, famine oedema, folic acid deficiency, liver disease and chronic diseases of (including coeliac disease) and operations on the gastro-intestinal tract, pellagra, pregnancy, tropical neuropathy, vitamin B_{12} neuropathy.

Acromegaly, diabetes, hyperinsulinism, myxoedema, porphyria, uraemia.

Neuropathy in A-alpha and beta-lipoproteinaemia and in dysglobulinaemia.

Neuropathy in polycythaemia vera, leukaemia, and haemorrhagic disorders.

3. INFECTIVE CONDITIONS

(a) *Local infection of nerves*: Brucellosis, leprosy, leptospirosis, and possibly infective mononucleosis, very rarely syphilis.

(b) *Polyneuritis complicating acute or chronic infections*: Dysentery, focal infection, gonorrhoea, influenza, malaria, measles, meningitis, mumps, paratyphoid, puerperal sepsis, scarlet fever, septicaemia, smallpox, syphilis, tuberculosis, typhoid, typhus.

(c) *Infections with organisms whose toxins have an affinity for the peripheral nerves*: Diphtheria, dysentery, tetanus.

4. POST-INFECTIVE (?ALLERGIC) POLYNEUROPATHY

(a) Acute post-infective polyradiculoneuropathy (the Guillain–Barré syndrome).

(b) Some cases of subacute and chronic polyneuropathy.

(c) ?Recurrent polyneuropathy.

5. TRAUMA

Physical injury and nerve entrapment, electric shock, and radiation injury.

6. CONNECTIVE TISSUE AND ALLIED DISORDERS

Giant-cell arteritis, polyarteritis nodosa, rheumatoid polyneuritis, sarcoidosis, systemic lupus erythematosus, systemic sclerosis, other vascular neuropathies including peripheral vascular disease.

7. GENETICALLY DETERMINED POLYNEUROPATHY

Peroneal muscular atrophy, the Roussy–Levy syndrome, progressive hypertrophic polyneuritis of Dejerine and Sottas, Refsum's syndrome, hereditary neuropathy with liability to pressure palsies, neuropathy in metachromatic leucodystrophy, in the Krabbe form of diffuse sclerosis and in other leukodystrophies and storage disorders, in primary amyloidosis, in porphyria, in Fabry's disease, in A-alpha and beta-lipoproteinaemia and various other obscure varieties of hereditary neuropathy including neuropathic arthrogryposis multiplex congenita, so-called 'globular' neuropathy, neuropathy with optic atrophy, nerve deafness and/or paraproteinaemia [see Bradley, 1974; Gardner-Medwin and Walton, 1974; Dyck et al., 1975, and pp. 669–711].

8. POLYNEURITIS OF OBSCURE ORIGIN

Recurrent polyneuritis. Chronic progressive polyneuritis.
Carcinomatous neuropathy, myelomatosis.

In some cases a toxin is introduced into the body from without. In others it is formed within the body as a result of bacterial action or of metabolic disturbances. Yet again the source may be impossible to define. Sometimes the toxin appears to possess a specific affinity for the peripheral nerves, and it has been suggested that it may combine with the phospholipids of the myelin sheaths. Many such toxins probably ascend the peripheral nerves. We thus encounter both a local neuritis involving the nerves supplying the region in which the toxin originates, for example, palatal paralysis in diphtheria, and also generalized polyneuritis, in which the toxin is disseminated in the blood stream and so reaches the peripheral nerves throughout the body, subsequently ascending them from their terminations.

The role of avitaminosis in the causation of polyneuritis is more complex than used to be thought and is discussed on page 844. In the infective disorders listed above, there is as yet little evidence, except in leprosy, to show that axons or myelin sheaths are directly damaged by the infecting organisms; in many such disorders the injury to the peripheral nerves is presumed to be either toxic or due to a hypersensitivity reaction, either cell-mediated or humoral in type. Certainly, both cytotoxic factors in serum and immunoglobulin abnormalities (Rosenberg et al., 1975) on the one hand and evidence of cell-mediated immunity to neural antigens on the other (Abramsky et al., 1975) have been found in different forms of polyneuropathy. In neuropathy secondary to the various connective tissue disorders, ischaemia resulting from damage to the vasa nervorum certainly plays an important role. In the group of genetically determined polyneuropathies the primary enzymatic defect which may be responsible for the storage of identifiable material in peripheral nerves as well as in other organs has been identified in some disorders as in Refsum's disease and several of the leukodystrophies [see pp. 647 and 651]. However, in most of these conditions the nature of the underlying abnormality is still unknown despite recent studies of the biochemical composition of normal and abnormal nerves (Bradley, 1974; Dyck *et al.*, 1975) and despite experimental studies in animals of the axoplasmic flow of radioactive protein in the normal state and in various forms of toxic neuropathy (Bradley and Williams, 1973).

PATHOLOGY

There have been important recent advances in knowledge concerning the pathology of peripheral neuropathy (polyneuritis) of various types. These have come partly from post-mortem studies but have been based more particularly on experimental studies in animals and upon nerve biopsy studies in patients (Thomas, 1970; Stevens *et al.*, 1973; Dyck *et al.*, 1975), utilizing techniques for the examination of single teased nerve fibres stained with osmic acid. Measurement of internodal length (the distance between nodes of Ranvier) in such teased fibres is an important part of the examination. Methods involving osmic acid staining of transverse sections of nerves in which fibres can be counted and their diameters measured have also made valuable contributions [FIGS. 138–41], as has electron microscopy. The sural nerve is the one most conveniently biopsied but has the occasional disadvantage that, being wholly sensory, it is not invariably diseased in neuropathies which are predominantly motor in type. The information derived from these studies must be carefully assessed in relation to known changes in fibre number and diameter and in internodal length observed in various peripheral nerves in subjects of varying age (Swallow, 1966; Lascelles and Thomas, 1966; O'Sullivan and Swallow, 1968; Ochoa and Mair, 1969 *a* and *b*). The ultrastructural abnormalities seen in both Wallerian degeneration (Thomas, 1964; Ballin and Thomas, 1969) and segmental demyelination (Weller and Nester, 1972) must also be carefully assessed with special techniques required to avoid artefact and in the knowledge of variations which may be observed in normal appearances. The importance of examining unmyelinated as well as myelinated fibres has recently been stressed (Peyronnard *et al.*, 1973; Behse *et al.*, 1975). Such studies have demonstrated that in many forms of neuropathy (in diphtheria, the Guillain-Barré syndrome, carcinomatous neuropathy, familial hypertrophic neuropathy, and metachromatic leucodystrophy) the disease process affects predominantly the Schwann cells and results in segmental demyelination of peripheral nerves, with a progressive shrinkage of the myelin away from the nodes of Ranvier and the eventual denuding of axons which frequently remain intact. In this phase, conduction in the affected nerves is markedly slowed. Occasionally in demyelination, sausage-shaped myelin swellings (so-called 'tomaculous neuropathy') are found, but the specificity of this change is in doubt (Madrid and Bradley, 1975). Recovery is accompanied by remyelination but the newly-formed myelin is often thinner than normal and the internodal distances are less than normal; however, nerve conduction velocity may recover eventually to normal. Repeated demyelination and remyelination may lead to Schwann cell proliferation, 'onion-bulb' formation [FIG. 142, p. 947] and ultimately to palpable hypertrophy of nerves (Thomas and Lascelles, 1967). In other forms of neuropathy (Gilliatt,

1966) including those due to alcoholism, porphyria, triorthocresylphosphate, isoniazid, vincristine, and thalidomide, the process appears to be one of axonal degeneration and segmental demyelination is slight or absent at first so that nerve conduction velocity is reduced comparatively little. In the neuropathies due to lead and acrylamide (Fullerton, 1966; Fullerton and Barnes, 1966) both the axons and their myelin sheaths may be affected simultaneously. In diabetes, too, segmental demyelination may come first but is quickly followed by axonal degeneration. Recent studies have plainly indicated that the distinction between demyelinating and axonal neuropathies is often less precise than was thought to be the case only a few years ago, especially when the process is advanced, as axonal degeneration is often followed quickly by secondary demyelination and vice versa (Bradley, 1974; Dyck *et al.*, 1975). Nevertheless, in early cases the distinction remains valid and is often of some diagnostic value.

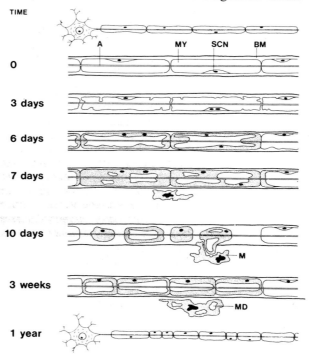

FIG. 138. Diagrammatic representation of the successive changes occurring during segmental demyelination and remyelination as in diphtheritic neuropathy. The axon (A) remains intact throughout but the myelin (MY) breaks down. There is activation of Schwann cells with division of their nuclei (SCN). Regeneration occurs within the basement membrane (BM). Both activated Schwann cells and macrophages (M) take part in the digestion of myelin debris (MD). Some internodes (sections of myelin between nodes of Ranvier) remain intact, others are damaged, and after remyelination abnormally short internodes are formed so that the nerve, after recovery, shows marked variation in internodal length. (Diagram reproduced from *Disorders of Peripheral Nerves* by W. G. Bradley, Blackwells, Oxford 1974, by kind permission of the author and publishers.)

SYMPTOMS AND PROGNOSIS

The symptoms and prognosis and further details of the pathology of the commoner and more important forms of polyneuropathy are described under their respective headings.

DIAGNOSIS

As a rule the diagnosis of polyneuritis is easy, owing to the characteristic symmetrical and peripheral distribution of the muscular weakness and wasting, pain, tenderness, and sensory impairment. The position is not so straight-forward

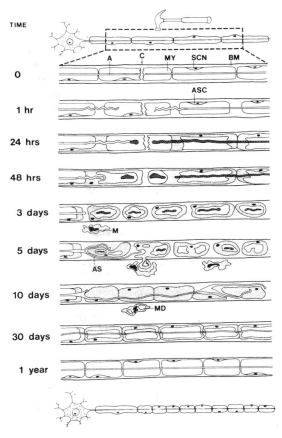

FIG. 139. Diagrammatic representation of changes occurring in a peripheral nerve distal to a traumatic lesion causing axonotmesis. At the level of the lesion (C) (e.g. a crush) there is disruption of the axon with fragmentation both of the axon and of the myelin sheath. The Schwann cells are activated and broken down myelin is digested by both Schwann cells and macrophages. The axon sprouts from the fifth day onwards and the Schwann cells begin to form new myelin sheaths from the tenth day. After regeneration, distal to the crush, all internodes are abnormally short (from Bradley (1974), reproduced by kind permission of the author and publishers)

H h

when the symptoms and signs are predominantly motor or sensory, or asymmetrical, or predominant in the lower limbs, or in those occasional cases in which proximal muscular weakness is more striking at first, when a variety of other neurological disorders may be mimicked. Electrical measurements of motor and sensory nerve conduction are invaluable in establishing the peripheral nerves as the site of the lesion and in indicating whether it is predominantly

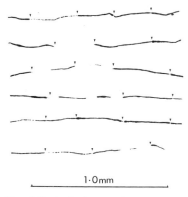

1·0mm

FIG. 140. A single teased nerve fibre, stained with osmic acid, from a case of hypertrophic neuropathy. Consecutive lengths of the single fibre are mounted below one another. Arrowheads mark the position of the nodes of Ranvier. None of the internodes is of normal length (about 1·0 mm in a fibre of 10 μm diameter) and there is extensive demyelination and remyelination with marked variation in internodal length (from Bradley (1974), reproduced by kind permission of the author and publishers)

demyelinating or axonal. The association of pain, ataxia, and loss of tendon reflexes in the lower limbs may simulate tabes. The pain of polyneuritis, however, when present, is of a persistent, burning character and is quite different from the lightning pains of tabes, and is associated with tenderness of the deep tissues on pressure, whereas in tabes these are insensitive. Although the pupillary reaction to light may be sluggish in polyneuritis, especially in the alcoholic and diabetic forms, a true Argyll Robertson pupil is never found (except, rarely, in peroneal muscular atrophy), and the V.D.R.L. reaction is negative, except in patients who happen to suffer both from syphilis and from polyneuritis. As stated elsewhere, some of the symptoms of subacute combined degeneration are due to an associated polyneuritis. The true cause of these symptoms, however, is usually easily established by the presence of extensor plantar responses, impairment of appreciation of vibration over the trunk as well as the limbs, and the presence of anaemia, glossitis, and gastric achylia, though the last may be present in patients suffering from polyneuritis due to other causes. When weakness predominates in proximal limb muscles as in some cases of the Guillain–Barré syndrome, diagnosis from polymyositis or motor neurone disease may not be easy clinically but is usually helped greatly by electromyography, nerve conduction velocity measurement, and examination of the CSF. When a diagnosis of polyneuritis has been made, the diagnosis of the cause is based upon distinctive features of the history and symptoms peculiar to the different varieties, and upon investigative findings which are described under their respective headings.

TREATMENT

The first step in treatment is the removal of the patient from exposure to the causal toxin, if this can be identified, and its elimination from the body, or the correction of abnormal metabolic states or vitamin deficiency. The necessary steps are described in the sections dealing with the various forms of polyneuritis. In certain acute forms of polyneuritis (e.g. the Guillain–Barré syndrome) assisted respiration and intensive care may be needed if the respiratory muscles are involved. Some varieties (as in connective tissue disease) are steroid-responsive and a course of treatment with prednisone or ACTH may reasonably be given in any case of subacute, predominantly demyelinating polyneuropathy

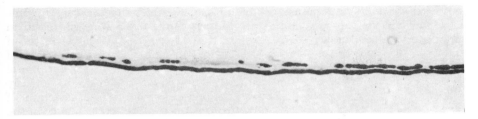

FIG. 141. A pair of teased myelinated nerve fibres stained with osmic acid. The upper fibre is fragmented into myelin ovoids as a result of axonal degeneration; the lower fibre is intact (from Bradley (1974), reproduced by kind permission of the author and publishers)

for which no cause can be found, especially if the protein content of the CSF is raised. The role of such treatment in the Guillain–Barré syndrome remains controversial (see below).

Rest in bed is essential only when the severity of the muscular weakness is such that the patient cannot walk or in those forms of polyneuritis (such as beriberi) in which the heart is also involved. In the more usual cases, continuing activity is important.

Local treatment consists of the prevention of muscular contractures, the maintenance of the nutrition of the muscles, and the promotion of the recovery of voluntary power. Wrist-drop and foot-drop must be prevented by the use of appropriate splints. As long as muscular tenderness is severe, splints cannot be borne, and the feet must then be supported by means of a sandbag placed beneath the soles, the weight of the bed-clothes being taken by a cradle. Later, aluminium or plastic night-shoes may be used to support the feet at a right angle. When contractures have already developed they must be overcome by appropriate physical means. Daily active and passive movements should be

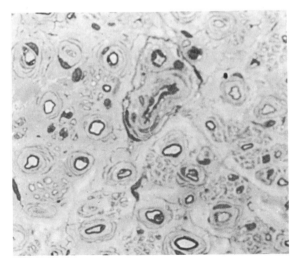

FIG. 142. Transverse section of a 1 μm araldite section of peripheral nerve stained with toluidine blue showing multiple 'onion-bulbs'; sural nerve biopsy from a case of hypertrophic neuropathy (kindly supplied by Dr. R. Madrid)

instituted as soon as the patient is able to bear them. Analgesic drugs will be required when the pain is severe. A useful review of the principles of treatment has been given by Bradley (1975).

REFERENCES

ABRAMSKY, O., WEBB, C., TEITELBAUM, D., and ARNON, R. (1975) Cell-mediated immunity to neural antigens in idiopathic polyneuritis and myeloradiculitis, *Neurology (Minneap.)*, **25,** 1154.

BALLIN, R. H. M., and THOMAS, P. K. (1969) Changes at the nodes of Ranvier during Wallerian degeneration: an electron microscope study, *Acta neuropath. (Berl.)*, **14,** 237.

BEHSE, F., BUCHTHAL, F., CARLSEN, F., and KNAPPEIS, G. G. (1975) Unmyelinated fibres and Schwann cells of sural nerve in neuropathy, *Brain*, **98,** 493.

BRADLEY, W. G. (1974) *Disorders of Peripheral Nerves*, Oxford.

BRADLEY, W. G. (1975) The treatment of polyneuropathy, *The Practitioner*, **215,** 452.

BRADLEY, W. G., and WILLIAMS, M. H. (1973) Axoplasmic flow in axonal neuropathies— I. Axoplasmic flow in cats with toxic neuropathies, *Brain*, **96,** 235.

DYCK, P. J., THOMAS, P. K., and LAMBERT, E. H. (1975) *Peripheral Neuropathy*, Philadelphia.

FULLERTON, P. M. (1966) Chronic peripheral neuropathy produced by lead poisoning in guinea-pigs, *J. Neuropath. exp. Neurol.*, **25,** 214.

FULLERTON, P. M., and BARNES, J. M. (1966) Peripheral neuropathy in rats produced by acrylamide, *Brit. J. industr. Med.*, **23,** 210.

GARDNER-MEDWIN, D., and WALTON, J. N. (1974) *Appendix to* The clinical examination of the voluntary muscles, in *Disorders of Voluntary Muscle*, 3rd ed., ed. Walton, J. N., p. 546, Edinburgh and London.

GILLIATT, R. W. (1966) Nerve conduction in human and experimental neuropathies, *Proc. roy. Soc. Med.*, **59,** 989.

LASCELLES, R. G., and THOMAS, P. K. (1966) Changes due to age in internodal length in the sural nerve in man, *J. Neurol. Neurosurg. Psychiat.*, **29,** 40.

MADRID, R., and BRADLEY, W. G. (1975) The pathology of neuropathies with focal thickening of the myelin sheath (tomaculous neuropathy), *J. neurol. Sci.*, **25,** 415.

MILLER, H. G. (1966) Polyneuritis, *Brit. med. J.*, **2,** 1219.

OCHOA, J., and MAIR, W. G. P. (1969 *a*) The normal sural nerve in man. I. Ultrastructure and numbers of fibres and cells, *Acta neuropath. (Berl.)*, **13,** 197.

OCHOA, J., and MAIR, W. G. P. (1969 *b*) The normal sural nerve in man. II. Changes in the axons and Schwann cells due to ageing, *Acta neuropath. (Berl.)*, **13,** 217.

O'SULLIVAN, D. J., and SWALLOW, M. (1968) The fibre size and content of the radial and sural nerves, *J. Neurol. Neurosurg. Psychiat.*, **31,** 464.

PEYRONNARD, J.-M., AGUAYO, A. J., and BRAY, G. M. (1973) Schwann cell internuclear distances in normal and regenerating unmyelinated nerve fibers, *Arch. Neurol. (Chic.)*, **29,** 56.

RESEARCH GROUP ON NEUROMUSCULAR DISEASES (1968) Classification of the neuro-muscular disorders, *J. neurol. Sci.*, **6,** 165.

ROSENBERG, R. N., AUNG, M. H., TINDALL, R. S. A., MOLENICH, S., BASKIN, F., CAPRA, J. D., and TOBEN, H. R. (1975) Idiopathic polyneuropathy associated with cytotoxic anti-neuroblastoma serum, *Neurology (Minneap.)*, **25,** 1101.

SIMPSON, J. A. (1962) The neuropathies, in *Modern Trends in Neurology*, 3rd series, ed. Williams, D., London.

SIMPSON, J. A. (1964) Biology and disease of peripheral nerves, *Brit. med. J.*, **2,** 709.

STEVENS, J. C., LOFGREN, E. P., and DYCK, P. J. (1973) Histometric evaluation of branches of peroneal nerve: technique for combined biopsy of muscle nerve and cutaneous nerve, *Brain Research*, **52,** 37.

SWALLOW, M. (1966) Fibre size and content of the anterior tibial nerve of the foot, *J. Neurol. Neurosurg. Psychiat.*, **29,** 205.

Thage, O., Trojaborg, W., and Buchthal, F. (1963) Electromyographic findings in polyneuropathy, *Neurology (Minneap.)*, **13**, 273.

Thomas, P. K. (1964) Changes in the endoneurial sheaths of peripheral myelinated nerve fibres during Wallerian degeneration, *J. Anat. (Lond.)*, **98**, 175.

Thomas, P. K. (1970) The quantitation of nerve biopsy findings, *J. neurol. Sci.*; **11**, 285.

Thomas, P. K., and Lascelles, R. G. (1967) Hypertrophic neuropathy, *Quart. J. Med.*, **36**, 223.

Weller, R. O., and Nester, B. (1972) Early changes at the node of Ranvier in segmental demyelination: histochemical and electron microscopic observations, *Brain*, **95**, 665.

ACUTE POST-INFECTIVE POLYNEURITIS

Synonyms. Acute infectious polyneuritis; febrile polyneuritis; Guillain–Barré syndrome; post-infective polyradiculoneuropathy.

Definition. An acute diffuse post-infective disease of the nervous system involving the spinal roots and peripheral nerves, and occasionally the cranial nerves.

AETIOLOGY

Acute post-infective polyneuritis or polyradiculoneuropathy is now one of the commonest forms of polyneuritis in Great Britain. A number of cases were observed among troops during the 1914–18 war (Guillain *et al.*, 1916; Holmes, 1917; Bradford *et al.*, 1918). The condition may occur in either sex and at any age but is uncommon in early childhood, and often has a peak incidence between 20 and 50 years of age (Marshall, 1963) but a bimodal age distribution has been noted in some reported series of cases (McFarland and Heller, 1966; Eisen and Humphreys, 1974) with one group occurring between 15 and 30 years, another between 40 and 65. In Olmsted County, Minnesota, the mean annual incidence was 1·6 per 100,000 of the population (Lesser *et al.*, 1973). Although this syndrome is clearly defined it is by no means certain that all cases are of uniform aetiology. In the past it was known as acute infective polyneuritis but no infecting organism has been isolated consistently from such cases though it has been known to follow a variety of specific and non-specific infective illnesses, and may arise apparently spontaneously. Associations with infectious mononucleosis (Raftery *et al.*, 1954) or subclinical Epstein-Barr virus infection (Grose and Feorino, 1972), measles (Lidin-Janson and Strannegard, 1972), cytomegalovirus infection (Leonard and Tobin, 1971), mycoplasma infection (*British Medical Journal*, 1975), and immune complex nephritis (Behan *et al.*, 1973) have been reported and the condition has been reported to follow surgical operations (Arnason and Asbury, 1968). The current view is that it is an inflammatory disorder due to allergy or hypersensitivity, perhaps as a result of a variety of unidentified allergens, but the possibility still exists that some cases could be due to the direct invasion of peripheral nerves by one or more viruses. Waksman and Adams (1955) produced a similar condition in animals by injecting an emulsion of peripheral nerve to which they had been sensitized, and Asbury and Arnason (1968), Pollard *et al.* (1975) and King *et al.* (1975), among others, have studied monophasic and relapsing or recurrent experimental allergic neuritis. Lymphocyte sensitization to human sciatic nerve extract and to muscle has been described in such cases (Caspary *et al.*, 1971) and immunocytes have been identified in the circulating blood (Whitaker *et al.*, 1970; Cook *et al.*, 1970), but sera obtained from such patients may produce demyelination of cultures of peripheral nervous tissue *in vitro* (Cook *et al.*, 1971; Hirano *et al.*, 1971) so that it seems possible that humoral as well as cellular immune processes play a part in pathogenesis. A similar disorder has been observed in dogs following the bite of a racoon, so-called 'coonhound paralysis' (Cummings and Haas, 1967).

PATHOLOGY

Naked-eye abnormalities are slight and consist of variable congestion of the meninges, and in fatal cases there may be petechial haemorrhages in the substance of the spinal cord. Microscopically the spinal cord may exhibit chromatolysis of the ganglion cells, both of the anterior horns and of the dorsal roots, with slight perivascular infiltration with small, round cells. The spinal roots and peripheral nerves show marked demyelination, with proliferation of Schwann cells of the neurilemma, and in some cases swelling and fragmentation of the axis cylinders. There is a marked focal, perivascular lymphocytic inflammatory exudate (Asbury *et al.*, 1969) with a net-like or vesicular pattern of myelin disruption with relative sparing of axons and phagocytosis of myelin by macrophages (Wisniewski *et al.*, 1969). In long-standing cases denervation atrophy is found in the muscles. Perivascular inflammatory infiltration has been observed in the brain, and infiltration with round cells may be present in the liver, kidneys, and lungs, the kidneys sometimes showing evidence of immune complex nephritis (Behan *et al.*, 1973).

SYMPTOMS AND SIGNS

There is often an initial febrile illness in which no nervous symptoms appear, followed by a period of latency, which may last from a few days to several weeks, at the end of which paralysis develops. More frequently the patient first comes under observation in the paralytic stage, symptoms of the initial stage being slight or absent. There is now increasing evidence to indicate that some cases of subacute or chronic polyneuropathy are aetiologically similar [see p. 954].

Rarely there may be headache, vomiting, slight pyrexia, and pains in the back and limbs, sometimes associated with a feeling of stiffness in the neck. More often the paralytic symptoms, which are often the first manifestations but sometimes develop after the prodromal symptoms described, come on suddenly. Less frequently the onset of the paralytic symptoms is gradual. The paralysis may affect all four limbs simultaneously or may begin in the lower limbs and spread to the upper. In contrast with other forms of polyneuritis all the muscles of a limb are usually affected, those of the proximal segments suffering as much as, or even more severely than, those of the distal segments. Occasionally weakness is even limited to proximal limb muscles and may be asymmetrical. In severe cases the muscles of the neck and trunk are also involved, and there is often paralysis of the facial muscles on both sides, though this is occasionally unilateral (Kimura, 1971). Dysphagia may occur as a result of pharyngeal paralysis, but the palate usually escapes; respiratory muscle involvement requiring assisted respiration is an important complication in severe cases (Hewer *et al.*, 1968). External ophthalmoplegia is occasionally seen. In occasional cases the affection is confined to the cranial nerves (cranial polyneuritis or polyneuritis cranialis). The paralysed muscles are flaccid, but severe wasting is exceptional. Superficial and deep reflexes are usually diminished or lost, but may be retained in spite of weakness of voluntary movement in the muscles concerned. The sensory symptoms characteristic of polyneuritis are usually but not invariably present, and in the early stages the patient may complain of pain, numbness, and tingling in the limbs. All forms of sensibility may be impaired over the peripheral segments of the limbs and the muscles may be tender but even in the presence of typical paraesthesiae sensory abnormalities on examination are often conspicuous by their absence. Bilateral optic neuritis leading to visual impairment is rare but papilloedema is seen occasionally and is usually attributed to the greatly increased protein content of the CSF: bilateral deafness is even rarer. The sphincters are rarely involved and never to a severe extent, though there may at times be slight retention of urine necessitating catheterization. Cerebral symptoms are usually absent and consciousness is unclouded throughout, but a confusional state rarely develops.

General symptoms of toxaemia may be present, including tachycardia and slight cardiac dilatation (Clarke *et al.*, 1954), and albuminuria and an erythematous rash. The blood may show a moderate polymorphonuclear leucocytosis. The characteristic change in the cerebrospinal fluid is a great excess of protein (occasionally up to 1 g per 100 ml) with either a normal cell count, or at most only a moderate excess of mononuclear cells. This is the 'dissociation albumino-cytologique' stressed by Guillain *et al.* (1916). The fluid may be yellow or brown and clot spontaneously. The high protein may persist for many weeks even after recovery. Nevertheless the same clinical picture may coexist with a spinal fluid that is virtually normal, particularly in the early stages.

DIAGNOSIS

Acute post-infective polyneuritis is readily distinguished from other forms of polyneuritis by the acute onset, the rapid development of the paralysis, and the severe involvement of the proximal limb muscles. It is distinguished from poliomyelitis by the symmetrical character of the paralysis, the presence of sensory loss, by the CSF changes, and by the slightness or absence of muscular wasting in the later stages. Measurement of motor and sensory conduction velocity (Buchthal and Rosenfalck, 1971; Eisen and Humphreys, 1974; Burke *et al.*, 1974) is an invaluable aid to diagnosis, demonstrating slowing of conduction in the great majority of cases soon after the onset, and abnormalities of the F-wave (Kimura and Butzer, 1975) may help to confirm that the central segments of the peripheral nerves are predominantly involved. Many acute cases have been diagnosed in the past as examples of Landry's paralysis but for reasons given previously [p. 782] this disorder is a syndrome of multiple aetiology and this diagnostic label should no longer be used. Acute myelitis, especially the ascending form, may also cause widespread flaccid paralysis, but in this condition the plantar reflexes are usually extensor, sensory loss is more extensive and involves the whole body below the level of the lesion, and sphincter disturbances are present.

PROGNOSIS

The mortality rate of the disease was high in the past in some epidemics, death usually occurring from paralysis of the respiratory muscles, with or without terminal bronchopneumonia. Slight remissions were not infrequent, but were often followed by severe relapses. In sporadic cases, however, the outlook is usually good, but improvement is slow and the paralysis, having reached its height, tends to remain stationary for some weeks. Sometimes recovery is incomplete. In the most favourable cases the patient is not likely to be convalescent in less than from three to six months and in occasional cases the condition may smoulder on for one or two years but may nevertheless recover completely. Pleasure *et al.* (1968) found that more than half of a series of 49 patients followed on average for 11 years showed some persistent evidence of peripheral nerve damage and 16 per cent had a significant residual disability. Oppenheimer and Spalding (1973) suggested that if recovery had not occurred within two years it was unlikely to take place, but Osuntokun and Agbebi (1973) reported that 27 of a series of 34 Nigerian patients recovered completely, two died, and five improved but appeared to be steroid-dependent.

TREATMENT

In the past, no effective treatment for the condition was known but, among others, Graveson (1957) and Jackson *et al.* (1957) suggested that the condition could be effectively controlled by cortisone or corticotrophin (ACTH). While many workers employ these drugs in all cases and there is an impression that ACTH (80 units daily intramuscularly at first, reducing gradually but continuing maintenance dosage for several months or even up to one or two years) is more effective than prednisone, though some prefer the latter (Newman and Nelson, 1974), others are equally adamant that such treatment does not modify the natural history of the illness (Goodall *et al.*, 1974). Undoubtedly some cases appear to respond dramatically, relapse after withdrawal and respond again, but some appear totally steroid-resistant and the use of immunosuppressive agents has not been strikingly successful in some cases (Drachman *et al.*, 1970) but others have found azathioprine helpful (Yuill *et al.*, 1970). The usual treatment of polyneuritis must be carried out [see p. 946]. Much depends upon good nursing. Bulbar and respiratory paralysis should be treated with intermittent positive pressure respiration as in poliomyelitis [see p. 505].

Complications including respiratory infections will demand appropriate antibiotics. Hypernatraemia with water retention which occurs in occasional cases may demand diuretics (Posner *et al.*, 1967).

REFERENCES

ARNASON, B. G., and ASBURY, A. K. (1968) Idiopathic polyneuritis after surgery, *Arch. Neurol. (Chic.)*, **18**, 500.

ASBURY, A. K., and ARNASON, B. G. (1968) Experimental allergic neuritis: a radioautographic study, *J. Neuropath. exp. Neurol.*, **27**, 581.

ASBURY, A. K., ARNASON, B. G., and ADAMS, R. D. (1969) The inflammatory lesion in idiopathic polyneuritis, *Medicine*, **48**, 173.

BEHAN, P. O., LOWENSTEIN, L. M., STILMANT, M., and SAX, D. S. (1973) Landry-Guillain-Barré-Strohl syndrome and immune-complex nephritis, *Lancet*, **i**, 850.

BRADFORD, J. B., BASHFORD, E. F., and WILSON, J. A. (1918-19) Acute infective polyneuritis, *Quart. J. Med.*, **12**, 88.

BRITISH MEDICAL JOURNAL (1975) Guillain-Barré syndrome, *Brit. med. J.*, **3**, 190.

BUCHTHAL, F., and ROSENFALCK, A. (1971) Sensory potentials in polyneuropathy, *Brain*, **94**, 241.

BURKE, D., SKUSE, N. F., and LETHLEAN, A. K. (1974) Sensory conduction of the sural nerve in polyneuropathy, *J. Neurol. Neurosurg. Psychiat.*, **37**, 647.

CASPARY, E. A., CURRIE, S., WALTON, J. N., and FIELD, E. J. (1971) Lymphocyte sensitization to nervous tissue and muscle in patients with the Guillain-Barré syndrome, *J. Neurol. Neurosurg. Psychiat.*, **34**, 179.

CLARKE, E. S., BAYLISS, R. I. S., and COOPER, R. (1954) Cardiovascular manifestations of the Guillain-Barré syndrome, *Brit. med. J.*, **2**, 1504.

COOK, S. D., DOWLING, P. C., MURRAY, M. R., and WHITAKER, J. N. (1971) Circulating demyelinating factors in acute idiopathic polyneuropathy, *Arch. Neurol. (Chic.)*, **24**, 136.

COOK, S. D., DOWLING, P. C., and WHITAKER, J. N. (1970) The Guillain-Barré syndrome: relationship of circulating immunocytes to disease activity, *Arch. Neurol. (Chic.)*, **22**, 470.

CUMMINGS, J. F., and HAAS, D. C. (1967) Coonhound paralysis. An acute idiopathic polyradiculoneuritis in dogs resembling the Landry-Guillain-Barré syndrome, *J. neurol. Sci.*, **4**, 51.

DRACHMAN, D. A., PATERSON, P. Y., BERLIN, B. S., and ROGUSKA, J. (1970) Immuno-suppression and the Guillain-Barré syndrome, *Arch. Neurol. (Chic.)*, **23**, 385.

EISEN, A., and HUMPHREYS, P. (1974) The Guillain-Barré syndrome: a clinical and electro-diagnostic study of 25 cases, *Arch. Neurol. (Chic.)*, **30**, 438.

GOODALL, J. A. D., KOSMIDIS, J. C., and GEDDES, A. M. (1974) Effect of corticosteroids on course of Guillain-Barré syndrome, *Lancet*, **i**, 524.

GRAVESON, G. S. (1957) Acute polyneuritis treated with cortisone, *Lancet*, **i**, 340.

GROSE, C., and FEORINO, P. M. (1972) Epstein-Barr virus and Guillain-Barré syndrome, *Lancet*, **ii**, 1285.

GUILLAIN, G., BARRÉ, J. A., and STROHL, A. (1916) Sur un syndrome de radiculo-névrite avec hyperalbuminose du liquide céphalorachidien sans réaction cellulaire. Remarques sur les caractères cliniques et graphiques des réflexes tendineux, *Bull. Soc. méd. Hôp. Paris*, **40**, 1462.

GUILLAIN, G. (1938) *Les polyradiculonévrites avec dissociation albuminocytologique et à évolution favorable*, Brussels.

HAYMAKER, W., and KERNOHAN, J. W. (1949) The Landry-Guillain-Barré syndrome, *Medicine (Baltimore)*, **28**, 59.

HEWER, R. L., HILTON, P. J., CRAMPTON SMITH, A., and SPALDING, J. M. K. (1968) Acute polyneuritis requiring artificial respiration, *Quart. J. Med.*, **37**, 479.

HIRANO, A., COOK, S. D., WHITAKER, J. N., DOWLING, P. C., and MURRAY, M. R. (1971) Fine structural aspects of demyelination *in vitro*. The effects of Guillain-Barré serum, *J. Neuropath. exp. Neurol.*, **30**, 249.

HOLMES, G. (1917) Acute febrile polyneuritis, *Brit. med. J.*, **2**, 37.

JACKSON, R. H., MILLER, H., and SCHAPIRA, K. (1957) Polyradiculitis (Landry-Guillain-Barré syndrome). Treatment with cortisone and corticotrophin, *Brit. med. J.*, **1**, 480.

JANEWAY, R., and KELLY, D. (1966) Papilloedema and hydrocephalus associated with recurrent polyneuritis, *Arch. Neurol. (Chic.)*, **15**, 507.

KIMURA, J. (1971) An evaluation of the facial and trigeminal nerves in polyneuropathy: electrodiagnostic study in Charcot-Marie-Tooth disease, Guillain-Barré syndrome, and diabetic neuropathy, *Neurology (Minneap.)*, **21**, 745.

KIMURA, J., and BUTZER, J. F. (1975) F-wave conduction velocity in Guillain-Barré syndrome, *Arch. Neurol. (Chic.)*, **32**, 524.

KING, R. H. M., POLLARD, J. D., and THOMAS, P. K. (1975) Aberrant remyelination in chronic relapsing experimental allergic neuritis, *Neuropath. Applied Neurobiol.*, **1**, 367.

LEONARD, J. C., and TOBIN, J. O'H. (1971) Polyneuritis associated with cytomegalovirus infections, *Quart. J. Med.*, **40**, 435.

LESSER, R. P., HAUSER, W. A., KURLAND, L. T., and MULDER, D. W. (1973) Epidemiologic features of the Guillain-Barré syndrome: experience in Olmsted County, Minnesota, 1935 through 1968, *Neurology (Minneap.)*, **23**, 1269.

LIDIN-JANSON, G., and STRANNEGARD, O. (1972) Two cases of Guillain-Barré syndrome and encephalitis after measles, *Brit. med. J.*, **2**, 572.

MCFARLAND, H. R., and HELLER, G. L. (1966) Guillain-Barré disease complex: a statement of diagnostic criteria and analysis of 100 cases, *Arch. Neurol. (Chic.)*, **14**, 196.

MARSHALL, J. (1963) The Landry-Guillain-Barré syndrome, *Brain*, **86**, 55.

NEWMAN, M. J., and NELSON, N. (1974) Treatment of subacute polyneuritis with corticosteroids, *Canad. J. neurol. Sci.*, **1**, 180.

OPPENHEIMER, D. R., and SPALDING, J. M. K. (1973) Late residua of acute idiopathic polyneuritis, *J. Neurol. Neurosurg. Psychiat.*, **36**, 978.

OSUNTOKUN, B. O., and AGBEBI, K. (1973) Prognosis of Guillain–Barré syndrome in the African: the Nigerian experience, *J. Neurol. Neurosurg. Psychiat.*, **36**, 478.

PLEASURE, D. E., LOVELACE, R. E., and DUVOISIN, R. C. (1968) The prognosis of acute polyradiculoneuritis, *Neurology (Minneap.)*, **18**, 1143.

POLLARD, J. D., KING, R. H. M., and THOMAS, P. K. (1975) Recurrent experimental allergic neuritis: an electron microscope study, *J. neurol. Sci.*, **24**, 365.

POSNER, J., ERTEL, N. H., KOSSMANN, R. J., and SCHEINBERG, L. C. (1967) Hyponatremia in acute polyneuropathy, *Arch. Neurol. (Chic.)*, **17**, 530.

RAFTERY, M., SCHUMACHER, E. E., GRAIN, G. O., and QUINN, E. L. (1954) Infectious mononucleosis and Guillain–Barré syndrome, *Arch. int. Med.*, **93**, 246.

WAKSMAN, B. H., and ADAMS, R. W. (1955) Allergic neuritis, an experimental disease of rabbits induced by the injection of peripheral nerve tissue and adjuvants, *J. exp. Med.*, **102**, 213.

WHITAKER, J. N., HIRANO, A., COOK, S. D., and DOWLING, P. C. (1970) The ultrastructure of circulating immunocytes in Guillain–Barré syndrome, *Neurology (Minneap.)*, **20**, 765.

WISNIEWSKI, H., TERRY, R. D., WHITAKER, J. N., COOK, S. D., and DOWLING, P. C. (1969) Landry–Guillain–Barré syndrome: a primary demyelinating disease, *Arch. Neurol. (Chic.)*, **21**, 269.

YUILL, G. M., SWINBURN, W. R., and LIVERSEDGE, L. A. (1970) Treatment of poly-neuropathy with azathioprine, *Lancet*, **ii**, 854.

RECURRENT AND RELAPSING POLYNEUROPATHY

Since Nattrass (1921) reported a case of recurrent hypertrophic neuritis in which the patient suffered recurrent acute episodes of polyneuropathy with apparent complete recovery between the episodes, there has been considerable controversy about the relationship of this syndrome and of subacute and chronic steroid-responsive demyelinating neuropathies leading eventually to peripheral nerve hypertrophy on the one hand and to the Guillain–Barré syndrome on the other. Austin (1958) reviewed the literature in detail and reported a patient who suffered 20 recurrent episodes of polyneuropathy over a five-year period, each apparently responding to steroid treatment. Certainly any recurrent demyelinating neuropathy, whatever its cause, may lead to peripheral nerve enlargement resulting from Schwann cell proliferation giving rise to 'onion-bulb' formation (Webster *et al.*, 1967; Zacks *et al.*, 1968; Dyck, 1969; Thomas *et al.*, 1975). It must also be noted that recurrent polyneuropathy or mono-neuropathy may sometimes be a dominantly inherited disorder (Roos and Thygesen, 1972) but this familial disorder does not usually result in peripheral nerve hypertrophy or an increase in the protein content of the CSF and it is probably related to the so-called familial recurrent palsies of peripheral nerves [p. 935]. Recurrent episodes of brachial plexus neuropathy (neuralgic amyotrophy) have also been reported sometimes to be familial (Taylor, 1960; Geiger *et al.*, 1974; Bradley *et al.*, 1975).

It must, however, be accepted that there exists a group of patients who present with either acute recurrent episodes of polyneuropathy or a subacute progressive syndrome, in whom peripheral nerve conduction is slowed, the CSF protein is raised, and nerve biopsy demonstrates segmental demyelination and often a hypertrophic process, and in whom there is an unequivocal response to steroid therapy so that some become steroid-dependent; a similar syndrome has been reported in a patient who showed evidence at autopsy of neurolymphomatosis (Borit and Altrocchi, 1971). Thomas *et al.* (1969) believe that this condition is a variant of the Guillain–Barré syndrome.

REFERENCES

AUSTIN, J. H. (1958) Recurrent polyneuropathies and their corticosteroid treatment, *Brain*, **81**, 157.

BORIT, A., and ALTROCCHI, P. H. (1971) Recurrent polyneuropathy and neurolymphomatosis, *Arch. Neurol. (Chic.)*, **24**, 40.

BRADLEY, W. G., MADRID, R., THRUSH, D. C., and CAMPBELL, M. J. (1975) Recurrent brachial plexus neuropathy, *Brain*, **98**, 381.

DYCK, P. J. (1969) Experimental hypertrophic neuropathy: pathogenesis of onion-bulb formations produced by repeated tourniquet applications, *Arch. Neurol. (Chic.)*, **21**, 73.

GEIGER, L. R., MANCALL, E. L., PENN, A. S., and TUCKER, S. H. (1974) Familial neuralgic amyotrophy—report of three families with review of the literature, *Brain*, **97**, 87.

NATTRASS, F. J. (1921) Recurrent hypertrophic neuritis, *J. Neurol. Psychopathol.*, **2**, 159.

ROOS, D., and THYGESEN, P. (1972) Familial recurrent polyneuropathy, *Brain*, **95**, 235.

TAYLOR, R. A. (1960) Heredofamilial mononeuritis multiplex with brachial predilection, *Brain*, **83**, 113.

THOMAS, P. K., LASCELLES, R. G., HALLPIKE, J. F., and HEWER, R. L. (1969) Recurrent and chronic relapsing Guillain–Barré polyneuritis, *Brain*, **92**, 589.

THOMAS, P. K., LASCELLES, R. G., and STEWART, G. (1975) Hypertrophic neuropathy, in *Handbook of Clinical Neurology*, ed. Vinken, P. J., and Bruyn, G. W., vol. 21, chap. 8, Amsterdam.

WEBSTER, H. DE F., SCHRÖDER, J. M., ASBURY, A. K., and ADAMS, R. D. (1967) The role of Schwann cells in the formation of 'onion bulbs' found in chronic neuropathies, *J. Neuropath. exp. Neurol.*, **26**, 276.

ZACKS, S. I., LIPSHUTZ, H., and ELLIOTT, F. (1968) Histochemical and electron microscopic observations on 'onion bulb' formations in a case of hypertrophic neuritis of 25 years duration with onset in childhood, *Acta Neuropath. (Berl.)*, **11**, 157.

ALCOHOLIC POLYNEUROPATHY

AETIOLOGY

The cause of alcoholic polyneuropathy is not fully understood. It has been thought to be a form of beriberi, the deficiency of thiamine being due to a combination of defective diet, impaired absorption owing to gastrointestinal irritation, and increased need caused by the high calorie value of the alcohol. It has been stated that if the deficiency of thiamine is repaired the patient may continue to improve though permitted to take alcohol. On the other hand, Brown (1941) found that the administration of thiamine did not hasten recovery. This, however, does not necessarily mean, as has been supposed, that the polyneuropathy is not initially due to thiamine deficiency, for chronic beriberi polyneuritis also responds poorly. Alcoholic beriberi with heart failure and oedema undoubtedly occurs: whether 'dry' alcoholic polyneuropathy is similarly caused is at present unsettled. However, Novak and Victor (1974) in a comprehensive neuropathological study, give cogent reasons for concluding first that thiamine deficiency is the primary factor and secondly that the pathological changes of alcoholic neuropathy are identical to those of beriberi. The sex and age incidence are those of alcoholic addiction, most patients being middle-aged, and males being affected more often than females.

PATHOLOGY

The changes in the nervous system are those of a predominantly axonal polyneuropathy of the 'dying-back' type (Prineas, 1970), involving the somatic peripheral nerves and sometimes the vagus and sympathetic nerves (Novak and Victor, 1974). However, the greater splanchnic nerve is usually spared (Low *et al.*, 1975) so that postural hypotension is rare and blood pressure control is usually normal. Although there is some slowing of conduction in peripheral nerves (Mawdsley and Mayer, 1965) this is rarely severe and there is little segmental demyelination (Gilliatt, 1966). Electrophysiological evidence confirms that the neuronal lesion is predominantly distal (Casey and Le Quesne, 1972). The affected neurones exhibit degenerative changes especially at the periphery, and chromatolysis is found in the ganglion cells of the anterior horns and dorsal root ganglia of the spinal cord, and of the motor nuclei of the cranial nerves. The changes in the muscles are those characteristic of degeneration of the lower motor neurones.

SYMPTOMS AND SIGNS

Sensory disturbances usually play a prominent part in the clinical picture. In the early stages the patient complains of numbness, tingling, and paraesthesiae in the hands and feet, and especially pain in the extremities. The pain may be very severe and is described as burning or 'like tearing flesh off the bones'. Cramp-like pains occur in the calves and are especially severe at night. Following the early sensory disturbances the limbs become weak, the lower limbs usually being more severely affected than the upper.

As is the rule in polyneuropathy, both motor and sensory symptoms affect predominantly the periphery of the limbs and in a symmetrical manner. In severe cases both wrist-drop and foot-drop are present, the latter causing a 'steppage' gait, and there is some wasting of the peripheral muscles of all four limbs. Weakness is most marked in the peripheral segments. If the patient can move his limbs, sensory ataxia can usually be demonstrated, and in one form of the disorder— the so-called pseudotabetic variety—ataxia is conspicuous in the lower limbs and is due to loss of postural sensibility. There is a blunting of all forms of sensibility in the periphery of the limbs, cutaneous anaesthesia, and analgesia usually extending up to the elbows and knees. Postural sensibility and appreciation of passive movements are impaired in the fingers and toes. At the same time pressure upon the muscles, especially those of the calves, is usually intensely painful, and scratching the sole may also evoke severe pain. In both cases pain may be delayed. Exceptionally pain and tenderness are slight or absent.

The tendon reflexes are diminished or lost, the ankle-jerks disappearing before the knee-jerks. The plantar reflexes may also be lost, but if present are flexor. The skin of the extremities is often oedematous and sweating. Muscular contractures develop in severe cases, especially in the flexors of the fingers, the hamstrings, and the calf muscles. The sphincters are usually unaffected.

Abnormalities in the cranial nerves are inconstant. The pupils tend to be contracted and may react sluggishly to light. Nystagmus is common. The cranial nerves may be affected, the vagus being most frequently involved, with a resulting tachycardia, and the facial next in frequency. Korsakow's psychosis, Wernicke's encephalopathy [see p. 846], or alcoholic dementia may complicate the picture. The cerebrospinal fluid may be normal, or its protein content may be moderately increased. A blood pyruvate estimation will be helpful in assessing thiamine deficiency. Other symptoms and signs of alcoholism (hepatic cirrhosis, gastritis) are often present. Myocardial failure due to alcoholic cardio-myopathy may also occur, and pulmonary tuberculosis is a not uncommon complication. The neurological picture and electromyographic findings are sometimes complicated by the presence of an associated alcoholic myopathy [p. 1037]. Patients are often obese and florid but are occasionally wasted due to malnutrition.

DIAGNOSIS

The diagnosis of polyneuropathy has been described on page 945.

PROGNOSIS

The prognosis of alcoholic polyneuropathy depends upon how early treatment is begun, and how far it is possible to remove or prevent the recurrence of the causal factor. When treatment can be begun early the prognosis is good, and in mild cases the symptoms disappear in a few weeks. In more severe cases recovery takes several months, and in long-standing cases recovery may be incomplete, especially in respect of return of power to the peripheral muscles. In some cases, in spite of early treatment and the withdrawal of alcohol, the disorder runs a rapidly progressive course with increasing mental confusion, terminating either by death in coma or heart failure or from an intercurrent pneumonia.

TREATMENT

Vitamin B₁ (thiamine) should certainly be given and may usefully be com-bined with other vitamins in an intramuscular injection of *Parentrovite* or of some similar multi-vitamin preparation. Subsequently a vitamin-rich diet is necessary but should for some time be supplemented by giving thiamine, 50 mg daily. The treatment of alcohol addiction must be combined with that of the polyneuropathy [see p. 946].

REFERENCES

BROWN, M. R. (1941) Alcoholic polyneuritis, *J. Amer. med. Ass.*, **116**, 1615.
CASEY, E. B., and LE QUESNE, P. M. (1972) Electrophysiological evidence for a distal lesion in alcoholic neuropathy, *J. Neurol. Neurosurg. Psychiat.*, **35**, 624.
GILLIATT, R. (1966) Nerve conduction in human and experimental neuropathies, *Proc. roy. Soc. Med.*, **59**, 989.
JOLLIFFE, N. (1938) The role of vitamin B₁ deficiency in the production of polyneuritis in the alcohol addict, *Brit. J. Inebr.*, **36**, 7.
LOW, P. A., WALSH, J. C., HUANG, C. Y., and McLEOD, J. G. (1975) The sympathetic nervous system in alcoholic neuropathy—a clinical and pathological study, *Brain*, **98**, 357.
MAWDSLEY, C., and MAYER, R. F. (1965) Nerve conduction in alcoholic polyneuropathy, *Brain*, **88**, 335.
NOVAK, D. J., and VICTOR, M. (1974) The vagus and sympathetic nerves in alcoholic polyneuropathy, *Arch. Neurol. (Chic.)*, **30**, 273.
PRINEAS, J. (1970) Peripheral nerve changes in thiamine-deficient rats, *Arch. Neurol. (Chic.)*, **23**, 541.
STRAUSS, M. B. (1938) The therapeutic use of vitamin B₁ in polyneuritis and cardio-vascular conditions, *J. Amer. med. Ass.*, **110**, 953.
VICTOR, M., and ADAMS, R. D. (1953) The effect of alcohol on the nervous system, *Res. Publ. Ass. nerv. ment. Dis.*, **32**, 526.

ISONIAZID NEUROPATHY

A sensorimotor neuropathy has been described in patients receiving isoniazid, usually in doses of 300 mg daily or more, for the treatment of tuberculosis, and may be accompanied by mental symptoms and skin changes similar to those of pellagra. It is believed to be due to a conditioned pyridoxine deficiency and can be prevented as a rule by the administration of pyridoxine, 25–50 mg daily. It has been shown that the neuropathy occurs in individuals who detoxicate isoniazid slowly and that the ability to detoxicate the drug slowly or rapidly is genetically determined. Sural nerve biopsy in such cases has confirmed that the neuropathy is predominantly axonal in type, involving myelinated and unmyelinated fibres (Ochoa, 1970).

REFERENCES

CARLSON, H. B., ANTHONY, E. M., RUSSELL, W. F., and MIDDLEBROOK, G. (1956) Prophylaxis of isoniazid neuropathy with pyridoxine, *New Engl. J. Med.*, **255**, 118.

CLARKE, C. A., PRICE EVANS, D. A., HARRIS, R., McCONNELL, R. B., and WOODROW, J. C. (1968) Genetics in medicine. A review. Part II. Pharmacogenetics, *Quart. J. Med.*, **37**, 183.

McCONNELL, R. B., and CHEETHAM, H. D. (1952) Acute pellagra during isoniazid therapy, *Lancet*, **ii**, 959.

OCHOA, J. (1970) Isoniazid neuropathy in man: quantitative electron microscope study, *Brain*, **93**, 831.

ARSENICAL POLYNEUROPATHY

AETIOLOGY

Polyneuropathy may follow either acute or chronic arsenical poisoning, more usually the latter. The arsenic may have been administered with intent to murder or in an attempt at suicide. For murderous purposes white arsenic or sodium arsenite, which is contained in certain rat-poisons and weed-killers, has usually been employed. Arsenic has also been obtained from fly-papers for this purpose. Accidental arsenical poisoning may occur in occupations involving handling arsenic (such as arsenical sprays used in agriculture—Heyman *et al.*, 1956), though this is rare, or as a result of taking food contaminated with arsenic, as in the Manchester epidemic in 1900, when poisoning was produced by the consumption of beer brewed with glucose containing arsenic. Poisoning has also been produced by the inhalation of arsenic from wallpapers, in which it has been used as a dye, as a result of licking golf balls when arsenical weedkiller has been used on the course, and from the ingestion of bootleg alcohol. Medicinal arsenical poisoning is rare today, but was more frequent in the past, when Fowler's solution was administered for long periods in the treatment of chorea, multiple sclerosis, and pernicious anaemia. Polyneuropathy was rare after treatment with arsenobenzene derivatives, once extensively used in the treatment of syphilis.

The observation that arsenical poisoning causes an accumulation of pyruvate in the blood suggests that arsenic, like other heavy metals, acts by reacting with a thiol group which is an essential component of co-enzyme A; this provides a link between arsenical polyneuropathy and polyneuropathy due to thiamine deficiency (Peters *et al.*, 1945).

A sensorimotor polyneuropathy virtually identical with that due to arsenic may be produced on occasion by other heavy metals including gold, mercury, zinc, bismuth, antimony, and thallium and the mechanism is believed to be similar. Thallium, which has been used commercially as a rat poison and as an insecticide or as a depilatory, has been responsible for a number of such cases [p. 809].

PATHOLOGY

This neuropathy is axonal in type as in thiamine deficiency.

SYMPTOMS AND SIGNS

The symptoms of arsenical polyneuropathy resemble those of the alcoholic variety. As in the latter, sensory symptoms are conspicuous, and pain is usually severe. Muscular weakness is usually more conspicuous in the lower than in the upper limbs. Korsakow's psychosis or a confusional state may be present. In the diagnosis of arsenical polyneuropathy the presence of abnormalities outside the nervous system assumes great importance. In chronic arsenical poisoning gastro-intestinal symptoms may be absent. Excessive salivation is not uncommon, and there is often a secondary anaemia. Cutaneous symptoms are usually present. These may consist of erythema or even of exfoliative dermatitis. In long-standing cases there is often cutaneous pigmentation. This is absent from the exposed parts and consists of a fine mottling of the skin, with patches of a light chocolate colour, the intervening areas being white. Hyperkeratosis of the palms and soles is often found, the thickened skin presenting a smooth, somewhat waxy appearance. Herpes zoster is a common complication. The blood pyruvate is raised and even when the resting level is normal, a pyruvate tolerance curve demonstrates that the serum pyruvate rises well above the normal upper limit of 1·3 mg per 100 ml after a loading dose of glucose.

DIAGNOSIS

The diagnosis of arsenical from other forms of polyneuropathy [p. 945] depends upon the presence of the abnormalities just described, especially the cutaneous symptoms of arsenical poisoning, and upon the demonstration by appropriate toxicological tests of arsenic in the hair, nails, urine, or faeces. The normal upper limit of arsenic in the hair is 0·1 mg/100 g hair (Heyman et al., 1956).

PROGNOSIS

The prognosis of arsenical polyneuropathy is good, provided the general symptoms of arsenical poisoning are not too far advanced when the patient comes under treatment. Recovery of voluntary power, however, is slow and may take one or two years.

TREATMENT

Dimercaprol was the first drug to be of value (Heyman et al., 1956); calcium versenate, another chelating agent, is also effective in promoting the excretion of arsenic but both have been supplanted by penicillamine (Simpson, 1962). In addition the general treatment of polyneuritis should be carried out [see p. 946].

REFERENCES

HASSIN, G. B. (1930) Symptomatology of arsenical polyneuritis, *J. nerv. ment. Dis.*, **72**, 628.
HEYMAN, A., PFEIFFER, J. B., WILLETT, R. W., and TAYLOR, H. M. (1956) Peripheral neuropathy caused by arsenical intoxication, *New Engl. J. Med.*, **254**, 401.
PETERS, R. A., STOCKEN, L. A., and THOMPSON, R. H. S. (1945) British Anti-Lewisite (BAL), *Nature (Lond.)*, **156**, 616.
SIMPSON, J. A. (1962) The neuropathies, in *Modern Trends in Neurology*, 3rd series, ed. Williams, D., London.

ORGANIC CHLORINE COMPOUNDS USED AS INSECTICIDES

Campbell (1952) reported 5 cases of polyneuritis and 3 of retrobulbar neuritis following the use of an insecticide containing ortho- and para-dichloro-benzene, DDT, and pentachlorophenol. He suggested that the last might be the toxic factor. For neurological complications of organophosphorus insecticides see page 815. Fullerton (1969) pointed out that whereas peripheral neuropathy is the predominant complication of industrial poisoning with lead, acrylamide, organophosphates, and thallium, substances such as tetrachlorethane, pentachlorophenol, and DDT produce polyneuropathy only after gross overdosage. Hexachlorophene, widely used as a skin antiseptic, may produce vacuolar degeneration in the central nervous system in infants [p. 809] but also causes demyelination in peripheral nerves in animals (de Jesus and Pleasure, 1973; Pleasure *et al.*, 1974) but no cases of human polyneuropathy due to this substance have yet been described.

REFERENCES

CAMPBELL, A. M. G. (1952) Neurological complications associated with insecticides and fungicides, *Brit. med. J.*, **2**, 415.
DE JESUS, P. V., and PLEASURE, D. E. (1973) Hexachlorophene neuropathy, *Arch. Neurol. (Chic.)*, **29**, 180.
FULLERTON, P. M. (1969) Toxic chemicals and peripheral neuropathy: clinical and epidemiological features, *Proc. roy. Soc. Med.*, **62**, 201.
PLEASURE, D. E., TOWFIGHT, J., SILBERBERG, D., and PARRIS, J. (1974) The pathogenesis of hexachlorophene neuropathy: in vivo and in vitro studies, *Neurology (Minneap.)*, **24**, 1068.

LEAD NEUROPATHY

Lead poisoning has been considered in detail on page 804. Lead may produce a predominantly motor type of polyneuropathy, often affecting predominantly those muscles in common use in the individual's occupation (e.g. wrist-drop in battery-makers). Subclinical neuropathy, identifiable by nerve conduction studies, is not uncommon in lead workers (Catton *et al.*, 1970). In experimental studies in the guinea-pig, Fullerton (1966) found that lead produced a combination of segmental demyelination and axonal degeneration but Lampert and Schochet (1968) found that demyelination and Schwann cell proliferation predominated.

REFERENCES

CATTON, M. J., HARRISON, M. J. G., FULLERTON, P. M., and KAZANTZIS, G. (1970) Sub-clinical neuropathy in lead workers, *Brit. med. J.*, **2**, 80.
FULLERTON, P. M. (1966) Chronic peripheral neuropathy produced by lead poisoning in guinea-pigs, *J. Neuropath. exp. Neurol.*, **25**, 214.
LAMPERT, P. W., and SCHOCHET, S. S. (1968) Demyelination and remyelination in lead neuropathy, *J. Neuropath. exp. Neurol.*, **27**, 527.

ORGANIC SOLVENTS

Trichloroethylene when used as an anaesthetic agent rarely if ever produces neurological complications, but its industrial use has been shown sometimes to cause polyneuropathy as well as other complications including confusion and even dementia (Mitchell and Parsons-Smith, 1969). *Carbon tetrachloride*, too, like carbon monoxide poisoning, has occasionally given rise to poly-neuropathy but the symptoms of poisoning by these agents are dominated by evidence of involvement of other organs (e.g. the liver or brain) (Fullerton, 1969 a). Industrial exposure to *methyl n-butyl ketone*, a solvent widely used in the printing of synthetic fabrics, has also been observed to cause an axonal dying-back type of neuropathy in animals (Spencer and Schaumburg, 1975; Spencer *et al.*, 1975) and caused moderately severe sensorimotor polyneuropathy in human subjects in a large industrial outbreak (Allen *et al.*, 1975).

n-Hexane, principally employed as a cement solvent, has caused poly-neuropathy in Japan and in the United States (Herskowitz *et al.*, 1971) and is also responsible for a predominantly motor type of polyneuropathy, though with minor sensory manifestations, which has been reported to follow the habitual inhalation of vapour produced from certain glues widely used in plastic modelling (glue-sniffer's neuropathy) (Goto *et al.*, 1974).

Acrylamide, a chemical widely used in the polymer industry, was reported to cause sensorimotor polyneuropathy in factory workers by Garland and Patterson (1967). Often the neurological manifestations are preceded by evidence of contact dermatitis on the hands followed by coldness and blueness and excessive sweating of the extremities (Spencer and Schaumburg, 1974 a and b). Severe ataxia is common and has been thought to indicate associated cerebellar damage (Fullerton, 1969 b). Electrophysiological and pathological studies in man and animals (Fullerton and Barnes, 1966; Bradley and Asbury, 1970; Hopkins and Gilliatt, 1971) suggest that this is predominantly a 'dying-back' type of axonal neuropathy.

In all of these disorders recovery usually occurs gradually after removal from exposure to the causal agent.

REFERENCES

ALLEN, N., MENDELL, J. R., BILLMAIER, D. J., FONTAINE, R. E., and O'NEILL, J. (1975) Toxic polyneuropathy due to methyl n-butyl ketone, *Arch. Neurol. (Chic.)*, **32**, 209.
BRADLEY, W. G., and ASBURY, A. K. (1970) Radioautographic studies of Schwann cell behavior: 1. Acrylamide neuropathy in the mouse, *J. Neuropath. exp. Neurol.*, **29**, 500.
FULLERTON, P. M. (1969 a) Toxic chemicals and peripheral neuropathy: clinical and epidemiological features, *Proc. roy. Soc. Med.*, **62**, 201.
FULLERTON, P. M. (1969 b) Electrophysiological and histological observations on peripheral nerves in acrylamide poisoning in man, *J. Neurol. Neurosurg. Psychiat.*, **32**, 186.

FULLERTON, P. M., and BARNES, J. M. (1966) Peripheral neuropathy in rats produced by acrylamide, *Brit. J. industr. Med.*, **23**, 210.

GARLAND, T. O., and PATTERSON, M. W. H. (1967) Six cases of acrylamide poisoning, *Brit. med. J.*, **4**, 134.

GOTO, I., MATSUMURA, M., INOUE, N., MURAI, Y., SHIDA, K., SANTA, T., and KUROIWA, Y. (1974) Toxic polyneuropathy due to glue sniffing, *J. Neurol. Neurosurg. Psychiat.*, **37**, 848.

HERSKOWITZ, A., ISHII, N., and SCHAUMBURG, H. (1971) n-Hexane neuropathy, *New Engl. J. Med.*, **285**, 82.

HOPKINS, A. P., and GILLIATT, R. W. (1971) Motor and sensory nerve conduction velocity in the baboon: normal values and changes during acrylamide neuropathy, *J. Neurol. Neurosurg. Psychiat.*, **34**, 415.

MITCHELL, A. B. S., and PARSONS-SMITH, B. G. (1969) Trichloroethylene neuropathy, *Brit. med. J.*, **1**, 422.

SPENCER, P. S., and SCHAUMBURG, H. H. (1974 a) A review of acrylamide neurotoxicity. Part I. Properties, uses and human exposure, *Canad. J. neurol. Sci.*, **1**, 143.

SPENCER, P. S., and SCHAUMBURG, H. H. (1974 b) A review of acrylamide neurotoxicity. Part II. Experimental animal neurotoxicity and pathologic mechanisms, *Canad. J. neurol. Sci.*, **1**, 152.

SPENCER, P. S., and SCHAUMBURG, H. H. (1975) Experimental neuropathy produced by 2,5-hexanedione—a major metabolite of the neurotoxic industrial solvent methyl n-butyl ketone, *J. Neurol. Neurosurg. Psychiat.*, **38**, 771.

SPENCER, P. S., SCHAUMBURG, H. H., RALEIGH, R. L., and TERHAAR, C. J. (1975) Nervous system degeneration produced by the industrial solvent methyl n-butyl ketone, *Arch. Neurol. (Chic.)*, **32**, 219.

THALIDOMIDE NEUROPATHY

Thalidomide, used some years ago as a hypnotic in Britain and in Europe was withdrawn from the market when it was found to produce phocomelia in the fetus if taken by the mother during the early months of pregnancy. After regular administration of the drug for several months many patients were found to develop a predominantly sensory neuropathy giving rise to unpleasant burning dysaesthesiae in the hands and feet accompanied by peripheral impairment of pain sensation often restricted to the digits (Fullerton and Kremer, 1961). While in milder cases slow recovery often occurred following withdrawal of the drug, in a number of severe cases painful paraesthesiae and sensory loss have persisted for many years. The neuropathy is due to selective involvement of large diameter fibres in the peripheral nerves and is predominantly axonal in type. In a follow-up study, Fullerton and O'Sullivan (1968) found that 50 per cent of patients (usually those most severely affected initially) remained unchanged for many years, but the others improved or recovered.

Recently it has been suspected that *methaqualone* (a constituent of *Mandrax*) may also cause peripheral neuropathy (*British Medical Journal*, 1973) but this is not yet certain.

REFERENCES

BRITISH MEDICAL JOURNAL (1973) Does methaqualone cause neuropathy?, *Brit. med. J.*, **3**, 307.

FULLERTON, P. M., and KREMER, M. (1961) Neuropathy after intake of thalidomide (Distaval), *Brit. med. J.*, **2**, 855.

FULLERTON, P. M., and O'SULLIVAN, D. J. (1968) Thalidomide neuropathy: a clinical, electrophysiological, and histological follow-up study, *J. Neurol. Neurosurg. Psychiat.*, **31**, 543.

POLYNEUROPATHY DUE TO TRIORTHOCRESYLPHOSPHATE

During the spring of 1930 thousands of cases of polyneuropathy, some of them fatal, occurred in the United States, owing to the consumption of fluid extract of ginger which was used in the manufacture of bootleg alcohol and was adulterated with triorthocresylphosphate. The condition became known as 'ginger paralysis'. Recent outbreaks of polyneuropathy in South Africa, Germany, Morocco, and the Merseyside area have been traced to cresyl esters in cooking-oil. The same toxic substance has been proved responsible for causing polyneuropathy in women who have taken apiol as an abortifacient. Triortho-cresylphosphate irreversibly inhibits pseudocholinesterase but since not all inhibitors of pseudocholinesterase produce degeneration of peripheral nerves some other factor would seem to be at work. There may also be inhibition of true cholinesterase (Hern, 1967).

Both in man and in experimental animals triorthocresylphosphate produces chromatolysis of the anterior horn cells of the spinal cord and of the ganglion cells of the motor nuclei of the pons and medulla, degeneration of the fasciculus gracilis and the corticospinal tracts in the spinal cord, and destruction of the myelin sheaths and axis cylinders of the peripheral nerves. Cavanagh (1953, 1964) showed that changes occur initially in those nerve fibres which are longest and of the greatest diameter, both in the peripheral and central nervous system and suggests that the primary pathological process is one of 'dying-back' of the axon. Symptoms of polyneuropathy developed from 10 to 20 days after the consumption of adulterated food or drink, and consisted of bilateral wrist-drop and foot-drop, with wasting of the distal muscles of the limbs. Pain in the limbs was common, but sensory loss was inconstant. In many cases the paralysis proved to be permanent. Acute retrobulbar neuritis has been described in apiol poisoning. For treatment see page 946.

REFERENCES

ARING, C. D. (1942) The systemic nervous affinity of triorthocresylphosphate (Jamaica ginger palsy), *Brain*, **65**, 34.

CAVANAGH, J. B. (1954) The toxic effects of tri-ortho-cresyl phosphate on the nervous system, *J. Neurol. Neurosurg. Psychiat.*, **17**, 163.

CAVANAGH, J. B. (1953) Organo-phosphorus neurotoxicity: a model 'dying back' process comparable to certain human neurological disorders, *Guy's Hosp. Rep.*, **112**, 303.

CAVANAGH, J. B. (1964) Peripheral nerve changes in ortho-cresyl phosphate poisoning in the cat, *J. Path. Bact.*, **87**, 365.

HERN, J. E. C. (1967) Inhibition of true cholinesterase in TOCP poisoning with potentiation by 'Tween 80', *Nature*, **215**, 963.

HOTSTON, R. D. (1946) Outbreak of polyneuritis due to orthotricresyl phosphate poisoning, *Lancet*, **i**, 207.

SMITH, M. I., ELVOLVE, E., and FRAZIER, W. H. (1930) Pharmacological action of certain phenol esters, with special reference to the etiology of so-called ginger paralysis, *Publ. Hlth Rep. (Wash.)*, **45**, 2509.

WEBER, M. L. (1936–7) Follow-up study of thirty-five cases of paralysis caused by adulterated Jamaica ginger extract, *Med. Bull. Veterans' Adm. (Wash.)*, **13**, 228.

NITROFURANTOIN NEUROPATHY

Nitrofurantoin (*Furadantin*) is a drug now widely used in the treatment of urinary infection. Cases have been reported in which a symmetrical sensori-motor peripheral neuropathy developed during treatment with this drug and was shown to occur only in those with severe impairment of renal function (Ellis, 1962; Loughridge, 1962). It is now clear that this drug should be used with great caution if the blood urea (or non-protein nitrogen) is above normal or if there are other indications of substantially impaired renal function. Even in normal persons the drug may cause reduction in motor and/or sensory nerve conduction velocity (Toole *et al.*, 1968) but clinical polyneuropathy is uncommon when the drug is given for short periods, when renal function is unimpaired.

REFERENCES

ELLIS, F. G. (1962) Acute polyneuritis after nitrofurantoin therapy, *Lancet*, **ii**, 1136.
LOUGHRIDGE, L. W. (1962) Peripheral neuropathy due to nitrofurantoin, *Lancet*, **ii**, 1133.
TOOLE, J. F., GERGEN, J. A., HAYES, D. M., and FELTS, J. H. (1968) Neural effects of nitro-furantoin, *Arch. Neurol. (Chic.)*, **18**, 680.

URAEMIC POLYNEUROPATHY

Since the original report of Asbury *et al.* (1962) it has become abundantly clear that a mixed sensorimotor polyneuropathy may occur frequently in patients who are uraemic as a result of chronic renal failure. 'Restless legs' (Ekbom, 1944) is an occasional manifestation (Banerji and Hurwitz, 1970; Thomas *et al.*, 1971). The neuropathy may be especially prominent in patients on dialysis who develop type B hepatitis (Davison *et al.*, 1972). In many cases improvement follows treatment of the renal disease, as by intermittent dialysis, but this is not invariable (Nielsen, 1974 *a*). Improvement or even recovery may, however, follow renal transplantation (Nielsen, 1974 *b*; Ibrahim *et al.*, 1974). The finding of slowing of motor and sensory nerve conduction velocity in such cases (Nielsen, 1973) and nerve biopsy studies have led to the conclusion that the neuropathy is demyelinating, but Dyck *et al.* (1971) give reasons for suggest-ing that in such cases the prominent demyelination is secondary to a primary axonal degeneration. Polyneuropathy has also been described as a complication of primary hyperoxaluria (Moorhead *et al.*, 1975).

REFERENCES

ASBURY, A. K., VICTOR, M., and ADAMS, R. D. (1962) Uremic polyneuropathy, *Trans. Amer. neurol. Ass.*, **87**, 100.
BANERJI, N. K., and HURWITZ, L. J. (1970) Restless legs syndrome, with particular reference to its occurrence after gastric surgery, *Brit. med. J.*, **4**, 774.
DAVISON, A. M., WILLIAMS, I. R., MAWDSLEY, C., and ROBSON, J. S. (1972) Neuropathy associated with hepatitis in patients maintained on haemodialysis, *Brit. med. J.*, **1**, 409.
DYCK, P. J., JOHNSON, W. J., LAMBERT, E. H., and O'BRIEN, P. C. (1971) Segmental demyelination secondary to axonal degeneration in uremic neuropathy, *Mayo Clin. Proc.*, **46**, 400.
EKBOM, K. (1944) Asthenia crurum paraesthetica (irritable legs), *Acta med. scand.*, **118**, 197.

IBRAHIM, M. M., BARNES, A. D., CROSLAND, J. M., DAWSON-EDWARDS, P., HONIGS-BERGER, L., NERMAN, C. E., and ROBINSON, B. H. B. (1974) Effect of renal transplantation on uraemic neuropathy, *Lancet*, **ii**, 739.

MOORHEAD, P. J., COOPER, D. J., and TIMPERLEY, W. R. (1975) Progressive peripheral neuropathy in patient with primary hyperoxaluria, *Brit. med. J.*, **2**, 312.

NIELSEN, V. K. (1973) The peripheral nerve function in chronic renal failure. V. Sensory and motor conduction velocity, *Acta med. scand.*, **194**, 445.

NIELSEN, V. K. (1974 *a*) The peripheral nerve function in chronic renal failure. VII. Longitudinal course during terminal renal failure and regular hemodialysis, *Acta med. scand.*, **195**, 155.

NIELSEN, V. K. (1974 *b*) The peripheral nerve function in chronic renal failure. IX. Recovery after renal transplantation. Electrophysiological aspects (sensory and motor nerve conduction), *Acta med. scand.*, **195**, 171.

THOMAS, P. K., HOLLINRAKE, K., LASCELLES, R. G., O'SULLIVAN, D. J., BAILLOD, R. A., MOORHEAD, J. F., and MACKENZIE, J. C. (1971) The polyneuropathy of chronic renal failure, *Brain*, **94**, 761.

CHLOROQUINE NEUROMYOPATHY

A motor polyneuropathy, unaccompanied by symptoms or signs of sensory dysfunction, may develop in patients receiving treatment with chloroquine, usually in doses of 500 mg daily or more for one year or longer. Histological studies indicate that the muscle fibres are also affected as they commonly show striking vacuolation which appears to be due to the accumulation of glycogen. The nerve lesion seems to affect mainly the terminal axons and recovery is usually rapid after withdrawal of the drug (Gérard *et al.*, 1973).

REFERENCES

GÉRARD, J. M., STROUPEL, N., COLLIER, A., and FLAMENT-DURAND, J. (1973) Morphologic study of a neuromyopathy caused by prolonged chloroquine treatment, *Europ. Neurol.*, **9**, 363.

WHISNANT, J. P., ESPINOSA, R. E., KIERLAND, R. R., and LAMBERT, E. H. (1963) Chloroquine neuromyopathy, *Mayo Clin. Proc.*, **38**, 501.

VINCRISTINE NEUROMYOPATHY

Vincristine sulphate, used increasingly of late for the treatment of leukaemia, of medulloblastoma in childhood, and of intracranial gliomas in adult life, has been found to produce in many cases a sensorimotor polyneuropathy (Sandler *et al.*, 1969; McLeod and Penny, 1969). Pathological and electrophysiological studies suggest that the damage is primarily axonal and of the 'dying-back' type (Casey *et al.*, 1973) but secondary demyelination with consequent slowing of nerve conduction also occurs (Gottschalk *et al.*, 1968; Bradley, 1970) and focal necrosis of muscle fibres is sometimes found (Bradley *et al.*, 1970). Intrathecal vincristine may produce extensive neuronal damage in the central nervous system (Schochet *et al.*, 1968).

REFERENCES

BRADLEY, W. G. (1970) The neuromyopathy of vincristine in the guinea pig: an electrophysiological and pathological study, *J. neurol. Sci.*, **10**, 133.

BRADLEY, W. G., LASSMAN, L. P., PEARCE, G. W., and WALTON, J. N. (1970) The neuromyopathy of vincristine in man, *J. neurol. Sci.*, **10**, 107.

CASEY, E. B., JELLIFFE, A. M., LE QUESNE, P. M., and MILLETT, Y. L. (1973) Vincristine neuropathy—clinical and electrophysiological observations, *Brain*, **96,** 69.

GOTTSCHALK, P. G., DYCK, P. J., and KIELY, J. M. (1968) Vinca alkaloid neuropathy: nerve biopsy studies in rats and in man, *Neurology (Minneap.)*, **18,** 875.

MCLEOD, J. G., and PENNY, R. (1969) Vincristine neuropathy: an electrophysiological and histological study, *J. Neurol. Neurosurg. Psychiat.*, **32,** 297.

SANDLER, S. G., TOBIN, W., and HENDERSON, E. S. (1969) Vincristine-induced neuropathy: a clinical study of fifty leukemic patients, *Neurology (Minneap.)*, **19,** 367.

SCHOCHET, S. S., LAMPERT, P. W., and EARLE, K. M. (1968) Neuronal changes induced by intrathecal vincristine sulfate, *J. Neuropath. exp. Neurol.*, **27,** 645.

DISULFIRAM NEUROPATHY

Sensorimotor polyneuropathy, improving slowly and often recovering completely after withdrawal of the drug, is an occasional complication of prolonged disulfiram (*Antabuse*) medication (Hayman and Wilkins, 1956; Bradley and Hewer, 1966). Optic neuritis occasionally occurs (Dent, 1950; Gardner-Thorpe and Benjamin, 1971).

REFERENCES

BRADLEY, W. G., and HEWER, R. L. (1966) Peripheral neuropathy due to disulfiram, *Brit. med. J.*, **2,** 449.

DENT, J. Y. (1950) Discussion following paper of A. S. Paterson.

GARDNER-THORPE, C., and BENJAMIN, S. (1971) Peripheral neuropathy after disulfiram administration, *J. Neurol. Neurosurg. Psychiat.*, **34,** 253.

HAYMAN, M., and WILKINS, P. A. (1956) Polyneuropathy as a complication of disulfiram therapy of alcoholism, *Quart. J. Stud. Alcohol*, **17,** 601.

PATERSON, A. S. (1950) Modern techniques for the treatment of acute and prolonged alcoholism, *Brit. J. Addict.*, **47,** 3.

DIPHENYLHYDANTOIN NEUROPATHY

Lovelace and Horwitz (1968) described the development of polyneuropathy in 26 patients after long-term administration of diphenylhydantoin for the treatment of epilepsy, and Eisen *et al.* (1974) have confirmed that in such epileptic patients, even in the absence of symptoms, there may be some slowing of motor and sensory nerve conduction velocity especially if the plasma level of the drug exceeds 20 μg/l. Fortunately this complication is uncommon and rarely clinically severe.

REFERENCES

EISEN, A., WOODS, J. F., and SHERWIN, A. L. (1974) Peripheral nerve function in long-term therapy with diphenylhydantoin, *Neurology (Minneap.)*, **24,** 411.

LOVELACE, R. E., and HORWITZ, S. J. (1968) Peripheral neuropathy in long-term diphenylhydantoin therapy, *Arch. Neurol. (Chic.)*, **18,** 69.

SODIUM CYANATE NEUROPATHY

When sickle cell anaemia is treated with sodium cyanate, polyneuropathy with evidence of axonal degeneration and demyelination may develop (Ohnishi *et al.*, 1975). It is possible that this condition may be related in certain respects to tropical ataxic neuropathy due to the ingestion of cyanogenetic glycosides [see Osuntokun *et al.*, 1974, and p. 851].

REFERENCES

OHNISHI, A., PETERSON, C. M., and DYCK, P. J. (1975) Axonal degeneration in sodium cyanate-induced neuropathy, *Arch. Neurol. (Chic.)*, **32**, 530.

OSUNTOKUN, B. O., MATTHEWS, D. M., HUSSEIN, H. A.-A., WISE, I. J., and LINNELL, J. C. (1974) Plasma and hepatic cobalamins in tropical ataxic neuropathy, *Clin. Sci. Molec. Med.*, **46**, 563.

NEURITIS COMPLICATING SEROTHERAPY

Neuritis is a rare sequel of serotherapy. It has been described after the administration of serum in the treatment of tetanus and diphtheria. Nervous symptoms usually occur two or three days after the onset of typical symptoms of serum sickness. The commonest lesion is radiculopathy, the fifth cervical spinal nerve being most commonly affected on one or both sides, with pain in the corresponding segmental distribution and paralysis of the muscles innervated, especially the deltoid. This syndrome is almost identical with that of 'shoulder-girdle neuritis' (neuralgic amyotrophy) [see p. 938]. Less frequently the whole brachial plexus may be involved, or a more diffuse polyneuritis may occur. Cerebral symptoms, probably resulting from encephalopathy, rarely occur. Optic neuritis has been described. Complete recovery usually occurs in from one to 18 months, though occasionally muscular weakness persists. Treatment appropriate to the situation of the lesion must be carried out.

REFERENCES

ALLEN, I. M. (1931) The neurological complications of serum therapy, with report of a case, *Lancet*, **ii**, 1128.

BARON, J. H. (1958) A.T.S. cervical polyradiculitis treated by cortisone, *Brit. med. J.*, **2**, 678.

POLYNEURITIS IN PREGNANCY

It is better to speak of polyneuritis in pregnancy than polyneuritis of pregnancy since any form of polyneuritis may occur in pregnancy. Persistent vomiting, unsuitable diet, and increased requirements due to the needs of the fetus may all contribute to nutritional deficiency in pregnancy, though whether of one or more factors is uncertain. Where beriberi is endemic, pregnancy appears to predispose to it. Bilateral retrobulbar neuritis resembling that ascribed by Moore to vitamin deficiency was observed by Ballantyne (1941) in hyperemesis gravidarum. Ungley (1933) described recurrent neuritis in pregnancy and the puerperium in three members of the same family.

When there is reason to suspect nutritional deficiency vitamin supplements should be given.

REFERENCES

BALLANTYNE, A. J. (1941) Ocular complications in hyperemesis gravidarum, *J. Obstet. Gynec.*, **48**, 206.

STRAUSS, M. B., and McDONALD, W. J. (1933) Polyneuritis of pregnancy, *J. Amer. med. Ass.*, **100**, 1320.

UNGLEY, C. C. (1933) Recurrent polyneuritis, *J. Neurol. Psychiat.*, **14**, 15.

UNGLEY, C. C. (1938) On some deficiencies of nutrition and their relation to disease, *Lancet*, **i**, 925.

DIABETIC POLYNEUROPATHY

AETIOLOGY

The aetiology of diabetic neuropathy is still controversial and has been reviewed by Thomas and Ward (1975). The incidence of this complication has varied enormously in different series. Goodman *et al.* (1953) noted pain and paraesthesiae in 40 per cent of cases but weakness and objective sensory loss was found in under 10 per cent. In other series the incidence has been substantially greater, and electrophysiological evidence of subclinical neuropathy can be detected in a large proportion of diabetic subjects. The condition is uncommon in childhood and its incidence rises steadily with increasing age. It is found in early-onset insulin-sensitive diabetes, in maturity-onset cases, and also in diabetes secondary to pancreatitis (Osuntokun, 1970) and haemochromatosis, and a hereditary predisposition has been postulated (Chopra *et al.*, 1969).

There has been considerable dispute concerning the relative role of metabolic factors on the one hand and of atherosclerosis of the vasa nervorum on the other; while the latter may play a role, especially in the pathogenesis of mononeuropathies, there is now general agreement that polyneuropathy is predominantly of metabolic origin in most cases. It cannot be correlated simply with hyperglycaemia, though neuropathy occurs in alloxan- or streptozotocin-induced diabetes in animals (Sharma and Thomas, 1974, 1975). Disorders of pantothenic acid (Bosanquet and Henson, 1957) and pyruvate (Butterfield and Thompson, 1957) metabolism have been found but do not correlate with the severity of the neuropathy. Abnormalities of lipid composition (Eliasson, 1966), of myelin protein (Palo *et al.*, 1972), or of the ionic permeability of nodal gap substance (Seneviratne and Weerasuriya, 1974) have been found in diabetic peripheral nerves, and there is also evidence of disordered sorbitol metabolism (Thomas and Ward, 1975), but no single causative biochemical abnormality has yet been identified.

PATHOLOGY

Motor and sensory nerve conduction studies and single-fibre electromyography (Downie and Newell, 1961; Gilliatt and Willison, 1962; Chopra and Hurwitz, 1969 *a*; Lamontagne and Buchthal, 1970; Thiele and Stålberg, 1975), and autopsy as well as sural nerve biopsy studies (Thomas and Lascelles, 1965; Chopra and Fannin, 1971) indicate that the neuropathy is demyelinating with Schwann cell abnormalities, reduction in the density of myelinated fibres of all sizes (Chopra and Hurwitz, 1969 *b*), and sometimes 'onion-bulb' hypertrophy (Ballin and Thomas, 1968). When isolated peripheral nerve lesions occur, however (mononeuropathy), especially in cranial nerves, pathological evidence has indicated that ischaemia with localized infarction of nerve trunks is the cause (Raff *et al.*, 1968).

SYMPTOMS

The main varieties of diabetic neuropathy which have been described include generalized sensorimotor polyneuropathy (the commonest, and often predominantly sensory), autonomic neuropathy, and mononeuropathy (of peripheral or cranial nerves).

Loss of tendon reflexes and of vibration sense in the lower limbs is very common in diabetes in the absence of other signs of neuropathy and in such cases nerve conduction is usually slowed. Severe polyneuropathy is exceptional but in such cases sensory symptoms usually predominate over motor, and the lower limbs are more affected than the upper. Pure sensory neuropathy may occur [p. 923]. Pain in the calves may be considerable, and loss of postural sensibility is often marked in the lower limbs, leading to severe ataxia. Charcot's arthropathy is rarely seen. 'Diabetic amyotrophy' (Garland, 1957; Casey and Harrison, 1972), characterized by pain, tenderness, and weakness of muscles, usually limited to the anterior aspect of one or both thighs, is due in most cases to a femoral nerve neuropathy. Isolated lesions of other peripheral nerves, particularly the lateral popliteal, also occur. Ocular palsies occurring in diabetes have been ascribed to neuritis of the oculomotor nerves, but are more probably mononeuropathies, due to vascular lesions involving the nerve trunks or mid-brain [see p. 169]. They usually resolve in three to six months. In elderly diabetics the pupils are often contracted and may react sluggishly to light ('diabetic pseudotabes'). Primary optic atrophy may occur. Absent circulatory reflexes, and particularly an abnormal response to the Valsalva manœuvre (Sharpey-Schafer and Taylor, 1960) are found in some cases and are due to autonomic neuropathy involving sympathetic fibres; postural hypotension is common (Low et al., 1975). In some cases, chronic diarrhoea, often nocturnal, and even steatorrhoea may occur; impotence is common and so too are disorders of sweating (British Medical Journal, 1974) including facial sweating after food (Watkins, 1973). Other complications of diabetes may be present, including impaired peripheral circulation, owing to arterial atheroma, which may lead to gangrene of the extremities or perforating ulcer.

DIAGNOSIS

The diagnosis of polyneuritis is described on page 945. The origin of the diabetic form is settled by the discovery of glycosuria and hyperglycaemia. The symptoms of metabolic neuropathy must be distinguished from those of vascular occlusion with resultant ischaemic neuropathy. Confusion is not likely to arise if the arterial pulse is carefully examined both in the proximal and peripheral parts of the limbs.

PROGNOSIS

The prognosis of diabetic neuropathy is good, provided that the patient responds satisfactorily to treatment for diabetes, that vascular degeneration is not severe, and that trophic lesions, such as gangrene and perforating ulcers, are absent.

TREATMENT

The usual treatment of diabetes must be carried out and it is clear that the adequacy of control can be closely correlated with arrest of, or actual improvement in, the symptoms and signs of polyneuropathy (The Lancet, 1972).

Measures appropriate to the usual management of polyneuritis may be indicated [p. 946].

REFERENCES

BALLIN, R. H. M., and THOMAS, P. K. (1968) Hypertrophic changes in diabetic neuropathy, Acta Neuropath. (Berl.), 11, 93.

BOSANQUET, F. D., and HENSON, R. A. (1957) Sensory neuropathy in diabetes mellitus, Psychiat. Neurol. Neurochirurg., 60, 107.

BRITISH MEDICAL JOURNAL (1974) Diabetic autonomic neuropathy, *Brit. med. J.*, **3**, 2.

BUTTERFIELD, W. J. H., and THOMPSON, R. H. S. (1957) The effect of dimercaprol (BAL) on blood sugar and pyruvate levels in diabetes mellitus, *Clin. Sci.*, **16**, 679.

CASEY, E. B., and HARRISON, M. J. G. (1972) Diabetic amyotrophy: a follow-up study, *Brit. med. J.*, **1**, 656.

CHOPRA, J. S., CONNON, J. J., and BANERJI, N. K. (1969) Diabetic neuropathy—clinical and electrophysiological study in synalbumin positive and synalbumin negative subjects, *Diabetologia*, **5**, 413.

CHOPRA, J. S., and FANNIN, T. (1971) Pathology of diabetic neuropathy, *J. Path.*, **104**, 175.

CHOPRA, J. S., and HURWITZ, L. J. (1969 a) A comparative study of peripheral nerve conduction in diabetes and non-diabetic chronic occlusive peripheral vascular disease, *Brain*, **92**, 83.

CHOPRA, J. S., and HURWITZ, L. J. (1969 b) Sural nerve myelinated fibre density and size in diabetics, *J. Neurol. Neurosurg. Psychiat.*, **32**, 149.

DOWNIE, A. W., and NEWELL, D. J. (1961) Sensory nerve conduction in patients with diabetes mellitus and controls, *Neurology (Minneap.)*, **11**, 876.

ELIASSON, S. G. (1966) Lipid synthesis in peripheral nerve from alloxan diabetic rats, *Lipids*, **1**, 237.

GARLAND, H. (1957) Diabetic amyotrophy, in *Modern Trends in Neurology* (2nd series), ed. Williams, D., p. 229, London.

GILLIATT, R. W., and WILLISON, R. G. (1962) Peripheral nerve conduction in diabetic neuropathy, *J. Neurol. Neurosurg. Psychiat.*, **25**, 11.

GOODMAN, J. I., BAUMOEL, S., FRANKEL, L., MARCUS, L. J., and WASSERMANN, S. (1953) *The Diabetic Neuropathies*, Springfield, Ill.

JORDAN, W. R. (1936) Neuritic manifestations in diabetes mellitus, *Arch. intern. Med.*, **57**, 307.

LAMONTAGNE, A., and BUCHTHAL, F. (1970) Electrophysiological studies in diabetic neuropathy, *J. Neurol. Neurosurg. Psychiat.*, **33**, 442.

THE LANCET (1972) Diabetic neuropathy: a preventable complication, *Lancet*, **ii**, 583.

LOW, P. A., WALSH, J. C., HUANG, C. Y., and McLEOD, J. G. (1975) The sympathetic nervous system in diabetic neuropathy—a clinical and pathological study, *Brain*, **98**, 341.

OSUNTOKUN, B. O. (1970) The neurology of non-alcoholic pancreatic diabetes mellitus in Nigerians, *J. neurol. Sci.*, **ii**, 17.

PALO, J., SAVOLAINEN, H., and HALTIA, M. (1972) Proteins of peripheral nerve myelin in diabetic neuropathy, *J. neurol. Sci.*, **16**, 193.

RAFF, M. C., SANGALANG, V., and ASBURY, A. K. (1968) Ischaemic mononeuropathy multiplex associated with diabetes mellitus, *Arch. Neurol. (Chic.)*, **18**, 487.

RUNDLES, R. W. (1945) Diabetic neuropathy, *Medicine (Baltimore)*, **24**, 111.

SENEVIRATNE, K. N., and WEERASURIYA, A. (1974) Nodal gap substance in diabetic nerve, *J. Neurol. Neurosurg. Psychiat.*, **37**, 502.

SHARMA, A. K., and THOMAS, P. K. (1974) Peripheral nerve structure and function in experimental diabetes, *J. neurol. Sci.*, **23**, 1.

SHARMA, A. K., and THOMAS, P. K. (1975) Peripheral nerve regeneration in experimental diabetes, *J. neurol. Sci.*, **24**, 417.

SHARPEY-SCHAFER, E. P., and TAYLOR, P. J. (1960) Absent circulatory reflexes in diabetic neuritis, *Lancet*, **i**, 559.

SIMPSON, J. A. (1962) The neuropathies, in *Modern Trends in Neurology* (3rd series), ed. Williams, D., London.

THIELE, B., and STÅLBERG, E. (1975) Single fibre EMG findings in polyneuropathies of different aetiology, *J. Neurol. Neurosurg. Psychiat.*, **38**, 881.

THOMAS, P. K., and LASCELLES, R. G. (1965) Schwann-cell abnormalities in diabetic neuropathy, *Lancet*, **i**, 1355.

THOMAS, P. K., and WARD, J. D. (1975) Diabetic neuropathy, in *Complications of Diabetes*, ed. Keen, H., and Jarrett, J., p. 151, London.

WATKINS, P. J. (1973) Facial sweating after food: a new sign of diabetic autonomic neuro-pathy, *Brit. med. J.*, **1**, 583.

WOLTMAN, H. W., and WILDER, R. M. (1929) Diabetes mellitus. Pathologic changes in the spinal cord and peripheral nerves, *Arch. intern. Med.*, **44**, 576.

HYPOGLYCAEMIC NEUROPATHY

In patients with an insulin-secreting pancreatic islet-cell adenoma, motor weakness may occur and can occasionally be accompanied by peripheral paraes-thesiae. It has been suggested that this syndrome is due to a peripheral neuro-pathy (Lambert *et al.*, 1960) but Tom and Richardson (1951) suggested that hyperinsulinism may damage the anterior horn cells of the spinal cord rather than the peripheral nerves. However, Danta (1969) reported two cases of sensori-motor polyneuropathy in patients with organic hyperinsulinism and found 22 other similar cases in the literature.

REFERENCES

DANTA, G. (1969) Hypoglycemic peripheral neuropathy, *Arch. Neurol. (Chic.)*, **21**, 121.

LAMBERT, E. H., MULDER, D. W., and BASTRON, D. W. (1960) Regeneration of peripheral nerves with hyperinsulinism neuropathy. Report of a case, *Neurology (Minneap.)*, **11**, 125.

TOM, M. I., RICHARDSON, J. C. (1951) Hypoglycaemia from islet-cell tumour of pancreas with amyotrophy and cerebrospinal nerve cell changes; a case report, *J. Neuropath.*, **10**, 57.

NEUROPATHY IN MYXOEDEMA AND PITUITARY DISORDERS

Bilateral compression of the median nerves in the carpal tunnels is a common complication of myxoedema (Murray and Simpson, 1958) but it has also been suggested that a symmetrical, predominantly sensory, neuropathy involving all four limbs may occur in such cases and responds to treatment with L-thyroxine (Nickel *et al.*, 1961). More recently Fincham and Cape (1968) and Dyck and Lambert (1970) have confirmed that a diffuse demyelinating sensorimotor neuropathy may indeed complicate hypothyroidism, and Shirabe *et al.* (1975) postulate a disorder of Schwann cell metabolism.

The carpal tunnel syndrome is also well known to complicate acromegaly but in this disorder, too, polyneuropathy has been described (Low *et al.*, 1974), as is also the case in thyrotropic hormone deficiency (Grabow and Chou, 1968) and pituitary gigantism (Lewis, 1972).

REFERENCES

DYCK, P. J., and LAMBERT, E. H. (1970) Polyneuropathy associated with hypothyroidism, *J. Neuropath. exp. Neurol.*, **29**, 631.

FINCHAM, R. W., and CAPE, C. A. (1968) Neuropathy in myxedema: a study of sensory nerve conduction in the upper extremities, *Arch. Neurol. (Chic.)*, **19**, 464.

GRABOW, J. D., and CHOU, S. M. (1968) Thyrotropin hormone deficiency with a peripheral neuropathy, *Arch. Neurol. (Chic.)*, **19**, 284.

LEWIS, P. D. (1972) Neuromuscular involvement in pituitary gigantism, *Brit. med. J.*, **2**, 499.

LOW, P. A., McLEOD, J. G., TURTLE, J. R., DONNELLY, P., and WRIGHT, R. G. (1974) Peripheral neuropathy in acromegaly, *Brain*, **97**, 139.

MURRAY, I. P. C., and SIMPSON, J. A. (1958) Acroparaesthesiae in myxoedema, *Lancet*, **i**, 1360.

NICKEL, S. N., FRAME, B., BEBIN, J., TOURTELOTTE, W. W., PARKER, J. A., and HUGHES, B. R. (1961) Myxoedema neuropathy and myopathy. A clinical and pathological study, *Neurology (Minneap.)*, **11**, 125.

SHIRABE, T., TAWARA, S., TERAO, A., and ARAKI, S. (1975) Myxoedematous polyneuropathy: a light and electron microscopic study of the peripheral nerve and muscle, *J. Neurol. Neurosurg. Psychiat.*, **38**, 241.

LIVER DISEASE AND POLYNEUROPATHY

Hepatic encephalopathy [p. 829] has been recognized for many years but the recognition of polyneuropathy as a complication of hepatic cirrhosis, active chronic hepatitis, and haemochromatosis (not secondary, in the latter condition, to diabetes) is comparatively recent (*British Medical Journal*, 1972). Knill-Jones *et al.* (1972) found evidence of an indolent, predominantly demyelinating polyneuropathy in 13 out of a series of 70 unselected patients with chronic liver disease, and Thomas and Walker (1965) described polyneuropathy resulting from xanthomatous deposits in peripheral nerves in primary biliary cirrhosis.

REFERENCES

BRITISH MEDICAL JOURNAL (1972) Peripheral neuropathy and chronic liver diseases, *Brit. med. J.*, **2**, 607.

KNILL-JONES, R. P., GOODWILL, C. J., DAYAN, A. D., and WILLIAMS, R. (1972) Peripheral neuropathy in chronic liver disease: clinical, electrodiagnostic, and nerve biopsy findings, *J. Neurol. Neurosurg. Psychiat.*, **35**, 22.

THOMAS, P. K., and WALKER, J. G. (1965) Xanthomatous neuropathy in primary biliary cirrhosis, *Brain*, **88**, 1079.

AMYLOID NEUROPATHY

Amyloidosis was in the past divided into primary and secondary forms. Secondary amyloidosis is associated with chronic suppuration, other chronic infective conditions and occasionally with malignant disease, particularly plasmacytoma. Primary amyloidosis occurs in the absence of any of these predisposing causes and is usually familial. So far as the amyloidosis is concerned it is doubtful whether the two forms differ, but in secondary amyloidosis the conspicuous features have usually been those of diffuse visceral involvement by the amyloid disease, while primary amyloidosis is likely to present more selectively, and not uncommonly with symptoms resulting from involvement of the peripheral nerves.

Three main varieties of inherited amyloid neuropathy, all of dominant inheritance (Andrade *et al.*, 1969, 1970), have been described. The commonest in many parts of the world is the so-called Portuguese type (Andrade, 1952) which presents as a rule with a diffuse polyneuropathy and has also been reported in Japan (Araki *et al.*, 1968). The so-called Indiana type (Rukavina *et al.*, 1956; Mahloudji *et al.*, 1969) usually presents with evidence of a bilateral carpal tunnel syndrome due to deposition of amyloid beneath the carpal ligament, a state of events which has also been described in amyloidosis secondary to myelomatosis (Dayan *et al.*, 1971). In the Iowa type (van Allen *et al.*, 1969) the affected family members showed evidence of progressive sensorimotor neuropathy, nephropathy, and peptic ulcer. The descriptions given below apply to the manifestations of the polyneuropathy as seen in the Portuguese and Iowa varieties.

The first symptoms are usually sensory, and consist of painful dysaesthesiae of the distal parts of the upper or lower limbs. The physical signs are those of a polyneuropathy with distal sensory loss, muscular wasting and weakness, and diminution or loss of the tendon reflexes. Hyperpathia is sometimes prominent and pain is more severely impaired than other forms of sensation (Dyck and Lambert, 1969). On the other hand, painless ulcers may occur. The peripheral nerves are characteristically thickened, and firmer than normal. Histological and electron microscopic studies have shown that deposits of amyloid are usually interfascicular but also occur in the endoneurium and perineurium and there is severe loss of unmyelinated axons and of smaller diameter myelinated fibres (Coimbra and Andrade, 1971 a and b; Thomas and King, 1974).

There may be an increase of protein or of the number of cells in the cerebro-spinal fluid.

Other symptoms of amyloid disease, notably macroglossia, myocardial involvement, and impairment of renal function may be present. Involvement of autonomic nerves commonly gives rise to gastro-intestinal symptoms, ortho-static hypotension, and impotence (Munsat and Poussaint, 1962).

The serum proteins may be low, with increased globulin and an abnormal protein found on electrophoresis. The Congo-red test may or may not be positive. Biopsy is the best method of confirming the diagnosis and may be carried out on the skin, gum, rectum or, most suitably in neurological cases, on a palpably thickened cutaneous nerve running from an area of abnormal sensation.

The diagnosis has to be made from other forms of peripheral neuropathy, especially those associated with thickening of the peripheral nerves, i.e. leprosy, and the various forms of hypertrophic neuropathy.

Death usually occurs in from one to five years from cardiac failure. Treatment is symptomatic.

REFERENCES

ANDRADE, C. (1952) A peculiar form of peripheral neuropathy, *Brain*, **75**, 408.
ANDRADE, C., ARAKI, S., BLOCK, W. D., COHEN, A. S., JACKSON, C. E., KUROIWA, Y., McKUSICK, V. A., NISSIM, J., SOHAR, E., and VAN ALLEN, M. W. (1970) Hereditary amyloidosis, *Arthritis and Rheumatism*, **13**, 902.
ANDRADE, C., CANIJO, M., KLEIN, D., and KAELIN, A. (1969) The genetic aspect of the familial amyloidotic polyneuropathy, *Humangenetik*, **7**, 163.
ARAKI, S., MAWATARI, S., OHTA, M., NAKAJIMA, A., and KUROIWA, Y. (1968) Polyneuritic amyloidosis in a Japanese family, *Arch. Neurol. (Chic.)*, **18**, 593.
CHAMBERS, R. A., MEDD, W. E., and SPENCER, H. (1958) Primary amyloidosis, *Quart. J. Med.*, **27**, 207.
COIMBRA, A., and ANDRADE, C. (1971 a) Familial amyloid polyneuropathy: an electron microscope study of the peripheral nerve in five cases. I. Interstitial changes, *Brain*, **94**, 199.
COIMBRA, A., and ANDRADE, C. (1971 b) Familial amyloid polyneuropathy: an electron microscope study of the peripheral nerve in five cases. II. Nerve fibre changes, *Brain*, **94**, 207.
DAYAN, A. D., URICH, H., and GARDNER-THORPE, C. (1971) Peripheral neuropathy and myeloma, *J. neurol. Sci.*, **14**, 21.
DYCK, P. J., and LAMBERT, E. H. (1969) Dissociated sensation in amyloidosis: compound action potential, quantitative histologic and teased-fiber, and electron microscopic studies of sural nerve biopsies, *Arch. Neurol. (Chic.)*, **20**, 490.

MAHLOUDJI, M., TEASDALL, R. D., ADAMKIEWICZ, J. J., HARTMAN, W. H., LAMBIRD, P. A., and McKUSICK, V. A. (1969) The genetic amyloidoses: with particular reference to hereditary neuropathic amyloidosis, type II (Indiana or Rukavina type), *Medicine (Baltimore)*, **48**, 1.

MUNSAT, T. L., and POUSSAINT, A. F. (1962) Clinical manifestations and diagnosis of amyloid polyneuropathy, *Neurology (Minneap.)*, **12**, 413.

RUKAVINA, J. G., BLOCK, W. D., JACKSON, C. E., FALLS, H. F., CAREY, J. H., and CURTIS, A. C. (1956) Primary systemic amyloidosis: a review and an experimental, genetic and clinical study of 29 cases with particular emphasis on the familial form, *Medicine (Baltimore)*, **35**, 239.

THOMAS, P. K., and KING, R. H. M. (1974) Peripheral nerve changes in amyloid neuropathy, *Brain*, **97**, 395.

VAN ALLEN, M. W., FROHLICH, J. A., and DAVIS, J. R. (1969) Inherited predisposition to generalized amyloidosis, *Neurology (Minneap.)*, **19**, 10.

PINK DISEASE

Synonyms. Erythroedema polyneuritis; acrodynia.

Definition. A disease affecting young children, now virtually unknown, characterized by irritability, photophobia, and red discoloration with slight swelling of the hands and feet, and symptoms of polyneuritis.

PATHOLOGY

The pathology of pink disease was investigated by Paterson and Greenfield (1924) and by Wyllie and Stern (1931) who found degeneration of peripheral nerves and chromatolysis of the anterior horn cells in the spinal cord. Histologically the cutaneous lesions consisted of hyperkeratosis, hypertrophy of the sweat glands, and lymphocytic infiltration of the corium, with oedema.

AETIOLOGY

The victims of the disease were young children between the ages of 4 months and 7 years, the onset usually occurring between the ages of 9 and 18 months. The disease used to be widely prevalent, especially in Australia and North America. Small local epidemics were characteristic. Most cases occurred between the autumn and early spring. Warkany and Hubbard (1948) suggested that mercury administered in teething powders or ointments was the causal agent. This is now established [see mercury poisoning, p. 808] and since the withdrawal of these powders and of calomel from the market, the disease has disappeared.

SYMPTOMS AND SIGNS

The earliest symptoms were usually those of a mild infection of the upper respiratory tract or of the alimentary canal. Shortly afterwards the child became miserable and irritable, and suffered from insomnia and loss of appetite. At the same time the hands and feet became bluish-red, slightly swollen, and cold. In addition there was often an erythematous rash over the face, trunk, and extremities. There was always excessive sweating, and desquamation occurred on the hands and feet. In severe cases trophic disturbances were present, including ulceration of the mouth, falling-out of teeth, nails and hair.

There was no paralysis, but the muscles were hypotonic, and in chronic cases the tendon reflexes were lost and analgesia of peripheral distribution was sometimes demonstrable. The pulse was rapid and the blood pressure often slightly raised. The urine often contained a trace of albumin and detectable amounts of mercury but the cerebrospinal fluid was normal.

DIAGNOSIS

The combination of symptoms and their occurrence in early childhood were unique, and the condition was, therefore, unlikely to be confused with any other.

PROGNOSIS

The mortality was low, approximately 5 per cent, death being due to cardiac failure, or more usually to an intercurrent infection, such as bronchopneumonia. The disease ran a chronic course and usually lasted from three months to a year.

TREATMENT

Treatment was mainly symptomatic. Bower (1954) found that ganglion-blocking drugs were worth a trial when autonomic symptoms predominated. Feeding often proved to be difficult on account of anorexia and irritability and sedatives were generally required. Slow improvement followed the withdrawal of drugs containing mercury and chelating agents were rarely required.

REFERENCES

BOWER, B. D. (1954) Pink disease: the autonomic disorder and its treatment with ganglion-blocking agents, *Quart. J. Med.*, N.S. **23**, 215.
PATERSON, D., and GREENFIELD, J. G. (1923–4) Erythroedema polyneuritis, *Quart. J. Med.*, **17**, 6 (contains 17 refs.).
WARKANY, J., and HUBBARD, D. M. (1948) Mercury in the urine of children with acrodynia, *Lancet*, **i,** 829.
WYLLIE, W. G., and STERN, R. O. (1931) Pink disease: its morbid anatomy, with a note on treatment, *Arch. Dis. Childh.*, **6,** 137.

METHYL MERCURY POISONING

The symptoms of methyl mercury poisoning in adults [p. 808] are usually dominated by manifestations of central nervous system damage but sensory symptoms in the extremities are common in such cases. However, electrophysiological studies have failed to show evidence of peripheral nerve damage and the sensory symptoms are therefore believed to be of central origin (Le Quesne *et al.*, 1974) though abnormalities of neuromuscular transmission have been found in some cases (Von Burg and Rustam, 1974).

REFERENCES

LE QUESNE, P. M., DAMLUJI, S. F., and RUSTAM, H. (1974) Electrophysiological studies of peripheral nerves in patients with organic mercury poisoning, *J. Neurol. Neurosurg. Psychiat.*, **37**, 333.
VON BURG, R., and RUSTAM, H. (1974) Electrophysiological investigations of methylmercury intoxication in humans. Evaluation of peripheral nerve by conduction velocity and electromyography, *Electroenceph. clin. Neurophysiol.*, **37,** 381.

DIPHTHERITIC NEUROPATHY

AETIOLOGY

Polyneuropathy is the commonest and most important of the nervous complications of diphtheria, the exotoxin of *Corynebacterium diphtheriae* having an affinity for the peripheral nerves. It is most frequently observed during childhood and is rare in adult life. Rolleston (1929) showed that the occurrence of paralysis bears a definite relationship to the severity of the local infection, which is usually faucial but may be extrafaucial. The introduction of antitoxin reduced greatly the incidence of paralysis, which is almost unknown in patients who receive antitoxin on the first day of their illness, and becomes progressively more frequent the longer such treatment is delayed.

Palatal paralysis is usually attributed to the ascent of the toxin from the common faucial site of infection to the medulla. Local ascent of the nerves by the toxin is responsible for the local development of paralysis following a cutaneous infection, the muscles paralysed being those supplied by the spinal segment from which the infected region is innervated (Walshe, 1918–19). Localized neuropathy in one or more extremities was noted after diphtheritic infection of wounds in the Middle East in the Second World War. Paralysis of accommodation and generalized polyneuropathy are due to the dissemination of the toxin by the blood stream to the ciliary muscle, and the peripheral nerves.

PATHOLOGY

The primary lesion in the peripheral nerves is segmental demyelination (Fisher and Adams, 1956; Morgan-Hughes, 1965, 1968) which is accompanied by characteristic slowing of motor nerve conduction, a finding which may persist for some time after clinical recovery. Secondary axonal degeneration may be produced in experimental animals (Bradley and Jennekens, 1971) and the demyelinated nerves are excessively sensitive to pressure (Hopkins and Morgan-Hughes, 1969). The neuropathic effects of the toxin have been shown experimentally to be dose-dependent; the toxin becomes unavailable for inactivation by antitoxin within one hour and small diameter nerve fibres are more severely affected (Cavanagh and Jacobs, 1964). Hemiplegia, a rare complication of diphtheria, appears usually to be due to a vascular lesion, either embolism or thrombosis of a cerebral artery, or to acute post-infective encephalitis.

SYMPTOMS AND SIGNS

Paralysis of the palate, which is usually the earliest nervous symptom, may occur within a few days of the onset of the infection. Usually, however, it develops during the second or third week. It is generally bilateral but may be unilateral. It causes the voice to acquire a nasal character and leads to regurgitation of fluids through the nose on swallowing. The palatal reflex is usually lost.

Paralysis of accommodation develops as a rule during the third or fourth week and leads to dimness of vision for near objects. It is usually bilateral, very rarely unilateral, and may pass unnoticed in myopic subjects who do not require to accommodate for near vision. The pupillary reactions to light and on convergence are unimpaired. Paresis of external ocular muscles is not very rare, the lateral rectus being most often affected.

The symptoms of generalized polyneuropathy, which are not always preceded by paralysis of the palate and of accommodation, do not develop until between the fifth and seventh week after infection. At this stage paralysis of the constrictors of the pharynx, of the intrinsic muscles of the larynx, associated with laryngeal anaesthesia, and paralysis of the diaphragm are the most serious complications, on account of the dysphagia and dyspnoea to which they lead. The adductors of the vocal cords are more often paralysed than the abductors. Paralysis of the neck muscles may occur.

The lower limbs are usually more severely affected than the upper, and movements of peripheral segments suffer more than those of proximal. Sensory loss is common, cutaneous anaesthesia and analgesia of the 'glove and stocking' distribution being associated with tenderness of the muscles on pressure. Postural sensibility is often grossly impaired, leading to marked ataxia, especially in the lower limbs, the so-called 'pseudotabetic form' of diphtheritic paralysis.

The tendon reflexes are lost early and may remain absent for months or even for years. Loss of the tendon reflexes may occur in the absence of other symptoms and, with or without palatal palsy, may constitute the only nervous symptoms of diphtheria. The plantar reflexes may be unobtainable but are usually flexor, though Rolleston drew attention to the occurrence of extensor plantar responses, an indication that the corticospinal tracts may rarely be involved. The sphincters are usually unaffected, but impotence has been described. The 'cardiac paralysis' of the early stages is probably due to the effect of the toxin on the myocardium, but at any stage tachycardia may occur as a result of vagal paralysis. The cerebrospinal fluid may be normal or its protein content may be increased.

Diphtheritic hemiplegia is fortunately rare. The symptoms are similar to those of other acquired forms of infantile hemiplegia [see p. 632]. Meningism is not uncommon in the acute stage. Cervical rigidity or opisthotonus may be associated with rigidity of the limbs, so-called 'spasmodic diphtheria'. The cerebrospinal fluid in such cases, though its pressure may be increased, is normal in composition. Permanent bulbar palsy is a rare sequel.

DIAGNOSIS

For the diagnosis of polyneuritis see page 945. The diphtheritic form is usually easily recognized on account of the age of the patient and the occurrence of such characteristic features as palatal paralysis and paralysis of accommodation. The diphtheria bacillus should always be sought at the site of infection, but may be absent.

PROGNOSIS

The prognosis of the paralysis is usually good if the child survives. Paralysis of the palate and of accommodation disappears in from three to six weeks, and recovery from limb paralysis is usually complete, though it may take several months. Paralysis of the pharynx, larynx, and diaphragm, though equally recoverable, is of more serious import owing to the risk of bronchopneumonia. Permanent paralysis of the limbs is fortunately very rare. Hemiplegia is a serious complication, as not only may it prove fatal, but in patients who survive recovery is usually incomplete, and epilepsy and mental defect may occur as sequels.

TREATMENT

The routine treatment of diphtheria includes injection of adequate doses of antitoxin as early as possible. If this has been carried out, the administration of further doses when paralysis develops is of doubtful value. Paralysis of the

I i

limbs should be treated on the lines laid down for the treatment of polyneuritis [see p. 936]. Paralysis of the pharynx and larynx necessitates special care in feeding. Food should be soft and semi-fluid, and if, in spite of this, coughing or choking occurs, it will be necessary to employ nasal feeding. Bulbar and respiratory paralysis should be treated as in poliomyelitis [see p. 505].

REFERENCES

BRADLEY, W. G., and JENNEKENS, F. G. I. (1971) Axonal degeneration in diphtheritic neuropathy, *J. neurol. Sci.*, **13**, 415.

CAVANAGH, J. B., and JACOBS, J. M. (1964) Some quantitative aspects of diphtheritic neuropathy, *Brit. J. exp. Path.*, **45**, 309.

FISHER, C. M., and ADAMS, R. D. (1956) Diphtheritic polyneuritis: a pathological study, *J. Neuropath. exp. Neurol.*, **15**, 243.

HOPKINS, A. P., and MORGAN-HUGHES, J. A. (1969) The effect of local pressure in diphtheritic neuropathy, *J. Neurol. Neurosurg. Psychiat.*, **32**, 614.

MAHER, R. M. (1948) Significance of palatal movements in diphtheria, *Lancet*, **i**, 57.

MORGAN-HUGHES, J. A. (1965) Changes in motor nerve conduction velocity in diphtheritic polyneuritis, *Rev. Pat. nerv. ment.*, **86**, 253.

MORGAN-HUGHES, J. A. (1968) Experimental diphtheritic neuropathy: a pathological and electrophysiological study, *J. neurol. Sci.*, **7**, 157.

ROLLESTON, J. D. (1913) Diphtheritic hemiplegia, *Clin. J.*, **42**, 12.

ROLLESTON, J. D. (1929) *Acute Infectious Diseases*, 2nd ed., London.

WALSHE, F. M. R. (1917–18) On the pathogenesis of diphtheritic paralysis, Part I, *Quart. J. Med.*, **11**, 191.

WALSHE, F. M. R. (1918–19) On the pathogenesis of diphtheritic paralysis, Part II, *Quart J. Med.*, **12**, 14.

POLYNEURITIS IN COLLAGEN DISORDERS

The occurrence of polyneuropathy in association with sarcoidosis, systemic lupus erythematosus, scleroderma, and rheumatoid arthritis raises problems of pathogenesis which are not yet completely solved (Hart and Golding, 1960; Kibler and Rose, 1960; Steinberg, 1960). In polyarteritis nodosa it is due to vascular lesions of the peripheral nerves, a mononeuritis multiplex and the same appears to be the case in systemic lupus (Bailey *et al.*, 1956). Indeed it seems probable that involvement of the vasa nervorum is a pathological process common to all of the disorders in this group. Dyck *et al.* (1972) described a neuropathy secondary to necrotizing angiitis in a patient with rheumatoid arthritis and found no essential difference between the lesions observed in this case and those seen in polyarteritis nodosa. Mononeuropathy may also occur in the necrotizing angiitis, virtually identical with polyarteritis nodosa, which may result from drug sensitivity or from the abuse of drugs such as amphetamine (Stafford *et al.*, 1975). Polyneuropathy secondary to sarcoidosis may be associated with sarcoid myopathy (Garcin and Lapresle, 1967). An inflammatory sensory perineuritis of unknown aetiology, principally involving cutaneous nerves, has also been described (Asbury *et al.*, 1972). In systemic lupus, systemic sclerosis, and polyarteritis nodosa the neuropathy may show some improvement with steroid drugs. In rheumatoid arthritis, Pallis and Scott (1965) identified five different types of peripheral neuropathy. Isolated lesions of major peripheral nerves in either the upper or lower limbs, digital neuropathy in the upper limbs and distal sensory neuropathy in the lower limbs are in their view relatively benign and often recover. However, the syndrome of distal sensorimotor polyneuropathy involving all four limbs carries a uniformly poor prognosis. It seems to arise more commonly in patients who have been treated with steroid drugs given for their rheumatoid disease and most affected individuals die of a diffuse vasculitis. Conn *et al.* (1972) pointed out that in such cases treated with steroids there was pathological evidence of proliferative endarteritis suggesting a healing process secondary to acute arteritis. In less severe cases of rheumatoid neuropathy there is evidence of segmental demyelination of peripheral nerves with less evidence of vascular damage (Weller *et al.*, 1970; Haslock *et al.*, 1970; Beckett and Dinn, 1972).

Whereas in many cases of polyneuropathy due to the causes listed above the nature of the primary disease is self-evident, in any subacute or chronic sensori-motor polyneuropathy with marked slowing of motor and/or sensory nerve conduction, particularly when the erythrocyte sedimentation rate is raised, the possibility of an underlying collagen or connective tissue disease should be considered.

REFERENCES

ASBURY, A. K., PICARD, E. H., and BARINGER, J. R. (1972) Sensory perineuritis, *Arch. Neurol. (Chic.)*, **26**, 302.

BAILEY, A. A., SAYRE, G. P., and CLARK, E. C. (1956) Neuritis associated with systemic lupus erythematosus, *Arch. Neurol. Psychiat. (Chic.)*, **75**, 251.

BECKETT, V. L., and DINN, J. J. (1972) Segmental demyelination in rheumatoid arthritis, *Quart. J. Med.*, **41**, 71.

CONN, D. L., McDUFFIE, F. C., and DYCK, P. J. (1972) Immunopathologic study of sural nerves in rheumatoid arthritis, *Arthritis and Rheumatism*, **15**, 135.

DYCK, P. J., CONN, D. L., and OKAZAKI, H. (1972) Necrotizing angiopathic neuropathy: three-dimensional morphology of fiber degeneration related to sites of occluded vessels, *Mayo Clin. Proc.*, **47**, 461.

GARCIN, R., and LAPRESLE, J. (1967) Syndrome multinévritique avec lésions de sarcoidose à la biopsie musculaire, *Neurological Problems*, p. 299, Paris.

HART, F. D., and GOLDING, J. R. (1960) Rheumatoid neuropathy, *Brit. med. J.*, **1**, 1594.

HASLOCK, D. I., WRIGHT, V., and HARRIMAN, D. G. F. (1970) Neuromuscular disorders in rheumatoid arthritis, *Quart. J. Med.*, **39**, 335.

KIBLER, R. F., and ROSE, F. C. (1960) Peripheral neuropathy in collagen diseases, *Brit. med. J.*, **1**, 1781.

PALLIS, C. A., and SCOTT, J. T. (1965) Peripheral neuropathy in rheumatoid arthritis, *Brit. med. J.*, **1**, 1141.

STAFFORD, C. R., BOGDANOFF, B. M., GREEN, L., and SPECTOR, H. B. (1975) Mononeuropathy multiplex as a complication of amphetamine angiitis, *Neurology (Minneap.)*, **25**, 570.

STEINBERG, V. L. (1960) Neuropathy in rheumatoid diseases, *Brit. med. J.*, **1**, 1600.

WELLER, R. O., BRUCKNER, F. E., and CHAMBERLAIN, M. A. (1970) Rheumatoid neuropathy: a histological and electrophysiological study, *J. Neurol. Neurosurg. Psychiat.*, **33**, 592.

LEPROUS NEURITIS

AETIOLOGY

Leprosy is due to infection with the *Mycobacterium leprae* of Hansen, an acidfast bacillus, staining like the tubercle bacillus by Ziehl-Neelsen's method. The mode of infection is uncertain, but the disease is certainly contagious. The organism has a predilection for the mucous membranes, skin, and peripheral nerves.

PATHOLOGY

The characteristic lesion is a granuloma, the leprous nodule, composed of large connective-tissue cells, the lepra-cells, containing the lepra bacilli and surrounded by epithelioid and plasma cells and fibroblasts. Two main varieties of pathological change have been described in the peripheral nerves. In tuberculoid neuritis, which may occur without skin lesions (Jopling and Morgan-Hughes, 1965), the powerful immune responses of the host represented by focal masses of epithelioid cells in the lesions keep the bacilli in abeyance, but the entire parenchyma of the nerve undergoes damage at sites of predilection so that there is extensive Wallerian degeneration distal to these lesions (Dastur and Dabholkar, 1974). In lepromatous neuritis, on the other hand, the immune response is suppressed, bacilli are present in large numbers, especially in Schwann cells, there are usually extensive associated skin lesions, and there is more diffuse damage to both peripheral nerve myelin and axons (Dastur, 1967). The dorsal root ganglia, the trigeminal ganglia, the sympathetic ganglia, and the anterior horns of the spinal cord may be invaded, and within the cord fibres derived from the dorsal root ganglia undergo degeneration.

SYMPTOMS

The onset of symptoms is gradual. Prodromal symptoms of a toxaemic nature may be present. These are followed by pains referred to the distribution of the peripheral nerves in the limbs and often by a sense of numbness of the extremities. Symptoms tend to be symmetrical, anaesthesia of the 'glove and stocking' distribution developing, together with atrophic paralysis of the muscles of the peripheral segments of the limbs. Pure neural tuberculoid leprosy without skin lesions is uncommon. In advanced lepromatous leprosy bizarre patterns of sensory impairment may occur in the skin of the upper extremities, with comparative sparing of sensation in the palm and antecubital fossa but dense sensory loss on the dorsum of the hand and forearm; this seems to be due to the fact that fine cutaneous nerve endings are most extensively damaged in cooler skin areas (Sabin, 1969). Facial anaesthesia and paralysis due to involvement of the fifth and seventh cranial nerves are often seen (Antia et al., 1966; Dastur et al., 1966). Trophic changes are conspicuous in the limbs. Bullae, ulceration, and necrosis of the phalanges occur, and the digits may ultimately be destroyed. Thickening of the peripheral nerves is usually, but not invariably, palpable.

DIAGNOSIS

Leprous neuritis must be distinguished from other forms of polyneuritis, especially from progressive hypertrophic polyneuritis, in which palpable thickening of the peripheral nerves may also occur, from syringomyelia, and from Raynaud's disease. Bacteriological examination and biopsy may be necessary.

PROGNOSIS

Modern chemotherapy with sulphone drugs has much improved the prognosis. Recovery is usually complete in a few years in cases treated early, though there may be evidence of residual nerve damage.

TREATMENT

For the treatment of leprosy the reader is referred to textbooks of tropical medicine. Shepard (1974) gives a useful review. Pressure-sensitive devices which are of value in management are discussed by Brand and Ebner (1969) and nerve grafting is helpful in selected cases (McLeod *et al.*, 1975).

REFERENCES

ANTIA, N. H., DIVEKAR, S. C., and DASTUR, D. K. (1966) The facial nerve in leprosy. 1. Clinical and operative aspects, *Int. J. Leprosy*, **34**, 103.
BRAND, P. W., and EBNER, J. D. (1969) Pressure sensitive devices for denervated hands and feet, *J. Bone Jt Surg.*, **51A**, 109.
COCHRANE, R. G. (1954) in *Modern Trends in Dermatology*, ed. MacKenna, R. M. B., p. 153, London.
DASTUR, D. K. (1967) The peripheral neuropathology of leprosy, in *Symposium on Leprosy*, ed. Antia, N. H., and Dastur, D. K., Bombay.
DASTUR, D. K., ANTIA, N. H., and DIVEKAR, S. C. (1966) The facial nerve in leprosy. 2. Pathology, pathogenesis, electromyography and clinical correlations, *Int. J. Leprosy*, **34**, 118.
DASTUR, D. K., and DABHOLKAR, A. S. (1974) Histochemistry of leprous nerves and skin lesions, *J. Path.*, **113**, 69.
JOPLING, W. H., and MORGAN-HUGHES, J. A. (1965) Pure neural tuberculoid leprosy, *Brit. med. J.*, **2**, 799.
JULIÃO, O. F. (1945) *Contribuição para o estudo do diagnóstico clínico da lepra nervosa*, São Paulo.
KHANOLKAR, V. R. (1951) Studies in the histology of early lesions of leprosy, *Indian Council of Med. Res. Spec. Rep. Series*, 19.
McLEOD, J. G., HARGRAVE, J. C., GYE, R. S., POLLARD, J. D., WALSH, J. C., LITTLE, J. M., and BOOTH, G. C. (1975) Nerve grafting in leprosy, *Brain*, **98**, 203.
SABIN, T. D. (1969) Temperature-linked sensory loss: a unique pattern in leprosy, *Arch. Neurol. (Chic.)*, **20**, 257.
SHEPARD, C. C. (1974) Leprosy, in *Harrison's Principles of Internal Medicine*, 7th ed., chap. 157, New York.

PROGRESSIVE HYPERTROPHIC POLYNEUROPATHY

Definition. A rare syndrome, frequently familial, characterized by conspicuous enlargement of the peripheral nerves, associated with symptoms of slowly progressive polyneuropathy, and sometimes other abnormalities. The condition was first described in 1889 by Gombault and Mallet, but is usually associated with the names of Dejerine and Sottas, who reported two cases in 1893. It must be noted that hypertrophy of peripheral nerves is simply the result of chronic recurrent demyelination and remyelination with Schwann cell hypertrophy. It may occur in relapsing steroid-responsive polyneuropathy [p. 954], in diabetes [p. 968], in leprosy, and in disorders in which abnormal metabolites are laid down within the nerves, as previously noted. Thus it is a typical feature of Refsum's disease [see Campbell and Williams (1967), Try (1969), and p. 651].

However, the term progressive hypertrophic polyneuropathy is usually used to identify a dominantly inherited disorder of unknown aetiology. There is now some doubt as to whether this condition can be distinguished clinically or pathologically from the hypertrophic variety of peroneal muscular atrophy [p. 699] or from the Roussy–Levy syndrome [p. 674 and Kriel *et al.*, 1974].

PATHOLOGY

There is a marked increase in the volume of the peripheral nerves, though some may be affected more than others. The sciatic nerve in a case reported by Harris and Newcomb (1929) measured 4 cm in diameter. In addition to the nerves of the limbs the cranial nerves may be involved, and similar changes have been described in the sympathetic nerves, the cauda equina, and the spinal roots. The thickening is principally due to hypertrophy and proliferation of the Schwann cells. This 'onion-bulb' hypertrophy has been studied with the electron microscope by Weller (1967), Thomas and Lascelles (1967), Weller and das Gupta (1968), and Weller and Herzog (1970), among others. The interfibrillar connective tissue of the nerve sheaths also undergoes hypertrophy, though to a lesser extent. There is extensive segmental demyelination with secondary damage to the axons (Dyck and Gomez, 1968; Dyck et al., 1974) and abnormalities of the lipid constitution of the peripheral nerves have been described in such cases (Dyck et al., 1970; Koeppen et al., 1971). Within the spinal cord degeneration of the posterior columns is frequently, but not invariably, present, and is probably secondary to the changes in the nerves. It is most marked in the lumbosacral region and in the cervical cord is confined to the fasciculus gracilis. Compression of the spinal cord giving rise to 'long tract signs' has been rarely reported in such cases and appears to be a mechanical effect produced by hypertrophied spinal roots (Symonds and Blackwood, 1962). The muscles exhibit a simple atrophy. The pathological changes in Refsum's syndrome are similar, and a cardiomyopathy has been described in the latter disease by Cammermeyer (1956) and Gordon and Hudson (1959).

AETIOLOGY

Although sporadic cases occur, the classical disease is invariably of dominant inheritance. Russell and Garland (1930) described fully developed or abortive cases in four generations of the same family. The onset of symptoms usually occurs in childhood, but exceptionally is deferred until adult life. Refsum's disease, by contrast, like many other inherited metabolic disorders, is a condition of autosomal recessive inheritance.

SYMPTOMS AND SIGNS

Symptoms may begin in childhood or adult life. Sensory symptoms are usually prominent in the early stages, and patients frequently complain of shooting pains in the limbs, which may be associated with a sense of numbness in the hands and feet. Difficulty in walking is often an early complaint. Muscular weakness and wasting develop symmetrically in the peripheral muscles of the limbs. Either the hands or the feet may be first affected, or both may suffer simultaneously. The wasting rarely extends above the knees or the elbows. Coarse fasciculation is frequently present in the affected muscles, which exhibit the reaction of degeneration. Claw-hand and claw-foot may follow the muscular atrophy, but pes cavus may be present as a congenital abnormality.

Cutaneous sensory loss of the 'glove and stocking' distribution is found, and postural sensibility is also impaired.

Argyll Robertson pupils have been described in a few cases, and the pupils, though reacting normally, may be small, probably on account of oculo-sympathetic paralysis. Nystagmus is frequently present and cataracts have been described (Gold and Hoganhuis, 1968). The deep reflexes are diminished or lost in the affected muscles; the plantar reflexes may be lost; exceptionally extensor plantar reflexes have been described but this is probably due to mechanical compression of the spinal cord (Symonds and Blackwood, 1962). Kyphoscoliosis is sometimes present, and arthropathic changes have been observed in the joints of the limbs. Palpable thickening of the peripheral nerves is a valuable diagnostic sign but is not invariably present. It is usually identified most easily in the ulnar or common peroneal nerves, in the greater auricular nerve or in cutaneous nerves crossing the sternomastoid when the head is turned to one side. The CSF protein may be raised.

DIAGNOSIS

There is little difficulty in making a correct diagnosis in a patient presenting the symptoms of a slowly progressive polyneuropathy and in whom the peripheral nerves are thickened. In neurofibromatosis, which may cause focal thickening of nerves, it is rare to find palpable thickening of the deep nerves, such as the ulnar, and polyneuritic symptoms are absent. Leprosy and sarcoidosis are unlikely to cause confusion. The inherited disorder must also be distinguished from the other forms of metabolic or post-infective polyneuritis (e.g. diabetic and amyloid neuropathy, Refsum's disease, and recurrent or post-infective polyneuritis) in which enlargement of nerves may occur. From these it can be differentiated by its familial incidence, and slow progressive course. Distinction from the hypertrophic variety of peroneal muscular atrophy may be impossible; indeed the two conditions may be variants of a single disease. In this condition, as in other forms of demyelinating neuropathy, nerve conduction is markedly slowed. Biopsy of a superficial cutaneous nerve may help to settle the diagnosis.

PROGNOSIS

The course of the disease is extremely slow and is usually steadily progressive, though remissions may occur. When the onset is in childhood patients usually survive to adult life, becoming increasingly crippled, and finally bedridden. Death occurs from some intercurrent disease.

TREATMENT

No treatment is known to influence the course of the disease, but treatment on the lines indicated for polyneuritis will help to maintain the power of the limbs as long as possible.

REFERENCES

CAMMERMEYER, J. (1956) Neuropathological changes in hereditary neuropathies: manifestations of the syndrome heredopathia atactica polyneuritiformis in the presence of interstitial hypertrophic polyneuritis, *J. Neuropath. exp. Neurol.*, **15,** 340.

CAMPBELL, A. M. G., and WILLIAMS, E. R. (1967) Natural history of Refsum's syndrome in a Gloucestershire family, *Brit. med. J.*, **3,** 777.

CROFT, P. B., and WADIA, N. H. (1957) Familial hypertrophic polyneuritis, *Neurology*, *(Minneap.)*, **7,** 356.

DEJERINE, J., and SOTTAS, J. (1893) Sur la névrite interstitielle hypertrophique et progressive de l'enfance, *C.R. Soc. Biol. (Paris)*, **50,** 63.

DYCK, P. J., ELLEFSON, R. D., LAIS, A. C., SMITH, R. C., TAYLOR, W. F., and VAN DYKE, R. A. (1970) Histologic and lipid studies of sural nerves in inherited hypertrophic neuropathy: preliminary report of a lipid abnormality in nerve and liver in Dejerine-Sottas disease, *Mayo Clin. Proc.*, **45,** 286.

DYCK, P. J., and GOMEZ, M. R. (1968) Segmental demyelinization in Dejerine-Sottas disease: light, phase-contrast, and electron microscopic studies, *Mayo Clin. Proc.*, **43,** 280.

DYCK, P. J., LAIS, A. C., and OFFORD, K. P. (1974) The nature of myelinated nerve fiber degeneration in dominantly inherited hypertrophic neuropathy, *Mayo Clin. Proc.*, **49,** 34.

GOLD, G. N., and HOGENHUIS, L. A. H. (1968) Hypertrophic interstitial neuropathy and cataracts, *Neurology (Minneap.)*, **18**, 526.

GORDON, N., and HUDSON, R. E. B. (1959) Refsum's syndrome—heredopathia atactica polyneuritiformis, *Brain*, **82**, 41.

HARRIS, W., and NEWCOMB, W. D. (1929) A case of relapsing interstitial hypertrophic polyneuritis, *Brain*, **52**, 108.

KOEPPEN, A. H., MESSMORE, H., and STEHBENS, W. E. (1971) Interstitial hypertrophic neuropathy: biochemical study of the peripheral nervous system, *Arch. Neurol. (Chic.)*, **24**, 340.

KRIEL, R. L., CLIFFER, K. D., BERRY, J., SUNG, J. H., and BLAND, C. S. (1974) Investigation of a family with hypertrophic neuropathy resembling Roussy-Levy syndrome, *Neurology (Minneap.)*, **24**, 801.

REFSUM, S. (1946) Heredopathia atactica polyneuritiformis, *Acta psychiat. scand.*, Suppl. 38.

RUSSELL, W. R., and GARLAND, H. G. (1930) Progressive hypertrophic polyneuritis, with case reports, *Brain*, **53**, 376.

SYMONDS, C. P., and BLACKWOOD, W. (1962) Spinal cord compression in hypertrophic neuritis, *Brain*, **85**, 251.

THOMAS, P. K., and LASCELLES, R. G. (1967) Hypertrophic neuritis, *Quart. J. Med.*, **36**, 223.

TRY, K. (1969) Heredopathia atactica polyneuritiformis (Refsum's disease): the diagnostic value of phytanic acid determination in serum lipids, *Europ. Neurol.*, **2**, 1.

WELLER, R. O. (1967) An electron microscopic study of hypertrophic neuropathy of Dejerine and Sottas, *J. Neurol. Neurosurg. Psychiat.*, **30**, 111.

WELLER, R. O., and DAS GUPTA, T. K. (1968) Experimental hypertrophic neuropathy: an electron microscope study, *J. Neurol. Neurosurg. Psychiat.*, **31**, 34.

WELLER, R. O., and HERZOG, I. (1970) Schwann cell lysosomes in hypertrophic neuropathy and in normal human nerves, *Brain*, **93**, 347.

OTHER INHERITED POLYNEUROPATHIES

Many inherited disorders of the central nervous system described elsewhere in this volume may also involve the peripheral nerves, giving manifestations of polyneuropathy. This is certainly the case in several of the leukodystrophies, especially metachromatic leukodystrophy [p. 647] and Krabbe's disease [p. 646]. Other rare degenerative diseases such as neuroaxonal dystrophy (Duncan et al., 1970 and p. 660) and Cockayne's syndrome (Moosa and Dubowitz, 1970 and p. 654) may also cause polyneuropathy. Loss of small sensory neurones is found in Fabry's disease (Ohnishi and Dyck, 1974 and p. 650) and sensory neuropathy has been reported in acrodermatitis chronica atrophicans (Hopf, 1975). Disorders of lipid metabolism, some clearly identifiable, such as Tangier disease or alpha-lipoprotein deficiency (Engel et al., 1967; Kocen et al., 1973 and p. 655) and some unidentified (Fessel, 1971) also give clinical manifestations of peripheral nerve disease. In the rare condition of giant axonal neuropathy (Carpenter et al., 1974; Igisu et al., 1975) the affected children show tight, curly, and pale scalp hair and progressive weakness and sensory loss in the lower extremities with difficulty in walking; sural nerve biopsy in such cases shows giant axons containing a massive increase in neurofilaments; the cause is unknown.

In the group of hereditary ataxias, peripheral nerve involvement is constant in peroneal muscular atrophy and other related disorders [pp. 699–704], and hereditary sensory neuropathy (Ohta et al., 1973; Murray, 1973 and see p. 669) which may be associated with increased synthesis of immunoglobulin A

(Whitaker *et al.*, 1974) is also well defined. While congenital insensitivity to pain is a disorder of multiple pathogenesis, being observed in dysautonomia [p. 1072] and in some cases being probably due to central nervous system dysfunction (Thrush, 1973), evidence of sensory peripheral neuropathy with abnormal Schwann cells has been reported (Appenzeller and Kornfeld, 1972).

Finally, in certain well-recognized metabolic disorders including porphyria (Ridley *et al.*, 1968; Ridley, 1969 and see p. 825), polyneuropathy is a well-recognized complication.

REFERENCES

APPENZELLER, O., and KORNFELD, M. (1972) Indifference to pain: a chronic peripheral neuropathy with mosaic Schwann cells, *Arch. Neurol. (Chic.)*, **27**, 322.

CARPENTER, S., KARPATI, G., ANDERMANN, F., and GOLD, R. (1974) Giant axonal neuropathy, *Arch. Neurol. (Chic.)*, **31**, 312.

DUNCAN, C., STRUB, R., McGARRY, P., and DUNCAN, D. (1970) Peripheral nerve biopsy as an aid to diagnosis in infantile neuroaxonal dystrophy, *Neurology (Minneap.)*, **20**, 1024.

ENGEL, W. K., DORMAN, J. D., LEVY, R. I., and FREDRICKSON, D. S. (1967) Neuropathy in Tangier disease. Alpha-lipoprotein deficiency manifesting as familial recurrent neuropathy and interstitial lipid storage, *Arch. Neurol. (Chic.)*, **17**, 1.

FESSEL, W. J. (1971) Fat disorders and peripheral neuropathy, *Brain*, **94**, 531.

HOPF, H. C. (1975) Peripheral neuropathy in acrodermatitis chronica atrophicans (Herxheimer), *J. Neurol. Neurosurg. Psychiat.*, **38**, 452.

IGISU, H., OHTA, M., TABIRA, T., HOSOKAWA, S., GOTO, I., and KUROIWA, Y. (1975) Giant axonal neuropathy: a clinical entity affecting the central as well as the peripheral nervous system, *Neurology (Minneap.)*, **25**, 717.

KOCEN, R. S., KING, R. H. M., THOMAS, P. K., and HAAS, L. F. (1973) Nerve biopsy findings in two cases of Tangier disease, *Acta neuropath. (Berl.)*, **26**, 317.

MOOSA, A., and DUBOWITZ, V. (1970) Peripheral neuropathy in Cockayne's syndrome, *Arch. Dis. Childh.*, **45**, 674.

MURRAY, T. J. (1973) Congenital sensory neuropathy, *Brain*, **96**, 387.

OHNISHI, A., and DYCK, P. J. (1974) Loss of small peripheral sensory neurons in Fabry disease, *Arch. Neurol. (Chic.)*, **31**, 120.

OHTA, M., ELLEFSON, R. D., LAMBERT, E. H., and DYCK, P. J. (1973) Hereditary sensory neuropathy, type II, *Arch. Neurol. (Chic.)*, **29**, 23.

RIDLEY, A. (1969) The neuropathy of acute intermittent porphyria, *Quart. J. Med.*, **38**, 307.

RIDLEY, A., HIERONS, R., and CAVANAGH, J. B. (1968) Tachycardia and the neuropathy of porphyria, *Lancet*, **ii**, 708.

THRUSH, D. C. (1973) Congenital insensitivity to pain—a clinical, genetic and neurophysiological study of four children from the same family, *Brain*, **96**, 369.

WHITAKER, J. N., FALCHUCK, Z. M., ENGEL, W. K., BLAESE, R. M., and STROBER, W. (1974) Hereditary sensory neuropathy: association with increased synthesis of immunoglobulin A, *Arch. Neurol. (Chic.)*, **30**, 359.

CHRONIC PROGRESSIVE POLYNEURITIS

The term 'chronic progressive polyneuritis' or 'slow chronic polyneuritis' (Harris, 1935) has been applied to rare cases of polyneuritis which cannot be attributed to any of the common toxic causes and which run a slowly progressive course. In all such cases, if the many causes of polyneuropathy as described above can reasonably be excluded, it is important to bear in mind the possibility, especially if the neuropathy is shown by electrophysiological studies to be predominantly of the axonal type, that it may be the manifestation of under-lying malignant disease [p. 871] or of a reticulosis or haematological disorder [p. 865]. However, it should be noted that whereas the neuropathy of multiple myeloma, for instance (Victor *et al.*, 1958; Walsh, 1971), which may recover after effective treatment of the primary disorder (Davis and Drachman, 1972), is, like other paraneoplastic neuropathies, predominantly axonal, that which may be the presenting symptom of Waldenström's macroglobulinaemia (Propp *et al.*, 1975) is predominantly demyelinating. Another possible cause of axonal neuropathy which should also be considered in obscure cases is occult intestinal malabsorption as in gluten sensitivity (Pallis and Lewis, 1974). Even if these and other obscure causes of polyneuropathy are considered, there remain some cases in which the cause of the neuropathy cannot be explained.

When the polyneuropathy, by contrast, proves to be predominantly demye-linating in type, with marked slowing of motor and sensory nerve conduction and especially if the protein content of the CSF is raised, or if there is peripheral nerve enlargement, the possibility must always be considered that the condition is related to recurrent or relapsing polyneuritis [p. 954]. The possibility of a response to treatment with steroid drugs is always to be considered and a thera-peutic trial with prednisone given in full dosage at least for several weeks or even, in diminishing dosage, for several months, monitoring progress by serial measurement of nerve conduction velocity, is usually justified. Measurement of serum immunoglobulin and complement (Whitaker *et al.*, 1973) may be of some limited value in identifying cases in which immune mechanisms are disordered.

REFERENCES

DAVIS, L. E., and DRACHMAN, D. B. (1972) Myeloma neuropathy: successful treatment of two patients and review of cases, *Arch. Neurol. (Chic.)*, **27**, 507.

HARRIS, W. (1935) Chronic progressive (endotoxic) polyneuritis, *Brain*, **58**, 368.

HYLAND, H. H., and RUSSELL, W. R. (1930) Chronic progressive polyneuritis, with report of a fatal case, *Brain*, **53**, 278.

PALLIS, C. A., and LEWIS, P. D. (1974) *The Neurology of Gastrointestinal Disease*, London.

PROPP, R. P., MEANS, E., DEIBEL, R., SHERER, G., and BARRON, K. (1975) Waldenström's macroglobulinemia and neuropathy, *Neurology (Minneap.)*, **25**, 980.

VICTOR, M., BANKER, B. Q., and ADAMS, R. D. (1958) The neuropathy of multiple myeloma, *J. Neurol. Neurosurg. Psychiat.*, **21**, 73.

WALSH, J. C. (1971) The neuropathy of multiple myeloma: an electrophysiological and histological study, *Arch. Neurol. (Chic.)*, **25**, 404.

WHITAKER, J. N., SCIABBARRASI, J., ENGEL, W. K., WARMOLTS, J. R., and STROBER, W. (1973) Serum immunoglobulin and complement (C3) levels, *Neurology (Minneap.)*, **23**, 1164.

POLYNEURITIS CRANIALIS

The term 'polyneuritis cranialis' has been used in two senses.

1. Certain of the cranial nerves may be involved in polyneuritis in association with the nerves of the limbs. The cranial nerves are commonly attacked in acute post-infective polyneuritis, but there is probably no form of polyneuritis in which cranial nerves may not suffer. They are usually symmetrically affected. The facial nerve is most frequently involved, leading to facial paralysis, which is usually bilateral, and next in frequency the bulbar nerves, leading to dysphagia, and the trigeminal. The oculomotor nerves are less frequently affected (Fisher,

1956), and the optic nerves usually escape, though bilateral optic neuritis may occur in severe polyneuritis. Exceptionally the cranial nerves may be affected alone in polyneuritis or there may be only slight involvement of the nerves of the limbs, indicated by paraesthesiae or diminution in the tendon reflexes.

2. The term 'polyneuritis cranialis' has also been applied to an inflammatory lesion of multiple cranial nerves within the skull. This usually follows osteomyelitis of the bones of the base of the skull or basal pachymeningitis secondary to nasal sinusitis or chronic otitis media. The lesion may involve the anterior group, the third, fourth, fifth, and sixth nerves on one or both sides, or the posterior group, the seventh to twelfth usually on one side only, but in some cases almost all the nerves may suffer. This condition must be distinguished from compression of multiple cranial nerves by neoplastic infiltration of the meninges. It must also be distinguished from the syndrome of multiple cranial nerve involvement, often beginning unilaterally, which may be seen in patients with nasopharyngeal carcinoma, in sarcoidosis or in other granulomatous meningitides including syphilis and torulosis. Unilateral or bilateral facial nerve palsy has been described as a complication of acute leukaemia and recurrent (often familial) unilateral or bilateral facial palsy, often associated with a congenitally fissured tongue, is often referred to as Melkersson's syndrome (Stevens, 1965).

REFERENCES

FISHER, M. (1956) An unusual variant of acute idiopathic polyneuritis (syndrome of ophthalmoplegia, ataxia and areflexia), New Engl. J. Med., 255, 57.

FORSTER, F. M., BROWN, M., and MERRITT, H. H. (1941) Polyneuritis with facial diplegia, New Engl. J. Med., 225, 51.

STEVENS, H. (1965) Melkersson's syndrome, Neurology (Minneap.), 15, 263.

TAYLOR, E. W., and McDONALD, C. A. (1932) The syndrome of polyneuritis with facial diplegia, Arch. Neurol. Psychiat. (Chic.), 27, 79.

VIETS, H. R. (1927) Acute polyneuritis with facial diplegia, Arch. Neurol. Psychiat. (Chic.), 17, 794.

YUDELSON, A. B. (1927) Facial diplegia in multiple neuritis, J. nerv. ment. Dis., 65, 30.

19

DISORDERS OF MUSCLE

THE ANATOMY AND PHYSIOLOGY OF MUSCLE

A VOLUNTARY muscle is composed of muscle fibres, each of which is a multi-nucleate cell, consisting of myofibrils, sarcoplasm, and a number of discrete intracellular organelles including mitochondria, ribosomes, and the sarcotubular system. Each fibre is enclosed within a sarcolemmal sheath, deep to which the muscle nuclei are situated and each has a motor end-plate in which the nerve fibre terminates. Under normal conditions muscle fibres never contract singly, but the functional unit of muscle activity is known as the motor unit, being that group of muscle fibres supplied by a single anterior horn cell and its motor nerve axon. Discharge of such a single anterior horn cell results in the simultaneous contraction of all of the muscle fibres which it innervates.

For many years it was thought (see Sissons, 1974) that the constituent fibres of motor units in mammalian skeletal muscle were gathered into groups or fasciculi, but the work of Edström and Kugelberg (1968) and others has shown that the fibres of a single unit are usually widely scattered throughout a muscle when examined in transverse section. Only after denervation and subsequent reinnervation by regenerating neurones are fibres innervated by a single anterior horn cell or by one of its axonal branches gathered together into groups (Kugelberg *et al.*, 1970). Contraction of the muscle fibres which make up a motor unit is preceded by electrical excitation of the fibre membranes. The appearance of this electrical activity in the electromyogram depends on physical factors such as the dimensions of the electrode used, as well as on the muscle chosen for examination. For example, in the biceps brachii of a healthy young adult, the electrical activity of a single motor unit usually appears as a di- or triphasic wave with a duration of 5–10 ms and an amplitude of less than 250 μV; however, the variation in form, amplitude, and duration is considerable (see Buchthal, 1957; Richardson and Barwick, 1974; Lenman, 1974). Recent evidence suggests that these so-called motor unit action potentials may on occasions be produced not by the electrical activity of the entire motor unit, but simply by the summated electrical activity of a number of its component fibres which may be regarded as constituting a sub-unit.

An important advance in our knowledge of the physiology of muscular contraction was the discovery of a humoral element in the transmission of the nerve impulse at the myoneural junction. It was Dale (1934) who first demonstrated that acetylcholine played an important part in this process. There is now good evidence to indicate that the synaptic vesicles in the motor nerve terminal are actually packets of acetylcholine. Single packets of acetylcholine are continually being released spontaneously and give rise to small depolarizations (miniature end-plate potentials) which can be recorded electrically with a micro-electrode in the region of the end-plate. The arrival of a nerve impulse at the motor end-plate results in the synchronous release of many packets of acetylcholine which produces a localized depolarization of the muscle fibre membrane in the region of the end-plate; this is the end-plate potential. When the end-plate potential reaches a certain critical size it triggers off an excitatory wave, the action potential, which then travels away from the end-plate along the surface membrane of the fibre (see Buller, 1974; Zaimis and Maclagan, 1974). At rest the inside of the fibre membrane is some 80 mV negative with respect to the outside, but during the action potential the polarization of the membrane momentarily reverses, so that for about one millisecond the inside of the fibre becomes positive. This reversal of electrical polarity is caused by increased sodium permeability of the fibre membrane. There is evidence that the wave of excitation spreads inwards into the substance of the muscle fibre along the transverse system of tubules, the 'T' system (see Huxley, 1964) and that the consequent mobilization of calcium ions in the sarcoplasmic reticulum initiates contraction of the myofibrils.

Ultrastructural investigations of skeletal muscle have demonstrated that the unit of structure of the individual myofibril is the sarcomere, extending from one Z-line (situated in the midst of the 'I'-band) to the next. Attached to each Z-line are a series of thin filaments of the protein actin. There is also a second type of filament which is rather thicker and is composed of myosin; these filaments correspond to the dark (birefringent) A-bands of the myofibrils. Each filament of myosin is surrounded by a hexagonal array of actin filaments; in addition, molecular cross-bridges reach out from the myosin to the actin filaments. It is thought that, during contraction, the cross-bridges repeatedly disengage and re-engage at successive sites on the actin filaments. The propulsion imparted to the actin filaments causes them to slide over the myosin filaments so as to interdigitate more fully with the latter; in this way the whole myofibril, and consequently its parent fibre, shortens. The biochemical changes which accompany muscle contraction are extremely complicated (for recent reviews see Peachey, 1968, and Gergely, 1974) but it is plain that among the many biochemical reactions which occur, creatine phosphate is broken down in the presence of calcium to creatine and phosphate, and adenosine triphosphate (ATP) is broken down to adenosine diphosphate (ADP). The release of high-energy phosphate bonds provides much of the energy required for muscular contraction.

It is also important to recognize that skeletal muscles are not homogeneous in that in man they contain at least two main types of muscle fibre which are morphologically and histochemically distinct. One type of fibre, the so-called Type I fibre, tends to be somewhat smaller than the second type; it contains myofibrils which are generally somewhat slender and a high concentration of mitochondria. Histochemical stains demonstrate that this type of fibre contains a high concentration of enzymes such as succinic dehydrogenase which are concerned with aerobic metabolism. In the larger Type II fibre, whose myofibrils are generally more coarse and more widely dispersed, there are fewer mitochondria and histochemical studies indicate that these fibres contain a higher concentration of glycogen and of enzymes such as phosphorylase and myofibrillar adenosine triphosphatase which are concerned with anaerobic metabolism. In man, all skeletal muscles contain an admixture of Type I and Type II fibres, so that in transverse sections stained histochemically, a characteristic checkerboard pattern is observed (see Dubowitz, 1968, 1974). Refinements of histochemical technique have shown that each of the major fibre types can be subdivided according to the intensity of staining demonstrated, for instance, with myofibrillar ATPase at varying pH (Dubowitz and Brooke, 1974). Physiological experiments also indicate that these fibres are functionally different. Thus in the animal kingdom it is known that there are certain muscles such as soleus which are made up predominantly of Type I fibres (so-called red muscle). These muscles are considered to be concerned largely with the maintenance of posture and, upon stimulation, are found to contract and relax relatively slowly. By contrast, other muscles concerned more directly with motor activity, such as the flexor digitorum longus, are made up predominantly of Type II fibres (white muscle) and are more rapidly contracting (fast 'twitch' muscles). Recent experiments (see Dubowitz, 1968, 1974) demonstrate that in some manner, as yet poorly understood, the motor nerve appears to control not only the physiological behaviour, but also the histochemical structure, of the muscle fibres in that transposition of the motor nerve supply from a fast muscle to a slow muscle, and vice versa, may completely alter the physiological and histochemical characteristics of the muscle fibres. Thus in a sense it is the neurones which control the behaviour of the muscle fibres which make up their motor units so that one can speak of Type I and Type II neurones. Thus when a group of muscle fibres which have lost their nerve supply are reinnervated by a sprouting neurone they become of uniform histochemical type (so-called 'type-grouping'—see Karpati and Engel, 1968 and Dubowitz and Brooke, 1974).

Finally, before commenting upon individual diseases of muscle, it is important to mention briefly a number of drugs which may act upon the neuromuscular junction. Acetylcholine (ACh), when released at the neuromuscular junction, is broken down by cholinesterase which is normally present in the subneural apparatus and can be demonstrated histochemically. The drug curare acts on the post-junctional membrane, where it reduces or prevents the depolarizing effect of the transmitter excited by the nerve impulse (Hunt and Kuffler, 1950; Riker, 1953). Drugs such as physostigmine and neostigmine destroy cholinesterase and allow ACh liberated at the myoneural junction to accumulate. Guanidine hydrochloride acts by increasing the output of acetylcholine at the nerve endings. Initially the accumulation of ACh produces muscular contraction as a result of depolarization of the muscle fibre membrane, but if this substance accumulates in excess, the depolarization persists and may result in blockage of the muscle action potential (depolarization block). Whereas drugs such as tubocurarine and gallamine compete with ACh for the end-plate chemical receptors and are thus known as competitive inhibitors, drugs such as decamethonium and suxamethonium produce muscle paralysis first as a result of depolarization block but subsequently also produce competitive block so that they are said to have a 'dual' action (see Zaimis and Maclagan, 1974).

REFERENCES

BUCHTHAL, F. (1957) *An Introduction to Electromyography*, Copenhagen.
BULLER, A. J. (1974) The physiology of the motor unit, in *Disorders of Voluntary Muscle*, ed. Walton, J. N., 3rd ed., Edinburgh and London.
DALE, H. (1934) Chemical transmission of the effects of nerve impulses, *Brit. med. J.*, **2**, 835.
DUBOWITZ, V. (1968) *Developing and Diseased Muscle*, London.
DUBOWITZ, V. (1974) Histochemical aspects of muscle disease, in *Disorders of Voluntary Muscle*, ed. Walton, J. N., 3rd ed., Edinburgh and London.
DUBOWITZ, V., and BROOKE, M. H. (1974) *Muscle Biopsy*, London.
EDSTRÖM, L., and KUGELBERG, E. (1968) Histochemical composition, distribution of fibres and fatiguability of single motor units, *J. Neurol. Neurosurg. Psychiat.*, **31**, 424.

GERGELY, J. (1974) Biochemical aspects of muscular structure and function, in *Disorders of Voluntary Muscle*, ed. Walton, J. N., 3rd ed., Edinburgh and London.

HUNT, C. C., and KUFFLER, S. W. (1950) Pharmacology of the neuromuscular junction, *Pharmacol. Rev.*, **2**, 96.

HUXLEY, A. F. (1964) Muscle, *Ann. Rev. Physiol.*, **26**, 131.

KARPATI, G., and ENGEL, W. K. (1968) 'Type grouping' in skeletal muscles after experimental reinnervation, *Neurology (Minneap.)*, **18**, 447.

KUGELBERG, E., EDSTRÖM, L., and ABBRUZZESE, M. (1970) Mapping of motor units in experimentally reinnervated rat muscle. Interpretation of histochemical and atrophic fibre patterns in neurogenic lesions, *J. Neurol. Neurosurg. Psychiat.*, **33**, 319.

LENMAN, J. A. R. (1974) Integration and analysis of the electromyogram and related techniques, in *Disorders of Voluntary Muscle*, ed. Walton, J. N., 3rd ed., Edinburgh and London.

PEACHEY, L. D. (1968) Muscle, *Ann. Rev. Physiol.*, **30**, 401.

RICHARDSON, A. T., and BARWICK, D. D. (1974) Clinical electromyography, in *Disorders of Voluntary Muscle*, ed. Walton, J. N., 3rd ed., Edinburgh and London.

RIKER, W. F. (1953) Excitatory and anti-curare properties of acetyl choline and related quaternary ammonium compounds at the neuromuscular junction, *Pharmacol. Rev.*, **5**, 1.

SISSONS, H. A. (1974) Anatomy of the motor unit, in *Disorders of Voluntary Muscle*, ed. Walton, J. N., 3rd ed., Edinburgh and London.

ZAIMIS, E., and MACLAGAN, J. (1974) General physiology and pharmacology of neuromuscular transmission, in *Disorders of Voluntary Muscle*, ed. Walton, J. N., 3rd ed., Edinburgh and London.

GENERAL COMMENTS ON DISORDERS OF MUSCLE

The past 25 years have seen increasing world-wide interest in diseases of muscle. A comprehensive classification of the neuromuscular disorders was produced by the Research Group on Neuromuscular Diseases of the World Federation of Neurology (1968) and has been modified by Gardner-Medwin and Walton (1974). It includes, however, many disorders which affect muscle through disease of the spinal cord, anterior horn cells, and peripheral nerves which have been dealt with in other parts of this volume (see CHAPTERS 13, 14, and 18). This chapter will therefore be concerned with those disorders which primarily affect voluntary muscle and the myoneural junction. The term 'myopathy' may reasonably be used (Walton, 1966) to define any disease or syndrome in which the patient's symptoms and/or physical signs can be attributed to pathological, biochemical, or electrophysiological changes which are occurring in the muscle fibres or in the interstitial tissues of the voluntary musculature and in which there is no evidence that the symptoms related to the muscular system are in any way secondary to disordered function of the central or peripheral nervous system. Within this group, therefore, are to be included many degenerative disorders which appear to be genetically determined, as well as others of a primary biochemical character and yet others in which the disease process appears to be essentially one of inflammation. The construction of this chapter will be different from many of the others in this book in that the clinical and genetic aspects of the various conditions to be considered are first described in turn, and the chapter concludes with commentaries upon differential diagnosis by means of clinical and investigative methods.

REFERENCES

GARDNER-MEDWIN, D., and WALTON, J. N. (1974) The clinical examination of the voluntary muscles, in *Disorders of Voluntary Muscle*, ed. Walton, J. N., 3rd ed., Edinburgh and London.

RESEARCH GROUP ON NEUROMUSCULAR DISEASES (1968) Classification of the neuromuscular disorders, *J. neurol. Sci.*, **6**, 165.

WALTON, J. N. (1966) Diseases of muscle, *Abstr. Wld Med.*, **40**, 1, 81.

PROGRESSIVE MUSCULAR DYSTROPHY

Muscular dystrophy can be defined as genetically-determined primary degenerative myopathy (Walton, 1966; Walton and Gardner-Medwin, 1974), but this definition can no longer be regarded as being entirely satisfactory as there are a number of myopathies, to which reference will be made in this chapter, which are genetically determined but which are not normally regarded as being muscular dystrophies in the accepted sense of the term. However, this definition may reasonably be retained, despite its defects, as the condition appears to be due to some factor or factors present in the individual's genetic constitution from birth; pathological and other evidence indicates that the disease is primarily one of the muscle cell and the process is at present classified as being degenerative as there is no evidence available to indicate its fundamental nature, though it is widely presumed that it may in the end prove to be the result of the absence of one or more enzymes within the muscle cell.

Much interest has been aroused in recent years by two new hypotheses advanced to explain the pathogenesis of muscular dystrophy, and particularly that of the Duchenne type. The 'neurogenic hypothesis', based in part upon the use of an electrophysiological technique developed in order to estimate the number of functioning motor units in certain distal limb muscles (McComas *et al.*, 1971) and in part upon other evidence (Dubowitz, 1975), assigned a primary pathogenetic role to dysfunction of the motor neurones, but the electrophysiological evidence upon which it is largely based has been challenged (Ballantyne and Hansen, 1974). The 'vascular hypothesis' (Mendell *et al.*, 1971) suggests that functional ischaemia of skeletal muscle is important in the pathogenesis of Duchenne muscular dystrophy but this view is not supported by muscle blood flow studies (Paulson *et al.*, 1974) or by morphological investigations of the muscle vasculature (Jerusalem *et al.*, 1974; Musch *et al.*, 1975). Certainly confusion has arisen from the fact, as will be seen, that chronic spinal muscular atrophy may closely mimic muscular dystrophy in all its forms and the overwhelming body of evidence still suggests that the primary muscular dystrophies are due to disease of the muscle cell itself, though the possibility of associated neuronal dysfunction must still be considered (Bradley, 1974).

CLASSIFICATION

Classification of the muscular dystrophies is by no means an academic matter as it is the only safe guide to prognosis and genetic counselling. The traditional clinico-anatomic classification of this group of diseases into the pseudohypertrophic, pelvic girdle atrophic, facioscapulohumeral, juvenile scapulohumeral, distal, ocular, late-life, and congenital forms has proved to be unsatisfactory both clinically and genetically, since if, for instance, one classifies all cases showing pseudohypertrophy into one group, this is then shown to be heterogeneous with several different forms of inheritance and little clinical uniformity. Important contributions to this problem have been made by Tyler and Wintrobe (1950), Stevenson (1953), Becker (1953, 1957), Walton and Nattrass (1954), Morton and Chung (1959), Dubowitz (1960), and Emery and Walton (1967). The most satisfactory clinico-genetic classification based upon current knowledge would appear to be that proposed by Walton and Gardner-Medwin (1974):

The 'pure' muscular dystrophies

 (a) X-linked muscular dystrophy
  Severe (Duchenne type)
  Benign (Becker type)
 (b) Autosomal recessive muscular dystrophy
  Limb-girdle types
  Childhood muscular dystrophy (except Duchenne)
  Congenital muscular dystrophies
 (c) Facioscapulohumeral muscular dystrophy
 (d) Distal muscular dystrophy
 (e) Ocular muscular dystrophy
 (f) Oculopharyngeal muscular dystrophy

Although this classification would seem to be the most satisfactory that can be devised based upon present knowledge, there are still a number of cases which are seen from time to time which are difficult to fit into any of the groups described. Many more detailed family studies will be required, using rigid clinical, genetic, and investigative criteria, before a final and definitive classification can be achieved. Though the nature of the pathological process causing muscular weakness and wasting in these cases is similar in character, though different in tempo, in the various groups, there are other features such as differences in the pattern of muscular involvement and in the degree to which enzymes such as creatine kinase leak into the serum in the different varieties, which strongly suggest that they may in the end prove to be different diseases from the aetiological standpoint.

It will now be convenient to consider the general clinical features of the muscular dystrophies, before describing the distinctive clinical characteristics of the various sub-varieties.

CLINICAL FEATURES OF THE MUSCULAR DYSTROPHIES

These depend upon which muscles are first involved by the disease process and upon the rate of progress of the disease. Weakness in the muscles around the pelvic girdle characteristically gives rise to slowness in walking, inability to run, frequent falling, difficulty in climbing stairs or in rising from the floor and eventually the patients develop accentuation of the lumbar lordosis and a characteristic waddling gait. Climbing up the legs on rising from the floor (Gowers' sign) is a characteristic feature of the condition [FIG. 143] but is by no means specific for muscular dystrophy, as it occurs in any condition in which pelvic girdle muscles are weakened and thus may be seen in various forms of spinal muscular atrophy, congenital myopathy, and polymyositis. Weakness in the shoulder girdles gives an unusually sloping appearance of the shoulders with a tendency for the scapulae to rise prominently when the patient attempts to abduct the arms. Many patients utilize trick movements by placing one hand beneath the other elbow in an attempt to lift the hand to the face or head. Facial weakness in its characteristic form, as seen in the facioscapulohumeral variety, causes inability to whistle and to pout the lips or to close the eyes, while distal weakness (as seen in the distal variety) gives rise to weakness of grip and of fine finger movements and foot-drop. Contractures are a common feature of all forms of muscular dystrophy in the late stages, but are seen particularly in the severe Duchenne type. They may result from weakness developing in a group of muscles whose antagonists remain comparatively powerful (this explains the partial foot-drop with turning in of the feet and toes which is seen in advancing cases of the Duchenne type and which typically causes the children to walk on their toes; it results from progressive weakness of the anterior tibial group

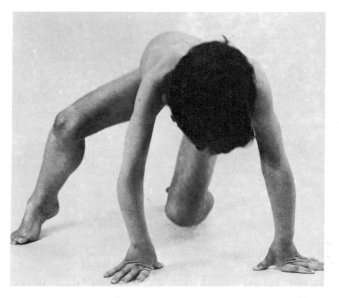

FIG. 143. A boy suffering from the Duchenne type muscular
dystrophy rising from the floor

at a time when the calf muscles remain powerful). Contractures may also be due to postural changes which develop in a patient confined to a wheelchair; in such a situation the biceps and hamstrings show a particular tendency to shorten. One of the most important clinical characteristics of all forms of muscular dystrophy is that muscles are picked out by the disease in a curiously selective manner and this is also one of the most difficult features to explain on any theory of pathogenesis. Though there are certain differences in the pattern of muscular involvement seen in the various sub-varieties, it is common in the upper limbs, for instance, to find that the serrati and pectoral muscles are weakened and atrophic, as are biceps and brachioradialis, while deltoid and triceps remain relatively powerful. In the lower limbs quadriceps and anterior tibials are particularly weakened and the calf muscles are spared, but in some cases of limb-girdle muscular dystrophy the hamstrings and quadriceps appear to be affected to an equal degree. Such a selective pattern of muscular involvement is very strongly suggestive of muscular dystrophy, but a similar affection of individual muscles with sparing of others may also be seen in some of the more benign varieties of spinal muscular atrophy [p. 706] though in many cases of the latter condition the pattern is somewhat different (e.g. the deltoid is often involved).

The Severe X-Linked (Duchenne) Type

Although it is clear that this condition is due to a sex-linked recessive gene, over half of the affected boys appear to be isolated cases and in these individuals the disease is presumed to have resulted from genetic mutation occurring perhaps in the cells of one segment of the ovary in either the patient's mother or maternal grandmother (Gardner-Medwin, 1970). The evidence indicating sex-linked recessive inheritance comes first from the inspection of pedigrees, secondly from the fact that several women have been known to have affected children by more than one male, and thirdly from the fact that three cases of the disease have now been reported in patients of female morphology suffering from Turner's syndrome (ovarian agenesis) with an XO chromosome constitution (Walton, 1956 a; Ferrier et al., 1965; Jalbert et al., 1966; Emery and Walton, 1967).

The condition usually first becomes clinically apparent towards the end of the third year of life with difficulty in walking, frequent falling, and difficulty in climbing stairs. The pelvic-girdle muscles are thus first affected, but involvement of the shoulder girdles soon follows. Enlargement of the calf muscles and sometimes of quadriceps, deltoids, and other muscles as well, occurs in about 90 per cent of cases at some stage but later disappears as the disease advances.

This enlargement has often been referred to as pseudohypertrophy in view of the fact that muscle biopsy may demonstrate, in some such muscles, a marked infiltration of fat, but there is good histological evidence now to suggest that in many cases this initial enlargement can be due to a true muscular hypertrophy with enlargement of individual muscle fibres. Most patients show slow progressive deterioration so that the majority are unable to walk by the time they are 10 years old. False or apparent clinical improvement may occur between the ages of 5 and 8 years, when the rate of deterioration due to the disease is apparently outstripped by the processes of normal physical development. Once the child is confined to a wheelchair, progressive deformity with muscular contractures and skeletal distortion and atrophy occur, and death usually results from inanition, respiratory infection, or cardiac failure towards the end of the second decade. Some of the children waste progressively, but some become excessively obese and no explanation for this discrepancy is forthcoming. Macroglossia is not infrequent and occasionally certain incisor teeth are absent. The intelligence quotient in these cases is 10 per cent or more lower than in a group of control children of comparable age and sex (Dubowitz, 1965; Murphy, et al., 1965). Marked skeletal atrophy and deformity occur and the shafts of long bones may become pencil-thin and fracture on minimal trauma (Walton and Warrick, 1954). Cardiac involvement is invariable in such cases, though it may not be detectable in the early stages. Persistent tachycardia is common and of particular importance is the characteristic electrocardiogram which shows tall R waves in the right precordial leads and deep Q waves in the limb leads and left precordial leads (Skyring and McKusick, 1961; Emery, 1972).

While as yet no effective treatment for this tragic progressive disorder has been discovered, and methods of management will be discussed later, an important recent advance has been the discovery that the female carriers of the gene can usually be detected by means of serum creatine kinase estimation, quantitative electromyography, and possibly muscle biopsy. Many more refined techniques of detection are now being tested including the measurement of protein synthesis by muscle polyribosomes *in vitro* (Ionasescu et al., 1971), the estimation of serum pyruvate kinase activity (Alberts and Samaha, 1974), and studies of phosphorylation in erythrocyte membranes (Roses et al., 1976), but serum creatine kinase estimation, employing Bayesian methods to determine the probability that the young woman is or is not a carrier (Emery and Morton, 1968) is still the most reliable. This fact is of particular importance to the sisters of dystrophic boys, who have approximately a 50–50 chance of being carriers. A carrier female, who may rarely show clinical evidence of minor degrees of muscle weakness and possibly enlargement of the calves, is likely to pass the disease on to half of her sons, and half her daughters will themselves be carriers; it is not, therefore, surprising that most young women who are found to be carriers decide not to have children. Selective abortion of male fetuses identified by amniocentesis (Emery et al., 1972) is an alternative worth considering. If all carriers can be detected and if most do not reproduce or produce male infants, then undoubtedly the incidence of the disease will fall in the future, though some cases will continue to arise as a result of genetic mutation. The principles of carrier detection and the recent literature on this topic have been reviewed by Gardner-Medwin (1968) and by Walton and Gardner-Medwin (1974).

The Benign X-Linked (Becker) Type of Muscular Dystrophy

The existence of a distinct benign X-linked recessive form of muscular dystrophy was first suggested by Becker and Kiener (1955) and subsequent reports have made it clear that the benign cases are distinct and not simply part of a spectrum of severity related to the Duchenne type. This disorder differs from the severe Duchenne variety in that the onset of the disease is usually between the fifth and twenty-fifth year, the disorder may be transmitted by affected males through carrier daughters to their grandsons, there is gradually progressive weakness and wasting of the pelvic and later of the pectoral muscles, and most patients become unable to walk 25 years or more after the onset. Cardiac involvement is common in these families (Markand et al., 1969), contractures and skeletal deformity occur late, if at all, and some such patients, though severely disabled, survive to a normal age. Crossing-over with deutan colour blindness and the Xg blood group has been described (Emery et al., 1969) and the locus for this form of X-linked dystrophy is probably different from that of the Duchenne gene. The detection of female carriers of this gene is sometimes possible (Emery et al., 1967) but is less precise than in the Duchenne type (Walton and Gardner-Medwin, 1974).

Limb-Girdle Muscular Dystrophy

This form of the disease occurs equally in the two sexes and usually begins in the second or third decade of life, but occasionally first appears in middle life. Though genetic evidence plainly indicates that in most families the condition is inherited by an autosomal recessive mechanism and that its incidence is therefore considerably increased by consanguinity, many cases are sporadic and it has been suggested that some may be due to manifestation in the heterozygote

(Morton and Chung, 1959; Chung and Morton, 1959). In about half the cases, muscle weakness begins in the shoulder-girdle muscles [FIG. 144] and may then remain limited to these for many years before eventually spreading to involve the pelvic girdle. In the other half, by contrast, the pelvic-girdle muscles are first involved and as a rule the weakness spreads to the shoulders in about 10 years. Enlargement of calf muscles is not uncommon in these cases. The severity of the disease varies a good deal from case to case and from family to family. Often muscular weakness and wasting are asymmetrical initially, and sometimes the disease process appears temporarily to arrest, but in most patients the degree of disability is severe within 20 years of the onset. There is some evidence to suggest that in the patients in whom weakness begins in the

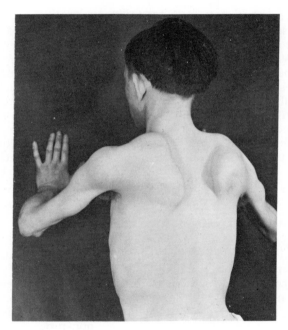

FIG. 144. A patient suffering from limb-girdle muscular
dystrophy, demonstrating bilateral winging of the scapulae

upper limbs the disease runs a more benign course than in those in whom the pelvic-girdle muscles are first involved. There may be considerable difficulty in distinguishing cases beginning in the pelvic girdle on purely clinical grounds from cases of benign spinal muscular atrophy and from other forms of myopathy of metabolic origin; electromyography and muscle biopsy are of particular value in making the distinction. Indeed a recent review of patients previously diagnosed as cases of limb-girdle muscular dystrophy in Newcastle upon Tyne, using quantitative electromyography, estimation of functioning motor units and histochemical studies applied to muscle biopsy sections, showed that half were in fact suffering from chronic spinal muscular atrophy of the Kugelberg–Welander type (Mastaglia and Walton, 1971; Walton, 1973) and in one case coming to autopsy (Tomlinson et al., 1974) the number of limb motor neurones in the spinal cord was greatly reduced, confirming the neuronal origin of the disorder. Contractures and skeletal deformity occur late in the course of this disease by comparison with the Duchenne type, but progress much more rapidly when the patient is unable to walk. Most sufferers are severely disabled in middle life and many die before the normal age.

Childhood Muscular Dystrophy with Autosomal Recessive Inheritance

This is one of the most difficult categories of muscular dystrophy to characterize. Proof of autosomal recessive inheritance is rarely possible and the arguments for the very existence of this condition have depended upon the occasional occurrence of muscular dystrophy in young girls and in a few families in which consanguinity of the parents has made autosomal recessive inheritance likely. Even though some cases previously reported (Kloepfer and Talley, 1958; Jackson and Carey, 1961; Johnston, 1964) have seemed reasonably convincing, few if any of those reported have been investigated in sufficient depth to exclude spinal muscular atrophy of the Kugelberg–Welander type (Penn et al., 1970; Mastaglia and Walton, 1971) which may sometimes mimic muscular dystrophy very closely, especially if there is extensive secondary myopathic change in the affected muscles superimposed upon evidence of the primary denervating process. Certainly cases so diagnosed have usually shown a more benign course than that demonstrated by males with typical Duchenne dystrophy. The onset may be in the second year or as late as the fourteenth, but is most often in the second half of the first decade. Progression is comparatively slow and patients usually become unable to walk in their early twenties, but sometimes as early as 15 years or as late as 43 years. The pattern of weakness may be very similar to that observed in the typical severe X-linked Duchenne type (Walton and Gardner-Medwin, 1974).

Congenital Muscular Dystrophy

It was Batten who in 1909 suggested that the syndrome of amyotonia congenita, as first described by Oppenheim (1900), might be due to a simple atrophic myopathy of congenital origin. However, he may well have been describing the condition which has been variously entitled benign congenital myopathy (Turner, 1940, 1949; Turner and Lees, 1962) or benign congenital hypotonia with incomplete recovery (Walton, 1956 b), a disorder which differs from the muscular dystrophies in its relatively non-progressive course and in the absence of specific histological abnormalities in the muscle fibres. However, Banker et al. (1957), Pearson and Fowler (1963), Gubbay et al. (1966), and Zellweger et al. (1967) described cases with congenital hypotonia and severe, but relatively non-progressive, muscular weakness in which the muscle histology was typical of muscular dystrophy. In several of these children there were widespread contractures suggesting arthrogryposis multiplex congenita. The proper nosological status of these non-progressive muscle disorders remains uncertain, but in a few cases congenital muscular dystrophy is rapidly progressive and terminates fatally within the first year of life (Wharton, 1965). Patients with congenital dystrophy intermediate in severity between the static and rapidly progressive groups make it unlikely that sub-division on the grounds of severity alone is justifiable.

The essential features of this disorder are severe hypotonia present from birth with the subsequent development of more or less progressive muscular wasting and weakness. The diagnosis from spinal muscular atrophy of infancy can only be made with confidence by means of electromyography, serum enzyme studies, and muscle biopsy. Sibs are not infrequently affected, but more definite evidence of autosomal recessive inheritance of this disorder is lacking.

Facioscapulohumeral Muscular Dystrophy

This form, which is inherited by an autosomal dominant mechanism (Tyler and Wintrobe, 1950; Stevenson, 1953), occurs equally in the two sexes and can begin at any age from childhood until adult life, though it is usually recognized first in adolescence. A possible autosomal recessive mode of inheritance has been suggested in certain families, but if this does occur it is very uncommon. Facial involvement is apparent at an early stage and is generally accompanied by weakness of shoulder-girdle muscles, which is often remarkably selective with bilateral winging of the scapulae and involvement of the pectoral muscles but with sparing of others. Biceps and brachioradiales are often selectively involved and there is difficulty in raising the arms above the head. Muscular hypertrophy or pseudo-hypertrophy is uncommon but may occasionally be seen in the calves and deltoids. In the lower extremities many such patients show selective involvement of the anterior tibial muscles with bilateral foot-drop and some few, showing unusually rapid progress, demonstrate a particularly severe accentuation of the lumbar lordosis at a comparatively early stage of the disease. The condition which has been referred to as scapuloperoneal muscular dystrophy may be no more than a variant of this form, but on the other hand most cases of scapuloperoneal muscular atrophy have been shown to be due to neuropathic, as distinct from myopathic, changes [p. 708]. In most patients with facio-scapulohumeral dystrophy the condition is benign, runs a prolonged course with periods of apparent arrest, and muscular contractures and skeletal deformity are late in developing. There are some patients in whom the disease process is apparently abortive and after certain muscles are selectively involved, the spread of weakness appears to cease spontaneously. Indeed, substantial variation in the severity of the condition in affected members in a single family is common. The patients tend to show a very characteristic pouting appearance of the lips with a typical transverse smile; most affected individuals survive and remain active until a normal age. Cardiac involvement is rare and the range of intelligence is normal.

As in limb-girdle muscular dystrophy, recent studies have shown that this condition is probably a syndrome of multiple aetiology rather than a single disease entity. Thus facio-scapulohumeral muscular atrophy has been described (Fenichel et al., 1967) and a recent study in Newcastle (Walton, 1973) showed evidence of denervation in a considerable proportion of patients. Inflammatory changes in muscle biopsy sections, resembling those of poly-myositis, have been reported in many cases (Munsat et al., 1972) but there is no clinical response to prednisone and this clinical syndrome may also be produced by a mitochondrial myopathy (Hudgson et al., 1972). In infancy, the so-called Möbius syndrome may be mimicked (Hanson and Rowland, 1971).

Distal Muscular Dystrophy

This form of the disease is rare in Britain and in the United States, but Welander (1951, 1957) has reported her experience of over 250 cases. In her experience the condition is inherited as an autosomal dominant character, begins usually between the ages of 40 and 60 years and affects both sexes, though it seems to be commoner in men than in women. Weakness begins in the small muscles of the hands and in the anterior tibial muscles and calves, but eventually spreads proximally, in contradistinction to the weakness observed in peroneal muscular atrophy (Charcot–Marie–Tooth disease) with which this disorder is most often confused. The condition in Sweden is comparatively benign and slowly progressive, but sporadic cases seen in other countries of the world tend to show a rather more rapid course and more severe disability (see Sumner *et al.*, 1971 and Walton and Gardner-Medwin, 1974).

Ocular Myopathy

This disorder usually begins with progressive bilateral ptosis (Hutchinson, 1879; Fuchs, 1890; Kiloh and Nevin, 1951). It used to be generally referred to in the literature as progressive nuclear ophthalmoplegia, but it has been shown that the condition is often due to a true myopathy of the external ocular muscles. However, Drachman *et al.* (1969) give reasons for suggesting that in some such cases the primary process may indeed be one of denervation, and Rosenberg *et al.* (1968), in reporting 28 cases, of which nine showed evidence of concomitant disease in the central nervous system (including ataxia, paraplegia, retinitis pigmentosa, and peripheral neuropathy), suggest that the condition is better called progressive ophthalmoplegia and that it is probably a syndrome of multiple pathogenesis. Certainly it is commonly associated with mito-chondrial abnormalities not only in ocular muscles (Zintz and Villiger, 1967) but also in the skeletal musculature (Olson *et al.*, 1972) in which the Type I muscle fibres may be of the so-called 'ragged-red' type, with excessive lipid droplets. Similar mitochondrial abnormalities may be found in cases of oculo-pharyngeal muscular dystrophy (see below) and have also been found in the cerebellum in cases of the Kearns–Sayre syndrome (Schneck *et al.*, 1973) in which ophthalmoplegia, retinitis pigmentosa, and cerebellar ataxia occur. Excessive curare sensitivity has also been reported in some cases of ocular 'myopathy' (Ross, 1963; Mathew *et al.*, 1970). Diplopia is rare and in most cases bilateral external ophthalmoplegia develops slowly and progressively over a period of many years. Usually there is also some weakness of the upper facial muscles and often the neck and shoulder-girdle muscles are affected to some extent. The facial weakness is particularly severe in the orbicularis oculi, but is not as intense as that seen in facioscapulohumeral muscular dystrophy.

Oculopharyngeal Muscular Dystrophy

Victor *et al.* (1962) separated those cases of ocular myopathy with dysphagia as a group to which they gave the name oculopharyngeal myopathy. Bray *et al.* (1965) supported this sub-division and defined the other distinguishing clinical features, of which the most valuable is the age of onset (mean 23 years for the ocular cases and 40 for the oculopharyngeal). Many of the reported cases have been of French-Canadian stock (see Barbeau, 1966) and occasional cases, often sporadic, have occurred elsewhere. The inheritance in familial cases is dominant. The disorder bears some slight resemblances to dystrophia myotonica, not only in some of its clinical and genetic features, but in the probable involvement of smooth muscle (Lewis, 1966) and reports of abnormalities of immunoglobulins (Russe *et al.*, 1969) in some families.

MYOTONIC DISORDERS

Myotonia, which occurs not only in man but also in certain goats (Brown and Harvey, 1939), is the continued active contraction of a muscle which persists after the cessation of voluntary effort or stimulation; an electrical after-discharge in the electromyogram (EMG) can be seen to accompany the phenomenon. Clinically, it is best demonstrated as a slowness in relaxation of the grip or by a persistent dimpling after a sharp blow on a muscle belly (e.g. in the thenar eminence or tongue). It appears to be due to an abnormality of the muscle fibre itself as it persists after section or blocking of the motor nerve and after curarization (Denny-Brown and Nevin, 1941). Three hereditary syndromes, all with autosomal dominant inheritance, have been described, namely myotonia congenita, dystrophia myotonica, and paramyotonia congenita. Only in one of these, namely dystrophia myotonica, are dystrophic changes observed within some of the affected muscles. Transitional cases may be seen suggesting a close relationship between the three disorders, and Maas and Paterson (1950) suggested that they may be different manifestations of the same disorder. However, the difference between the course and prognosis of typical cases of dystrophia myotonica on the one hand and of myotonia congenita on the other, and the fact that in most families the conditions breed true, suggest that they are different diseases. The evidence on this question was reviewed by Caughey and Myrianthopoulos (1963). Further nosological problems arise over the close relationship between paramyotonia and the periodic paralyses. It seems clear that all of these disorders are more closely related to each other than they are to the pure muscular dystrophies.

In a rare and little-understood syndrome, sometimes called neuromyotonia, a clinically similar but probably distinct phenomenon is associated with myokymia (benign coarse fasciculation), cramps, hyperhidrosis, and sometimes muscle wasting (Gamstorp and Wohlfart, 1959; Greenhouse et al., 1967). The cases of continuous muscle fibre activity described by Isaacs (1967) and Mertens and Zschocke (1965) seem to be similar. Although the failure of relaxation in these cases is similar to myotonia, no dimple is induced by percussion and electromyography shows that the after-discharge is different in form. Phenytoin is often beneficial in such cases (Gardner-Medwin and Walton, 1969; Wallis et al., 1970).

Myotonia may also be produced experimentally by the administration of diazocholesterol and dichlorophenoxyacetic acid (Kuhn and Stein, 1966; Somers and Winer, 1966; Schröder and Kuhn, 1968; Wallis et al., 1970).

MYOTONIA CONGENITA

Myotonia congenita (Thomsen, 1876; Nissen, 1923; Thomasen, 1948) usually begins at birth but symptoms may be delayed until the end of the first or even into the second decade. Myotonia is usually generalized, giving painless stiffness which is accentuated by rest and cold and gradually relieved by exercise. It is particularly easy to demonstrate this phenomenon by asking the patient to grip firmly and then to relax, when difficulty in opening the hand will be experienced. The phenomenon can also be demonstrated by percussion of affected muscles and is often well seen in the thenar eminence and tongue; percussion in either situation results in the formation of a dimple in the muscle which only slowly disappears. Diffuse hypertrophy of muscles usually persists throughout life in these cases, though the myotonia tends to improve. There has been evidence of an associated psychosis in some individuals and families (Johnson, 1967). Rarely myotonia may increase during exertion (myotonia paradoxa) when it must be distinguished from the cramping stiffness of McArdle's disease. Hypertrophia musculorum vera (Friedreich, 1863; Spiller, 1913) may well be a variant of this condition.

Recessively inherited myotonia congenita (Becker, 1966; Harper and Johnston, 1972) may well prove to be commoner than dominantly inherited Thomsen's disease and may account for most of those cases in which symptoms and signs are not present at birth but develop in late infancy or childhood. In these cases myotonia may be more severe than in classical Thomsen's disease.

DYSTROPHIA MYOTONICA

Dystrophia myotonica (myotonia atrophica) was described by Steinert (1909) and Batten and Gibb (1909) and has been reviewed by Thomasen (1948) and Caughey and Myrianthopoulos (1963). It is a diffuse systemic disorder in which myotonia and distal muscular atrophy are accompanied by cataracts, frontal baldness in the male [Fig. 145], gonadal atrophy, cardiomyopathy, impaired

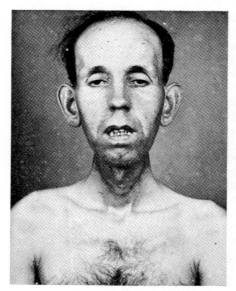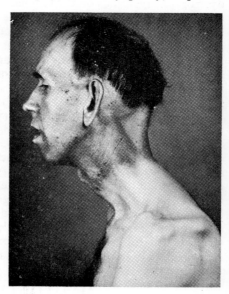

Fig. 145. Dystrophia myotonica. Note the frontal alopecia, myopathic facies, and wasting of the sternomastoids

pulmonary ventilation, mild endocrine anomalies, bone changes, mental defect or dementia, hypersomnia and abnormalities of the serum immunoglobulins. The affected families show progressive social decline in successive generations, diminished fertility, and an increased infantile mortality rate. The presenting symptom of the condition is usually weakness in the hands, difficulty in walking and frequent falling and myotonia is only rarely obtrusive. Poor vision, loss of weight, impotence or loss of libido, ptosis and increased sweating are common. The condition is usually observed to begin between the ages of 20 and 50 but clinical features of the disorder may be recognized in offspring of affected individuals in the second decade. Recently it has become apparent that the condition may present in infancy and childhood with severe muscular weakness and hypotonia and delay in walking and these children may erroneously be regarded as examples of benign congenital hypotonia unless the existence of myotonic dystrophy in other members of the family is recognized (Dodge *et al.*, 1965; Pruzanski, 1966). The fact that infantile hypotonia due to myotonic dystrophy occurs almost exclusively with affected female rather than male parents argues in favour of a maternal environmental factor (Harper and Dyken, 1972; Dyken and Harper, 1973).

The facial appearance is characteristic [FIG. 145]; ptosis is usual and involvement of other external ocular muscles may be seen. Wasting of the masseters, temporal muscles, and sternomastoids is almost invariable and in the extremities there is distal weakness and wasting involving mainly forearm muscles, the anterior tibial group and the calves and peronei. Slit-lamp examination reveals cataracts in about 90 per cent of cases. Cardiac involvement is very common (Kennel *et al.*, 1974) and the pulmonary vital capacity and maximum expiratory pressure are often impaired (Kilburn *et al.*, 1959; Kaufman, 1965); as a result, many patients tolerate barbiturate anaesthesia poorly and hypersomnia may occur (Coccogna *et al.*, 1975). Disordered oesophageal contraction can often be demonstrated by contrast radiography or manometry (Gleeson *et al.*, 1967). The testes are usually small and histologically the changes in these organs resemble those of Klinefelter's syndrome though the nuclear sex is male. Irregular menstruation and infertility and prolonged parturition are common in affected females. Pituitary function is usually normal but there may be a selective failure of adrenal androgenic function and occasionally thyroid activity and glucose utilization are impaired (Marshall, 1959; Caughey and Myrianthopoulos, 1963). Hyperostosis of the skull vault, localized or diffuse, and a small sella turcica are frequent radiological findings (Jequier, 1950; Walton and Warrick, 1954). Both mental defect and progressive dementia occur. Rosman and Kakulas (1966) have described neuronal heterotopias in the brain at autopsy in four cases and investigation in life may reveal a high incidence of abnormality in the electro-encephalogram (Barwick *et al.*, 1965; Lundervold *et al.*, 1969) or progressive cerebral ventricular enlargement (Refsum *et al.*, 1967). Excessive catabolism of immunoglobulin-G has been demonstrated in these patients by Wochner *et al.* (1966) and Jensen *et al.* (1971). Abnormalities of insulin secretion have also been described in such cases (Walsh *et al.*, 1970) and in recent years abnormalities in the sensitivity of blood platelets to adrenaline (Bousser *et al.*, 1975) and of the erythrocyte membrane (Roses and Appel, 1973; Butterfield *et al.*, 1974) have aroused considerable interest.

In genetic counselling the early recognition of affected individuals, if possible before they have a family, is of considerable importance. Slit-lamp examination and electromyography in addition to a careful clinical examination are the most useful methods (Bundey *et al.*, 1970; Polgar *et al.*, 1972; Harper, 1973). The demonstration of linkage between the gene responsible for myotonic dystrophy, ABH secretor, and the Lutheran blood group (Harper *et al.*, 1971, 1972) has allowed antenatal diagnosis by amniocentesis in some families, but unfortunately linkage is not close enough for this method to be universally applicable.

Most patients show progressive deterioration and become severely disabled and unable to walk within 15 to 20 years of the onset. Death from respiratory infection or cardiac failure usually occurs well before the normal age.

PARAMYOTONIA CONGENITA

This condition, first described by Eulenburg (1886), is characterized by myotonia which is apparent only on exposure to cold, and in addition the patients experience attacks of generalized muscular weakness similar to those of familial periodic paralysis. The condition is closely related to hyperkalaemic periodic paralysis or adynamia episodica hereditaria (Gamstorp, 1956). Resnick and Engel (1967) have, however, described patients with myotonia who suffered attacks of periodic paralysis of the hypokalaemic variety. Thus although the nosological status of paramyotonia congenita remains confused (Pratt, 1967) it remains a useful diagnostic category for patients in whom myotonia and weakness are induced by cold, so long as it is recognized that the particular precipitants and any associated electrolyte changes in each family must be worked out if useful advice and treatment are to be given (Thrush et al., 1972).

CHONDRODYSTROPHIC MYOTONIA (THE SCHWARTZ-JAMPEL SYNDROME)

This rare syndrome, presumed to be of autosomal recessive inheritance, is characterized by generalized myotonia, dwarfism, skeletal abnormalities with hip contractures or dislocations and a peculiar facial appearance with tense puckering of the mouth, blepharospasm, and narrow palpebral fissures (Schwartz and Jampel, 1962; Aberfeld et al., 1965, 1970). Intelligence is usually normal; the myotonia may be relieved by procaine amide (Huttenlocher et al., 1969).

TREATMENT

Muscular Dystrophy

Regrettably there is no evidence that any form of drug treatment has any influence upon the course of muscular dystrophy. Many remedies have been tried in the past and have been found wanting and none is to be recommended for routine administration, though complications such as respiratory infection may demand appropriate antibiotics. There is good evidence to suggest that physical exercise is of value in delaying the march of the weakness and the onset of contractures and it is advisable to institute a regular programme of exercise, which may be started under the supervision of a skilled physiotherapist and subsequently continued at home by the patients, who, like their parents and other relatives, should be given appropriate instructions. Passive stretching of those tendons, such as the tendons of Achilles, which show a tendency to shorten, should also be carried out regularly, particularly in Duchenne type cases. In certain selected cases the wearing of light spinal supports is helpful in delaying skeletal deformity and occasionally calipers and night-splints are successful in helping affected individuals to walk for longer periods than they would otherwise be able to do. Recent evidence suggests that surgical division of the Achilles tendons in selected cases, a procedure which has long been regarded as being contra-indicated, and certain other surgical procedures may be beneficial in selected cases, provided these are followed by immediate mobilization of the patient in walking plasters or calipers (Siegel et al., 1968; Siegel, 1972). Immobilization of patients with muscular dystrophy is in general to be avoided as far as ever possible as this frequently causes deterioration. Walton and Gardner-Medwin (1974) point out that the use of radical surgical measures is controversial. Certainly patients with Duchenne dystrophy may be helped to walk for two or three years longer than without surgery, but many at this stage take to a wheelchair with relief and the time comes when adjustment to a wheelchair life may be preferred to aggressive physiotherapeutic measures. Not least in importance is the psychological management of these patients which may demand considerable reserves of patience and understanding on the part of parents, doctors, nurses, and social workers. Optimism and encouragement, however unjustifiable in the face of continuing deterioration, are greatly needed.

Myotonia

In dystrophia myotonica, no treatment is known which will influence the progressive muscular wasting and weakness which eventually develops. In paramyotonia, the treatment of the attacks of periodic paralysis is similar to that required in patients with familial periodic paralysis and depends upon whether the paralysis is shown to be hypo- or hyperkalaemic in type. Myotonia itself may, however, be substantially relieved by means of appropriate drugs. These are particularly valuable in patients with myotonia congenita, but are also helpful in some with myotonic dystrophy in whom the myotonia is severe. Of drugs used in the past, including quinine, prednisone, and procainamide, the latter is probably the most successful in a dosage of 250–500 mg three or four times daily, depending upon tolerance (Leyburn and Walton, 1959). Recently it has been shown (Munsat, 1967) that, if anything, hydantoin sodium (*Epanutin* or *Dilantin*) is sometimes even more successful in a dosage of 100 mg three times daily.

REFERENCES

ABERFELD, D. C., HINTERBUCHNER, L. P., and SCHNEIDER, M. (1965) Myotonia, dwarfism, diffuse bone disease and unusual ocular and facial abnormalities (a new syndrome), *Brain*, **88**, 313.

ABERFELD, D. C., NAMBA, T., VYE, M. V., and GROB, D. (1970) Chondrodystrophic myotonia: report of two cases, *Arch. Neurol. (Chic.)*, **22**, 455.

ALBERTS, M. C., and SAMAHA, F. J. (1974) Serum pyruvate kinase in muscle disease and carrier states, *Neurology (Minneap.)*, **24**, 462.

BALLANTYNE, J. P., and HANSEN, S. (1974) Myopathies: the neurogenic hypothesis, *Lancet*, **ii**, 588.

BANKER, B. O., VICTOR, M., and ADAMS, R. D. (1957) Arthrogryposis multiplex due to congenital muscular dystrophy, *Brain*, **80**, 319.

BARBEAU, A. (1966) The syndrome of hereditary late onset ptosis and dysphagia in French Canada, in *Progressive Muskeldystrophie, Myotonie, Myasthenie*, ed. Kuhn, E., New York.

BARWICK, D. D., OSSELTON, J. W., and WALTON, J. N. (1965) Electroencephalographic studies in hereditary myopathy, *J. Neurol. Neurosurg. Psychiat.*, **28**, 109.

BATTEN, F. E. (1909) The myopathies or muscular dystrophies; critical review, *Quart. J. Med.*, **3**, 313.

BATTEN, F. E., and GIBB, H. P. (1909) Myotonia atrophica, *Brain*, **32**, 187.

BECKER, P. E. (1953) *Dystrophia Musculorum Progressiva*, Stuttgart.

BECKER, P. E. (1957) Neue Ergebnisse der Genetik der Muskeldystrophien, *Acta Genet. med. (Roma)*, **7**, 303.

BECKER, P. E. (1966) Zur Genetik der Myotonien. In *Progressive Muskeldystrophie, Myotonie, Myasthenie*, p. 247, Berlin.

BECKER, P. E., and KIENER, F. (1955) Eine neue x-chromosomale Muskeldystrophie, *Arch. Psychiat. Nervenkr.*, **193**, 427.

BOUSSER, M. G., CONRAD, J., LECRUBIER, C., and SAMAMA, M. (1975) Increased sensitivity of platelets to adrenaline in human myotonic dystrophy, *Lancet*, **ii**, 307.

BRADLEY, W. G. (1974) State of play in the neural hypothesis of muscular dystrophy, *Nature (Lond.)*, **250**, 285.

BRAY, G. M., KAARSOO, M., and ROSS, R. T. (1965) Ocular myopathy with dysphagia, *Neurology (Minneap.)*, **15**, 678.

BROWN, G. L., and HARVEY, A. M. (1939) Congenital myotonia in the goat, *Brain*, **62**, 341.

BUNDEY, S., CARTER, C. O., and SOOTHILL, J. F. (1970) Early recognition of heterozygotes for the gene for dystrophia myotonica, *J. Neurol. Neurosurg. Psychiat.*, **33**, 279.

BUTTERFIELD, D. A., CHESNUT, D. B., ROSES, A. D., and APPEL, S. H. (1974) Electron spin resonance studies of erythrocytes from patients with myotonic muscular dystrophy, *Proc. Nat. Acad. Sci.*, **71**, 909.

CAUGHEY, J. E., and MYRIANTHOPOULOS, N. C. (1963) *Dystrophia Myotonica and Related Disorders*, Springfield, Ill.

CHUNG, C. S., and MORTON, N. E. (1959) Discrimination of genetic entities in muscular dystrophy, *Amer. J. hum. Genet.*, **11**, 339.

COCCAGNA, G., MANTOVANI, M., PARCHI, C., MIRONI, F., and LUGARESI, E. (1975) Alveolar hypoventilation and hypersomnia in myotonic dystrophy, *J. Neurol. Neurosurg. Psychiat.*, **38**, 977.

DENNY-BROWN, D., and NEVIN, S. (1941) The phenomenon of myotonia, *Brain*, **64**, 1.

DODGE, P. R., GAMSTORP, I., BYERS, R. K., and RUSSELL, P. (1965) Myotonic dystrophy in infancy and childhood, *Pediatrics*, **35**, 3.

DRACHMAN, D. A., WETZEL, N., WASSERMAN, M., and NAITO, H. (1969) Experimental denervation of ocular muscles, *Arch. Neurol. (Chic.)*, **21**, 170.

DUBOWITZ, V. (1960) Progressive muscular dystrophy of the Duchenne type in females and its mode of inheritance, *Brain*, **83**, 432.

DUBOWITZ, V. (1965) Intellectual impairment in muscular dystrophy, *Arch. Dis. Childh.*, **40**, 296.

DUBOWITZ, V. (1975) Neuromuscular disorders in childhood: old dogmas, new concepts, *Arch. Dis. Childh.*, **50**, 335.

DYKEN, P. R., and HARPER, P. S. (1973) Congenital dystrophia myotonica, *Neurology (Minneap.)*, **23**, 465.

EMERY, A. E. H. (1972) Abnormalities of the electrocardiogram in hereditary myopathies, *J. med. Genet.*, **9**, 8.

EMERY, A. E. H., CLACK, E. R., and TAYLOR, J. L. (1967) Detection of carriers of benign X-linked muscular dystrophy, *Brit. med. J.*, **4**, 522.

EMERY, A. E. H., and MORTON, R. (1968) Genetic counselling in lethal X-linked disorders, *Acta genet. (Basel)*, **18**, 534.

EMERY, A. E. H., SMITH, C. A. B., and SANGER, R. (1969) The linkage relations of the loci for benign (Becker type) X-borne muscular dystrophy, colour blindness and the Xg blood groups, *Ann. Hum. Genet. (Lond.)*, **32**, 261.

EMERY, A. E. H., and WALTON, J. N. (1967) The genetics of muscular dystrophy, in *Progress in Medical Genetics*, ed. Steinberg, A. G., and Bearn, A. G., vol. V, New York.

EMERY, A. E. H., WATT, M. S., and CLACK, E. R. (1972) The effects of genetic counselling in Duchenne muscular dystrophy, *Clin. Genet.*, **3**, 147.

EULENBERG, A. (1886) Ueber eine familiäre, durch sechs Generationen verfolgbare Form congenitaler Paramyotonie, *Neurol. Zbl.*, **5**, 265.

FENICHEL, G. M., EMERY, E. S., and HUNT, P. (1967) Neurogenic atrophy simulating facioscapulohumeral muscular dystrophy: a dominant form, *Arch. Neurol. (Chic.)*, **17**, 257.

FERRIER, P., BAMATTER, F., and KLEIN, D. (1965) Muscular dystrophy (Duchenne) in a girl with Turner's syndrome, *J. med. Genet.*, **2**, 38.

FRIEDREICH, N. (1863) Ueber congenitale halbseitige Kopfhypertrophie, *Virchows Arch. path. Anat.*, **38**, 474.

FUCHS, E. (1890) Ueber isolierte doppelseitige Ptosia, *Arch. Ophthal. (Chic.)*, **36**, 234.

GAMSTORP, I. (1956) Adynamia episodica hereditaria, *Acta paediat. (Uppsala)*, Suppl. 108.

GAMSTORP, I., and WOHLFART, G. (1959) A syndrome characterised by myokymia, myotonia, muscular wasting and increased perspiration, *Acta psychiat. scand.*, **34**, 181.

GARDNER-MEDWIN, D. (1968) Studies of the carrier state in the Duchenne type of muscular dystrophy. 2. Quantitative electromyography as a method of carrier detection, *J. Neurol. Neurosurg. Psychiat.*, **31**, 124.

GARDNER-MEDWIN, D. (1970) Mutation rate in Duchenne type of muscular dystrophy, *J. med. Genet.*, **7**, 334.

GARDNER-MEDWIN, D., and WALTON, J. N. (1969) Myokymia with impaired muscular relaxation, *Lancet*, **i**, 127.

GLEESON, J. A., SWANN, J. C., HUGHES, D. T. D., and LEE, F. I. (1967) Dystrophia myotonica—a radiological survey, *Brit. J. Radiol.*, **40**, 96.

GREENHOUSE, A. H., BICKNELL, J. M., PESCH, R. N., and SEELINGER, D. F. (1967) Myotonia, myokymia, hyperhidrosis and wasting of muscle, *Neurology (Minneap.)*, **17**, 263.

GUBBAY, S. S., WALTON, J. N., and PEARCE, G. W. (1966) Clinical and pathological study of a case of congenital muscular dystrophy, *J. Neurol. Neurosurg. Psychiat.*, **29**, 500.

HANSON, P. A., and ROWLAND, L. P. (1971) Möbius syndrome and facioscapulohumeral muscular dystrophy, *Arch. Neurol. (Chic.)*, **24**, 31.

HARPER, P. S. (1973) Pre-symptomatic detection and genetic counselling in myotonic dystrophy, *Clin. Genet.*, **4**, 1.

HARPER, P. S., BIAS, W. B., HUTCHINSON, J. R., and McKUSICK, V. A. (1971) ABH secretor status of the fetus: a genetic marker identifiable by amniocentesis, *J. med. Genet.*, **8**, 438.

HARPER, P. S., and DYKEN, P. R. (1972) Early-onset dystrophia myotonica: evidence supporting a maternal environmental factor, *Lancet*, **ii**, 53.

HARPER, P. S., and JOHNSTON, D. M. (1972) Recessively inherited myotonia congenita, *J. med. Genet.*, **9**, 213.

HARPER, P. S., RIVAS, M. L., BIAS, W. B., HUTCHINSON, J. R., DYKEN, P. R., and McKUSICK, V. A. (1972) Genetic linkage confirmed between the locus for myotonic dystrophy and the ABH-secretion and Lutheran blood group loci, *Amer. J. hum. Genet.*, **24**, 310.

HUDGSON, P., BRADLEY, W. G., and JENKISON, M. (1972) Familial 'mitochondrial' myopathy: a myopathy associated with disordered oxidative metabolism in muscle fibres. Part I—Clinical, electrophysiological and pathological findings, *J. neurol. Sci.*, **16**, 343.

HUTCHINSON, J. (1879) An ophthalmoplegia externa or symmetrical immobility (partial) of the eye with ptosis, *Trans. med.-chir. Soc. Edinb.*, **62**, 307.

HUTTENLOCHER, P. R., LANDWIRTH, J., HANSON, V., GALLACHER, B. B., and BENSCH, K. (1969) Ostochondro-muscular dystrophy: a disorder manifested by multiple skeletal deformities, myotonia and dystrophic changes in muscle, *Pediatrics*, **44**, 945.

IONASESCU, V., ZELLWEGER, H., and CONWAY, T. W. (1971) A new approach for carrier detection in Duchenne muscular dystrophy, *Neurology (Minneap.)*, **21**, 703.

ISAACS, H. (1967) Continuous muscle fibre activity in an Indian male with additional evidence of terminal motor fibre abnormality, *J. Neurol. Neurosurg. Psychiat.*, **30**, 126.

JACKSON, C. E., and CAREY, J. H. (1961) Progressive muscular dystrophy: autosomal recessive type, *Pediatrics*, **28**, 77.

JALBERT, P., MOURIQUAND, C., BEAUDOING, A., and JALLIARD, M. (1966) Myopathie progressive de type Duchenne et mosaique XO/XX/XXX: Considerations sur la genèse de la fibre musculaire striée, *Ann. Génét.*, **9**, 104.

JENSEN, H., JENSEN, K. B., and JARNUM, S. (1971) Turnover of IgG and IgM in myotonic dystrophy, *Neurology (Minneap.)*, **21**, 68.

JEQUIER, M. (1950) Dystrophie myotonique et hyperostose cranienne, *Schweiz. med. Wschr.*, **80**, 593.

JERUSALEM, F., ENGEL, A. G., and GOMEZ, M. R. (1974) Duchenne dystrophy—I. Morphometric study of the muscle microvasculature, *Brain*, **97**, 115.

JOHNSON, J. (1967) Myotonia congenita (Thomsen's disease) and hereditary psychosis, *Brit. J. Psychiat.*, **113**, 1025.

JOHNSTON, H. A. (1964) Severe muscular dystrophy in girls, *J. med. Genet.*, **1**, 79.

KAUFMAN, L. (1965) Respiratory function in muscular dystrophy, in *Research in Muscular Dystrophy*, 2nd series, London.

KENNEL, A. J., TITUS, J. L., and MERIDETH, J. (1974) Pathologic findings in the atrioventricular conduction system in myotonic dystrophy, *Mayo Clin. Proc.*, **49**, 838.

KILBURN, K. H., EAGAN, J. T., SIEKER, H. O., and HEYMAN, A. (1959) Cardiopulmonary insufficiency in myotonic and progressive muscular dystrophy, *New Engl. J. Med.*, **261**, 1089.

KILOH, L. G., and NEVIN, S. (1951) Progressive dystrophy of external ocular muscles (ocular myopathy), *Brain*, **74**, 115.

KLOEPFER, H. W., and TALLEY, C. (1958) Autosomal recessive inheritance of Duchenne type muscular dystrophy, *Ann. hum. Genet.*, **22**, 138.

KUHN, E., and STEIN, W. (1966) Modellmyotonie nach 2,4-dichlorphenoxyacetat (2,4-D), *Klin. Wschr.*, **44**, 700.

LEWIS, I. (1966) Late-onset muscular dystrophy: oculopharyng-oesophageal variety, *Canad. med. Ass. J.*, **95**, 146.

LEYBURN, P., and WALTON, J. N. (1959) The treatment of myotonia: a controlled trial, *Brain*, **82**, 81.

LUNDERVOLD, A., REFSUM, S., and JACOBSEN, W. (1969) The EEG in dystrophia myotonica, *Europ. Neurol.*, **2**, 279.

MAAS, O., and PATERSON, A. S. (1950) The identity of myotonia congenita, dystrophia myotonica and paramyotonia, *Brain*, **73**, 318.

McCOMAS, A. J., SICA, R. E. P., and CAMPBELL, M. J. (1971) 'Sick' motoneurones: a unifying concept of muscle disease, *Lancet*, **i**, 321.

MARKAND, O. N., NORTH, R. R., D'AGOSTINO, A. N., and DALY, D. D. (1969) Benign sex-linked muscular dystrophy, *Neurology (Minneap.)*, **19**, 617.

MARSHALL, J. (1959) Observations on endocrine function in dystrophia myotonica, *Brain*, **82**, 221.

MASTAGLIA, F. L., and WALTON, J. N. (1971) Histological and histochemical changes in skeletal muscle from cases of chronic juvenile and early adult spinal muscular atrophy (the Kugelberg-Welander syndrome), *J. neurol. Sci.*, **12**, 15.

MATHEW, N. T., JACOB, J. C., and CHANDY, J. (1970) Familial ocular myopathy with curare sensitivity, *Arch. Neurol. (Chic.)*, **22**, 68.

MENDELL, J. R., ENGEL, W. K., and DERRER, E. C. (1971) Duchenne muscular dystrophy: functional ischemia reproduces its characteristic lesions, *Science*, **172**, 1143.

MERTENS, H. G., and ZSCHOCKE, S. (1965) Neuromyotonie, *Klin. Wschr.*, **43**, 917.

MORTON, N. E., and CHUNG, C. S. (1959) Formal genetics of muscular dystrophy, *Amer. J. hum. Genet.*, **11**, 360.

MUNSAT, T. L. (1967) Therapy of myotonia: a double-blind evaluation of diphenylhydantoin, procainamide and placebo, *Neurology (Minneap.)*, **17**, 359.

MUNSAT, T. L., PIPER, D., CANCILLA, P., and MEDNICK, J. (1972) Inflammatory myopathy with facioscapulohumeral distribution, *Neurology (Minneap.)*, **22**, 335.

MURPHY, E. G., THOMPSON, M. W., COREY, P. N. J., and CONEN, P. E. (1965) Varying manifestations of Duchenne muscular dystrophy in a family with affected females, in *Muscle*, ed. Paul, W. M., Daniel, E. E., Kay, C. M., and Monckton, G., New York.

MUSCH, B. C., PAPAPETROPOULOS, T. A., McQUEEN, D. A., HUDGSON, P., and WEIGHTMAN, D. (1975) A comparison of the structure of small blood vessels in normal, denervated and dystrophic human muscle, *J. neurol. Sci.*, **26**, 221.

NISSEN, K. (1923) Beiträge zur Kenntnis der Thomsen'schen Krankheit (myotonia congenita) mit besonderer Berücksichtigung des hereditären Momentes und seiner Beziehungen zu den Mendelschen Vererbungsregeln, *Z. klin. Med.*, **96**, 58.

OLSON, W., ENGEL, W. K., WALSH, G. O., and EINAUGLER, R. (1972) Oculocraniosomatic neuromuscular disease with 'ragged-red' fibers: histochemical and ultrastructural changes in limb muscles of a group of patients with idiopathic progressive external ophthalmoplegia, *Arch. Neurol. (Chic.)*, **26**, 193.

OPPENHEIM, H. (1900) Ueber allgemeine und localisierte Atonie der Muskulatur (myatonie) in frühen Kindesalter, *Mschr. Psychiat. Neurol.*, **8**, 232.

PAULSON, O. B., ENGEL, A. G., and GOMEZ, M. R. (1974) Muscle blood flow in Duchenne type muscular dystrophy, limb-girdle dystrophy, polymyositis, and in normal controls, *J. Neurol. Neurosurg. Psychiat.*, **37**, 685.

PEARSON, C. M., and FOWLER, W. G. (1963) Hereditary non-progressive muscular dystrophy inducing arthrogryposis syndrome, *Brain*, **86**, 75.

PENN, A. S., LISAK, R. P., and ROWLAND, L. P. (1970) Muscular dystrophy in young girls, *Neurology (Minneap.)*, **20**, 147.

POLGAR, J. G., BRADLEY, W. G., UPTON, A. R. M., ANDERSON, J., HOWAT, J. M. L., PETITO, F., ROBERTS, D. F., and SCOPA, J. (1972) The early detection of dystrophia myotonica, *Brain*, **95**, 761.

PRATT, R. T. C. (1967) *The Genetics of Neurological Disorders*, London.

PRUZANSKI, W. (1966) Variants of myotonic dystrophy in pre-adolescent life (the syndrome of myotonic dysembryoplasia), *Brain*, **89**, 563.

REFSUM, S., LOUNUM, A., SJAASTAD, O., and ENGESET, A. (1967) Dystrophia myotonica: repeated pneumoencephalographic studies in ten patients, *Neurology (Minneap.)*, **17**, 345.

RESNICK, J. S., and ENGEL, W. K. (1967) Myotonic lid lag in hypokalaemic periodic paralysis, *J. Neurol. Neurosurg. Psychiat.*, **30**, 47.

ROSENBERG, R. N., SCHOTLAND, D. L., LOVELACE, R. E., and ROWLAND, L. P. (1968) Progressive ophthalmoplegia, *Arch. Neurol. (Chic.)*, **19**, 362.

ROSES, A. D., and APPEL, S. H. (1973) Protein kinase activity in erythrocyte ghosts of patients with myotonic muscular dystrophy, *Proc. Nat. Acad. Sci.*, **70**, 1855.

ROSES, A. D., ROSES, M. J., MILLER, S. E., HULL, K. L., and APPEL, S. H. (1976) Carrier detection in Duchenne muscular dystrophy, *New Engl. J. Med.*, **294**, 193.

ROSMAN, N. P., and KAKULAS, B. A. (1966) Mental deficiency associated with muscular dystrophy. A neuropathological study, *Brain*, **89**, 769.

ROSS, R. T. (1963) Ocular myopathy sensitive to curare, *Brain*, **86**, 67.

RUSSE, H., BUSEY, H., and BARBEAU, A. (1969) Immunoglobulin changes in oculopharyngeal muscular dystrophy, *Proc. 2nd Internat. Congr. Neurogenetics*, Montreal.

SCHNECK, L., ADACHI, M., BRIET, P., WOLINTZ, A., and VOLK, B. W. (1973) Ophthalmoplegia plus with morphological and chemical studies of cerebellar and muscle tissue, *J. neurol. Sci.*, **19**, 37.

SCHRÖDER, J. M., and KUHN, E. (1968) Zur Ultrastruktur der Muskelfaser bei der experimentellen 'Myotonie' mit 20,25-Diazacholesterin, *Virchows Arch. Abt. A Path. Anat.*, **344**, 181.

SCHWARTZ, O., and JAMPEL, R. S. (1962) Congenital blepharophimosis associated with a unique generalized myopathy, *Arch. Ophthalmol.*, **68**, 52.

SIEGEL, I. (1972) Equinocavovarus in muscular dystrophy: its treatment by percutaneous tarsal medullostomy and soft tissue release, *Arch. Surg.*, **104**, 644.

SIEGEL, I., MILLER, J. E., and RAY, R. D. (1968) Subcutaneous lower limb tenotomy in the treatment of pseudohypertrophic muscular dystrophy, *J. Bone Jt. Surg.*, **50-A**, 1437.

SKYRING, A., and McKUSICK, V. A. (1961) Clinical, genetic and electrocardiographic studies in childhood muscular dystrophy, *Amer. J. med. Sci.*, **242**, 534.

SOMERS, J. E., and WINER, N. (1966) Reversible myopathy and myotonia following administration of a hypocholesterolemic agent, *Neurology (Minneap.)*, **16**, 761.

SPILLER, W. G. (1913) The relation of the myopathies, *Brain*, **36**, 75.

STEINERT, H. (1909) Myopathologische Beiträge: I. Ueber das klinische und anatomische Bild des Muskelschwunds der Myotoniker, *Dtsch Z. Nervenheilk.*, **37**, 58.

STEVENSON, A. C. (1953) Muscular dystrophy in Northern Ireland, *Ann. Eugen. (Lond.)*, **18**, 50.

SUMNER, D., CRAWFURD, M. D'A., and HARRIMAN, D. G. F. (1971) Distal muscle dystrophy in an English family, *Brain*, **94**, 51.

THOMASEN, E. (1948) *Thomsen's Disease, Paramyotonia, Dystrophia Myotonica*, Aarhus.

THOMSEN, J. (1876) Tonische Krämpfe in willkürlich beweglichen Muskeln in Folge von ererbter psychischer Disposition (ataxia muscularis?), *Arch. Psychiat. Nervenkr.*, **6**, 706.

K k

THRUSH, D. C., MORRIS, C. J., and SALMON, M. V. (1972) Paramyotonia congenita—a clinical, histochemical and pathological study, *Brain*, **95**, 536.

TOMLINSON, B. E., WALTON, J. N., and IRVING, D. (1974) Spinal cord limb motor neurones in muscular dystrophy, *J. neurol. Sci.*, **22**, 305.

TURNER, J. W. A. (1940) The relationship between amyotonia congenita and congenital myopathy, *Brain*, **63**, 163.

TURNER, J. W. A. (1949) On amyotonia congenita, *Brain*, **72**, 25.

TURNER, J. W. A., and LEES, F. (1962) Congenital myopathy—a fifty year follow-up, *Brain*, **85**, 733.

TYLER, F. H., and WINTROBE, M. M. (1950) Studies in disorders of muscle. I. The problem of progressive muscular dystrophy, *Ann. intern. Med.*, **32**, 72.

VICTOR, M., HAYES, R., and ADAMS, R. D. (1962) Oculopharyngeal muscular dystrophy. A familial disease of late life characterised by dysphagia and progressive ptosis of the eyelids, *New Engl. J. Med.*, **267**, 1267.

WALLIS, W. E., VAN POZNAK, A., and PLUM, F. (1970) Generalized muscular stiffness, fasciculations, and myokymia of peripheral nerve origin, *Arch. Neurol. (Chic.)*, **22**, 430.

WALSH, F. B. (1957) *Clinical Neuro-ophthalmology*, 2nd ed., London.

WALSH, J. C., TURTLE, J. R., MILLER, S., and McLEOD, J. G. (1970) Abnormalities of insulin secretion in dystrophia myotonica, *Brain*, **93**, 731.

WALTON, J. N. (1956 a) The inheritance of muscular dystrophy: further observations, *Ann. hum. Genet.*, **21**, 40.

WALTON, J. N. (1956 b) Amyotonia congenita: a follow-up study, *Lancet*, **i**, 1023.

WALTON, J. N. (1966) Diseases of muscle, *Abstr. Wld. Med.*, **40**, 1, 81.

WALTON, J. N. (1973) Some changing concepts in neuromuscular disease, in *Clinical Studies in Myology* (Proceedings of the Second International Congress on Muscle Diseases, Part 2), ed. Kakulas, B. A., p. 429, Amsterdam.

WALTON, J. N., and GARDNER-MEDWIN, D. (1974) Progressive muscular dystrophy and the myotonic disorders, in *Disorders of Voluntary Muscle*, ed. Walton, J. N., 3rd ed., Edinburgh and London.

WALTON, J. N., and NATTRASS, F. J. (1954) On the classification, natural history and treatment of the myopathies, *Brain*, **77**, 169.

WALTON, J. N., and WARRICK, C. K. (1954) Osseous changes in myopathy, *Brit. J. Radiol.*, **27**, 1.

WELANDER, L. (1951) Myopathia distalis tarda hereditaria, *Acta med. scand.*, Suppl. 264, 1.

WELANDER, L. (1957) Homozygous appearance of distal myopathy, *Acta Genet. med. (Roma)*, **7**, 321.

WHARTON, B. A. (1965) An unusual variety of muscular dystrophy, *Lancet*, **i**, 603.

WOCHNER, R. D., DREWS, G., STROBER, W., and WALDMANN, T. A. (1966) Accelerated breakdown of immunoglobulin G (IgG) in myotonic dystrophy: a hereditary error of immunoglobulin catabolism, *J. clin. Invest.*, **45**, 321.

ZELLWEGER, H., AFIFI, A., McCORMICK, W. F., and MERGNER, W. (1967) Severe congenital muscular dystrophy, *Amer. J. Dis. Child.*, **114**, 591.

ZINTZ, VON R., and VILLIGER, W. (1967) Elektronenmikroskopische Befunde bei 3 Fällen von chronisch progressiver okulärer Muskeldystrophie, *Ophthalmologica (Basel)*, **153**, 439.

INFLAMMATORY DISORDERS OF MUSCLE

SPECIFIC INFECTIONS

Voluntary muscle may be involved as a secondary effect of suppuration arising in skin, bone, or connective tissue and widespread necrosis frequently occurs following trauma as a result of infection with the anaerobic organism of gas gangrene. Some viral infections may give rise to an acute myositis; this is particularly common in infection with certain viruses of the Coxsackie type. Thus in the syndrome often called Bornholm disease, pain in the muscles of the trunk and diaphragmatic involvement, giving pain on deep breathing and coughing, are frequently seen but the disorder is self-limiting and usually recovers within a few days. Acute myositis has also been described in influenza (Middleton *et al.*, 1970). Muscle is only rarely involved in parasitic infestations, but muscular pain and weakness may occur in toxoplasmosis (Chandar *et al.*, 1968), in South American trypanosomiasis, and in trichinosis, which usually develops after the ingestion of infested pork. Fleeting muscle pain and tenderness may be accompanied by peri-orbital oedema and *Trichinella spiralis* may be detected on muscle biopsy (Adams, 1975).

MUSCULAR INVOLVEMENT IN COLLAGEN OR CONNECTIVE TISSUE DISEASES AND SARCOIDOSIS

In cases of rheumatoid arthritis, pathological examination of muscle biopsy sections often demonstrates foci of inflammatory cell infiltration, but this focal nodular myositis is rarely accompanied by any specific muscular wasting and weakness save for that resulting secondarily from joint disease. In sarcoidosis, however, muscular involvement may be so widespread that occasional patients with this affliction present with a subacute weakness and wasting of proximal muscles and typical sarcoid granulomas may be observed on muscle biopsy (see Pearson and Currie, 1974). Sometimes this course of events is seen in patients with established sarcoidosis (Silverstein and Sitzbach, 1969; Jerusalem and Imbach, 1970; Douglas *et al.*, 1973). However, it has recently become clear that a diffuse granulomatous myopathy, often with histological changes in the muscle indistinguishable from those of sarcoidosis, may occur without any other clinical or investigative evidence of the latter condition (Gardner-Thorpe, 1972; Hewlett and Brownell, 1975) and the possibility that this granulomatous disorder may on occasion be a form of polymyositis unrelated to sarcoidosis has been raised. In polyarteritis nodosa, severe localized muscle pain, subcutaneous oedema, and tenderness may occur as a result of muscle infarction. Focal nodular myositis may also occur in disseminated lupus erythematosus, but in occasional cases muscular involvement is more severe and diffuse and this syndrome may reasonably then be identified as one of polymyositis, although in occasional such cases histological investigation reveals a vacuolar myopathy (Pearson and Yamazaki, 1958). The diffuse muscular involvement commonly seen in patients with progressive systemic sclerosis is undoubtedly due to an associated polymyositis (see below) and indeed some children and adolescents with polymyositis show features of acrosclerosis with associated dysphagia and a Raynaud's syndrome. Localized muscular abnormalities indistinguishable from those of polymyositis may also be noted in the muscles underlying areas of linear morphoea or scleroderma (Stern *et al.*, 1975).

POLYMYOSITIS

The classification and nosological status of polymyositis remains somewhat controversial. This name is usually given to identify a group of cases in which muscular wasting and weakness occur and are sometimes associated with local

muscle pain, tenderness and wasting or with evidence of some form of connective tissue or collagen disease. Muscle biopsy generally demonstrates areas
of muscle fibre necrosis accompanied by interstitial or perivascular cellular
infiltrates or both, though these are not invariable. The term is commonly used
to include cases with florid skin change, which are more properly called dermatomyositis; it is usually taken to indicate the so-called idiopathic syndrome and
excludes disorders such as polymyalgia rheumatica (see below) and also acute
myositis resulting from infections with micro-organisms and viruses. The
relationship of the myopathies seen in sarcoidosis, Sjogren's disease, and
bronchogenic carcinoma to polymyositis is still somewhat obscure (Pearson and
Currie, 1974), though with the exception of the specific myasthenic-myopathic
syndrome (see below) which is sometimes observed in patients with lung cancer,
it seems probable that some cases of so-called carcinomatous myopathy in
reality belong with the syndrome of polymyositis (Rose and Walton, 1966).
Denny-Brown (1960) and Shy (1962) suggested that such polymyopathies
should be identified according to their aetiology and pathological characteristics.
However, Walton and Adams (1958), Barwick and Walton (1963), and Rose and
Walton (1966) concluded that the term 'polymyositis' should be retained as in
many cases the aetiology of the condition remains obscure despite full investigation. Furthermore, a response to steroid therapy, suggesting a relationship to
diseases of the connective tissue group, occurs in many patients in whom
muscle biopsy findings are non-specific. There is evidence to suggest that in
occasional cases of polymyositis, involvement of distal branches of peripheral
nerves occurs, possibly within the muscle, and these cases may reasonably be
described as examples of neuromyositis (McEntee and Mancall, 1965). It must
also be noted that polymyositis and polyneuritis are both well-recognized manifestations of systemic lupus erythematosus and may occur together.

AETIOLOGY

The work of Dawkins (1965), Kakulas (1966), and Currie (1971) demonstrating that polymyositis may be produced in animals by the injection of muscle
homogenates with Freund's adjuvant supports the view that this syndrome in
the human may well be the result of cell-mediated delayed hypersensitivity.
It is thus possible to suggest that polymyositis in which there is no clinical
evidence to suggest that any tissue other than muscle is involved may be an
organ-specific auto-immune disease, while in cases showing involvement of skin
or joints it may be regarded as being a feature of a non-organ-specific auto-
immune disease. The clear-cut relationship between polymyositis and dermatomyositis on the one hand, and malignant disease on the other, also suggests that
the condition may sometimes be the result of a conditioned auto-immune
response in patients suffering from cancer. Attempts to demonstrate antimuscle
antibodies in the serum of patients with polymyositis failed to confirm the
presumed auto-immune character of the disease (Stern et al., 1967). The close
relationship of the condition to other disorders of the connective tissue group
can, however, be underlined by the occurrence of certain cases which may
successively present manifestations of polymyositis, disseminated lupus
erythematosus, and/or scleroderma or systemic sclerosis.

Increasing evidence has recently emerged to support the auto-immune
hypothesis. Thus Currie et al. (1971) found an increased incidence of lymphocyte
transformation in response to muscle antigen in cells obtained from cases of
polymyositis and demonstrated that these cells were cytotoxic to muscle cells

in tissue culture; confirmatory evidence has been reported by Mastaglia and Currie (1971), Esiri *et al.* (1973), and Haas and Arnason (1974), though Lisak and Zweiman (1975) reported contrary findings. Whitaker and Engel (1972) found vascular deposits of immunoglobulin and complement in muscle biopsies obtained from such patients and Dawkins and Zilko (1975) found evidence of subtle immunodeficiency in patients with both polymyositis and myasthenia gravis.

There have also been several reports of the detection of picornavirus (Chou and Gutmann, 1970), myxovirus (Chou, 1968; Sato *et al.*, 1971), and Coxsackie virus-like (Mastaglia and Walton, 1971) particles in muscle biopsies from such patients. Thus it seems likely that polymyositis is due to lymphocyte-mediated delayed hypersensitivity and that viral infection may be one factor which is capable of initiating this process.

CLASSIFICATION

The clinical classification proposed by Walton and Adams (1958), as modified by Rose and Walton (1966), seems reasonably satisfactory for clinical assessment and is given below:

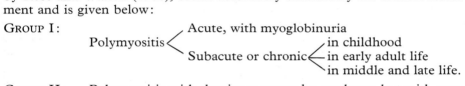

GROUP I: Polymyositis — Acute, with myoglobinuria
Subacute or chronic — in childhood / in early adult life / in middle and late life.

GROUP II: Polymyositis with dominant muscular weakness but with some evidence of an associated collagen disease or dermatomyositis with severe muscular disability and with minimal or transient skin changes.

GROUP III: Polymyositis complicating severe collagen disease, e.g. rheumatoid arthritis, or dermatomyositis with florid skin changes and minor muscle weakness.

GROUP IV: Polymyositis complicating malignant disease (including 'carcinomatous myopathy' and dermatomyositis occurring in patients with malignant disease).

It must be accepted that some of the cases classified arbitrarily in these groups, and particularly some with myoglobinuria, as well as progressive cases of late onset, may be due to metabolic abnormalities unrelated aetiologically to the group of collagen or connective tissue disorders to which most cases of polymyositis rightfully belong.

INCIDENCE

Polymyositis is world-wide, occurs in many races and appears to be commoner in men. It is more common in adult life than muscular dystrophy, but is less common than the latter in childhood. About 15 per cent of cases occur under the age of 15, another 15 per cent between the ages of 16 and 30, about 25 per cent between 31 and 45, and 30 per cent between the ages of 46 and 60. The condition usually occurs spontaneously, but may follow a variety of febrile illnesses and has been known to develop after the administration of various drugs, including sulphonamides and penicillamine (Schraeder *et al.*, 1972) or following exposure to sunlight. It is rarely familial (Lewkonia and Buxton, 1973).

CLINICAL MANIFESTATIONS

Detailed analyses of the clinical manifestations of polymyositis have been given by many authors (Eaton, 1954; Garcin et al., 1955; Pearson and Rose, 1960; Barwick and Walton, 1963; Pearson and Currie, 1974). Muscle pain and tenderness occur in approximately 50 per cent of cases, as does dysphagia. Cutaneous manifestations are seen in about two-thirds of all patients and may take the form of widespread erythema with desquamation seen particularly on the face and on other exposed areas of the trunk, but occasionally involving almost the whole body. A particularly characteristic heliotrope erythema around the eyes, together with periorbital oedema, is seen in some patients, as is congestion of the nail beds. In some cases the skin changes are slight and may take the form of no more than a faint butterfly-type rash on the face, while in others, particularly in childhood, there may be ulceration over bony prominences with subcutaneous calcification; the latter on occasion can be very extensive (calcinosis universalis). Raynaud's syndrome is a common association and many younger patients develop thickening and loss of elasticity of the skin over the fingers, face, and anterior chest wall resembling those of generalized scleroderma or acrosclerosis.

In about a quarter of the patients joint pain and stiffness may be observed. Proximal limb muscles are almost invariably involved and it is characteristic that the neck muscles are weak in many cases so that patients may have difficulty in holding up the head. Specific involvement of distal limb muscles, without proximal weakness, is uncommon, but weakness may be generalized in about a third of all cases, and in under a third contractures eventually develop. Facial weakness and involvement of external ocular muscles occur rarely (Rothstein et al., 1971; Bates et al., 1973; Susac et al., 1973). Occasionally myasthenic fatigability is striking and is partially responsive to edrophonium or neostigmine, but treatment with these and related drugs usually produces only temporary improvement. The deep tendon reflexes may be depressed in the affected muscles but are often surprisingly brisk despite the severity of the muscular weakness.

Pulmonary involvement with chronic respiratory insufficiency has been described (Camp et al., 1972) and myocardial damage with pericarditis also occurs rarely (Walton and Adams, 1958), but these and other forms of visceral affection are usually indicative of associated systemic sclerosis or systemic lupus.

PROGNOSIS

Even without treatment the course of the illness is variable. Sometimes it runs a fluctuating course with spontaneous exacerbations and remissions; progressive deterioration with a fatal termination within a few weeks or months of the onset is seen particularly in acute dermatomyositis, but in some patients spontaneous arrest has been seen. However, before the introduction of steroid drugs, the over-all mortality of the disease was about 50 per cent. Slow insidious progression is seen, particularly in middle age, but spontaneous recovery may occur in childhood (Nattrass, 1954; Rose, 1974).

In a review of 89 cases observed and studied in north-east England, Rose and Walton (1966) found that 16 per cent of their patients had associated malignant disease. Seventy-five patients in their series had received adequate steroid therapy and in the great majority the treatment was followed by subjective and objective clinical improvement accompanied by a progressive reduction in serum enzyme activity. Withdrawal of treatment during the first two years after the onset sometimes resulted in relapse. Most patients required treatment for at least three years and no deaths occurred under the age of 30. Most of the children and young adults recovered completely, but after the age of 30 a number of patients went on to develop evidence of diffuse connective tissue disease unresponsive to treatment, while after the age of 50 malignant disease which was present in a high proportion of cases adversely affected the prognosis. An even more extensive follow-up study reported by De Vere and Bradley (1975) has amply confirmed the benefits of steroid treatment.

TREATMENT

The condition should usually be treated with 60 mg of prednisone daily, given for two or three weeks, thereafter reducing the dose to 40 mg daily when clinical improvement appears and subsequently regulating the maintenance dose according to the level of serum creatine kinase activity and the clinical response. Occasionally even higher doses of prednisone (up to 120 mg daily) may be required for short periods, and in resistant cases ACTH, 80 units daily, is worth trying as an alternative and has the advantage in childhood of having less effect in the suppression of growth. Once there is an adequate clinical response, alternate day treatment has considerable advantages. Maintenance therapy may have to be continued for many years before the drug can be withdrawn. There is now increasing evidence that immunosuppressive remedies such as cyclophosphamide or azathioprine, 100 mg daily, may be useful when combined with maintenance doses of prednisone, especially in resistant cases, and many authorities now combine prednisone and immunosuppressive treatment from the onset (Currie and Walton, 1971; Haas, 1973; De Vere and Bradley, 1975). Respiratory and urinary infection should be treated with appropriate antibiotics and in occasional severe cases intermittent positive pressure respiration is necessary. Following the acute stage, active and passive movements carried out under the supervision of a skilled physiotherapist are valuable.

POLYMYALGIA RHEUMATICA

Polymyalgia rheumatica (Bagratuni, 1953; Gordon, 1960; Todd, 1961; Hart, 1969) occurs almost always in elderly patients whose principal complaint is one of widespread muscular pain, often with local tenderness, minor constitutional upset, and sometimes general malaise. Muscle weakness is not present as a rule, though pain may be so severe that movement is restricted and many patients are wrongly diagnosed as suffering from polymyositis. Difficulty in getting out of a bath or out of a low chair without help is characteristic. Muscle biopsy usually reveals normal muscle. Some patients go on to develop rheumatoid arthritis and Paulley and Hughes (1960) and others have suggested that there is a close relationship between this condition and cranial arteritis, which may develop in others. Indeed, there is increasing evidence that a diffuse giant-cell arteritis is present in many cases and subclinical hepatic dysfunction, improving with treatment, has been described (Long and James, 1974). In all patients the erythrocyte sedimentation rate is substantially raised, but the electromyogram, serum enzyme studies, and muscle biopsy are usually negative. The response to steroid therapy is usually immediate and dramatic.

REFERENCES

ADAMS, R. D. (1975) *Diseases of Muscle*, 3rd ed., New York.

BAGRATUNI, L. (1953) Polymyalgia rheumatica, *Ann. rheum. Dis.*, **12**, 98.

BARWICK, D. D., and WALTON, J. N. (1963) Polymyositis, *Amer. J. Med.*, **35**, 646.

BATES, D., STEVENS, J. C., and HUDGSON, P. (1973) 'Polymyositis' with involvement of facial and distal musculature: one form of the facioscapulohumeral syndrome?, *J. neurol. Sci.*, **19**, 105.

CAMP, A. V., LANE, D. J., and MOWAT, A. G. (1972) Dermatomyositis with parenchymal lung involvement, *Brit. med. J.*, **1**, 155.

CHANDAR, K., MAIR, H. J., and MAIR, N. S. (1968) Case of toxoplasma polymyositis, *Brit. med. J.*, **1**, 158.

CHOU, S.-M. (1968) Myxovirus-like structures and accompanying nuclear changes in chronic polymyositis, *Arch. Path.*, **86**, 649.

CHOU, S.-M., and GUTMANN, L. (1970) Picornavirus-like crystals in subacute polymyositis, *Neurology (Minneap.)*, **20**, 205.

CURRIE, S. (1971) Experimental myositis: the in-vivo and in-vitro activity of lymph-node cells, *J. Path.*, **105**, 169.

CURRIE, S., SAUNDERS, M., KNOWLES, M., and BROWN, A. E. (1971) Immunological aspects of polymyositis: the in-vitro activity of lymphocytes on incubation with muscle antigen and with muscle cultures, *Quart. J. Med.*, **40**, 63.

CURRIE, S., and WALTON, J. N. (1971) Immunosuppressive therapy in polymyositis, *J. Neurol. Neurosurg. Psychiat.*, **34**, 447.

DAWKINS, R. L. (1965) Experimental myositis associated with hypersensitivity to muscle, *J. Path. Bact.*, **90**, 619.

DAWKINS, R. L., and ZILKO, P. J. (1975) Polymyositis and myasthenia gravis: immunodeficiency disorders involving skeletal muscle, *Lancet*, **i**, 200.

DENNY-BROWN, D. (1960) The nature of polymyositis and related muscular diseases, *Trans. Coll. Phycns Philad.*, **28**, 14.

DEVERE, R., and BRADLEY, W. G. (1975) Polymyositis: its presentation, morbidity and mortality, *Brain*, **98**, 637.

DOUGLAS, A. C., MCLEOD, J. G., and MATTHEWS, J. D. (1973) Symptomatic sarcoidosis of skeletal muscle, *J. Neurol. Neurosurg. Psychiat.*, **36**, 1034.

EATON, L. M. (1954) The perspective of neurology in regard to polymyositis; study of 41 cases, *Neurology (Minneap.)*, **4**, 245.

ESIRI, M. M., MACLENNAN, I. C. M., and HAZLEMAN, B. L. (1973) Lymphocyte sensitivity to skeletal muscle in patients with polymyositis and other disorders, *Clin. exp. Immunol.*, **14**, 25.

GARCIN, R., LAPRESLE, J., GRUNER, J., and SCHERRER, J. (1955) Les polymyosites, *Rev. Neurol.*, **92**, 465.

GARDNER-THORPE, C. (1972) Muscle weakness due to sarcoid myopathy, *Neurology (Minneap.)*, **22**, 917.

GORDON, I. (1960) Polymyalgia rheumatica, *Quart. J. Med.*, **116**, 473.

HAAS, D. C. (1973) Treatment of polymyositis with immunosuppressive drugs, *Neurology (Minneap.)*, **23**, 55.

HAAS, D. C., and ARNASON, B. G. W. (1974) Cell-mediated immunity in polymyositis, *Arch. Neurol. (Minneap.)*, **31**, 192.

HART, F. D. (1969) Polymyalgia rheumatica, *Brit. med. J.*, **2**, 99.

HEWLETT, R. H., and BROWNELL, B. (1975) Granulomatous myopathy: its relationship to sarcoidosis and polymyositis, *J. Neurol. Neurosurg. Psychiat.*, **38**, 1090.

JERUSALEM, F., and IMBACH, P. (1970) Granulomatöse myositis und muskelsarkoidose, *Dtsch med. Wschr.*, **43**, 2184.

KAKULAS, B. A. (1966) Destruction of differentiated muscle cultures by sensitized cells, *J. Path. Bact.*, **91**, 495.

LEWKONIA, R. M., and BUXTON, P. H. (1973) Myositis in father and daughter, *J. Neurol. Neurosurg. Psychiat.*, **36**, 820.

LISAK, R. P., and ZWEIMAN, B. (1975) Mitogen and muscle extract induced in vitro proliferative responses in myasthenia gravis, dermatomyositis, and polymyositis, *J. Neurol. Neurosurg. Psychiat.*, **38**, 521.

LONG, R., and JAMES, O. (1974) Polymyalgia rheumatica and liver disease, *Lancet*, **i**, 77.

MCENTEE, W. J., and MANCALL, E. L. (1965) Neuromyositis: a reappraisal, *Neurology (Minneap.)*, **15**, 69.

MASTAGLIA, F. L., and CURRIE, S. (1971) Immunological and ultrastructural observations on the role of lymphoid cells in the pathogenesis of polymyositis, *Acta neuropath. (Berl.)*, **18**, 1.

MASTAGLIA, F. L., and WALTON, J. N. (1971) Coxsackie virus-like particles in skeletal muscle from a case of polymyositis, *J. neurol. Sci.*, **11**, 593.

MIDDLETON, P. J., ALEXANDER, R. M., and SZYMANSKI, M. T. (1970) Severe myositis during recovery from influenza, *Lancet*, **ii**, 533.

NATTRASS, F. J. (1954) Recovery from muscular dystrophy, *Brain*, **77**, 549.

PAULLEY, J. W., and HUGHES, J. P. (1960) Giant-cell arteritis, or arteritis of the aged, *Brit. med. J.*, **2**, 1562.

PEARSON, C. M., and CURRIE, S. (1974) Polymyositis and related disorders, in *Disorders of Voluntary Muscle*, ed. Walton, J. N., 3rd ed., Edinburgh and London.

PEARSON, C. M., and ROSE, A. S. (1960) Myositis, the inflammatory disorders of muscle, *Res. Publ. Ass. nerv. ment. Dis.*, **38**, 422.

PEARSON, C. M., and YAMAZAKI, J. N. (1958) Vacuolar myopathy in systemic lupus erythematosus, *Amer. J. clin. Path.*, **29**, 455.

ROSE, A. L. (1974) Childhood polymyositis. A follow-up study with special reference to treatment with corticosteroids, *Amer. J. Dis. Child.*, **127**, 518.

ROSE, A. L., and WALTON, J. N. (1966) Polymyositis: a survey of 89 cases with particular reference to treatment and prognosis, *Brain*, **89**, 747.

ROTHSTEIN, T. L., CARLSON, C. B., and SUMI, S. M. (1971) Polymyositis with facio-scapulohumeral distribution, *Arch. Neurol. (Chic.)*, **25**, 313.

SATO, T., WALKER, D. L., PETERS, H. A., REESE, H. H., and CHOU, S.-M. (1971) Chronic polymyositis and myxovirus-like inclusions, *Arch. Neurol. (Chic.)*, **24**, 409.

SCHRAEDER, P. L., PETERS, H. A., and DAHL, D. S. (1972) Polymyositis and penicillamine, *Arch. Neurol. (Chic.)*, **27**, 456.

SHY, G. M. (1962) The late onset myopathy, *Wld Neurol.*, **3**, 149.

SILVERSTEIN, A., and SITZBACH, L. E. (1969) Muscle involvement in sarcoidosis, *Arch. Neurol. (Chic.)*, **21**, 235.

STERN, G. M., ROSE, A. L., and JACOBS, K. (1967) Circulating antibodies in polymyositis, *J. neurol. Sci.*, **5**, 181.

STERN, L. Z., PAYNE, C. M., ALVAREZ, J. T., and HANNAPEL, L. K. (1975) Myopathy associated with linear scleroderma, *Neurology (Minneap.)*, **25**, 114.

SUSAC, J. O., GARCIA-MULLIN, R., and GLASER, J. S. (1973) Ophthalmoplegia in dermato-myositis, *Neurology (Minneap.)*, **23**, 305.

TODD, J. W. (1961) Polymyalgia rheumatica, *Lancet*, **ii**, 1111.

WALTON, J. N., and ADAMS, R. D. (1958) *Polymyositis*, Edinburgh.

WHITAKER, J. N., and ENGEL, W. K. (1972) Vascular deposits of immunoglobulin and complement in idiopathic inflammatory myopathy, *New Engl. J. Med.*, **286**, 333.

MYASTHENIA GRAVIS

Definition. A chronic disease with a tendency to remit and to relapse, characterized by abnormal muscular fatigability which may for a long time be confined to, or predominant in, an isolated group of muscles and is later associated in many cases with permanent weakness of some muscles. The fatigability is due to a disorder of conduction at the myoneural junction which can be temporarily relieved by neostigmine and similar drugs, and in some cases permanently benefited by removal of the thymus gland. Early descriptions were given by Wilks (1877) and Erb (1879), while the present name was coined by Jolly (1895). Walker (1934) was the first to describe the beneficial effect of physostigmine, and the first successful thymectomy was performed by Blalock in 1936.

CLASSIFICATION

As Simpson (1974) points out, the symptom of myasthenia is not peculiar to one disease. Similar fatigability can be observed in muscles affected by polymyositis, systemic lupus, dermatomyositis, and one type of carcinomatous myopathy (see below). However, a therapeutic response to anticholinesterase drugs is necessary for the definition of true myasthenia gravis, and although some response may be found in the symptomatic myasthenias, it is rarely dramatic and often fails within a few weeks. Myasthenia gravis is therefore a clearly-recognizable disease in which the response to appropriate drugs is dramatic and sustained and it is one which has an individual natural history and pathology.

INCIDENCE AND NATURAL HISTORY

Myasthenia occurs in all races and affects both sexes, but is seen in women twice as often as in men (Osserman, 1958). Its prevalence in Finland is 50–75 cases per million of the population. Only occasionally is it seen in more than one member of the same family but it has been reported in twins (Namba et al., 1971 a), and there is a form showing an onset in early childhood which may be of autosomal recessive inheritance (Bundey, 1972). Jacob et al (1968) found no familial incidence in a series of 70 cases, but others (Namba et al., 1971 b) have found a substantially increased familial incidence and noted that familial cases generally showed a much earlier age of onset.

Recent evidence suggests a possible relationship with HL-A8 antigen (in women), of HL-A3 (in some older males), and of HL-A2 (in patients with thymoma) and evidence is accumulating to suggest that the disease may occur in several forms which are clinically, immunologically, and genetically different (Feltkamp et al., 1974; Fritze et al., 1974). The mean age of onset is about 26 years in women and 30 years in men, but the condition may sometimes arise for the first time in childhood and occasionally as late as 80 years. It often arises without apparent cause, but occasionally follows emotional upset, physical stress, febrile illness, or pregnancy. Most remissions occur within the first 5 years of the disease process, and most deaths also occur within this period. After the disease has been in progress for 10 years, death from myasthenia itself is rare and in some instances the disease is apparently burnt out by this stage (Simpson, 1974).

There is a close relationship between myasthenia gravis and thyrotoxicosis and the two diseases occur in combination in the same individual far more often than can be accounted for by chance (Schlezinger and Corin, 1968; Namba and Grob, 1971). The condition which has been called acute thyrotoxic bulbar palsy is almost certainly due in most cases to myasthenia affecting bulbar muscles in a thyrotoxic individual.

Neonatal myasthenia is seen in about one in seven of the children born to myasthenic mothers, but in those who survive it usually recovers in between a week and three months after birth and does not recur (Wise and McQuillen, 1970; Namba et al., 1970). Myasthenia has also been reported in dogs (Fraser et al., 1970), and a myasthenic syndrome in man has been noted during the administration of various drugs including phenytoin (Brumlik and Jacobs,

1974), antibiotics, especially streptomycin (Hokkanen and Toivakka, 1969), kanamycin and colistimethate (McQuillen *et al.*, 1968; Decker and Fincham, 1971), and penicillamine (Bucknall *et al.*, 1975).

SYMPTOMS AND SIGNS

The muscles most often affected by the disease are the external ocular, bulbar, neck and shoulder-girdle muscles in this descending order, but it is not uncommon to find that those of respiration and the proximal muscles of the lower extremities are also involved. The onset is usually gradual and ptosis of one or both upper lids is often the first symptom and is soon associated with diplopia due to paralysis of one or more of the external ocular muscles. These symptoms typically appear in the evening when the patient is tired and disappear after a night's rest. When the bulbar muscles are first involved, difficulty in swallowing and/or in chewing is described, again most evident in the course of a meal, and speech may become indistinct when the patient is tired.

On examination unilateral or bilateral ptosis is often found and is intensified by asking the patient to gaze upwards. Weakness of the external ocular muscles is usually asymmetrical and may progress to complete external ophthalmoplegia of one or both eyes. Occasionally conjugate ocular movements appear to be affected, but more often there is no functional relationship between the muscles involved in the two eyes and weakness of a single muscle (e.g. lateral rectus) is not uncommon. Paresis of accommodation has been described and the pupillary reflexes are usually normal but may be sluggish or exhibit fatigability.

The facial muscles are almost always seen to be affected [FIG. 146]. Weakness

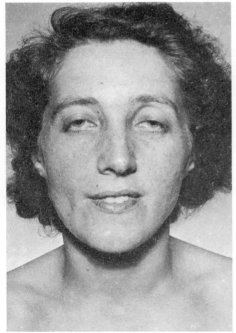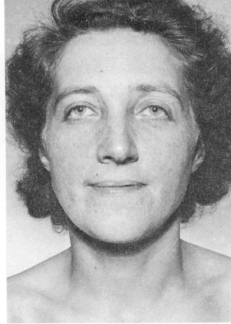

FIG. 146. Myasthenia gravis. *Left*, bilateral ptosis and weakness of facial muscles; *right*, the change in facial expression after an injection of neostigmine (from *An Atlas of Clinical Neurology* by J. D. Spillane, Oxford University Press, 2nd ed., 1975, reproduced by kind permission of the author and publishers)

of the orbicularis oculi is a relatively constant sign; in the lower face the rectrac-
tors of the angles of the mouth tend to suffer more than the elevators, so that
a characteristic myasthenic snarling appearance on smiling is seen. Weakness
of the jaw muscles leads to difficulty in chewing and weakness of the muscles
of the soft palate, pharynx, tongue, and larynx to difficulty in swallowing and in
articulation. The characteristic fatigability of speech may be demonstrated
by asking the patient to count up to 50, during which time speech becomes
progressively less distinct and palatal weakness may give a nasal character to the
voice and occasional regurgitation of fluids through the nose on swallowing.
Typically, weakness of the neck muscles tends to cause the head to fall forward,
a sign seen most often in myasthenia gravis but also observed in some cases of
polymyositis. In severe cases the weakness of the upper limbs is such that the
hands cannot be lifted to the mouth and it is characteristic that muscle power
may initially be reasonably satisfactory, but after testing a particular movement
on several occasions, the strength rapidly declines. Breathlessness is always
a sinister symptom in patients with myasthenia, as respiratory weakness may
develop rapidly and may even cause sudden death. Sudden respiratory failure
is often called a myasthenic crisis (Szobor, 1970).

Muscular wasting is not usually observed in the early stages, but in long-
standing cases of myasthenia it is common to find permanent weakness and
wasting, irreversible by drugs, in the external ocular muscles and in certain limb
muscles, particularly the triceps brachii. The term 'myasthenic myopathy' is
sometimes used to identify this irreversible muscular weakness, but as the term
is also utilized to describe rare cases of myopathy of undetermined cause in
whom weakness is improved, if only partially or transiently, by neostigmine,
its meaning is imprecise (Rowland et al., 1973). While in the majority of cases
muscular weakness eventually becomes widespread throughout the muscles of
the head and neck, trunk and limbs, Grob (1953) and Ferguson et al. (1955)
showed that in some cases the disease appears to remain limited to the external
ocular muscles and never spreads to those of the bulb or limbs.

It is a notable feature of myasthenia gravis that the tendon reflexes almost
always remain brisk, even in the presence of severe weakness.

DIAGNOSIS

The diagnosis of myasthenia depends first upon the characteristic clinical
picture and secondly upon the fatigability which may be demonstrated electrically by means of repetitive supramaximal stimulation of a nerve such as the
ulnar, with simultaneous recording of the evoked muscle potential from the
hypothenar muscles. These and other electrophysiological tests of neuromuscular transmission [FIGS. 147 and 148] are reviewed by Johns et al. (1955),
Slomić et al. (1968), Desmedt and Borenstein (1970), and Brown (1974).
Ocular tonometry (Campbell et al., 1970; Wray and Pavan-Langston, 1971)
or nystagmography (Spector et al., 1975) carried out before and after the
injection of edrophonium are of particular value in the diagnosis of ocular
myasthenia.

However, the single most useful diagnostic test is assessment of the clinical
response to an injection of neostigmine or edrophonium hydrochloride. The
quick-acting edrophonium hydrochloride (Tensilon), which is given initially
in a dosage of 2 mg, followed immediately by a further 8 mg intravenously if
there is no severe reaction, has now supplanted neostigmine for diagnostic
purposes (Osserman and Kaplan, 1953). Provocative tests designed to increase

myasthenia, utilizing such drugs as curare and quinine, may be dangerous and are rarely required. However, methods involving the regional perfusion with curare of certain muscle groups are much safer and are valuable in some doubtful cases (Brown and Charlton, 1975; Brown *et al.*, 1975; Horowitz *et al.*, 1975). Churchill-Davidson and Richardson (1952) showed that myasthenic patients are abnormally resistant to the action of depolarizing neuromuscular blocking drugs such as decamethonium and that tolerance is particularly marked in clinically unaffected muscles. However, depolarization block, if it occurs at all, is brief and soon changes to a longer competitive (curare-like) type of block. This dual response in the child or adult is characteristic of

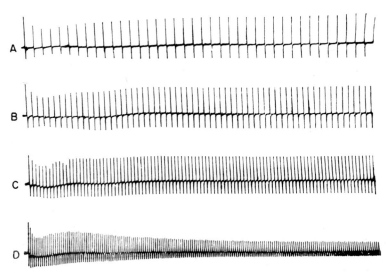

FIG. 147. Neuromuscular transmission in myasthenia gravis. The muscle action potentials recorded from the hypothenar muscles during supramaximal stimulation of the ulnar nerve at different frequencies. A, stimulus frequency 5 Hz; B, 10 Hz; C, 25 Hz; D, 50 Hz. The response to the initial stimulus measures 6·2 mV. (Illustration kindly provided by Dr. R. J. Johns, reproduced with permission from *Bull. Johns Hopk. Hosp.*, **99**, 129, 1956.)

myasthenia gravis, though the response obtained in normal neonates is similar (Churchill-Davidson and Wise, 1963). This particular provocative test is rarely necessary for diagnosis.

An important point in clinical management is to remember the frequency with which myasthenia gravis may be associated with either benign or malignant thymoma (Goldman *et al.*, 1975) so that tomography of the anterior mediastinum is an essential investigation in all cases. Radiographs of the chest should also be done to exclude bronchial carcinoma, but the myasthenic syndrome which may complicate malignant disease (see below) shows clinical and electro-physiological features which are in many respects different from those of myasthenia gravis. Tests designed to exclude associated thyrotoxicosis or other auto-immune disorders (Hausmanowa-Petrusewicz *et al.*, 1969), including rheumatoid arthritis (Aarli *et al.*, 1975) may also be indicated.

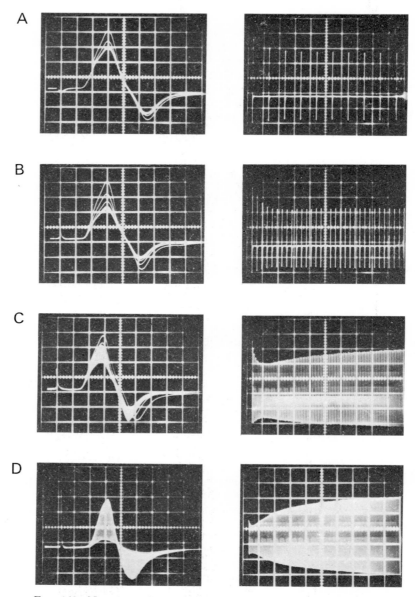

Fig. 148. Neuromuscular transmission in the Eaton–Lambert syndrome. Recording of motor unit action potentials from one hypothenar eminence during supramaximal stimulation of the ulnar nerve. A, stimulus frequency 1 Hz; B, 3 Hz; C, 10 Hz; D, 30 Hz. At each frequency the left panel represents superimposed responses, with each horizontal division representing 2 ms; on the right are sequential responses, each horizontal division representing 1 s. On the vertical scale each division in A, B, and C represents 1 mV, in D 5 mV. (Illustration kindly provided by Dr. J. C. Brown.)

AETIOLOGY

Simpson (1960) drew attention to the interrelationship between myasthenia gravis and a number of other diseases, including thyroid disorders, diabetes, rheumatoid arthritis, systemic lupus, and sarcoidosis. He suggested that myasthenia was probably an auto-immune disorder and that the thymus might produce an antibody against muscle end-plate protein. Strauss et al. (1960) demonstrated a muscle-binding globulin in myasthenic serum and Marshall and White (1961) showed that direct injection of bacterial antigen into the guinea-pig thymus produced a histological reaction similar to that of myasthenia. Goldstein and Hofmann (1968) claimed to have produced a syndrome resembling myasthenia in animals by the injection of thymus extract producing an auto-immune thymitis, but Vetters et al. (1969) failed to confirm these findings. Desmedt (1957, 1966) suggested that the lesion is presynaptic as the disorder of function is closely simulated by the administration of hemicholinium which impairs acetylcholine synthesis, while Dahlbäck et al. (1961) demonstrated in their studies of isolated intercostal muscles removed from myasthenic and control patients, that there appeared to be a disturbance of transmitter formation or release. There are now many reports of the finding of circulating antibodies to muscle (Namba and Grob, 1966; Namba et al., 1967; Oosterhuis et al., 1968) and to neuronal extracts (Kornguth et al., 1970; Martin et al., 1974), of lymphocyte transformation in response to muscle antigens (Kott et al., 1973), and to acetylcholine receptor (Abramsky et al., 1975) in patients with myasthenia. The role of T lymphocytes has been studied extensively (Armstrong et al., 1973); experimental myasthenia has been induced in monkeys by purified acetylcholine receptor (Tarrab-Hazdai et al., 1975) and humoral antibodies to this receptor have been found in the serum of patients with myasthenia (Aharonov et al., 1975). These and many other observations suggest that some kind of auto-immune response may prevent the proper release or formation of acetylcholine at the motor end-plate or that there is some abnormality of the acetylcholine receptor site. Despite all these advances and many more, the exact role of auto-immune mechanisms is still unclear (Lisak, 1975). The presence of morphological abnormalities in terminal nerve endings in myasthenic muscle (Coërs and Desmedt, 1959; Bickerstaff and Woolf, 1960) is as yet unexplained; abnormalities of the fine structure and geometry of the motor end-plates (Simpson, 1971; Santa et al., 1972 a) and evidence of neurogenic muscular atrophy (Brownell et al., 1972; Oosterhuis and Bethlem, 1973) have also been reported. The suggestion that neonatal myasthenia must be due to a circulating toxin, possibly released from the thymus (Wilson et al., 1953) receives some support from the finding of a factor in serum from patients with myasthenia which modifies the rosette-forming cells present in the spleen of adult thymectomized mice (Bach et al., 1972). Thus it appears that both cellular immunity, mediated by T lymphocytes of thymic origin, and humoral factors play a part in pathogenesis.

TREATMENT

The standard treatment for myasthenia gravis is still neostigmine or the closely related drug pyridostigmine (*Mestinon*). The usual dosage of neostigmine is to begin by giving a 15 mg tablet three or four times a day, and almost always it is necessary to give in addition atropine, 0·6 mg twice daily, to overcome the muscarinic side-effects of the drug. Recent evidence suggests that the long-acting *Mestinon*, which has been used by many workers in the past in combination with neostigmine which has seemed to act more quickly, is probably preferable as the standard medication and the initial dosage is 60 mg three or four times daily, again with atropine or propantheline. The dosage is then steadily increased until maximum benefit is obtained. Some patients find that it is best to take the tablets every two hours, while some require them three-hourly. Other drugs which have been utilized in recent years include ambenonium hydrochloride (*Mytelase*) of which the usual dosage is 10–25 mg three or four times daily and aldosterone inhibitors but these remedies seem to have no advantage over the traditional medication and adjuvants commonly employed including potassium chloride and ephedrine (see Simpson, 1974) add little of value.

Occasional cases of myasthenia with failure to respond to cholinergic drugs have been described (Black *et al.*, 1973) and long-term treatment has even been thought to be a possible factor in causing irreversible myopathy (Fenichel *et al.*, 1972) and changes in the motor end-plates (Engel *et al.*, 1973). There has also been increasing interest in the use of ACTH and prednisone. At first, 10-day courses of 100–160 units of ACTH daily were advised (Namba *et al.*, 1971 *c*) and were sometimes found to produce temporary worsening of the condition with progressive improvement after completion of the course of treatment. Maintenance treatment with ACTH has also been advised (Cape and Utterback, 1972). More recently similar short intensive courses of prednisolone have been recommended (Brunner *et al.*, 1972) but much evidence is now emerging to suggest that long-term alternate-day treatment with 100 mg of prednisone is equally or more effective (Warmolts and Engel, 1972; Pinelli *et al.*, 1974). Immunosuppressive drugs (Mertens *et al.*, 1969) and thoracic duct drainage (Bergström *et al.*, 1975) have also been tried. Not all patients respond to steroids but alternate-day prednisone with pyridostigmine is probably now the initial treatment of choice in patients without thymoma.

The differential diagnosis between myasthenic and cholinergic crises, in which rapidly increasing muscular weakness occurs and in which serious respiratory weakness may threaten life, can be a matter of considerable difficulty. The most useful single test is to give an intravenous injection of edrophonium. If this increases muscle power, then it is likely that the weakness is myasthenic and requires more treatment, while if it reduces muscle power it is likely that the weakness is cholinergic and that treatment must be reduced. Any hint of impending respiratory insufficiency may be an indication for withdrawal of all drugs and for assisted respiration with positive pressure apparatus and tracheostomy. Unfortunately some patients show a differential sensitivity of different muscles to various drugs. It is not unknown to find that a dose of pyridostigmine which improves power in the limb muscles may be sufficient to cause cholinergic paralysis of the diaphragm.

The place of thymectomy is still in some doubt. Simpson (1958, 1974) has reviewed the problem in detail and has pointed out that thymectomy benefits both sexes but that the extent of improvement is greatest in women, who would otherwise have a worse prognosis than men. Benefit following the operation may occur at any time, but the results are best in young women with a short history suffering from severe myasthenia. They are also good in juvenile myasthenia (Hansson *et al.*, 1972). Perlo *et al.* (1971) found remission or improvement after operation in 76 per cent of a series of 267 patients and it is now apparent that those patients without germinal centres in the thymus respond best and more rapidly, and operation carried out early rather than late also produces better results (*British Medical Journal*, 1975). However, it would appear that any patient who is deteriorating despite optimum medication has nothing to lose in the hands of an experienced surgeon and may improve. The prognosis for life seems to be worse if a thymoma is present and radiotherapy is generally recommended to the thymus in these cases before operation. Even after thymectomy, two out of three patients with a thymoma die within five years, but the survivors may benefit to the same extent as those without a tumour. As some thymomas are malignant, death is sometimes due to metastases, but even a non-neoplastic thymus may regrow after operation (Joseph and Johns, 1973).

THE MYASTHENIC-MYOPATHIC SYNDROME (THE EATON-LAMBERT SYNDROME)

This syndrome is generally associated with oat-cell carcinoma of the bronchus, though it has been occasionally described in patients with carcinoma in other sites and has been reported rarely to present with the clinical picture of a sub-acute proximal myopathy in young patients without malignant disease (Brown and Johns, 1974) [and see p. 872]. The clinical picture is usually one of subacute muscular fatigability with weakness and wasting affecting the proximal parts of the limbs and trunk, but occasionally the external ocular and bulbar muscles are involved (Rooke *et al.*, 1960; Oh, 1974). The weakness is often myasthenic in the sense that the patient complains of increased enfeeblement after exertion, but it has been observed in many such cases that muscle power may in fact increase after brief exercise, a reversed myasthenic effect. In contrast to true myasthenia gravis, the condition is only slightly improved by treatment with neostigmine or pyridostigmine, though there may be definite improvement in strength after an injection of edrophonium hydrochloride. However, the tendon reflexes in this condition, unlike those in true myasthenia, are almost always depressed or absent. In contrast to the findings in true myasthenia gravis, repetitive stimulation of motor nerves at tetanic rates may cause an increase in the amplitude of the evoked potentials in the hypothenar muscles and these patients are excessively sensitive to decamethonium. The ultrastructural appearances of the motor end-plates in this condition are different from those seen in myasthenia gravis (Santa *et al.*, 1972 *b*). Occasional cases with electro-physiological features of both myasthenia gravis and the myasthenic syndrome occur (Schwartz and Stalberg, 1975) but in general the findings are distinctive and tests of neuromuscular transmission [FIG. 148] are mandatory whenever this condition is suspected. Not only is the progressive potentiation in muscular strength which follows an initial period of fatigue after exercise a distinguishing feature of this condition, but it has been shown (McQuillen and Johns, 1966) that the muscular weakness and fatigability may be greatly improved by the administration of guanidine, which has no convincing effect in true myasthenia gravis. Guanidine hydrochloride is given orally in a dose of 20–50 mg/kg body weight (Lambert, 1966; Oh and Kim, 1973).

REFERENCES

AARLI, J. A., MILDE, E.-J., and THUNOLD, S. (1975) Arthritis in myasthenia gravis, *J. Neurol. Neurosurg. Psychiat.*, **38**, 1048.

ABRAMSKY, O., AHARONOV, A., TEITELBAUM, D., and FUCHS, S. (1975) Myasthenia gravis and acetylcholine receptor, *Arch. Neurol. (Chic.)*, **32**, 684.

AHARONOV, A., ABRAMSKY, O., TARRAB-HAZDAI, R., and FUCHS, S. (1975) Humoral antibodies to acetylcholine receptor in patients with myasthenia gravis, *Lancet*, **ii**, 340.

ARMSTRONG, R. M., NOWAK, R. M., and FALK, R. E. (1973) Thymic lymphocyte function in myasthenia gravis, *Neurology (Minneap.)*, **23**, 1078.

BACH, J.-F., DARDENNE, M., PAPIERNIK, M., BAROIS, A., LEVASSEUR, P., and LE BRIGAND, H. (1972) Evidence for a serum-factor secreted by the human thymus, *Lancet*, **ii**, 1056.

BERGSTRÖM, K., FRANKSSON, C., MATELL, G., NILSSON, B. Y., PERSSON, A., VON REIS, G., and STENSMAN, R. (1975) Drainage of thoracic duct lymph in twelve patients with myasthenia gravis, *Europ. Neurol.*, **13**, 19.

BICKERSTAFF, E. R., and WOOLF, A. L. (1960) The intramuscular nerve endings in myasthenia gravis, *Brain*, **83**, 10.

BLACK, J. T., BRAIT, K. A., DEJESUS, P. V., HARNER, R. N., and ROWLAND, L. P. (1973) Myasthenia gravis lacking response to cholinergic drugs, *Neurology (Minneap.)*, **23**, 851.

BRITISH MEDICAL JOURNAL (1975) Early thymectomy for myasthenia gravis, *Brit. med. J.*, **3**, 262.

BROWN, J. C. (1974) Repetitive stimulation and neuromuscular transmission studies, in *Disorders of Voluntary Muscle*, ed. Walton, J. N., 3rd ed., Edinburgh and London.

BROWN, J. C., and CHARLTON, J. E. (1975) Study of sensitivity to curare in myasthenic disorders using a regional technique, *J. Neurol. Neurosurg. Psychiat.*, **38**, 27.

BROWN, J. C., CHARLTON, J. E., and WHITE, D. J. K. (1975) A regional technique for the study of sensitivity to curare in human muscle, *J. Neurol. Neurosurg. Psychiat.*, **38**, 18.

BROWN, J. C., and JOHNS, R. J. (1974) Diagnostic difficulties encountered in the myasthenic syndrome sometimes associated with carcinoma, *J. Neurol. Neurosurg. Psychiat.*, **37**, 1214.

BROWNELL, B., OPPENHEIMER, D. R., and SPALDING, J. M. K. (1972) Neurogenic muscle atrophy in myasthenia gravis, *J. Neurol. Neurosurg. Psychiat.*, **35**, 311.

BRUMLIK, J., and JACOBS, R. S. (1974) Myasthenia gravis associated with diphenyl-hydantoin therapy for epilepsy, *Canad. J. neurol. Sci.*, **1**, 127.

BRUNNER, N. G., NAMBA, T., and GROB, D. (1972) Corticosteroids in management of severe, generalized myasthenia gravis, *Neurology (Minneap.)*, **22**, 603.

BUCKNALL, R. C., DIXON, A. ST. J., GLICK, E. N., WOODLAND, J., and ZUTSHI, D. W. (1975) Myasthenia gravis associated with penicillamine treatment for rheumatoid arthritis, *Brit. med. J.*, **1**, 600.

BUNDEY, S. (1972) A genetic study of infantile and juvenile myasthenia gravis, *J. Neurol. Neurosurg. Psychiat.*, **35**, 41.

CAMPBELL, M. J., SIMPSON, E., CROMBIE, A. L., and WALTON, J. N. (1970) Ocular myasthenia: evaluation of Tensilon tonography and electronystagmography as diagnostic tests, *J. Neurol. Neurosurg. Psychiat.*, **33**, 639.

CAPE, C. A., and UTTERBACK, R. A. (1972) Maintenance adrenocorticotropic hormone (ACTH) treatment in myasthenia gravis, *Neurology (Minneap.)*, **22**, 1160.

CHURCHILL-DAVIDSON, H. C., and RICHARDSON, A. T. (1952) The action of decamethonium iodide (C.10) in myasthenia gravis, *J. Neurol. Neurosurg. Psychiat.*, **15**, 129.

CHURCHILL-DAVIDSON, H. C., and WISE, R. P. (1963) Neuromuscular transmission in the newborn infant, *Anaesthesiology*, **24**, 271.

COËRS, C., and DESMEDT, J. E. (1959) Mise en évidence d'une malformation caractéristique de la jonction neuromusculaire dans la myasthénie, *Acta neurol. belg.*, **59**, 539.

DAHLBACK, O., ELMQVIST, D., JOHNS, T. R., RADNER, S., and THESLEFF, S. (1961) An electrophysiologic study of the neuromuscular junction in myasthenia gravis, *J. Physiol. (Lond.)*, **156**, 336.

DECKER, D. A., and FINCHAM, R. W. (1971) Respiratory arrest in myasthenia gravis with colistimethate therapy, *Arch. Neurol. (Chic.)*, **25**, 141.

DESMEDT, J. E. (1957) Bases physiopathologiques du diagnostic de la myasthénie par le test de Jolly, *Rev. neurol.*, **96**, 505.

DESMEDT, J. E. (1966) Presynaptic mechanisms in myasthenia gravis, *Ann. N.Y. Acad. Sci.*, **135**, 209.

DESMEDT, J. E., and BORENSTEIN, S. (1970) The testing of neuromuscular transmission, in *Handbook of Clinical Neurology*, ed. Vinken, P. J., and Bruyn, G. W., vol. 7, p. 104, Amsterdam.

ENGEL, A. G., LAMBERT, E. H., and SANTA, T. (1973) Study of long-term anticholinesterase therapy: effects on neuromuscular transmission and on motor end-plate fine structure, *Neurology (Minneap.)*, **23**, 1273.

ERB, W. H. (1879) Ueber einen eigenthumlichen bulbaren (?) Symptomcomplex, *Arch. Psychiat. Nervenkr.*, **60**, 172.

FELTKAMP, T. E. W., VAN DEN BERG-LOONEN, P. M., NIJENHUIS, L. E., ENGELFRIET, C. P., VAN ROSSUM, A. L., VAN LOGHEM, J. J., and OOSTERHUIS, H. J. G. H. (1974) Myasthenia gravis, autoantibodies, and HL-A antigens, *Brit. med. J.*, **1**, 131.

FENICHEL, G. M., KIBLER, W. B., OLSON, W. H., and DETTBARN, W.-D. (1972) Chronic inhibition of cholinesterase as a cause of myopathy, *Neurology (Minneap.)*, **22**, 1026.

FERGUSON, F. R., HUTCHINSON, E. C., and LIVERSEDGE, L. A. (1955) Myasthenia gravis. Results of medical management, *Lancet*, **ii**, 636.

FRASER, D. C., PALMER, A. C., SENIOR, J. E. B., PARKES, J. D., and YEALLAND, M. F. T. (1970) Myasthenia gravis in the dog, *J. Neurol. Neurosurg. Psychiat.*, **33**, 431.

FRITZE, D., HERRMANN, C., NAEIM, F., SMITH, G. S., and WALFORD, R. L. (1974) HL-A antigens in myasthenia gravis, *Lancet*, **i**, 240.

GOLDMAN, A. J., HERRMANN, C., KEESEY, J. C., MULDER, D. G., and BROWN, W. J. (1975) Myasthenia gravis and invasive thymoma: a 20-year experience, *Neurology (Minneap.)*, **25**, 1021.

GOLDSTEIN, G., and HOFMANN, W. W. (1968) Electrophysiological changes similar to those of myasthenia gravis in rats with experimental autoimmune thymitis, *J. Neurol. Neurosurg. Psychiat.*, **31**, 453.

GROB, D. (1953) Course and management of myasthenia gravis, *J. Amer. med. Ass.*, **153**, 529.

HANSSON, O., JOHANSSON, L., STALBERG, E., and WESTERHOLM, C.-J. (1972) Thymectomy in juvenile myasthenia gravis, *Neuropädiatrie*, **3**, 429.

HAUSMANOWA-PETRUSEWICZ, I., CHORZELSKI, T., and STRUGALSKA, H. (1969) Three-year observation of a myasthenic syndrome concurrent with other autoimmune syndromes in a patient with thymoma, *J. neurol. Sci.*, **9**, 273.

HOKKANEN, E., and TOIVAKKA, E. (1969) Streptomycin-induced neuromuscular fatigue in myasthenia gravis, *Ann. Clin. Res.*, **1**, 220.

HOROWITZ, S. H., GENKINS, G., KORNFELD, P., and PAPATESTAS, A. E. (1975) Regional curare test in evaluation of ocular myasthenia, *Arch. Neurol. (Chic.)*, **32**, 84.

JACOB, A., CLACK, E. R., and EMERY, A. E. H. (1968) Genetic study of sample of 70 patients with myasthenia gravis, *J. med. Genet.*, **5**, 257.

JOHNS, R. J., GROB, D., and HARVEY, A. McG. (1955) Electromyographic changes in myasthenia gravis, *Amer. J. Med.*, **19**, 679.

JOLLY, F. (1895) Ueber Myasthenia Gravis Pseudoparalytica, *Klin. Wschr.*, **32**, 1.

JOSEPH, B. S., and JOHNS, T. R. (1973) Recurrence of nonneoplastic thymus after thymectomy for myasthenia gravis, *Neurology (Minneap.)*, **23**, 109.

KORNGUTH, S. E., HANSON, J. C., and CHUN, R. W. M. (1970) Antineuronal antibodies in patients having myasthenia gravis, *Neurology (Minneap.)*, **20**, 749.

KOTT, E., GENKINS, G., and RULE, A. H. (1973) Leukocyte response to muscle antigens in myasthenia gravis, *Neurology (Minneap.)*, **23**, 374.

LAMBERT, E. H. (1966) Defects of neuromuscular transmission in syndromes other than myasthenia gravis, *Ann. N.Y. Acad. Sci.*, **135**, 367.

LISAK, R. P. (1975) Immunologic aspects of myasthenia gravis, *Ann. Clin. Lab. Sci.*, **5**, 288.

McQUILLEN, M. P., CANTOR, H. E., and O'ROURKE, J. R. (1968) Myasthenic syndrome associated with antibiotics, *Arch. Neurol. (Chic.)*, **18**, 402.

McQUILLEN, M. P., and JOHNS, R. J. (1966) The nature of the defect in the Eaton–Lambert syndrome, *Neurology (Minneap.)*, **17**, 527.

MARSHALL, A. H. E., and WHITE, R. G. (1961) Experimental thymic lesions resembling those of myasthenia gravis, *Lancet*, **i**, 1030.

MARTIN, L., HERR, J. C., WANAMAKER, W., and KORNGUTH, S. (1974) Demonstration of specific antineuronal nuclear antibodies in serà of patients with myasthenia gravis, *Neurology (Minneap.)*, **24**, 680.

MERTENS, H. G., BALZEREIT, F., and LEIPERT, M. (1969) The treatment of severe myasthenia gravis with immunosuppressive agents, *Europ. Neurol.*, **2**, 321.

NAMBA, T., BROWN, S. B., and GROB, D. (1970) Neonatal myasthenia gravis: report of two cases and review of the literature, *Pediatrics*, **45**, 488.

NAMBA, T., SHAPIRO, M. S., BRUNNER, N. G., and GROB, D. (1971 *a*) Myasthenia gravis occurring in twins, *J. Neurol. Neurosurg. Psychiat.*, **34**, 531.

NAMBA, T., BRUNNER, N. G., BROWN, S. B., MUGURUMA, M., and GROB, D. (1971 *b*) Familial myasthenia gravis: report of 27 patients in 12 families and review of 164 patients in 73 families, *Arch. Neurol. (Chic.)*, **25**, 49.

NAMBA, T., BRUNNER, N. G., SHAPIRO, M. S., and GROB, D. (1971 *c*) Corticotropin therapy in myasthenia gravis: effects, indications, and limitations, *Neurology (Minneap.)*, **21**, 1008.

NAMBA, T., and GROB, D. (1966) Autoantibodies and myasthenia gravis, with special reference to muscle ribonucleoprotein, *Ann. N.Y. Acad. Sci.*, **135**, 606.

NAMBA, T., and GROB, D. (1971) Myasthenia gravis and hyperthyroidism occurring in two sisters, *Neurology (Minneap.)*, **21**, 377.

NAMBA, T., HIMEI, H., and GROB, D. (1967) Complement fixing and tissue binding serum globulins in patients with myasthenia gravis, and their relation to muscle ribonucleoprotein, *J. Lab. Clin. Med.*, **70**, 258.

OH, S. J. (1974) The Eaton–Lambert syndrome in ocular myasthenia gravis, *Arch. Neurol. (Chic.)*, **31**, 183.

OH, S. J., and KIM, K. W. (1973) Guanidine hydrochloride in the Eaton–Lambert syndrome, *Neurology (Minneap.)*, **23**, 1084.

OOSTERHUIS, H. J. G. H., and BETHLEM, J. (1973) Neurogenic muscle involvement in myasthenia gravis, *J. Neurol. Neurosurg. Psychiat.*, **36**, 244.

OOSTERHUIS, H. J. G. H., BETHLEM, J., and FELTKAMP, T. E. W. (1968) Muscle pathology, thymoma, and immunological abnormalities in patients with myasthenia gravis, *J. Neurol. Neurosurg. Psychiat.*, **31**, 460.

OSSERMAN, K. E. (1958) *Myasthenia Gravis*, New York.

OSSERMAN, K. E., and KAPLAN, L. I. (1953) Studies in myasthenia gravis. Use of edrophonium chloride (Tensilon) in differentiating myasthenic from cholinergic weakness, *Arch. Neurol. Psychiat. (Chic.)*, **70**, 385.

PERLO, V. P., ARNASON, B., POSKANZER, D., CASTLEMAN, B., SCHWAB, R. S., OSSERMAN, K. E., PAPATESTIS, A., ALPERT, L., and KARK, A. (1971) The role of thymectomy in the treatment of myasthenia gravis, *Ann. N.Y. Acad. Sci.*, **183**, 308.

PINELLI, P., TONALI, P., and SCOPPETTA, C. (1974) Long-term treatment of myasthenia gravis with alternate-day prednisone, *Europ. Neurol.*, **12**, 129.

ROOKE, E. D., EATON, L. M., LAMBERT, E. H., and HODGSON, C. H. (1960) Myasthenia and malignant intrathoracic tumor, *Med. Clin. N. Amer.*, **44**, 977.

ROWLAND, L. P., LISAK, R. P., SCHOTLAND, D. L., DEJESUS, P. V., and BERG, P. (1973) Myasthenic myopathy and thymoma, *Neurology (Minneap.)*, **23**, 282.

SANTA, T., ENGEL, A. G., and LAMBERT, E. H. (1972 *a*) Histometric study of neuromuscular junction ultrastructure. I. Myasthenia gravis, *Neurology (Minneap.)*, **22**, 71.

SANTA, T., ENGEL, A. G., and LAMBERT, E. H. (1972 *b*) Histometric study of neuromuscular junction ultrastructure. II. Myasthenic syndrome, *Neurology (Minneap.)*, **22**, 370.

SCHLEZINGER, N. S., and CORIN, M. S. (1968) Myasthenia gravis associated with hyperthyroidism in childhood, *Neurology (Minneap.)*, **18**, 1217.

SCHWARTZ, M. S., and STALBERG, E. (1975) Myasthenia gravis with features of the myasthenic syndrome, *Neurology (Minneap.)*, **25**, 80.

SIMPSON, J. A. (1958) An evaluation of thymectomy in myasthenia gravis, *Brain*, **81**, 112.

SIMPSON, J. A. (1960) Myasthenia gravis: a new hypothesis, *Scot. med. J.*, **5**, 419.

SIMPSON, J. A. (1971) A morphological explanation of the transmission defect in myasthenia gravis, *Ann. N.Y. Acad. Sci.*, **183**, 241.

SIMPSON, J. A. (1974) Myasthenia gravis and myasthenic syndromes, in *Disorders of Voluntary Muscle*, ed. Walton, J. N., 3rd ed., Edinburgh and London.

SLOMIĆ, A., ROSENFALCK, A., and BUCHTHAL, F. (1968) Electrical and mechanical responses of normal and myasthenic muscle, with particular reference to the staircase phenomenon, *Brain Research*, **10**, 1.

SPECTOR, R. H., DAROFF, R. B., and BIRKETT, J. E. (1975) Edrophonium infrared optokinetic nystagmography in the diagnosis of myasthenia gravis, *Neurology (Minneap.)*, **25**, 317.

STRAUSS, A. J. L., SEEGAL, B. C., HSU, K. C., BURKHOLDER, P. M., NASTUK, W. L., and OSSERMAN, K. E. (1960) Immunofluorescence demonstration of a muscle binding, complement-fixing serum globulin fraction in myasthenia gravis, *Proc. Soc. exp. Biol. (N.Y.)*, **105**, 184.

SZOBOR, A. (1970) *Crises in Myasthenia Gravis*, Budapest.

TARRAB-HAZDAI, R., AHARONOV, A., SILMAN, I., and FUCHS, S. (1975) Experimental autoimmune myasthenia induced in monkeys by purified acetylcholine receptor, *Nature (Lond.)*, **256**, 128.

VETTERS, J. M., SIMPSON, J. A., and FOLKARDE, A. (1969) Experimental myasthenia gravis, *Lancet*, **ii**, 28.

WALKER, M. B. (1934) Treatment of myasthenia gravis with physostigmine, *Lancet*, **i**, 1200.

WARMOLTS, J. R., and ENGEL, W. K. (1972) Benefit from alternate-day prednisone in myasthenia gravis, *New Engl. J. Med.*, **286**, 17.

WILKS, S. (1877) Bulbar paralysis; fatal; no disease found, *Guy's Hosp. Rep.*, **37**, 54.

WILSON, A., OBRIST, A. R., and WILSON, H. (1953) Some effects of extracts of thymus glands removed from patients with myasthenia gravis, *Lancet*, **ii**, 368.

WISE, G. A., and McQUILLEN, M. P. (1970) Transient neonatal myasthenia, *Arch. Neurol. (Chic.)*, **22**, 556.

WRAY, S. H., and PAVAN-LANGSTON, D. (1971) A reevaluation of edrophonium chloride (Tensilon) tonography in the diagnosis of myasthenia gravis, *Neurology (Minneap.)*, **21**, 586.

ENDOCRINE AND METABOLIC MYOPATHIES

ENDOCRINE MYOPATHIES

DISORDERS OF THE THYROID GLAND

Thyrotoxic Myopathy

Chronic thyrotoxic myopathy was first described by Bathurst in 1895 and it is well recognized that in severe cases of thyrotoxicosis weakness and wasting of proximal limb muscles, particularly in the upper extremities, may occur and may resolve when the thyroid disease is effectively treated. Ramsay (1965) described clinical and electromyographic studies carried out on 54 consecutive unselected patients with proven thyrotoxicosis and demonstrated that while few complained of muscular weakness, clinical examination showed demonstrable weakness in over 80 per cent and the electromyogram showed a reduced mean action potential duration and a higher percentage of polyphasic potentials in more than 90 per cent of cases. Four months after treatment of the thyrotoxicosis the EMG had returned to normal in most patients. Similar findings were reported by Satoyoshi *et al.* (1963) who also found that weakness sometimes improved when oral potassium was given. These findings suggest that in thyrotoxicosis there is almost always a reversible abnormality of muscle function and that electromyography, using an objective technique, is probably the most sensitive indicator of this change.

Exophthalmic Ophthalmoplegia (Ophthalmic Graves' Disease)

Exophthalmic ophthalmoplegia, endocrine exophthalmos, or as it is now more often called, ophthalmic Graves' disease, must be mentioned as the principal effect of this disorder is upon the external ocular muscles, which are greatly increased in bulk, as are the orbital contents as a whole. The subject is reviewed in detail by Brain (1959), by Hales and Rundle (1960), and by Hall *et al.* (1970). The main symptoms are exophthalmos and diplopia and the degree of ophthalmoplegia is usually proportional to the severity of the exophthalmos. Sometimes the latter is so great [FIG. 149] that the eyelids cannot be closed and corneal ulceration ensues. Papilloedema may occur and, if not relieved, may

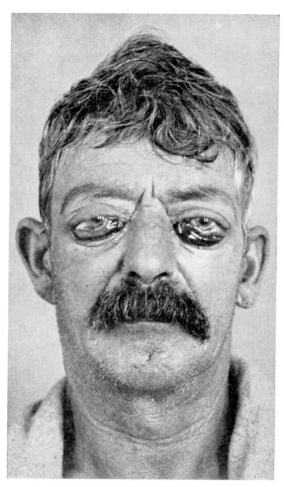

FIG. 149. Severe endocrine exophthalmos (ophthalmic Graves' disease)

progress to optic atrophy and blindness. In severe cases surgical decompression of the orbit is required and sometimes must be carried out as an emergency (MacCarty *et al.*, 1970). Some patients are mildly thyrotoxic, others first develop the syndrome after treatment of thyrotoxicosis, and the condition may occur in association with myxoedema but most individuals are euthyroid and have a high titre of thyroglobulin antibodies. An exophthalmos-producing substance distinct from the long-acting thyroid stimulator is believed to be responsible (Hall *et al.*, 1970). Hormonal treatment is usually disappointing; radiotherapy to the orbit is sometimes helpful but high dosage steroid treatment is usually the most successful method of reducing exophthalmos quickly. In milder cases not requiring either steroids or surgery, little can be done and the results of treatment of associated thyrotoxicosis with iodine-131 are unpredictable (Jones *et al.*, 1969), but the condition is often self-limiting, improving spontaneously in many cases after some years or ultimately becoming stabilized. Guanethidine eye-drops are useful in reducing lid retraction in some cases (Martin and Jay, 1969).

In differential diagnosis the orbital pseudotumour syndrome, often due to orbital myositis responsive to prednisone and presumed to be due to a connective tissue disorder involving orbital muscles (Jellinek, 1969) must be considered as must proptosis, often asymmetrical, due to mucocele of the ethmoid sinus and other orbital lesions [p. 169].

Thyrotoxicosis and Myasthenia Gravis

About 5 per cent of myasthenic patients have, or later develop, thyrotoxicosis (McArdle, 1974). Engel (1961) noted that myasthenia may become worse when hyperthyroidism increases. Both conditions must be treated in the usual manner, but it should be noted that the risks of thyroidectomy are greatly increased in patients suffering from myasthenia gravis.

Thyrotoxic Periodic Paralysis

An association between thyrotoxicosis and periodic paralysis has been observed, particularly among the Chinese and Japanese, and may be dominantly inherited (McFadzean and Yeung, 1969). Okinaka and his colleagues (1957), in a study of 6,333 cases of hyperthyroidism, found that 8·9 per cent of the males and 0·4 per cent of the females had had attacks of periodic paralysis which were of hypokalaemic type. Adequate treatment of the hyperthyroidism results in the disappearance of the periodic attacks of weakness or in a marked decrease in their number and severity (Norris *et al.*, 1968; Brody and Dudley, 1969).

Myopathy in Hypothyroidism

Muscular hypertrophy with weakness and slowness of muscular contraction and relaxation has been described in children suffering from sporadic cretinism (Debré and Semelaigne, 1935; Spiro *et al.*, 1970). When a similar condition occurs in adults it is known as Hoffman's syndrome (Hoffman, 1896) and Wilson and Walton (1959) described cases in which the clinical evidence of hypothyroidism was relatively unobtrusive and the muscular symptoms predominated. This syndrome may superficially resemble myotonia and has then been called pseudomyotonia (Crispell and Parson, 1954) but it has also been shown that sometimes hypothyroidism may be superimposed upon a pre-existing and virtually symptomless myotonia congenita (Jarcho and Tyler, 1958). Astrom *et al.* (1961) suggested that myxoedema may occasionally be associated with a girdle myopathy causing mild proximal weakness and wasting similar to that seen in chronic thyrotoxic myopathy. In their cases improvement was observed on treatment with thyroxin. Salick *et al.* (1968) also reported a case of myxoedematous myopathy and Takamori *et al.* (1972) described abnormalities of neuromuscular transmission resembling those of the Eaton–Lambert syndrome in two cases of hypothyroidism.

DISORDERS OF THE PITUITARY AND ADRENAL GLANDS

In acromegaly and pituitary gigantism, generalized muscular weakness may be observed but is rarely an outstanding feature (Adams *et al.*, 1962). Similarly, widespread weakness with some atrophy has been described in hypopituitarism (Walton, 1960), but the exact nature of the myopathic change in such cases is unclear (Shy, 1960). However, the clinical, electromyographic, and histological features of the myopathy of acromegaly have now been elucidated (Mastaglia *et al.*, 1970; Pickett *et al.*, 1975). General weakness is also seen in some cases of Addison's disease and is probably the result of the changes in plasma and muscle water and electrolytes. Treatment of the condition leads to a rapid improvement in muscular strength and no permanent muscle changes have been described in this disorder, though Witts *et al.* (1938) and Thorn (1949) noted contractures at the elbows and knees occurring in occasional cases of Addison's disease and suggested that these were due to changes of unknown nature occurring in the fasciae and tendons.

Cushing's Syndrome and Steroid Myopathy

In 1959 Müller and Kugelberg (1959) described six patients with Cushing's syndrome of whom five had weakness of the muscles of the pelvic girdle and thighs. Electromyography demonstrated myopathic changes in the affected muscles, and in the same year Perkoff *et al.* (1959) reported cases of muscle weakness and wasting occurring in patients under treatment with steroids. Since then both the naturally-occurring myopathy and the iatrogenic disorder have been frequently reported (Shy, 1960), and it seems that the latter is most often caused by steroids such as triamcinolone which have a fluorine atom in the 9α position (Harman, 1959; Williams, 1959). A similar syndrome has been described in patients receiving dexamethasone and betamethasone (Golding *et al.*, 1961); usually in such cases weakness resolves when prednisone is substituted, though occasional cases have been reported (Perkoff *et al.*, 1959) in which the latter drug was responsible. Coomes (1965) examined electromyographically 50 patients receiving corticosteroid drugs and compared his findings with those obtained in a series of control individuals. He found that the mean action potential duration of motor action potentials obtained from one deltoid muscle was markedly reduced in patients showing striking side-effects of steroid therapy. He concluded that corticosteroid myopathy is commonest in those patients who show most side-effects of the treatment and that measurement of the mean action potential duration in the EMG recorded from an appropriate muscle appears to be a reliable method of detecting early myopathic change. Current evidence suggests that the myopathy quickly resolves once the steroid treatment is withdrawn and Pleasure *et al.* (1970) also describe resolution of the myopathy of Cushing's disease after effective treatment. Muscle biopsy typically demonstrates atrophy of Type II muscle fibres in both the naturally occurring and iatrogenic disorders and the potassium content of the muscle is reduced.

ACTH Myopathy

Prineas *et al.* (1968) reported proximal muscle weakness and wasting developing in a series of pigmented patients who had undergone adrenalectomy for the treatment of Cushing's disease. Investigation demonstrated that these patients were suffering from a myopathy and muscle biopsy sections showed a striking accumulation of fat within individual muscle fibres. It was concluded that this myopathy was the result of excessive circulating ACTH.

METABOLIC MYOPATHIES

Myopathy in Metabolic Bone Disease

Prineas *et al.* (1965) described two patients with chronic muscular weakness, one of whom had a parathyroid adenoma and the other was found to be suffering from osteomalacia and idiopathic steatorrhoea. The main clinical features were proximal muscular wasting and weakness, pain and discomfort on movement, with hypotonia and brisk tendon reflexes. They suggested that in these cases a disturbance of vitamin D metabolism could interfere with the excitation-contraction coupling involving the entry of calcium into the muscle fibre during contraction. Similar cases have been described by Smith and Stern (1967). Myopathy in osteomalacia due to anticonvulsant medication has also been described (Marsden *et al.*, 1973) and muscular weakness was also the presenting feature of three cases of hypophosphataemic osteomalacia (Schott and Wills, 1975).

Myopathy in Chronic Renal Failure

Floyd *et al.* (1974) reported 11 cases of proximal myopathy occurring in patients with end-stage renal failure, in four of whom osteomalacia was discovered and in these there was some improvement in muscular weakness with vitamin D. In the other seven, weakness improved dramatically after renal transplantation or dialysis.

Glycogen Storage Disease of Muscle

In 1951 McArdle described the case of a man of 30 who had generalized muscular pain and stiffness which increased during slight exertion. He showed that the blood lactate and pyruvate levels failed to rise after exercise and suggested that the disorder was due to a defect of glucose utilization. In 1959 two additional cases were reported (Schmid and Mahler, 1959; Mommaerts *et al.*, 1959) and one of these also showed myoglobinuria. In both cases the muscle glycogen content was increased and myophosphorylase activity was absent. Mellick *et al.* (1962) described another case of myophosphorylase deficiency in which there was permanent muscular weakness in the girdle muscles, and Schmid and Hammaker (1961) described three cases in a single family in which the pattern of inheritance suggested an autosomal recessive mechanism; Adamson *et al.* (1967) described three cases of variable severity in a single family. Engel *et al.* (1963) described two patients, one of whom had severe muscular weakness and wasting without cramps developing in late life, while a second, also in middle age, developed cramps after exercise without weakness and wasting and both patients showed a partial defect of muscle phosphorylase activity with a normal total glycogen content in the muscle. While oral fructose may improve exercise tolerance in some patients, no form of treatment is consistently successful in relieving the symptoms of this relatively benign but disabling disorder which is best diagnosed by carrying out estimations of lactate in venous blood before and after ischaemic exercise and in which physiological contracture of muscles and myoglobinuria often follow exertion (McArdle, 1974).

It has become increasingly apparent in recent years that other forms of muscle glycogenosis, though rare, are more common than was at one time realized. In a child of 4 with a diffuse myopathy, Thomson *et al.* (1963) demonstrated a defect of phosphoglucomutase, and more recently Tarui *et al.* (1965), Layzer *et al.* (1967), Bonilla and Schotland (1970), and Tobin *et al.* (1973) have also described a myopathic disorder closely resembling McArdle's disease which is due to phosphofructokinase deficiency. It has been well recognized that the condition now called limit dextrinosis (Illingworth *et al.*, 1956) gives glycogen storage in liver, skeletal muscle, and in heart and is due to a deficiency of debranching enzyme (amylo-1,6-glucosidase). This condition, however, like Pompe's disease which gives rise to glycogen storage in the heart, skeletal muscles, and central nervous system and which is due to amylo-1,4-glucosidase (acid maltase) deficiency, is usually incompatible with survival beyond the first few years of life. Antenatal diagnosis of Pompe's disease by amniocentesis is now possible (Galjaard *et al.*, 1973). However, it has become apparent quite recently that acid maltase deficiency may be much less grave in its prognosis and several cases are now on record in which the patients presented with an apparently progressive myopathy of girdle muscles in late childhood or in adult life (Zellweger *et al.*, 1965; Courtecuisse *et al.*, 1965; Hudgson *et al.*, 1968; Engel, 1970). Thus the possible diagnosis of glycogen storage disease of muscle must now be considered in all cases of suspected limb-girdle muscular dystrophy arising in middle life, and muscle biopsy may be diagnostic as striking vacuolation of muscle fibres is usually thereby revealed and the vacuoles contain large quantities of glycogen. It seems more than probable that in the years to come, many more specific myopathic disorders related to individual enzyme defects may well be defined. Unfortunately none of these conditions yet appears to be amenable to any form of effective treatment, although attempts to treat Pompe's disease with purified acid maltase isolated from human placenta are now being made.

It should also be mentioned that myopathy resulting from severe and prolonged hypoglycaemia has been described in patients suffering from islet cell adenoma of the pancreas (Mulder *et al.*, 1956).

PERIODIC PARALYSIS SYNDROMES

Hypokalaemic Periodic Paralysis

The classical hypokalaemic variety of periodic paralysis has been well recognized for many years and has been reviewed by McArdle (1974). This condition gives rise to attacks of flaccid weakness of the voluntary muscles but those of speech, swallowing, and respiration are usually spared. Attacks most often begin in the second decade and are most frequent in early adult life. Commonly they last for several hours and often start early in the morning on waking, after a period of rest following exertion, or after a heavy carbohydrate meal. During attacks the plasma potassium level is usually found to be low (less than 3 mEq/l); there is positive balance of potassium and some or all of the retained potassium seems to pass into the muscle cell (Grob *et al.*, 1957; Zierler and Andres, 1957). Shy *et al.* (1961) showed that the resting membrane potential is normal during an attack of paralysis, and these authors and Pearce (1964) demonstrated that electron microscopy of muscle biopsy specimens taken during an attack shows vacuoles resulting from dilatation of the sarcoplasmic reticulum. Conn and Streeten (1960) suggested that this form of periodic paralysis might be due to intermittent aldosteronism, as it is well recognized that patients with primary aldosteronism due to tumours of the adrenal (Conn, 1955) do have attacks of muscular weakness. However, aldosteronism can be distinguished from periodic paralysis by the associated hypertension, alkalosis, and hypernatraemia and by the persistence of the hypokalaemia between the attacks; furthermore, in familial periodic paralysis increased aldosterone excretion is not usually found. A similar syndrome has been described in Papua and New Guinea due to dietary potassium/sodium imbalance (Duggin and Price, 1974).

Exercise or peripheral nerve stimulation have been found to abort or postpone attacks of weakness (Campa and Sanders, 1974). Administration of potassium chloride, 4–6 g daily, has been used in treating attacks of the hypokalaemic type but rarely seems to shorten the episodes of weakness. Spironolactone, 25 mg four times daily, and other aldosterone antagonists have been found, however, to reduce greatly their frequency and severity (Poskanzer and Kerr, 1961 a). More recently acetazolamide 250 mg four times daily has been found to be an even more effective prophylactic treatment (Resnick et al., 1968), as the metabolic acidosis induced by this drug appears to lower the rate of entry of potassium into the muscle cell (Vroom et al., 1975). Occasionally in these cases muscular weakness is curiously localized to one or more muscle groups and sometimes after frequent episodes of weakness permanent atrophy of muscles develops (Dyken et al., 1969), but on the whole the patients tend to improve spontaneously as they grow older.

Hyperkalaemic Periodic Paralysis (Adynamia Episodica Hereditaria)

In 1951 Tyler et al. described a group of cases in which the serum potassium level did not fall during the attacks and the patients were made worse by potassium chloride. Helweg-Larsen et al. (1955) described a similar condition and Gamstorp (1956) described two families containing such cases and entitled the condition adynamia episodica hereditaria (hyperkalaemic periodic paralysis is probably a more satisfactory title (Klein et al., 1960)). This condition is closely related to paramyotonia (Lundberg et al., 1974) for some of the patients show definite myotonia (Drager et al., 1958; Van der Meulen et al., 1961) though in others the myotonia seems curiously limited to the muscles around the eye and can be evoked by placing ice-bags on the eyelids, a manœuvre which tends to give a remarkable degree of lid-lag. Van't Hoff (1962) has referred to such cases as examples of myotonic periodic paralysis. In affected individuals the attacks are usually much shorter in duration than in the hypokalaemic variety, lasting on an average 30–40 minutes, and they may be precipitated immediately by exercise. Cardiac arrhythmia is an occasional complication (Lisak et al., 1972) and some patients develop muscular wasting (Saunders et al., 1968) with histological evidence of myopathy with tubular aggregates on electron microscopy (Macdonald et al., 1968). Commonly there is a rise in the serum potassium level, though some patients have severe weakness when the level is no higher than 4 mEq/l, whereas in normal people a level of 8 mEq/l is needed as a rule before weakness develops. Abbott et al. (1962) and McComas et al. (1968) showed that the muscle fibre membrane potential is lowered during the attacks in such cases. The attacks may be cut short by the intravenous administration of calcium gluconate or by the inhalation of salbutamol (Wang and Clausen, 1976), while acetazolamide, 250 mg two or three times daily, hydrochlorothiazide, 25 mg two or three times daily, and dichlorphenamide have all been used successfully for prophylaxis (McArdle, 1974; Hoskins *et al.*, 1975).

Sodium-responsive Normokalaemic Periodic Paralysis

The third type of periodic paralysis, entitled provisionally the so-called sodium-responsive normokalaemic variety (Poskanzer and Kerr, 1961 b) is probably a variant of the hyperkalaemic type, except for the fact that in these cases the attacks have been seen occasionally to last for days or weeks and have often developed at night. Nevertheless in these patients paralysis is always increased by the administration of potassium and improved by large doses of sodium chloride. It is in cases of this type that Shy *et al.* (1966) described the appearance of increased numbers of mitochondria in muscle biopsy sections examined with the electron microscope and referred to this change as pleoconial myopathy. Meyers *et al.* (1972) found frequent tubular aggregates in muscle sections, attributed to proliferation of the sarcoplasmic reticulum. Poskanzer and Kerr (1961 b) found that acetazolamide combined with 9-alpha-fluoro-hydrocortisone, 0·1 mg daily, prevented the attacks.

Clearly, therefore, careful investigation of every case of periodic paralysis is necessary in order to establish the nature of the patient's illness. Attempts to demonstrate a primary enzyme defect or a specific disorder of carbohydrate metabolism in such cases have been unsuccessful, but empirical treatment, both given prophylactically or in order to cut short the attacks, has proved to be successful once the character of the patient's attacks has been carefully defined.

MYOGLOBINURIA

Myoglobin may appear in the urine as a result of acute crush injury of muscle (Bywaters and Stead, 1945) and in localized ischaemic muscular necrosis, while, as already mentioned, it can occur in certain acute forms of polymyositis. It has also been described in poisoning as a result of eating quails (Ouzounellis, 1968, 1970) and as an occasional consequence of other toxins and drugs (Rowland *et al.*, 1964).

A specific syndrome of paroxysmal myoglobinuria of unknown aetiology has also been described and is also called idiopathic rhabdomyolysis (Savage *et al.*, 1971); this is characterized by acute attacks of severe cramp-like muscle pain and tenderness associated with weakness or paralysis which are accompanied, within a few hours, by myoglobinuria. The condition usually clears up within two to three days with rest, but occasional cases show such severe and widespread muscle damage that death ensues. Korein *et al.* (1959) distinguished two types, of which Type I occurs predominantly in males in late adolescence or early adult life; the pain and myoglobinuria follow exercise, which must be curtailed as the recurrent attacks may eventually cause permanent weakness and wasting. Some such cases may be due to carnitine palmityl transferase deficiency (Cumming *et al.*, 1976). In cases of Type II, which are seen particularly in childhood, an acute infection often precedes the muscle pain and myoglobinuria; the attacks are severe, with fever and leucocytosis, but tend to occur at progressively longer intervals and usually clear up with the passage of time. Widespread muscle fibre necrosis and regeneration are seen in muscle biopsy sections (Schutta *et al.*, 1969).

MALIGNANT HYPERPYREXIA

This rare condition gives a rapid rise in body temperature during surgical anaesthesia and has often proved fatal. It may be precipitated by many anaesthetic agents, and although it is commonest in patients anaesthetized with halothane and/or suxamethonium, no anaesthetic agent has been shown to be absolutely safe (Harriman et al., 1973). The hyperpyrexia is accompanied by extreme muscular rigidity, tachycardia, tachypnoea, cyanosis, and respiratory and metabolic acidosis (King et al., 1972). The susceptibility is often dominantly inherited (King et al., 1972; Bradley et al., 1973 a) and in many affected patients and families evidence of overt or subclinical myopathy is found (Steers et al., 1970) and sometimes features superficially resembling myotonia congenita. A similar condition has been described in Landrace and Pietrain pigs (Hall et al., 1972; Lister, 1973). There is evidence of abnormality of the muscle fibre membrane and sarcoplasmic reticulum in such cases (Harriman et al., 1973; Denborough et al., 1974) and intravenous procaine may be of some value in prophylaxis (Moulds and Denborough, 1972). While the resting activity of creatine kinase in the serum is raised in some susceptible individuals, this alone is insufficient as a predictive screening test, and muscle biopsy under local anaesthesia followed by in vitro study of the halothane-induced contracture may be needed to identify the individuals liable to develop the typical reaction to anaesthesia (Ellis et al., 1972, 1975; Isaacs et al., 1975).

MYOPATHY DUE TO VARIOUS TOXINS AND DRUGS

Widespread muscle necrosis leading to renal tubular necrosis is a rare complication of carbon monoxide poisoning (Loughridge et al., 1958). Severe myalgia and muscular stiffness can occur in patients receiving clofibrate (Smith et al., 1970). Among other drugs known to cause myopathy are chloroquine (Hughes et al., 1971), emetine (Duane and Engel, 1970), and polymyxin E (Vanhaeverbeek et al., 1974). Severe muscle fibrosis with contractures (myosclerosis) may be rarely seen in spinal muscular atrophy or polymyositis (Bradley et al., 1973 b) but has also been described as a consequence of the repeated intramuscular injection of meperidine (Aberfeld et al., 1968), pethidine (Mastaglia et al., 1971), and pentazocine (Steiner et al., 1973).

ALCOHOLIC MYOPATHY

Acute and widespread muscle necrosis with local pain, tenderness, and oedema, sometimes leading to renal damage and oliguria, is now well known to occur in some chronic alcoholic patients following a debauch (Hed et al., 1962). In some patients with an acute alcoholic myopathy associated with muscle cramps, impairment of myophosphorylase activity with results of an ischaemic lactate test similar to those observed in McArdle's disease have been described, and myoglobinuria may occur (Perkoff et al., 1967). In addition, however, a subacute, progressive, proximal myopathy has been reported in alcoholic individuals (Hed et al., 1962; Klinkerfuss et al., 1967), and while undoubtedly some cases so diagnosed have proved to be suffering from alcoholic neuropathy involving motor axons predominantly (Faris and Reyes, 1971), the existence of a subacute or chronic myopathy due to alcohol is now well established (Pittman and Decker, 1971; McArdle, 1974) and may be associated with hypokalaemia (Martin et al., 1971). Gradual recovery usually follows the withdrawal of alcohol. Cardiomyopathy is also well recognized (British Medical Journal, 1972).

XANTHINURIA

Symptomatic myopathy in a patient with inherited xanthine oxidase deficiency giving rise to xanthinuria was reported by Chalmers *et al.* (1969 *a* and *b*) and by Parker *et al.* (1969) and crystals of xanthine were demonstrated in skeletal muscle by electron microscopy. Similar crystals without clinical evidence of muscle disease may be found in patients with gout treated with allopurinol (Watts *et al.*, 1971).

LIPID STORAGE MYOPATHY

In 1970 Engel *et al.* described twin 18-year-old sisters who experienced muscle cramps and occasional episodes of myoglobinuria and in whom a defect in the utilization of long-chain fatty acids was demonstrated. Bradley *et al.* (1969) described a patient with a subacute proximal myopathy associated with the massive deposition of fat in Type I muscle fibres, and Engel and Siekert (1972) reported a similar case in which improvement followed prednisone treatment. It is now known that this condition is due to an inherited deficiency of carnitine (Engel and Angelini, 1973; Karpati *et al.*, 1975; Vandyke *et al.*, 1975) and that in such cases vacuolation of leukocytes may be found (Markesbery *et al.*, 1974). Marked improvement may follow treatment with carnitine (Karpati *et al.*, 1975; Agelini, 1975). A similar syndrome but more often presenting with muscle cramps provoked by exercise and myoglobinuria may result from carnitine palmityl transferase deficiency (Cumming *et al.*, 1976).

HYPERMETABOLIC MYOPATHY

Ernster *et al.* (1959) and Luft *et al.* (1962) described a woman who was not thyrotoxic but in whom there was severe hypermetabolism with a very large increase in basal metabolic rate. Her muscle mitochondria showed morphological abnormalities and loose coupling of oxidative phosphorylation. Several similar cases have subsequently been reported; the relationship of this condition to the other 'mitochondrial myopathies' is uncertain [see p. 1045].

REFERENCES

ABBOTT, B. C., CREUTZFELDT, O., FOWLER, B., and PEARSON, C. M. (1962) Membrane potentials in human muscles, *Fed. Proc.*, **21**, 318.

ABERFELD, D. C., BIENENSTOCK, H., SHAPIRO, M. S., NAMBA, T., and GROB, D. (1968) Diffuse myopathy related to meperidine addiction in a mother and daughter, *Arch. Neurol. (Chic.)*, **19**, 384.

ADAMS, R. D., DENNY-BROWN, D., and PEARSON, C. M. (1962) *Diseases of Muscle: A Study in Pathology*, 2nd ed., New York.

ADAMSON, D. C., SALTER, R. H., and PEARCE, G. W. (1967) McArdle's syndrome (myophosphorylase deficiency), *Quart. J. Med.*, **36**, 565.

ANGELINI, C. (1975) Carnitine deficiency, *Lancet*, **ii**, 554.

ASTROM, K. E., KUGELBERG, E., and MÜLLER, R. (1961) Hypothyroid myopathy, *Arch. Neurol. (Chic.)*, **5**, 472.

BATHURST, L. W. (1895) A case of Graves' disease associated with idiopathic muscular atrophy, *Lancet*, **ii**, 529.

BONILLA, E., and SCHOTLAND, D. L. (1970) Histochemical diagnosis of muscle phosphofructokinase deficiency, *Arch. Neurol. (Chic.)*, **22**, 8.

BRADLEY, W. G., HUDGSON, P., GARDNER-MEDWIN, D., and WALTON, J. N. (1969) Myopathy associated with abnormal lipid metabolism in skeletal muscle, *Lancet*, **i**, 495.

BRADLEY, W. G., HUDGSON, P., GARDNER-MEDWIN, D., and WALTON, J. N. (1973 b) The syndrome of myosclerosis, *J. Neurol. Neurosurg. Psychiat.*, **36**, 651.

BRADLEY, W. G., WARD, M., MURCHISON, D., HALL, L., and WOOLF, N. (1973 a) Clinical, electrophysiological and pathological studies on malignant hyperpyrexia, *Proc. roy. Soc. Med.*, **66**, 67.

BRAIN, W. R. (1959) Pathogenesis and treatment of endocrine exophthalmos, *Lancet*, **i**, 109.

BRITISH MEDICAL JOURNAL (1972) Alcoholic cardiomyopathy, *Brit. med. J.*, **2**, 247.

BRODY, I. A., and DUDLEY, A. W. (1969) Thyrotoxic hypokalemic periodic paralysis, *Arch. Neurol. (Chic.)*, **21**, 1.

BYWATERS, E. G. L., and STEAD, J. K. (1945) Thrombosis of the femoral artery with myoglobinuria and low serum potassium concentration, *Clin. Sci.*, **5**, 195.

CAMPA, J. F., and SANDERS, D. B. (1974) Familial hypokalemic periodic paralysis, *Arch. Neurol. (Chic.)*, **31**, 110.

CHALMERS, R. A., JOHNSON, M., PALLIS, C., and WATTS, R. W. E. (1969 a) Xanthinuria with myopathy, *Quart. J. Med.*, **38**, 493.

CHALMERS, R. A., WATTS, R. W. E., BITENSKY, L., and CHAYEN, J. (1969 b) Microscopic studies on crystals in skeletal muscle from two cases of xanthinuria, *J. Path.*, **99**, 45.

CONN, J. W. (1955) Primary aldosteronism, a new clinical syndrome, *J. lab. clin. Med.*, **45**, 661.

CONN, J. W., and STREETEN, D. H. P. (1960) in *The Metabolic Basis of Inherited Disease*, ed. Stanbury, J. B., Wyngaarden, J. B., and Fredrickson, D. S., New York.

COOMES, E. N. (1965) Corticosteroid myopathy, *Ann. rheum. Dis.*, **24**, 465.

COURTECUISSE, V., ROYER, P., HABIB, R., MONNIER, C., and DEMOS, J. (1965) Glycogenose musculaire par déficit d'alpha-1,4-glucosidase simulant une dystrophie musculaire progressive, *Arch. franç. Pédiat.*, **22**, 1153.

CRISPELL, K. R., and PARSON, W. (1954) Occurrence of myotonia in 2 patients following thyroidectomy for hyperthyroidism, *Trans. Amer. Goiter Ass.*, 399.

CUMMING, W. J. K., HARDY, M., HUDGSON, P., and WALLS, J. (1976) Carnitine-palmityl-transferase deficiency, *J. neurol. Sci.*. **30**, 247.

DEBRÉ, R., and SEMELAIGNE, G. (1935) Syndrome of diffuse muscular hypertrophy in infants causing athletic appearance: its connection with congenital myxedema, *Amer. J. Dis. Child.*, **50**, 1351.

DENBOROUGH, M. A., WARNE, G. L., MOULDS, R. F. W., TSE, P., and MARTIN, F. I. R. (1974) Insulin secretion in malignant hyperpyrexia, *Brit. med. J.*, **3**, 493.

DRAGER, G. A., HAMILL, J. F., and SHY, G. M. (1958) Paramyotonia congenita, *Arch. Neurol. Psychiat. (Chic.)*, **80**, 1.

DUANE, D. D., and ENGEL, A. G. (1970) Emetine myopathy, *Neurology (Minneap.)*, **20**, 733.

DUGGIN, G. G., and PRICE, M. A. (1974) Hypokalaemic muscular paresis in migratory Papua/New Guineans, *Lancet*, **i**, 649.

DYKEN, M., ZEMAN, W., and RUSCHE, T. (1969) Hypokalemic periodic paralysis, *Neurology (Minneap)*, **19**, 691.

ELLIS, F. R., CLARKE, I. M. C., MODGILL, M., CURRIE, S., and HARRIMAN, D. G. F. (1975) Evaluation of creatine phosphokinase in screening patients for malignant hyperpyrexia, *Brit. med. J.*, **3**, 511.

ELLIS, F. R., KEANEY, N. P., HARRIMAN, D. G. F., SUMNER, D. W., KYEI-MENSAH, K., TYRRELL, J. H., HARGREAVES, J. B., PARIKH, R. K., and MULROONEY, P. L. (1972) Screening for malignant hyperpyrexia, *Brit. med. J.*, **3**, 559.

ENGEL, A. G. (1961) Thyroid function and myasthenia gravis, *Arch. Neurol. (Chic.)*, **4**, 663.

ENGEL, A. G. (1970) Acid maltase deficiency in adults: studies in four cases of a syndrome which may mimic muscular dystrophy or other myopathies, *Brain*, **93**, 599.

ENGEL, A. G., and ANGELINI, C. (1973) Carnitine deficiency of human skeletal muscle with associated lipid storage myopathy: a new syndrome, *Science*, **173**, 899.

ENGEL, A. G., and SIEKERT, R. G. (1972) Lipid storage myopathy responsive to prednisone, *Arch. Neurol. (Chic.)*, **27**, 174.

ENGEL, W. K., EYERMAN, E. L., and WILLIAMS, H. E. (1963) Late onset type of skeletal muscle phosphorylase deficiency. A new familial variety with completely and partially affected subjects, *New Engl. J. Med.*, **268**, 135.

ENGEL, W. K., VICK, N. A., GLUECK, C. J., and LEVY, R. I. (1970) A skeletal-muscle disorder associated with intermittent symptoms and a possible defect of lipid metabolism, *New Engl. J. Med.*, **282**, 697.

ERNSTER, L., IKKOS, D., and LUFT, R. (1959) Enzymic activities of human skeletal muscle mitochondria: a tool in clinical metabolic research, *Nature (Lond.)*, **184**, 1851.

FARIS, A. A., and REYES, M. G. (1971) Reappraisal of alcoholic myopathy, *J. Neurol. Neurosurg. Psychiat.*, **34**, 86.

FLOYD, M., AYYAR, D. R., BARWICK, D. D., HUDGSON, P., and WEIGHTMAN, D. (1974) Myopathy in chronic renal failure, *Quart. J. Med.*, **43**, 509.

GALJAARD, H., MEKES, M., DE JOSSELIN DE JONG, J. E., and NIERMEIJER, M. F. (1973) A method for rapid prenatal diagnosis of glycogenosis II (Pompe's disease), *Clin. Chim. Acta*, **49**, 361.

GAMSTORP, I. (1956) Adynamia episodica hereditaria, *Acta paediat. (Uppsala)*, (Suppl.), **108**, 1.

GOLDING, D. N., MURRAY, S., PEARCE, G. W., and THOMPSON, M. (1961) Corticosteroid myopathy, *Ann. phys. Med.*, **6**, 171.

GROB, D., LILJESTRAND, A., and JOHNS, R. J. (1957) Potassium movement in patients with familial periodic paralysis, *Amer. J. Med.*, **23**, 356.

HALES, I. B., and RUNDLE, F. F. (1960) Ocular changes in Graves' disease, *Quart. J. Med.*, **29**, 113.

HALL, L. W., TRIM, C. M., and WOOLF, N. (1972) Further studies of porcine malignant hyperthermia, *Brit. med. J.*, **2**, 145.

HALL, R., DONIACH, D., KIRKHAM, K., and EL KABIR, D. (1970) Ophthalmic Graves' disease, *Lancet*, **i**, 375.

HARMAN, J. B. (1959) Muscular wasting and corticosteroid therapy, *Lancet*, **i**, 887.

HARRIMAN, D. G. F., SUMNER, D. W., and ELLIS, F. R. (1973) Malignant hyperpyrexia myopathy, *Quart. J. Med.*, **42**, 639.

HED, R., LUNDMARK, C., FAHLGREN, H., and ORELL, S. (1962) Acute muscular syndrome in chronic alcoholism, *Acta med. scand.*, **171**, 585.

HELWEG-LARSEN, H. F., HAUGE, M., and SAGILD, U. (1955) Hereditary transient muscular paralysis in Denmark: genetic aspects of family periodic paralysis and family periodic adynamia, *Acta genet. (Basel)*, **5**, 263.

HOFFMAN, J. (1896) Ein Fall von Thomsen'scher Krankheit, compliciert durch Neuritis multiplex, *Dtsch Z. Nervelheilk.*, **9**, 272.

HOSKINS, B., VROOM, F. Q., and JARRELL, M. A. (1975) Hyperkalemic periodic paralysis, *Arch. Neurol. (Chic.)*, **33**, 519.

HUDGSON, P., GARDNER-MEDWIN, D., WORSFOLD, M., PENNINGTON, R. J. T., and WALTON, J. N. (1968) Adult myopathy in glycogen storage disease due to acid maltase deficiency, *Brain*, **91**, 435.

HUGHES, J. T., ESIRI, M., OXBURY, J. M., and WHITTY, C. W. M. (1971) Chloroquine myopathy, *Quart. J. Med.*, **40**, 85.

ILLINGWORTH, B., CORI, G. T., and CORI, C. F. (1956) Amylo-1,6-glucosidase in muscle tissue in generalized glycogen storage disease, *J. biol. Chem.*, **218**, 123.

ISAACS, H., HEFFRON, J. J. A., and BADENHORST, M. (1975) Predictive tests for malignant hyperpyrexia, *Brit. J. Anaesth.*, **47**, 1075.

JARCHO, L. W., and TYLER, F. H. (1958) Myxoedema, pseudomyotonia and myotonia congenita, *Arch. intern. Med.*, **102**, 357.

JELLINEK, E. H. (1969) The orbital pseudotumour syndrome and its differentiation from endocrine exophthalmos, *Brain*, **92**, 35.

JONES, D. I. R., MUNRO, D. S., and WILSON, G. M. (1969) Observations on the course of exophthalmos after ^{131}I therapy, *Proc. roy. Soc. Med.*, **62**, 15.

KARPATI, G., CARPENTER, S., ENGEL, A. G., WATTERS, G., ALLEN, J., ROTHMAN, S., KLASSEN, G., and MAMER, O. A. (1975) The syndrome of systemic carnitine deficiency, *Neurology (Minneap.)*, **25**, 16.

KING, J. O., DENBOROUGH, M. A., and ZAPF, P. W. (1972) Inheritance of malignant hyperpyrexia, *Lancet*, **i**, 365.

KLEIN, R., EGAN, T., and USHER, P. (1960) Changes in sodium, potassium and water in hyperkalaemic periodic paralysis, *Metabolism*, **9**, 1005.

KLINKERFUSS, G., BLEISCH, V., DIOSO, M. M., and PERKOFF, G. T. (1967) A spectrum of myopathy associated with alcoholism. II. Light and electron microscopic observations, *Ann. intern. Med.*, **67**, 493.

KOREIN, J., CODDON, D. R., and MOWREY, F. H. (1959) The clinical syndrome of paroxysmal paralytic myoglobinuria, *Neurology (Minneap.)*, **9**, 767.

LAYZER, R. B., ROWLAND, L. P., and RANNEY, H. M. (1967) Muscle phosphofructokinase deficiency, *Arch. Neurol. (Chic.)*, **17**, 512.

LISAK, R. P., LEBEAU, J., TUCKER, S. H., and ROWLAND, L. P. (1972) Hyperkalemic periodic paralysis and cardiac arrhythmia, *Neurology (Minneap.)*, **22**, 810.

LISTER, D. (1973) Correction of adverse response to suxamethonium of susceptible pigs, *Brit. med. J.*, **1**, 208.

LOUGHRIDGE, L. W., LEADER, L. P., and BOWEN, D. A. L. (1958) Acute renal failure due to muscle necrosis in carbon-monoxide poisoning, *Lancet*, **ii**, 349.

LUFT, R., IKKOS, D., PALMIERI, G., ERNSTER, L., and AFZELIUS, B. (1962) A case of severe hypermetabolism of nonthyroid origin with a defect in the maintenance of mitochondrial respiratory control: a correlated clinical, biochemical and morphological study, *J. clin. Invest.*, **41**, 1776.

LUNDBERG, P. O., STALBERG, E., and THIELE, B. (1974) Paralysis periodica paramyotonica: a clinical and neurophysiological study, *J. neurol. Sci.*, **21**, 309.

MCARDLE, B. (1951) Myopathy due to a defect in muscle glycogen breakdown, *Clin. Sci.*, **10**, 13.

MCARDLE, B. (1974) Metabolic and endocrine myopathies, in *Disorders of Voluntary Muscle*, ed. Walton, J. N., 3rd ed., Edinburgh and London.

MACCARTY, C. S., KENEFICK, T. P., MCCONAHEY, W. M., and KEARNS, T. P. (1970) Ophthalmopathy of Graves' disease treated by removal of roof, lateral walls and lateral sphenoid ridge: review of 46 cases, *Mayo Clin. Proc.*, **45**, 488.

MCCOMAS, A. J., MROZEK, K., and BRADLEY, W. G. (1968) The nature of the electrophysiological disorder in adynamia episodica, *J. Neurol. Neurosurg. Psychiat.*, **31**, 448.

MACDONALD, R. D., REWCASTLE, N. B., and HUMPHREY, J. G. (1968) The myopathy of hyperkalemic periodic paralysis, *Arch. Neurol. (Chic.)*, **19**, 274.

MCFADZEAN, A. J. S., and YEUNG, R. (1969) Familial occurrence of thyrotoxic periodic paralysis, *Brit. med. J.*, **1**, 760.

MARKESBERY, W. R., MCQUILLEN, M. P., PROCOPIS, P. G., HARRISON, A. R., and ENGEL, A. G. (1974) Muscle carnitine deficiency, *Arch. Neurol. (Chic.)*, **31**, 320.

MARSDEN, C. D., REYNOLDS, E. H., PARSONS, V., HARRIS, R., and DUCHEN, L. (1973) Myopathy associated with anticonvulsant osteomalacia, *Brit. med. J.*, **4**, 526.

MARTIN, B., and JAY, B. (1969) Use of guanethidine eye drops in dysthyroid lid retraction, *Proc. roy. Soc. Med.*, **62**, 18.

MARTIN, J. B., CRAIG, J. W., ECKEL, R. E., and MUNGER, J. (1971) Hypokalemic myopathy in chronic alcoholism, *Neurology (Minneap.)*, **21**, 1160.

MASTAGLIA, F. L., BARWICK, D. D., and HALL, R. (1970) Myopathy in acromegaly, *Lancet*, **ii**, 907.

MASTAGLIA, F. L., GARDNER-MEDWIN, D., and HUDGSON, P. (1971) Muscle fibrosis and contractures in a pethidine addict, *Brit. med. J.*, **4**, 532.

MELLICK, R. S., MAHLER, R. F., and HUGHES, B. P. (1962) McArdle's syndrome: phosphorylase-deficient myopathy, *Lancet*, **i**, 1045.

MEYERS, K. R., GILDEN, D. H., RINALDI, C. F., and HANSEN, J. L. (1972) Periodic muscle weakness, normokalemia and tubular aggregates, *Neurology (Minneap.)*, **22**, 269.

MOMMAERTS, W. F. H. M., ILLINGWORTH, B., PEARSON, C. M., GUILLORY, R. J., and SERAYDARIAN, K. (1959) A functional disorder of muscle associated with the absence of phosphorylase, *Proc. nat. Acad. Sci. (Wash.)*, **46**, 791.

MOULDS, R. F. W., and DENBOROUGH, M. A. (1972) Procaine in malignant hyperpyrexia, *Brit. med. J.*, **4**, 526.

MULDER, D. W., BASTRON, J. A., and LAMBERT, E. H. (1956) Hyperinsulin neuronopathy, *Neurology (Minneap.)*, **6**, 627.

MÜLLER, R., and KUGELBERG, E. (1959) Myopathy in Cushing's syndrome, *J. Neurol. Neurosurg. Psychiat.*, **22**, 314.

NORRIS, F. H., PANNER, B. J., and STORMONT, B. M. (1968) Thyrotoxic periodic paralysis, *Arch. Neurol. (Chic.)*, **19**, 88.

OKINAKA, S., SHIZUME, K., IINO, S., WATANABE, A., IRIE, M., NOGUCHI, A., KUMA, S., KUMA, K., and ITO, T. (1957) The association of periodic paralysis and hyperthyroidism in Japan, *J. clin. Endocr.*, **17**, 1454.

OUZOUNELLIS, T. I. (1968) Myoglobinuries par ingestion de cailles, *Presse Méd.*, **76**, 1863.

OUZOUNELLIS, T. I. (1970) Some notes on quail poisoning, *J. Amer. med. Ass.*, **211**, 1186.

PARKER, R., SNEDDEN, W., and WATTS, R. W. E. (1969) The mass-spectrometric identification of hypoxanthine and xanthine ('oxypurines') in skeletal muscle from two patients with congenital xanthine oxidase deficiency (xanthinuria), *Biochem. J.*, **115**, 103.

PEARCE, G. W. (1964) Tissue culture and electron microscopy, in *Disorders of Voluntary Muscle*, ed. Walton, J. N., 1st ed., London.

PERKOFF, G. T., DIOSO, M. M., BLEISCH, V., and KLINKERFUSS, G. (1967) A spectrum of myopathy associated with alcoholism, I. Clinical and laboratory findings, *Ann. intern. Med.*, **67**, 481.

PERKOFF, G. T., SILBER, R., TYLER, F. H., CARTWRIGHT, G. E., and WINTROBE, M. M. (1959) Studies in disorders of muscle. XII. Myopathy due to the administration of therapeutic amounts of 17-hydroxycortico-steroids, *Amer. J. Med.*, **26**, 891.

PICKETT, J. B. E., LAYZER, R. B., LEVIN, S. R., SCHNEIDER, V., CAMPBELL, M. J., and SUMNER, A. J. (1975) Neuromuscular complications of acromegaly, *Neurology (Minneap.)*, **25**, 638.

PITTMAN, J. G., and DECKER, J. W. (1971) Acute and chronic myopathy associated with alcoholism, *Neurology (Minneap.)*, **21**, 293.

PLEASURE, D. E., WALSH, G. O., and ENGEL, W. K. (1970) Atrophy of skeletal muscle in patients with Cushing's syndrome, *Arch. Neurol. (Chic.)*, **22**, 118.

POSKANZER, D. C., and KERR, D. N. S. (1961 a) Periodic paralysis with response to spironolactone, *Lancet*, **ii**, 511.

POSKANZER, D. C., and KERR, D. N. S. (1961 b) A third type of periodic paralysis with normokalaemia and favourable response to sodium chloride, *Amer. J. Med.*, **31**, 328.

PRINEAS, J. W., HALL, R., BARWICK, D. D., and WATSON, A. J. (1968) Myopathy associated with pigmentation following adrenalectomy for Cushing's syndrome, *Quart. J. Med.*, **37**, 63.

PRINEAS, J. W., MASON, A. S., and HENSON, R. A. (1965) Myopathy in metabolic bone disease, *Brit. med. J.*, **1**, 1034.

RAMSAY, I. D. (1965) Electromyography in thyrotoxicosis, *Quart. J. Med.*, **34**, 255.

RESNICK, J. S., ENGEL, W. K., GRIGGS, R. C., and STAM, A. C. (1968) Acetazolamide prophylaxis in hypokalemic periodic paralysis, *New Engl. J. Med.*, **278**, 582.

ROWLAND, L. P., FAHN, S., HIRSCHBERG, E., and HARTER, D. H. (1964) Myoglobinuria, *Arch. Neurol. (Chic.)*, **10**, 537.

SALICK, A. I., COLACHIS, S. C., and PEARSON, C. M. (1968) Myxedema myopathy: clinical, electrodiagnostic, and pathologic findings in advanced cases, *Arch. phys. Med.*, **49**, 230.

SATOYOSHI, E., MURAKAMI, K., KOWA, H., KINOSHITA, M., NOGUCHI, K., HOSHINA, S., NISHIYAMA, Y., and ITO, K. (1963) Myopathy in thyrotoxicosis, *Neurology (Minneap.)*, **13**, 645.

SAUNDERS, M., ASHWORTH, B., EMERY, A. E. H., and BENEDIKZ, J. E. G. (1968) Familial myotonic periodic paralysis with muscle wasting, *Brain*, **91**, 295.

SAVAGE, D. C. L., FORBES, M., and PEARCE, G. W. (1971) Idiopathic rhabdomyolysis, *Arch. Dis. Childh.*, **46**, 594.

SCHMID, R., and HAMMAKER, L. (1961) Hereditary absence of muscle phosphorylase (McArdle's syndrome), *New Engl. J. Med.*, **264**, 223.

SCHMID, R., and MAHLER, R. (1959) Chronic progressive myopathy with myoglobinuria: demonstration of a glycogenolytic defect in the muscle, *J. clin. Invest.*, **38**, 1044.

SCHOTT, G. D., and WILLS, M. R. (1975) Myopathy in hypophosphataemic osteomalacia presenting in adult life, *J. Neurol. Neurosurg. Psychiat.*, **38**, 297.

SCHUTTA, H. S., KELLY, A. M., and ZACKS, S. I. (1969) Necrosis and regeneration of muscle in paroxysmal idiopathic myoglobinuria: electron microscopic observations, *Brain*, **92**, 191.

SHY, G. M. (1960) Some metabolic and endocrinological aspects of disorders of striated muscle, *Res. Publ. Ass. nerv. ment. Dis.*, **38**, 274.

SHY, G. M., GONATAS, N. K., and PEREZ, M. C. (1966) Two childhood myopathies with abnormal mitochondria—1. Megaconial myopathy. 2. Pleoconial myopathy, *Brain*, **89**, 133.

SHY, G. M., WANKO, T., ROWLEY, P. T., and ENGEL, A. G. (1961) Studies in familial periodic paralysis, *Exp. Neurol.*, **3**, 53.

SMITH, A. F., MacFIE, W. G., and OLIVER, M. F. (1970) Clofibrate, serum enzymes, and muscle pain, *Brit. med. J.*, **2**, 86.

SMITH, R., and STERN, G. M. (1967) Myopathy, osteomalacia and hyperparathyroidism, *Brain*, **90**, 593.

SPIRO, A. J., HIRANO, A., BEILIN, R. L., and FINKELSTEIN, J. W. (1970) Cretinism with muscular hypertrophy (Kocher-Debré-Semelaigne syndrome), *Arch. Neurol. (Chic.)*, **23**, 340.

STEERS, A. J. W., TALLACK, J. A., and THOMPSON, D. E. A. (1970) Fulminating hyperpyrexia during anaesthesia in a member of a myopathic family, *Brit. med. J.*, **2**, 341.

STEINER, J. C., WINKELMAN, A. C., and DE JESUS, P. V. (1973) Pentazocine-induced myopathy, *Arch. Neurol. (Chic.)*, **28**, 408.

TAKAMORI, M., GUTMANN, L., CROSBY, T. W., and MARTIN, J. D. (1972) Myasthenic syndromes in hypothyroidism: electrophysiological study of neuromuscular transmission and muscle contraction in two patients, *Arch. Neurol. (Chic.)*, **26**, 326.

TARUI, S., OKUNA, G., IKURA, Y., TANAKA, T., SUDA, M., and NISHIKAWA, M. (1965) Phosphofructokinase deficiency in skeletal muscle. A new type of glycogenosis, *Biochem. biophys. Res. Commun.*, **19**, 517.

THOMSON, W. H. S., MacLAURIN, J. C., and PRINEAS, J. W. (1963) Skeletal muscle glycogenosis; an investigation of two dissimilar cases, *J. Neurol. Neurosurg. Psychiat.*, **26**, 60.

THORN, G. W. (1949) *The Diagnosis and Treatment of Adrenal Insufficiency*, p. 144, Springfield, Ill.

TOBIN, W. E., HUIJING, F., PORRO, R. S., and SALZMAN, R. T. (1973) Muscle phosphofructokinase deficiency, *Arch. Neurol. (Chic.)*, **28**, 128.

TYLER, F. H., STEPHENS, F. E., GUNN, F. D., and PERKOFF, G. T. (1951) Studies on disorders of muscle. VII. Clinical manifestations and inheritance of a type of periodic paralysis without hypopotassaemia, *J. clin. Invest.*, **30**, 492.

VAN DER MEULEN, J. P., GILBERT, G. J., and KANE, C. A. (1961) Familial hyperkalaemic paralysis with myotonia, *New Engl. J. Med.*, **264**, 1.

VANDYKE, D. H., GRIGGS, R. C., MARKESBERY, W., and DiMAURO, S. (1975) Hereditary carnitine deficiency of muscle, *Neurology (Minneap.)*, **25**, 154.

VANHAEVERBEEK, M., ECTORS, M., VANHAELST, L., and FRANKEN, L. (1974) Myopathy caused by polymyxin E: functional disorder of the cell membrane, *J. Neurol. Neurosurg. Psychiat.*, **37**, 1343.

VAN'T HOFF, W. (1962) Familial myotonic periodic paralysis, *Quart. J. Med.*, **31**, 385.

VROOM, F. Q., JARRELL, M. A., and MAREN, T. H. (1975) Acetazolamide treatment of hypokalemic periodic paralysis, *Arch. Neurol. (Chic.)*, **32**, 385.

WALTON, J. N. (1960) Muscular dystrophy and its relation to the other myopathies, *Res. Publ. Ass. nerv. ment. Dis.*, **38**, 378.

WANG, P., and CLAUSEN, T. (1976) Treatment of attacks in hyperkalaemic familial periodic paralysis by inhalation of salbutamol, *Lancet*, **i**, 221.

WATTS, R. W. E., SCOTT, J. T., CHALMERS, R. A., BITENSKY, L., and CHAYEN, J. (1971) Microscopic studies on skeletal muscle in gout patients treated with allopurinol, *Quart. J. Med.*, **40**, 1.

WILLIAMS, R. S. (1959) Triamcinolone myopathy, *Lancet*, **i**, 698.

WILSON, J., and WALTON, J. N. (1959) Some muscular manifestations of hypothyroidism, *J. Neurol. Neurosurg. Psychiat.*, **22**, 320.

WITTS, L. J., LAKIN, C. E., and THOMPSON, A. P. (1938) Discussion on Addison's disease at the Association of Physicians, *Quart. J. Med.*, **7**, 590.

ZELLWEGER, H., BROWN, B. I., McCORMICK, W., and TU, J. B. (1965) A mild form of muscular glycogenosis in two brothers with alpha-1,4-glucosidase deficiency, *Ann. paediat.*, **205**, 413.

ZIERLER, K. L., and ANDRES, R. (1957) Movement of potassium into skeletal muscle during spontaneous attack in family periodic paralysis, *J. clin. Invest.*, **36**, 730.

THE FLOPPY INFANT SYNDROME

It is well recognized that generalized muscular hypotonia in infancy can be due to a variety of causes. In a survey of 111 floppy infants, Paine (1963) found that 48 were suffering from various forms of cerebral palsy, 28 from mental retardation, 3 from cerebral degenerative disease, and 1 from brain tumour. There were 4 cases of spinal muscular atrophy and 4 of myopathy, while 18 were found to have a condition which could only be entitled 'benign congenital hypotonia' (Walton, 1956, 1957). Congenital muscular dystrophy as a cause of such a syndrome has already been considered [see p. 998]. The term 'benign congenital hypotonia' can still reasonably be reserved for those floppy infants in whom hypotonia is not demonstrated to be the result of any specific metabolic disorder or to be secondary to mental defect or central nervous disease and in whom full investigation, including electromyography and muscle biopsy, fails to demonstrate any specific abnormality of the muscle fibres other than, in some cases, an over-all decrease in their diameter, a failure of differentiation into the usual histochemical types or congenital fibre type disproportion (see Dubowitz and Brooke, 1973). While recent work has clearly indicated a remarkable variability in the clinical course of spinal muscular atrophy in infancy and childhood (Byers and Banker, 1961; Dubowitz, 1964; Gardner-Medwin *et al.*, 1967; and see p. 706) it has recently become apparent that some floppy infants may be suffering from certain apparently specific though benign disorders of muscle which are relatively non-progressive. The syndrome of arthrogryposis multiplex congenita (variable muscular weakness and wasting with contractures, especially in the extremities, present from birth) may be due to congenital muscular dystrophy [p. 998], to denervation due either to failure of development of neurones or fetal spinal muscular atrophy (Bharucha *et al.*, 1972; Dastur *et al.*, 1972), or to congenital peripheral neuropathy (Pena *et al.*, 1968; Hooshmand *et al.*, 1971; Yuill and Lynch, 1974). Some cases are attributed to excessive intrauterine pressure (Lloyd-Roberts and Lettin, 1970). There remain, however, a substantial number of hypotonic infants who show gradual improvement and in whom no other diagnostic label than one of benign congenital hypotonia can yet be applied, since modern methods of investigation fail to demonstrate any cause for the widespread muscular hypotonia which they manifest. It must, however, be appreciated that this condition is no more than a syndrome, almost certainly of multiple aetiology. A number of the more specific forms of benign and relatively non-progressive myopathy which have been described in recent years will now be mentioned.

CENTRAL CORE DISEASE

In 1956 Shy and Magee described a family of children in which the affected individuals did not walk until about the age of 4 years. The patients showed profound and widespread muscular hypotonia and muscle biopsy revealed large muscle fibres, most of which showed one or sometimes two central cores which had different staining properties from other fibrils. Further cases have been described by Bethlem and Meyjes (1960) and by Engel et al. (1961). Dubowitz and Pearse (1960) found the central core to be devoid of oxidative enzymes and of phosphorylase activity and suggested that it was non-functioning. The condition is plainly benign and genetically determined, being probably the result of an autosomal recessive gene, but as in the several other conditions described below, its pathogenesis remains obscure. Muscle cramps after exercise have been described in such cases (Bethlem et al., 1966) and multicore formation within a single fibre is not uncommon (Engel et al., 1971). The finding of multicores in an acquired myopathy beginning in adult life (Bonnette et al., 1974) has raised some doubts about the specificity of central cores in relation to congenital myopathy.

NEMALINE MYOPATHY

In 1963 Shy et al. described another congenital non-progressive myopathy in which curious collections of rod-shaped bodies were found within the muscle fibres. It is now apparent that in some such cases the clinical diagnosis can be suspected as these patients usually show not only evidence of a diffuse myopathy, but also facial weakness, a high arched palate, prognathism of the lower jaw, and skeletal changes resembling those of arachnodactyly, though none of the other stigmata of Marfan's syndrome are present (Ford, 1960; Conen et al., 1963; Engel et al., 1964). Examination of muscle from such cases with the electron microscope (Price et al., 1965; Hudgson et al., 1967; Shafiq et al., 1967) has shown that the subsarcolemmal rods appear to be due to a selective swelling and degeneration of Z-bands with consequent destruction of myofilaments in the adjacent part of the muscle fibre.

Recently the specificity of nemaline rods has been called into question, as these structures may be produced experimentally in muscle by tenotomy (Engel et al., 1966) and may be found from time to time in muscle biopsies from patients with a variety of neuromuscular disorders (Karpati et al., 1972). Type I fibre atrophy (Kinoshita and Satoyoshi, 1974) and virtual absence of Type II fibres (Karpati et al., 1971) have each been described in association with nemaline bodies and the myopathy which often accompanies the fully developed Marfan syndrome (Goebel et al., 1973) may not give rise to rod body formation.

MITOCHONDRIAL MYOPATHIES

Shy and Gonatas (1964) and Shy et al. (1966) described an 8-year-old white female with evidence of a slowly progressive myopathy beginning at the age of three years in whom a muscle biopsy showed enormously enlarged mitochondria measuring up to 5 μm in length and containing rectangular crystalline-like inclusions of high density; they called this condition 'megaconial myopathy'.

Subsequently under the title of 'pleoconial myopathy' Shy *et al.* (1966) described patients with symptoms resembling those of normokalaemic periodic paralysis in whom muscle biopsy showed enormous numbers of rounded mitochondria within muscle fibres.

Subsequently it has become apparent that these morphological abnormalities of the mitochondria are non-specific. Thus 'megaconial' mitochondria, often associated with 'ragged-red' Type I muscle fibres, seen clearly on histochemical study of muscle biopsies, are commonly found in limb muscles in patients with ocular or oculopharyngeal myopathy [p. 1000] or so-called oculocraniosomatic neuromuscular disease (Olson *et al.*, 1972; Tamura *et al.*, 1974). Abnormal mitochondria are also seen in muscle biopsy sections from patients with hyper-metabolic myopathy [p. 1038], and sometimes in lipid storage myopathy, hypothyroidism, polymyositis, McArdle's disease, and denervation atrophy. Nevertheless there do seem to be a group of patients with subacute proximal myopathy, sometimes with facial involvement suggesting facioscapulohumeral muscular dystrophy, and often inherited, in whom striking mitochondrial abnormalities associated with variable abnormalities of oxidative metabolism in the muscle fibres are found (Hudgson *et al.*, 1972; Worsfold *et al.*, 1973).

FINGERPRINT BODY MYOPATHY

In a 5-year-old girl with non-progressive muscular weakness present from infancy, Engel *et al.* (1972) found hypertrophy of Type II muscle fibres and the Type I fibres showed fingerprint-like inclusions clearly demonstrable by electron microscopy. Similar changes were found by Gordon *et al.* (1974) in a woman aged 55 years with a history suggesting that she had had a myopathy since birth, but have also been reported in dystrophia myotonica (Tomé and Fardeau, 1973). The pathogenesis of this change, and of the crystalline intra-nuclear inclusions noted by Jenis *et al.* (1969) in another case of congenital myopathy, remain to be determined.

MYOTUBULAR MYOPATHY

In a 9-year-old child with a form of Möbius disease characterized by facial diplegia, external ocular palsies, a decrease in muscle mass, moderate symmetrical muscle weakness, and poor development of all somatic muscles, Spiro *et al.* (1966) found changes which may represent the first example of cellular develop-mental arrest in the human. Most of the muscle fibres contained central nuclei, often lying in chains, and the appearances in the muscle were very similar to those of the so-called myotubes seen in the normal fetus in the early months of intra-uterine life. Subsequent reports, reviewed by Campbell *et al.* (1969), by van Wijngaarden *et al.* (1969), and by Bradley *et al.* (1970), have, however, shown many differences between these structures and fetal myotubes, so that although this condition appears to be a clinical and morphological entity, its pathogenesis is still a matter of speculation. The central nuclei are confined to the Type I muscle fibres in some cases (Engel *et al.*, 1968) and some cases are familial. The condition generally runs a benign course and gradual improve-ment in muscle power usually occurs (Tizard, 1974).

It may be concluded that although it is too early to be certain that the syn-dromes mentioned represent separate specific disorders of muscle, in the field of benign congenital myopathy new advances are taking place with great rapidity and many interesting histological abnormalities of the muscle fibre are being demonstrated by histochemical, biochemical, and ultrastructural techniques.

REFERENCES

BETHLEM, J., and MEYJES, F. E. P. (1960) Congenital non-progressive central core disease of Shy and Magee, *Psychiat. Neurol. Neurochir. (Amst.)*, **63**, 246.

BETHLEM, J., VAN GOOL, J., HÜLSMANN, W. C., and MEIJER, A. E. F. H. (1966) Familial non-progressive myopathy with muscle cramps after exercise, *Brain*, **89**, 569.

BHARUCHA, E. P., PANDYA, S. S., and DASTUR, D. K. (1972) Arthrogryposis multiplex congenita. Part 1: Clinical and electromyographic aspects, *J. Neurol. Neurosurg. Psychiat.*, **35**, 425.

BONNETTE, H., ROELOFS, R., and OLSON, W. H. (1974) Multicore disease: report of a case with onset in middle age, *Neurology (Minneap.)*, **24**, 1039.

BRADLEY, W. G., PRICE, D. L., and WATANABE, C. K. (1970) Familial centronuclear myopathy, *J. Neurol. Neurosurg. Psychiat.*, **33**, 687.

BYERS, R. K., and BANKER, B. Q. (1961) Infantile muscular atrophy, *Arch. Neurol. (Chic.)*, **5**, 140.

CAMPBELL, M. J., REBEIZ, J. J., and WALTON, J. N. (1969) Myotubular, centronuclear or pericentronuclear myopathy?, *J. neurol. Sci.*, **8**, 425.

CONEN, P. E., MURPHY, E. G., and DONOHUE, W. L. (1963) Light and electron microscopic studies on 'myogranules' in a child with hypotonia and muscle weakness, *Canad. med. Ass. J.*, **89**, 983.

DASTUR, D. K., RAZZAK, Z. A., and BHARUCHA, E. P. (1972) Arthrogryposis multiplex congenita. Part 2: Muscle pathology and pathogenesis, *J. Neurol. Neurosurg. Psychiat.*, **35**, 435.

DUBOWITZ, V. (1964) Infantile muscular atrophy. A prospective study with particular reference to a slowly progressive variety, *Brain*, **87**, 707.

DUBOWITZ, V., and BROOKE, M. H. (1973) *Muscle Biopsy*, London.

DUBOWITZ, V., and PEARSE, A. G. E. (1960) Oxidative enzymes and phosphorylase in central-core disease of muscle, *Lancet*, **ii**, 23.

ENGEL, A. G., ANGELINI, C., and GOMEZ, M. R. (1972) Fingerprint body myopathy: a newly recognized congenital muscle disease, *Mayo Clin. Proc.*, **47**, 377.

ENGEL, A. G., GOMEZ, M. R., and GROOVER, R. V. (1971) Multicore disease: a recently recognized congenital myopathy associated with multifocal degeneration of muscle fibers, *Mayo Clin. Proc.*, **46**, 666.

ENGEL, W. K., BROOKE, M. H., and NELSON, P. G. (1966) Histochemical studies of denervated or tenotomized cat muscle, *Ann. N.Y. Acad. Sci.*, **138**, 160.

ENGEL, W. K., FOSTER, J. B., HUGHES, B. P., HUXLEY, H. E., and MAHLER, R. (1961) Central core disease—an investigation of a rare muscle cell abnormality, *Brain*, **84**, 167.

ENGEL, W. K., GOLD, G. N., and KARPATI, G. (1968) Type I fiber hypotrophy and central nuclei, *Arch. Neurol. (Chic.)*, **18**, 435.

ENGEL, W. K., WANKO, T., and FENICHEL, G. M. (1964) Nemaline myopathy: a second case, *Arch. Neurol. (Chic.)*, **11**, 22.

FORD, F. R. (1960) Congenital universal muscle hypoplasia, in *Diseases of the Nervous System in Infancy, Childhood and Adolescence*, Oxford.

GARDNER-MEDWIN, D., HUDGSON, P., and WALTON, J. N. (1967) Benign spinal muscular atrophy arising in childhood and adolescence, *J. neurol. Sci.*, **5**, 121.

GOEBEL, H. H., MULLER, J., and DeMYER, W. (1973) Myopathy associated with Marfan's syndrome: fine structural and histochemical observations, *Neurology (Minneap.)*, **23**, 1257.

GORDON, A. S., REWCASTLE, N. B., HUMPHREY, J. G., and STEWART, B. M. (1974) Chronic benign congenital myopathy: fingerprint body type, *Canad. J. neurol. Sci.*, **1**, 106.

HOOSHMAND, H., MARTINEZ, A. J., and ROSENBLUM, W. I. (1971) Arthrogryposis multiplex congenita. Simultaneous involvement of peripheral nerve and skeletal muscle, *Arch. Neurol. (Chic.)*, **24**, 561.

HUDGSON, P., BRADLEY, W. G., and JENKISON, M. (1972) Familial 'mitochondrial' myopathy: a myopathy associated with disordered oxidative metabolism in muscle fibres. Part 1. Clinical, electrophysiological and pathological findings, *J. neurol. Sci.*, **16**, 343.

HUDGSON, P., GARDNER-MEDWIN, D., FULTHORPE, J. J., and WALTON, J. N. (1967) Nemaline myopathy, *Neurology (Minneap.)*, **17**, 1125.

JENIS, E. H., LINDQUIST, R. R., and LISTER, R. C. (1969) New congenital myopathy with crystalline intranuclear inclusions, *Arch. Neurol. (Chic.)*, **20**, 281.

KARPATI, G., CARPENTER, S., and ANDERMANN, F. (1971) A new concept of childhood nemaline myopathy, *Arch. Ophthalmol.*, **85**, 291.

KARPATI, G., CARPENTER, S., and EISEN, A. A. (1972) Experimental core-like lesions and nemaline rods, *Arch. Neurol. (Chic.)*, **27**, 237.

KINOSHITA, M., and SATOYOSHI, E. (1974) Type I fiber atrophy and nemaline bodies, *Arch. Neurol. (Chic.)*, **31**, 423.

LLOYD-ROBERTS, G. C., and LETTIN, A. W. F. (1970) Arthrogryposis multiplex congenita, *J. Bone Jt Surg.*, **52B**, 494.

MCARDLE, B. (1974) Endocrine and metabolic myopathies, in *Disorders of Voluntary Muscle*, ed. Walton, J. N., 3rd ed., Edinburgh and London.

OLSON, W., ENGEL, W. K., WALSH, G. O., and EINAUGLER, R. (1972) Oculocraniosomatic neuromuscular disease with 'ragged-red' fibers, *Arch. Neurol. (Chic.)*, **26**, 193.

PAINE, R. S. (1963) The future of the 'floppy infant', *Develop. Med. Child Neurol.*, **5**, 115.

PEÑA, C. E., MILLER, F., BUDZILOVICH, G. N., and FEIGIN, I. (1968) Arthrogryposis multiplex congenita: a report of two cases of a radicular type with familial incidence, *Neurology (Minneap.)*, **18**, 926.

PRICE, H. M., GORDON, G. B., PEARSON, C. M., MUNSAT, T. L., and BLUMBERG, J. M. (1956) New evidence for excessive accumulation of Z-band material in nemaline myopathy, *Proc. nat. Acad. Sci. (Wash.)*, **54**, 1398.

SHAFIQ, S. A., DUBOWITZ, V., PETERSON, H. DE C., and MILHORAT, A. T. (1967) Nemaline myopathy: report of a fatal case, with histochemical and electron microscopic studies, *Brain*, **90**, 817.

SHY, G. M., ENGEL, W. K., SOMERS, J. E., and WANKO, T. (1963) Nemaline myopathy, a new congenital myopathy, *Brain*, **86**, 793.

SHY, G. M., and GONATAS, N. K. (1964) Human myopathy with giant abnormal mitochondria, *Science*, **145**, 493.

SHY, G. M., GONATAS, N. K., and PEREZ, M. C. (1966) Two childhood myopathies with abnormal mitochondria—1. Megaconial myopathy, 2. Pleoconial myopathy, *Brain*, **89**, 133.

SHY, G. M., and MAGEE, K. R. (1956) A new congenital non-progressive myopathy, *Brain*, **79**, 610.

SPIRO, A. J., SHY, G. M., and GONATAS, N. K. (1966) Myotubular myopathy, *Arch. Neurol. (Chic.)*, **14**, 1.

TAMURA, K., SANTA, T., and KUROIWA, Y. (1974) Familial oculocranioskeletal neuromuscular disease with abnormal muscle mitochondria, *Brain*, **97**, 665.

TIZARD, J. P. M. (1974) Neuromuscular disorders in infancy and early childhood, in *Disorders of Voluntary Muscle*, ed. Walton, J. N., 3rd ed., Edinburgh and London.

TOMÉ, F. M. S., and FARDEAU, M. (1973) 'Fingerprint inclusions' in muscle fibres in dystrophia myotonica, *Acta neuropath. (Berl.)*, **24**, 62.

VAN WIJNGAARDEN, G. K., FLEURY, P., BETHLEM, J., and MEIJER, A. E. F. H. (1969) Familial 'myotubular' myopathy, *Neurology (Minneap.)*, **19**, 901.

WALTON, J. N. (1956) Amyotonia congenita—a follow-up study, *Lancet*, **i**, 1023.

WALTON, J. N. (1957) The limp child, *J. Neurol. Neurosurg. Psychiat.*, **20**, 144.

WORSFOLD, M., PARK, D. C., and PENNINGTON, R. J. (1973) Familial 'mitochondrial' myopathy: a myopathy associated with disordered oxidative metabolism in muscle fibres. Part 2. Biochemical findings, *J. neurol. Sci.*, **19**, 261.

YUILL, G. M., and LYNCH, P. G. (1974) Congenital non-progressive peripheral neuropathy with arthrogryposis multiplex, *J. Neurol. Neurosurg. Psychiat.*, **37**, 316.

SOME MISCELLANEOUS DISORDERS OF MUSCLE

RESTLESS LEGS

The aetiology of this condition, reviewed in detail by Ekbom (1960), is unknown. There is no evidence that it is a primary muscular disorder, but it gives rise to unpleasant aching in the muscles of the lower limbs when the patient rests in a chair and the symptoms are often particularly troublesome in bed. They may be associated with muscular cramps so that they interfere with sleep and after a period of restless shuffling the patient may be compelled to get up and to walk the floor to obtain relief. The syndrome of 'painful legs and moving toes' described by Spillane et al. (1971) may simply be an unusually severe variant of this disorder. There are no abnormal physical signs on examination and no lesions within the muscles or peripheral nerves have been discovered (Harriman et al., 1970). The aetiology of this troublesome syndrome is totally unexplained, but some patients are greatly helped by treatment with chlorpromazine given in a dosage of 50–100 mg at night, and perhaps 25 mg three times a day as well. Diazepam and hydantoinates are sometimes helpful in relieving the associated muscle cramps which occur in some cases.

TIBIALIS ANTERIOR SYNDROME

Severe boring pain in the tibialis anterior muscle, particularly in adults undertaking unaccustomed exercise is typical of this syndrome. The condition is probably due to ischaemia followed by swelling of the tibialis anterior and its associated muscles lying within a tight fascial compartment. In rare cases the pain may be intense, and widespread necrosis of the anterior tibial muscles may occur, and can even be fatal as a result of myoglobinuria. In mild chronic cases recurrent pain in the appropriate distribution occurs whenever the patient exerts himself. Relief may then be obtained by means of surgical decompression of the anterior crural compartment (Sirbou et al., 1944; British Medical Journal, 1975).

PROGRESSIVE MYOSITIS OSSIFICANS

Although localized myositis ossificans may occur as a result of the ossification of certain muscles as a result of their repeated involvement in the trauma of certain exercises or occupations and may occasionally occur in muscles in the region of the hip joint (particularly the adductors) following paraplegia or paraparesis, as after partial recovery from transverse myelitis, there is a genetically-determined progressive disorder in which widespread ossification of muscles occurs. Most of these patients are children who often have associated anomalies of their great toes or other digits and it seems that the ossification in muscle is preceded by sclerosis of intramuscular connective tissue (McKusick, 1956). This rare disorder, which is probably transmitted by a dominant gene which often shows incomplete penetrance (Tünte et al., 1967), often begins by giving rise to swelling or swellings in the neck which mimic congenital torticollis and eventually in most cases the muscles of the back, shoulder, and pelvic girdles become ossified. The overlying skin may ulcerate and in the terminal stages aspiration pneumonia and/or asphyxia may occur. There is some recent evidence that diphosphonate treatment may promote resorption of bone in such cases (Russell et al., 1972).

THE STIFF-MAN SYNDROME

In 1956 Moersch and Woltman reported on 14 patients who had suffered a progressive fluctuating muscular rigidity and spasm and used the term 'stiff-man syndrome' to describe this condition. The condition predominantly affects male adults who, after a prodromal phase of aching and tightness of the axial muscles, go on to develop a symmetrical continuous stiffness of the skeletal muscles upon which painful muscular spasms are superimposed; these may be precipitated by movement. The cause of the condition is unknown but there is evidence to suggest that it may be due to overactivity in a central norepinephrine neuronal system with increased excitability of spinal cord motor neurones (Schmidt et al., 1975). Diazepam (Howard, 1963) may be remarkably successful in controlling the symptoms. It must be distinguished from the syndrome of myokymia with continuous muscle fibre activity (Isaacs and Heffron, 1974; and see p. 1001) which responds to phenytoin.

REFERENCES

BRITISH MEDICAL JOURNAL (1975) Acute muscle compartment compression syndromes, *Brit. med. J.*, **3**, 193.

EKBOM, K. A. (1960) Restless legs syndrome, *Neurology (Minneap.)*, **10**, 868.

FOSTER, J. B. (1974) The clinical features of some miscellaneous neuromuscular disorders, in *Disorders of Voluntary Muscle*, ed. Walton, J. N., 3rd ed., Edinburgh and London.

HARRIMAN, D. G. F., TAVERNER, D., and WOOLF, A. L. (1970) Ekbom's syndrome and burning paraesthesiae. A biopsy study by vital staining and electron microscopy of the intramuscular innervation with a note on age changes in motor nerve endings in distal muscles, *Brain*, **93**, 393.

HOWARD, F. M. (1963) A new and effective drug in the treatment of stiff-man syndrome, *Mayo Clin. Proc.*, **38**, 203.

ISAACS, H., and HEFFRON, J. J. A. (1974) The syndrome of 'continuous muscle-fibre activity' cured: further studies, *J. Neurol. Neurosurg. Psychiat.*, **37**, 1231.

MCKUSICK, V. (1956) *Heritable Disorders of Connective Tissue*, p. 184, St. Louis, Mo.

MOERSCH, F. P., and WOLTMAN, H. W. (1956) Progressive muscular rigidity and spasm (stiff-man syndrome), *Mayo Clin. Proc.*, **31**, 421.

RUSSELL, R. G. G., SMITH, R., BISHOP, M. C., PRICE, D. A., and SQUIRE, C. M. (1972) Treatment of myositis ossificans progressiva with a diphosphonate, *Lancet*, **i**, 10.

SCHMIDT, R. T., STAHL, S. M., and SPEHLMANN, R. (1975) A pharmacologic study of the stiff-man syndrome, *Neurology (Minneap.)*, **25**, 622.

SIRBOU, A. B., MURPHY, M. J., and WHITE, A. S. (1944) Soft tissue complications of fractures of the leg, *Calif. west Med.*, **60**, 53.

SPILLANE, J. D., NATHAN, P. W., KELLY, R. E., and MARSDEN, C. D. (1971) Painful legs and moving toes, *Brain*, **94**, 541.

TÜNTE, W., BECKER, P. E., and KNORRE, G. (1967) Zur Genetik der Myositis ossificans progressiva, *Humangenetik*, **4**, 320.

DIFFERENTIAL DIAGNOSIS

The differential diagnosis of muscle disease depends first upon the clinical history and examination, secondly upon electromyographic and other neuro-physiological evidence, thirdly upon the biochemical findings, and fourthly upon pathological changes in muscle as revealed by biopsy.

CLINICAL DIAGNOSIS

In the characteristic case of muscular dystrophy showing the usual slowly progressive pattern of increasing muscular weakness and selective atrophy of the proximal limb muscles, diagnosis is rarely in doubt. On the other hand, in an infant or child showing a picture of relatively diffuse non-progressive atrophy and weakness, it may be apparent that the condition belongs to one of the group of so-called benign congenital myopathies. There are, however, some cases in which differential diagnosis between a congenital non-progressive myopathy and progressive muscular dystrophy of early onset may be an extremely difficult matter on purely clinical grounds and may then depend upon ancillary investigations.

If the pattern of muscular weakness and wasting is obscured by subcutaneous fat or when muscular involvement is predominantly distal, as in myotonic dystrophy and distal myopathy, it may not always be easy to distinguish muscular dystrophy from neuropathic disorders such as progressive muscular atrophy, polyneuropathy, and peroneal muscular atrophy. Usually, however, the associated neurological signs, including fasciculation, and the sensory abnormalities which generally occur in polyneuropathy and peroneal muscular atrophy are sufficient to clarify the position. In early life, fasciculation is a useful sign, both in the tongue and in limb muscles, which may help to identify benign or pseudomyopathic forms of spinal muscular atrophy, and electromyography is of particular value in distinguishing the latter disorder from muscular dystrophy, as the classical features of central denervation are almost always found.

Usually, therefore, it is comparatively easy to distinguish myopathy from neuropathy on clinical grounds alone, but it may be much more difficult to separate cases of sporadic muscular dystrophy from other forms of myopathy. The possibility of an endocrine cause for the muscular weakness must always be considered, and associated signs of endocrine disease and/or of metabolic bone disease should be sought carefully. It must also be noted that in untreated myasthenia gravis fatigability of muscles may not always be immediately apparent, and in any patient with proximal muscular weakness of comparatively recent onset, even when there is no involvement of ocular and bulbar muscles, a diagnostic injection of edrophonium chloride is indicated. Equivocal improvement following such an injection is sometimes seen in polymyositis and a more striking response may be observed in the myasthenic-myopathic syndrome complicating bronchial carcinoma, in which, however, the tendon reflexes are usually absent, whereas in true myasthenia they are brisk, and electrophysiological tests of neuromuscular transmission will usually be helpful in making the distinction. It should also be noted that in cases of periodic paralysis and of myoglobinuria, permanent muscular atrophy may eventually supervene, though in such cases there is invariably a clear-cut history of episodic attacks of weakness or of muscle pain and the diagnosis will then be elucidated by clinical methods.

The differential diagnosis between muscular dystrophy and subacute or chronic polymyositis may be an extremely difficult matter. Among the criteria of value in differential diagnosis are first, the rapidity of onset and occasional remissions which occur in polymyositis; secondly, the global weakness and wasting which occur in this disease, unlike the selective pattern which is more characteristic of dystrophy; thirdly, a positive family history, if present, clearly indicates a genetically-determined disorder of muscle; fourthly, the almost constant involvement of neck muscles and the frequent occurrence of dysphagia strongly favour polymyositis, while these features are rare in muscular dystrophy except in the oculopharyngeal variety (it should also be recalled that myasthenia may selectively involve the neck muscles in occasional cases); finally, associated phenomena such as skin changes and the Raynaud phenomenon are found to be present in many cases of polymyositis.

Even with the help of these and other clinical guides, there are nevertheless cases in which diagnosis remains in doubt and must then depend upon investigative findings.

ELECTROMYOGRAPHY [also see p. 882]

In neuropathic disorders, spontaneous fibrillation potentials may be recorded from a muscle undergoing an active process of denervation, while the pattern of motor unit activity on volition, though reduced from normal, clearly indicates that the surviving motor unit action potentials are either normal or increased in size. Measurement of motor and sensory nerve conduction velocity may assist in identifying the nature and site of the lesion in the motor neurones [p. 886]. In myopathic disorders, by contrast, spontaneous activity in the form of fibrillation potentials is uncommon, though fibrillation has been found in some cases and is more frequently seen in polymyositis than in muscular dystrophy (Walton and Adams, 1958). In the myotonic disorders a characteristic discharge taking the form of chains of oscillations of high frequency, is seen, and similar spontaneous discharges evoked by movement of the exploring electrode, which, however, do not show the classical waxing and waning of the myotonic discharge but which continue at a constant frequency and then cease spontaneously, may be recorded in various forms of non-myotonic myopathy including polymyositis and have been called pseudomyotonic discharges. Volitional activity in the myopathic disorders, and particularly in muscular dystrophy and polymyositis, demonstrates a break-down of the motor unit action potentials corresponding to patchy degeneration of muscle fibres and as a result there is an increase in the proportion of short-duration and polyphasic motor unit action potentials (Kugelberg, 1947; Walton, 1952). Buchthal *et al.* (1960) showed that a decrease in mean action potential amplitude and duration, together with a reduced motor unit territory and fibre density, is seen particularly often in the Duchenne type of muscular dystrophy. In myotonic dystrophy and polymyositis they found that motor unit territory and the mean duration of the motor unit potentials were similarly reduced, but normal amplitudes were maintained. In polymyositis Buchthal and Pinelli (1953) found that the mean duration of the motor unit action potential was decreased by up to 60 per cent and the incidence of polyphasic potentials was increased three times. In the more benign forms of muscular dystrophy (the limb-girdle and facioscapulo-humeral types) similar but less conclusive quantitative changes may be observed (Buchthal, 1962; Richardson and Barwick, 1974). Changes in the motor unit action potentials similar to those observed in muscular dystrophy are found in thyrotoxic myopathy (Havard *et al.*, 1963), in steroid myopathy (Müller and Kugelberg, 1959), in the myopathies of Addison's disease and sarcoidosis (Buchthal, 1962), and in other metabolic myopathies. Farmer *et al.* (1959) found that the absolute refractory period of voluntary muscle was reduced in cases of muscular dystrophy.

More specialized techniques of electromyographic examination including integration and analysis of the electromyogram and single fibre electromyography are reviewed by Lenman (1974) and methods of intracellular recording by McComas and Johns (1974). The electrophysiological technique of estimating the number of functioning motor units in the extensor digitorum brevis muscle of the foot, as developed by McComas *et al.* (1971), has suggested that motor unit dysfunction may play a role in the pathogenesis of muscular dystrophy but this 'neurogenic hypothesis' has been challenged. Nevertheless, this method of identifying motor units has proved to be of considerable diagnostic value (Lenman, 1974).

In myasthenia gravis the electromyogram may be entirely normal, except that a myopathic pattern, as described above, may be obtained from fatigued muscle. A progressive diminution in the amplitude of the action potentials in myasthenic muscle obtained in response to supramaximal stimulation of its motor nerve at rates of 3 Hz and detected by surface electrodes (Harvey and Masland, 1941) is a useful diagnostic sign of myasthenia, but only occurs as a rule in muscles which are clinically affected by the disease (Botelho et al., 1952; Brown, 1974). At tetanic rates of stimulation (50 Hz) the amplitude of the evoked muscle action potential usually increases greatly in cases of the myasthenic-myopathic syndrome complicating lung cancer (Lambert et al., 1956; Brown, 1974) but a similar, though less striking, increment (Simpson, 1974) is occasionally seen in myasthenia gravis. No specific electromyographic appearances have been described in cases of familial periodic paralysis, but in patients with various forms of benign congenital myopathy the electromyogram may again reveal a myopathic pattern without any specific features (see Richardson and Barwick, 1974).

BIOCHEMICAL DIAGNOSIS

Many biochemical tests can be employed in differentiating the various forms of myopathy. Thus in the endocrine myopathies various tests apposite to the diagnosis of the individual endocrine deficiencies may well be required in certain cases. In the periodic paralysis syndromes, in addition to serial estimations of the serum potassium level and measures designed to precipitate attacks for diagnostic purposes, there are certain cases in which measurement of sodium and potassium output in the urine, and even of sodium and potassium balance, may be needed. In cases of severe generalized muscle pain and weakness, a search for myoglobin in the urine is essential, while in those patients who develop muscle pain after effort it is usually necessary to exclude certain forms of glycogen storage disease by the measurement of lactate and pyruvate in venous blood distal to a tourniquet following a period of ischaemic work; estimation of phosphorylase and of other glycolytic enzymes by histochemical and chemical methods applied to muscle biopsy samples, as well as the estimation of the total glycogen content of muscle, may also be needed (see McArdle, 1974).

In polymyositis the erythrocyte sedimentation rate is raised in about half the cases and there may be an elevation of the serum gamma-globulin level which can be demonstrated by electrophoresis (Barwick and Walton, 1963). Tests for circulating antibodies in the serum of such patients have been disappointing (Caspary et al., 1964). Antimyosin antibody is found not only in some cases of polymyositis and in myasthenia gravis, but also in some patients with muscular dystrophy and neurogenic atrophy and in a proportion of normal individuals. Antinuclear factor is present, however, in a higher proportion of cases of polymyositis than of controls. Positive LE-cell preparations are occasionally seen in such cases (Pearson and Currie, 1974) but such examinations as the latex fixation and Rose-Waaler tests are of little diagnostic value. The more sophisticated immunological methods which may be of value in the diagnosis of polymyositis, myasthenia gravis, and the Guillain–Barré syndrome are respectively reviewed on pages 1012, 1023, and 949.

Many other relatively non-specific biochemical findings have been described in cases of myopathy and have been reviewed by Pennington (1974). Thus an excessive output of creatine and a diminished creatininuria have been observed in many forms of myopathy but have little diagnostic significance. Amino-aciduria is also seen in a proportion of cases, while changes observed in serum lipid and protein levels lack specificity. Abnormalities of protein composition and turnover in dystrophic muscle, though of considerable research interest (Rowland et al., 1968; Samaha and Gergely, 1969; Penn et al., 1972; Ionasescu et al., 1972, 1973; Samaha, 1973), as well as disorders of carbohydrate metabolism (Ellis and Strickland, 1972) are not yet of value in diagnosis, but recent observations of erythrocyte deformation (Brown et al., 1967; Lumb and Emery, 1975; and see p. 1003) may ultimately add precision to diagnosis. Of the greatest diagnostic value, however, have been changes in serum enzyme activities. Sibley and Lehninger (1949) first demonstrated that the serum aldolase level was raised in patients with various muscle diseases including progressive muscular dystrophy. Subsequently many authors have used the assay of this enzyme in the diagnosis of muscular dystrophy and it has been found that its activity in the serum is raised to about ten times the normal upper limit in early cases of Duchenne type muscular dystrophy, while less striking increases are observed in the more benign varieties. Pearson (1957) showed that similar though less striking increases occurred in the serum activity of the transaminases (amino-transferases) and pointed out that a substantial rise in enzyme activity might occur long before overt clinical signs of Duchenne type dystrophy appeared—that is, in the preclinical phase of the disease. In 1959 Ebashi et al. reported a pronounced increase in creatine kinase activity in the serum of patients with muscular dystrophy and demonstrated that in early cases of the Duchenne type this increase might even be three hundredfold. It is now apparent that estimation of this enzyme in the serum is much the most sensitive early diagnostic test for this form of muscular dystrophy, and Pearce et al. (1964) among others have confirmed that it is increased in preclinical cases. It is well recognized that the activity of this and other enzymes (see Pennington, 1974) which leak out of the diseased muscle into the serum is at its highest in the early stages of all forms of muscle disease and tends to decline as the disease advances. In the Duchenne type dystrophy, activity is probably highest at about the second or third year of life and declines progressively after the age of 10. Similar reductions are seen during the course of limb-girdle and facioscapulohumeral dystrophy and in myotonic dystrophy, although in these three disorders the initial increases are very much less striking. In polymyositis the activity is highest in acute cases before treatment, but a rapid decline occurs following treatment, particularly if it is effective. The activity of this enzyme in the serum has been reported to increase markedly four to six hours after a test dose of prednisone in patients with muscular dystrophy but not in polymyositis (Takahashi et al., 1975). Estimation of serum creatine kinase activity has recently been shown to be the most useful single test for the identification of the carrier state in female relatives of patients suffering from X-linked muscular dystrophy [p. 996], but other enzymes such as pyruvate kinase, and adenylate kinase are now being tested (Pennington, 1974).

HISTOLOGICAL DIAGNOSIS

Traditionally, muscle biopsy has been one of the standard methods employed in the differential diagnosis of the various myopathies (Adams et al., 1962). Many pathological changes have been described in muscle and detailed reviews have been given by Bethlem (1970), Dubowitz and Brooke (1973), Adams (1974), and Hudgson and Mastaglia (1974), among others. Percutaneous muscle biopsy of the quadriceps (Edwards, 1971) is sometimes useful, especially when repeated biopsy is needed, though the specimen obtained is small. Increasing knowledge has led to decreasing confidence concerning the specificity of pathological changes seen in muscle biopsy specimens in so far as the differential diagnosis of myopathy is concerned. Although techniques such as intravital staining of the motor end-plates (Woolf and Coërs, 1974), histochemistry, tissue culture, and electron microscopy have been of considerable interest from the research standpoint, they have begun only recently to add precision to the histological diagnosis of the myopathies especially in such conditions as the congenital and metabolic myopathies.

Among the most characteristic histological features observed in cases of muscular dystrophy of all types (Adams *et al.*, 1962; Pearce and Walton, 1962; Pearson, 1973) are such changes as marked variations in fibre size, fibre splitting, the central migration of sarcolemmal nuclei [FIG. 150], areas of fibre atrophy, the formation of nuclear chains, areas of necrosis with phagocytosis of necrotic sarcoplasm [FIG. 151], and basophilia of sarcoplasm with an enlargement of sarcolemmal nuclei [FIG. 152] which show prominent nucleoli (changes construed as being due to abortive regeneration); infiltration with fat cells and connective tissue is also observed. Scattered hyaline fibres seen in transverse section with others which are necrotic, interspersed with clumps of regenerating fibres, are the histological hallmark of Duchenne muscular dystrophy in the early or preclinical stages (Pearson, 1962; Cullen and Fulthorpe, 1975). When changes of the type described are uniformly distributed throughout the muscle sections, it is not usually difficult to accept that the diagnosis is one of muscular dystrophy. On the other hand, similar changes may be seen in polymyositis (Walton and Adams, 1958; Pearson, 1974; Adams, 1974), in which condition, however, signs of muscle fibre destruction and repair (necrosis, phagocytosis, and regenerative activity) are usually more striking and widespread, though they may be surprisingly slight even in acute cases. Most important in the diagnosis of polymyositis, but often scanty and only very rarely observed in muscular dystrophy except in some cases of the facioscapulohumeral syndrome [p. 999], are interstitial or perivascular infiltrations of inflammatory cells such as lymphocytes and plasma cells [FIG. 153]. It is also important to note that whereas chronic denervation atrophy, as in the spinal muscular atrophies of childhood, chronic polyneuropathy and motor neurone disease, usually gives groups of uniformly atrophic fibres lying alongside groups of fibres which are normal in size or even hypertrophied [FIG. 155], with so-called 'type-grouping' or large fields of fibres of uniform histochemical type (see Dubowitz and Brooke, 1973; Dubowitz, 1974; and p. 990), in disseminated neurogenic atrophy the atrophic fibres, often sharply angulated and containing dark pyknotic nuclei, may occur in groups of only four or five fibres and are easily overlooked. Furthermore there is increasing evidence that in chronic denervation many muscles show secondary myopathic change (Drachman *et al.*, 1967; Mastaglia and Walton, 1971) with muscle fibre necrosis, phagocytosis and regenerative activity so that the unwary may be led to diagnose a primary myopathy. Undoubtedly this error has led often in the past to a mistaken diagnosis of muscular dystrophy in patients with spinal muscular atrophy.

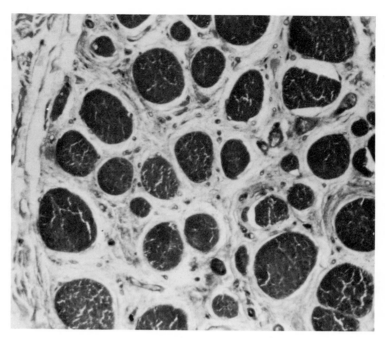

Fig. 150. Transverse section of biceps brachii biopsy from a case of advanced limb-girdle dystrophy showing rounding of fibres, random variation in size, central nuclei, fibre-splitting, and infiltration with connective tissue. H & E, ×240

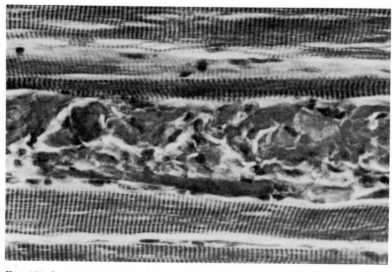

Fig. 151. Longitudinal section of quadriceps biopsy from a case of Duchenne type muscular dystrophy demonstrating focal necrosis and phagocytosis of a segment of muscle fibre. Picro-Mallory, ×640

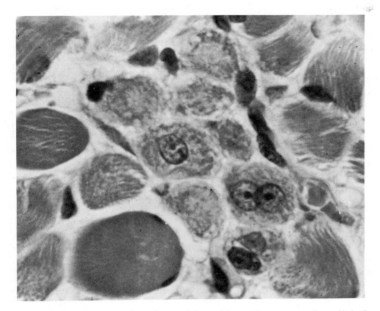

FIG. 152. Transverse section of a quadriceps biopsy from a case of preclinical Duchenne type dystrophy. H & E, ×640. Note the group of central fibres with sparse myofibrils and large vesicular nuclei with prominent nucleoli, demonstrating regenerative activity

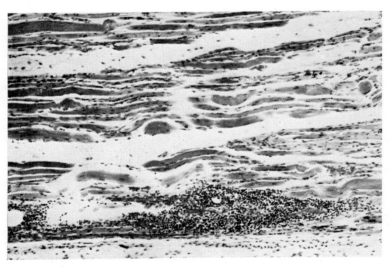

FIG. 153. Muscle in acute polymyositis

If, therefore, in a muscle section there is gross variation in fibre size with fibre-splitting, infiltration with fat and connective tissue and little phagocytosis or regenerative activity and no evidence of groups of tiny atrophic fibres, one may reasonably assume that the process is probably, but not certainly, dystrophic. If, by contrast, there is widespread necrosis and phagocytosis of muscle fibres with some, though not excessive, variation in fibre size, with profuse regenerative activity and massive infiltration of inflammatory cells between fibres and around blood vessels, it is not difficult to decide that one is probably dealing with a case of polymyositis. In between these two extremes, however, there is a considerable overlapping of the types of change which may be seen in dystrophy on the one hand and polymyositis on the other. Furthermore, in some cases of myasthenia gravis (Russell, 1953) degenerative changes are observed within muscle fibres, and lymphorrhages (collections of lymphocytes) may be seen around blood vessels or occasionally between fibres. Changes are often less striking in cases of the myasthenic-myopathic syndrome complicating bronchial carcinoma (Croft and Wilkinson, 1965), and although the pathological changes in muscle in cases of thyrotoxic and other endocrine myopathies may certainly be construed as being myopathic in the broadest sense, they are often slight and difficult to define.

The finding of striated annulets or so-called ringbinden (Wohlfart, 1951; Greenfield et al., 1957) in which striated myofibrils are seen to be encircling muscle fibres cut in transverse section, is often regarded as being diagnostic of myotonic dystrophy [FIG. 154], though this is not absolutely so as these

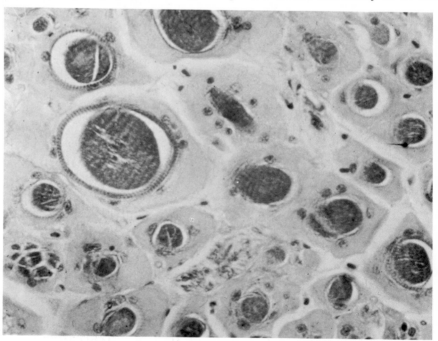

FIG. 154. Transverse section of quadriceps, obtained at autopsy from a case of dystrophia myotonica, PTAH, × 480, demonstrating ringbinden and/or sarcoplasmic masses surrounding the transversely-sectioned central myofibrils of virtually every muscle fibre. (By kind permission of Dr. G. W. Pearce)

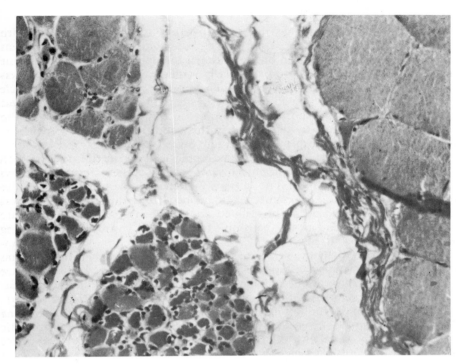

FIG. 155 (a)

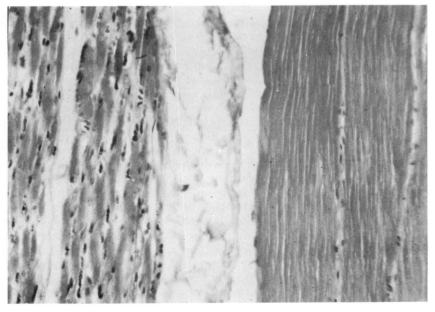

FIG. 155 (b). Grouped atrophy of denervation demonstrated in a biopsy of tibialis anterior from a patient with peroneal muscular atrophy. (a) Transverse section, H & E, ×640. (b) Longitudinal section, H & E, ×640

abnormalities may occasionally be seen in other muscle diseases and are probably due to the fracture of peripherally-situated myofibrils which then wind around the intact portion of the fibre. In myotonic dystrophy, chains of nuclei within muscle fibres are particularly striking and the nuclei are often small and pyknotic, unlike the large vesicular nuclei occurring in chains which are seen in some cases of Duchenne type dystrophy and of polymyositis and which probably indicate abortive regenerative activity. Abnormalities of the muscle spindles are often more striking in this condition than in other neuro-muscular diseases (Cazzato and Walton, 1968; Swash and Fox, 1975). Peripheral masses of palely-staining homogeneous sarcoplasm lying in the periphery of muscle fibres (so-called sarcoplasmic masses) are also characteristically seen in myotonic cases [FIG. 154]. The 'myopathic' changes described can, in the great majority of cases, be readily distinguished from those of denervation atrophy [FIG. 155] except, as mentioned above, when secondary myopathic change is widespread and grouped atrophic fibres are few; histochemical studies may be especially useful here.

Vacuolar change within muscle fibres is another pathological change of some interest. Massive vacuoles within the substance of muscle fibres and often lying in a subsarcolemmal position, and shown by alcoholic PAS staining to contain glycogen, are characteristic of the various forms of glycogen storage disease of muscle [FIG. 156] including Pompe's disease (Hudgson et al., 1968) and McArdle's disease (Salter et al., 1968). Widespread but less striking vacuolar change can also be seen with the light microscope within the muscle fibres of patients with periodic paralysis during attacks, and electron microscopy (Shy et al., 1961) has confirmed that these vacuoles are due to dilatation of the endoplasmic reticulum. Pearson and Yamazaki (1958) suggested that vacuolar change in muscle may also be characteristic of disseminated lupus erythematosus, and similar histological abnormalities may be seen in the myopathy which may result from the long-continued administration of chloroquine (see Kakulas, 1974). Vacuolar changes may also be noted with the light microscope in lipid storage myopathy due to carnitine deficiency (Bradley et al., 1969; Engel and Siekert, 1972) but this condition is much better identified in frozen sections using stains for neutral fat. Histochemistry is also of great value in the recognition of 'ragged-red' fibres in the mitochondrial myopathies, in confirming the absence of phosphorylase in McArdle's disease, in identifying Type II fibre atrophy in steroid myopathy and many other conditions and fibre type disproportion in some cases of benign congenital hypotonia, and in demonstrating the 'type-grouping' of many chronic denervating processes, to name only a few of its contributions (see Dubowitz and Brooke, 1973; Dubowitz, 1974). Indeed, histochemical study is now an essential technique in the examination of muscle biopsy specimens. It should finally be mentioned that in cases of so-called benign congenital myopathy or hypotonia in which myopathic changes have been observed in the electromyogram, examination of muscle biopsy specimens under the light microscope has been singularly disappointing (Walton, 1957), and it is only since particular attention has been paid to these cases, using histochemical stains and electron microscopy, that entities such as central core disease, nemaline myopathy [FIGS. 157 and 158], and myotubular myopathy [FIG. 159] and the various mitochondrial myopathies have been recognized. It is more than likely that the use of these highly-specialized techniques will in the future identify many more specific syndromes within this relatively difficult and little-understood group.

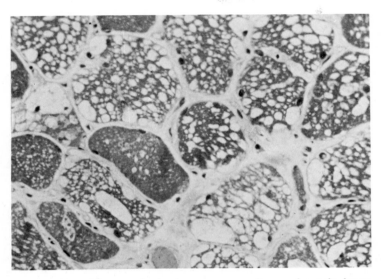

FIG. 156. Vacuolar myopathy in glycogen storage disease of muscle due to acid maltase deficiency. Transverse section of quadriceps biopsy. H & E, ×640

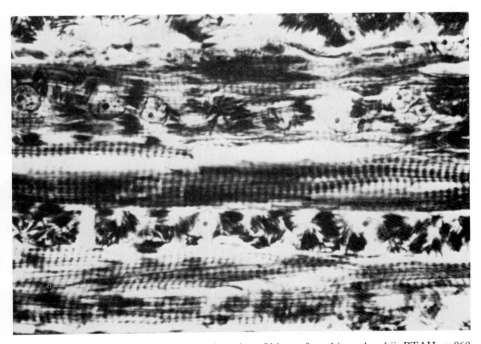

FIG. 157. Nemaline myopathy; longitudinal section of biopsy from biceps brachii, PTAH, ×960. Note the collections of rods lying between the fibres. (From Hudgson, P., Gardner-Medwin, D., Fulthorpe, J. J., and Walton, J. N. (1967), *Neurology (Minneap.)*, **17**, 1125. By kind permission of the Editor)

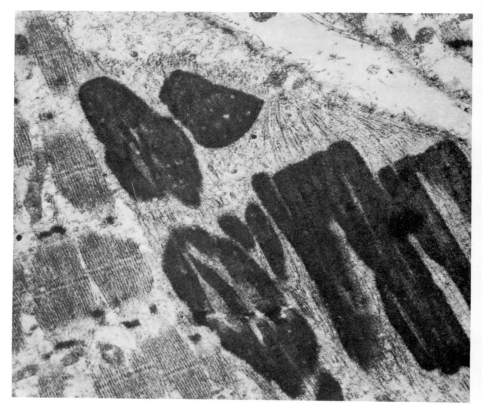

FIG. 158. Electron micrograph of longitudinal section of biceps brachii biopsy, ×25,000, demonstrating electron-dense nemaline rods, lying in the sub-sarcolemmal portion of a muscle fibre. (From Hudgson, P., Gardner-Medwin, D., Fulthorpe, J. J., and Walton, J. N. (1967), *Neurology (Minneap.)*, **17**, 1125. By kind permission of the Editor)

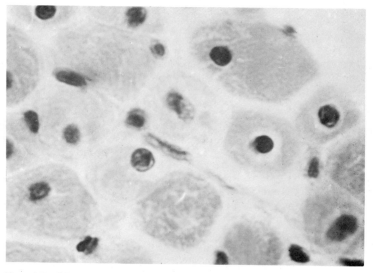

FIG. 159. Myotubular or centronuclear myopathy, transverse section of quadriceps biopsy. H & E, ×960. Note the central nuclei surrounded by clear 'halos' in several muscle fibres

REFERENCES

ADAMS, R. D. (1974) Pathological reactions of the skeletal muscle fibre in man, in *Disorders of Voluntary Muscle*, ed. Walton, J. N., 3rd ed., Edinburgh and London.

ADAMS, R. D. (1975) *Diseases of Muscle*, 3rd ed., New York.

ADAMS, R. D., DENNY-BROWN, D., and PEARSON, C. M. (1962) *Diseases of Muscle, A Study in Pathology*, 2nd ed., New York.

BARWICK, D. D., and WALTON, J. N. (1963) Polymyositis, *Amer. J. Med.*, **35**, 646.

BETHLEM, J. (1970) *Muscle Pathology*, Amsterdam.

BOTELHO, S. Y., DEATERLY, C. F., AUSTIN, S., and COMROE, J. H. (1952) Evaluation of the electromyogram of patients with myasthenia gravis, *Arch. Neurol. Psychiat. (Chic.)*, **67**, 441.

BRADLEY, W. G., HUDGSON, P., GARDNER-MEDWIN, D., and WALTON, J. N. (1969) Myopathy associated with abnormal lipid metabolism in skeletal muscle, *Lancet*, **i**, 495.

BROWN, H. D., CHATTOPADHYAY, S. K., and PATEL, A. B. (1967) Erythrocyte abnormality in human myopathy, *Science*, **157**, 1577.

BROWN, J. C. (1974) Repetitive stimulation and neuromuscular transmission studies, in *Disorders of Voluntary Muscle*, ed. Walton, J. N., 3rd ed., Edinburgh and London.

BUCHTHAL, F. (1962) The electromyogram, *Wld Neurol.*, **3**, 16.

BUCHTHAL, F., and PINELLI, P. (1953) Muscle action potentials in polymyositis, *Neurology (Minneap.)*, **3**, 424.

BUCHTHAL, F., ROSENFALCK, P., and ERMINIO, F. (1960) Motor unit territory and fibre density in myopathies, *Neurology (Minneap.)*, **10**, 398.

CASPARY, E. A., GUBBAY, S. S., and STERN, G. M. (1964) Circulating antibodies in polymyositis and other muscle-wasting disorders, *Lancet*, **ii**, 941.

CAZZATO, G., and WALTON, J. N. (1968) The pathology of the muscle spindle: a study of biopsy material in various muscular and neuromuscular diseases, *J. neurol. Sci.*, **7**, 15.

CROFT, P. B., and WILKINSON, M. (1965) The incidence of carcinomatous neuromyopathy in patients with various types of carcinoma, *Brain*, **88**, 427.

CULLEN, M. J., and FULTHORPE, J. J. (1975) Stages in fibre breakdown in Duchenne muscular dystrophy. An electron microscopic study, *J. neurol. Sci.*, **24**, 179.

DRACHMAN, D. B., MURPHY, S. R., NIGAM, M. P., and HILLS, J. R. (1967) 'Myopathic' changes in chronically denervated muscle, *Arch. Neurol. (Chic.)*, **16**, 14.

DUBOWITZ, V. (1974) Histochemical aspects of muscle disease, in *Disorders of Voluntary Muscle*, ed. Walton, J. N., 3rd ed., Edinburgh and London.

DUBOWITZ, V., and BROOKE, M. H. (1973) *Muscle Biopsy*, London.

EBASHI, S., TOYOKURA, Y., MOMOI, H., and SUGITA, H. (1959) High creatine phosphokinase activity of sera of progressive muscular dystrophy, *J. Biochem. (Tokyo)*, **46**, 103.

EDWARDS, R. H. T. (1971) Percutaneous needle-biopsy of skeletal muscle in diagnosis and research, *Lancet*, **ii**, 593.

ELLIS, D. A., and STRICKLAND, J. M. (1972) Differences in the metabolism of glucose between normal and dystrophic human muscle, *Biochem. J.*, **130**, 17.

ENGEL, A. G., and SIEKERT, R. G. (1972) Lipid storage myopathy responsive to prednisone, *Arch. Neurol. (Chic.)*, **27**, 174.

ENGEL, W. K. (1965) Muscle biopsy, in *Clinical Orthopaedics and Related Research*, ed. De Palma, A. F., London.

FARMER, T. W., BUCHTHAL, F., and ROSENFALCK, P. (1959) Refractory and irresponsive periods of muscle in progressive muscular dystrophy and paresis due to lower motor neurone involvement, *Neurology (Minneap.)*, **9**, 747.

GREENFIELD, J. G., SHY, G. M., ALVORD, E. C., and BERG, L. (1957) *An Atlas of Muscle Pathology in Neuromuscular Diseases*, Edinburgh.

HARVEY, A. M., and MASLAND, R. L. (1941) A method for the study of neuromuscular transmission in human subjects, *Bull. Johns Hopk. Hosp.*, **69**, 1.

HAVARD, C. W. H., CAMPBELL, E. D. R., ROSS, H. B., and SPENCE, A. W. (1963) Electromyographic and histological findings in the muscles of patients with thyrotoxicosis, *Quart. J. Med.*, **32**, 145.

HUDGSON, P., GARDNER-MEDWIN, D., WORSFOLD, M., PENNINGTON, R. J. T., and WALTON, J. N. (1968) Adult myopathy in glycogen storage disease due to acid maltase deficiency, *Brain*, **91**, 435.

HUDGSON, P., and MASTAGLIA, F. L. (1974) Ultrastructural studies of diseased muscle, in *Disorders of Voluntary Muscle*, ed. Walton, J. N., 3rd ed., Edinburgh and London.

IONASESCU, V., ZELLWEGER, H., McCORMICK, W. F., and CONWAY, T. W. (1973) Comparison of ribosomal protein synthesis in Becker and Duchenne muscular dystrophies, *Neurology (Minneap.)*, **23**, 245.

IONASESCU, V., ZELLWEGER, H., SHIRK, P., and CONWAY, T. W. (1972) Abnormal protein synthesis in facioscapulohumeral muscular dystrophy, *Neurology (Minneap.)*, **22**, 1286.

KAKULAS, B. A. (1974) Experimental myopathies, in *Disorders of Voluntary Muscle*, ed. Walton, J. N., 3rd ed., Edinburgh and London.

KUGELBERG, E. (1947) Electromyogram in muscular dystrophy, *J. Neurol. Neurosurg. Psychiat.*, **10**, 122.

LAMBERT, E. H., EATON, L. M., and ROOKE, E. D. (1956) Defect of neuromuscular conduction associated with malignant neoplasms, *Amer. J. Physiol.*, **187**, 612.

LENMAN, J. A. R. (1974) Integration and analysis of the electromyogram and related techniques, in *Disorders of Voluntary Muscle*, ed. Walton, J. N., 3rd ed., Edinburgh and London.

LUMB, E. M., and EMERY, A. E. H. (1975) Erythrocyte deformation in Duchenne muscular dystrophy, *Brit. med. J.*, **3**, 467.

McARDLE, B. (1974) Metabolic and endocrine myopathies, in *Disorders of Voluntary Muscle*, ed. Walton, J. N., 3rd ed., Edinburgh and London.

McCOMAS, A. J., CAMPBELL, M. J., and SICA, R. E. P. (1971) Electrophysiological study of dystrophia myotonica, *J. Neurol. Neurosurg. Psychiat.*, **34**, 132.

McCOMAS, A. J., and JOHNS, R. J. (1974) Potential changes in the normal and diseased muscle cell, in *Disorders of Voluntary Muscle*, ed. Walton, J. N., 3rd ed., Edinburgh and London.

MASTAGLIA, F. L., and WALTON, J. N. (1971) Histological and histochemical changes in skeletal muscle from cases of chronic juvenile and early adult spinal muscular atrophy (the Kugelberg–Welander syndrome), *J. neurol. Sci.*, **12**, 15.

MÜLLER, R., and KUGELBERG, E. (1959) Myopathy in Cushing's syndrome, *J. Neurol. Neurosurg. Psychiat.*, **22**, 314.

PEARCE, G. W. (1965) Histopathology of voluntary muscle, *Postgrad. med. J.*, **41**, 294.

PEARCE, G. W., and WALTON, J. N. (1962) Progressive muscular dystrophy: the histopathological changes in skeletal muscle obtained by biopsy, *J. Path. Bact.*, **83**, 535.

PEARCE, J. M. S., PENNINGTON, R. J. T., and WALTON, J. N. (1964) Serum enzyme studies in muscle disease—Part II: Serum creatine kinase activity in muscular dystrophy and in other myopathic and neuropathic disorders, *J. Neurol. Neurosurg. Psychiat.*, **27**, 96.

PEARSON, C. M. (1957) Serum enzymes in muscular dystrophy and certain other muscular and neuromuscular diseases. I. Serum glutamic oxalacetic transaminase, *New Engl. J. Med.*, **256**, 1069.

PEARSON, C. M. (1962) Histopathological features of muscle in the preclinical stages of muscular dystrophy, *Brain*, **85**, 109.

PEARSON, C. M. (1973) *The Striated Muscle*, Baltimore.

PEARSON, C. M., and CURRIE, S. (1974) Polymyositis and related disorders, in *Disorders of Voluntary Muscle*, ed. Walton, J. N., 3rd ed., Edinburgh and London.

PEARSON, C. M., and YAMAZAKI, J. N. (1958) Vacuolar myopathy in systemic lupus erythematosus, *Amer. J. clin. Path.*, **29**, 455.

PENN, A. S., CLOAK, R. A., and ROWLAND, L. P. (1972) Myosin from normal and dystrophic human muscle, *Arch. Neurol. (Chic.)*, **27**, 159.

PENNINGTON, R. J. T. (1974) Biochemical aspects of muscle disease, in *Disorders of Voluntary Muscle*, ed. Walton, J. N., 3rd ed., Edinburgh and London.

RICHARDSON, A. T., and BARWICK, D. D. (1974) Clinical electromyography, in *Disorders of Voluntary Muscle*, ed. Walton, J. N., 3rd ed., Edinburgh and London.

ROWLAND, L. P., DUNNE, P. B., PENN, A. S., and MAHER, E. (1968) Myoglobin and muscular dystrophy: electrophoretic and immunochemical study, *Arch. Neurol. (Chic.)*, **18**, 141.

RUSSELL, D. S. (1953) Histological changes in the striped muscles in myasthenia gravis, *J. Path. Bact.*, **65**, 279.

SALTER, R. H., ADAMSON, D. G., and PEARCE, G. W. (1968) McArdle's syndrome (myophosphorylase deficiency), *Quart. J. Med.*, **36**, 565.

SAMAHA, F. J. (1973) Actomyosin alterations in Duchenne muscular dystrophy, *Arch. Neurol. (Chic.)*, **28**, 405.

SAMAHA, F. J., and GERGELY, J. (1969) Biochemistry of normal and myotonic dystrophic human myosin, *Arch. Neurol. (Chic.)*, **21**, 200.

SHY, G. M., WANKO, T., ROWLEY, P. T., and ENGEL, A. G. (1961) Studies in familial periodic paralysis, *Exp. Neurol.*, **3**, 53.

SIBLEY, J. A., and LEHNINGER, A. L. (1949) Aldolase in the serum and tissues of tumour-bearing animals, *J. nat. Cancer Inst.*, **9**, 303.

SIMPSON, J. A. (1974) Myasthenia gravis and the myasthenic syndromes, in *Disorders of Voluntary Muscle*, ed. Walton, J. N., 3rd ed., Edinburgh and London.

SWASH, M., and FOX, K. P. (1975) Abnormal intrafusal muscle fibres in myotonic dystrophy: a study using serial sections, *J. Neurol. Neurosurg. Psychiat.*, **38**, 91.

TAKAHASHI, K., OIMOMI, M., SHINKO, T., SHUTTA, K., MATSUO, B., TAKAI, T., and IMURA, H. (1975) Response of serum creatine phosphokinase to steroid hormone, *Arch. Neurol. (Chic.)*, **32**, 89.

WALTON, J. N. (1952) The electromyogram in myopathy: analysis with the audio-frequency spectrometer, *J. Neurol. Neurosurg. Psychiat.*, **15**, 219.

WALTON, J. N. (1957) The limp child, *J. Neurol. Neurosurg. Psychiat.*, **20**, 144.

WALTON, J. N., and ADAMS, R. D. (1958) *Polymyositis*, Edinburgh.

WOHLFART, G. (1951) Dystrophia myotonica and myotonia congenita. Histopathological studies with special reference to changes in muscles, *J. Neuropath. exp. Neurol.*, **10**, 109.

WOOLF, A. L., and COËRS, C. (1974) Pathological anatomy of the intramuscular nerve endings, in *Disorders of Voluntary Muscle*, ed. Walton, J. N., 3rd ed., Edinburgh and London.

20

DISORDERS OF THE AUTONOMIC NERVOUS SYSTEM

THE AUTONOMIC NERVOUS SYSTEM

THE 'autonomic' or 'vegetative' nervous system is the term applied to that part of the nervous system which is concerned in the innervation of unstriated muscle and many of the secretory glands. Physiologically it is divisible into two parts— the sympathetic and the parasympathetic, which to a large extent are mutually antagonistic in function, and employ anatomically separate pathways.

ANATOMY OF THE AUTONOMIC PERIPHERAL NERVES

In the case of both the sympathetic and the parasympathetic nerves two neurones intervene between the central nervous system and the innervated viscus, the efferent path being interrupted at a ganglion. The first neurone, which runs between the central nervous system and the ganglion, is termed *preganglionic*. The second neurone, which runs from the ganglion to the viscus, is termed *postganglionic*.

SYMPATHETIC FIBRES
Efferent Paths

The sympathetic outflow from the central nervous system is limited to the region of the spinal cord lying between the first thoracic and the first lumbar segments inclusive, although rarely there may be sympathetic nerves arising as high as C8 or as low as L3 (Johnson and Spalding, 1974).

Preganglionic Fibres. The preganglionic neurones are ganglion cells situated in the lateral horn of the grey matter of the spinal cord between these levels. The axons of these ganglion cells leave the spinal cord by the corresponding ventral roots and spinal nerves, from which they pass to the corresponding ganglia of the sympathetic chain. The preganglionic fibres are myelinated, and the root by which they pass from the ventral root to the sympathetic ganglion is known as a white ramus. Arrived at the sympathetic ganglion, some preganglionic fibres terminate in the ganglion corresponding to the segment at which they leave the cord. Others pass upwards or downwards in the sympathetic chain, to terminate in ganglia above or below. Others again, passing through the ganglia of the sympathetic chain, emerge to terminate in more peripheral ganglia, the collateral sympathetic ganglia, or sympathetic plexuses, which are usually situated in close relationship with the blood vessels supplying the principal viscera. The most important of such nerves are the splanchnic nerves. The greater splanchnic nerve is derived from the ganglia of the sympathetic chain, from the fifth to the ninth or tenth thoracic segments, and runs to the coeliac plexus; the lesser splanchnic nerve, from the tenth and eleventh thoracic ganglia, goes to the aorticorenal plexus, and the lowest splanchnic nerve, from the eleventh thoracic ganglion, to the renal plexus.

The Sympathetic Chain. The sympathetic chain, which lies close to the vertebral column on either side, consists of a series of sympathetic ganglia possessing for the most part a segmental arrangement, linked together by sympathetic fibres. There are three cervical ganglia—superior, middle, and inferior—eleven thoracic, four lumbar, and four sacral ganglia, all paired, together with one unpaired coccygeal ganglion. Although all the preganglionic fibres emerge from the thoracic and first lumbar segments of the cord, by means of the sympathetic chain they are brought into relationship with spinal nerves throughout the whole length of the vertebral column.

Postganglionic Fibres. The postganglionic sympathetic fibres are unmyelinated. Some arise from ganglion cells in each of the ganglia of the sympathetic chain and pass to the corresponding spinal nerve by a grey ramus, to be distributed to the tissues innervated by this nerve. Other postganglionic fibres take origin in collateral ganglia and pass to the various viscera.

Afferent Paths

Afferent sympathetic fibres, both myelinated and unmyelinated, enter the nervous system by the dorsal roots at all levels, having their ganglion cells in the thoracic root ganglia. There has been much dispute about the function of these 'autonomic afferent' fibres (Johnson and Spalding, 1974) which travel along the efferent fibres, and their very existence has been called into question as much autonomic function is affected by activity in somatic afferent fibres. For practical clinical purposes, the autonomic system is best regarded as being wholly efferent.

PARASYMPATHETIC FIBRES

The parasympathetic is also known as the craniosacral autonomic nervous system because its outflow is situated in the cranial and sacral regions. Unlike the sympathetic system, the ganglia of the parasympathetic are situated in the immediate neighbourhood of the innervated viscera. Thus the preganglionic fibres are long, and the postganglionic short. The principal preganglionic fibres of the cranial parasympathetic pass through the third nerve to the ciliary ganglion, through the seventh to the geniculate, pterygopalatine, submaxillary, and otic ganglia, through the ninth to the otic ganglion, and through the vagus to the ganglia of the thoracic and abdominal viscera supplied by this nerve. The vagus is the most important parasympathetic nerve. Its dorsal motor nucleus is the site of origin of the fibres which innervate the viscera it supplies. The sacral autonomic outflow is derived from the second and third sacral segments, and passes to the vesical plexus by the pelvic splanchnic nerves. The sacral parasympathetic outflow also supplies the enteric plexus of the large gut from the splenic flexure to the anus. The principal afferent fibres of the parasympathetic reach the central nervous system through the vagus nerve, having their ganglion cells in the inferior ganglion of that nerve.

PHYSIOLOGY

The physiology of the autonomic nervous system in respect of various organs is considered below. Certain generalizations which have been made concerning the functions of the sympathetic and the parasympathetic, and their mutual antagonism, must be mentioned.

The sympathetic dilates the pupil, widens the palpebral fissure, and in animals causes proptosis; it increases the heart rate and the conductivity of the atrio-ventricular bundle; it constricts most blood vessels, especially those of the skin and the splanchnic viscera, but dilates the coronary arteries and causes contraction of the spleen; it thus causes a rise of blood pressure and an increased blood flow, especially through the heart, lungs, brain, and muscles; it inhibits peristalsis in the alimentary canal, and promotes contraction of some at least of the sphincters; it is inhibitory to the detrusor muscle of the bladder; it causes erection of the hairs of the skin, and sweating; it excites the secretion of adrenaline, which, by stimulating the sympathetic nerve endings, in turn reinforces sympathetic action, and also raises the blood sugar by liberating sugar from the liver.

The parasympathetic, on the other hand, constricts the pupil, retards the heart and diminishes conductivity in the atrioventricular bundle, dilates the blood vessels of the skin and viscera, constricts the bronchioles, excites the secretion of tears and saliva, promotes peristalsis and inhibits the action of some at least of the alimentary sphincters, promotes contraction of the bladder, through the pelvic splanchnic nerves plays the principal part in sexual activity, and excites secretion of insulin, which lowers the blood sugar.

Whereas most sympathetic nerves are adrenergic (i.e. they act through the release of adrenaline at their nerve endings) and most parasympathetic nerves are cholinergic (acting through the release of acetylcholine) it seems that sudomotor sympathetic nerves (which cause sweating) are cholinergic.

The antagonism between the sympathetic and the parasympathetic was stressed especially by Cannon, who pointed out that the changes produced by sympathetic stimulation are an appropriate preparation for violent activity. The sympathetic has thus been described as an activator for flight or fight, while the parasympathetic presides over anabolic, excretory, and reproductive activities. This is a fair generalization, though in some respects it oversimplifies the facts. Contrary to the long-held view that the intracranial blood vessels are uninfluenced by autonomic activity, evidence is emerging to suggest that the cerebral autonomic nerves may have a homeostatic function, participating in autoregulation by modulating the myogenic tone of the intracranial vessels in response to altered perfusion pressures and distal circulatory demands (Sundt, 1973); for example, a possible role in the pathogenesis of the intracranial arterial spasm which is a common complication of subarachnoid haemorrhage is postulated.

SYMPATHETIC DENERVATION OF THE SKIN

The sympathetic nerve supply to the skin may be interrupted by lesions or surgical division of the outflow from the spinal cord in the white rami or ganglia, or of the peripheral nerves. In either case the area of skin denervated shows loss of (1) pilomotor, (2) vasomotor, and (3) sudomotor activity. (1) The pilomotor reflex consists of the appearance of gooseflesh by the application of cold or the scratch of a pin. (2) Vasomotor paralysis causes flushing, as a result of which the temperature of the denervated area becomes higher than that of the corresponding area on the normal side. This difference may be palpable or may require special methods of thermometry for its determination. (3) Loss of sweating may also be palpable, but is best investigated by applying to the skin a colour-indicator such as chinizarin 2–6-disulphonic acid. The patient is given 300–600 mg of acetylsalicylic acid with one or two cups of hot tea and put under a radiant heat cradle. Where sweating occurs the skin becomes violet, the dry areas remaining light. (For details of this test see Guttmann, 1940.) Alternatively the skin may be painted with the following solution: chemically pure iodine, 1·5–2 g, castor oil, 10 ml, and absolute alcohol to 100 ml, after which fine rice starch powder is dusted on and the test continued as above.

HYPERHIDROSIS

Excessive sweating, e.g. from the palms, may be a congenital abnormality. Localized hyperhidrosis may occur on the face during eating, especially spicy foods—gustatory reflex sweating. Boswell says of Johnson: 'While in the act of eating the veins of his forehead swelled and generally a strong perspiration was visible.' Such gustatory sweating, which may affect only one half of the face, can occur as a congenital abnormality or may sometimes develop for no apparent cause during adult life; it can often be relieved by the use of propantheline. The 'syndrome of crocodile tears', in which lacrimation occurs during eating, may follow facial paralysis and is presumed to be due to the fact that during nerve fibre regeneration, parasympathetic fibres intended for the salivary glands are misdirected to the lacrimal gland. Flushing and hyperhidrosis in the temple may occur after injury in the region of the parotid gland—the auriculotemporal syndrome. Hyperhidrosis is also seen in the distribution of a cutaneous nerve which is the site of a partial lesion, as in causalgia. Cerebral lesions causing hemiplegia may lead to excessive sweating on the paralysed half of the body.

When necessary, hyperhidrosis can be treated by sympathectomy.

CLINICAL TESTS OF AUTONOMIC FUNCTION

Tests in common clinical use in order to assess the integrity of the autonomic nervous system are reviewed in detail by Johnson and Spalding (1974). Among those in common use are the following:

Sympathetic Nervous System

The sweating response to an induced rise in body temperature is described above; this does not test the afferent side of the reflex arc concerned with sympathetic sudomotor activity and is not a reliable test for integrity of the sympathetic nervous system as a whole as sudomotor activity may be intact when vasomotor activity is impaired and vice versa.

Much more important therefore in determining whether there is widespread reflex vasomotor paralysis are tests involving the accurate measurement of arterial blood pressure and its response to various stresses, including change in posture (in the normal individual the blood pressure usually rises slightly on assuming the erect posture, while in patients with sympathetic denervation there is a marked fall). Valsalva's manœuvre (a deep inspiration followed by an attempted forcible expiration against a closed glottis) produces a four-phase response in normal individuals and this is blocked and normally replaced simply by a temporary fall in blood pressure in patients with autonomic failure (as in orthostatic hypotension—see below).

In attempting to determine whether the afferent or efferent pathways of the sympathetic reflex arc are involved, recording of blood pressure after a sudden loud noise, during intense mental concentration, or after the application of an ice-pack to the skin may sometimes be helpful, as a rise in response to any of these stimuli indicates that the efferent pathway is functioning and that any lesion is likely to be on the afferent side. These tests, however, are not very reliable, as a negative response to each stimulus is sometimes obtained in normal individuals.

The 'flare' response, which is particularly useful in determining the site of the lesion in injury to spinal roots or peripheral nerves, is described on page 895. Investigation of thermoregulatory mechanisms and especially of bodily adaptation to extremes of heat or cold requires sophisticated equipment and can rarely be utilized in clinical practice.

The Parasympathetic Nervous System

As the arterial blood pressure rises, the heart rate usually falls due to a parasympathetic baroreceptor reflex and its integrity can be well tested by carrying out Valsalva's manœuvre (see above) during which the heart rate and blood pressure show an inverse relationship. The integrity of vagal function upon the heart may also be tested by pressure upon the carotid sinus or eyeball which normally produces reflex bradycardia (though these tests must be used with caution as cardiac arrest rarely occurs) or by the use of drugs such as atropine which inhibit vagal activity.

REFERENCES

GUTTMANN, L. (1940) Topographic studies of disturbances of sweat secretion after complete lesions of peripheral nerves, *J. Neurol. Psychiat.*, N.S., **3**, 197.
JOHNSON, R. H., and SPALDING, J. M. K. (1974) *Disorders of the Autonomic Nervous System*, Oxford.
SUNDT, T. M. (1973) The cerebral autonomic nervous system: a proposed physiologic function and pathophysiologic response in subarachnoid hemorrhage and in focal cerebral ischemia, *Mayo Clin. Proc.*, **48**, 127.

DISORDERS OF AUTONOMIC FUNCTION

Among the disorders of autonomic function which are seen from time to time in clinical practice are drug-induced syndromes occurring, for instance, during the treatment of Parkinsonism, page 593; abnormalities of the pupils such as Adie's syndrome, page 94; conditions such as Hirschsprung's disease due to lesions of the myenteric plexus; autonomic manifestations of polyneuropathy including the autonomic neuropathy of diabetes; and five types of disorder or phenomena deserving brief attention here, including autonomic dysfunction in lesions of the spinal cord, the role of the autonomic nervous system in the mechanisms of referred pain, familial dysautonomia, idiopathic orthostatic hypotension, and acute autonomic neuropathy.

DISTURBANCES OF THE FUNCTIONS OF THE AUTONOMIC NERVOUS SYSTEM AFTER LESIONS OF THE SPINAL CORD

The difference in the distribution of the sympathetic and somatic nervous outflow from the spinal cord accounts for the occurrence in many cases of a difference in the distribution of the sympathetic and somatic (motor and sensory) disturbances after lesions of the spinal cord. Since the sympathetic outflow to the whole body leaves the cord below the eighth cervical spinal segment, lesions at and above this level may cause a disturbance of sympathetic function over the whole body, though the motor and sensory innervation of the head and neck and of a part of the upper limbs remains undisturbed. At the mid-thoracic level of the cord the upper levels of the sympathetic and somatic disturbances approximately coincide. When the lesion of the cord is situated below the first lumbar spinal segment the somatic innervation is alone affected, the sympathetic outflow leaving the cord entirely above the lesion. The following disturbances of sympathetic function are found in cases of complete transection of the cord and in cases of less severe lesions which interrupt the intraspinal paths of the sympathetic. The pilomotor reflex elicited by a massive stimulus applied to the skin above the level of the lesion does not extend to areas innervated by parts of the cord below the lesion, but the reflex is excitable from these regions after the disappearance of spinal shock. The cutaneous temperature over the paralysed parts is higher than over normal parts of the body and vasoconstriction in response to exposure of the whole body to cold is diminished below the level of the lesion. Dermographism is diminished at the level of the lesion but usually somewhat increased below. Orthostatic hypotension may occur in cervical cord lesions but adaptation to repeated changes in posture frequently occurs (Johnson et al., 1969). [See also section on Compression of the Spinal Cord, p. 744.]

SWEATING

Excessive sweating after complete division of the spinal cord usually appears over parts of the body which are thus separated from the control of higher autonomic centres. Such sweating develops *pari passu* with the recovery of other reflex functions in the divided cord. It varies in intensity from time to time and may be reflexly excited by cutaneous stimuli, flexor spasms of the lower limbs, distension of the bladder, and exposure to heat.

Disturbances of sweating are rarely observed after partial lesions of the spinal cord, except in syringomyelia. In this disease loss of sweating may occur when the sympathetic ganglion cells in the lateral horns of grey matter are destroyed, and is most often seen over the face and upper limb. Excessive sweating with a similar distribution may, however, occur, sometimes spontaneously and sometimes being excited reflexly when the patient takes hot or highly seasoned food.

THE AUTONOMIC NERVOUS SYSTEM AND PAIN

REFERRED PAIN

Since most viscera are innervated only by the autonomic nervous system, it follows that the sensation of visceral pain must be mediated by afferent autonomic fibres, or at least by afferent fibres which travel with the sympathetic nerves. The remarkable lack of definitive information about the afferent functions of the autonomic nervous system and about the role played by the sympathetic in pain syndromes is underlined by Melzack (1972) who concluded that 'the sympathetic nervous system *contributes*, in some way, to all of these pain states'. The most potent cause of visceral pain is an increase in the tension of the viscus. Visceral pain is a diffuse and poorly localized sensation, and is frequently associated with pain referred to, and tenderness of, the superficial tissues of the body over an area which is innervated by the same segments of the nervous system as the painful viscus. The physiological explanation of referred pain is uncertain. It has been attributed to a heightened excitability of the fibres and synapses concerned in pain conduction in the spinal cord, which receives impulses from the segments innervating the viscus, and also to a branching of axons, so that the same fibre supplies both somatic and visceral structures (Sinclair *et al.*, 1948). The 'gate theory' [see p. 39 and Melzack, 1973] provides an even more plausible explanation but remains unproven. Referred pain may or may not be accompanied by cutaneous 'hyperalgesia'.

One of the commonest examples of referred pain is that associated with disease of the coronary arteries, such as occurs in angina pectoris. In angina, pain is usually referred into the third, fourth, and fifth cervical and first, second, and third thoracic segments on the left side and often into the same or a somewhat similar area on the right side. Sometimes the pain is referred to the lower jaw.

The autonomic nervous system sometimes provides an alternative path for painful sensations from areas deprived of their somatic sensory nerves. When pain can be evoked in such circumstances the painful impulse may be conducted to the central nervous system by somatic afferents which accompany the autonomic nerves supplying the blood vessels. Certainly the pain sensation which occurs as a consequence of the vasodilatation of intracranial or extracranial arteries (as in migraine) is conveyed by somatic afferent fibres from the walls of the blood vessels. Sympathectomy is also performed for causalgia; the pathogenesis of this disorder is considered on page 891. Similarly, sympathectomy relieves pain in the disorder variously referred to as 'the shoulder-hand syndrome' or 'reflex dystrophy of the upper extremity' (Pak *et al.*, 1970) in which painful swelling of the hand, often with atrophy of bone (Sudeck's atrophy) occurs, usually in association with pericapsulitis of the shoulder joint (a 'frozen shoulder').

REFERENCES

JOHNSON, R. H., SMITH, A. C., and SPALDING, J. M. K. (1969) Blood pressure response to standing and to Valsalva's manœuvre: independence of the two mechanisms in neurological diseases including cervical cord lesions, *Clin. Sci.*, **36,** 77.

JOHNSON, R. H., and SPALDING, J. M. K. (1974) *Disorders of the Autonomic Nervous System*, Oxford.

MELZACK, R. (1972) Mechanisms of pathological pain, in *Scientific Foundations of Neurology*, ed. Critchley, M., O'Leary, J. L., and Jennett, W. B., London.

MELZACK, R. (1973) *The Puzzle of Pain*, Harmondsworth, Middlesex.

PAK, T. J., MARTIN, G. M., MAGNESS, J. L., and KAVANAUGH, G. L. (1970) Reflex sympathetic dystrophy. Review of 140 cases, *Minn. Med.*, **53,** 507.

SINCLAIR, D. C., WEDDELL, G., and FEINDEL, W. H. (1948) Referred pain and associated phenomena, *Brain*, **71,** 184.

FAMILIAL DYSAUTONOMIA

Familial dysautonomia (the Riley–Day syndrome) is a rare disorder occurring mainly in Jewish children and inherited by an autosomal recessive mechanism. Clinically it is characterized by defective lacrimation, hyperhidrosis, episodic hypertension, hyperpyrexia and vomiting, and attacks of epilepsy. Most patients also show dysphagia, ageusia, areflexia and a relative insensitivity to pain sensation and they die as a rule from respiratory infection or uraemia in infancy or childhood. The condition appears to be due to an inborn error of catecholamine metabolism which results in the excretion of homovanillic acid in the urine (Smith *et al.*, 1963). The presence of parasympathetic denervation is confirmed by the instillation of 2·5 per cent methacholine into the eye; this produces miosis (Dancis and Smith, 1966). An abnormality of sensory nerve conduction, with two discrete peaks of differing latency, has been described in such cases (Brown and Johns, 1967); on sural nerve biopsy there is a marked reduction in the number of unmyelinated fibres and of heavily myelinated fibres (Aguayo *et al.*, 1971) and at autopsy there may be focal demyelination in the posterior roots and posterior columns of the spinal cord (Fogelson *et al.*, 1967).

REFERENCES

AGUAYO, A. J., NAIR, C. P. V., and BRAY, G. M. (1971) Peripheral nerve abnormalities in the Riley–Day syndrome, *Arch. Neurol. (Chic.)*, **24**, 106.

BROWN, J. C., and JOHNS, R. J. (1967) Nerve conduction in familial dysautonomia (Riley–Day syndrome), *J. Amer. med. Ass.*, **201**, 200.

DANCIS, J., and SMITH, A. A. (1966) Familial dysautonomia, *New Engl. J. Med.*, **274**, 207.

FOGELSON, M. H., RORKE, L. B., and KAYE, R. (1967) Spinal cord changes in familial dysautonomia, *Arch. Neurol. (Chic.)*, **17**, 103.

RILEY, C. M., DAY, R. L., GREELY, D. M., and LANGFORD, N. S. (1949) Central autonomic dysfunction with defective lacrimation. Report of five cases, *Pediatrics*, **3**, 468.

SMITH, A. A., TAYLOR, T., and WORTIS, S. B. (1963) Abnormal catechol amine metabolism in familial dysautonomia, *New Engl. J. Med.*, **268**, 705.

IDIOPATHIC ORTHOSTATIC HYPOTENSION

This condition (the so-called Shy–Drager syndrome) has already been mentioned on page 321. The most striking clinical manifestations of this disorder are postural hypotension with syncope on standing and loss of the normal autonomic reflexes (Chokroverty *et al.*, 1969; Thomas and Schirger, 1970). Anhidrosis, impotence, dysuria, and disorders of bowel function are common (Martin *et al.*, 1968), there may be undue sensitivity to nicotine (Graham and Oppenheimer, 1972), an increased plasma renin accounting for supine hypertension (Love *et al.*, 1971), and evidence of cerebral dysautoregulation (Meyer *et al.*, 1973). Many patients also show Parkinsonian features or cerebellar ataxia and dementia develops rarely. Pathologically there is degeneration of dorsal vagal nuclei and of the cells of the intermediolateral column in the spinal cord, while Lewy bodies identical with those seen in idiopathic Parkinsonism are found in some cases in the substantia nigra (Vanderhaeghen *et al.*, 1970; Thapedi *et al.*, 1971; Bannister and Oppenheimer, 1972) and the pathological changes of striatonigral degeneration have also been reported (Schober *et al.*, 1975).

REFERENCES

BANNISTER, R., and OPPENHEIMER, D. R. (1972) Degenerative diseases of the nervous system associated with autonomic failure, *Brain*, **95**, 457.

CHOKROVERTY, S., BARRON, K. D., KATZ, F. H., DEL GRECO, F., and SHARP, J. T. (1969) The syndrome of primary orthostatic hypotension, *Brain*, **92**, 743.

GRAHAM, J. G., and OPPENHEIMER, D. R. (1969) Orthostatic hypotension and nicotine sensitivity in a case of multiple system atrophy, *J. Neurol. Neurosurg. Psychiat.*, **32**, 28.

LOVE, D. R., BROWN, J. J., CHINN, R. H., JOHNSON, R. H., LEVER, A. F., PARK, D. M., and ROBERTSON, J. I. S. (1971) Plasma renin in idiopathic orthostatic hypotension: differential response in subjects with probable afferent and efferent autonomic failure, *Clin. Sci.*, **41**, 289.

MARTIN, J. B., TRAVIS, R. H., and VAN DEN NOORT, S. (1968) Centrally mediated orthostatic hypotension, *Arch. Neurol. (Chic.)*, **19**, 163.

MEYER, J. S., SHIMAZU, K., FUKUUCHI, Y., OHUCHI, T., OKAMOTO, S., KOTO, A., and ERICSSON, A. D. (1973) Cerebral dysautoregulation in central neurogenic orthostatic hypotension (Shy–Drager syndrome), *Neurology (Minneap.)*, **23**, 262.

SCHOBER, R., LANGSTON, J. W., and FORNO, L. S. (1975) Idiopathic orthostatic hypotension: biochemical and pathologic observations in 2 cases, *Europ. Neurol.*, **13**, 177.

THAPEDI, I. M., ASHENHURST, E. M., and ROZDILSKY, B. (1971) Shy–Drager syndrome: report of an autopsied case, *Neurology (Minneap.)*, **21**, 26.

THOMAS, J. E., and SCHIRGER, A. (1970) Idiopathic orthostatic hypotension: a study of its natural history in 57 neurologically affected patients, *Arch. Neurol. (Chic.)*, **22**, 289.

VANDERHAEGHEN, J. J., PERIER, O., and STERNON, J. E. (1970) Pathological findings in idiopathic orthostatic hypotension: its relationship with Parkinson's disease, *Arch. Neurol. (Chic.)*, **22**, 207.

ACUTE AUTONOMIC NEUROPATHY

This rare, unexplained disorder (Thomashefsky *et al.*, 1972; Hopkins *et al.*, 1974), has been described as presenting in childhood or adult life with an acute onset and variable features of autonomic paralysis including postural hypotension, paralysis of accommodation, anhidrosis, loss of lacrimation, and urinary and faecal retention. Most reported cases have shown spontaneous recovery after a few weeks or months. Young *et al.* (1975) described such a case under the title of 'pure pan-dysautonomia with recovery'.

REFERENCES

HOPKINS, A., NEVILLE, B., and BANNISTER, R. (1974) Autonomic neuropathy of acute onset, *Lancet*, **i**, 769.

THOMASHEFSKY, A. J., HORWITZ, S. J., and FEINGOLD, M. H. (1972) Acute autonomic neuropathy, *Neurology (Minneap.)*, **22**, 251.

YOUNG, R. R., ASBURY, A. K., CORBETT, J. L., and ADAMS, R. D. (1975) Pure pan-dysautonomia with recovery—description and discussion of diagnostic criteria, *Brain*, **98**, 613.

AUTONOMIC AND METABOLIC CENTRES

Recent increase in knowledge has made this subject a vast and complex one. For details readers are referred to reviews by Harris and Donovan (1966), Blackwell and Guilliman (1973), Handler and Orloff (1973), Hayward (1975), Daniel and Prichard (1975), and Guyton (1976). Here it is possible to give only a brief summary, and to deal more particularly with points of special clinical importance.

ANATOMY

The autonomic nervous system and many metabolic functions are under the control of nerve centres, many of which are situated in the hypothalamus. This is the region of the brain lying ventrally to the thalamus and constituting the floor of the third ventricle. The most important part of the hypothalamus is the tuber cinereum, which forms part of the floor of the third ventricle and extends from the optic chiasm anteriorly to the corpora mammillaria behind. In the centre of the tuber is the infundibulum, from which rises the stalk of the pituitary. The hypothalamus contains a large number of scattered ganglion cells, which have been differentiated into a number of nuclei. The nuclei themselves are arranged in three groups and there is some evidence that a functional differentiation corresponds to this anatomical arrangement. The following are the principal nuclei of the preoptic area and the hypothalamus (Le Gros Clark, 1948):

Preoptic Area   Medial Preoptic nucleus.
                                  Lateral Preoptic nucleus.

Hypothalamus—
Pars Supraoptica
Hypothalami   Nucleus Supraopticus.
                                  Nucleus Paraventricularis.
                                  Nucleus Suprachiasmaticus.

Nucleus Hypothalamicus Anterior

Pars Tuberalis
Hypothalami   Nucleus Hypothalamicus Dorsomedialis.
                                  Nucleus Hypothalamicus Ventromedialis.
                                  Nucleus Arcuatus.
                                  Nucleus Hypothalamicus Lateralis.

Nucleus Hypothalamicus Posterior

Pars Mammillaris
Hypothalami   Nucleus Mammillaris Medialis.
                                  Nucleus Mammillaris Lateralis.
                                  Nucleus Intercalatus.
                                  Nucleus Premammillaris.
                                  Nucleus Supramammillaris.

The projections of the hypothalamus are not yet completely known. The following tracts, however, are probably of special importance. From the supraoptic nucleus arises a tract which terminates in the pars intermedia and the posterior lobe of the hypophysis. The fornix system runs from the hippocampus to the mammillary region and the mammillothalamic tract (bundle of Vicq d'Azyr) runs from the mammillary body to the anterior nucleus of the thalamus. There are also both efferent and afferent tracts running between the mammillary body and the midbrain.

The hypothalamus is richly supplied with blood from the vessels of the circle of Willis.

The importance of the frontal lobe for autonomic function has recently been established. Its anatomical relations with the hypothalamus are described by Le Gros Clark (1948): their functional relationships are discussed by Fulton (1949) and Jacobson (1972). Respiratory and vasomotor changes can be evoked from area 13, incision of the posterior part of area 14 on both sides causes 'sham rage' in monkeys [see p. 1146], and removal of area 24, the anterior cingulate gyrus, renders monkeys unusually tame and alters their social adjustments [see FIG. 160 and p. 1147]. In man there is evidence of descending input from the hippocampus, amygdala, and cingulate cortex as well as from the frontal corticohypothalamic fibres (Jacobson, 1972).

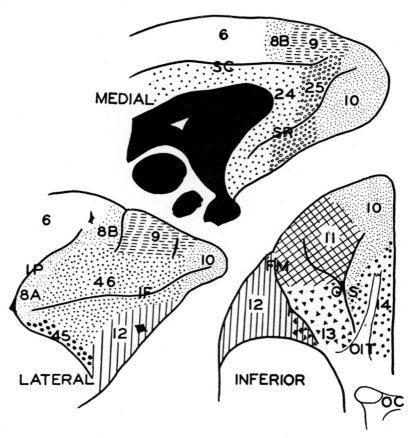

FIG. 160. A map of the cyto-architectural areas of the prefrontal cortex (from Walker, 1940)

THE FUNCTIONS OF THE HYPOTHALAMUS

The functions of the hypothalamus have been investigated by means of stimulation and experimental lesions. The posterior and lateral hypothalamus is an important centre for the activity of the sympathetic nervous system—the dynamogenic or ergotropic zone of Hess (1954). Stimulation of the posterior hypothalamus causes an increase of the heart rate, rise of blood pressure, dilatation of the pupil, erection of the hair, and inhibition of movements of the gut and of the tone of the bladder. The nuclei of the posterior hypothalamus are also responsible for the massive reaction known as 'sham rage' which occurs in animals when this region has been released from higher control. Destruction of this area, on the other hand, causes lethargy and parasomnia.

The nuclei of the tuber, on the other hand, appear to be concerned with the functions of the parasympathetic—the endophylactic or trophotropic zone of Hess. Stimulation of this region causes slowing of the heart rate and increase in the atrioventricular conduction time. There is also an increase in the peristaltic movements of the stomach and of the tone of the bladder. Lesions of this region may cause haemorrhagic erosions of the mucosa of the body of the stomach. The hypothalamus influences the release of gonadotrophic hormones from the pituitary, and adiposogenital dystrophy, characterized by great obesity and genital atrophy, may be produced by experimental lesions of the tuber.

The hypothalamus is also concerned with the regulation of the temperature of the body, in which shivering, sweating, vasoconstriction, and vasodilatation as well as other factors play a part. In the anterior hypothalamus there is a centre for regulating heat loss, and lesions in this area may cause hyperthermia. There is a centre concerned with regulating heat production and conservation so that lesions in this area may produce a state in which the body temperature of the individual matches that of the environment, thus varying according to the ambient temperature (poikilothermia). The role of the hypothalamus in carbohydrate metabolism is not completely understood, but glycosuria, which is usually transitory, may follow lesions of this region. The hypothalamus is also concerned in water and sleep regulation. Thus it appears that cells of the supraoptic nuclei form antidiuretic hormone (ADH) (or its precursors) which then travels down the axons into the posterior pituitary, being subsequently stored in the gland in the form of neurosecretory granules. The hypothalamus exerts its control over the sleep cycle by virtue of its input from the cerebral cortex and its output to the reticular system. The posterior hypothalamus, including the mammillary body, is important in this regard and lesions here may cause hypersomnia or reversal of the sleep rhythm, while anterior hypothalamic lesions may give insomnia (see Haymaker et al., 1969; Jacobson, 1972).

The Relationship between the Hypothalamus and the Pituitary (Hypophysis)

An important part of the influence of the hypothalamus upon bodily functions is exerted through the pituitary. Its anterior lobe is thus under nervous control though it has no nerve supply. This paradox is explained by the hypophysial portal venous system, through which humoral substances secreted by nerve cells in the hypothalamus are conveyed to, and excite, the pituitary. Thus electrical stimulation of the hypothalamus excites gonadotrophic, adrenocorticotrophic, somatotrophic, lactogenic, and thyrotrophic hypophysial secretion while direct electrical stimulation of the gland itself has no such effect. The posterior lobe of the pituitary gland (the neurohypophysis), unlike the anterior, is under direct nervous control, receiving a direct input from the paraventricular nuclei concerned especially with autonomic activity as described above, and from the supraoptic nucleus which is especially concerned with the secretion of vasopressin (antidiuretic hormone). Oxytocin is also produced in the periventricular nucleus and is carried down the axons of the hypothalamo-hypophyseal tract into the posterior hypophysis. Secretion of this hormone stimulates contraction of the lactating mammary gland and of the pregnant uterus; it also has a mild antidiuretic effect.

Disorders of the anterior lobe of the pituitary have been reviewed recently by Nelson (1974) and those of the neurohypophysis by Dingman and Thorn (1974).

SYNDROMES OF THE HYPOTHALAMUS

ADIPOSITY

Adiposity, which is generally associated with genital hypoplasia or atrophy, may occur as a symptom of a variety of pathological states involving either the hypothalamus or the hypophysis, or both of these structures.

1. *Chromophobe adenoma of the pituitary* may produce it [see p. 276].
2. *Tumours above the pituitary*, especially craniopharyngiomas [see p. 278].
3. *Internal hydrocephalus* from any cause may lead to obesity and genital hypoplasia as a result of distension of the floor of the third ventricle which compresses the sella turcica and the pituitary. In this way the syndrome may result from a tumour remote from the sella turcica, for example a tumour of the cerebellum. More often, however, it is secondary to aqueduct stenosis or communicating hydrocephalus.

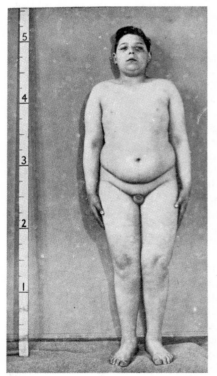

FIG. 161. Adiposogenital dystrophy in a boy aged 11; weight, 70 kg

4. The syndrome may be produced by *infective conditions of the nervous system*, especially by encephalitis lethargica and, rarely, basal syphilitic meningitis. Granulomatous meningitis, say in sarcoidosis, may have a similar effect.

5. *Idiopathic adiposogenital dystrophy.* In most cases of this syndrome, including those in which the disturbance of function is most marked, none of the above causes can be held responsible. The disorder appears to be present from birth, and it is usually noticed at an early age that the child is exceptionally fat [FIG. 161]. Both sexes are affected, though boys appear to suffer more often than girls. The cheeks are rosy, and the skin is soft and hairless, except on the scalp. In these cases obesity is often associated with skeletal overgrowth, the child being unusually tall as well as exceptionally fat. There is often a marked genital hypoplasia, though exceptionally genital function may be normal. This is the case more often in females than in males. Sugar tolerance is usually increased. Polyuria, lethargy, and narcolepsy are infrequent associated symptoms. There is no evidence of a lesion involving the visual paths and the sella turcica is radiographically normal. These negative findings,

together with the early onset, render it possible to distinguish the idiopathic variety of adiposogenital dystrophy (Fröhlich's syndrome) from other conditions of which similar disturbances are symptomatic.

CACHEXIA (DIENCEPHALIC WASTING)

Cachexia is much less frequently encountered as a symptom of a lesion of the hypothalamus than obesity. It is occasionally produced, however, by suprasellar tumours and is common in the advanced stages of Parkinsonism due to encephalitis lethargica. A hypothalamic syndrome causing severe wasting in infancy and childhood has also been described (Russell, 1951; White and Ross, 1963; Gamstorp, 1972). Symptoms appear as a rule in the first two years of life; the child shows rapid longitudinal growth with emaciation and almost total lack of subcutaneous fat despite an adequate food intake and no evidence of malabsorption. The children are alert, often hyperactive and sometimes euphoric with retraction of the upper eyelids and a 'surprised' expression (Gamstorp, 1972). Often the CSF protein content is raised and in most cases a tumour of the diencephalon is found, or an optic nerve glioma extending posteriorly, but the syndrome has been reported without a demonstrable tumour (Bain et al., 1966).

SEXUAL FUNCTIONS

Failure of the sexual functions to develop at the normal age, or retrogression after normal development, may be the result of lesions either of the hypothalamus or of the hypophysis. Sexual infantilism, or, in the adult, impotence or amenorrhoea, according to sex, is then usually associated with obesity as described in the last section.

Sexual precocity is much rarer. It may be a symptom either of endocrine or of nervous disorder. In the endocrine sphere it may be produced by tumours of the ovary, testis, or suprarenal. Pineal tumours cause sexual precocity in a proportion of cases, almost exclusively in males [see p. 275], but sexual precocity may also be produced by other tumours of the midbrain and by hydrocephalus from any cause. It has also been reported after encephalitis lethargica and in association with tuberous sclerosis and suprasellar tumours, as well as in rare cases of glioma of the hypothalamus.

So far we have been considering bodily changes in the reproductive organs resulting from disease of the nervous system. Loss of sexual desire without concurrent bodily change may be encountered in patients with a tumour involving the base of the brain and sometimes occurs after head injury, and in association with extensive destructive cerebral lesions of any kind. Excessive libido, on the other hand, may be experienced by patients in whom a tumour or a more diffuse lesion, such as general paresis in an early stage, diminishes inhibition.

Impotence implies a condition in the male in which sexual desire is normal but the patient cannot achieve an erection of the penis adequate for sexual intercourse. Erection of the penis and ejaculation of semen depend in the first instance upon the integrity of reflex arcs at the sacral level of the spinal cord. Injury to these reflex arcs, such as may occur in tabes, spina bifida, or a tumour or injury of the cauda equina, may cause impotence. Since, however, higher centres also play a part in the sexual act, impotence may be produced by lesions of the spinal cord at a higher level, as, for example, in multiple sclerosis. If the nervous system is normal and there is no debilitating general disease, impotence is usually neurotic in origin. Simple anxiety may cause impotence, which may be associated with ejaculatio praecox, which is explained by the fact that the sympathetic nervous system, which is over-active during anxiety, is inhibitory to erection of the penis but motor to the vesiculae seminales. Often, however, the cause of neurotic impotence lies deeply in the personality and can only be exposed by psychological analysis.

DIABETES INSIPIDUS

Mode of Production. It has been shown experimentally that diabetes insipidus follows bilateral destruction of the supra-optic nuclei, or removal of the posterior lobe of the pituitary and its stalk. The subject has been reviewed by Kuhlenbeck (1954), who discussed the complex relations between the hypothalamus, the hypophysis, and the hypophysioportal circulation, by Campbell and Dickinson (1960) and by Dingman and Thorn (1974). The antidiuretic hormone (ADH) is produced by the nerve cells of the supra-optic and paraventricular nuclei, and reaches the neurohypophysis by their descending tracts. The hormone is necessary for the resorption of water by the renal tubules. There are two separate hormones secreted by the neurosecretory granules of the posterior pituitary, namely vasopressin and oxytocin. Vasopressin has substantial pressor (blood-pressure raising) and antidiuretic effects and mild oxytocic effects, while oxytocin, as mentioned above, causes ejection of milk from the breast and uterine contraction but is also mildly antidiuretic. Commercial pituitary extracts (e.g. Pitocin) contain both oxytocin and vasopressin. The peptide structure of both hormones is now known and both have been synthesized (de Vigneaud, 1956). When we speak of ADH we normally mean vasopressin, but often the term is used to apply to situations in which both vasopressin and oxytocin are acting. However, diabetes insipidus strictly means vasopressin deficiency.

The secretion of ADH is excited by an increase in plasma osmolality, and by a reduction in the circulating blood volume, and emotional stimuli: it is inhibited by a decrease in plasma osmolality and a rise in circulating blood volume.

Aetiology. Diabetes insipidus usually occurs as a result of lesions involving either the tuber cinereum or the neurohypophysis, though in the latter case the polyuria is usually less severe than in the former. Tuberal lesions responsible for diabetes insipidus include trauma, ranging from gunshot wounds of the suprahypophysial region to closed head injury with concussion, basal meningitis, which is usually syphilitic but may be due to sarcoidosis, torula or a variety of other causes, epidemic encephalitis, cerebral malaria, internal hydrocephalus, and tumours of the third ventricle; and the syndrome may be produced by primary and secondary neoplasms and tuberculoma of the hypophysis. It may also occur in essential xanthomatosis.

Symptoms. Diabetes insipidus causes extreme thirst and the passage of large volumes of urine of low specific gravity, amounting in severe cases to several gallons a day. Sleep is disturbed by thirst and the necessity for frequent micturition. Excessive hunger is a rare accompaniment. There are several tests for diabetes insipidus (see Campbell and Dickinson, 1960), of which the simplest is that water deprivation does not lead to release of ADH and hence the specific gravity of the urine does not rise above 1,014. Full details of the dehydration test, the vasopressin test, and the hypertonic saline test are given by Dingman and Thorn (1974). The nicotine test, which involves assessment of the antidiuretic effect of smoking cigarettes after a period of initial hydration, in order to assess the stimulant effect of nicotine upon the cells of the supraoptic nucleus, is also helpful in some cases.

Diagnosis. The polyuria of diabetes insipidus must be distinguished from that which occurs in other conditions, especially renal failure, hereditary nephrogenic diabetes insipidus [p. 837], and psychogenic compulsive water-drinking (de Wardener and Barlow, 1958). The last is prone to occur in middle-aged women, who show a low plasma osmolality in contrast to the high one of diabetes insipidus, and fail to respond to vasopressin.

Prognosis. The prognosis of diabetes insipidus is considerably influenced by the nature of the causative lesion. Polyuria following encephalitis lethargica was rarely severe. There were often marked fluctuations in the urinary output from day to day, and spontaneous recovery often occurred. In syphilitic cases and in sarcoidosis benefit may follow appropriate treatment. When the cause is tumour or hydrocephalus, relief may follow if the primary disorder can be treated surgically.

Prognosis in traumatic cases is uncertain. Some patients improve or recover after a few months: in others the disorder is permanent.

Treatment. In severe cases, pitressin (partially purified vasopressin) affords the only palliative treatment. Nasal insufflation of posterior lobe extract may be tried but is sometimes ineffective. Often it is necessary to inject vasopressin (0·1–0·2 ml of a preparation containing 20 I.U. of pressor activity/ml) sub-cutaneously to obtain a few hours' relief from the polyuria and thirst. It may be necessary to give more than one dose during the day. If one dose only is given, it should be administered at bedtime, in order to ensure several hours' sleep. Vasopressin tannate in oil, of which the usual nocturnal dose is 1 ml (containing 5 I.U.) given by intramuscular injection, is more slowly acting.

DISTURBANCES OF SLEEP

The role of the hypothalamus in the normal regulation of sleep is still uncertain, but clinical experience shows that lesions in the region of the tuber cinereum may lead either to persistent somnolence or to paroxysmal attacks of sleep similar to those occurring in idiopathic narcolepsy [see p. 1154].

It has been suggested that a syndrome of periodic hypersomnolence and megaphagia which usually occurs in adolescent males (the Kleine-Levin syndrome, see p. 1157) is of hypothalamic origin but the aetiology is not yet known. The physiopathology of sleep disorders has recently been reviewed by Dement et al. (1975). Sleep-like coma has been reported due to lesions of the posterior hypothalamus (Plum and Posner, 1972).

OTHER HYPOTHALAMIC DISTURBANCES

Sugar Metabolism. The disturbances of sugar metabolism which have been produced by experimental lesions of the hypothalamus find a clinical counter-part in the occurrence of glycosuria as a result of lesions of this part of the brain. Glycosuria is most often seen in patients with a tumour in the region of the hypothalamus or the fourth ventricle. It is more often due to a lowered renal threshold than to hyperglycaemia. 'Cerebral glycosuria' may also occur after head injury and spontaneous subarachnoid haemorrhage, and in meningitis and encephalitis.

Temperature Regulation. Irregular pyrexia may occur in patients with a lesion in the region of the tuber cinereum, and the hyperpyrexia which not uncommonly follows operations in this region is probably the result of injury to a hypothalamic temperature-regulating mechanism [see p. 1077].

Ulceration of the Alimentary Canal. Many years ago Schiff demonstrated that lesions in the neighbourhood of the hypothalamus were followed by acute ulceration of the upper part of the alimentary canal, and this has since been confirmed. Perforating ulcers may thus be produced in the oesophagus, stomach, and duodenum of experimental animals. Cushing drew attention to the occurrence of similar ulceration in man, as a rare sequel of head injury and cerebral operations, and it may also follow operation on the spinal cord.

Respiratory Disturbances. There is evidence that abnormalities in the rate and amplitude of respiration may be produced by lesions of the hypothalamus, and it is probable that this is the explanation of the respiratory disturbances which were sometimes seen as sequels of encephalitis lethargica.

REFERENCES

APPENZELLER, O. (1970) The Autonomic Nervous System, Amsterdam.

BAIN, H. W., DARTE, J. M. M., KEITH, W. S., and KRUYFF, E. (1966) The diencephalic syndrome of early infancy due to silent brain tumor. With special reference to treatment, Pediatrics, **38,** 473.

BANNISTER, R., ARDILL, L., and FENTEM, P. (1967) Defective autonomic control of blood vessels in idiopathic orthostatic hypotension, Brain, **90,** 725.

BARD, P. (1929) The central representation of the sympathetic system, Arch. Neurol. Psychiat. (Chic.), **22,** 230.

BEATTIE, J., BROW, G. R., and LONG, C. N. H. (1930) Physiological and anatomical evidence for the existence of nerve tracts connecting the hypothalamus with spinal sympathetic centres, Proc. roy. Soc. B, **106,** 253.

BLACKWELL, R. E., and GUILLEMIN, R. (1973) Hypothalamic control of adenohypophyseal secretions, Ann. Rev. Physiol., **35,** 357.

CAMPBELL, E. J. M., and DICKINSON, G. (1960) Clinical Physiology, Oxford.

CLARK, W. E. LE G. (1948) The connexions of the frontal lobes of the brain, Lancet, **i,** 353.

CLARK, W. E. LE G., BEATTIE, J., RIDDOCH, G., and DOTT, N. M. (1938) The Hypothalamus, London.

DANIEL, P. M., and PRICHARD, M. M. L. (1975) Studies of the Hypothalamus and the Pituitary Gland, Oxford.

DE VIGNEAUD, V. (1956) Trail of sulfur research: from insulin to oxytocin, Science, **123,** 967.

DE WARDENER, H. E., and BARLOW, E. D. (1958) Compulsive water-drinking, Quart. J. Med., **27,** 567.

DEMENT, W., GUILLEMINAULT, C., and ZARCONE, V. (1975) The pathologies of sleep; a case series approach, in The Nervous System, vol. 2, The Clinical Neurosciences, ed. Chase, T. N., New York.

DINGMAN, J. F., and THORN, G. W. (1974) Diseases of the neurohypophysis, in Harrison's Principles of Internal Medicine, 7th ed., chap. 84, New York.

FULTON, J. F. (1949) Functional Localization in the Frontal Lobes and Cerebellum, Oxford.

GAMSTORP, I. (1972) Neurological disorders and growth disturbances in infancy and childhood, Europ. Neurol., **7,** 1.

GLEES, P. (1961) Experimental Neurology, chap. xii, Oxford.

GUYTON, A. C. (1976) Textbook of Medical Physiology, 5th ed., Philadelphia.

HANDLER, J. S., and ORLOFF, J. (1973) The mechanism of action of antidiuretic hormone, in Handbook of Physiology, ed. Orloff, F., and Berlener, R. W., sec. 8, Baltimore.

HARRIS, G. W., and DONOVAN, B. T. (1966) *The Pituitary Gland*, vols. 1–3, Berkeley, Calif.

HAYMAKER, W., ANDERSON, E., and NAUTA, W. J. H. (1969) *The Hypothalamus*, Springfield, Ill.

HAYWARD, J. N. (1975) Neural control of the posterior pituitary, *Ann. Rev. Physiol.*, **37**, 191.

HEAD, H. On disturbances of sensation with especial reference to the pain of visceral disease. Part I, *Brain*, 1893, **16**, 1; Part II, *Brain*, 1894, **17**, 339; Part III, *Brain*, 1896, **19**, 153.

HESS, W. R. (1954) *Diencephalon*, New York.

JACOBSON, S. (1972) Hypothalamus and autonomic nervous system, in *An Introduction to the Neurosciences*, ed. Curtis, B. A., Jacobson, S., and Marcus, E. M., Philadelphia.

KUHLENBECK, H. (1954) *The Human Diencephalon*, Basel.

LE MARQUAND, H. S., and RUSSELL, D. S. (1934–5) A case of pubertas praecox (macrogenitosomia praecox) in a boy associated with a tumour in the floor of the third ventricle, *Roy. Berks. Hosp. Rep.*, p. 31.

LEWIS, T. (1937) The nocifensor system of nerves and its reactions, *Brit. med. J.*, **1**, 431.

LEWIS, T. (1938) Suggestions relating to the study of somatic pain, *Brit. med. J.*, **1**, 321.

LIST, C. F., and PEET, M. M. (1938) Sweat secretion in man. IV. Sweat secretion of the face and its disturbances, *Arch. Neurol. Psychiat. (Chic.)*, **40**, 442.

MUNCH-PETERSON, C. J. (1931) Glycosurias of cerebral origin, *Brain*, **54**, 72.

NELSON, D. H. (1974) Diseases of the anterior lobe of the pituitary gland, in *Harrison's Principles of Internal Medicine*, 7th ed., chap. 83, New York.

PLUM, F., and POSNER, J. B. (1972) *Diagnosis of Stupor and Coma*, 2nd ed., Philadelphia.

RANSON, S. W. (1926) Anatomy of the sympathetic nervous system with reference to sympathectomy and ramisection, *J. Amer. med. Ass.*, **86**, 1886.

RICHTER, C. P. (1930) Experimental diabetes insipidus, *Brain*, **53**, 76.

RUSSELL, A. (1951) A diencephalic syndrome of emaciation in infancy and childhood, *Arch. Dis. Childh.*, **26**, 274.

SACHS, E., and MACDONALD, M. E. (1925) Blood sugar studies in experimental pituitary and hypothalamic lesions, with a review of literature, *Arch. Neurol. Psychiat. (Chic.)*, **13**, 335.

SINCLAIR, D. C., WEDDELL, G., and FEINDEL, W. H. (1948) Referred pain and associated phenomena, *Brain*, **71**, 184.

WALKER, A. E. (1940) A cyto-architectural study of the prefrontal area of the macaque monkey, *J. comp. Neurol.*, **73**, 59.

WALSH, E. G. (1964) *Physiology of the Nervous System*, 2nd ed., chap. 12, London.

WECHSLER, I. S. (1956) Hypothalamic syndromes, *Brit. med. J.*, **2**, 375.

WHITE, J. C., and SMITHWICK, R. H. (1942) *The Autonomic Nervous System: Anatomy, Physiology and Surgical Application*, 2nd ed., London.

WHITE, P. T., and ROSS, A. T. (1963) Inanition syndrome in infants with anterior hypothalamic neoplasms, *Neurology (Minneap.)*, **13**, 974.

21

DISEASES OF THE BONES OF THE SKULL

OSTEITIS DEFORMANS

Synonym. Paget's disease.

Definition. A chronic disease of the bones characterized by absorption and new bone formation and leading to enlargement of the skull, deformity of the vertebral column, and bowing of the clavicles and long bones of the extremities, and in some cases to nervous symptoms secondary to the bony changes.

AETIOLOGY AND PATHOLOGY

Osteitis deformans is a rare disease of unknown aetiology developing in middle life and affecting both sexes.

Histologically, the changes in the bones consist of resorption and softening of bone followed by replacement with a poorly mineralized osteoid matrix with increased vascularity, accompanied by considerable fibrosis; enlargement of bones results from the laying down of osteoid both beneath the periosteum and on the inner side of the corticalis. Deformities result from softening of the bones. The skull becomes thickened, and the distinction between the inner and the outer tables and the diploë is obliterated. The cranial cavity is increased in breadth and to a lesser extent in length, but its vertical diameter becomes diminished. The base tends to sink relatively to the region of the foramen magnum, which is supported by the vertebral column, and platybasia or basilar impression may result [see p. 1090]. Thickening of the skull also leads to a reduction of the size of the vascular and neural foramina and may thus be responsible for symptoms of compression of cerebral hemispheres, cerebellum, and cranial nerves. Similar changes in the bones of the vertebral column lead to kyphosis and reduction in the height of the patient, and sometimes to compression of the spinal cord. The clavicles and the long bones of the limbs may also become softened, thickened, and bowed. Increased blood flow through newly formed arteriovenous channels may rarely cause high output cardiac failure.

OSSEOUS SYMPTOMS

The onset of the disease is insidious, the patient usually complaining first of pains in the head and limbs. The gradual enlargement of the skull necessitates an increase in hat size, and deformities of the spine and long bones are noted, together with a resulting diminution in height, which in extreme cases may amount to as much as 30 cm. The enlarged skull bulges in the frontal and parietal regions. Affected bones often feel unusually warm to the touch. Radiographs show a characteristic appearance, the thickened bone being mottled and 'woolly': rarely there are large islands of osteoporosis in the skull [FIG. 162].

NERVOUS SYMPTOMS

Mental deterioration and epileptiform attacks may occur as a result of compression of the cerebral hemispheres, and symptoms of cerebellar deficiency

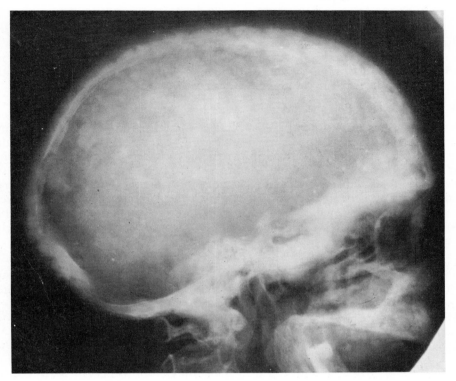

FIG. 162. Paget's disease of the skull. Lateral radiograph demonstrating thickening and the typical 'woolly' appearance of the skull vault with some platybasia. (Kindly provided by Dr. G. L. Gryspeerdt.)

have also been observed as well as obstructive hydrocephalus (Friedman *et al.*, 1971).

Any of the cranial nerves may be compressed owing to reduction in the calibre of their foramina, the olfactory, optic, and vestibulocochlear nerves being most often affected. Unilateral optic atrophy, paralysis of one lateral rectus, trigeminal neuralgia and hemifacial spasm have all been described (Friedman *et al.*, 1971) as have dysarthria and dysphagia. In spite of deformity of the spine associated with vertebral collapse, symptoms of compression of the spinal roots are rare, but compression of the cord itself has been reported in a number of cases and may be associated with cranial nerve lesions, such as optic atrophy. Symptoms of spinal compression are described on page 736. Retinitis pigmentosa may be present.

DIAGNOSIS

The diagnosis is readily made by X-ray examination of the bones, and this should always be carried out in middle-aged patients who complain of obscure pains in the head or limbs or exhibit unexplained cranial nerve palsies or paraplegia. A systolic bruit, due to increased blood flow through the affected bone, may be heard over the skull or spine. The serum alkaline phosphatase is usually raised.

PROGNOSIS

Osteitis deformans is an extremely chronic and slowly progressive disease. Local sarcoma of bone sometimes occurs as a complication.

Rarely, in severe cases, owing to multiple arteriovenous communications in the affected bones, 'high-output' cardiac failure occurs and an association with atheroma and cardiac infarction has been postulated.

TREATMENT

Treatment is unsatisfactory. Analgesics are often required and radiotherapy has been said to relieve bone pain in some cases. Calcium and vitamin D should probably be given. Intravenous infusions of mithramycin have been recommended (Ryan et al., 1970) but Friedman et al. (1971) found this treatment to be poorly tolerated and ineffective. Laminectomy is necessary when the spinal cord is compressed; and when platybasia causes compression of the lower medulla or upper spinal cord, decompression at the foramen magnum may be indicated but operation is invariably difficult as the affected bone is excessively vascular.

REFERENCES

BOGAERT, L. VAN (1933) Über eine hereditäre und familiäre Form der Pagetschen Ostitis deformans mit Chorioretinitis pigmentosa, Z. ges. Neurol. Psychiat., **147,** 327.

BOLL, J. (1946-7) Paget's disease of the skull with platybasia, Proc. roy. Soc. Med., **40,** 85.

FRIEDMAN, P., SKLAVER, N., and KLAWANS, H. L. (1971) Neurologic manifestations of Paget's disease of the skull, Dis. nerv. Syst., **32,** 809.

GREGG, D. (1926) Neurologic symptoms in osteitis deformans (Paget's disease), Arch. Neurol. Psychiat. (Chic.), **15,** 613.

GRÜNTHAL, E. (1931) Über den Hirnbefund bei Pagetscher Krankheit des Schädels, Z. ges. Neurol. Psychiat., **136,** 656.

GURDJIAN, E. S., WEBSTER, J. E., and LATIMER, F. R. (1952) Paget's disease of the spine with compression of the spinal cord, Trans. Amer. neurol. Ass., **77,** 243.

KAUFMAN, M. R. (1929) Psychosis in Paget's disease, Arch. Neurol. Psychiat. (Chic.), **21,** 828.

PAGET, J., FRICKER, G., and VER BRUGGHEN, A. (1950) Osteitis fibrosa cystica localisata of the skull, J. Neurosurg., **7,** 447.

RYAN, W. G., SCHWARTZ, T. B., and NORTHROP, G. (1970) Experiences in the treatment of Paget's disease of bone with mithramycin, J. Amer. med. Ass., **213,** 1153.

WYLLIE, W. G. (1923) The occurrence in osteitis deformans of lesions of the central nervous system, with a report of four cases, Brain, **46,** 336.

LEONTIASIS OSSEA AND POLYOSTOTIC FIBROUS DYSPLASIA

Leontiasis ossea is characterized by hyperostoses of the bones of the face and skull; sometimes all of the bones of the skull and face are involved and the condition is then similar clinically and pathologically to Paget's disease, but in other cases the overgrowth is limited to one or both cranial bones or to one or both jaws. The name of the condition derives from the leonine facial appearance of many cases. Unlike typical Paget's disease, the condition, which may give rise to convulsions due to compression of the brain, or to cranial nerve palsies, usually begins in childhood and is slowly progressive.

Polyostotic fibrous dysplasia (Albright's syndrome) is limited as a rule to young girls; changes in the long bones, cutaneous pigmentation, and precocious puberty may be accompanied by cranial nerve palsies and/or optic atrophy due to involvement of the bones of the skull base. It is now generally believed that leontiasis ossea is merely a variant of polyostotic fibrous dysplasia in which the bones of the skull and face are selectively involved (Krane, 1974). The patches of cutaneous pigmentation often show a jagged outline (coast of Maine) unlike those of smooth outline seen in neurofibromatosis.

REFERENCES

ALBRIGHT, F. (1947) Polyostotic fibrous dysplasia, *J. clin. Endocr.*, **7,** 307.
KRANE, S. M. (1974) Hyperostosis, neoplasms and other disorders of bone and cartilage, in *Harrison's Principles of Internal Medicine*, 7th ed., chap. 354, New York.
SMITH, A. G., and ZAVALETA, A. (1952) Osteoma, ossifying fibroma and fibrous dysplasia of the facial and cranial bones, *Arch. Path.*, **54,** 507.

CRANIOSTENOSIS

Synonyms. Oxycephaly; acrocephaly; turricephaly; tower skull.

Definition. A congenital abnormality of the skull due to premature synostosis of the sutures and characterized by an abnormal shape of the head, exophthalmos, optic atrophy, and symptoms of increased intracranial pressure.

AETIOLOGY AND PATHOLOGY

It is generally agreed that craniostenosis is due to premature synostosis of the skull bones. This usually begins in the coronal, sagittal, and lambdoid sutures, but variations are encountered, and the synostosis may be asymmetrical. It has been attributed to displacement of the centres of ossification towards the sutures. Mann (1937) considered that it is due to a localized arrest of development of the post-optic visceral mesoderm (maxillary process) possibly of atavistic significance. The condition is congenital and sometimes hereditary. Though the sutures are closed, the brain continues to grow at the usual rate. Compensatory enlargement of the skull occurs by means of expansion where the sutures are not united and by thinning of the bone—convolutional atrophy—from pressure of the growing brain. The ultimate breakdown of this compensatory process leads to symptoms of increased intracranial pressure. The optic atrophy has been attributed to various causes, including compression of the optic nerves by narrowing of their canals, stretching of the nerves by elongation, pressure upon them by the brain, and papilloedema due to increased intracranial pressure. Probably different factors operate in different cases, and the optic nerves may be damaged in more than one of these ways simultaneously. The exophthalmos appears to be due to abnormal shallowness of the orbits.

Craniostenosis is a feature of the acrocephalosyndactyly of Apert, in which oxycephaly is associated with syndactyly, and of the craniofacial dysostosis of Crouzon.

SYMPTOMS

Since craniostenosis is due to a congenital abnormality, the deformity of the skull may be present at birth, but the patient may not come under observation until other symptoms, such as headache and failing vision, develop, which usually occur in childhood.

The skull is brachycephalic and dome-shaped, with a high forehead, and there may be flattening of the maxillae or asymmetrical facial deformity. The short upper lip is highly characteristic. Owing to the shallowness of the orbits the eyes are prominent, and may even become spontaneously dislocated, and a divergent squint and nystagmus are common. Papilloedema may be present or optic atrophy, either primary or secondary, with impairment of vision, which may reach complete blindness. Other symptoms due either directly to the bone changes or indirectly to increased intracranial pressure include anosmia and

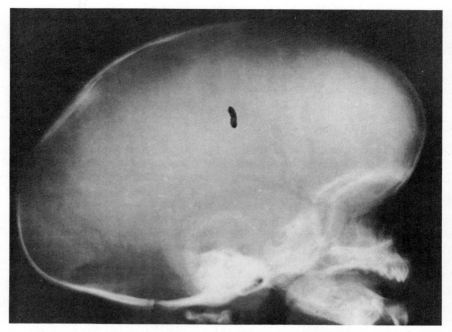

Fig. 163. Scapulocephaly due to premature synostosis of the sagittal suture; note the abnormal shape of the skull and the thinning of the calvarium

deafness. The mental state is usually normal. Radiographs of the skull show the premature synostosis of the sutures and compensatory enlargement, with marked thinning of the calvarium, especially in the frontal region [Fig. 163].

Craniofacial Dysostosis. This disorder, described by Crouzon, is closely related to craniostenosis, and is usually hereditary. The forehead recedes to the high, rather pointed vertex—trigonocephaly. There are also hyperplasia of the maxillae and relative prognathism, together with exophthalmos, divergent squint, and in some cases optic atrophy.

DIAGNOSIS

The condition is usually recognized at a glance from the shape of the skull. In microcephaly the abnormally small skull size is secondary to hypoplasia of the brain, and symptoms of increased intracranial pressure are absent. In hydrocephalus the skull is enlarged in all its diameters and its total volume, which in craniostenosis tends to be subnormal, is increased. Craniostenosis is not likely to be confused with other causes of increased intracranial pressure if attention is paid to the shape of the skull and to the X-ray appearances.

PROGNOSIS

In mild cases compensatory enlargement of the skull may be adequate to prevent the development of symptoms. When, however, headache is present or vision is threatened, no improvement can be anticipated, and the patient's condition is likely to become worse.

TREATMENT

Only surgical treatment is effective. Attempts have been made to deal radically with the cause by opening the sutures and paring their edges. Since in some cases it is possible that the optic nerves are directly compressed in their canals, radiographs of the optic canals should be taken, and if they appear to be unusually small their surgical enlargement should be considered. King (1938) reviewed the surgical treatment and described a new technique, and reviews of modern surgical methods of treatment have been given by Pemberton and Freeman (1962) and Anderson and Geiger (1965).

REFERENCES

ANDERSON, F. M., and GEIGER, L. (1965) Craniosynostosis. A survey of 204 cases, *J. Neurosurg.*, **22**, 229.
CROUZON, O. (1929) *Études sur les maladies familiales nerveuses et dystrophique*, Paris.
DAVIS, F. A. (1925) Tower skull, oxycephalus, *Amer. J. Ophthal.*, **8**, 513.
KING, J. E. J. (1938) Oxycephaly: a new operation and its results, *Arch. Neurol. Psychiat. (Chic.)*, **40**, 1205.
MANN, I. C. (1937) *Developmental Abnormalities of the Eye*, London.
PEMBERTON, J. W., and FREEMAN, J. M. (1962) Craniosynostosis. A review of experience with forty patients with particular reference to ocular aspects and comments on operative indications, *Amer. J. Ophthal.*, **54**, 641.
SAETHRE, H. (1931) Ueber den Turmschädel, seine Erblichkeit, Pathogenese und neuropsychiatrischen Symptome, *Acta psychiat. (Kbh.)*, **6**, 405.
WORMS, G., and CARILLON, R. (1930) Oxycephaly, *Rev. Oto-neuro-ophthal.*, **8**, 736.

CLEIDOCRANIAL DYSOSTOSIS

In this rare developmental disorder absence of part or the whole of both clavicles is accompanied by an increase in the width of the forehead. Sometimes there is an associated absence of one or more shoulder-girdle muscles but there are no associated neurological manifestations except in occasional cases in which there are also congenital malformations of the brain and/or other parts of the nervous system.

HYPERTELORISM

In this developmental disorder the distance between the eyes is increased; there is a vertical ridge on the forehead and the bridge of the nose is excessively broad. Usually there is no neurological defect but in occasional rare and severe cases associated maldevelopment of the forebrain gives rise to mental deficiency.

REFERENCES

CURRARINO, G., and SILVERMAN, F. N. (1960) Orbital hypertelorism, arhinencephaly and trigonocephaly, *Radiology*, **74,** 206.
KLEMMER, R. N., SNOKE, P. O., and COOPER, H. K. (1931) Cleidocranial dysostosis, *Amer. J. Roentgenol.*, **25,** 710.

BASILAR IMPRESSION AND OTHER CRANIOVERTEBRAL ANOMALIES

Basilar impression is an abnormality of the base of the skull in which the angle between the basisphenoid and the basilar portion of the occipital bone—normally between 110 and 140 degrees—is widened [FIG. 164]. In the congenital form the foramen magnum is deformed and the medulla is unusually low, so that it and the upper part of the cervical spinal cord may be compressed by the dens. In a lateral radiograph the line drawn from the posterior end of the hard palate to the posterior lip of the foramen magnum normally lies above the cervical spine, but in basilar impression it crosses the odontoid process at some point (Chamberlain, 1939); Bull *et al.* (1955) point out that the plane of the axis relative to that of the hard palate is a more reliable guide. Normally these

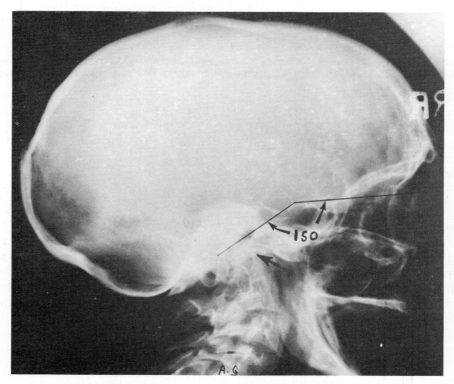

FIG. 164. Basilar impression associated with developmental anomalies of the cervical spine. The angle between the basisphenoid and the basilar portion of the occipital bone (small arrows) is 150 degrees, indicating platybasia. The large arrow points to the odontoid peg which is well above Chamberlain's line

are roughly parallel: in basilar impression they form an acute angle. The condition is often identified, particularly in the American literature, by the term 'platybasia', but the latter term, which simply means a flat base of skull, can equally be applied to the changes in the skull base which occur, for instance, in Paget's disease. Spillane *et al.* (1957) point out that basilar impression may be present without platybasia. Basilar impression is the name best reserved for the congenital disorder in which, perhaps because of a congenital abnormality of the occipital bone, the posterior part of the atlas vertebra is partially invaginated into the cranial cavity.

Basilar impression is therefore congenital and may be associated with fusion of the bodies of some cervical vertebrae—the Klippel–Feil syndrome—or it may be due to osteogenesis imperfecta (Hurwitz and McSwiney, 1960). The Klippel–Feil syndrome may, of course, occur without associated craniovertebral malformation; some such patients show 'mirror movements' in the upper extremities so that a voluntary movement carried out with one hand is mimicked spontaneously with the other (Gunderson and Solitare, 1968).

Basilar impression may lead to hydrocephalus and, as Gustafson and Oldberg (1940) suggested, may be responsible for the Arnold–Chiari syndrome, but these are more probably associated congenital abnormalities. The spinal cord may exhibit hydromyelia but there is also a clear association with syringomyelia (Foster *et al.*, 1969; Barnett *et al.*, 1974). In adults the clinical picture may resemble mu̇ 'tiple sclerosis, syringomyelia, or high cervical tumour. The commonest clinical features are those of a spastic tetraparesis with marked impairment of position and joint sense in both hands and to a lesser extent in the legs, but in some cases there are also signs of involvement of lower cranial nerves, cerebellar ataxia and/or hydrocephalus due to obstruction to the outflow of CSF from the fourth ventricle (O'Connell and Aldren Turner, 1950; Michie and Clark, 1968). Symptoms suggesting dysfunction of the C8–T1 segments of the spinal cord in some such cases have been attributed to venous obstruction and stagnant hypoxia in the cervical cord (Taylor and Byrnes, 1974). The head is sometimes mushroom-shaped and the neck abnormally short, but the diagnosis can only be made by X-ray examination. If symptoms occur the treatment is surgical decompression (Gordon, 1969).

Achondroplasia may cause not only spinal cord compression but also internal hydrocephalus without platybasia or basilar impression, possibly due to shortening of the skull base (Spillane, 1952). Symptoms of high cervical cord compression may result from atlanto-axial subluxation with separation of the odontoid process of the axis; this may be a congenital malformation or the result of trauma but can also occur spontaneously in rheumatoid arthritis (Stevens *et al.*, 1971). The radiology of the craniovertebral anomalies has been reviewed in detail by Wackenheim (1974).

REFERENCES

BARNETT, H. J. M., FOSTER, J. B., and HUDGSON, P. (1974) *Syringomyelia*, London.

BULL, J., NIXON, W. L. B., and PRATT, R. T. C. (1955) The radiological criteria and familial occurrence of primary basilar impression, *Brain*, **78**, 229.

CHAMBERLAIN, W. E. (1939) Basilar impression (platybasia), *Yale J. Biol. Med.*, **11**, 487.

FOSTER, J. B., HUDGSON, P., and PEARCE, G. W. (1969) The association of syringomyelia and congenital cervico-medullary anomalies: pathological evidence, *Brain*, **92**, 25.

GORDON, D. S. (1969) Neurological syndromes associated with craniovertebral anomalies, *Proc. roy. Soc. Med.*, **62**, 725.

GUNDERSON, C. H., and SOLITARE, G. B. (1968) Mirror movements in patients with the Klippel–Feil syndrome, *Arch. Neurol. (Chic.)*, **18,** 675.

GUSTAFSON, W. A., and OLDBERG, E. (1940) Neurologic significance of platybasia, *Arch. Neurol. Psychiat. (Chic.)*, **44,** 84.

HURWITZ, L. J., and McSWINEY, R. R. (1960) Basilar impression and osteogenesis imperfecta in a family, *Brain*, **83,** 138.

MICHIE, I., and CLARK, M. (1968) Neurological syndromes associated with cervical and craniocervical anomalies, *Arch. Neurol. (Chic.)*, **18,** 241.

O'CONNELL, J. E. A., and ALDREN TURNER, J. W. (1950) Basilar impression of the skull, *Brain*, **73,** 405.

SPILLANE, J. D. (1952) Three cases of achondroplasia with neurological complications, *J. Neurol. Neurosurg. Psychiat.*, **15,** 246.

SPILLANE, J. D., PALLIS, C., and JONES, A. M. (1957) Developmental abnormalities in the region of the foramen magnum, *Brain*, **80,** 11.

STEVENS, J. C., CARTLIDGE, N. E. F., SAUNDERS, M., APPLEBY, A., HALL, M., and SHAW, D. A. (1971) Atlanto-axial subluxation and cervical myelopathy in rheumatoid arthritis, *Quart. J. Med.*, **40,** 391.

TAYLOR, A. R., and BYRNES, D. P. (1974) Foramen magnum and high cervical cord compression, *Brain*, **97,** 473.

WACKENHEIM, A. (1974) *Roentgen Diagnosis of the Craniovertebral Region*, Berlin.

22

PAROXYSMAL AND CONVULSIVE DISORDERS

EPILEPSY

Definition. Epilepsy is a paroxysmal and transitory disturbance of the functions of the brain which develops suddenly, ceases spontaneously, and exhibits a conspicuous tendency to recurrence. Though in its most typical forms it is characterized by the sudden onset of loss of consciousness, which may or may not be associated with tonic spasm and clonic contractions of the muscles, many varieties of epileptic attack occur, their distinctive features depending upon differences in the site of origin, extent of spread, and nature of the disturbance of function. Epilepsy is thus a symptom. In some cases a local lesion of the brain plays the chief part in causation; in others hereditary predisposition seems the important factor: in others again the cause is unknown. A generalized attack has long been known as 'grand mal', an attack characterized by momentary loss of consciousness only without falling and without, as a rule, motor accompaniments, as 'petit mal'. However, as will be seen, the term petit mal is best reserved for a specific variety of epilepsy which begins in childhood and there are other varieties of minor epilepsy which are different aetiologically which give only transient impairment of consciousness but yet differ from true petit mal. Attacks of epilepsy are often known as 'fits' or 'seizures'.

THE PHYSIOLOGICAL NATURE OF EPILEPSY

The invention of electroencephalography [see p. 1110], though it has posed many problems which are still unsolved, has thrown much new light upon the nature of epilepsy. The electroencephalograms obtained in epilepsy are described in more detail later. For our present purpose it is sufficient to say that epileptic attacks are usually accompanied by abnormal changes in the electrical potentials of the brain; hence epilepsy has been described as 'paroxysmal cerebral dysrhythmia' (Gibbs *et al.*, 1937). In spite of this advance many problems remain unsolved, for cortical dysrhythmias similar to those found in epilepsy may be present in patients suffering from disorders other than epilepsy, and also in non-epileptic relatives of epileptics. Furthermore, in certain unquestionable attacks of epilepsy, EEG recordings taken through the intact skull may show no abnormality.

Nevertheless, this work supports the view that the physiological basis of a convulsion is a discharge of neurones rather than a primary impairment or loss of cortical function. Experimentally it can be shown in animals that convulsant drugs induce fits, the pattern of which can be modified by the successful removal of different levels of the nervous system from the cortex downwards. Moreover, electrical stimulation of the cortex in man, as shown especially by Foerster, results in convulsions which can only be satisfactorily interpreted as the expression of a regional cortical discharge. Transitory post-epileptic symptoms, whether loss or disorder of consciousness, paralysis, or sensory loss, have been interpreted as being due to temporary exhaustion of neurones which have been the site of discharge. However, Efron (1961) has given cogent reasons for suggesting that an active process of inhibition rather than 'exhaustion', resulting from persistent subclinical epileptic discharge, is a more probable explanation for post-epileptic paralysis (Todd's paralysis).

Excitation, however, is not the most likely explanation of loss of consciousness occurring as the sole, or almost the sole, manifestation of epilepsy, as in petit mal. The bilaterally synchronous wave-and-spike cortical discharge which charac-terizes petit mal appears to originate at a subcortical centre, perhaps the inter-thalamic nuclei (Jasper and Droogleever-Fortuyn, 1947) and the resulting impairment of consciousness was interpreted by Grey Walter (1947) as the result of an abnormal synchronization of cortical rhythms, and by Williams (1950) as indicating a blockage of afferent impulses to the cortex. In the light of experimental work and the behaviour of the EEG in man, Gastaut and Fischer-Williams (1960) put forward the hypothesis that 'a grand mal seizure seems to depend on a thalamic discharge which involves the non-specific reticular struc-tures and is projected to the cortex in what may be considered a generalized recruiting response transmitted along the diffuse cortical projection pathways'. They compared 'the hypersynchronous discharge of generalized epilepsy' with a sort of 'paroxysmal sleep' localized to the thalamocortical system and provok-ing a functional exclusion of this system; if it be supposed that the same factor also precipitates hypersynchrony of the reticular formation, it is possible to explain all the features of a grand mal attack, the thalamic discharge being responsible for the loss of consciousness and the discharge of the brain stem reticular formation for the tonic and clonic element in the convulsions. Accord-ing to the same authors petit mal may be explained as the result of a thalamic discharge occurring in a subject with a very effective inhibitory mechanism. The lack of convulsions may depend on the fact that the reticular formation is rhythmically inhibited. The site of origin of the myoclonic jerks which occur in some forms of epilepsy was also studied by Gastaut and Fischer-Williams. Such jerks may be evoked by sensory stimuli, especially after the administration of convulsant drugs, and appear to originate in the mesencephalon and thalamus. The disturbances of consciousness, mood, and behaviour which occur as a result of discharges originating in the temporal lobe have been interpreted as disorders of a specific integrating role in respect of consciousness played by this part of the brain (Penfield and Jasper, 1954).

Epilepsy, then, is to be regarded as an uncontrolled neural discharge, that is, as an abnormal conversion of the potential energy of the neurones into kinetic energy. Fundamentally, therefore, it is a physico-chemical disturbance, and it is to be expected that the causative abnormal physico-chemical state of the neurones should be produced by a wide variety of agencies. How they operate is most likely to be elucidated by study of the physiological disorder underlying the onset and cessation of a focal attack. Symonds (1959) considered possible regulatory biochemical factors. He suggested that gamma-aminobutyric acid (GABA) may be 'a natural anticonvulsant' formed in the brain. Local lesions may cause seizures either by allowing the accumulation of an excitatory sub-stance or by depressing the tonic inhibitory control of afferent impulses. Recent experimental work has shown that the application of acetylcholine to the cerebral cortex may provoke focal convulsions, while generalized fits may follow the intravenous injection of this substance; thus fits may be due to exogenous or endogenous factors which influence its local or generalized release in excess of the normal quantities required for synaptic transmission. GABA and acetyl-choline have opposite effects upon brain excitability so that an imbalance between these two substances within the brain could be one factor predisposing to seizure production (Jurgelsky and Thomas, 1966). It is also evident that the excitability of individual neurones may be influenced by the activity of the sodium pump which affects the concentration gradient of Na^+ across the neuronal membrane; if the gradient increases the neurone is hyperpolarized and difficult to excite, while if it is diminished neuronal excitability increases. The so-called 'burst' firing patterns of single cortical neurones which may be recorded with microelectrodes in experimental epilepsy in animals and which are presumed to play a part in the genesis of the epileptic spike discharge in the EEG are described by Ward (1972). The balance between acetylcholine (excitatory) and GABA (inhibitory) may be upset, for instance, by pyridoxine deficiency as the latter substance is essential for the synthesis of GABA (see Sutherland *et al.*, 1974). These delicate and interrelated factors may be affected not only by the effects of focal cerebral lesions but also by a variety of metabolic factors including pyrexia, hypoxia, hypocalcaemia, hypoglycaemia, water intoxication, and alkalosis but also by the effects of various drugs and toxins or drug withdrawal. A low serum magnesium without hypocalcaemia has been found in some children with convulsions (Wong and Teh, 1968) but seems unlikely to be a primary aetiological factor. During convulsions cerebral metabolism increases and the brain's need for oxygen and glucose increases, while in animals with experimentally induced convulsions brain lactate increases markedly (Posner *et al.*, 1969; Beresford *et al.*, 1969).

It must also be accepted that virtually every individual is potentially epileptic if the provocation, whether physical or pharmacological, is sufficient, but in some, presumed to have a very high 'epileptic threshold' this provocation must be intense, while in others in whom seizures occur without apparent precipitating factors it is presumed that the 'convulsive threshold' is low. It follows that if one accepts this concept of the 'threshold' there is a continuum between the epileptic and normal populations varying between the majority in whom substantial provocation is needed to produce a fit and the severe epileptics who have frequent attacks without evident cause. The margin between the two populations is clearly indistinct.

AETIOLOGY

The following classification of some of the principal causes of epilepsy is for convenience arranged schematically, but it must be remembered that the precise way in which a cause operates is often obscure and in some instances a single pathological condition might be placed in more than one category.

1. *Local Causes*

    (*a*) Focal intracranial lesions sometimes associated with increased intracranial pressure:

        Intracranial tumour; cerebral abscess; subdural haematoma; angioma or haematoma.

    (*b*) Inflammatory and demyelinating conditions:

        Meningitis; all forms of acute and subacute encephalitis; toxoplasmosis; neurosyphilis; multiple sclerosis; cerebral cysticercosis.

    (*c*) Trauma:

        Perinatal brain injury and/or haemorrhage; head injuries of later life.

(*d*) Congenital abnormalities:
Congenital diplegia; tuberous sclerosis; porencephaly.

(*e*) Degenerations and inborn errors of metabolism:
The cerebral lipidoses; diffuse sclerosis and the leukodystrophies; encephalopathies of infancy and childhood, including 'infantile spasms'; Pick's disease; Alzheimer's disease; progressive myoclonic epilepsy; subacute spongiform encephalopathy; Creutzfeldt–Jakob disease.

(*f*) Vascular disorders:
Cerebral atheroma, intracranial haemorrhage, thrombosis, embolism; eclampsia; hypertensive encephalopathy; cerebral complications of 'connective tissue' or 'collagen diseases'; polycythaemia; intracranial aneurysm; acute cerebral ischaemia from any cause.

2. *General Causes*

(*a*) Exogenous poisons:
Alcohol; absinthe; thujone; cocaine; strychnine; lead; chloroform; ether; insulin; amphetamines; camphor; *Metrazol*, organophosphorus and organochlorine compounds used as insecticides, and fluoracetic acid derivatives; amine-oxidase inhibitors, imipramine and its derivatives; and *withdrawal* of alcohol, barbiturates, and other drugs.

(*b*) Anoxia:
Asphyxia; carbon monoxide poisoning; nitrous oxide anaesthesia; profound anaemia.

(*c*) Disordered metabolism:
Uraemia; hepatic failure; hypo-adrenalism; water intoxication; porphyria; hypoglycaemia; hyperpyrexia; alkalosis; pyridoxine deficiency.

(*d*) Endocrine disorders:
Parathyroid tetany; idiopathic hypoparathyroidism and pseudohypoparathyroidism.

(*e*) Conditions associated particularly with childhood:
Rickets; acute infections ('febrile convulsions').

3. *Psychological Factors*

These are relatively unimportant. It is doubtful if psychological factors alone are sufficient to cause epileptiform convulsions. In individuals otherwise predisposed, however, fright or anxiety may precipitate attacks.

4. *Constitutional Epilepsy*

When all the above factors have been excluded there remains a large group of patients who suffer from convulsions for which no local or general cause can be found. We are, therefore, compelled to regard these individuals as suffering from a predisposition to convulsions, the nature of which is not yet understood, except in terms of the epileptic or convulsive threshold as mentioned above. It must also be borne in mind that the distinction between constitutional and symptomatic epilepsy is not clear-cut. There is an intermediate group of patients in whom predisposition determines the development of epilepsy after a focal cerebral lesion such as a head injury. (See Lennox's (1947) study of twin pairs with seizures.) Thus while a division of cases of epilepsy into symptomatic and idiopathic ('constitutional' or 'cryptogenic' or 'centrencephalic') groups is of some clinical value it should be recognized that, in a sense, to make a diagnosis of idiopathic epilepsy is a confession of failure as it simply implies that even with modern methods of investigation the cause of the epilepsy cannot be demonstrated.

The History of Patients Suffering from Epilepsy

The following inquiries should be made of a patient suffering from convulsions.

When did the first attack occur? Was it precipitated by an accident or associated with an acute illness? How soon was it followed by the second? What is the usual interval between the attacks? Are they increasing in frequency? Do the attacks occur in bouts? Has the patient had a series of attacks without recovering consciousness? Do the attacks occur at any special time of the day? Do they occur only by day or only by night? In the case of a woman, are they related to the menstrual periods? Is any factor known to precipitate the attacks? Does the patient have any warning? If so, what, and by how long does it precede the attack? How does an attack begin? Is its onset local or general, gradual or sudden? Is consciousness lost? Do convulsive movements occur in the attack? If so, are they symmetrical or asymmetrical? Has the patient injured himself in an attack? Does he bite his tongue and pass urine? How long do the attacks last? What is his condition afterwards? Are the attacks followed by headache, sleepiness, paralysis, or mental disturbance, such as automatism? What treatment has he had and how has he responded to it? Has he at any time suffered from head injury? If the attacks did not begin in infancy, did he suffer from infantile convulsions? Is there a family history of epilepsy or of fainting fits or of mental disorder?

Heredity

Inherited predisposition plays a considerable part in the aetiology of epilepsy. In a series of 200 epileptics there was a family history of the disease in 28 per cent. We must distinguish, however, between the inheritance of a predisposition and the inheritance of epilepsy. What seems to be inherited is the physical or neurophysiological basis of a 'dysrhythmia', but only a small proportion of those with such a 'dysrhythmia' become epileptic. Lennox et al. (1940) studied the EEG in the parents of epileptics; only in 5 per cent were both normal; in 35 per cent both were abnormal. The same authors stated that an abnormal EEG is six times as common among the relatives of epileptics as in controls, and this was true both of 'symptomatic' and 'idiopathic' epileptics. However, clinical evidence indicates that a history of epilepsy in other members of the family is obtained twice as commonly in patients with idiopathic epilepsy as in those whose seizures are symptomatic. Lennox (1947) believed that the 'dysrhythmia' is inherited as a Mendelian dominant. For the reasons given above, it is difficult to estimate the liability of an epileptic parent to transmit the disorder to his or her offspring, since it often remains latent and the condition reappears in a collateral line. Not more than one in thirty-six of the children of a mixed group of epileptics develops epilepsy, but in some families the incidence is higher. The risk is greater if there are several cases in the family and if the non-epileptic conjugal partner has a family history of epilepsy or an unstable EEG.

Trauma

The role of trauma in causing epilepsy is difficult to estimate. It is well known that severe head injuries may be followed by epilepsy [p. 398]. In adults, post-traumatic epilepsy rarely follows closed head injury unless the latter was severe enough to cause 24 hours of post-traumatic amnesia or unless 'early fits' occurred within the first 48 hours after the injury, in which case the development of post-traumatic epilepsy subsequently is much more common (Jennett, 1961). The incidence is much greater after penetrating wounds of the brain and in young children in whom less severe closed head injuries may be followed by fits. After missile injury the incidence rose from 11·4 per cent between one and two years to 33·3 per cent between three and five years in one series (Adeloye and Odeku, 1971), while after closed head injury Jennett *et al.* (1973) found that fits began within the first year in only half of those who ulti- mately developed post-traumatic epilepsy and they were able to devise a statistical method of determining the percentage risk in individual cases depending upon such factors as the duration of post-traumatic amnesia, the presence or absence of a dural tear, and the occurrence of early epilepsy. The presence of an acute traumatic intracranial haematoma significantly increases the incidence of both early and late traumatic epilepsy (Jennett, 1975). Epilepsy is relatively commoner among firstborn children than among later members of the family, and this may be explained by the increased liability of the firstborn to head injury during birth.

Other Local Cerebral Lesions

There is evidence also that other lesions of the nervous system predispose to epileptic attacks, for example, infantile hemiplegia. That minor cerebral lesions are also of some aetiological importance is indicated by the frequency with which slight abnormalities are found in the nervous system in epileptics. For example, Hodskins and Yakovlev (1930) found a completely normal nervous system in only 17 per cent of 300 epileptics in an institution. In addition to a wide range of congenital abnormalities, cerebral birth lesions, and lesions caused by encephalitis in childhood, certain other disorders predispose towards epilepsy which may, however, be delayed for many years. These include eclampsia and hypertension complicating pregnancy, otitis media and mastoid- itis, probably only when complicated by cortical venous thrombosis. Among the many lesions found at autopsy in some cases have been 'chronic localized encephalitis' (Rasmussen *et al.*, 1958) and focal cortical dysplasia (Taylor *et al.*, 1971). However, it must be remembered that the anoxia and other metabolic changes consequent upon repeated convulsions may themselves produce neuro- pathological abnormalities in the brain (Meldrum and Brierley, 1972, 1973). Epilepsy is associated with rheumatic heart disease more frequently than can be explained by chance. In mitral stenosis a small cerebral embolus may cause epilepsy, as may a small asymptomatic infarct in patients with intracranial atheroma (Dodge *et al.*, 1954).

Metabolic and Endocrine Factors

Prolonged search has not revealed any constant metabolic abnormality in epileptic patients, though hints are not wanting that some metabolic disturbance may play a part in the production of the fits. Generalized convulsions may occur in tetany due either to alkalosis, to destruction of the parathyroids, or to idio- pathic hypoparathyroidism, and in epileptics a fit can often be precipitated if alkalosis is induced by over-breathing. There is no evidence, however, that alkalosis is normally responsible for the attacks. Attacks may be induced in some epileptics by water retention (Ansell and Clarke, 1956) or by excessive alcohol consumption. The role of menstruation in precipitating attacks in women is unexplained, but supports the importance in some cases of hormonal and metabolic factors. Pregnancy may also influence the attacks. It is not uncommon for an epileptic woman to be free from attacks during pregnancy. Others, again, are worse when pregnant. The truth probably is that epilepsy may be influenced for better or worse by many different factors.

Febrile Convulsions

Convulsions accompanying febrile illnesses in infancy and early childhood have been regarded by some authorities as carrying a good prognosis. Certainly some infants may have one or two such attacks and no more but many go on to develop spontaneous fits later and a proportion have definite epileptic discharges in the EEG (Frantzen et al., 1968). Often there is a history of similar febrile convulsions occurring in some other member of the family (Frantzen et al., 1970). Attacks so classified occur only in children of less than nine years of age and usually in the first five years of life (Shaw et al., 1972; Lennox-Buchthal, 1974), although fever may occasionally precipitate seizures in adult epileptics (British Medical Journal, 1972). The attacks are occasionally fatal and if frequent may lead to permanent structural brain damage (British Medical Journal, 1975 a). While some regard febrile convulsions as representing a specific clinical syndrome, others believe that these attacks constitute merely one form of idiopathic epilepsy of childhood. There has been much dispute about the benefits of prophylactic treatment after the first attack and phenytoin has been found ineffective (Melchior et al., 1971) but many workers recommend phenobarbitone for at least twelve months (Lennox-Buchthal, 1974).

Neonatal Fits and Benign Focal Epilepsy of Childhood

Neonatal fits may occur in the first 48 hours after birth, usually due to cerebral birth injury, or between the fifth and sixth day when they are generally consequent upon hypocalcaemia (British Medical Journal, 1974). Benign focal epilepsy of childhood (Lerman and Kivity, 1975; British Medical Journal, 1975 b) is a syndrome delineated comparatively recently in which the patients show typical brief hemifacial seizures which tend to become generalized if they occur during sleep. The EEG usually shows slow, diphasic, high voltage temporal spikes, often followed by slow waves. In all of a series of 100 cases (Lerman and Kivity, 1975) the attacks ceased and the EEG changes disappeared before adult life.

Migraine

While loss of consciousness during an attack of migraine or at the height of the headache is usually syncopal, there is a slightly increased incidence of epilepsy in migraine sufferers, even in those who have no evidence of a cerebral lesion (such as an angioma) of which both the migraine and the epilepsy could be symptomatic. A possible role for tyramine in the physiological mechanism of the two disorders has been postulated by Scott et al. (1972).

Sex and Age Incidence

Females have been said to suffer from epilepsy slightly more frequently than males. In Gowers' series of 3,000 cases the ratio of females to males was 13:12. However, the sex incidence may be changing as Lennox and Lennox (1960) found that whereas under the age of 5 years there were 105 females for every

100 affected males, over the age of 20 years the male:female incidence was 100:59. The number of epileptics in the United Kingdom has been estimated to be about 300,000 with 35,000 new cases arising annually (Pond *et al.*, 1960; Brewis *et al.*, 1966; Office of Health Economics, 1971). The commonest age of onset is 0–4 years, with the first fit occurring in many more patients between 5 and 24 years of age; the incidence of initial attacks then declines steadily throughout adult life with a further slight peak, especially in males, over the age of 65 years (Office of Health Economics, 1971). Similar figures have been reported from many other countries including Switzerland, Holland, and the United States.

PATHOLOGY

There is no constant pathological change to be found in the brains of epileptics, though abnormalities are common. The difficulty is to determine which pathological changes may be the cause of epilepsy and which may result from the seizures that, if severe and frequent, may undoubtedly cause cerebral anoxia. In patients with symptomatic epilepsy secondary to identifiable organic disease of the brain little difficulty will usually arise but the interpretation of minor abnormalities in cases of presumed idiopathic epilepsy is much more difficult (Meyer, 1963). Probably in most such cases loss of nerve cells in the cortex and cerebellum, a finding described by many authors, is the result, rather than the cause of the epilepsy but small areas of cortical dysplasia, especially in the temporal lobe, may be causative in some cases (Taylor *et al.*, 1971). Microscopically much attention has been directed to focal lesions in Ammon's horn. When recent these consist of foci of tissue destruction with prominent neuronal loss, especially in Sommer's sector, which are later followed by gliosis. Such changes appear to be responsible for temporal lobe epilepsy in a high proportion of cases and Earle *et al.* (1953) suggested that hippocampal herniation at birth is an aetiological factor of great importance. However, similar pathological changes in Ammon's horn and in the region of the amygdala may be a sequel of anoxia. Certainly they may be the consequence of prolonged or recurrent seizures experimentally induced in animals (Meldrum and Brierley, 1972, 1973) or of a variety of processes inducing anoxia in man (Corsellis, 1957). It now seems possible that in many cases such lesions may be due to one or more febrile convulsions occurring in infancy and that the mesial temporal sclerosis so induced then acts as the focus of epileptic discharge which results in temporal lobe epilepsy developing subsequently (Falconer, 1974). Perinatal cerebral infarction due to occlusion of branches of the posterior cerebral artery may be another aetiological factor in some cases (Remillard *et al.*, 1974). Cavanagh (1958) reported eight cases of temporal lobe epilepsy of many years' standing associated with small tumours, considered most likely to be hamartomas, but a few showing early evidence of neoplastic transformation. In a large series of temporal lobes removed from patients with epilepsy, Falconer (1971) found mesial temporal sclerosis in one-half, between one-fifth and a quarter showed hamartomas or developmental anomalies, one-tenth scars or infarcts, and no specific pathological change was found in the remainder.

THE CLINICAL CLASSIFICATION OF SEIZURES

Traditionally (Janz, 1969), attacks of epilepsy, whether idiopathic or symptomatic, have been divided into major epilepsy (grand mal), minor epilepsy (petit mal), focal epilepsy (Jacksonian epilepsy), temporal lobe epilepsy (psychomotor epilepsy), and myoclonic attacks, and these traditional terms will be generally utilized in this chapter. However, increasing knowledge has shown that this descriptive classification is unsatisfactory for a variety of reasons. Thus there are many forms of minor epilepsy, with or without transient impairment of consciousness, which are not true petit mal; in epilepsy of focal onset, depending upon the site of origin in the brain, a variety of motor, sensory, behavioural, and psychomotor manifestations may be noted but if the epileptic discharge spreads rapidly to become generalized, a major attack may occur and the focal symptoms then constitute merely the aura of the major attack. Temporal lobe epilepsy is now becoming more generally known as complex partial epilepsy (Penry and Daly, 1975). A more up-to-date classification, modified from the International League Against Epilepsy (1969) and Sutherland *et al.* (1974), is given below:

1. *Generalized Seizures*

   Bilaterally symmetrical seizures without local onset:
   (*a*) Absences (petit mal)
   (*b*) Bilateral myoclonus
   (*c*) Infantile spasms
   (*d*) Clonic seizures
   (*e*) Tonic seizures
   (*f*) Tonic–clonic seizures
   (*g*) Akinetic seizures

2. *Partial Seizures*

   Seizures beginning locally with:
   (*a*) Elementary symptomatology
       motor ⎱
       sensory ⎰ Jacksonian epilepsy
       autonomic
   (*b*) Complex symptomatology
       impaired consciousness ⎫
       complex hallucinations ⎬ temporal lobe epilepsy
       affective symptoms ⎪
       automatism ⎭
   (*c*) Partial seizures becoming generalized
       tonic-clonic seizures

3. *Unclassified Seizures*

   Seizures which cannot be classified because of incomplete data.

SYMPTOMS

Major Epilepsy (Grand Mal)

Pre-convulsive Symptoms. Epileptic patients frequently exhibit symptoms which precede an attack for hours, or even for a day or two, and which enable those about them to recognize that a fit is likely to occur. These pre-convulsive symptoms include mental changes such as irritability and depression, abnormal feelings referred to the head, giddiness, and sudden myoclonic twitches.

Precipitating Factors. Usually these are absent. Rarely the kind of stimulus which more often causes syncope may precipitate an epileptic attack [see p. 321].

Severe coughing may do so (so-called laryngeal epilepsy). Eating, or drinking alcohol, sometimes brings on an attack. There are also the varieties of evoked or reflex epilepsy [see p. 1106].

The Aura. The aura, or warning of the attack, occurs in up to three-fifths of all cases. It is a symptom produced by the beginning of the epileptic discharge and perceived by the patient before consciousness is lost. In the remaining cases the patient experiences no warning, but becomes unconscious at the onset. An aura is less common in idiopathic major epilepsy than in those in which there is a focal onset. Since the focus of origin of the fit may be situated in a variety of localities within the brain there is a corresponding variety of auras. In temporal lobe epilepsy, the aura may take the form of a complex mental state, such as a feeling of unreality (*jamais vu*) or, on the other hand, of familiarity (*déjà vu*), as though events being experienced have happened before. The patient may feel that he is disembodied, or he may experience an intense but inexplicable fear. This last aura is sometimes associated with running, the patient running several yards before falling unconscious—'cursive epilepsy'. If the discharge begins in the anterior temporal region, the aura may be referred to one of the special senses and olfactory and gustatory hallucinations may occur; if more posterior, there may be visual auras consisting of complex scenes (formed visual hallucinations) or simple flashes of light or balls of fire (crude visual hallucinations); auditory auras may take the form of hallucinations of hearing words or phrases uttered, or may consist merely of crude sounds. Vertigo or subjective giddiness is a common aura. Sensory auras may consist of sensations of numbness, tingling or electric shocks referred to part of the body, or there may be a sensation as though a limb were shrivelling up. Painful sensory auras occur, but are rare. Abnormal visceral sensations frequently constitute the aura in temporal lobe attacks, the patient experiencing a peculiar sensation ('butterflies' in the stomach) or sometimes even pain in the epigastrium. There are many forms of motor aura. There may be a strong impulse to speak associated with a feeling of inability to do so or else chewing or 'smacking' of the lips may occur, again usually in seizures originating in the temporal lobe. The fit may begin with spasm or clonic movement of part of the body, for example turning of the head to one side (an adversive attack) or flexion of the upper limb, and the patient may be aware of the movement before he loses consciousness. Sometimes the whole body is rotated to one side.

Frequently the aura is so brief and takes the form of no more than a transient indefinable sensation that the patient is unable to describe it though he knows that he has a warning of insufficient duration for him to be able to reach a place of safety.

The Convulsion. The convulsion may begin with the epileptic cry, a harsh scream due to forcible expiration of air through the partly closed vocal cords, but this is more often absent than present. Consciousness is lost either immediately after the aura or at the very beginning of the attack, and the patient falls to the ground. He usually has no recollection of falling. In the fall he may injure himself, and permanent scars on the face, limbs or trunk from this cause are common in epileptics. The first motor manifestation of the convulsion proper is usually a phase of tonic spasm of the muscles. This is for the most part symmetrical on the two sides of the body, though it is common for the head and eyes to be rotated to one side and for the mouth to be drawn to one side by asymmetry in the degree of facial spasm. The upper limbs are usually adducted at the shoulders and flexed at the elbows and wrists. The fingers are flexed at the metacarpophalangeal and extended at the interphalangeal joints, the thumb being adducted. The lower limbs are usually extended, with the feet inverted. The respiratory and trunk muscles partake in the spasm, and respiration is arrested. The tonic phase may last only a few seconds and rarely endures more than half a minute.

It is followed by the clonic phase, in which sustained tonic contraction of the muscles gives place to sharp, short, interrupted jerks. The tonic phase may be so intense that occasionally compression fracture of the body of one or more thoracic vertebrae may occur in a fit and this should be borne in mind if the patient complains of pain in the back after recovery.

In the clonic phase the tongue may be bitten if it is caught between the teeth when the jaw is closed. Foaming at the mouth may occur, and the saliva may be blood-stained if the tongue has been bitten. Incontinence of urine often occurs: incontinence of faeces is less common.

At the onset of an epileptic fit the patient may be either pale or flushed. He becomes progressively cyanosed during the arrest of respiratory movements which occurs in the tonic stage, the cyanosis passing off when respiration is re-established in the clonic stage. Subconjunctival or cutaneous petechial haemorrhages may occur. There is often profuse sweating. The pupils become dilated at the beginning of the attack and the reaction to light is usually lost. The corneal reflexes are also lost in a severe attack; the tendon reflexes may be abolished and the plantar reflexes may be extensor for a short time after the attack.

The Post-convulsive Phase. Towards the end of the clonic phase the intervals between the muscular contractions become longer and the jerks finally cease. The patient remains unconscious for a variable time, usually from a few minutes to half an hour and on recovering consciousness often sleeps for several hours. Headache is common after an attack. Usually after recovering consciousness the patient is mentally normal. Exceptionally, however, a convulsion is followed by an abnormal mental state which may last a few minutes or even for several hours. In post-epileptic automatism the patient, though apparently conscious, may carry out a series of complex actions which are often inappropriate to the circumstances and of which he subsequently has no recollection. Sometimes the epileptic attack is followed by a period of hysterical behaviour. Rarely the epileptic patient may become maniacal after a convulsion. Post-epileptic mental aberration follows temporal lobe epilepsy more frequently than it does major epilepsy.

Minor Epilepsy

Minor epilepsy is a term often applied to slight epileptic attacks in which transient impairment or loss of consciousness is the most prominent symptom.

Petit Mal

Whereas in the past the term petit mal was often used to identify all forms of minor epilepsy unaccompanied by convulsions, the term is now reserved for transient minor 'absences' or 'blank spells' which invariably begin in childhood and never in adult life though in occasional cases, having begun in a child, they may continue for many years (Gibberd, 1972). In the present state of knowledge, true petit mal is invariably idiopathic, never symptomatic. The child, without warning, stares blankly into space, the eyes may roll up beneath the upper lids, and for a second or two he will stop talking or whatever he is doing and then will continue with his activity, often unaware that an attack has taken place. Occasionally a single myoclonic twitch of the head and upper limbs may accompany such episodes. Falling does not occur and the attacks often occur many times in the day. Some patients with attacks of petit mal also have major seizures or develop these as they grow older. Attacks of true petit mal are usually accompanied by 3 Hz generalized wave and spike discharges in the EEG [p. 1112]. Rarely prolonged mental confusion or even stupor in childhood or much less commonly in adult life may result from 'petit mal status' (Brett, 1966; Schwartz and Scott, 1971).

An epileptic encephalopathy in childhood characterized by frequent tonic seizures and atypical absences, a low I.Q. and an interictal EEG with frequent diffuse spike and slow wave discharges occurring at 2–2·5 Hz has been called the Lennox–Gastaut syndrome or petit mal variant; in such cases benzodiazepine, paradoxically, may precipitate status epilepticus (Tassinari et al., 1971).

Other Forms of Minor Epilepsy

These may occur at any age and may be idiopathic or symptomatic, the pattern depending upon the origin and spread of the epileptic discharge. Some such attacks, occurring either in childhood or in adult life, may be clinically indistinguishable from true petit mal.

The slightest form of minor epilepsy, often described by the patient as a 'sensation', consists of a disturbance of consciousness often similar to the aura of a major attack, and sometimes associated with giddiness. In a 'sensation' consciousness may not be completely lost. Next in severity comes complete loss of consciousness, preceded or not by an aura, but the motor and postural functions of the brain are so little affected that the patient remains standing and does not fall. He looks somewhat dazed and stares as in an attack of petit mal. After a few seconds he recovers and may continue what he was doing before the attack. In more severe attacks the motor and postural functions are affected, and the patient, besides losing consciousness, may fall to the ground or may exhibit slight muscular rigidity or carry out a brief stereotyped movement. Attacks in which falling occurs but in which there are no convulsive movements are often called akinetic epilepsy. Transitory pallor may occur in minor epilepsy. Incontinence of urine may occur, though it is less frequent than in major attacks. There is no post-ictal coma.

Temporal Lobe Epilepsy. The clinical picture of temporal lobe epilepsy depends upon whether the epileptic discharge remains localized to the temporal lobe (in which case focal features related to temporal lobe dysfunction are consistently noted) or whether it spreads rapidly throughout the remainder of the brain, in which case there may be a major fit with a 'temporal lobe aura' or even a major fit without an aura which is then indistinguishable from an attack of idiopathic grand mal. The EEG is of considerable value in the diagnosis. In these attacks the patient may become confused, often anxious and negativistic, and sometimes carries out movements of a highly organized but semi-automatic character (automatism).

Automatism may take various forms; sometimes it is purposeless, occasionally purposive (e.g. undressing in public) and, rarely, aggressive or violent behaviour can occur. In such cases the epileptic discharge appears to originate in the peri-amygdaloid region (Feindel and Penfield, 1954). Only very rarely can violent behaviour occurring during such a period of automatism be accepted as the cause of violent crime (Gunn and Fenton, 1971), but outbursts of rage due to this cause are well documented (Holden, 1957). Gelastic epilepsy, in which outbursts of laughing occur during the attack (Gumpert et al., 1970), may occur in association with cursive epilepsy (running at the onset) (Chen and Forster, 1973); these too are forms of automatism. Attacks may last for only a few seconds or for minutes or longer, whether or not a major convulsion follows the aura. Varied disturbances of the content of consciousness may occur: these include hallucinations of smell and taste (uncinate epilepsy), vision and hearing, perceptual illusions, disordered sense of reality or of the body, disturbances of memory, and paroxysms of fear. Recurring nightmares may represent one form of attack (Boller et al., 1975). Visual phenomena may include formed hallucinations, macropsia and micropsia, while depersonalization (*jamais vu* or unreality) suggests to the patient a dream or 'trance-like' state and *déjà vu*, an intense feeling of familiarity, may be accompanied by vivid visual or auditory memory patterns which the patient is subsequently unable to recall though remembering that they were familiar and a constantly recurring pattern of his attack. Differential diagnosis from the phobic anxiety–depersonalization syndrome, often presenting with agarophobia in middle-aged women ('the house-bound house-wife') may give rise to difficulty in differential diagnosis but the EEG may be very helpful (Harper and Roth, 1962). Depression is also an occasional feature. Impaired sexual drive is common (Taylor, 1969) and hypergraphia (compulsive writing) has been described (Waxman and Geschwind, 1974). Uncinate attacks are characterized by hallucinations of smell or taste. They are often accompanied by movements of the lips, tongue, and jaw, for example, those of tasting or chewing, and are commonly associated with a disturbance of memory (Currie et al., 1971). Uncinate attacks are usually the result of organic disease in the region of the uncus [see p. 1100].

Jacksonian Epilepsy. Jacksonian epilepsy usually begins in one of three foci, the thumb and index finger, the angle of the mouth, or the great toe. A convulsion with such a focal onset and the type of spread described on page 23 is almost always a symptom of organic disease of the brain in the region of the precentral gyrus. A similar focal onset is not unknown in presumed idiopathic epilepsy, particularly in children, but in such cases the spread of the convulsion is often more rapid than in a typical Jacksonian attack and consciousness is lost early. However, benign focal epilepsy in childhood [see p. 1099] has been identified as a distinctive syndrome.

Sensory Epilepsy. This is the sensory equivalent of motor Jacksonian epilepsy and consists of paraesthesiae, such as tingling or 'electric shocks', less frequently of painful sensation, involving usually a part or the whole of one side of the body. The attacks may occur without loss of consciousness and are usually the result of a lesion in the opposite parietal lobe.

Epilepsia Partialis Continua. This is a rare form of focal convulsion in which Jacksonian epilepsy, confined to a limited part of the body, continues for hours, days, weeks, or rarely months, without stopping. It is invariably due to a focal lesion of the brain though the nature of the lesion may not be immediately apparent.

N n

Adversive Attacks. These begin with turning of the head and eyes and sometimes of the body to the opposite side: they originate in front of the precentral gyrus in the region of the so-called frontal eye field (Brodmann's area 8).

Inhibitory Epilepsy. This is a very rare form of attack in which transitory loss of power occurs in a limb or in one-half of the body without precedent tonic spasm or clonic movements. It may or may not be associated with impairment or loss of consciousness.

'Drop' Attacks. In these the patient falls to the ground without warning. The only evidence for loss of consciousness is unawareness of the fall itself. The patient can get up at once. There are two varieties of these: (1) a form of akinetic epilepsy (see above); and (2) sudden falls occurring chiefly in middle-aged or elderly women. It is unlikely that the latter attacks are epileptic; they seem often to be a symptom of atheromatous ischaemia of the brain stem (vertebro-basilar insufficiency). However, Stevens and Matthews (1973), confirming that this type of attack is almost totally confined to women and that, in contradistinction to akinetic epilepsy, consciousness is fully retained, were not convinced that ischaemia is a satisfactory explanation, but could suggest no satisfactory alternative.

'Tonic Epilepsy.' These attacks consist of episodes of muscular rigidity associated with loss of consciousness, but not followed by clonic movements. In the usual form of tonic convulsion the posture of the body differs from that of the tonic phase of a major epileptic attack. The head is extended, the upper limbs are thrown out in front of the patient, extended at the elbows, internally rotated and hyperpronated, with the fingers somewhat flexed. The lower limbs are extended. This type of fit is usually the result of organic disease of the brain [see p. 1095] but occurs occasionally in idiopathic epilepsy. Focal 'tonic fits' in which similar attacks may involve one or two limbs without loss of consciousness have been described in multiple sclerosis and have been attributed to the presence of a brain stem lesion (Matthews, 1954).

Diencephalic Epilepsy

Epilepsy of diencephalic origin, characterized by a variety of phenomena indicating transient autonomic dysfunction, including spontaneous periodic hypothermia (Fox *et al.*, 1973), has been postulated but there is still controversy as to whether such periodic diencephalic phenomena are truly epileptic.

Vestibular and Vestibulogenic Attacks. Behrman and Wyke (1958) distinguished two varieties of attack both with an aura of vertigo. They suggested that vestibular attacks originate in the cortical vestibular centre in the mid-temporal region and that vestibulogenic attacks are excited by labyrinthine discharge, often from an abnormal labyrinth, which excites discharge from neurones in the brain stem reticular system.

Evoked or Reflex Epilepsy. It occasionally happens that a convulsion may be excited by some form of external stimulation (*British Medical Journal*, 1975 c). This may be a sudden loud noise—*acoustico-motor epilepsy*—or music—*musicogenic epilepsy*—or a visual—*photic*—or cutaneous stimulus. The precipitation of attacks by reading is well recognized ('*reading epilepsy*') (Bingel, 1957; Stoupel, 1968), but in one such case they were also precipitated by speaking and writing (*language-induced epilepsy*) (Geschwind and Sherwin,

1967). It is uncertain as to whether in reading epilepsy the attacks are precipitated by the written or printed word, by the eye movements involved in reading, or by some other mechanism (Brooks and Jirauch, 1971). So-called *'television epilepsy'* has also been increasingly recognized in recent years. Both childhood petit mal but more particularly grand mal in children and less commonly in adults may be precipitated by watching television, particularly when the set is flickering or poorly adjusted so that flickering lines appear. Sometimes a voluntary movement will precipitate an attack. In such cases sudden movement is particularly likely to induce a type of 'tonic fit' in the limb which is moved (Lishman *et al.*, 1962). Numerous activities which may act in this way are described by Symonds (1959). Coughing may precipitate an attack (*cough seizures*), presumably as a consequence of a transient reduction in cerebral blood flow due to a reduced venous return to the heart; this is especially liable to occur in patients with overt or unsuspected cerebral vascular disease (Morgan-Hughes, 1966). So-called carotid sinus epilepsy (Behrman and Knight, 1956) is almost certainly carotid sinus syncope leading to epileptiform manifestations in the attacks. An attack may be self-induced; this particularly occurs in children with petit mal who may rapidly move their fingers between their eyes and the sun to induce an attack (Hutchison *et al.*, 1958; Whitty, 1960).

There may be visceral concomitants; not only may gastric distension precipitate an attack, but in some patients the onset is always associated with diarrhoea.

Reflex inhibition of a fit is an allied phenomenon. When a convulsion has a focal onset and begins with movement, for example, of one limb, a strong stimulus, such as a firm grip, rubbing, or passive movement applied to the limb, will often abort an attack, if it is begun immediately after the onset. Efron (1956, 1957) has shown that uncinate attacks may sometimes be arrested by smelling a powerful odour.

Pyknolepsy. Pyknolepsy is a term once applied to a syndrome characterized by very frequent attacks of petit mal. As the condition is in no way different from petit mal the term has now been discarded.

Infantile Spasms

This name has been given to brief attacks, beginning almost invariably in infants within the first few months of life, in which there is a sudden shock-like flexion of the arms and often flexion of the head, neck, and trunk with drawing up of the knees (so-called salaam attacks). These momentary attacks may occur many times in the day; their development sometimes in infants who appear to be of normal intellect is followed by progressive mental deterioration so that when they eventually cease the child is often left spastic and severely retarded. The EEG usually shows a pattern of almost continuous irregular slow spike-and-wave activity which has been called hypsarrhythmia (Gibbs and Gibbs, 1952; Bower and Jeavons, 1959; Kiloh *et al.*, 1972). In most cases coming to autopsy the degenerative changes seen in the cortex and white matter of the cerebrum are non-specific but in some there may be evidence of dysmyelination and the syndrome has been observed in children with hypoglycaemia, phenylketonuria, cerebral birth injury, and tuberous sclerosis (della Rovere *et al.*, 1964). Abnormalities of dendritic development in the pyramidal neurones of the frontal cortex have also been described (Huttenlocher, 1974). While anticonvulsants are relatively ineffective, ACTH or steroid drugs, if given early enough, may arrest the process in some cases.

Myoclonus Epilepsy. See page 1132.

The Time-relationship of Attacks

Individuals differ greatly in respect of the frequency of their attacks. At one extreme are those who have only one, or perhaps two, in a lifetime; at the other, those who convulse several times a day.

As Gowers pointed out, there are three common modes of onset of the convulsions. A child may have petit mal for a long period before beginning to have major fits. Alternatively, the first attack may be a severe one and thereafter major fits may occur at short intervals, with or without attacks of petit mal in addition; or there may be major attacks separated by long intervals of months or even years. In 76 per cent of Gowers' cases the intervals between attacks were less than one month. Some patients always have attacks in groups of two or more within a few hours.

Time of day is an important factor in determining the occurrence of fits. In 42 per cent of a series of cases attacks occurred by day only, in 24 per cent by night only, and in the remainder both by day and by night. When the attacks were confined to the day they occurred only half as frequently as in the other two groups. Nocturnal fits are most likely to occur shortly after going to sleep and between 4 and 5 a.m., while the commonest time for diurnal attacks is during the first hour after awakening. Recently, Gibberd and Bateson (1974), in a review of 645 cases, found that only 38 had attacks which occurred only during sleep and of those beginning with nocturnal attacks only, the proportion who subsequently developed diurnal attacks increased year by year. Sleep deprivation may also precipitate attacks (Gunderson *et al.*, 1973). Menstruation markedly influences the occurrence of fits in women. Many women have attacks only at the menstrual period, usually just before the period begins, less frequently during or immediately after (Laidlaw, 1956). 'Long-distance rhythms', i.e. the regular recurrence of attacks at intervals of many months, have been studied by Griffiths and Fox (1938).

Status Epilepticus. An epileptic patient may have a succession of convulsions with recovery of consciousness between the attacks—serial epilepsy. In some cases, however, one attack follows another without any intervening period of consciousness—status epilepticus. Unless the convulsions can be arrested, coma deepens, and pyrexia, or even hyperpyrexia, develops, and death occurs. Some patients exhibit a special tendency to develop status epilepticus, and do so on many occasions.

Status epilepticus occurs more often in symptomatic than idiopathic epilepsy and there seems to be a clear association with frontal lobe lesions and possibly cerebral oedema (Janz, 1964; Oxbury and Whitty, 1971). While status in early post-traumatic epilepsy in adults usually implies that the brain injury has been severe, paradoxically it seems to be rare after severe head injury and much commoner after minor or even trivial head injury in childhood (Grand, 1974). Prolonged confusion due to petit mal status has been described in childhood (Brett, 1966) and subclinical 'electrical status epilepticus' occurring during sleep with almost continuous spike and wave discharge which ceases on waking, in mentally retarded children who suffer occasional diurnal petit mal and nocturnal grand mal, has been described (Patry *et al.*, 1971).

Status epilepticus in animals is accompanied first by marked rises in arterial and cerebral venous pressure with severe metabolic and respiratory acidosis, hyperglycaemia, and reduced arteriovenous (AV) differences for oxygen and carbon dioxide. In the later stages blood pressure is low, cerebral AV differences for O_2 and CO_2 are enhanced, and there is usually hyperpyrexia, hyperkalaemia, and hypoglycaemia (Meldrum and Horton, 1973).

Mental and Physical Abnormalities

No mental or physical abnormalities are constantly associated with epilepsy, and many epileptic patients exhibit neither. As already indicated, however, there are a number of organic or metabolic disorders of the brain which may produce both dementia and epilepsy. Epilepsy is sometimes associated with mental deficiency, and one easily recognizable type of mentally defective, epileptic child is excitable, noisy, destructive, and difficult to control ('the hyperkinetic syndrome'). The cause of the progressive mental deterioration which sometimes accompanies epilepsy is obscure. It may not always be a direct result of the fits, since it can be absent in patients having frequent severe attacks, but recurrent anoxia occurring in major fits and giving rise to progressive brain damage is certainly the cause in most cases.

Behaviour disorders, with aggressive outbursts and paranoid traits, are particularly common in some adults and children with severe temporal lobe epilepsy. Furthermore, epilepsy is known to occur occasionally in patients suffering from psychotic illnesses, particularly paranoid schizophrenia, while spontaneous fits may develop following electroconvulsive therapy.

Thus it may be concluded that epilepsy itself does not *produce* mental changes unless the fits are severe or frequent enough to produce anoxic damage to the brain, in which case there may be sudden mental deterioration, especially in childhood (Illingworth, 1955) or else progressive dementia may develop. Mental dullness and lack of concentration with a deteriorating performance in school or at work is sometimes due to the drugs being given to treat the epilepsy rather than to the condition itself and folic-acid deficiency as a result of anticonvulsant therapy should be considered as a possible aetiological factor in causing mental deterioration (Neubauer, 1970). Petit mal status should also be excluded in children (Brett, 1966).

Physical signs which have been described in some cases of epilepsy in previous reports, including nystagmus, dysarthria, and ataxia, are in most instances due to the treatment rather than to the disease. Other features such as evidence of pyramidal tract disease, when present, should invariably suggest that the epilepsy is symptomatic of some underlying organic lesion of the brain.

No constant endocrine abnormality has been found to be associated with epilepsy, though minor disorders of skeletal growth and genital development are common. Some adolescent epileptics are exceptionally tall for their age. Obesity of the hypopituitary and eunuchnoid type is sometimes seen, together with a heterosexual distribution of pubic hair, but these changes, as well as coarsening of the facial features (Falconer and Davidson, 1973) are more probably due to the anticonvulsant therapy, especially with phenytoin. Facial naevus may suggest an intracranial angioma on the same side, which may cause an audible bruit on auscultation of the skull. In spite of numerous investigations no constant metabolic abnormality has been generally recognized in cases of 'idiopathic' epilepsy. Frequent major fits, mental backwardness and tetany, associated sometimes with intracranial calcification, may occur in cases of idiopathic hypoparathyroidism and in pseudohypoparathyroidism (Simpson, 1952; Glaser and Levy, 1960); the fits may be improved by treatment with dihydrotachysterol (*A.T. 10*) given in an initial dosage of 1·25 mg three times daily until the serum calcium is normal, and then a smaller maintenance dose is required.

Investigative Findings

In 'idiopathic' epilepsy the cerebrospinal fluid is normal except that during or after frequent fits or an attack of status epilepticus there may be a rise in pressure to above 200 mm of fluid and a modest rise in protein content of the fluid. A consistently raised CSF protein and a pleocytosis should suggest that the epilepsy is symptomatic. Air encephalography and/or ventriculography usually give normal findings but in some cases of long-standing epilepsy and epilepsy of late onset signs of ventricular dilatation and cortical atrophy are apparent (Hunter *et al.*, 1962). It is not certain as to whether these findings indicate that the cortical atrophy is the result of frequent fits or whether an unspecified degenerative process causing the cortical atrophy is also the cause of the attacks. The radiological abnormalities resulting from neoplasms, hamartomas, focal scarring, mesial temporal sclerosis, and the other numerous causes of temporal lobe epilepsy have been reviewed recently by Newcombe and Shah (1975); dilatation of, or a filling defect in, one temporal horn, often requiring tomography for its demonstration, is the commonest finding.

Gamma encephalography [p. 148] and computerized transaxial tomography (CTT, or the EMI scan) [p. 151] are likely to play an increasing role in the investigation of epileptic patients, particularly in adult life, in order to exclude the presence of a cerebral lesion of which the epilepsy may be symptomatic. Thus Wallace (1974) who studied 132 patients with late-onset epilepsy, using gamma-encephalography found that 26 had abnormal scans, due to tumour, abscess, infarction, or trauma. Similarly Bogdanoff *et al.* (1975) in a study of 50 unselected cases of focal epilepsy using the CTT scan found porencephalic cysts in six, diffuse cerebral atrophy in five, cerebellar hemiatrophy in three, focal cortical atrophy in two, neoplasms in two, hydrocephalus in one, and cerebellar hypoplasia in one.

Electroencephalography

The diagnostic importance of the EEG in epilepsy lies in the fact that an abnormal record obtained in the interval between the attacks may establish the diagnosis when this is otherwise in doubt. Further, the effect of different drugs upon the abnormal rhythms, and the general response to treatment can be studied. It is important to stress the present limitations of electroencephalography in the diagnosis of epilepsy. From 10 to 20 per cent of epileptics have a normal EEG, and the percentage is higher in those having grand mal only and after the age of 40. A normal EEG, therefore, does not exclude epilepsy. Patients with petit mal usually exhibit the wave-and-spike pattern [see FIG. 165] or a three Hz wave, but the abnormal rhythm may be present only after over-ventilation. These rhythms, however, are not pathognomonic of petit mal, but may occur in other forms of epilepsy. Grand mal is not associated with any single characteristic form of EEG, but paroxysmal diffuse multiple spikes in rapid rhythm or isolated generalized paroxysmal outbursts of spike or sharp-wave activity are usually associated with grand mal. Temporal lobe epilepsy is often identified by means of focal spike or sharp wave discharges arising in one or other temporal region or by paroxysmal outbursts of rhythmical slow theta activity which are similarly located. These discharges may only become apparent during early sleep so that sleep recordings induced by sedative drugs may be helpful. Recording with sphenoidal or pharyngeal electrodes before, during, and after thiopentone-induced sleep is a valuable technique and the unilateral absence of barbiturate-induced fast activity over one temporal lobe is a valuable guide to the presence of a focal epileptogenic lesion. Focal epileptogenic cortical lesions in other areas are often similarly associated with corresponding focal, abnormal EEG discharges. With the possible exception of the wave-and-spike pattern and its fast and slow variants there is no abnormal EEG which is pathognomonic of epilepsy, and non-specific abnormalities may be found in epilepsy, psychoneurosis, psychopathy, or psychosis. It follows that an abnormal EEG can be interpreted only in relation to the clinical history of the patient (Gibbs *et al.*, 1937, 1938, 1943; Jasper and Kershman, 1941; Williams, 1941; Kiloh *et al.*, 1972). An epileptic dysrhythmia is much more likely to be detected during sleep than during waking life (Gibbs and Gibbs, 1947) and may be evoked by an injection of leptazol (*Metrazol*) or bemegride (*Megimide*) (Ziskind and Bercel, 1947; Hill and Parr, 1963). Electrocorticography is used for the precise localization of an epileptic focus at operation, and telemetering, a technique by means of which the electroencephalogram can be conveyed from small transistorized transmitters attached to the mobile patient to a static recorder, can be used for continuous recording during diurnal activity and during sleep. The latter technique, if combined with videotape recording, is particularly useful in relating the patient's behaviour on the one hand to cerebral electrical events on the other.

DIAGNOSIS

The diagnosis of epilepsy falls into two parts. It is first necessary to distinguish epileptic attacks from other paroxysmal disturbances, and secondly, to decide whether the attacks are symptomatic of organic disease or metabolic disorder, or whether the patient is suffering from constitutional or idiopathic epilepsy.

Diagnosis of the Nature of the Attack

Both minor and major attacks must be distinguished from *syncope*. Syncope usually occurs in individuals with vasomotor instability or as the result of exhaustion, haemorrhage, an emotional shock, sudden change of posture, standing for long periods, or disease of the autonomic nervous system [see pp. 321 and 1073]. Both the onset and the cessation of syncopal attacks are more gradual than is usually the case in epilepsy, and the former is usually preceded by a feeling of faintness. In syncope also the patient is limp, whereas the occurrence of slight rigidity is in favour of epilepsy; on the other hand, transient rigidity and twitching and even incontinence may occur in severe syncope. Perspiration and severe pallor favour a diagnosis of fainting. Nevertheless, in some individuals pressure upon the carotid sinus or circumstances which usually induce syncope may precipitate an epileptic attack. For a discussion of the relationship between syncope and epilepsy, see page 324.

In *narcolepsy* consciousness is lost, but convulsive movements are absent and the patient, unlike the epileptic, shows all the features of natural sleep and can be immediately roused. In *cataplexy* voluntary power is lost but consciousness is retained.

Aural vertigo may be confused with minor and major epilepsy, in which vertigo may also occur, often as a transient aura. In vertigo of aural origin, however, consciousness is retained and other symptoms of aural disease, such as tinnitus and deafness, are usually present. Though an attack of aural vertigo may be brief, it usually lasts longer than a minor attack or an aura, and passes away more gradually. But the relationship between the labyrinth and epilepsy is complex [see p. 1106].

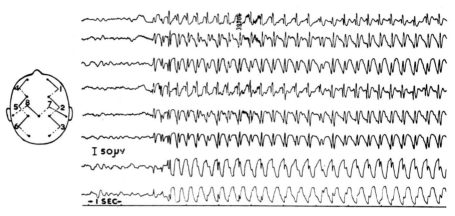

FIG. 165. Male, aged 18. Generalized, bilaterally synchronous and symmetrical 3 Hz wave-and-spike discharges during a petit mal attack

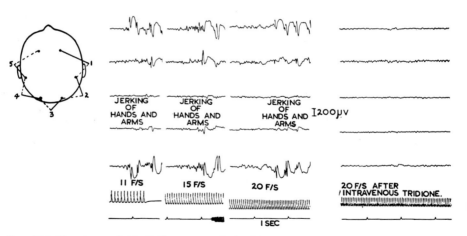

FIG. 166. Female, aged 19. Epilepsy, myoclonic. Photo-myoclonic response at various flash frequencies and subsequent effect of intravenous tridione

Hysterical convulsions are usually easily distinguished from epileptic attacks if the patient is seen when convulsing. Their onset is usually gradual, and they usually occur only in the presence of an audience. Consciousness is not completely lost, for the patient can usually be roused by forcible measures, and an attempt to elicit the corneal reflex usually evokes a vigorous contraction of the orbicularis oculi. If the patient cries out during the attack he usually articulates words or phrases, and laughing and crying may occur. The movements which constitute an hysterical convulsion are not clonic jerks as in epilepsy, but such as can be carried out voluntarily, for example, clutching at objects in the neighbourhood. The tongue is not bitten, nor does incontinence of urine usually occur in an hysterical attack. However, there is a particular type of hysterical attack which occurs usually in young females, less often in males, in which

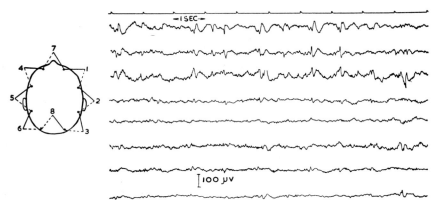

Fig. 167. Male, aged 30. Temporal lobe epilepsy. Focal sharp and slow waves in the right temporal region

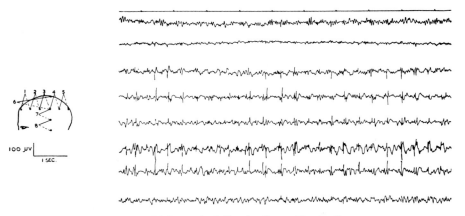

Fig. 168. Male, aged 14. Focal epilepsy. Focal spikes

sudden falling without convulsive movements occurs and the picture may be indistinguishable from that of akinetic epilepsy. After being asked frequently by one or more doctors the patient may oblige by passing urine in an attack. These attacks are often very frequent, occur particularly at times of stress, appear to cause the patient little concern and show virtually no response to anti-convulsant drugs. The difficulty of differential diagnosis is increased by the fact that epileptic and hysterical attacks may coexist in the same individuals. A similar type of attack occasionally occurs in a medicolegal context in adults after trivial head injury and frequently ceases abruptly after settlement of a compensation claim.

Anxiety attacks are occasionally confused with epilepsy. In these consciousness is not lost, but the predominant symptom is an intense sense of anxiety, which is often associated with a feeling of giddiness, palpitation, and sweating.

The panic attacks of the phobic anxiety-depersonalization syndrome (Harper and Roth, 1962) may be readily confused with temporal lobe epilepsy as in these episodes mounting panic and angor animi (fear of 'impending doom') are often associated with a sense of intense depersonalization or unreality and if there is associated hyperventilation, syncope sometimes occurs or even tetany. Usually, however, consciousness remains unimpaired and there are associated phobias about going out of the house alone, crossing roads or entering crowded places, which are not a feature of epilepsy. Similar symptoms sometimes occur in depressive illness.

Under the term *vasovagal attacks*, Gowers (1907) described 'prolonged seizures, the symptoms of which consist chiefly in disturbance of some of the functions of the pneumo-gastric'. The patient complained of gastric, respiratory, or cardiac discomfort, and these symptoms were often associated with vaso-constriction and coldness of the extremities. Women were more subject to these paroxysms than men. They were distinguished from epilepsy by their gradual onset and longer duration, and by the usual absence of loss of consciousness. It is doubtful if they represent a nosological entity; most were probably syncopal, some were probably due to anxiety and others were in all probability episodes of temporal lobe epilepsy, properly falling, as Gowers suggested, into the 'borderland of epilepsy'.

Migraine is a paroxysmal disturbance which may simulate epilepsy. The onset of an attack of migraine, however, is gradual. Consciousness is not lost, and headache usually occurs. It must be remembered, however, that the same individual may suffer from both migraine and epilepsy, and that very exceptionally a severe attack of migraine may terminate in an epileptic fit.

When it has been established that a patient suffers from epileptiform attacks, it remains to exclude the various focal and metabolic causes of convulsions enumerated on pages 1095–6.

Diagnosis of the Cause

Gross organic lesions such as *hydrocephalus* and *infantile hemiplegia* give rise to no difficulty.

Tuberous sclerosis can be diagnosed as a cause of epilepsy associated with mental defect only when adenoma sebaceum is present, when there are phako-mata to be seen in the retina or by the characteristic X-ray changes.

Renal disease and *hypertensive encephalopathy* may be excluded by examination of the cardiovascular system, including the blood pressure, and of the urine and the blood urea but it must be noted that hyperuricaemia with acute renal failure has been described as a sequel of status epilepticus or recurrent grand mal (Warren *et al.*, 1975).

The diagnosis of *syphilis* can be established by means of the history, the presence of signs of the infection of the nervous system, and a positive V.D.R.L. reaction in the blood or cerebrospinal fluid.

When *alcohol* or *amphetamines* or *drug intoxication* or *withdrawal* is the cause of the convulsions a history of alcoholism or of drug-taking can usually be obtained.

Heart block offers little difficulty in diagnosis if the possibility of its occurrence is borne in mind. If an attack is witnessed it is found to coincide with cardiac asystole and flushing usually accompanies the return of consciousness. When complete atrioventricular block is established the pulse rate is usually about 30. Even if the pulse rate is normal between the attacks, impaired conduction in the atrioventricular bundle can usually be demonstrated by an electrocardiogram.

Spontaneous hypoglycaemia may cause syncopal or epileptic attacks, or in milder cases, fatigability, anxiety, sweating, giddiness, diplopia, or mental confusion. The subject was well reviewed by Conn (1947). Apart from gross disease of the liver, hypophysis, or adrenals, the two chief causes are: (1) adenoma, carcinoma, or hyperplasia of the islet cells of Langerhans of the pancreas; and (2) reactive hyperinsulinism. The former is the more likely to give rise to epilepsy, which is commonly nocturnal, when the blood sugar is at its lowest. The diagnosis is based upon the low fasting blood sugar in the former, and abnormal sugar tolerance tests and the correlation between the attacks and the low blood sugar in both (Wauchope, 1933; Prunty, 1944; Conn, 1947).

Special consideration must be given to two common causes of convulsions developing after the age of 30, namely intracranial tumour and cerebral arteriosclerosis. In *intracranial tumour* convulsions may precede other symptoms by months or years, and when this is the case the cause can often only be suspected. Though convulsions due to cerebral tumour may be generalized, a focal origin for the attacks should suggest tumour, especially when they are followed by temporary aphasia or paresis. Sooner or later headache and other symptoms of increased intracranial pressure make their appearance, together with signs of a progressive cerebral lesion. The EEG may suggest the presence of a focal lesion, radiographs of the skull or echo-encephalography may indicate a 'shift' of midline structures and gamma-encephalography, computerized transaxial tomography, air encephalography, ventriculography, or angiography may be required. Epileptiform attacks due to *cerebral arteriosclerosis* usually occur in late middle life and old age. They may follow upon clinically evident episodes of cerebral infarction (post-hemiplegic epilepsy), but sometimes the cause of the attacks is a previous asymptomatic minor cortical infarct. Vascular abnormality is usually demonstrable in the arteries of the retina, and the blood pressure may be raised.

Cysticercosis should be considered when epilepsy begins in adult life in men who have lived abroad, especially in India, and a search should be made for subcutaneous cysts. Calcified cysts may be demonstrated radiographically in the muscles and less often in the brain.

PROGNOSIS

The risk that death will occur during an epileptic attack is relatively slight, except in status epilepticus, in which condition the patient's life is always threatened until consciousness returns, and death may occur even after recovery of consciousness. However, death is well recognized to occur in febrile convulsions in infancy (Lennox-Buchthal, 1974) and there have been many reports of unexpected, unexplained death in young and otherwise physically fit epileptic subjects; many are found dead in bed but others die after seizures which were witnessed and showed no unusual characteristics (Hirsch and Martin, 1971). Autopsy examination usually fails to demonstrate the cause of death (Terrence *et al.*, 1975). However, some patients are shown to have died from asphyxia due to a nocturnal fit in which the patient's face may become buried in a pillow and drowning due to a convulsion in the bath has also been described. Mortality and morbidity data have been comprehensively reviewed by Kurtzke (1972).

Minor accidents resulting from the attacks include injuries induced by the fall, though these are rarely serious, but dislocation of the shoulder, which is produced by muscular action, is not uncommon; once having occurred, it is liable to recur in subsequent attacks. The violence of the convulsions may cause compression fracture of vertebral bodies, usually in the thoracic region, a possibility which should always be considered when the patient complains of pain in the back after a fit. Fractures of limb bones occur less frequently.

The prognosis as to recovery from the attacks depends upon a number of factors. To achieve recovery it is necessary to abolish the attacks by means of treatment for a sufficient length of time for the tendency to be permanently suppressed. Persevering and thorough treatment is therefore essential, and must be continued for at least three years after the attacks have ceased and in many cases indefinitely. Treatment should always be withdrawn gradually but even so, fits recur, even after three or more years of freedom in up to 30 per cent of cases. The sooner the treatment can be begun after the first fit, the better the outlook. Holowach et al. (1972) followed up 148 epileptic children, all of whom had been free from attacks for four years on anticonvulsant medication, for 5–12 years after drug withdrawal. Seizures recurred in 24 per cent; there was no relation between relapse on the one hand and sex, race, heredity, puberty, or seizure frequency on the other. With an early age of onset and prompt control of seizures the relapse rate was only 13 per cent; it was higher in cases of later onset or prolonged duration and in those with neurological, psychological, or marked electroencephalographic abnormalities. In adult epileptics, the relapse rate after withdrawal of anticonvulsants is higher, approaching 40 per cent (*The Lancet*, 1972 a). Individuals suffering from frequent severe attacks are least likely to be completely cured. The outlook is often best when the attacks occur only during sleep, and treatment is most likely to be successful when they take place at a regular time of the day or of the month, so that intensive treatment can be timed so as to avert them. Marked mental deterioration makes the outlook worse. Thus few patients in institutions become free from attacks, and the death rate among institutional epileptics is four times that of the general population. Probably about 30 per cent of non-institutional epileptics are cured, in the sense of remaining free from attacks indefinitely but in over 60 per cent the attacks can be completely controlled with treatment (Bridge *et al.*, 1947; Frantzen, 1961; Rodin, 1972).

There has been some controversy concerning the prognosis of childhood petit mal. Lees and Liversedge (1962) suggested that in many children with this form of minor epilepsy attacks continued into adult life. However, Livingston *et al.* (1965) found that the attacks eventually ceased in adolescence in over three-quarters of their cases, but grand mal eventually developed in 54 per cent of those who started with 'pure' petit mal seizures.

TREATMENT

General Management

Symptomatic epilepsy, resulting, say, from an intracranial tumour, is best treated by curing the condition of which the epilepsy is but a symptom, but this is only rarely possible and thus, in many symptomatic cases, the same treatment as that given for idiopathic epilepsy must be employed.

It is desirable that an epileptic patient should as far as possible live a normal life. Children should attend school and should be subjected to ordinary discipline. Measures useful in the prevention of attacks, of secondary handicaps, and of reducing the stigma which is still too often attached to the diagnosis of epilepsy, are reviewed by Taylor and Bower (1971), while vocational and educational problems have been considered in detail by Rodin *et al.* (1972) and social adjustment by Bagley (1972). Adults should carry on an occupation, though certain trades will necessarily be ruled out. Occupations involving working at heights, or near dangerous machinery, or driving vehicles are obviously unsuitable, and sufferers from epilepsy were in the past precluded by law from obtaining a motor-driver's licence in Great Britain. After a single fit, however, for which investigation demonstrated no obvious cause, many neurologists were prepared to recommend that driving should be banned for one year only and that anticonvulsant drugs should only be taken for the first six months of this period. Maxwell and Leyshon (1971), among others, found that many epileptics had, in the past, obtained driving licences through false declarations on their application forms. All neurologists are aware of serious, sometimes fatal, road accidents which have occurred as a result of a driver suffering a fit. Since 1968, in Great Britain, an epileptic patient may, on the presentation of medical evidence, have his driving licence restored after three years of total freedom from attacks, provided he is prepared to continue anticonvulsant therapy indefinitely. If he prefers to attempt withdrawal of anticonvulsant drugs, accepting a 40 per cent relapse rate, even after three years of freedom from attacks, a further period of one year of freedom from attacks will normally be required before it is reasonable to certify that the patient no longer suffers from epilepsy and that it is safe for him to drive. Those who wish to attempt withdrawal of treatment should be warned that if a further attack occurs, then another period of three years of freedom from attacks on treatment will be required before he can drive. It is also possible to recommend restoration of a licence to an individual certified, over a three-year period, as suffering from nocturnal attacks only. In general, a history of epilepsy, even if controlled, is sufficient to debar any individual permanently from driving a heavy goods vehicle or a public service vehicle or from flying an aeroplane. Regulations in various parts of the United States and in other countries vary from state to state and from country to country but are broadly similar (Stock *et al.*, 1970).

Children should be allowed to take part in sports; an individual decision must be made in every case depending upon the frequency and severity of the attacks but the riding of horses or of bicycles can often be allowed if the attacks are well controlled. A regular occupation is a considerable prophylactic against attacks. Certain risks of everyday life must be explained to the patient and his friends, but it is difficult, if not impossible, to guard him against them all. The water in his bath should be shallow, and he should not swim in deep water unaccompanied. Institutional treatment may be necessary for mentally handicapped patients, and those having severe and frequent fits, if adequate home care is not available. Those in whom the disorder renders an ordinary occupation impossible often do well in special residential centres (Reid, 1972).

No general rule can be laid down concerning the marriage of epileptics. There is no evidence that marriage affects the tendency to fits either beneficially or adversely, though pregnancy may prove either beneficial or the reverse. The risk of transmitting the disorder to children must be individually assessed in each case. This risk is clearly greatest when there is a family history of epilepsy or when an EEG shows that the non-epileptic parent has an abnormal record, and least when a focal lesion of the brain can be held partly responsible for the attacks. Even when the epileptic tendency is hereditary it is exceptional for a patient to transmit the disorder in the direct line, and the chances are thirty-five to one against any individual child of an epileptic parent developing epilepsy.

Careful attention must be paid to general hygiene in epilepsy. Moderate exercise is desirable; attacks rarely occur during exercise but may follow violent exertion. Any factor adversely affecting the general health should receive attention. Alcohol is best avoided, as over-indulgence, or even a modest intake, may precipitate attacks.

The Investigation of Epilepsy of Late Onset

In many centres there has been a vogue which has demanded the full investigation with contrast radiological studies of all patients over the age of 30 years who develop epilepsy. However, under 20 per cent of such individuals eventually prove to have intracranial tumours and in the early stages such tumours, most of which are gliomas, are often not revealed by angiography or air encephalography. However, as relatively innocuous non-invasive techniques such as gamma-encephalography and computerized transaxial tomography become more widely available on an out-patient basis, they are likely to be used increasingly in such cases. Indications for full investigation include symptoms of raised intracranial pressure and clinical or electroencephalographic indications of a focal cerebral lesion. Otherwise patients with late-onset epilepsy should be treated in the same way as any case of presumed idiopathic epilepsy arising in childhood or early adult life until or unless such manifestations develop.

Treatment of the Epileptic Attack

Treatment of a patient in an epileptic attack consists merely in preventing him from injuring himself. A gag should be placed between the teeth and an airway maintained. The attack is self-limited, and no immediate treatment will shorten its course.

Surgical Treatment

From the most ancient times trephining the skull played a part in the treatment of epilepsy. Certainly if a surgically accessible intracranial tumour is demonstrated to be the cause, it can be removed. When there is clear evidence of an organic lesion of the brain, especially one of traumatic origin, and the attacks have a focal onset which can be related to the lesion, and the site of which can be demonstrated by electrocorticography, excision of the affected area may abolish the attacks (Penfield and Jasper, 1954). Hemispherectomy has had a considerable vogue in the management of epilepsy secondary to severe infantile hemiplegia (Krynauw, 1950 and see p. 635) and even in the presence of other gross destructive cerebral lesions, cortical excisions following upon electrocorticography have often proved beneficial (Rasmussen and Gossman, 1963). Surgical treatment is, however, indicated only, as a rule, when the attacks are intractable and inadequately controlled by drugs (because the surgeon in removing one scar must leave another) and when the lesion is situated in an area of the brain which, when excised, is unlikely to result in permanent and severe neurological deficit. Even in temporal lobe epilepsy, in which good results have followed anterior temporal lobectomy in appropriate cases (Penfield and Flanigin, 1950; Falconer and Serefitinides, 1963; Bengzon et al., 1968; Taylor and Falconer, 1968; Falconer, 1970; Engel et al., 1975), probably less than one per cent of cases require, and are suitable for, surgical treatment. The results appear to be best in children in whom mesial temporal sclerosis (in Ammon's horn) is found at operation (Falconer and Taylor, 1968; Falconer, 1972; Davidson and Falconer, 1975). However, it is now the general experience in neurological and neurosurgical units that with the increasing efficacy of modern anticonvulsant drugs, fewer and fewer patients are referred for surgical treatment. In some patients with intractable epilepsy, repetitive cerebellar stimulation has been used and shown to be helpful, but this method is still experimental (Grabow et al., 1974).

Treatment with Drugs

Certain drugs have been found to diminish the severity and frequency of epileptic attacks and in favourable cases to abolish them completely (see below). When the attacks occur regularly at the same hour of the day or period of the month, the doses are timed correspondingly so as to produce their maximal effect when the attack is expected. Thus when the attacks are nocturnal or occur in the early morning, a single dose at bedtime may be sufficient. When they occur only at the monthly periods, medication can sometimes be increased in the previous and subsequent weeks. When the fits are irregular a dose may be taken two or three times a day. Perseverance in treatment is essential, and the patient must continue to take the effective drug for at least three years after the attacks cease, if a relapse is to be avoided. Electroencephalography may prove helpful in assessing the results of treatment, but even if the EEG remains abnormal and the patient is free from attacks after three years, withdrawal of treatment should be attempted, subject to the provisos, especially those related to driving, mentioned above.

Bromides. For many years the bromides were the most effective drugs in the treatment of epilepsy, but they are now outmoded.

DRUG TREATMENT
General Principles

These are fully reviewed by Woodbury et al. (1972), Eadie and Tyrer (1974), and Calne (1975). It is first important to recognize that one group of drugs, including the barbiturates, hydantoinates, and acetylureas, together with a number of modern synthetic remedies, are effective in major epilepsy (whether idiopathic or symptomatic) and also in focal epilepsy (including the temporal lobe variety) as well as in some cases of myoclonic epilepsy (see below) but not in petit mal. A second group, including the diones and suximides, may control petit mal but on occasion may even seem to make associated major epilepsy worse or may appear to precipitate major attacks in patients with petit mal who have never suffered such episodes before (Gastaut, 1964; Wilson, 1969). There is also some recent evidence to indicate that the prognosis of petit mal in the long-term is better if the child is treated with at least one drug effective in the control of major epilepsy (usually a hydantoin derivative) as well as with one or more of those which are effective in petit mal.

In all cases patients or their parents must be warned not to discontinue treatment without medical advice as this may precipitate dangerous episodes of status epilepticus. Difficulties which arise in the management of epilepsy are one of the major justifications for the existence of neurological follow-up clinics, as regular and careful supervision of such patients, and patient regulation and alteration in anticonvulsant medication and dosage, may pay considerable dividends. In general, combined tablets, containing more than one drug, are to be condemned, as when using these remedies it is not possible to adjust the dosage of the individual constituents of the tablet independently.

An important recent development has been the discovery that the serum levels of many anticonvulsant drugs produced by standard doses vary widely from patient to patient, and that low serum levels may be correlated with poor control of seizures and excessively high levels with symptoms of toxicity. Patients who are slow inactivators of isoniazid may also have difficulty in metabolizing phenytoin (Brennan *et al.*, 1970). If serum levels can be estimated regularly, usually with the aid of gas liquid chromatography, the dose can be adjusted to suit the individual in order to achieve better control of the seizures and to lessen side-effects (Gibberd *et al.*, 1970; Buchanan and Allen, 1971; Gardner-Medwin, 1973; Richens and Dunlop, 1975; *The Lancet*, 1975). A desirable serum concentration of phenytoin is 60–80 μmol/l (15–20 μg/ml).

Major and Focal Epilepsy

The principle must be to give the minimum dose of drugs sufficient to control the attacks for as long as may be necessary. Occasionally a single drug suffices but more often it is necessary to give a combination of at least two, and occasionally of three or more drugs in combination, in order to achieve maximum control, bearing in mind the fact that often one drug may potentiate the effect of another, but always remembering that not only are the therapeutic effects of these remedies additive but also that the same may apply to their side-effects. Sometimes, therefore, the addition of a new drug to the patient's existing medication may result in psychomotor retardation and a paradoxical increase in the number of fits. Thus sulthiame added to phenytoin has been found to produce symptoms of phenytoin intoxication (Houghton and Richens, 1974). All of the drugs in common use tend to produce some slowing of mental processes to a greater or lesser extent but this is particularly true of the barbiturates and occasionally satisfactory control of the attacks is only achieved at the expense of a disabling degree of drowsiness. It must, however, be remembered that as patients become accustomed to their medication such side-effects may noticeably diminish with the passage of time so that these symptoms are not invariably an indication for a reduction in treatment if attacks are under control.

However, all of the drugs to be considered below, apart from toxic effects common to the individual remedy, which will be mentioned, have a tendency at times to produce an unacceptable degree of drowsiness, dysarthria and ataxia, often with nystagmus, blurred vision, and even diplopia. These manifestations often develop relatively suddenly in a patient who has been receiving a stable regimen of treatment for some time; the patient has a 'drugged' and almost drunken appearance which is virtually diagnostic but may be misconstrued by the unwary as being due to organic intracranial disease. Such toxic effects are particularly common in those taking primidone and hydantoinates; complete withdrawal of these remedies is not as a rule necessary as the level of dosage at which they appear is finely balanced in the individual and a reduction in dosage of a single tablet or capsule per day sometimes results in rapid amelioration of these symptoms, though more often a more substantial reduction in daily dosage is required. Estimation of serum levels may be of particular value in monitoring the dosage required to abolish side-effects. Tyrer *et al.* (1970) reported an outbreak of phenytoin intoxication resulting from the fact that a different excipient was used in making tablets containing phenytoin, so that factors other than the patient's own ability to absorb and metabolize the drug must be borne in mind. Macrocytic anaemia due to folic acid deficiency has long been recognized to be an occasional complication of anticonvulsant therapy but recent evidence (Reynolds, 1968) suggests that such a deficiency may also account for some other side-effects of these drugs and that improvement may follow the regular administration of folic acid, 5 mg daily. Paradoxically, however, this remedy sometimes results in an increase in the number of seizures. Hunter *et al.* (1969) suggested that the administration of folic acid sometimes caused a reduction in the serum vitamin B_{12}. Reynolds *et al.* (1968) found that the behaviour of epileptic patients improved with folic acid even when fits increased in frequency, but Ralston *et al.* (1970) and Norris and Pratt (1971) found no effect of this remedy upon fit frequency, mental state, or serum B_{12} levels. The abnormality of folate metabolism, which may be due either to inhibition of intestinal conjugases (Baugh and Krumdieck, 1969) or to hepatic enzyme induction (Maxwell *et al.*, 1972) is thought to be one factor accounting for the peripheral neuropathy which occasionally results from long-term phenytoin treatment (Lovelace and Horwitz, 1967; Horwitz *et al.*, 1968). Irreversible Purkinje cell damage with cerebellar ataxia is an occasional complication of severe intoxication (Utterback *et al.*, 1958; Hofmann, 1958). Drug rashes also occur not infrequently in patients receiving phenobarbitone and hydantoinates; they can sometimes be controlled with antihistamine drugs but more often necessitate withdrawal of the offender and the substitution of another remedy.

Other important side-effects of anticonvulsant drugs, and especially phenytoin, include involuntary movements (Ahmad *et al.*, 1975), defects of blood coagulation (Solomon *et al.*, 1972), renal insensitivity to frusemide (Ahmad, 1974), disorders of cerebral monoamine metabolism (Chadwick *et al.*, 1975), and disordered calcium metabolism leading to osteomalacia, possibly due to an accelerated breakdown of vitamin D resulting from hepatic enzyme induction (Dent *et al.*, 1970; Richens and Rowe, 1970; Christiansen *et al.*, 1972; *The Lancet*, 1972 b). Christiansen *et al.* (1974) suggest that all epileptics receiving anticonvulsant therapy should also be given prophylactic vitamin D. During episodes of severe intoxication the CSF protein may be raised (Rawson, 1968).

A possible teratogenic effect of phenytoin has also been postulated. Speidel and Meadow (1972) found that major congenital malformations including congenital heart disease, cleft lip and palate, and microcephaly occurred twice as often in the children born to epileptic mothers as would have been expected in the general population, and similar findings have been reported by Fedrick (1973) and Loughnan *et al.* (1973). The effect is not a powerful one but clearly warrants further investigation.

The Treatment Routine

It is usual to begin in an adult with phenobarbitone, 30 mg twice daily, increasing if need be to three times a day, or to give 15 mg daily in a tablet or elixir to a young child. However, other workers prefer phenytoin or even carbamazepine, especially in childhood, as the initial remedy (Lerman and Kivity-Ephraim, 1974). Phenobarbitone is contra-indicated in mentally-defective and hyperkinetic children in whom the hyperkinesis may be accentuated. A few adults may tolerate up to 60 mg three times a day but even smaller doses may produce intolerable drowsiness. Less soporific in its effects and occasionally useful as an alternative anticonvulsant is methylphenobarbitone

(*Prominal, Phemitone*) which is given in a dosage of 100–200 mg two or three times daily.

If modest doses of phenobarbitone are insufficient to control the attacks it is usual to add phenytoin sodium (*Epanutin, Dilantin*) in a dosage of 100 mg two or three times a day (the dose suitable for a child is 50 mg twice or three times daily); few patients can take more than four such daily doses without developing the side-effects mentioned above. Strandjord and Johannessen (1974) pointed out that a single daily dose produced satisfactory levels of the drug in the serum over the subsequent 24 hours so that a single larger dose may prove to be more convenient and just as satisfactory as daily divided doses. In a high proportion of patients phenobarbitone and phenytoin in combination will produce an acceptable degree of attack control but when seizures continue it is then reasonable gradually to substitute primidone (*Mysoline*) for the phenobarbitone, while continuing the phenytoin. This powerful drug is given in a dosage of 250 mg three or four times daily (125 mg twice daily for a young child). Even on low dosage some patients develop nausea and vomiting and others drowsiness and ataxia; more patients fail to tolerate this drug than any other but, by contrast, some individuals find that they can take up to six tablets a day without ill-effect. Usually the combined use of primidone and pheno-barbitone is contra-indicated because of their combined sedative effects.

In patients whose seizures continue to resist treatment with the standard and established remedies mentioned above, there are a number of newer drugs which may usefully be given in addition. One of the most useful is sulthiame (*Ospolot*) which is given in a dosage of 200 mg, two, three, or four times daily (50 mg tablets are available for children). In some cases of major and temporal lobe epilepsy it is an effective adjuvant to the more traditional remedies and it often improves behaviour in epileptic children (Liu, 1966). It has few side-effects (apart from occasional irritating paraesthesiae in the extremities) and can often be given in maximum dosage along with other remedies. However, Green *et al.* (1974) suggest that the principal effect of this drug is to increase serum levels of phenytoin given concomitantly, and that this may explain much of its beneficial effect. Also valuable in some cases are other hydantoins including methoin (*Mesontoin*) (which has unfortunately been known to produce marrow aplasia) and the rather less toxic ethotoin (*Peganone*); the dose of the former is 100 mg two or three times a day and of the latter 250–500 mg two or three times daily for an adult, with correspondingly lower doses for children. While these drugs can be added in modest dosage to primidone and phenytoin sodium, they may produce additive side-effects. Commonly used in the past was phenyl-acetylurea (*Phenurone*), particularly in temporal lobe and myoclonic epilepsy, but this drug is particularly toxic, producing nausea and vomiting in many patients, liver and renal damage in some, and carrying the risk of marrow aplasia. More recently introduced and much less toxic is phenylethylacetylurea (*Pheneturide*) of which the adult dose is 200 mg three times a day (Vas and Parsonage, 1967). When sulthiame is ineffective it can usefully be tried as an adjuvant remedy along with phenobarbitone, hydantoinates and/or primidone. An alternative powerful new anticonvulsant, which some believe to be the initial remedy of choice, is carbamazepine (*Tegretol*) of which the adult dose is also 200 mg three times a day.

Drugs with weaker anticonvulsant effects when given by mouth, but worthy of a trial along with established remedies in resistant cases, include chlordiaze-poxide (*Librium*), 5–10 mg three times daily, diazepam (*Valium*), 2–5 mg three times daily, and beclamide (*Nydrane*), 500 mg three or four times daily. The latter drug is very non-toxic, and like sulthiame, has proved to be of some value in children with behaviour disorders (Beley *et al.*, 1962; Price and Spencer, 1967).

Remedies introduced even more recently include clonazepam, which has been shown to be effective in all forms of epilepsy, including petit mal, in total daily doses varying from 1·0 mg to 10·0 mg (Fazio *et al.*, 1975) and sodium valproate, which appears to inhibit GABA transaminase, thus increasing the cerebral concentration of GABA. The latter remedy is most effective in petit mal but also seems to be of some value in controlling major and focal seizures as well as in potentiating the effects of other anticonvulsant drugs; the dose, regardless of age, is 200 mg twice daily, increasing to 600 mg daily after three days (Jeavons and Clark, 1974). Less widely used, but sometimes of value in intractable epilepsy in childhood is a ketogenic diet (Wilder, 1921); ketosis may be effectively induced by the administration of medium-chain triglycerides (Huttenlocher *et al.*, 1971).

Petit Mal

As already mentioned it is now regarded as essential in children with petit mal to give, in addition to the specific remedies for this form of epilepsy, another remedy (usually phenytoin, 50 mg twice daily) in order to guard against the immediate or subsequent development of major seizures.

The drug of choice is now ethosuximide (*Zarontin*) which can be given, even to young children, in a dosage of 250 mg two, three, or four times daily (Browne *et al.*, 1975). Often the attacks cease abruptly but sometimes petit mal is remarkably resistant and it may be necessary to add one or two other remedies, also in full dosage, in order to achieve control of the attacks. These include the older remedies trimethadione (*Tridione*) and paramethadione (*Paradione*) each of which is given in a dosage of 300 mg three times a day. Sometimes these two drugs produce an unpleasant visual glare phenomenon, and agranulocytosis, aplastic anaemia, nephrosis, and liver damage have been described but are all rare. Their mode of action is different from that of many other anticonvulsants and they have a depressant effect upon cortical inhibitory pathways (Fromm and Kohli, 1972). Routine regular white blood cell counts were once advised in patients receiving these drugs but are of little value; it is wiser to advise the parents to seek medical advice if the child under treatment develops a sore throat or high temperature.

Other suximide drugs which may be tried in petit mal in place of ethosuximide and possibly with one or both of the dione drugs, but which are usually less effective are phensuximide (*Milontin*), 250–500 mg three or four times daily, and methsuximide (*Celontin*), 300 mg up to three or four times a day. In occasional cases, for reasons which are not clearly understood, chlortetracycline (*Aureomycin*), 250 mg three times a day, is effective in petit mal and so, too, are diuretics including frusemide (*Lasix*) (but regular measurement of serum potassium is necessary with this drug and is inconvenient), and acetazolamide (*Diamox*), 250–500 mg once or twice daily. Clonazepam, given in a dosage of 1·0 to 10·0 mg daily, has recently been shown to be an effective remedy (Dreifuss *et al.*, 1975) as has sodium valproate, 400–600 mg daily (Jeavons and Clark, 1974). Somewhat paradoxically, imipramine which has a convulsant effect in animals and which may precipitate major fits in adults, seems to be an effective anticonvulsant in some patients with intractable petit mal in a dosage of 1·3 mg/kg body weight daily (Fromm *et al.*, 1972).

Amphetamine sulphate and dextroamphetamine sulphate in a dosage of 5–10 mg at 8 a.m. and 12 noon were sometimes found to be of value in patients with petit mal and were also of some benefit in patients with major or temporal lobe epilepsy when drowsiness due to medication was a problem but have now been largely discarded. Paradoxically, a small dose of amphetamine, tried with caution, may improve and sedate some hyperkinetic children and those with aggressive behaviour disorders.

In the treatment of petit mal, toxic side-effects of medication are in general less of a problem, because of the character of the drugs being used, than in the management of major and temporal lobe epilepsy. In all forms of epilepsy, however, the aim must be to achieve a balance between the control of the attacks on the one hand and the preservation of mental capacity, concentration, and alertness on the other.

Treatment of Status Epilepticus

For many years paraldehyde was regarded as the most effective drug, being given in doses of 10 ml intramuscularly to an adult and repeated as necessary. In an emergency it could be given by intravenous drip in a dosage of 0·05 to 0·1 ml per kg of body weight in normal saline. Unfortunately the intramuscular injections were painful and occasionally gave abscess formation while phlebitis usually followed intravenous administration. In mild cases the patient may respond to 120–250 mg of phenobarbitone sodium intramuscularly followed by 120 mg every hour for several hours. Intravenous phenytoin given by continuous infusion at a rate not exceeding 50 mg per minute may also be effective, but continuous electrocardiographic monitoring is needed because of the depressant effect of the drug upon cardiac function (Janz and Kautz, 1964; Wallis *et al.*, 1968). Chlormethiazole, also given by intravenous infusion at a rate of 0·7 g/hour, has also been found to control status in some cases (Harvey *et al.*, 1975). General anaesthetics have long been used; thiopentone has been used by intravenous drip (Mortimer, 1961) and in severe cases muscle relaxants and positive pressure respiration have been employed. Probably the single most effective remedy is diazepam (*Valium*) (Gastaut *et al.*, 1965), which is given intravenously in a drip in successive 10 mg doses every 15 minutes until control is achieved or until 50–60 mg has been given over one or two hours. EEG monitoring is valuable to show when the cerebral epileptic discharge has been controlled (James and Whitty, 1961; Mortimer, 1961).

Nasal feeding should be used if unconsciousness is prolonged. The patient should be nursed flat and preferably in the semiprone position.

Petit mal status, which may give prolonged disorientation, accompanied by almost continuous spike-and-wave activity in the child's EEG, is best treated by ethosuximide (*Zarontin*), in a dosage of 250 mg four-hourly but phenytoin (*Epanutin*) should be given as well (at least 50 mg two or three times daily) to guard against the development of major seizures. ACTH has also been recommended in such cases (80 units daily intramuscularly for a week).

Psychotherapy

There is no reason to regard epilepsy as primarily a psychological disorder. In a few cases, however, mental stress and emotional difficulties appear to precipitate attacks. Depression, anxiety, and hysterical manifestations may also occur in epileptic individuals. When such subordinate causes can be found, benefit may result from appropriate treatment. Help is often obtained by the addition of antidepressive and/or tranquillizing remedies to the patient's anticonvulsant medication, always remembering that certain antidepressive drugs (particularly imipramine) may potentiate epileptic discharges whereas some tranquillizers (e.g. chlordiazepoxide and diazepam) have an anticonvulsant effect.

REFERENCES

ADELOYE, A., and ODEKU, E. L. (1971) Epilepsy after missile wounds of the head, *J. Neurol. Neurosurg. Psychiat.*, **34**, 98.

AHMAD, S. (1974) Renal insensitivity to frusemide caused by chronic anticonvulsant therapy, *Brit. med. J.*, **3**, 657.

AHMAD, S., LAIDLAW, J., HOUGHTON, G. W., and RICHENS, A. (1975) Involuntary movements caused by phenytoin intoxication in epileptic patients, *J. Neurol. Neurosurg. Psychiat.*, **38**, 225.

ANSELL, B., and CLARKE, E. (1956) Epilepsy and menstruation. The role of water retention, *Lancet*, **ii**, 1232.

BAGLEY, C. (1972) Social prejudice and the adjustment of people with epilepsy, *Epilepsia*, **13**, 33.

BALDWIN, M., and BAILEY, P. (1958) *Temporal Lobe Epilepsy*, Springfield, Ill.

BAUGH, C. M., and KRUMDIECK, C. L. (1969) Effects of phenytoin on folic-acid conjugases in man, *Lancet*, **ii**, 519.

BEHRMAN, S., and KNIGHT, G. (1956) Carotid sinus epilepsy and its treatment by denervation, *Brit. med. J.*, **ii**, 1522.

BEHRMAN, S., and WYKE, B. D. (1958) Vestibulogenic seizures, *Brain*, **81**, 529.

BELEY, A., GIRARD, C., LEROY, C., and PINEL, J. P. (1962) Studies on the effects of N-benzyl-beta-chloropropionamide (Nydrane) in behaviour disorders in children, *Rev. de Neuropsychiatrie Infantile*, **10**, 9.

BENGZON, A. R. A., RASMUSSEN, T., GLOOR, P., DUSSAULT, J., and STEPHENS, M. (1968) Prognostic factors in the surgical treatment of temporal lobe epileptics, *Neurology (Minneap.)*, **18**, 717.

BERESFORD, H. R., POSNER, J. B., and PLUM, F. (1969) Changes in brain lactate during induced cerebral seizures, *Arch. Neurol. (Chic.)*, **20**, 243.

BINGEL, A. (1957) Reading epilepsy, *Neurology (Minneap.)*, **7**, 752.

BIRD, C. A. K., GRIFFIN, B. P., MIKLASZEWSKA, J. M., and GALBRAITH, A. W. (1966) Tegretol (carbamazepine): a controlled trial of a new anticonvulsant, *Brit. J. Psychiat.*, **112**, 737.

BOGDANOFF, B. M., STAFFORD, C. R., GREEN, L., and GONZALEZ, C. F. (1975) Computerized transaxial tomography in the evaluation of patients with focal epilepsy, *Neurology (Minneap.)*, **25**, 1013.

BOLLER, F., WRIGHT, D. G., CAVALIERI, R., and MITSUMOTO, H. (1975) Paroxysmal 'nightmares': sequel of a stroke responsive to diphenylhydantoin, *Neurology (Minneap.)*, **25**, 1026.

BOWER, B. D., and JEAVONS, P. M. (1959) Infantile spasms and hypsarrhythmia, *Lancet*, **i**, 605.

BRAIN, W. R. (1925-6) The inheritance of epilepsy, *Quart. J. Med.*, **19**, 299.

BRENNAN, R. W., DEHEJIA, H., KUTT, H., VEREBELY, K., and McDOWELL, F. (1970) Diphenylhydantoin intoxication attendant to slow inactivation of isoniazid, *Neurology (Minneap.)*, **20**, 687.

BRETT, E. M. (1966) Minor epileptic status, *J. neurol. Sci.*, **3**, 52.

BREWIS, M., POSKANZER, D. C., ROLLAND, C., and MILLER, H. (1966) Neurological disease in an English city, *Acta neurol. scand.*, **42**, Suppl. 24.

BRIDGE, E. M., KAJDI, L., and LIVINGSTON, S. (1947) A fifteen year study of epilepsy in children, *Res. Publ. Ass. nerv. ment. Dis.*, **26**, 451.

BRITISH MEDICAL JOURNAL (1972) Febrile convulsions in early childhood, *Brit. med. J.*, **2**, 608.

BRITISH MEDICAL JOURNAL (1974) Fits in the newborn, *Brit. med. J.*, **1**, 127.

BRITISH MEDICAL JOURNAL (1975 *a*) More about febrile convulsions, *Brit. med. J.*, **1**, 591.

BRITISH MEDICAL JOURNAL (1975 *b*) Benign focal epilepsy of childhood, *Brit. med. J.*, **3**, 451.

BRITISH MEDICAL JOURNAL (1975 *c*) 'Reflex' epilepsy, *Brit. med. J.*, **3**, 338.

BROOKS, J. E., and JIRAUCH, P. M. (1971) Primary reading epilepsy: a misnomer, *Arch. Neurol. (Chic.)*, **25**, 97.

BROWNE, T. R., DREIFUSS, F. E., DYKEN, P. R., GOODE, D. J., PENRY, J. K., PORTER, R. J., WHITE, B. G., and WHITE, P. T. (1975) Ethosuximide in the treatment of absence (petit mal) seizures, *Neurology (Minneap.)*, **25**, 515.

BUCHANAN, R. A., and ALLEN, R. J. (1971) Diphenylhydantoin (Dilantin) and phenobarbital blood levels in epileptic children, *Neurology (Minneap.)*, **21**, 866.

CALNE, D. B. (1975) *Therapeutics in Neurology*, Oxford.

CAVANAGH, J. B. (1958) On certain small tumours—encountered in the temporal lobe, *Brain*, **81**, 389.

CHADWICK, D., JENNER, P., and REYNOLDS, E. H. (1975) Amines, anticonvulsants, and epilepsy, *Lancet*, **i**, 473.

CHEN, R.-C., and FORSTER, F. M. (1973) Cursive epilepsy and gelastic epilepsy, *Neurology (Minneap.)*, **23**, 1019.

CHRISTIANSEN, C., KRISTENSEN, M., and RØDBRO, P. (1972) Latent osteomalacia in epileptic patients on anticonvulsants, *Brit. med. J.*, **3**, 738.

CHRISTIANSEN, C., RØDBRO, P., and SJÖ, O. (1974) 'Anticonvulsant action' of vitamin D in epileptic patients? A controlled pilot study, *Brit. med. J.*, **2**, 258.

CONN, J. W. (1947) The diagnosis and management of spontaneous hypoglycaemia, *J. Amer. med. Ass.*, **134**, 130.

CORSELLIS, J. A. N. (1957) The incidence of Ammon's horn sclerosis, *Brain*, **80**, 193.

COX, P. J. N., and MARTIN, E. (1959) Infantile spasms and hypsarrhythmia, *Lancet*, **i**, 1099.

CURRIE, S., HEATHFIELD, K. W. G., HENSON, R. A., and SCOTT, D. F. (1971) Clinical course and prognosis of temporal lobe epilepsy: a survey of 666 patients, *Brain*, **94**, 173.

DAVIDSON, S., and FALCONER, M. A. (1975) Outcome of surgery in 40 children with temporal-lobe epilepsy, *Lancet*, **i**, 1260.

DAVIS, J. P., and LENNOX, W. G. (1947) The effect of trimethyloxazolidine dione and dimethylethyloxazolidine dione on seizures and the blood, *Res. Publ. Ass. nerv. ment. Dis.*, **26**, 423.

DENT, C. E., RICHENS, A., ROWE, D. J. F., and STAMP, T. C. B. (1970) Osteomalacia with long-term anticonvulsant therapy in epilepsy, *Brit. med. J.*, **4**, 69.

DODGE, P. R., RICHARDSON, E. P., and VICTOR, M. (1954) Recurrent convulsive seizures as a sequel to cerebral infarction, *Brain*, **77**, 610.

DREIFUSS, F. E., PENRY, J. K., ROSE, S. W., KUPFERBERG, H. J., DYKEN, P., and SATO, S. (1975) Serum clonazepam concentrations in children with absence seizures, *Neurology (Minneap.)*, **25**, 255.

EADIE, M. J., and TYRER, J. H. (1974) *Anticonvulsant Therapy*, Edinburgh and London.

EARLE, K. M., BALDWIN, M., and PENFIELD, W. (1953) Incisural sclerosis and temporal lobe seizures produced by hippocampal herniation at birth, *Arch. Neurol. Psychiat. (Chic.)*, **69**, 27.

EFRON, R. (1956) The effect of olfactory stimuli in arresting uncinate fits, *Brain*, **79**, 267.

EFRON, R. (1957) The conditioned inhibition of uncinate fits, *Brain*, **80**, 251.

EFRON, R. (1961) Post-epileptic paralysis. Theoretical critique and report of a case, *Brain*, **84**, 381.

ENGEL, J., DRIVER, M. V., and FALCONER, M. A. (1975) Electrophysiological correlates of pathology and surgical results in temporal lobe epilepsy, *Brain*, **98**, 129.

FALCONER, M. A. (1970) Significance of surgery for temporal lobe epilepsy in childhood and adolescence, *J. Neurosurg.*, **33**, 233.

FALCONER, M. A. (1971) Genetic and related aetiological factors in temporal lobe epilepsy, *Epilepsia*, **12**, 13.

FALCONER, M. A. (1972) Place of surgery for temporal lobe epilepsy during childhood, *Brit. med. J.*, **2**, 631.

FALCONER, M. A. (1974) Mesial temporal (Ammon's horn) sclerosis as a common cause of epilepsy: aetiology, treatment, and prevention, *Lancet*, **ii**, 767.

FALCONER, M. A., and DAVIDSON, S. (1973) Coarse features in epilepsy as a consequence of anticonvulsant therapy, *Lancet*, **ii**, 1112.

FALCONER, M. A., and SEREFITINIDES, F. A. (1963) A follow-up study in temporal lobe epilepsy, *J. Neurol. Neurosurg. Psychiat.*, **26**, 154.

FALCONER, M. A., and TAYLOR, D. C. (1968) Surgical treatment of drug-resistant epilepsy due to mesial temporal sclerosis, *Arch. Neurol. (Chic.)*, **19**, 353.

FAZIO, C., MANFREDI, M., and PICCINELLI, A. (1975) Treatment of epileptic seizures with clonazepam, *Arch. Neurol. (Chic.)*, **32**, 304.

FEDRICK, J. (1973) Epilepsy and pregnancy: a report from the Oxford record linkage study, *Brit. med. J.*, **2**, 442.

FEINDEL, W., and PENFIELD, W. (1954) Localization of discharge in temporal lobe automatism, *Arch. Neurol. Psychiat. (Chic.)*, **72**, 605.

FOX, R. H., WILKINS, D. C., BELL, J. A., BRADLEY, R. D., BROWSE, N. L., CRANSTON, W. I., FOLEY, T. H., GILBY, E. D., HEBDEN, A., JENKINS, B. S., and RAWLINS, M. D. (1973) Spontaneous periodic hypothermia: diencephalic epilepsy, *Brit. med. J.*, **2**, 693.

FRANTZEN, E. (1961) An analysis of the results of treatment in epileptics under ambulatory supervision, *Epilepsia*, **2**, 207.

FRANTZEN, E., LENNOX-BUCHTHAL, M., and NYGAARD, A. (1968) Longitudinal EEG and clinical study of children with febrile convulsions, *Electroenceph. clin. Neurophysiol.*, **24**, 197.

FRANTZEN, E., LENNOX-BUCHTHAL, M., NYGAARD, A., and STENE, J. (1970) A genetic study of febrile convulsions, *Neurology (Minneap.)*, **20**, 909.

FROMM, G. H., AMORES, C. Y., and THIES, W. (1972) Imipramine in epilepsy, *Arch. Neurol. (Chic.)*, **27**, 198.

FROMM, G. H., and KOHLI, C. M. (1972) The role of inhibitory pathways in petit mal epilepsy, *Neurology (Minneap.)*, **22**, 1012.

GARDNER-MEDWIN, D. (1973) Why should we measure serum levels of anticonvulsant drugs in epilepsy?, *Clin. Electroenceph.*, **4**, 132.

GARLAND, H., and SUMNER, D. (1964) Sulthiame in treatment of epilepsy, *Brit. med. J.*, **1**, 454.

GASTAUT, H. (1964) Certain basic concepts concerning the treatment of the epilepsies, *Brit. J. Clin. Practice*, **18**, 26.

GASTAUT, H., and FISCHER-WILLIAMS, M. (1960) The physiopathology of epileptic seizures, in *Handbook of Physiology*, ed. Field, J., Sect. 1, vol. 1, p. 329, Washington, D.C.

GASTAUT, H., NAQUET, R., POIRE, R., and TASSINARI, C. A. (1965) Treatment of status epilepticus with diazepam (Valium), *Epilepsia (Amst.)*, **6**, 167.

GESCHWIND, N., and SHERWIN, I. (1967) Language-induced epilepsy, *Arch. Neurol. (Chic.)*, **16**, 25.

GIBBERD, F. B. (1972) The prognosis of petit mal in adults, *Epilepsia (Amst.)*, **13**, 171.

GIBBERD, F. B., and BATESON, M. C. (1974) Sleep epilepsy: its pattern and prognosis, *Brit. med. J.*, **2**, 403.

GIBBERD, F. B., DUNNE, J. F., HANDLEY, A. J., and HAZLEMAN, B. L. (1970) Supervision of epileptic patients taking phenytoin, *Brit. med. J.*, **1**, 147.

GIBBS, E. L., and GIBBS, F. A. (1947) Sleep records in epilepsy, *Res. Publ. Ass. nerv. ment. Dis.*, **26**, 366.

GIBBS, F. A., and GIBBS, E. L. (1952) *Atlas of Electroencephalography*, vol. 2, p. 24, Cambridge, Mass.

GIBBS, F. A., GIBBS, E. L., and LENNOX, W. G. (1937) Epilepsy: a paroxysmal cerebral dysrhythmia, *Brain*, **60**, 377.

GIBBS, F. A., GIBBS, E. L., and LENNOX, W. G. (1938) Cerebral dysrhythmias of epilepsy. Measures for their control, *Arch. Neurol. Psychiat. (Chic.)*, **34**, 298.

GIBBS, F. A., GIBBS, E. L., and LENNOX, W. G. (1943) Electroencephalographic classification of epileptic patients and control subjects, *Arch. Neurol. Psychiat. (Chic.)*, **1**, 111.

GIBBS, F. A., LENNOX, W. G., and GIBBS, E. L. (1936) The electroencephalogram in diagnosis and in localization of epileptic seizures, *Arch. Neurol. Psychiat. (Chic.)*, **36**, 1225.

GIRDWOOD, R. H. (1959) The role of folic acid in blood disorders, *Brit. med. Bull.*, **15**, 17.

GLASER, G. H., and LEVY, L. L. (1960) Seizures and idiopathic hypoparathyroidism, *Epilepsia (Amst.)*, **1**, 454.

GOWERS, W. R. (1901) *Epilepsy and Other Chronic Convulsive Diseases*, London.

GOWERS, W. R. (1907) *The Borderland of Epilepsy*, London.

GRABOW, J. D., EBERSOLD, M. J., ALBERS, J. W., and SCHIMA, E. M. (1974) Cerebellar stimulation for the control of seizures, *Mayo Clin. Proc.*, **49**, 759.

GRAND, W. (1974) The significance of post-traumatic status epilepticus in childhood, *J. Neurol. Neurosurg. Psychiat.*, **37**, 178.

GREEN, J. R., TROUPIN, A. S., HALPERN, L. M., FRIEL, P., and KANAREK, P. (1974) Sulthiame: evaluation as an anticonvulsant, *Epilepsia*, **15**, 329.

GRIFFITHS, G. M., and FOX, J. T. (1938) Rhythm in epilepsy, *Lancet*, **ii**, 409.

GUMPERT, J., HANSOTIA, P., and UPTON, A. (1970) Gelastic epilepsy, *J. Neurol. Neurosurg. Psychiat.*, **33**, 479.

GUNDERSON, C. H., DUNNE, P. B., and FEHER, T. L. (1973) Sleep deprivation seizures, *Neurology (Minneap.)*, **23**, 678.

GUNN, J., and FENTON, G. (1971) Epilepsy, automatism, and crime, *Lancet*, **i**, 1173.

HARPER, M., and ROTH, M. (1962) Temporal lobe epilepsy and the phobic anxiety-depersonalization syndrome. Part I: A comparative study, *Comprehens. Psychiat.*, **3**, 129.

HARVEY, P. K. P., HIGENBOTTAM, T. W., and LOH, L. (1975) Chlormethiazole in treatment of status epilepticus, *Brit. med. J.*, **2**, 603.

HAWKINS, C. F., and MEYNELL, M. J. (1958) Macrocytosis and macrocytic anaemia caused by anti-convulsant drugs, *Quart. J. Med.*, **27**, 45.

HILL, J. D. N., and PARR, G. (1963) *Electroencephalography*, 2nd ed., London.

HIRSCH, C. S., and MARTIN, D. L. (1971) Unexpected death in young epileptics, *Neurology (Minneap.)*, **21**, 682.

HODSKINS, M. B., and YAKOVLEV, P. I. (1930) Neurosomatic deterioration in epilepsy, *Arch. Neurol. Psychiat. (Chic.)*, **23**, 986.

HOFMANN, W. W. (1958) Cerebellar lesions after parenteral Dilantin administration, *Neurology (Minneap.)*, **8**, 210.

HOLDEN, J. C. (1957) Temporal-lobe epilepsy associated with severe behavioural disturbances, *Lancet*, **ii**, 724.

HOLOWACH, J., THURSTON, D. L., and O'LEARY, J. (1972) Prognosis in childhood epilepsy: follow-up study of 148 cases in which therapy had been suspended after prolonged anticonvulsant control, *New Engl. J. Med.*, **286**, 169.

HORWITZ, S. J., KLIPSTEIN, F. A., and LOVELACE, R. E. (1968) Relation of abnormal folate metabolism to neuropathy developing during anticonvulsant drug therapy, *Lancet*, **i**, 563.

HOUGHTON, G. W., and RICHENS, A. (1974) Phenytoin intoxication induced by sulthiame in epileptic patients, *J. Neurol. Neurosurg. Psychiat.*, **37**, 275.

HUNTER, R., BARNES, J., and MATTHEWS, D. M. (1969) Effect of folic-acid supplement on serum-vitamin-B$_{12}$ levels in patients on anticonvulsants, *Lancet*, **ii**, 666.

HUNTER, R., HURWITZ, L. J., FULLERTON, P. M., NIEMAN, E. A., and DAVIES, H. (1962) Unilateral ventricular enlargement. A report of 75 cases, *Brain*, **85**, 295.

HUTCHISON, J. H., STONE, F. H., and DAVIDSON, J. R. (1958) Photogenic epilepsy induced by the patient, *Lancet*, **i**, 243.

HUTTENLOCHER, P. R. (1974) Dendritic development in neocortex of children with mental defect and infantile spasms, *Neurology (Minneap.)*, **24**, 203.

HUTTENLOCHER, P. R., WILBOURN, A. J., and SIGNORE, J. M. (1971) Medium-chain triglycerides as a therapy for intractable childhood epilepsy, *Neurology (Minneap.)*, **21**, 1097.

ILLINGWORTH, R. S. (1955) Sudden mental deterioration with convulsions in infancy, *Arch. Dis. Childh.*, **30**, 529.

INTERNATIONAL BUREAU FOR EPILEPSY (1966) *Epilepsy and Driving Licences*, Social studies in epilepsy, No. 4 Supplement to *British Epilepsy Association Journal*, London.

JACKSON, J. H. (1931) Epilepsy and epileptiform convulsions, *Selected Writings*, vol. 1, London.

JAMES, J. L., and WHITTY, C. W. M. (1961) The electroencephalogram as a monitor of status epilepticus suppressed peripherally by curarisation, *Lancet*, **ii**, 239.

JANZ, D. (1964) Status epilepticus and frontal lobe lesions, *J. neurol. Sci.*, **1**, 446.

JANZ, D. (1969) *Die Epilepsien*, Stuttgart.

JANZ, D., and KAUTZ, G. (1964) The aetiology and treatment of status epilepticus, *German Medical Monthly*, **9**, 451.

JASPER, H. H., and DROOGLEEVER-FORTUYN, J. (1947) Experimental studies on the functional anatomy of petit mal epilepsy, *Res. Publ. Ass. nerv. ment. Dis.*, **26**, 272.

JASPER, H. H., and KERSHMAN, J. (1941) Electro-encephalographic classification of the epilepsies, *Arch. Neurol. Psychiat. (Chic.)*, **45**, 903.

JEAVONS, P. M., and CLARK, J. E. (1974) Sodium valproate in treatment of epilepsy, *Brit. med. J.*, **2**, 584.

JENNETT, W. B. (1961) *Late Epilepsy after Blunt Head Injury*, Hunterian Lecture to Royal College of Surgeons, London.

JENNETT, W. B. (1975) Epilepsy and acute traumatic intracranial haematoma, *J. Neurol. Neurosurg. Psychiat.*, **38**, 378.

JENNETT, W. B., TEATHER, D., and BENNIE, S. (1973) Epilepsy after head injury: residual risk after varying fit-free intervals since injury, *Lancet*, **ii**, 652.

JURGELSKY, W., and THOMAS, J. A. (1966) The *in vivo* protection of gamma-amino-butyric acid against organic phosphate inhibition of ACHE, *Life Sci.*, **5**, 1525.

KILOH, L. G., McCOMAS, A. J., and OSSELTON, J. W. (1972) *Clinical Electroencephalography*, 3rd ed., London.

KRYNAUW, R. A. (1950) Infantile hemiplegia treated by removing one cerebral hemisphere, *J. Neurol. Neurosurg. Psychiat.*, **13**, 243.

KURTZKE, J. F. (1972) Mortality and morbidity data on epilepsy, in *The Epidemiology of Epilepsy*, ed. Alter, M., and Hauser, W. A., NINDS Monograph No. 14, Bethesda.

LAIDLAW, J. (1956) Catamenial epilepsy, *Lancet*, **ii**, 1235.

THE LANCET (1972 *a*) Withdrawal of anticonvulsant drugs in epilepsy, *Lancet*, **i**, 478.

THE LANCET (1972 *b*) Anticonvulsant osteomalacia, *Lancet*, **ii**, 805.

THE LANCET (1975) Drug levels in epilepsy, *Lancet*, **ii**, 264.

LEES, F., and LIVERSEDGE, L. A. (1962) The prognosis of petit mal and minor epilepsy, *Lancet*, **ii**, 797.

LENNOX, W. G. (1945) The petit mal epilepsies, *J. Amer. med. Ass.*, **129**, 1069.

LENNOX, W. G. (1947) Sixty-six twin pairs affected by seizures, *Res. Publ. Ass. nerv. ment. Dis.*, **26**, 11.

LENNOX, W. G., GIBBS, E. L., and GIBBS, F. A. (1940) The inheritance of epilepsy as revealed by the electro-encephalogram, *Arch. Neurol. Psychiat. (Chic.)*, **44**, 1155.

LENNOX, W. G., and LENNOX, M. A. (1960) *Epilepsy and Related Disorders*, Boston, Mass.

LENNOX-BUCHTHAL, M. A. (1974) Febrile convulsions, in *Handbook of Clinical Neurology*, ed. Vinken, P. J., and Bruyn, G. W., vol. 15, chap. 12, Amsterdam.

LERMAN, P., and KIVITY, S. (1975) Benign focal epilepsy of childhood, *Arch. Neurol. (Chic.)*, **32**, 261.

LERMAN, P., and KIVITY-EPHRAIM, S. (1974) Carbamazepine sole anticonvulsant for focal epilepsy of childhood, *Epilepsia*, **15**, 229.

LISHMAN, W. A., SYMONDS, C. P., WHITTY, C. W. M., and WILLISON, R. G. (1962) Seizures induced by movement, *Brain*, **85**, 93.

LIU, M. C. (1966) Clinical experience with sulthiame (Ospolot), *Brit. J. Psychiat.*, **112**, 621.

LIVINGSTON, S., TORRES, I., PAULI, L. L., and RIDER, R. V. (1965) Petit mal epilepsy. Results of a prolonged follow-up study of 117 patients, *J. Amer. med. Ass.*, **194**, 227.

LOUGHNAN, P. M., GOLD, H., and VANCE, J. C. (1973) Phenytoin teratogenicity in man, *Lancet*, **i**, 70.

LOVELACE, R. E., and HORWITZ, S. J. (1967) Peripheral neuropathy in long-term diphenylhydantoin therapy, *Trans. Amer. Neurol. Ass.*, **92**, 262.

MATTHEWS, W. B. (1954) Tonic seizures in multiple sclerosis, *Brain*, **81**, 193.

MAXWELL, J. D., HUNTER, J., STEWART, D. A., ARDEMAN, S., and WILLIAMS, R. (1972) Folate deficiency after anticonvulsant drugs: an effect of hepatic enzyme induction?, *Brit. med. J.*, **1**, 297.

MAXWELL, R. D. H., and LEYSHON, G. E. (1971) Epilepsy and driving, *Brit. med. J.*, **3**, 12.

MELCHIOR, J. C., BUCHTHAL, F., and LENNOX-BUCHTHAL, M. (1971) The ineffectiveness of diphenylhydantoin in preventing febrile convulsions in the age of greatest risk, under three years, *Epilepsia (Amst.)*, **12**, 55.

MELDRUM, B. S., and BRIERLEY, J. B. (1972) Neuronal loss and gliosis in the hippocampus following repetitive epileptic seizures induced in adolescent baboons by allyglycine, *Brain Research*, **48**, 361.

MELDRUM, B. S., and BRIERLEY, J. B. (1973) Prolonged epileptic seizures in primates, *Arch. Neurol. (Chic.)*, **28**, 10.

MELDRUM, B. S., and HORTON, R. W. (1973) Physiology of status epilepticus in primates, *Arch. Neurol. (Chic.)*, **28**, 1.

MEYER, A. (1963) Epilepsy, in *Greenfield's Neuropathology*, 2nd ed., ed. Blackwood, W., McMenemey, W. H., Meyer, A., Norman, R. M., and Russell, D. S., London.

MORGAN-HUGHES, J. A. (1966) Cough seizures in patients with cerebral lesions, *Brit. med. J.*, **2**, 494.

MORTIMER, P. L. F. (1961) The encephalogram as a monitor of status epilepticus, *Lancet*, **ii**, 776.

NEUBAUER, C. (1970) Mental deterioration in epilepsy due to folate deficiency, *Brit. med. J.*, **2**, 759.

NEWCOMBE, R. L., and SHAH, S. H. (1975) Radiological abnormalities in temporal lobe epilepsy with clinicopathological correlations, *J. Neurol. Neurosurg. Psychiat.*, **38**, 279.

NORRIS, J. W., and PRATT, R. F. (1971) A controlled study of folic acid in epilepsy, *Neurology (Minneap.)*, **21**, 659.

OFFICE OF HEALTH ECONOMICS (1971) *Epilepsy in Society*, London.

OXBURY, J. M., and WHITTY, C. W. M. (1971) Causes and consequences of status epilepticus in adults, *Brain*, **94**, 733.

PATRY, G., LYAGOUBI, S., and TASSINARI, A. (1971) Subclinical 'electrical status epilepticus' induced by sleep in children, *Arch. Neurol. (Chic.)*, **24**, 242.

PENFIELD, W., and FLANIGIN, H. (1950) Surgical therapy of temporal lobe seizures, *Arch. Neurol. Psychiat. (Chic.)*, **64**, 491.

PENFIELD, W., and JASPER, H. (1954) *Epilepsy and the Functional Anatomy of the Human Brain*, Boston.

PENRY, J. K., and DALY, D. D. (1975) *Complex Partial Seizures and Their Treatment*, vol. 11 in Advances in Neurology series, New York.

POND, D. A., BIDWELL, B. H., and STEIN, L. (1960) A survey of epilepsy in fourteen general practices. I. Demographic and medical data, *Psychiat. Neurol. Neurochir.*, **63**, 217.

POSNER, J. B., PLUM, F., and POZNAK, A. VAN (1969) Cerebral metabolism during electrically induced seizures in man, *Arch. Neurol. (Chic.)*, **20**, 388.

PRICE, S. A., and SPENCER, D. A. (1967) A trial of beclamide (Nydrane) in mentally subnormal patients with disorders of behaviour, *J. Ment. Subnormal.*, **13**, 75.

PRUNTY, F. T. G. (1944) Reactive hyperinsulinism, *Brit. med. J.*, **2**, 398.

RALSTON, A. J., SNAITH, R. P., and HINLEY, J. B. (1970) Effects of folic acid on fit-frequency and behaviour in epileptics on anticonvulsants, *Lancet*, **i**, 867.

RASMUSSEN, T., and GOSSMAN, H. (1963) Epilepsy due to gross destructive brain lesions, *Neurology (Minneap.)*, **13**, 659.

RASMUSSEN, T., OLSZEWSKI, J., and LLOYD-SMITH, D. (1958) Focal seizures due to chronic localized encephalitis, *Neurology (Minneap.)*, **8**, 435.

RAWSON, M. D. (1968) Diphenylhydantoin intoxication and cerebrospinal fluid protein, *Neurology (Minneap.)*, **18**, 1009.

REID, J. J. A. (1972) The need for special centres for epilepsy in England and Wales, *Epilepsia (Amst.)*, **13**, 211.

REMILLARD, G. M., ETHIER, R., and ANDERMANN, F. (1974) Temporal lobe epilepsy and perinatal occlusion of the posterior cerebral artery, *Neurology (Minneap.)*, **24**, 1001.

REYNOLDS, E. H. (1968) Mental effects of anticonvulsants and folic acid metabolism, *Brain*, **91**, 197.

REYNOLDS, E. H., CHANARIN, I., and MATTHEWS, D. M. (1968) Neuropsychiatric aspects of anticonvulsant megaloblastic anaemia, *Lancet*, **i**, 394.

RICHENS, A., and DUNLOP, A. (1975) Serum-phenytoin levels in management of epilepsy, *Lancet*, **ii**, 247.

RICHENS, A., and ROWE, D. J. F. (1970) Disturbance of calcium metabolism by anti-convulsant drugs, *Brit. med. J.*, **4**, 73.

RODIN, E. A. (1972) Medical and social prognosis in epilepsy, *Epilepsia (Amst.)*, **13**, 121.

RODIN, E. A., RENNICK, P., DENNERLL, R., and LIN, Y. (1972) Vocational and educational problems of epileptic patients, *Epilepsia (Amst.)*, **13**, 149.

ROVERE, M. DELLA, HOARE, R. D., and PAMPIGLIONE, G. (1964) Tuberose sclerosis in children, an E.E.G. study, *Develop. med. Child. Neurol.*, **6**, 149.

SCHWARTZ, M. S., and SCOTT, D. F. (1971) Isolated petit-mal status presenting de novo in middle age, *Lancet*, **ii**, 1399.

SCOTT, D. F., MOFFETT, A., and SWASH, M. (1972) Observations on the relation of migraine and epilepsy, *Epilepsia (Amst.)*, **13**, 365.

SHAW, R. F., GALL, J. C. Jun., and SCHUMAN, S. H. (1972) Febrile convulsions as a problem in waiting times, *Epilepsia (Amst.)*, **13**, 305.

SIMPSON, J. A. (1952) Neurological manifestations of hypoparathyroidism, *Brain*, **75**, 76.

SLATER, E., and BEARD, A. W. (1963) The schizophrenia-like psychoses of epilepsy, *Brit. J. Psychiat.*, **109**, 95.

SOLOMON, G. E., HILGARTNER, M. W., and KUTT, H. (1972) Coagulation defects caused by diphenylhydantoin, *Neurology (Minneap.)*, **22**, 1165.

SPEIDEL, B. D., and MEADOW, S. R. (1972) Maternal epilepsy and abnormalities of the fetus and newborn, *Lancet*, **ii**, 839.

STEVENS, D. L., and MATTHEWS, W. B. (1973) Cryptogenic drop attacks: an affliction of women, *Brit. med. J.*, **1**, 439.

STOCK, M. S., BURG, F. D., LIGHT, W. O., and DOUGLASS, J. M. (1970) Licensing the driver with alterations of consciousness, *Arch. Neurol. (Chic.)*, **23**, 210.

STOUPEL, N. (1968) On the reflex epilepsies: epilepsy caused by reading, *Electroenceph. clin. Neurophysiol.*, **25**, 416.

STRANDJORD, R. E., and JOHANNESSEN, S. I. (1974) One daily dose of diphenylhydantoin for patients with epilepsy, *Epilepsia (Amst.)*, **15**, 317.

SUTHERLAND, J. M., TAIT, H., and EADIE, M. J. (1974) *The Epilepsies: Modern Diagnosis and Treatment*, 2nd ed., Edinburgh and London.

SYMONDS, C. (1959) Excitation and inhibition in epilepsy, *Brain*, **82**, 133.

TASSINARI, C. A., GASTAUT, H., DRAVET, C., and ROGER, J. (1971) A paradoxical effect: status epilepticus induced by benzodiazepines, *Electroenceph. clin. Neurophysiol.*, **31**, 182.

TAYLOR, D. C. (1969) Sexual behavior and temporal lobe epilepsy, *Arch. Neurol. (Chic.)*, **21**, 510.

TAYLOR, D. C., and BOWER, B. D. (1971) Prevention in epileptic disorders, *Lancet*, **ii**, 1136.

TAYLOR, D. C., and FALCONER, M. A. (1968) Clinical, socio-economic, and psychological changes after temporal lobectomy for epilepsy, *Brit. J. Psychiat.*, **114**, 1247.

TAYLOR, D. C., FALCONER, M. A., BRUTON, C. J., and CORSELLIS, J. A. N. (1971) Focal dysplasia of the cerebral cortex in epilepsy, *J. Neurol. Neurosurg. Psychiat.*, **34**, 369.

TERRENCE, C. F. Jun., WISOTZKEY, H. M., and PERPER, J. A. (1975) Unexpected, unexplained death in epileptic patients, *Neurology (Minneap.)*, **25**, 594.

TYRER, J. H., EADIE, M. J., SUTHERLAND, J. M., and HOOPER, W. D. (1970) Outbreak of anticonvulsant intoxication in an Australian city, *Brit. med. J.*, **4**, 271.

UTTERBACK, R. A., OJEMAN, R., and MALEK, J. (1958) Parenchymatous cerebellar degeneration with Dilantin intoxication, *J. Neuropath. exp. Neurol.*, **17**, 516.

VAS, C. J., and PARSONAGE, M. J. (1967) Treatment of intractable temporal lobe epilepsy with pheneturide, *Acta neurol. scand.*, **43**, 580.

WALLACE, J. C. (1974) Radionuclide brain scanning in investigation of late-onset seizures, *Lancet*, **ii**, 1467.

WALLIS, W., KUTT, H., and McDOWELL, F. (1968) Intravenous diphenylhydantoin in treatment of acute repetitive seizures, *Neurology (Minneap.)*, **18**, 513.

WALTER, W. G. (1947) Analytical means of discovering the origin and nature of epileptic disturbances, *Res. Publ. Ass. nerv. ment. Dis.*, **26**, 237.

WARD, A. A. Jun. (1972) Basic mechanisms of the epilepsies, in *Scientific Foundations of Neurology*, ed. Critchley, M., O'Leary, J. L., and Jennett, W. B., London.

WARREN, D. J., LEITCH, A. G., and LEGGETT, R. J. E. (1975) Hyperuricaemic acute renal failure after epileptic seizures, *Lancet*, **ii**, 385.

WAUCHOPE, G. M. (1933) Hypoglycaemia, *Quart. J. Med.*, N.S. **2**, 117.

WAXMAN, S. G., and GESCHWIND, N. (1974) Hypergraphia in temporal lobe epilepsy, *Neurology (Minneap.)*, **24**, 629.

WHITTY, C. W. M. (1960) Photic and self-induced epilepsy, *Lancet*, **i**, 1207.

WILDER, R. M. (1921) Effect of ketonuria on course of epilepsy, *Mayo Clin. Bull.*, **2**, 307.

WILLIAMS, D. (1941) The significance of an abnormal electroencephalogram, *J. Neurol. Psychiat.*, N.S. **4**, 257.

WILLIAMS, D. (1950) New orientation in epilepsy, *Brit. med. J.*, **1**, 685.

WILSON, J. (1969) Drug treatment of epilepsy in childhood, *Brit. med. J.*, **4**, 475.

WILSON, J., WALTON, J. N., and NEWELL, D. J. (1959) Beclamide in intractable epilepsy: a controlled trial, *Brit. med. J.*, **1**, 1275.

WONG, H. B., and TEH, Y. F. (1968) An association between serum-magnesium and tremor and convulsions in infants and children, *Lancet*, **ii**, 18.

WOODBURY, D. M., PENRY, J. K., and SCHMIDT, R. P. (1972) *Antiepileptic Drugs*, New York.

ZISKIND, E., and BERCEL, N. A. (1947) Preconvulsive paroxysmal electro-encephalographic changes after metrazol injection, *Res. Publ. Ass. nerv. ment. Dis.*, **26**, 487.

MYOCLONUS

The term 'myoclonus' is applied to a brief, shock-like muscular contraction which may involve a whole muscle or may rarely be limited to a small number of muscle fibres. Myoclonus may be confined to a single muscle or may involve many muscles, either successively or simultaneously. Frequently contractions occur symmetrically in muscles on the opposite sides of the body. The contraction may be too slight to cause movement of a segment of the limb, or may cause such violent movements as to throw the patient to the ground. The contraction never involves groups of muscles which are normally synergically associated, nor does it as a rule affect mutually antagonistic muscles.

The situation of the disorder of function responsible for myoclonus has been much discussed. When myoclonus is associated with epilepsy the disturbance appears to arise at a situation deeply placed which is able to activate both cerebral hemispheres and it seems likely that it originates in the reticular substance of the

brain stem. There is also evidence that myoclonus without epilepsy may be caused by disorders of the olivo-dentate system. Myoclonus may occur without any demonstrable pathological lesion—essential myoclonus. Bradshaw (1954) and Aigner and Mulder (1960) have reviewed this topic and it has been shown that no fewer than 30 different entities have been described in which myoclonus may occur.

The Causes of Myoclonus

While the sharp, transient muscular contractions or 'jerks' which constitute the myoclonic phenomena are in most cases to be regarded as representing a type of transient epileptic discharge arising in cerebral or brain stem neurones, other forms of epileptic attack are not invariably associated with myoclonus. Myoclonic jerks which occur on falling asleep in the 'drifting' stage are physiological and probably depend upon a transient reactivation of reticular system neurones. When, however, nocturnal myoclonus continues during deep sleep, it is often found that major fits, possibly nocturnal, eventually occur in such cases and this syndrome is undoubtedly to be regarded as a form of epilepsy. Recurrent myoclonic jerks in the early morning after waking, causing the patient to spill the breakfast tea or coffee or even to 'throw' cutlery across the room, is not infrequently seen in some children with idiopathic epilepsy, and a single myoclonic jerk in the upper limbs occasionally occurs in an attack of petit mal. 'Jerking' or 'jumping' of the limbs and trunk in response to a sudden noise may sometimes be so intense as to be undoubtedly pathological. It has been called hyperekplexia or the 'essential startle disease' (Gastaut and Villeneuve, 1967), is occasionally familial and may be indistinguishable from myoclonus, except that it is always precipitated by noise. Physiological evidence which suggests that evoked potentials may easily be recorded in scalp EEG recordings as a result of peripheral sensory stimuli suggests that perhaps in patients with the benign forms of myoclonus, inhibitory mechanisms in the brain stem reticular substance are defective.

In Unverricht's progressive myoclonic epilepsy degenerative changes have been described in cortical ganglion cells and in cerebellar dentate nuclei. Myoclonus may occur also in encephalitis lethargica, subacute sclerosing panencephalitis, and the cerebral lipidoses. Jones and Nevin (1954) described it as a symptom of subacute spongiform encephalopathy and it is now accepted as a common manifestation of Creutzfeldt–Jakob disease [see p. 697]. The olivodentate form may be the result of an abiotrophic degeneration, as in Hunt's dyssynergia cerebellaris myoclonica, vascular lesions, tumours, and multiple sclerosis. Action myoclonus may be a sequel of cerebral anoxia (see below). Myoclonus in the legs has been described as a result of pathological changes in the spinal cord (Campbell and Garland, 1956).

Myoclonus is thus a symptom which may be produced by a variety of different lesions, and in some cases the nature of the underlying disorder of function is still obscure. The classification of varieties of myoclonus is, therefore, necessarily somewhat arbitrary.

VARIETIES OF MYOCLONUS

FACIAL MYOCLONUS

This name has been given, erroneously, by some authors to hemifacial spasm [see p. 185].

MYOCLONUS IN ENCEPHALOMYELITIS AND OTHER SPINAL LESIONS

Myoclonus is a somewhat uncommon symptom of encephalitis lethargica. It occurred with special frequency in some epidemics [see p. 487]. It may also occur in subacute sclerosing panencephalitis and in Creutzfeldt–Jakob disease which is now known to be due to a slow virus infection. It has also been reported in cervical herpes zoster, especially in those cases in which there is evidence that the infection has spread in the spinal cord beyond the first sensory neurone. Rhythmical myoclonus in one upper limb has been described as the result of a cervical cord tumour (Garcin *et al.*, 1968). Campbell and Garland (1956) described a condition which they called progressive myoclonic spinal neuronitis in which myoclonic jerking in the lower limbs was followed by the development of a progressive paraplegia. Rhythmical myoclonus in the lower part of the body, sometimes involving the abdominal wall, coming on acutely and resolving after diazepam treatment, was thought by Hopkins and Michael (1974) possibly to be due to viral invasion of the spinal cord, and Whiteley *et al.* (1976) described two patients with encephalomyelitis giving rise to rigidity and stimulus-sensitive muscular spasms of the lower limbs. The latter authors postulate a possible relationship between spinal myoclonus and the 'stiff-man' syndrome.

PALATO-PHARYNGO-LARYNGO-OCULO-DIAPHRAGMATIC MYOCLONUS

This syndrome, as its name implies, is characterized by the synchronous occurrence of a rhythmical myoclonus of the soft palate, pharynx, larynx, eyes, and diaphragm, and sometimes of other muscles. The distribution of the myoclonus may be unilateral or bilateral. The palatal movement has been described as 'nystagmus of the soft palate'. The rate of the movements varies from 80 to 180 to the minute, and is usually about 120 to 130 contractions to the minute. It is uninfluenced by drugs, and apparently by sleep, but may be inhibited at first by voluntary effort, and disappears if paralysis supervenes in the myoclonic muscles. It appears to be due to a degenerative process of unknown cause in most cases, but has been observed in multiple sclerosis and as a sequel to brain stem infarction. The disorder appears to be one of the olivo-cerebellar modulatory projection on to the rostral brain stem (Herrmann and Brown, 1967).

PARAMYOCLONUS MULTIPLEX

The term 'paramyoclonus multiplex' and its synonyms, myoclonus simplex and essential myoclonus, should be reserved for the syndrome first described by Friedreich in 1881 and characterized by the onset during adult life of frequent myoclonic muscular contractions. These are most frequently observed in the facial muscles and in the biceps, triceps, and brachioradialis in the upper limbs and in the quadriceps, and to a lesser extent in the adductors of the hip, biceps, and semitendinosus in the lower limbs. The muscular contraction involves the whole muscle or groups of muscles and occurs regularly with a frequency varying from 10 to 50 times a minute. The jerking movements are increased by tension and anxiety and may be inhibited by volitional contraction; though they may affect symmetrically muscles on the two sides of the body, these do not contract synchronously. The myoclonic movements disappear during sleep. The electrical reactions of the muscles are normal, sensation is unimpaired, and the

only associated abnormality is an exaggeration of the tendon reflexes. The disorder is a benign and chronic one which does not threaten life, and in some cases recovery occurs. These patients do not as a rule develop epileptic seizures, dementia, or ataxia; no consistent pathological changes have been discovered in the brain in this condition, which Mahloudji and Pikielny (1967) suggest should be called 'hereditary essential myoclonus'. Treatment with sedative drugs is on the same lines as for epilepsy but there is recent evidence to suggest that diazepam may be the most effective remedy.

ACTION MYOCLONUS

In 1963 Lance and Adams described a syndrome of action myoclonus occurring as a sequel of hypoxic encephalopathy. They said that 'The essential clinical picture was that of an arrhythmic fine or coarse jerking of a muscle or group of muscles in disorderly fashion, excited mainly by muscular activity particularly when a conscious attempt at precision was required, worsened by emotional arousal, suppressed by barbiturates and superimposed upon a mild cerebellar ataxia'. Many additional cases have now been reported and diazepam has been shown to be the most effective drug for controlling the jerking (Lance, 1968; Sherwin and Redmon, 1969). Clonazepam, which raises brain levels of serotonin (Chadwick et al., 1975), may prove to be even more effective.

INFANTILE MYOCLONIC ENCEPHALOPATHY (POLYMYOCLONIA)

This rare condition, also described under the heading of dancing eyes and dancing feet (Dyken and Kolář, 1968), has been mentioned on page 539. It begins suddenly in infancy with opsoclonus, limb myoclonus, and irritability and runs a protracted but relatively non-progressive course with exacerbations and remissions. Its cause is unknown but an auto-immune encephalopathy has been postulated.

PROGRESSIVE FAMILIAL MYOCLONIC EPILEPSY

Myoclonic contractions are common in patients suffering from idiopathic epilepsy, occurring between the epileptic attacks and usually becoming intensified before the attack occurs. In addition epileptic attacks have been described rarely in patients regarded as suffering from paramyoclonus multiplex, though it is difficult to say on what grounds such cases are distinguished from idiopathic epilepsy with myoclonus. The term 'progressive familial myoclonus epilepsy' is best reserved for the rare but well-defined syndrome first described by Unverricht in 1891, and later carefully studied by Lundborg (1903). Recent reports are by Harriman and Millar (1955), Noad and Lance (1960), Harenko and Toivakka (1961), and Rallo et al. (1968). Myoclonus epilepsy thus defined is usually familial, and occurs in several sibs, being inherited as an autosomal recessive disorder.

The distinctive pathological feature is the presence of inclusion bodies in the cytoplasm of the nerve cells. Harriman and Millar describe two types: (1) the Lafora bodies staining like amyloid; and (2) lipid inclusions resembling those of amaurotic family idiocy. The most striking pathological changes are observed in cerebral cortical neurones and in the dentate nuclei of the cerebellum. Millar and Neill (1959) found that in such cases an abnormal mucoprotein may be detected in the serum. Yokoi et al. (1968) showed that isolated Lafora bodies contain insoluble aggregates of an unusual polyglucosan and suggest that

progressive myoclonic epilepsy should be regarded as one of the 'glycogen deposition diseases'. However, Dastur *et al.* (1966), while agreeing that the disorder is probably one of glycoprotein storage, described atypical inclusion bodies in affected adults, and Matthews *et al.* (1969) found no Lafora or other inclusion bodies in a clinically typical case at autopsy. Ultrastructural changes are described by Brown *et al.* (1968). Several recent reports have shown, however, that in many cases typical Lafora bodies, identifiable as membrane-bound spaces containing mucopolysaccharide, may be demonstrated in muscle biopsy sections examined with the electron microscope (Carpenter *et al.*, 1974; Neville *et al.*, 1974; Coleman *et al.*, 1974). Lafora body disease has also been shown rarely to give a syndrome resembling presenile dementia in adult life (Suzuki *et al.*, 1971).

The onset of symptoms occurs as a rule between the ages of 6 and 16, usually when the patient is about 10, development up to that point having been normal. Generalized epileptiform attacks with loss of consciousness appear first, and, to begin with, frequently occur only at night. After several years the characteristic myoclonic contractions develop. These are shock-like muscular contractions simultaneously involving symmetrical muscles on both sides of the body, sufficiently strong to produce movements of the limb segments. They involve the muscles of the face, trunk, and of both upper and lower limbs. They disappear during sleep and are intensified by emotional excitement. They often increase in severity before a generalized epileptic attack but are not attended by loss of consciousness. Myoclonus may occur in the ocular muscles, the lips, and the tongue, interfering with speech and with swallowing. In the limbs the flexors are more often attacked than the extensors. Writing may become impossible, and sudden contractions of the flexors of the lower limbs when the patient is standing or walking may throw him violently to the ground. After some years, during which myoclonic and epileptic attacks are associated, a progressive dementia develops, and the patient passes into the third stage of the disease, in which the epileptic attacks tend to disappear, though myoclonus continues. Dysarthria and dysphagia increase, and death follows progressive cachexia. Noad and Lance (1960) reported a family with signs of cerebellar disorder. The EEG shows bilaterally synchronous sharp waves associated with the myoclonus, which Harriman and Millar think indicates that the discharge originates in the brain stem. Noad and Lance found that the EEG discharge resembled that seen in the lipidoses.

The relationship of this condition to Hunt's dyssynergia cerebellaris myoclonica [p. 677] is uncertain but in the latter disorder myoclonus and cerebellar ataxia, rather than major fits and dementia, predominate. The two disorders also differ pathologically (de Barsy *et al.*, 1969).

Treatment is merely palliative. The usual treatment of epilepsy may control the generalized epileptic attacks, but has less influence upon the myoclonus. Diazepam or clonazepam may have some effect upon the myoclonus but not upon the progressive dementia.

REFERENCES

AIGNER, B. R., and MULDER, D. W. (1960) Myoclonus, *Arch. Neurol. (Chic.)*, **2**, 600.

BARSY, T. DE, MYLE, G., TROCH, C., MATTHYS, R., and MARTIN, J. J. (1969) La dyssynergie cérébelleuse myoclonique (R. Hunt): affection autonome ou variante du type dégénératif de l'épilepsie myoclonique progressive (Unverricht-Lundborg) (approche anatomo-chimique), *J. neurol. Sci.*, **8**, 111.

BRADSHAW, J. P. P. (1954) A study of myoclonus, *Brain*, **77**, 138.

BROWN, W. J., KOTORII, K., and RIEHL, J.-L. (1968) Ultrastructural studies in myoclonus epilepsy, *Neurology (Minneap.)*, **18**, 427.

CAMPBELL, A. M. G., and GARLAND, H. G. (1956) Progressive myoclonic spinal neuronitis, *J. Neurol. Neurosurg. Psychiat.*, **19**, 268.

CARPENTER, S., KARPATI, G., ANDERMANN, F., JACOB, J. C., and ANDERMANN, E. (1974) Lafora's disease: peroxisomal storage in skeletal muscle, *Neurology (Minneap.)*, **24**, 531.

CHADWICK, D., HARRIS, R., JENNER, P., REYNOLDS, E. H., and MARSDEN, C. D. (1975) Manipulation of brain serotonin in the treatment of myoclonus, *Lancet*, **ii**, 434.

COLEMAN, D. L., GAMBETTI, P., DI MAURO, S., and BLUME, R. E. (1974) Muscle in Lafora disease, *Arch. Neurol. (Chic.)*, **31**, 396.

DASTUR, D. K., SINGHAL, B. S., GOOTZ, M., and SEITELBERGER, F. (1966) Atypical inclusion bodies with myoclonic epilepsy, *Acta Neuropathy. (Berl.)*, **7**, 16.

DYKEN, P., and KOLÁŘ, O. (1968) Dancing eyes, dancing feet: infantile polymyoclonia, *Brain*, **91**, 305.

GARCIN, R., RONDOT, P., and GUIOT, G. (1968) Rhythmic myoclonus of the right arm as the presenting symptom of a cervical cord tumour, *Brain*, **91**, 75.

GASTAUT, H., and VILLENEUVE, A. (1967) The startle disease or hyperekplexia, *J. neurol. Sci.*, **5**, 523.

GUILLAIN, G. (1937-8) The syndrome of synchronous and rhythmic palato-pharyngo-laryngo-oculo-diaphragmatic myoclonus, *Proc. roy. Soc. Med.*, **31**, 1031.

HARENKO, A., and TOIVAKKA, E. I. (1961) Myoclonus epilepsy (Unverricht-Lundborg) in Finland, *Acta neurol. scand.*, **37**, 282.

HARRIMAN, D. G. F., and MILLAR, J. H. D. (1955) Progressive familial myoclonic epilepsy in three families; its clinical features and pathological basis, *Brain*, **78**, 325.

HERMANN, C., Jun., and BROWN, J. W. (1967) Palatal myoclonus: a reappraisal, *J. neurol. Sci.*, **5**, 473.

HOPKINS, A. P., and MICHAEL, W. F. (1974) Spinal myoclonus, *J. Neurol. Neurosurg. Psychiat.*, **37**, 1112.

JACQUIN, G., and MARCHAND, L. (1913) Myoclonie épileptique progressive, *Encéphale*, **8** (1), 205.

JONES, D. P., and NEVIN, S. (1954) Rapidly progressive cerebral degeneration (subacute vascular encephalopathy with mental disorder, focal disturbances, and myoclonic epilepsy), *J. Neurol. Neurosurg. Psychiat.*, **17**, 148.

LANCE, J. W. (1968) Myoclonic jerks and falls: aetiology, classification and treatment, *Med. J. Aust.*, **1**, 113.

LANCE, J. W., and ADAMS, R. D. (1963) The syndrome of intention or action myoclonus as a sequel to hypoxic encephalopathy, *Brain*, **86**, 111.

LUNDBORG, H. (1903) *Die progressive Myoklonus-Epilepsie*, Uppsala.

MAHLOUDJI, M., and PIKIELNY, R. T. (1967) Hereditary essential myoclonus, *Brain*, **90**, 669.

MATTHEWS, W. B., HOWELL, D. A., and STEVENS, D. L. (1969) Progressive myoclonus epilepsy without Lafora bodies, *J. Neurol. Neurosurg. Psychiat.*, **32**, 116.

MILLAR, J. H. D., and NEILL, D. W. (1959) Serum mucoproteins in progressive familial myoclonic epilepsy, *Epilepsia*, **1**, 115.

NEVILLE, H. E., BROOKE, M. H., and AUSTIN, J. H. (1974) Studies in myoclonus epilepsy (Lafora body form). IV. Skeletal muscle abnormalities, *Arch. Neurol. (Chic.)*, **30**, 466.

NOAD, K. B., and LANCE, J. W. (1960) Familial myoclonic epilepsy and its association with cerebellar disturbance, *Brain*, **83**, 618.

RALLO, E., MARTIN, F., INFANTE, F., BEAUMANOIR, A., and KLEIN, D. (1968) Epilepsie myoclonique progressive maligne (maladie de Lafora), *Acta neurol. belg.*, **68**, 356.

SHERWIN, I., and REDMON, W. (1969) Successful treatment in action myoclonus, *Neurology (Minneap.)*, **19**, 846.

O O

SUZUKI, K., DAVID, E., and KUTSCHMAN, B. (1971) Presenile dementia with 'Lafora-like' intraneuronal inclusions, *Arch. Neurol. (Chic.)*, **25,** 69.
UNVERRICHT, H. (1891) *Die Myoclonie*, Leipzig.
WHITELEY, A. M., SWASH, M., and URICH, H. (1976) Progressive encephalomyelitis with rigidity: its relation to subacute myoclonic spinal neuronitis and to the stiff-man syndrome, *Brain*, **99,** 27.
YOKOI, S., AUSTIN, J., WITMER, F., and SAKAI, M. (1968) Studies in myoclonus epilepsy (Lafora body form), *Arch. Neurol. (Chic.)*, **19,** 15.

TETANY

Definition. Tetany, or carpopedal spasm, is a form of muscular spasm beginning in, and sometimes remaining limited to, the peripheral muscles of the limbs. It is associated with an increased excitability of the neuromuscular apparatus to all forms of stimuli. It is a symptom of a variety of disorders which either reduce the calcium content of the blood or increase its alkalinity.

AETIOLOGY

Modern investigations of the metabolism of calcium and of the biochemistry of the blood have rendered it possible to reduce the immediate causes of tetany to two. It is probable that in all cases the patient is suffering from either a subnormal calcium content of the blood, or from an alkalosis, though a few conditions remain which have not yet been sufficiently investigated to enable them to be placed in either class. An attempt has been made to attribute all forms of tetany to calcium deficiency, on the hypothesis that alkalosis diminishes the amount of ionized calcium in the blood, even though its total calcium content remains normal. This at present, however, remains unproved, and there are indications that tissue anoxia may be of some importance. Tetany may, in fact, occur rarely in metabolic acidosis if there are associated hyperphosphataemia and hypocalcaemia; if bicarbonate is given to correct the acidosis this may precipitate tetany due to the associated hypocalcaemia but this complication can usually be prevented by giving calcium gluconate (see Welt, 1974).

Conditions characterized by a Subnormal Blood Calcium

Parathyroid Deficiency. The important role of the parathyroids in the metabolism of calcium and their influence upon the calcium content of the blood are well recognized. Hyperparathyroidism due to a parathyroid tumour causes the blood calcium content to rise above its normal figure of between 9 and 11 mg per 100 ml. Hypoparathyroidism leads to a subnormal blood-calcium content which may be as low as 4 or 5 mg per 100 ml, and in such cases tetany may occur—tetania parathyreopriva. Hypoparathyroidism, which is rare, is usually the result of accidental removal of the parathyroid glands during thyroidectomy but may rarely follow I_{131} treatment of thyrotoxicosis, presumably as a result of irradiation of the parathyroids (see Potts, 1974). Tetany may also occur in idiopathic hypoparathyroidism (of unknown cause) and pseudo-hypoparathyroidism (due to a deficient end-organ response to endogenous parathyroid hormone).

Defective Intestinal Calcium Absorption. Fatty diarrhoea, when severe and of long duration, may lead to a fall in the blood calcium content sufficient to cause tetany. Thus tetany may occur in sprue, in cases of idiopathic steatorrhoea, and, exceptionally, in tuberculous enteritis. The low blood calcium in

such cases has been attributed to loss of calcium from the intestine in combination with fatty acids in the form of soaps. It appears, however, that the chief cause of the calcium defect is a failure to absorb vitamin D (Hunter, 1930). No hard and fast line can be drawn between defective absorption and excessive loss. Tetany is also an occasional manifestation of acute pancreatitis; the hypocalcaemia which rarely occurs in this condition is unexplained (see Snodgrass, 1974).

Rickets and Osteomalacia. In the past, dietary deficiency of vitamin D or lack of exposure to sunlight was the commonest cause of rickets which often gave rise to infantile tetany (spasmophilia). About 10 per cent of such cases also suffered epileptic seizures. The widespread use of vitamin supplements in infancy has virtually abolished rickets due to dietary deficiency but a number of forms of vitamin-D resistant rickets have been described; in one of these, hypophosphatasia, a single enzyme defect has been identified (Fraser, 1957; Krane, 1974). Some cases of adult osteomalacia are due to an inadequate dietary intake of calcium and vitamin D (Dent and Smith, 1969).

Increased Demand for Calcium. Pregnancy and lactation may cause tetany, owing to the increased demand which they make upon the calcium resources of the mother. The likelihood of this occurring is much increased when the intake of vitamin D and calcium is subnormal, as in osteomalacia.

High Urinary Calcium Loss. Chronic renal failure may lead to tetany as a result of hypocalcaemia and raised serum phosphate, which is present also in hypoparathyroidism, but this complication is rare, presumably because of the associated acidosis. A raised blood potassium may be a contributory factor.

Conditions characterized by Alkalosis

Alkalosis occurs when the ratio of acid to base in the blood is diminished, with the result that the pH, normally between 7·3 and 7·5, rises as does the serum bicarbonate. This may occur in the following conditions:

Excessive Ingestion of Alkali. Overdosage with sodium bicarbonate and other alkalis used in the treatment of dyspepsia may cause alkalosis and hence tetany, especially if the power of the kidney to excrete alkali is diminished by nephritis.

Hyperpnoea. Overbreathing, by washing out CO_2 from the blood, may lead to alkalosis and hence to tetany. Tetany may thus be induced by voluntary or hysterical overbreathing, or by hyperpnoea occurring as a result of disturbance of function of the respiratory centre, for example in encephalitis.

High Intestinal Obstruction. It has long been known that tetany may complicate disorders associated with repeated vomiting—gastric tetany—and McCallum suggested that in such cases alkalosis was produced by a loss of acid from the body in the vomit. Since, however, alkalosis may occur in cases of pyloric obstruction due to carcinoma of the stomach, in which the vomit may be free from acid, this hypothesis cannot be the whole explanation. It has been shown experimentally that high intestinal obstruction in itself leads to a fall in the chloride content and a rise in the bicarbonate content of the blood.

Other Causes of Tetany

So-called idiopathic tetany was once described in an epidemic form in some of the countries of central Europe, usually in the spring months. Tetany also occurs in association with a low blood potassium, e.g. in hyperaldosteronism.

PATHOPHYSIOLOGY

The pathophysiology of tetany has been reviewed by Alajouanine *et al.* (1958). They believe that it is essentially a functional disorder of the peripheral sensorimotor fibres resulting from various metabolic disturbances. Electrically the nerves show hyperexcitability, diminished capacity for accommodation, and a tendency to show repetitive responses to single stimuli. These authors discount a cerebral origin for tetany, a point discussed by Matthews (1958).

SYMPTOMS

An attack of tetany is usually preceded by tingling sensations in the periphery of the limbs, especially in the hands, and there are often similar paraesthesiae with a sense of stiffness in the lips and tongue. The attack itself consists of muscular spasm which develops spontaneously, but its intensity may be increased by external stimuli, such as manipulation of the limbs. In mild cases the spasm is confined to the hands and feet, or even to the hands. The tonic contraction of the interossei of the hands leads to a typical attitude—*le main d'accoucheur*. The fingers are slightly flexed at the metacarpophalangeal joints and extended at the interphalangeal joints. They are strongly adducted, and the thumb is similarly adducted and usually extended. The cause of the limitation of the muscular spasm in mild cases to the small muscles of the hands is unknown. Exceptionally the fingers become flexed at all joints. The characteristic attitude of the feet is one of plantar-flexion at the ankle and adduction of the toes.

In severe attacks the muscular spasm spreads to the proximal muscles of the limbs. In the upper limbs it predominates as a rule in the flexors of the elbow and in the adductors of the shoulder. In the lower limbs the knees are usually extended and the hips adducted. In such cases the muscles of the head may also go into spasm, the masseters closing the jaw and the angles of the mouth being retracted in a *risus sardonicus*. The eyes may be partly closed and the bulbar muscles may also be affected, especially those of the larynx. Laryngospasm with resultant stridor has been described, particularly in children with rickets. Dysarthria and dyspnoea may thus be produced. Spasm of the trunk muscles may also occur, leading to slight opisthotonus. Generalized convulsions have been described, especially in childhood.

Though slight attacks of tetany are painless, considerable cramp-like pain attends the more violent spasms. Sweating and tachycardia and even rise of temperature may occur in severe attacks.

The increased excitability of the neuromuscular apparatus is demonstrable in the response to certain tests, even in the absence of actual attacks of tetany. *Chvostek's sign* consists of a brisk contraction of the facial muscles in response to a light tap over the facial nerve in front of the ear. Pressure upon the main artery supplying a limb or upon the peripheral nerves may precipitate an attack of tetany—*Trousseau's sign*. This test is simply applied by means of the cuff of a sphygmomanometer. The response to electrical stimulation of the nerves is also abnormal with increased excitability of the motor nerves. Electromyographic changes are discussed by Alajouanine *et al.* (1958).

In hypoparathyroidism generalized epileptiform convulsions associated with loss of consciousness may occur, but are rare except in children with idiopathic hypoparathyroidism in whom mental backwardness is usual [p. 837]. Confusion and intellectual blunting may occur in acquired hypoparathyroidism while papilloedema may develop, with or without cataract, in the idiopathic form.

The EEG may show spikes and slow waves in the frontal areas. X-rays of the skull may demonstrate calcification in the basal ganglia and dentate nuclei. For a discussion of this see Roberts (1959) and Glaser and Levy (1960).

DIAGNOSIS

The symptoms of tetany are so striking that they are not likely to be confused with other conditions. The onset of the muscular spasm in the hands and feet and the associated signs of increased neuromuscular excitability are pathognomonic. Tetanus is distinguished by the fact that in this disease muscular spasm, though subject to exacerbations, is constant and not, as in tetany, intermittent. Moreover, in tetanus the *main d'accoucheur* attitude does not occur and spasm of the masseters as a rule develops early, whereas in tetany this is a late symptom occurring only in severe attacks. Hysteria may be associated with tetany when the latter is produced by hysterical hyperpnoea. In addition hysterical muscular rigidity may simulate tetany. Other hysterical symptoms, such as anaesthesia, are usually to be found in such cases, and the patient's emotional reaction to her symptoms is characteristic.

In every case of tetany the underlying cause must be ascertained. This is usually easy if the common causes are borne in mind and appropriate inquiries are made. It is always, however, desirable that the pH and bicarbonate content of the blood plasma and the calcium and phosphate content of the serum should be ascertained in order to determine whether the condition is due to a low blood calcium or alkalosis.

PROGNOSIS

Recovery from an attack of tetany is almost invariable, though death may occur in a severe attack, owing to laryngeal or bronchial spasm. The prognosis as to cessation of the attacks depends upon the nature of their cause and the efficiency of treatment.

TREATMENT

In hypocalcaemic tetany the blood calcium may be raised by administering calcium lactate as a powder taken in repeated doses up to a total of 10 to 30 g daily together with calciferol in the dose appropriate to the individual. Effervescent calcium tablets may be more palatable and convenient than calcium lactate. Dihydrotachysterol (*A.T. 10*), has a more rapid effect and is given in a dosage of 1·25 mg three times daily until the serum calcium is normal after which a single daily maintenance dose may suffice. A severe attack may be cut short by slowly injecting 20 ml of a 5 per cent solution of calcium gluconate intravenously.

In tetany due to steatorrhoea the dietary fat intake should be restricted to a minimum and the patient should be given calciferol. This vitamin, with or without irradiation with ultraviolet light, is all that is required in the treatment of tetany associated with rickets, and the same treatment should be given in osteomalacia and when tetany occurs in pregnancy, together with calcium by mouth and a calcium-rich diet. Parathyroid extract should not be given in these conditions, since it raises the blood calcium by withdrawing calcium from the bones.

When tetany is due to vitamin-resistant rickets or some other inborn error of metabolism the appropriate treatment will depend upon the identification of the underlying biochemical disorder.

REFERENCES

ALAJOUANINE, T., CONTAMIN, F., and CATHALA, H. P. (1958) *Le Syndrome Tétanie*, Paris.

DENT, C. E., and SMITH, R. (1969) Nutritional osteomalacia, *Quart. J. Med.*, **38,** 195.

FOLEY, J. (1951) Calcification in a family, *J. Neurol. Neurosurg. Psychiat.*, N.S. **14,** 253.

FRASER, D. (1957) Hypophosphatasia, *Amer. J. Med.*, **22,** 730.

GLASER, G. H., and LEVY, L. L. (1960) Seizures and idiopathic hypoparathyroidism, *Epilepsia*, **1,** 454.

GRANT, D. K. (1953) Papilloedema and fits in hypoparathyroidism, *Quart. J. Med.*, N.S. **22,** 243.

HUNTER, D. (1930) Goulstonian Lectures. The significance to clinical medicine of studies in calcium and phosphorus metabolism, *Lancet*, **i,** 897, 947, 999.

KRANE, S. M. (1974) Metabolic bone disease, in *Harrison's Principles of Internal Medicine*, 7th ed., chap. 352, New York.

MATTHEWS, W. (1958) Tonic seizures in disseminated sclerosis, *Brain*, **81,** 193.

POTTS, J. T. Jun. (1974) Disorders of parathyroid glands, in *Harrison's Principles of Internal Medicine*, 7th ed., chap. 350, New York.

ROBERTS, P. D. (1959) Familial calcification of the basal ganglia and its relation to hypoparathyroidism, *Brain*, **82,** 599.

SALVESEN, H. A. (1930, 1931) Observations on human tetany. I. Spontaneous tetany in adults, *Acta med. scand.*, **73,** 511; II. Postoperative tetany, *Brain*, **74,** 13.

SNODGRASS, P. J. (1974) Diseases of the pancreas, in *Harrison's Principles of Internal Medicine*, 7th ed., chap. 302, New York.

WELT, L. G. (1974) Acidosis and alkalosis, in *Harrison's Principles of Internal Medicine*, 7th ed., chap. 265, New York.

WEST, R. (1935) Studies in the neurological mechanism of parathyroid tetany, *Brain*, **58,** 1.

23

PSYCHOLOGICAL ASPECTS OF NEUROLOGY

THE growth of medical psychology has rendered it necessary to restrict the scope of the psychological section of a textbook of neurology. Much of psychiatry and psychotherapy falls outside the province of neurology. Nevertheless, since the brain is the organ of the mind the neurologist has unique opportunities of observing the effects of nervous disease upon mental functions, and in particular of studying disorders of perception, memory, and emotion. He is also concerned with the psychoses and psychoneuroses in the differential diagnosis of organic nervous disease. This section, therefore, deals with psychological medicine primarily from the standpoint of the neurologist. But since the neurologist is a doctor it falls to his lot to treat large numbers of patients suffering from psychological disorders. He cannot avoid, therefore, being at times a psychotherapist; hence some consideration of the relationships between neurology and psychiatry is called for in this chapter.

ANATOMY AND PHYSIOLOGY

GENERAL CONSIDERATIONS

The principal difference between the human and the subhuman brain consists in the great development of the cerebral cortex in man. The cortex is, in the first instance, an end-station at which are received nervous impulses derived from the eyes, the ears, and other sensory organs. The corresponding regions of the cortex are linked by association paths by means of which the sensations which form the raw material of perception evoke memories and become enriched with meanings, which can be communicated to others by means of speech, writing, and gesture (Critchley, 1975). The function of the cerebral cortex, therefore, as Head pointed out in relation to sensation, is primarily discriminative, and the massive development of the cortex in man compared with that in the lower animals is paralleled by the great enhancement of the range of his discriminative faculties, which has occurred in spite of there having been little improvement, and in some cases an actual retrogression, of his sensory acuity.

By contrast there is far less difference between man and the lower animals in respect of the development of subcortical centres, and in particular of the thalamus and hypothalamus. It is these regions of the brain, basal alike in situation and in function, which are intimately concerned with the affective element in feeling, with the emotional and instinctive life, and the regulation of the autonomic nervous system and to some extent of metabolic and endocrine function. The brain, however, works as a whole and there is a constant interplay between cortical and subcortical functions. Perception evokes emotion and, conversely, emotion provides the interest which activates perception.

There is another aspect, however, of the relationship between the cerebral cortex and subcortical function. Discrimination, the function of the cortex,

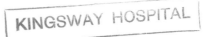

implies inhibition, for, if an organism is to react appropriately to a stimulus, inappropriate modes of reaction must be simultaneously inhibited. This is true even at the level of a simple reflex arc; it is far more essential when the range both of potential stimuli and of potential reactions has been so greatly enlarged by the development of the cerebral cortex. The cortex, therefore, acquires inhibitory functions as the complement of its discriminative functions.

Anatomy and Physiology of the Diencephalon

As Pribram (1958) showed, it is convenient to begin with the thalamus which seems in many ways both physiologically and anatomically basic to the organization of animal behaviour. The dorsal thalamus is divided into an external portion and an internal core. Each of these has nuclei which receive impulses from outside the thalamus and other nuclei which, as far as is known, do not. These are distinguished as extrinsic and intrinsic nuclei. The extrinsic nuclei of the external division receive the somatic sensory tracts, and the optic and auditory pathways: the intrinsic nucleus is the posterior nucleus. The extrinsic nuclei of the internal core receive impulses from the posterior hypothalamus and the central reticular formation: the intrinsic nucleus is the medial. Turning now to the projections from these nuclei we find that the extrinsic nuclei of the external portion project to the primary sensory cortical areas concerned with somatic sensibility, hearing, and vision in the parietal, temporal, and occipital lobes, while the intrinsic, posterior, nucleus projects to the rest of the parieto-temporo-occipital cortex. The extrinsic nuclei of the internal core project to the limbic areas of the medial aspect of the frontal and parietal lobes and to the anterior rhinencephalon and the basal ganglia, and the medial, the intrinsic, nucleus projects to the antero-frontal cortex. There is an important corticofugal pathway (the medial forebrain bundle) running from the mediobasal part of the frontal lobe to the thalamus and the hypothalamic nuclei, including the corpora mammillaria.

Experimental stimulation and destruction of these regions in animals leads to the following conclusions. The projections from the extrinsic nuclei of the external part of the dorsal thalamus are the familiar sensory afferent pathways, and interference with them causes sensory loss in the corresponding modalities. Damage to the parts of the cerebral cortex supplied by the projections from the intrinsic nuclei of the external part lead to a failure to differentiate and respond to patterns of sensory stimuli—a condition resembling that known in man as agnosia. These nuclei, their projections and the corresponding cortical areas must therefore be regarded as constituting a higher-level perceptual discriminative mechanism.

On the other hand, ablations and stimulations of the anatomical systems represented by the nuclei of the internal core of the thalamus, and their projections through the medial and basal telencephalon, affect feeding (eating and drinking), fighting and aggression, fleeing and avoidance, mating, and maternal behaviour: they are therefore concerned with what may in the broadest sense be termed instinctive behaviour. All such activities, when they occur in man, are linked with emotion to a greater or a lesser extent, and it seems a reasonable inference that the same is true of animals.

The role of various hypothalamic nuclei in controlling activity in the autonomic nervous system has already been described [pp. 1076–83]; emotional disorders and altered autonomic activity are closely interlinked and it is now apparent that the hypothalamus, brain stem reticular system, parts of the thalamus, the hippocampus, amygdala, fornix, and, in particular, the cingulate gyrus are closely interlinked and play a fundamental integrating role in controlling emotion as well as memory and behaviour. Even though in strictly anatomical terms, parts of the hypothalamus and brain stem reticular substance are not strictly part of the limbic system, functionally they are so closely related that it is reasonable to regard all of these structures as forming the limbic brain [FIG. 169].

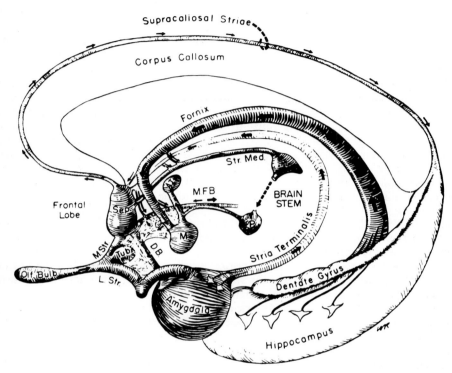

FIG. 169. The limbic system. (From Smythies, J. R. (1966) *The Neurological Foundations of Psychiatry*, by kind permission of the author and Blackwell Scientific Publications)

In the hypothalamus, in addition to the anterior and posterior nuclei concerned with temperature and cardiovascular control and with endocrine activity, and the supraoptic nucleus which produces ADH, the perifornical nucleus, if stimulated, causes hunger, increased blood pressure and sometimes rage, the ventromedial nucleus satiety, the lateral hypothalamic area thirst and hunger, and the mammillary body feeding reflexes (see Guyton, 1976). Many of these functions appear to be mediated through the brain stem reticular formation.

The Limbic System: Behavioural Functions

Recent neurophysiological studies in primates have shown that many hypothalamic and other limbic centres are especially concerned with sensations which have an emotional content and are either pleasant (rewarding) or painful, probably in an emotional rather than a physical sense (punishment or aversion).

Thus centres in the septum, hypothalamic ventromedial nuclei, and medial forebrain bundle may produce such a feeling of reward on stimulation that if an indwelling electrode is inserted and the animal can then apply stimuli himself he will do so repeatedly. By contrast, stimulation of the perifornical nucleus of the hypothalamus and of the mesencephalic central grey matter gives manifestations suggestive of pain, displeasure, and punishment, and will outweigh the effects of simultaneous stimulation of a reward centre (Herd, 1972; Isaacson, 1974; Weil, 1974). Physiologically, both habituation (diminishing response) and reinforcement have been shown with different stimulus patterns; pharmacologically both reward and punishment can be suppressed by various tranquillizing drugs (Cooper *et al.*, 1974). It seems probable that much human behaviour is dependent upon the balance of activity in reward and punishment centres.

In animals it has also been shown that intense stimulation of the punishment centres (e.g. the perifornical nucleus) may produce a rage response, while stimulation more rostrally gives manifestations of fear and anxiety; by contrast, repeated stimulation of reward centres will result in docility and tranquillity. The influence of the hypothalamus upon the reticular system in relation to sleep and waking can be shown by the fact that stimulation dorsal to the mammillary bodies gives excessive wakefulness and excitement with evidence of sympathetic overactivity, while stimulation in parts of the septum, anterior hypothalamus, or in some points of the thalamic reticular nuclei causes somnolence and sometimes actual sleep (see Guyton, 1976).

The Limbic Lobe and Emotion

Psychophysiologically, emotion implies a number of factors: there is (1) some external object which excites it. (2) There are specific feelings characteristic of particular emotions, and (3) the emotion tends to find expression in some characteristic action. Accompanying the feelings and the motor activities there are (4) certain other physiological states in which the autonomic nervous system and endocrine activity play an important part. And, finally, there is often (5) a pre-existing physiological state which is necessary if the appetite, or emotional need, is to be experienced. This is most obvious in the case of hunger, thirst, and the sexual impulse.

Papez in 1937 suggested that the cortical control of emotional processes began in the hippocampus and that the information was then transferred via the fornix to the mammillary body and anterior thalamic nuclei. This 'Papez circuit' [FIG. 169], as Smythies (1966) showed, was the forerunner conceptually of the limbic system which controls not only the emotions but also memory and much of behaviour. Unfortunately, however, the functions we are considering are often so subjective that the functions of many parts of the limbic system are poorly understood and what little we know has been derived from experiments involving electrical stimulation.

Stimulation of the *amygdala* (Smythies, 1970; Isaacson, 1974) can cause changes in heart rate and blood pressure, defaecation and micturition, pupillary dilatation, and an increased output of various anterior pituitary hormones. In other areas involuntary movements (tonic or circling movements, chewing or lip-smacking) may be elicited or alternatively an arrest reaction, in which the animal 'freezes' in one posture. Yet other areas, if stimulated, give manifestations of rage, fear, reward, or punishment as described above, while elsewhere stimuli produce sexual activity including erection, ejaculation, copulatory movements, ovulation, or uterine contraction. Thus many of the emotional and behavioural manifestations of temporal lobe epilepsy, including fear (Williams, 1956) or hypersexuality (Green, 1958) may be reproduced.

The *hippocampus* distributes many outgoing signals to the hypothalamus and other parts of the limbic system via the fornix (Guyton, 1976). Apart from its olfactory function, its other major role appears to be in relation to memory (see below). Stimulation of other parts of the limbic cortex (the cingulate gyrus and orbitofrontal cortex) may give changes in respiratory and cardiac rate and blood pressure, facilitation of movements induced by cortical stimulation elsewhere, licking, swallowing, changes in gastro-intestinal motility and secretion, and various affective reactions (e.g. rage or docility, increased or diminished awareness). Ablation of the cingulate gyri may give tameness in animals and suppression of previous rage reactions, while bilateral ablations of the orbitofrontal cortex may cause insomnia and motor restlessness (Hyvarinen, 1973). In man, cingulectomy and various other ablations of limbic cortex have been used as psychosurgical procedures for the treatment of obsessional states, hypersexuality and other behaviour disorders (Winter, 1971).

Memory

Clinical, behavioural, and neuropathological evidence clearly indicates, as mentioned above, that the recording of and registration of information occurs in the hippocampus and its connections (Barbizet, 1963; Lance and McLeod, 1975) but the storage of the memory trace or engram plainly involves a considerable part of the limbic system. Severe loss of recent memory with inability to record and retain new impressions occurs as a consequence of lesions of the mammillary bodies in the Wernicke–Korsakoff syndrome or after surgery (Kahn and Crosby, 1972). Remote memory is sometimes impaired in these subjects to a greater extent than is generally realized (Sanders and Warrington, 1971). However, division of the fornix (Whitty, 1962) and extensive bilateral frontal lobe damage (Denny-Brown, 1951) do not as a rule affect memory, while bilateral anterior cingulectomy produces only transient memory impairment (Whitty and Lewin, 1960); however, the effects of bilateral lesions of the thalamic dorsomedial nuclei in animals upon learning tasks may be more profound (Schulman, 1964). Sweet *et al.* (1959) reported a case in which memory was impaired as a result of surgical division of the anterior pillars of the fornix during removal of a colloid cyst of the third ventricle, but it is possible that structures other than the fornix were also damaged. In the 'split-brain' animal each hemisphere can be trained to store information, so that the corpus callosum is not essential for information processing, storage, and retrieval (Sperry, 1961). However, after commissurotomy in man (Zaidel and Sperry, 1974), some defects of memory were found, suggesting that 'processes mediating the initial encoding of engrams and the retrieval and read-out of contralateral engram elements involve interhemispheric cooperation'. Work carried out in flatworms (McConnell, 1962) suggested that cellular RNA was concerned in the memory process and that acquired information could be transferred to another worm which ingested the RNA derived from one which had succeeded in learning a task. Much more work upon the transfer of memory by such chemical means has been done, with results which have often been conflicting. As Cooper *et al.* (1974) have said, 'There is evidence that protein and RNA synthesis may occur along with learning but the experiment has yet to be designed which explicitly relates these two events'. For the present, therefore, it is reasonable that we should still regard memory as being a process which can be explained and controlled by neurophysiological mechanisms and disordered by many diseases which affect the structure and/or function of the brain.

A great deal of information has now accumulated to indicate that in clinical practice it is lesions of the anterior temporal lobe and particularly of the hippo-campus which most often impair memory. The so-called Kluver–Bucy syndrome, resulting from bilateral anterior temporal lobectomy in cats, usually involving the amygdala in whole or in part, gives loss of fear, tameness, and diminished aggression and a change in dietary habits, sexual overactivity, and sometimes 'psychic blindness' (Simpson, 1969), but, contrary to a widely held belief, no impairment of memory (see Guyton, 1976). However, Penfield and Jasper (1954) and Penfield (1958), in the course of their investigations of temporal lobe epilepsy, showed that memories could be evoked by hippocampal stimula-tion, and Bickford et al. (1958) produced a temporary loss of memory for recent events by electrical stimulation in this region. Scoville and Milner (1957) observed persistent, profound, and generalized loss of recent memory in 10 cases of bilateral hippocampal excision, the amnesia being unrelated to any deterioration of the intellect or personality of the subject and de Jong et al. (1969) described such a case following bilateral hippocampal infarction. Milner (1958, 1966) and Walker (1957) both reported cases of recent memory impair-ment after *unilateral* temporal lobe lesions. It was suggested that in such cases the corresponding area on the opposite side must previously have been damaged, and in fact, recent neuropathological studies (Brierley, 1966; van Buren and Borke, 1972; Penfield and Mathieson, 1974) have confirmed this hypothesis. However, the use of new and precise techniques of cognitive function, involving dichotic learning tasks and other methods of assessing auditory inattention (*British Medical Journal*, 1972; Heilman et al., 1974) have shown that a unilateral defect of 'auditory memory' may follow unilateral anterior temporal lobectomy performed for temporal lobe epilepsy (Blakemore and Falconer, 1967). Hence there is no doubt that bilateral hippocampal lesions are likely to cause permanent and continuing loss of memory for recent events, and this disability was also observed by Rose and Symonds (1960) and by Brierley et al. (1960) in patients who had suffered from encephalitis, which had selectively damaged the limbic brain, including the hippocampus. The important area seems to lie from 5·5 cm to 8 cm behind the tip of the temporal lobe. Such memory loss may be particularly prominent after recovery from herpes simplex encephalitis [p. 495].

The syndrome of *transient global amnesia*, which gives a sudden impairment of recent memory, often with retrograde amnesia for several days or weeks which subsequently is reduced to an hour or two at most after recovery, which usually occurs in a few hours (Steinmetz and Vroom, 1972) is described on page 1174. All the available evidence suggests that this syndrome, which may recur, is usually due to bilateral temporal lobe ischaemia due to atherosclerosis (Heathfield et al., 1973).

The Functions of the Frontal Lobe

Pribram pointed out that in animals experimental damage to the frontal cortex which derives its thalamic input from the medial nuclear group affects the ability of the animal to solve problems which depend upon the use of past experience. It has long been believed that the frontal lobes play a particularly important part in the control of intellect, initiative, personality and social consciousness. Penfield and Evans (1935) found that the maximum amputation of the right or left frontal lobe produced little change except for some impairment of those processes necessary for planned initiative, and Jefferson (1937) concluded from 8 cases of unilateral frontal lobectomy that the role of the frontal lobes was quantitative rather than qualitative. Rylander (1939) reported 32 cases of operation on the frontal lobe. Emotional changes consisted of diminished inhibition of affective responses and a tendency to euphoria, less often to depression. Changes in psychomotor activity took the form either of restlessness or lack of initiative and interest. In the intellectual life the more automatic forms of intelligence were relatively well preserved, together with attention and memory, but the higher forms of reasoning, thinking in symbols, and judgement had deteriorated. All of these features were exhibited by Brickner's (1936, 1939) patient who was observed for eight years after bilateral frontal lobectomy.

The operation of prefrontal leucotomy or lobotomy threw new light upon the functions of the frontal lobes which may be summarized as follows: 'According to Freeman and Watts, the prefrontal regions in man are concerned with foresight, imagination and the apperception of the self. These psychological functions are invested with emotion by way of the association fibres that link the hippocampus and cingulate gyrus with the thalamus and the hypothalamus. It would seem, then, that the functions of the prefrontal lobes are concerned with the adjustment of the personality as a whole to future contingencies. The imagination, therefore, in the pure sense of the term, may be said to reside in the prefrontal areas. Pure intellection in the sense of analysis, synthesis, and selectivity does not appear to require the integrity of the frontal and prefrontal areas to the extent that was previously thought necessary' (Brain and Strauss, 1945). This view received support from the observations of Hebb and Penfield (1940) and Hebb (1941) that extensive resection of one or both frontal lobes is not necessarily followed by intellectual deterioration, though Penfield (1948) in a later study found a slight drop in general intelligence after frontal gyrectomy and lobotomy, which he attributed to the patients' greater distractibility. But, as Smythies (1966) pointed out, despite much speculation and the virtual certainty that the frontal lobe is concerned with storage of certain social behaviour patterns, its exact functions are still poorly understood (Meyer, 1974). Disturbances of micturition, including frequency, urgency, and incontinence, are well recognized to occur in some bifrontal lesions (Andrew and Nathan, 1964) and less often as a consequence of a unilateral frontal tumour (Maurice-Williams, 1974). However, as Humphrey (1972) has pointed out, it may reasonably be inferred that the frontal lobes possess a regulating function, shaping the development of intellectual resources and the pursuit of long-term goals. The effect upon personality of massive bifrontal lesions was well demonstrated by the celebrated case of Phineas Gage who in 1848 had a crowbar driven through the front of his skull. He was described as 'fitful, irreverent, indulging at times in the greatest profanity . . . manifesting but little deference for his fellows, impatient of restraint or advice when it conflicts with his desires, at times pertinaciously obstinate, yet capricious and vacillatory'. Thus, a 'frontal lobe syndrome' has come to be recognized; an affected individual previously capable of judgement and sustained application and organization of his life, may thus become aimless and improvident, with loss of tact, sensitivity, and self control with impulsiveness and a failure to appreciate the consequences of reckless behaviour.

Destruction of the dorsomedial nuclei of the thalamus has been shown to produce similar effects to those of frontal leucotomy and the syndrome may follow stereotaxic surgery for Parkinsonism. Since the efferent frontothalamic pathways are comparatively scanty it has been suggested that leucotomy works by interrupting the afferent pathways from the dorsomedial nuclei to the frontal cortex and from the anteromedial nuclei to the cingulate gyri. Because the standard prefrontal operation all too often gave relief from stress at the cost of lethargy, social incompetence, and other manifestations of the frontal lobe syndrome (Partridge, 1950) it has now been discarded in favour of more selective procedures such as undercutting of the orbital cortex, cingulectomy, frontal tractotomy, and various stereotaxic techniques (Knight, 1964; Bond, 1972) which aim at producing relief of emotional tension or behaviour disorder with minimal effects upon intellect and personality.

REFERENCES

ANDREW, J., and NATHAN, P. W. (1964) Lesions of the anterior frontal lobes and disturbances of micturition and defaecation, *Brain*, **87,** 233.

BARBIZET, J. (1963) Defect of memorizing of hippocampal–mammillary origin: a review, *J. Neurol. Neurosurg. Psychiat.*, **26,** 127.

BARD, P. (1928) A diencephalic mechanism for the expression of rage with special reference to the sympathetic nervous system, *Amer. J. Physiol.*, **84,** 490.

BICKFORD, R. C., MULDER, D. W., DODGE, H. W., Jun., SVIEN, H. J., and ROME, H. P. (1958) Changes in memory function induced by electrical stimulation of the temporal lobe in man, *Res. Publ. Ass. nerv. ment. Dis.*, **36,** 227.

BLAKEMORE, C. F., and FALCONER, M. A. (1967) Long-term effects of anterior temporal lobectomy on certain cognitive functions, *J. Neurol. Neurosurg. Psychiat.*, **30,** 364.

BOND, M. R. (1972) Psychosurgery, in *Scientific Foundations of Neurology*, ed. Critchley, M., O'Leary, J. L., and Jennett, W. B., London.

BRAIN, W. R., and STRAUSS, E. B. (1945) *Recent Advances in Neurology and Neuropsychiatry*, London.

BRICKNER, R. M. (1936) *The Intellectual Functions of the Frontal Lobes*, New York.

BRICKNER, R. M. (1939) Bilateral frontal lobectomy. Follow-up report of case, *Arch. Neurol. Psychiat. (Chic.)*, **41,** 580.

BRIERLEY, J. B. (1966) The neuropathology of amnesic states, in *Amnesia*, ed. Whitty, C. W. M., and Zangwill, O. L., London.

BRIERLEY, J. B., and BECK, E. (1958) The effects upon behaviour of lesions in the dorsomedial and anterior thalamic nuclei of cat and monkey, *Ciba Foundation Symposium on the Neurological Basis of Behaviour*, p. 90, London.

BRIERLEY, J. B., CORSELLIS, J. A. N., HIERONS, R., and NEVIN, S. (1960) Subacute encephalitis of later adult life, *Brain*, **83,** 357.

BRITISH MEDICAL JOURNAL (1972) Auditory inattention, *Brit. med. J.*, **2,** 178.

COOPER, J. B., BLOOM, F. E., and ROTH, R. H. (1974) *The Biochemical Basis of Neuropharmacology*, 2nd ed., New York.

CRITCHLEY, M. (1975) *Silent Language*, London.

DEJONG, R. N., ITABASHI, H. H., and OLSON, J. R. (1969) Memory loss due to hippocampal lesions, *Arch. Neurol. (Chic.)*, **20,** 339.

DENNY-BROWN, D. (1951) The frontal lobes and their functions, in *Modern Trends in Neurology*, ed. Feiling, A., p. 13, London.

DENNY-BROWN, D., and CHAMBERS, R. A. (1958) The parietal lobe and behavior, *Res. Publ. Ass. nerv. ment. Dis.*, **36,** 35.

GREEN, J. D. (1958) The rhinencephalon and behaviour, *Ciba Foundation Symposium on the Neurological Basis of Behaviour*, p. 222, London.

GUYTON, A. C. (1976) *Textbook of Medical Physiology*, 5th ed., Philadelphia.

HEATHFIELD, K. W. G., CROFT, P. B., and SWASH, M. (1973) The syndrome of transient global amnesia, *Brain*, **96,** 729.

HEBB, D. O. (1941) Human intelligence after removal of cerebral tissue from the right frontal lobe, *J. genet. Psychol.*, **25,** 257.

HEBB, D. O., and PENFIELD, W. (1940) Human behavior after extensive bilateral removal from the frontal lobes, *Arch. Neurol. Psychiat. (Chic.)*, **44**, 421.

HEILMAN, K. M., WATSON, R. T., and SCHULMAN, H. M. (1974) A unilateral memory defect, *J. Neurol. Neurosurg. Psychiat.*, **37**, 790.

HERD, J. A. (1972) Physiology of strong emotions, *Physiologist*, **17**, 5.

HUMPHREY, M. E. (1972) Personality, in *Scientific Foundations of Neurology*, ed. Critchley, M., O'Leary, J. L., and Jennett, W. B., London.

HYVARINEN, J. (1973) CNS: afferent mechanisms with emphasis on physiological and behavioral correlations, *Ann. Rev. Physiol.*, **35**, 243.

ISAACSON, R. L. (1974) *The Limbic System*, New York.

JEFFERSON, G. (1937) Removal of right and left frontal lobes in man, *Brit. med. J.*, **2**, 199.

KAHN, E. A., and CROSBY, E. C. (1972) Korsakoff's syndrome associated with surgical lesions involving the mammillary bodies, *Neurology (Minneap.)*, **22**, 117.

KLÜVER, H. (1958) 'The temporal lobe syndrome' produced by bilateral ablations, *Ciba Foundation Symposium on the Neurological Basis of Behaviour*, p. 175, London.

KNIGHT, G. (1964) The orbital cortex as an objective in the surgical treatment of mental illness, *Brit. J. Surg.*, **51**, 114.

LANCE, J. W., and McLEOD, J. G. (1975) *A Physiological Approach to Clinical Neurology*, 2nd ed., London.

LASHLEY, K. (1960) The thalamus and emotion, in *The Neuropsychology of Lashley*, ed. Beach, F. A., Hebb, D. O., Morgan, C. T., and Nissen, H. W., New York.

McCONNELL, J. V. (1962) Memory transfer through cannibalism in planarians, *J. Neuropsychiat.*, **3**, Suppl. 1, 42.

MAURICE-WILLIAMS, R. S. (1974) Micturition symptoms in frontal tumours, *J. Neurol. Neurosurg. Psychiat.*, **37**, 431.

MEYER, A. (1974) The frontal lobe syndrome, the aphasias and related conditions—a contribution to the history of cortical localization, *Brain*, **97**, 565.

MILNER, B. (1958) Psychological defects produced by temporal lobe excision, *Res. Publ. Ass. nerv. ment. Dis.*, **36**, 244.

MILNER, B. (1966) Amnesia following operations on the temporal lobe, in *Amnesia*, ed. Whitty, C. W. M., and Zangwill, O. L., London.

PAPEZ, J. W. (1937) A proposed mechanism of emotion, *Arch. Neurol. Psychiat. (Chic.)*, **38**, 725.

PARTRIDGE, M. A. (1950) *Prefrontal Leucotomy*, Oxford.

PENFIELD, W. (1948) Bilateral frontal gyrectomy and postoperative intelligence, *Res. Publ. Ass. nerv. ment. Dis.*, **27**, 519.

PENFIELD, W. (1958) The role of the temporal cortex in the recall of past experiences and interpretation of the present, *Ciba Foundation Symposium on the Neurological Basis of Behaviour*, p. 149, London.

PENFIELD, W., and EVANS, J. (1935) The frontal lobes in man. A clinical study of maximum removals, *Brain*, **58**, 115.

PENFIELD, W., and JASPER, H. (1954) *Epilepsy and the Functional Anatomy of the Human Brain*, Boston.

PENFIELD, W., and MATHIESON, G. (1974) Memory. Autopsy findings and comments on the role of hippocampus in experiential recall, *Arch. Neurol. (Chic.)*, **31**, 145.

PRIBRAM, K. (1958) Comparative neurology and the evolution of behavior, in *Behavior and Evolution*, ed. Roe, A., and Simpson, G. G., New Haven.

ROSE, F. C., and SYMONDS, C. P. (1960) Persistent memory defect following encephalitis, *Brain*, **83**, 195.

RYLANDER, G. (1939) *Personality Changes after Operations on the Frontal Lobes*, Copenhagen.

SANDERS, H. I., and WARRINGTON, E. K. (1971) Memory for remote events in amnesic patients, *Brain*, **94**, 661.

SCHULMAN, S. (1964) Impaired delayed response from thalamic lesions, *Arch. Neurol. (Chic.)*, **11**, 477.

SCOVILLE, W. B., and MILNER, B. (1957) Loss of recent memory after bilateral hippocampal lesions, *J. Neurol. Neurosurg. Psychiat.*, **20**, 11.

SIMPSON, J. A. (1969) The clinical neurology of temporal lobe disorders, in *Current Problems in Neuropsychiatry*, ed. Herrington, R. N., Ashford, Kent.

SMYTHIES, J. R. (1966) *The Neurological Foundations of Psychiatry*, Oxford.

SMYTHIES, J. R. (1970) *Brain Mechanisms and Behavior*, New York.

SPERRY, R. W. (1961) Cerebral organization and behaviour, *Science*, **133**, 1749.

STEINMETZ, E. F., and VROOM, F. Q. (1972) Transient global amnesia, *Neurology (Minneap.)*, **22**, 1193.

SWEET, W. H., TALLAND, G. A., and ERWIN, F. R. (1959) Loss of recent memory following section of the fornix, *Trans. Amer. neurol. Ass.*, **84**, 76.

TALLAND, G. A. (1958) Psychological studies of Korsakow's psychosis. II. Perceptual functions, *J. nerv. ment. Dis.*, **127**, 197.

TALLAND, G. A. (1959) The interference theory of forgetting and the amnesic syndrome, *J. abnorm. soc. Psychol.*, **59**, 10.

TALLAND, G. A., and EKDAHL, M. (1959) Psychological studies of Korsakow's psychosis. IV. The rate and mode of forgetting narrative material, *J. nerv. ment. Dis.*, **129**, 391.

VAN BUREN, J. M., and BORKE, R. C. (1972) The mesial temporal substratum of memory, *Brain*, **95**, 599.

WALKER, A. E. (1957) Recent memory impairment in unilateral temporal lobe lesions, *Arch. Neurol. Psychiat. (Chic.)*, **78**, 543.

WEIL, J. L. (1974) *A Neurophysiological Model of Emotional and Intentional Behavior*, Springfield, Ill.

WHITTY, C. W. M. (1962) The neurological basis of memory, in *Modern Trends in Neurology—3*, p. 314, London.

WHITTY, C. W. M., and LEWIN, W. (1960) A Korsakoff syndrome in the post-cingulectomy confusional state, *Brain*, **83**, 648.

WILLIAMS, D. (1956) The structure of emotions reflected in epileptic experiences, *Brain*, **79**, 29.

WINTER, A. (Ed.) (1971) *The Surgical Control of Behavior*, Springfield, Ill.

ZAIDEL, D., and SPERRY, R. W. (1974) Memory impairment after commissurotomy in man, *Brain*, **97**, 263.

CONSCIOUSNESS AND UNCONSCIOUSNESS

The Neural Basis of Consciousness

Consciousness is a primary element in experience and cannot be defined in terms of anything else. Neurology lends support to the distinction between the content of consciousness and the state of consciousness itself. The content of consciousness consists of sensations, emotions, images, memories, ideas, and similar experiences, and these depend upon the activities of the cerebral cortex and the thalamus and the relations between them, in the sense that lesions of these structures alter the content of consciousness without as a rule changing the state of consciousness as such. However, it has been shown that other structures, particularly that part of the central reticular formation of the brain stem, which is known as the ascending reticular activating system and which extends at least from the lower border of the pons to the ventromedial thalamus, profoundly influence the state of consciousness. The cells of this system occupy a paramedian area in the brain stem from the lower part of the pons to a rostral level including the posterior hypothalamus, the thalamic intralaminar nuclei, and the septal area. Magoun and his collaborators (Magoun, 1952), and Gellhorn (1954) showed that, in Gellhorn's words, 'the cortex receives at least two kinds of afferent impulses, those which alter the activity of the greater part or the whole of the cortex and those which activate specific cortical projection areas (visual, auditory, &c.)', and, again quoting Gellhorn, 'destruction of the reticulo-hypothalamic system does not interfere with the action of the sensory impulses on a specific projection area, but it eliminates the tonic impulses from the hypothalamic-reticular system on the cortex as a whole. Under these conditions no conscious processes are elicited.' There is evidence that drugs which tend to produce unconsciousness, such as anaesthetics and hypnotics, selectively depress the ascending reticular alerting system, while those which cause wakefulness have the opposite, facilitatory effect upon it.

In valuable reviews, Plum (1972) and Plum and Posner (1972) have summarized the position as follows:

1. Lesions which destroy the reticular formation below the lower third of the pons do not produce coma.
2. Above this level a lesion must destroy both sides of the paramedian reticulum to interrupt consciousness.
3. The arousal effects of reticular stimulation upon behaviour and the EEG are separable in that bilateral lesions of the pontine tegmentum producing coma may be associated with a normal 'waking' EEG.
4. Sleep is an active physiological process, not a mere failure of arousal and is clearly separable from stupor and coma.
5. Sleeping and waking can occur in man even after total bilateral destruction of the cerebral hemispheres.

Hence a lesion or dysfunction of the reticular system will only produce stupor or coma if it

(*a*) affects both sides of the brain stem;
(*b*) is located between the lower third of the pons and the posterior diencephalon; and
(*c*) is either of acute onset or large in its extent.

SLEEP

Sleep is to be regarded as a periodical physiological depression of function of those parts of the brain concerned with consciousness, induced by the appropriate state of the reticulo-hypothalamic system. Electroencephalography shows that as sleep deepens there is a transition from normal alpha waves to a phase of bursts of more rapid waves (spindles) and then the development of slow random waves. Dreams have been shown to be associated with a burst of alpha waves in the second stage of sleep. As Plum and Posner (1972) point out, sleep is an active physiological process during which some neurones show decreased activity while in others activity is increased. Normal sleep has been shown to have several stages, one of which is the so-called 'rapid eye-movement' (R.E.M.) phase during which most dreams occur. This phase, also called 'paradoxical sleep', occurs shortly after falling asleep and again shortly before waking and seems to be the most important stage of sleep in relieving fatigue. Paradoxical sleep occupies in total about 20–25 per cent of a night's sleep in the healthy adult and itself possesses tonic and phasic features. The tonic features include an EEG of fairly low voltage, devoid of spindles and slow waves, penile erection, and loss of muscle tone. Phasic features include changes in blood pressure, heart rate, and respiration, increased cerebral blood flow, occasional myoclonic jerks, and bursts of conjugate eye movement (Oswald, 1972). While severe nightmares usually occur during paradoxical sleep, sleep walking, enuresis, and night terrors in childhood more often occur during orthodox sleep. Recent work has shown that a disordered relationship between the R.E.M. and non-R.E.M. phases of sleep may occur in various disorders of brain function (Jouvet, 1962). Insomnia, particularly in the elderly, is usually associated with brief awakenings and with a reduction in the proportion of paradoxical sleep (Kales, 1969). In drug withdrawal syndromes (e.g. delirium tremens), the patient tends to alternate between wakefulness and fitful sleep of which up to 100 per cent is paradoxical (Oswald, 1972). Barbiturate anaesthetics produce EEG changes similar to those accompanying normal sleep. Though sleep-like states can be induced by electrical stimulation of an area in the diencephalon it is an oversimplification to regard this as a 'sleep centre'. Sleep is the result of complex processes whereby, facilitated by fatigue, the withdrawal of afferent impulses leads to a reversible depression of the alerting system, which inactivates the cerebral cortex (see Wolstenholme and O'Connor, 1961; Kales, 1969).

During sleep not only is consciousness lost, but certain bodily changes occur. The pulse rate, blood pressure, and the respiratory rate fall as a rule in orthodox sleep but rise in the paradoxical phase; the eyes usually deviate upwards, the pupils are contracted, but usually react to light, but slowly; the tendon reflexes are abolished and the plantar reflexes may become extensor.

NARCOLEPSY AND OTHER SLEEP DISTURBANCES

Narcolepsy is sleep which is abnormal by reason that its onset is irresistible, though the circumstances may be inappropriate and excessive fatigue is absent. The patient can be roused from the narcoleptic attack as from normal sleep.

It is necessary to consider with narcolepsy four other forms of sleep disturbance which, since they may be associated with narcolepsy or with each other in the same patient, are closely related to one another. These are cataplexy, sleep paralysis, hallucinatory states associated with sleep, and somnambulism. The first case of narcolepsy was described by Westphal in 1877, but the term 'narcolepsy' was first used by Gélineau (1880).

Narcolepsy

The irresistible attacks of sleep characteristic of narcolepsy may be very numerous, occurring many times a day. It has been estimated that there may be 100,000 narcoleptics in the United States (Guilleminault et al., 1974; British Medical Journal, 1975b). In the attacks the patient quickly falls asleep but can be aroused immediately by appropriate stimuli. The attacks are most likely to occur in circumstances normally conducive to drowsiness, such as after a heavy meal, during a lecture, in the cinema, in church, or during a monotonous occupation, especially when driving a car. They are usually worse in the afternoon. They are occasionally precipitated by strong emotion. The sleep is usually brief, lasting only for seconds or minutes, but if the patient remains undisturbed he may sleep for hours. Typically in such cases the patient lapses at once into paradoxical sleep for about 15 minutes in contrast to the course of events in normal sleep (Roth et al., 1969); vivid dreams are common even in very brief episodes. Nocturnal recordings from such patients often show an abnormal relationship between R.E.M. and non-R.E.M. (orthodox) sleep (Dement et al., 1966). Measurement of pupillary size has been shown to correlate with degrees of wakefulness and to be a useful means of assessing the response of narcoleptic subjects to treatment (Yoss et al., 1969) and Birchfield *et al.* (1958) found mild hypoxia and hypercapnia in narcoleptic subjects when awake, comparable to the findings in normal subjects during sleep.

Cataplexy

By cataplexy is understood an attack to which sufferers from narcolepsy are liable, but which differs from sleep in that, though the patient suddenly loses all power of movement and of maintaining posture, consciousness is preserved. Sometimes tremor of the head or muscular twitching occurs at the onset, but these may be absent. The patient sinks limply to the ground with the eyes closed. The muscles are hypotonic, the pupils may fail to react to light, the tendon reflexes may be diminished or lost, and during the attacks the plantar reflexes may be extensor. Though completely unable to move or to utter a sound, the patient is fully aware of all that is happening. Cataplectic attacks usually last less than a minute and recovery is rapid. They are commonly precipitated by strong emotion, pleasurable or otherwise, especially by laughter or excitement, and the patient may be unable to move until he has controlled his emotion (Guilleminault *et al.*, 1974).

Sleep Paralysis

Sleep paralysis resembles cataplexy except that instead of being precipitated during the day by emotion, it usually occurs during the period of falling asleep or of awakening. The patient, though fully conscious, is unable to move hand or foot and often experiences intense anxiety. A touch will rapidly disperse the paralysis. So-called 'night-nurse's paralysis' is undoubtedly a similar phenomenon.

Hallucinatory States associated with Sleep

Sufferers from narcolepsy sometimes experience vivid hallucinations. These, which are more often visual than auditory, may occur as the patient is falling asleep, when they are termed hypnagogic hallucinations. Sometimes, however, they occur during the night, when the patient is apparently awake. These hallucinations are often elaborate and terrifying, and though they seem real at the time their true character is readily recognized during normal waking life. The night-terrors of childhood appear to be of a similar nature.

Somnambulism

Somnambulism may be regarded as the reciprocal of cataplexy in that the patient, though partly asleep, is able to stand and walk in an automatic fashion. It is rarely associated with narcolepsy, but more often occurs in adolescents who are of a neurotic disposition but otherwise normal. It may occur as an isolated incident following exposure to unusual stress (e.g. during examinations).

The Nature of Narcolepsy and Allied Disorders

Contrary to the views proposed early in the twentieth century, it is now clear that these phenomena are unrelated to epilepsy. Narcolepsy is to be regarded as paradoxical sleep of sudden and irresistible onset, and cataplexy as a form of localized sleep affecting the centres concerned in movement and posture only. Sleep paralysis, which is also associated with paradoxical sleep, is the outcome of a failure of uniform spread of sleep over the reticular system, the parts concerned with consciousness remaining awake when the parts concerned with motor and postural control have fallen asleep, or, conversely, have awakened before them. The hallucinatory states appear to be the product of a dissociation of consciousness, akin to dreaming, or to the evocation of memory engrams when the subject is partially awake; and somnambulism, the converse of cataplexy, is a condition associated with orthodox rather than paradoxical sleep in which the highest levels are asleep, but lower levels concerned with the control of organized movement are awake. Thus an imbalance of activity in the various parts of the reticular activating mechanism may be postulated.

The Causes of Narcolepsy

True narcolepsy is always idiopathic but abnormal states of drowsiness or hypersomnia may follow head injury or may be due to cerebral arteriosclerosis, neurosyphilis, encephalitis, or intracranial tumour involving the posterior part of the hypothalamus. Narcolepsy has been thought to be due to lesions in, but is more probably a disturbance of function of, the reticular system, and an inborn error of metabolism affecting the metabolism of serotonin and other brain amines has been postulated (Parkes *et al.*, 1974). Males are more subject to idiopathic narcolepsy than females and the onset usually occurs during adolescence or, at any rate, under the age of 30. It can probably be regarded in the true sense as a functional disorder, that is, a disturbance of function consisting of an exaggeration of a normal tendency to drowsiness. In patients with pathological somnolence or hypersomnia, in which sleep is usually orthodox and not paradoxical, physical abnormalities indicative of disorder of other functions of the hypothalamus may be present, especially obesity, with or without genital atrophy. The Pickwickian syndrome is a name which has been given to a syndrome, believed to be of hypothalamic origin, characterized by obesity, pathological daytime somnolence (orthodox sleep), and nocturnal periodic breathing with hypercapnia (Kuhlo, 1968).

DIAGNOSIS

Both narcolepsy and cataplexy are so distinctive that diagnosis usually presents no difficulty. Narcolepsy is distinguished from both epilepsy and syncope by the circumstances in which the attacks occur and by the fact that when consciousness is lost the patient can immediately be aroused. Cataplexy is distinguished from these disorders by the preservation of consciousness. As pathological drowsiness or hypersomnia is sometimes difficult to distinguish from idiopathic narcolepsy, however, it may be useful to record the EEG and eye movements during episodes of sleep (see above) and it is usually wise to exclude as far as possible organic disease involving the hypothalamus. The skull should be X-rayed as a routine to make certain that there is no enlargement of the sella or parasellar calcification.

PROGNOSIS

The disorder does not threaten life unless the patient should be unfortunate enough to have an attack in a dangerous situation. The response to treatment is sometimes disappointing and the attacks usually continue indefinitely, though occasionally they cease spontaneously. Epilepsy has been reported rarely to develop in patients with a long history of narcolepsy but the relationship may well be coincidental.

TREATMENT

The sufferer from narcolepsy will necessarily be debarred from occupations in which an attack of sleep may endanger him, and should not usually be allowed to drive a car if his attacks are severe. Traditionally amphetamine and its derivatives have been recommended for the treatment of both narcolepsy and cataplexy. While barbiturates reduce selectively the proportion of paradoxical sleep but prolong orthodox sleep, amphetamines reduce the duration of both and doses of dextroamphetamine sulphate given on waking and again at midday, graduated according to need, will certainly control narcolepsy in many cases. When narcolepsy or cataplexy by day are associated with disturbances of nocturnal sleep it may be wise to give a nightly dose of a barbiturate or nitrazepam. Recent work suggests that imipramine (*Tofranil*) in a dosage of 25–50 mg three times a day, is effective in some cases, but desmethylimipramine (*Pertofran*) in similar dosage is even more effective in controlling cataplexy; it may have to be given along with amphetamine for full control of narcolepsy (Hishikawa *et al.*, 1966). With increasing concern being expressed about the illegal use of amphetamines and their derivatives, and recent evidence that clomipramine 75 mg daily may be more effective still in both narcolepsy and cataplexy (Guilleminault *et al.*, 1974; *British Medical Journal*, 1975 *a* and *b*) it seems that the latter is now the drug of choice in most cases and it is also helpful in controlling hypnagogic hallucinations.

PERIODIC SOMNOLENCE AND MORBID HUNGER

Kleine (1925) and Levin (1936) described a rare disorder characterized by periodic attacks of excessive appetite followed by profound sleepiness which may last for days. During this phase the patient's personality may be profoundly altered, but in the intervals between the attacks he is usually normal. In the attacks of prolonged somnolence the patient awakens only as a rule to eat ravenously (often of a wide variety of unusual foods) and abnormal sexual behaviour with frequent masturbation and hypersexuality may be seen (Critchley, 1962; Garland *et al.*, 1965). The condition is almost invariably seen in adolescent males but a case in a young female has been described (Duffy and Davison, 1968). Depression, delusions and amnesia may be noted temporarily after an attack. The cause is unknown and in my experience no abnormality, clinical, biochemical, or electroencephalographic can be discovered during the attack. Amphetamine has been used with some success (Gallinek, 1954) in the treatment of the condition and Duffy and Davison (1968) found that intravenous methedrine cut short the attacks. Imipramine and its derivatives, especially clomipramine (Parkes *et al.*, 1974), may prove to be even more successful.

REFERENCES

BIRCHFIELD, R. I., SIEKER, H. O., and HEYMAN, A. (1958) Alterations in blood gases during natural sleep and narcolepsy, *Neurology (Minneap.)*, **8**, 107.
BRAIN, W. R. (1939) Sleep normal and pathological, *Brit. med. J.*, **2**, 51.
BRAIN, W. R. (1958) The physiological basis of consciousness, *Brain*, **81**, 426.
BRITISH MEDICAL JOURNAL (1975 *a*) Treatment of cataplexy, *Brit. med. J.*, **1**, 233.
BRITISH MEDICAL JOURNAL (1975 *b*) Narcolepsy, *Brit. med. J.*, **1**, 477.
CAIRNS, H. (1952) Disturbances of consciousness with lesions of the brain-stem and diencephalon, *Brain*, **75**, 109.
CRITCHLEY, M. (1962) Periodic hypersomnia and megaphagia in adolescent males, *Brain*, **85**, 627.
DANIELS, L. E. (1934) Narcolepsy, *Medicine (Baltimore)*, **13**, 1 (contains 268 references).

DEMENT, W., RECHTSHAFFEN, A., and GULEVICH, G. (1966) The nature of the narcoleptic sleep attack, *Neurology (Minneap.)*, **16**, 18.

DUFFY, J. P., and DAVISON, K. (1968) A female case of the Kleine-Levin syndrome, *Brit. J. Psychiat.*, **114**, 77.

GALLINEK, A. (1954) The syndrome of episodes of hypersomnia, bulimia and abnormal mental states, *J. Amer. med. Ass.*, **154**, 1081.

GARLAND, H., SUMNER, D., and FOURMAN, P. (1965) The Kleine-Levin syndrome. Some further observations, *Neurology (Minneap.)*, **15**, 1161.

GÉLINEAU (1880) De la narcolepsie, *Gaz. Hop. (Paris)*, **53**, 626 and 635.

GELLHORN, E. (1954) Physiological processes related to consciousness and perception, *Brain*, **67**, 401.

GUILLEMINAULT, C., WILSON, R. A., and DEMENT, W. C. (1974) A study on cataplexy, *Arch. Neurol. (Chic.)*, **31**, 255.

HISHIKAWA, Y., IDA, H., NAKAI, K., and KANEKO, Z. (1966) Treatment of narcolepsy with imipramine (Tofranil) and desmethylimipramine (Pertofran), *J. neurol. Sci.*, **3**, 453.

JOUVET, M. (1962) Recherches sur les structures nerveuses et les méchanismes responsables des différentes phases du sommeil physiologique, *Arch. ital. Biol.*, **100**, 125.

KALES, E. (Ed.) (1969) *Sleep : Physiology and Pathology*, Philadelphia.

KLEINE, W. (1925) Periodische Schlafsucht, *Mschr. Psychiat. Neurol.*, **57**, 285.

KLEITMAN, N. (1929) Sleep, *Physiol. Rev.*, **9**, 624.

KUHLO, W. (1968) Neurophysiologische und klinische Untersuchungen beim Pickwick-Syndrom, *Arch. Psychiat. Neurol.*, **211**, 170.

LEVIN, M. (1932) Cataplexy, *Brain*, **55**, 397.

LEVIN, M. (1936) Periodic somnolence and morbid hunger: a new syndrome, *Brain*, **59**, 494.

MAGOUN, H. W. (1952) The ascending reticular activating system, *Res. Publ. Ass. nerv. ment. Dis.*, **30**, 480.

OSWALD, I. (1972) Sleep, in *Scientific Foundations of Neurology*, ed. Critchley, M., O'Leary, J. L., and Jennett, W. B., London.

PARKES, J. D., FENTON, G., STRUTHERS, G., CURZON, G., KANTAMANENI, B. D., BUXTON, B. H., and RECORD, C. (1974) Narcolepsy and cataplexy. Clinical features, treatment and cerebrospinal fluid findings, *Quart. J. Med.*, **43**, 525.

PLUM, F. (1972) Organic disturbances of consciousness, in *Scientific Foundations of Neurology*, ed. Critchley, M., O'Leary, J. L., and Jennett, W. B., London.

PLUM, F., and POSNER, J. B. (1972) *Stupor and Coma*, 2nd ed., Philadelphia.

RANSON, S. W. (1939) Somnolence caused by hypothalamic lesions in the monkey, *Arch. Neurol. Psychiat. (Chic.)*, **41**, 1.

ROTH, B., BRUHOVÁ, S., and LEHOVSKY, M. (1969) REM sleep and NREM sleep in narcolepsy and hypersomnia, *Electroenceph. clin. Neurophysiol.*, **26**, 176.

WALTER, W. G., GRIFFITHS, G. M., and NEVIN, S. (1939) The electroencephalogram in a case of pathological sleep due to hypothalamic tumour, *Brit. med. J.*, **1**, 107.

WILSON, S. A. K. (1928) The narcolepsies, *Brain*, **51**, 63.

WOLSTENHOLME, G., and O'CONNOR, M. (1961) *Ciba Foundation Symposium on the Nature of Sleep*, London.

YOSS, R. E., MOYER, N. J., and OGLE, K. N. (1969) The pupillogram and narcolepsy, *Neurology (Minneap.)*, **19**, 921.

STUPOR AND COMA

In the past the term hypersomnia has been used to describe a state in which the patient has been thought to be pathologically sleepy, the resemblance to sleep lying in the fact that he can be to some extent aroused by the kind of stimuli which arouse a healthy person from sleep. Since, however, the mental state of such patients when aroused is often far from normal Jefferson proposed the term parasomnia for this condition. Between full consciousness and pathological complete unconsciousness or coma there exist states which differ not only in degree but also in quality, but much work remains to be done before they can be completely differentiated. At present it is convenient to distinguish broadly two different states of unconsciousness, namely, coma and stupor. In coma the patient cannot be aroused by any stimulus however vigorous and painful. Semi-coma can be defined as complete loss of consciousness with a response only at the reflex level, while less severe degrees of impairment of consciousness have been entitled severe, moderate, and mild confusion (Medical Research Council, 1941). The Glasgow coma scale (Teasdale and Jennett, 1974) in which four grades of eye opening, five of the 'best verbal response' and five of the 'best motor response' are charted in individual cases has been found to be of even greater practical value. Lethargy is a state of drowsiness and indifference in which increased stimulation may be needed to obtain a response, while stupor is a term used to define a state 'from which the subject can only be aroused by vigorous and continuous external stimulation' (Plum and Posner, 1972). Para-somnia may be regarded as one variety of stupor. *Akinetic mutism*, another state of stupor described by Cairns, resembled sleep in being associated with general muscular relaxation, but differed from sleep in that, although the patient's eyes remained apparently alert to moving objects, strong afferent stimuli were incapable of arousing him. So-called 'coma vigil' is similar. According to Plum and Posner (1972), in akinetic mutism the patient, though usually lying with his eyes closed, retains cycles of self-sustained arousal, giving the appearance of vigilance but vocalizing little or not at all. He is totally incontinent and makes only the most rudimentary movements even in response to noxious stimuli. The state is thus one of 'motionless, mindless wakefulness' or one cause of 'mute of malady' (*British Medical Journal*, 1973) and despite the patient's immobility there are few signs of damage to descending motor pathways.

By contrast, in the so-called de-efferented state or '*locked-in syndrome*', the patient is fully aware of his surroundings and is conscious and alert, but usually tetraplegic, aphonic, and anarthric so that he can communicate only through blinking or by carrying out various ocular movements voluntarily (Nordgren et al., 1971; Feldman, 1971; Hawkes, 1974). It is therefore most important to distinguish this state, in which the patient can hear and respond, despite exten-sive paralysis, from akinetic mutism. The EEG may be helpful, showing a reactive alpha or theta rhythm consistent with consciousness (Hawkes and Bryan-Smith, 1974).

Lesions Responsible for Stupor and Coma

The clinico-pathological studies of Cairns (1952) and French (1952) estab-lished that stupor or coma could occur as a result of lesions involving the central portion of the brain stem between the anterior end of the third ventricle and the lower pons. A wide range of pathological processes may therefore be responsible, the chief of which are head injury, tumour, vascular and inflammatory lesions, and it may well be that toxic states lead to unconsciousness primarily through their effect upon this part of the brain.

In Cairns's (1952) original description, akinetic mutism resulted from a craniopharyngioma compressing the walls of the third ventricle. Skultety (1968), as a result of experimental work in animals and clinicopathological observations in man, found that bilateral lesions of the periaqueductal grey matter of the upper brain stem were alone insufficient to cause this state and Plum and Posner (1972) review reports of this state developing as a consequence of bilateral frontal lobe infarction, diffuse cortical or white matter damage due to anoxia, hypoglycaemia, head injury or demyelination, hydrocephalus, bilateral destruction of corpus striatum, globus pallidus or thalamus, paramedian lesions of the brain stem reticular substance, and brain stem compression secondary to cerebellar haemorrhage. Nevertheless, dysfunction of the reticular system or of its afferent or efferent connections was probably a common factor.

The *locked-in syndrome*, by contrast, is clearly related to bilateral destruction of the medulla or basis pontis with sparing of the tegmentum, usually as a consequence of demyelination (e.g. in central pontine myelinolysis) or infarction (Adams *et al.*, 1959; Kemper and Romanul, 1967). However, it has been described as a consequence of bilateral infarction of the lateral two-thirds of the cerebral peduncles (Karp and Hurtig, 1974).

THE CAUSES OF UNCONSCIOUSNESS

In this section we shall discuss the principal causes of unconsciousness as a necessary preliminary to considering how the cause is to be discovered in any particular case. It will be noted that even though the cause of unconsciousness may be described in general terms, it is often impossible to say in detail how that cause operates, or it may act in so complex a way that one cannot say which of a number of factors is the more important.

CEREBRAL VASCULAR LESIONS

A cerebral vascular lesion is one of the commonest causes of coma. Usually the unconsciousness is due to the fact that the cerebral vascular lesion directly or indirectly interferes with the functions of the ascending reticular alerting formation. Ischaemia of this structure may be the result either of a rise in intracranial pressure or of local pressure upon the diencephalon or brain stem, or impairment of blood supply secondary to pathological narrowing of the relevant arteries. The conditions most likely to produce these results are: (1) a massive subarachnoid haemorrhage; (2) a subarachnoid haemorrhage invading one cerebral hemisphere; (3) a massive intracerebral or intracerebellar haemorrhage, or one rupturing into a cerebral ventricle; (4) an area of cerebral infarction in one hemisphere large enough to cause considerable oedema of the hemisphere; (5) brain stem haemorrhage or infarction due to vertebro-basilar atheroma; and (6) hypertensive encephalopathy. The symptomatology of these lesions is described elsewhere, but in general a vascular cause for unconsciousness is suggested by the presence of atheroma or hypertension, a sudden or relatively sudden onset of the symptoms, focal signs corresponding to those produced by a vascular lesion, or signs of meningeal irritation of sudden onset. The presence of red blood cells or xanthochromia and a raised protein in the cerebrospinal fluid would support the diagnosis. [See also p. 337.]

SPACE-OCCUPYING LESIONS

Unconsciousness due to intracranial tumour or abscess usually comes on much more slowly than that due to a cerebral vascular lesion, though occasionally haemorrhage into a tumour or the sudden development of oedema or of tentorial or cerebellar herniation may cause rapid loss of consciousness. A history of symptoms of increased intracranial pressure, especially headache increasing in severity, is therefore usually obtainable, and papilloedema is likely to be present.

Signs of vascular disease are usually absent, but the diagnosis may be difficult when a tumour develops late in life in a patient who suffers from hypertension or atheroma. Subdural haematoma is most commonly encountered in the middle-aged or elderly, in whom it may develop without discoverable cause or insidiously after a minor head injury. Headache is usually a prominent symptom, and unconsciousness, when it develops, often fluctuates strikingly in depth. Papilloedema and signs of focal cerebral compression are present only rarely.

HEAD INJURY

When unconsciousness is due to head injury, there is usually a history of the injury, and there may be bruising of the scalp or signs of fracture of the vault or of the base of the skull. It must be remembered, however, that a patient who becomes unconscious from some other cause may injure his head in falling, and that a head injury may indirectly affect the brain, for example, by leading to thrombosis of one internal carotid artery. Traumatic intracranial arterial haemorrhage leads to progressively deepening coma, with signs of a focal lesion of one hemisphere, often beginning with convulsions and producing hemiplegia. Herniation of the medial portion of the temporal lobe through the tentorial hiatus will often cause compression of the third nerve as it crosses the free border of the tentorium and as a result the pupil on the same side becomes fixed and dilated and other signs of a third nerve palsy on the same side may develop later. By contrast, cerebellar tonsillar herniation due to a space-occupying lesion (whether haemorrhage, tumour, or abscess) in the posterior fossa usually gives occipital headache and neck stiffness, possibly with bradycardia and depression of respiration due to brain stem compression. However, it may be impossible clinically to distinguish between traumatic intracranial arterial haemorrhage and a rapidly progressive subdural haematoma or haemorrhage from a cerebral laceration.

MENINGITIS AND ENCEPHALITIS

When meningitis is the cause of coma, the onset of symptoms is usually subacute, and before losing consciousness the patient complains of intense headache, which is associated with fever, cervical rigidity, and Kernig's sign. The diagnosis is confirmed by the discovery of the characteristic changes in the cerebrospinal fluid, from which it may be possible to isolate the causal organism. The onset of encephalitis is also usually subacute, and associated with fever, though herpes simplex encephalitis [p. 495] may be explosive in onset, leading to coma within a few hours. The physical signs are those of more or less diffuse damage to the brain, and in many cases also the spinal cord, the precise distribution and character of which varies in relation to the aetiology. Signs of meningeal irritation are present in some but by no means all, and there is often, but not invariably, a pleocytosis in the CSF.

OTHER BRAIN DISEASES

Among the many other diseases which may from time to time cause coma and which must be distinguished by their age of onset and specific clinical features are the leukodystrophies and cerebral diffuse sclerosis, multiple sclerosis with extensive cerebral demyelination (rarely), central pontine myelinolysis, deficiency disorders such as Wernicke's encephalopathy, degenerative or toxic encephalopathies, and slow virus disorders such as multifocal leukoencephalopathy or Creutzfeldt–Jakob disease.

METABOLIC DISORDERS

Uraemic Coma. Uraemic coma may occur in acute or chronic renal failure. The metabolic changes so produced are complex, and it is probable that a raised blood urea, though an important index of their severity, is not in itself the main cause of unconsciousness. There is usually metabolic acidosis, accompanied by complex disturbances of the body sodium and potassium. Water intoxication, due to fluid retention, with a serum osmolality of less than 260 mOsm/l, is a factor in some cases. The blood calcium may be subnormal and the administration of alkalis to correct the acidosis may precipitate tetany. There is usually a raised blood pyruvate, and the cerebral consumption of oxygen is reduced. Headache, vomiting, dyspnoea, mental confusion, drowsiness or restlessness, and insomnia are early symptoms, and later muscular twitchings or generalized convulsions are likely to precede the coma. The raised blood urea establishes the diagnosis. A fatal encephalopathy of undetermined cause, often associated with spongiform change in the brain, which gives rise to progressive dysarthria, mental changes, an abnormal EEG, and often ultimately seizures, myoclonus, asterixis, apraxia, and focal neurological signs with eventual coma has been described in patients with renal failure under treatment with chronic haemodialysis (Burks *et al.*, 1976).

Diabetic Coma. Diabetic coma is usually associated with ketoacidosis, a blood sugar greater than 250 mg/100 ml, and massive ketonuria. However, lactic acidosis without ketonuria is an occasional cause of metabolic acidosis in diabetic subjects, especially after treatment with hypoglycaemic agents, and must be distinguished from the lactic acidosis which may result from severe anoxia or from poisoning with methyl alcohol or paraldehyde. Hyperosmolality due to hyperglycaemia (hyperglycaemic nonketonic diabetic coma) has also been described (Gerich *et al.*, 1971) and a similar syndrome has been described in non-diabetic patients with severe burns (Rosenberg *et al.*, 1965). The patient is usually wasted, pale, and dehydrated. Both the rate and amplitude of the respirations are increased, and the ocular tension is very low. The pulse is rapid and feeble, and the blood pressure tends to fall. The tendon reflexes are sometimes depressed due to the presence of an associated diabetic neuropathy but may be normal, and the plantar responses are usually flexor until the patient is actually comatose. The breath has the characteristic odour of acetone. Large quantities of sugar and acetone are demonstrable in the urine in ketotic cases, and the blood sugar is much raised.

Hypoglycaemic Coma. Hypoglycaemic coma is not difficult to recognize if it is due to an overdose of insulin which the patient is known to be taking. The presence of sugar in the urine does not exclude this, since the urine may have been excreted before the patient became hypoglycaemic. Spontaneous hypoglycaemia sufficient to cause coma is usually the result in an adult of the excessive production of insulin by a tumour composed of cells of the islets of Langerhans in the pancreas. In such cases fainting fits or convulsions or periods of mental disorder may precede the onset of coma by weeks or months. On the other hand, the coma may occur without warning in a patient apparently previously healthy, and the patient may then live on in an unconscious state for weeks or months. Hypoglycaemia may also occur spontaneously in early infancy and may then be responsible for severe brain damage if not recognized and treated early, and in adult life it has been observed to arise spontaneously in patients with liver disease, in alcoholism, hypopituitarism, and Addison's disease. At the time of the onset the hypoglycaemic patient sweats profusely, the pupils are dilated, the tendon reflexes increased, and the plantar reflexes may be extensor. Hypothermia sometimes occurs; in occasional cases there are symptoms and signs of focal cerebral dysfunction (a 'stroke-like' presentation) (Montgomery and Pinner, 1964). The diagnosis can be made by examination of the blood sugar, which is found to be extremely low, in the region of 30 or 40 mg per 100 ml or even much lower.

Unless treated promptly and effectively, hypoglycaemia can result in irreversible brain damage and the pathological changes, affecting the Purkinje cells of the cerebellum, the cerebral cortex, basal ganglia, and hippocampus, are similar to those of severe anoxia. Dementia and cerebellar ataxia are the main clinical features of this syndrome.

Heat Stroke. After prolonged exertion in hot surroundings (as in racing cyclists) the normal rise in body temperature with profuse sweating can be followed by an ominous clinical picture of hyperpyrexia, an abrupt cessation of sweating, the rapid onset of coma, convulsions, and death. The condition may be precipitated by the use of amphetamine drugs. Hyperpyrexia may also be seen in tetanus and a result of lesions involving the floor of the third ventricle (such as intraventricular haemorrhage) or pons (e.g. pontine haemorrhage). Many patients who survive heat stroke are left with permanent neurological sequelae including paraparesis, cerebellar ataxia, or dementia (Salem, 1966).

Hypothermia. An abnormally low body temperature may give rise to deepening coma. While hypothermia has been described in cases of myxoedema and hypopituitarism (see below) accidental hypothermia can result from a failure of the normal temperature-regulating mechanism of the body, the reverse of that which occurs in heat stroke. It can result from prolonged exposure in cold conditions (as in mountaineers or fell-walkers) and has also been described in elderly patients, often suffering from disorders such as arthritis or Parkinsonism which reduce mobility, who live in unheated rooms in winter conditions (Rosin and Exton-Smith, 1964). Drugs such as chlorpromazine may also precipitate hypothermic coma which can be fatal. Often there is generalized rigidity and muscle fasciculation may be seen but true shivering is absent; hypoxia and CO_2 retention are common (McNicol and Smith, 1964). The mortality rate is high but in those patients who respond to gradual warming (and treatment for hypothyroidism when appropriate) complete recovery is usual.

Hepatic Coma. The cause of hepatic coma is still incompletely understood [see p. 829]. The diagnosis is not usually difficult when the patient is known to be suffering from liver failure. Jaundice, however, may be absent. In patients with liver disease coma tends to be precipitated by gastro-intestinal haemorrhage, hypotension, infection, the rapid removal of large quantities of ascitic fluid, the use of certain diuretics, the administration of some sedatives, particularly morphine, and the ingestion of high protein foods or ammonium compounds. Except when it is of sudden onset, hepatic coma is usually preceded by the neurological symptoms of hepatic insufficiency, especially asterixis or flapping tremor [see p. 830]. Otherwise the diagnosis rests upon the presence of physical signs of liver disease, including hepatic foetor, and biochemical evidence of disturbed liver function.

Porphyria. Porphyria is an occasional cause of coma.

Pulmonary Disease. Hypoventilation due to chronic pulmonary disease may give an encephalopathy leading ultimately to coma, especially in patients with cor pulmonale in whom coma may occasionally follow the prolonged administration of oxygen. The syndrome of alveolar hypoventilation [p. 840] is usually characterized by dull headache followed by drowsiness and, if unchecked, the patient may ultimately lapse into coma. Hypoxia is accompanied by hypercarbia (see below) with a chronic insensitivity of the respiratory centre. Asterixis and myoclonus are not uncommon in such cases (Plum and Posner, 1972).

Anoxia. Apart from that which may result from carbon monoxide poisoning, cerebral anoxia may result from suffocation, drowning, severe anaemia, ischaemia due to cardiac arrest, complications of open-heart surgery, heart disease, pulmonary embolism, fat embolism (after severe limb fractures), or diffuse embolism or other disease of the large cerebral arteries or smaller cerebral vessels (as in thrombotic microangiopathy or disseminated intravascular coagulation), to name but a few causes. Plum and Posner (1972) divide anoxia into the anoxic, anaemic, and ischaemic varieties. Cerebral malaria is a rare cause of ischaemic anoxia.

Disorders of Osmolality. Hyponatraemia or water intoxication has been increasingly recognized as a cause of delirium, leading often to coma. It is most often due to inappropriate ADH secretion, due to bronchial carcinoma, or to organic lesions in the region of the hypothalamus and/or pituitary, but sometimes occurring without evident cause (Goldberg, 1963). Sometimes it results from compulsive water drinking in psychotic or alcoholic individuals or may complicate renal failure.

Hypernatraemia may cause delirium, less often coma, and is seen in children with severe diarrhoea, or adults with diabetes insipidus, but may also be iatrogenic due to excess saline administration. These causes of delirium, drowsiness, or coma are recognized by measurement of the serum osmolality.

COMA OF ENDOCRINE ORIGIN

This may present a difficult diagnostic problem when it occurs in patients in whom the pre-existing endocrine disease has not been recognized.

Hypopituitary Coma. In hypopituitary coma again the unconsciousness appears to be the result of complex interacting factors, of which the most important would appear to be hypoglycaemia, hypotension, diminished suprarenal cortical function and occasionally hypothermia. The onset may be sudden, for example, if it is precipitated by an infection. The patient is usually a woman who exhibits the endocrine changes of hypopituitarism. The blood pressure and blood sugar are likely to be low, and the body temperature may be subnormal or above normal. The thyroid gland is likely to be impalpable, while the urinary excretion of 17-ketosteroids and the serum cortisol are very low. The syndrome of pituitary apoplexy [p. 278] must be remembered as a possible cause of sudden collapse and coma in patients with pituitary neoplasms who may also exhibit signs of hypopituitarism.

Coma in Myxoedema. A myxoedematous patient may gradually become comatose, more usually in the winter months. The characteristic feature is profound hypothermia, temperatures of 26–31 °C being by no means uncommon.

A low-reading thermometer must be used to record these and on suspicion the temperature should be taken rectally. The patient presents the usual clinical and biochemical features of myxoedema.

Suprarenal Cortical Failure. Coma from this cause may be difficult to recognize if it occurs suddenly as the result of stress, for example, in a patient not known to be suffering from Addison's disease. The low blood pressure, and electrolyte disturbances, however, are characteristic. Mild delirium is not uncommon in untreated Addison's disease, but as Plum and Posner (1972) point out, stupor and coma only occur as a rule in Addisonian crises. Papilloedema, presumably due to cerebral oedema, has been described (Jefferson, 1956). Acute adrenal failure due to meningococcal septicaemia (the Fredericksen–Waterhouse syndrome) is now a rare cause of sudden collapse and coma in infants and young children.

Abnormalities of Blood Calcium. Hypercalcaemia as a cause of mental confusion or coma may be missed if the blood calcium is not routinely examined. Hypercalcaemia may be due to parathyroid tumour, carcinoma, with or without bone secondaries, myelomatosis, or sarcoidosis (Lemann and Donatelli, 1964; Watson, 1963; Dent and Watson, 1964). Hypocalcaemia, due to spontaneous hypoparathyroidism, may also cause coma, but much less often (Plum and Posner, 1972); tetany and/or convulsions are the more usual manifestations but cerebral oedema with papilloedema has been reported (Grant, 1953).

CARBON DIOXIDE INTOXICATION

Carbon dioxide retention may be the result of acute or chronic pulmonary disease, or respiratory failure of neuromuscular origin in, for example, motor neurone disease, poliomyelitis, polyneuritis, myopathy, and myasthenia. It causes a fall in the pH and a rise in the pCO_2 in the blood. Though the patient is hypoxic, the state of consciousness is related to the level of CO_2 in the blood. In chronic CO_2 retention the respiratory centre fails to react to the raised level of CO_2 and respiration is then maintained by the receptors which respond to oxygen lack. Consequently, administering oxygen to such patients may remove the stimulus to respiration, raise the blood CO_2 still further, and precipitate coma. The same result may be produced by sedatives, particularly morphine, or even by barbiturates. Milder degrees of CO_2 intoxication cause drowsiness and confusion. In some cases there is papilloedema due to cerebral oedema. Estimation of the pCO_2 in arterial blood will usually confirm the diagnosis.

CARBON MONOXIDE INTOXICATION

In carbon monoxide intoxication there is almost always a history of exposure to coal-gas or the exhaust fumes of a motor-car, or some other source of carbon monoxide. In doubtful cases the diagnosis can be made by the spectroscopic examination of the blood.

NARCOTIC AND SEDATIVE DRUGS

When a narcotic drug is the cause of coma, there is usually evidence of this, sometimes in the patient's own statement before becoming unconscious, sometimes in the fact that he or she is known to have had a supply of such a drug. In practice the drugs most commonly taken for suicidal purposes are aspirin and barbiturates, less frequently pethidine, methadone, morphine, or heroin. Drugs which may produce coma as the result of a therapeutic overdosage include the barbiturates, any of the drugs generally used in the treatment of epilepsy, the tranquillizers and antidepressive remedies.

When alcohol is the cause of coma, this can usually be established from the history; the face is flushed, the conjunctivae congested, the pulse rapid, and the blood pressure low. The size of the pupils varies according to the toxic agent: they tend to be dilated in alcoholic coma, contracted in coma due to morphine, but in the case of other drugs are intermediate in size. The reaction to light is usually sluggish, and may be lost. The tendon reflexes tend to be diminished or lost, and the plantar reflexes extensor. Respiration is shallow, and the pulse rapid and of low tension. The drug responsible should be sought in the stomach washings, and its level estimated in the blood.

EPILEPSY

In the case of post-epileptic coma there is usually a history of epilepsy, or at least of the attack which preceded the coma. In the absence of this information, scars on the face or a bitten tongue may provide a clue. Focal signs of a cerebral lesion are usually absent, but the plantar reflexes may be extensor. After a single epileptic attack the period of unconsciousness is usually short, not more than from half an hour to an hour, but status epilepticus may be followed by prolonged coma. Prolonged drowsiness or confusion may rarely result from petit mal status in childhood, rarely in adults [p. 1104]. In elderly patients with symptomatic epilepsy due to cerebral scarring resulting, for instance, from previous infarction, post-epileptic stupor and subsequent delirium may be unusually prolonged due to the cerebral metabolic demand consequent upon one or more prolonged seizures as well as the resultant hypoxia.

HYSTERIA

In hysterical trance the patient, though apparently unconscious, usually shows some response to external stimuli. For example, an attempt to elicit the corneal reflex may cause a vigorous contraction of the orbicularis oculi. Rigidity of the hysterical type may be present, and signs of organic disease are absent. The nystagmus evoked by cold water injected into one or both ears is normal, and the EEG is generally normal. The diagnosis of catatonic stupor as a cause of psychogenic unresponsiveness may be more difficult as in such cases the EEG is often abnormal (Plum and Posner, 1972); catatonia (the limbs maintain a posture passively imposed by the examiner) is often a helpful sign in such cases.

THE INVESTIGATION OF THE UNCONSCIOUS PATIENT

The patient who presents with coma will require a most detailed and systematic examination, since any part of the body may provide a clue to the cause of the unconsciousness.

THE HEAD

The head should be examined for evidence of injury indicated by cuts or abrasions. The skull should be palpated for a depressed fracture, and the ears and nose examined for haemorrhage and leakage of cerebrospinal fluid. The ears should also be investigated for infection of the middle ear. Scars on the face may point to injuries received in previous epileptic attacks, and the tongue should be examined to see if it has been recently bitten or is the site of similar scars.

THE BREATH

The smell of the breath may provide a clue, for example, in alcoholic intoxication the characteristic odour of alcohol can be detected, and that of acetone in diabetic coma. In hepatic coma there is the characteristic foetor, but the smell of the breath in uraemia may be simulated by that present in many unconscious patients with oral infection.

THE NECK

An attempt should be made gently to flex the cervical spine. Cervical rigidity may indicate meningitis or subarachnoid haemorrhage. Gross inequality in the pulsation of the internal carotid arteries or a systolic bruit would suggest atheroma or thrombosis of the one on the side of the diminished pulsation or murmur as a possible cause of cerebral infarction.

THE SKIN

Cyanosis will be present when coma is due to CO_2 intoxication, while carbon monoxide poisoning causes a cherry-red colour. Patients with Addison's disease will show the characteristic brown pigmentation. Multiple telangiectases are found in hereditary telangiectasia, in which condition a cerebral telangiectasis may give rise to cerebral haemorrhage, and spider naevi over the upper part of the body are characteristic of hepatic disease. Purpura may be associated with an intracranial haemorrhage in thrombocytopenic purpura or other haemorrhagic disorders, with a cerebral embolus in subacute infective endocarditis, and also with meningococcal meningitis. The characteristic skin changes of myxoedema and hypopituitarism (with loss of body hair) will be present in patients suffering from coma due to those conditions. The scars of injections may be found in diabetics and drug addicts.

RESPIRATION

After voluntary hyperventilation patients with diffuse metabolic or structural brain disease may demonstrate post-hyperventilation apnoea (Plum and Posner, 1972) but the performance of this test demands that the patient should be sufficiently conscious to be able to perform it. Periodic (Cheyne-Stokes) respiration in which hyperpnoea alternates with apnoea usually occurs in patients with central cerebral or high brain stem lesions. Central neurogenic hyperventilation (Plum and Swanson, 1959) has been described in patients with dysfunction of the brain stem tegmentum while brain stem lesions may also give apneustic breathing (a pause at full inspiration—Plum and Alvord, 1964) or ataxic, irregular respiration with random deep and shallow breaths; the latter pattern occurs particularly with medullary lesions (Plum and Swanson, 1958). At its worst, in some medullary lesions, the respiratory centre becomes so insensitive to normal chemical stimuli, but conversely so sensitive to sedative drugs that the patient, who can breathe adequately when commanded to do so, hypoventilates progressively and may even stop breathing completely when asleep (Plum and Posner, 1972). Autonomous breathing (Newsom Davis, 1974) is a rare syndrome which may occur as a consequence of a lesion at the cervicomedullary junction giving paralysis of the chest and limbs but with retention of spontaneous breathing; however, the patient is unable to take a breath or to stop breathing voluntarily.

THE PUPILS

Plum and Posner (1972) have summarized the pupillary changes which may occur in comatose patients. Midbrain tectal lesions give round, regular, medium-sized pupils which do not react to light but may show hippus; nuclear midbrain lesions also as a rule give medium-sized pupils, fixed to all stimuli, which are often irregular and unequal. A third nerve lesion distal to the nucleus gives a fixed, dilated pupil on the side of the lesion. Tegmental lesions in the pons give bilaterally small pupils which in pontine haemorrhage may be pinpoint. A lateral medullary lesion may give an ipsilateral Horner's syndrome, while the pupil on the side of an occluded carotid artery giving cerebral infarction is often small. Bilateral pupillary dilatation during neck flexion can be a sign of uncal herniation (Norris and Fawcett, 1965). Drugs such as atropine, and cerebral anoxia dilate the pupils, morphine constricts, and many metabolic encephalopathies give small pupils with a normal light reflex.

OCULAR MOVEMENTS

In unconscious patients with bilateral or diffuse disorders of the cerebrum the eyes look straight ahead, oculocephalic movements (on head rotation) are brisk, and caloric stimulation gives sustained deviation of the eyes. A frontal lobe lesion may cause deviation of the eyes towards the side of the lesion, while a lateral pontine lesion may cause conjugate deviation to the opposite side with absence of oculocephalic and caloric responses. Skew deviation results from a dorsolateral pontine lesion. Conjugate deviation downwards means a midbrain lesion, while dysconjugate ocular deviation means a structural brain stem lesion if strabismus can be excluded. Oculocephalic and caloric responses are normal in metabolic disorders unless severe (Plum and Posner, 1972).

OTHER SYSTEMS

The examination of other parts of the nervous system is obviously of special importance in view of the large number of nervous disorders which give rise to coma. Special attention should be paid to the fundi where papilloedema will indicate increased intracranial pressure, or may be associated with hypertensive retinopathy. The cardiovascular system may yield evidence of hypertension, atheroma, or mitral stenosis and atrial fibrillation, a common cause of cerebral embolism. The lungs may yield evidence of the cause of CO_2 retention. X-rays of the lungs will be necessary to exclude a primary carcinoma. The abdomen may show the venous congestion and hepatomegaly of chronic liver disease, or the renal enlargement of polycystic kidneys, or one of the abdominal or pelvic organs may be the site of a neoplasm.

LABORATORY INVESTIGATIONS

Routine investigations of the urine and blood should be carried out. In addition, the blood sugar and blood urea should always be examined, and the blood electrolytes, calcium, osmolality, $p(O_2)$ and $p(CO_2)$ will also need to be investigated if it is thought that the coma is the result of their derangement, and to make sure that they are maintained at a normal level in the management of the unconscious patient. Provided there is no special contra-indication such as the signs of uncal or cerebellar herniation as described, examination of the cerebrospinal fluid may be indicated. This is essential to establish the diagnosis of meningitis or subarachnoid haemorrhage.

OTHER INVESTIGATIONS

Other investigations which may be necessary include X-rays of the skull, electroencephalography, gamma-encephalography or computerized transaxial tomography, cerebral angiography, and electrocardiography.

The EEG in Coma

The EEG may be of value in the diagnosis of coma in several ways: (1) it may indicate the presence of a focal lesion as opposed to a diffuse inflammatory or metabolic cause for the coma; (2) it may provide some evidence as to the probable nature of the focal lesion, as described elsewhere in the relevant sections of this book; (3) if there is a diffuse disturbance, the EEG may throw some light on its nature, distinguishing, for example, between some forms of encephalitis, epilepsy, and a metabolic disorder; and (4) changes in the degree of abnormality, and particularly in a metabolic disorder, may provide evidence of improvement or deterioration in the patient's condition.

THE DIAGNOSIS OF BRAIN DEATH

This problem has assumed increasing importance in recent years, first because of the increasing difficulty of deciding in patients with brain damage whether it is justifiable to maintain life indefinitely with assisted respiration and other supportive means, and secondly because of the difficult question of deciding when it may be concluded that the cerebral lesion is irreversible, that death is imminent, and that preparations may be made to remove viable organs, especially the kidneys, for subsequent transplantation. Plum (1972) has given a series of clinical criteria of brain death currently employed at the Cornell–New York Hospital Medical Center, and while this question continues to be a fertile source of ethical and medicolegal controversy, these represent a reasonable guide to current practice:

1. The Nature and Duration of Coma

(a) The cause must be unequivocally structural disease (e.g. trauma, neoplasm, etc.) or of clearly known anoxic origin.

(b) There must be no chance that depressant drugs or hypothermia contribute to the clinical picture.

(c) Signs of absent brain function must persist at least 12 hours under direct observation.

2. Cerebral Cortical Function must be Absent

(a) Behavioural or reflex responses above the foramen magnum level must be lacking to noxious stimuli applied anywhere on the body.

(b) The EEG properly recorded must be isoelectric for 60 min at an amplitude of 50 μV/cm.

3. Brain Stem Function must be Absent

(a) The pupils must be fixed to a strong light stimulus and without evidence of peripheral third nerve injury.

(b) Oculovestibular responses must be absent.

(c) There must be no motor activity whatever in structures innervated by cranial nerves.

(d) Spontaneous respiration must be absent. If the patient is on a respirator, there must be no breathing movements despite being removed from the respirator

P p

for 3 min (receiving diffusion oxygen) and having a normal arterial $p(CO_2)$ at the start.

(*e*) The circulation may be intact.

(*f*) Purely spinal reflex responses may be retained.

THE MANAGEMENT OF THE UNCONSCIOUS PATIENT

During recent years improvements in the technique of dealing with the unconscious patient have been so great that it is now possible to maintain unconscious patients in a condition of otherwise good health indefinitely.

Nursing. The unconscious patient should be nursed on his side with the head on a thin pillow, and turned at least every two hours, the usual attention being paid to the care of the skin, especially the pressure areas. If the foot of the bed is raised 15–22 cm so that the trachea is horizontal, the need for tracheostomy (see below) may be reduced (Atkinson, 1970).

The Respiratory Tract. The mouth and pharynx should be cleansed regularly by means of a swab held in forceps, and mucus and saliva prevented from accumulating in the pharynx by clearing the mouth periodically with a soft rubber catheter attached to a mechanical sucker. Regular turning of the patient will improve the ventilation of the lungs, and a physiotherapist should where necessary supervise postural drainage. If there are signs of pulmonary collapse the patient will require bronchoscopy in order that an obstructed bronchus may be cleared by suction. An oral airway will be required by a deeply unconscious patient, and if there is severe respiratory depression artificial respiration will also be necessary. This is usually best carried out by a positive pressure mechanical respirator combined with tracheal intubation, or tracheostomy. The latter measure is preferable if unconsciousness is likely to be prolonged, and a cuffed tracheostomy tube has the advantage of preventing the aspiration of food or saliva. Penicillin should be given regularly as a prophylactic against pneumonia, but if chest infection occurs a broad-spectrum antibiotic should be substituted.

Feeding. A patient who is unconscious for more than a few hours will require both food and drink, and since he cannot swallow this must be given by an oesophageal tube. This, however, is not a complete safeguard against the aspiration of food, since a feed may be regurgitated and vomiting may occur. These risks reinforce the need for tracheostomy in the majority of cases. Many nutritious commercial preparations are available for tube feeding, providing not only an adequate caloric intake but also the necessary vitamin and mineral supplements.

The Blood Electrolytes. There are several ways in which the blood electrolytes may become disordered in the unconscious patient. When the unconsciousness is itself the result of a metabolic disturbance the biochemical changes which that produces will be present. The blood biochemistry may also be disordered as the result of an excessive or inadequate intake of water, or an excessive amount of protein in the diet. A cerebral lesion may itself lead to hypernatraemia as the result of disorder of the thirst mechanisms, or hyponatraemia unresponsive to corticosteroids which may sometimes be due to inappropriate secretion of antidiuretic hormone (ADH). The fluid intake and output of the unconscious patient should therefore be carefully recorded, and from time to time also the blood urea, sodium, potassium, chloride, and glucose. It may also be necessary to estimate the urinary sugar, sodium, potassium, chloride, and nitrogen.

The Sphincters. The unconscious patient will have retention or incontinence of urine, and this is best dealt with by the use of a self-retaining catheter which should be changed every three days. The urine should be examined for infection. Constipation is best dealt with by enemas.

HALLUCINATIONS AND ALLIED DISORDERS OF PERCEPTION

Hallucinations may be defined as mental impressions of sensory vividness occurring without external stimulus, but appearing to be located, or to possess a cause located, outside the subject. An illusion is defined as a misinterpretation of an external stimulus, but illusions in some cases are closely related to hallucinations and may occur as symptoms of hallucinatory states. A delusion, by contrast, is an idea or thought (such as a false concept of persecution) which has no substance in fact; in contrast to visual and auditory hallucinations, it is purely a thought process with no sensory content, but hallucinations and delusions may occur together in various toxic/confusional states and in psychotic illnesses such as schizophrenia. Psychophysiologically, though hallucinations manifest themselves as changes in the content of consciousness, there is considerable evidence that they are often the result of disordered function of the reticulo-hypothalamic and associated pathways concerned with the state of consciousness as a whole.

The principal circumstances in which hallucinations may occur are: (1) in dreaming and the hypnagogic state; (2) in the pathological disturbances of sleep; (3) as a result of organic disease of the sense organs or of the central nervous system (including focal epilepsy); (4) in states of intoxication, particularly after the administration of certain drugs such as mescaline and lysergic acid or after withdrawal of alcohol, amphetamines, or barbiturates; and (5) in certain psychoses.

Lhermitte (1951) reviewed the subject of hallucinations with particular reference to those resulting from nervous disease. Visual hallucinations may occur in patients suffering from severe visual loss as a result of disease of the eyes, or with lesions in any part of the visual pathways as well as elsewhere in the nervous system. When a hemianopia is present the hallucinations may be seen in the normal half fields or in the blind half fields. Lhermitte himself described what he termed peduncular hallucinosis, namely the occurrence of hallucinations, especially visual hallucinations, as a result of lesions of the upper part of the brain stem. Lhermitte interpreted these hallucinations as an expression of a dissociation of the state of sleep in which, although bodily activity remains awake, mental processes are disturbed or memory engrams are evoked permitting the appearance of images analogous to those which normally occur only in dreams. Clearly any explanation of hallucinations occurring in association with organic lesions of the sense organs or the central nervous system must also take into account the mental state of the patient as a whole.

Hallucinations involving various sensory modalities, together with perceptual illusions and other disorders of consciousness, are particularly liable to occur as a result of lesions of the temporal lobes. The perceptual illusions include disordered visual perception, for example macropsia or micropsia and a similar alteration in auditory perception, feelings of unreality of the self or the surroundings, and disturbances of awareness of the body. Visual hallucination of the self has been described in which the individual feels that he is observing his own body from outside his physical self; this unusual phenomenon has some affinities with sensations of intense depersonalization or unreality. Visual hallucinations may occur on occasion as a result of epileptic discharge arising in the posterior part of the temporal lobe or in the parieto-occipital region and, when 'formed', invariably indicate the presence of a focal cortical lesion when toxic causes can be excluded.

REFERENCES

ADAMS, R. D., VICTOR, M., and MANCALL, E. L. (1959) Central pontine myelinolysis, *Arch. Neurol. Psychiat.*, **81,** 154.

ATKINSON, W. J. (1970) Posture of the unconscious patient, *Lancet*, **i,** 404.

BRAIN, W. R. (1947) Some observations on visual hallucinations and central metamorphopsia, *Acta psychiat. scand.*, Suppl. 46.

BRITISH MEDICAL JOURNAL (1973) Mute of malady, *Brit. med. J.*, **1,** 755.

BURKS, J. S., ALFREY, A. C., HUDDLESTONE, J., NORRENBERG, M. D., and LEWIN, E. (1976) A fatal encephalopathy in chronic haemodialysis patients, *Lancet*, **i,** 764.

CAIRNS, H. (1952) Disturbances of consciousness with lesions of the brain-stem and diencephalon, *Brain*, **75,** 109.

CRITCHLEY, M. (1939) Neurological aspects of visual and auditory hallucinations, *Brit. med. J.*, **2,** 634.

DENT, C. E., and WATSON, L. C. A. (1964) Hyperparathyroidism and cancer, *Brit. med. J.*, **2,** 218.

FELDMAN, M. H. (1971) Physiological observations in a chronic case of 'locked-in' syndrome, *Neurology (Minneap.)*, **21,** 459.

FRENCH, J. B. (1952) Brain lesions associated with prolonged unconsciousness, *Arch. Neurol. Psychiat. (Chic.)*, **68,** 727.

GERICH, J. E., MARTIN, M. M., and RECANT, L. (1971) Clinical and metabolic characteristics of hyperosmolar nonketotic coma, *Diabetes*, **20,** 228.

GOLDBERG, M. (1963) Hyponatraemia and the inappropriate secretion of antidiuretic hormone, *Amer. J. Med.*, **35,** 293.

GRANT, D. K. (1953) Papilloedema and fits in hypoparathyroidism, *Quart. J. Med.*, **22,** 243.

HAWKES, C. H. (1974) 'Locked-in' syndrome: report of seven cases, *Brit. med. J.*, **4,** 379.

HAWKES, C. H., and BRYAN-SMITH, L. (1974) The electroencephalogram in the 'locked-in' syndrome, *Neurology (Minneap.)*, **24,** 1015.

JEFFERSON, A. (1956) Clinical correlation between encephalopathy and papilloedema in Addison's disease, *J. Neurol. Neurosurg. Psychiat.*, **19,** 21.

KARP, J. S., and HURTIG, H. I. (1974) 'Locked-in' state with bilateral midbrain infarcts, *Arch. Neurol. (Chic.)*, **30,** 176.

KEMPER, T. L., and ROMANUL, F. C. A. (1967) State resembling akinetic mutism in basilar artery occlusion, *Neurology (Minneap.)*, **17,** 74.

LEMANN, J., and DONATELLI, A. A. (1964) Calcium intoxication due to primary hyperparathyroidism: a medical and surgical emergency, *Ann. intern. Med.*, **60,** 447.

LHERMITTE, J. (1951) *Les Hallucinations*, Paris.

McNICOL, M. W., and SMITH, R. (1964) Accidental hypothermia, *Brit. med. J.*, **1,** 19.

MEDICAL RESEARCH COUNCIL (1941) *A Glossary of Psychological Terms Commonly Used in Cases of Head Injury*, London.

MONTGOMERY, B. M., and PINNER, C. A. (1964) Transient hypoglycaemic hemiplegia, *Arch. intern. Med.*, **114,** 680.

NEWSOM DAVIS, J. (1974) Autonomous breathing, *Arch. Neurol. (Chic.)*, **30**, 480.

NORDGREN, R. E., MARKESBERY, W. R., FUKUDA, K., and REEVES, A. G. (1971) Seven cases of cerebromedullospinal disconnection: the 'locked-in' syndrome, *Neurology (Minneap.)*, **21**, 1140.

NORRIS, F. H., and FAWCETT, J. (1965) A sign of intracranial mass with impending uncal herniation, *Arch. Neurol. (Chic.)*, **12**, 381.

PLUM, F. (1972) Organic disturbances of consciousness, in *Scientific Foundations of Neurology*, ed. Critchley, M., O'Leary, J. L., and Jennett, W. B., London.

PLUM, F., and ALVORD, E. C., Jun. (1964) Apneustic breathing in man, *Arch. Neurol. (Chic.)*, **10**, 101.

PLUM, F., and POSNER, J. B. (1972) *Stupor and Coma*, 2nd ed., Philadelphia.

PLUM, F., and SWANSON, A. G. (1958) Abnormalities in the central regulation of respiration in acute and convalescent poliomyelitis, *Arch. Neurol. Psychiat. (Chic.)*, **80**, 267.

PLUM, F., and SWANSON, A. G. (1959) Central neurogenic hyperventilation in man, *Arch. Neurol. Psychiat. (Chic.)*, **81**, 535.

ROSENBERG, S. A., BRIEF, D. K., KINNEY, J. M., HERRERA, M. G., WILSON, R. E., and MOORE, F. D. (1965) The syndrome of dehydration, coma and severe hyperglycaemia without ketosis in patients convalescing from burns, *New Engl. J. Med.*, **272**, 931.

ROSIN, A. J., and EXTON-SMITH, A. N. (1964) Clinical features of accidental hypothermia, with some observations on thyroid function, *Brit. med. J.*, **1**, 16.

SALEM, S. N. (1966) Neurological complications of heat stroke in Kuwait, *Ann. Trop. Med. Parasitol.*, **60**, 393.

SKULTETY, F. M. (1968) Clinical and experimental aspects of akinetic mutism, *Arch. Neurol. (Chic.)*, **19**, 1.

TEASDALE, G., and JENNETT, W. B. (1974) Assessment of coma and impaired consciousness, *Lancet*, **ii**, 81.

WATSON, L. C. A. (1963) Hypercalcaemia and cancer, *Postgrad. med. J.*, **39**, 646.

DISORDERS OF MEMORY

Memory may be defined as the power to retain and recall past experiences. A little reflection, however, will show that memory thus defined includes functions of differing complexity. Perhaps the simplest form of memory is that involved in remembering a series of digits or a passage of meaningless jargon. In such an act of recollection or mechanical memory there is little emphasis upon the 'pastness' of what is recollected. The emphasis is rather upon the persistence into the present of a series of acts which have become habitual, perhaps through repetition. In such an act of remembering there is nothing more than the three fundamental elements of memory—registration, retention, and recall. Compare this, however, with the recollection, evoked by a place or a scent, of a single past experience fraught with strong emotion. Such an act is initiated by an associative process and there is considerable emphasis upon the 'pastness' of the experience by contrast with a present in which it is no longer occurring. Moreover, one of two such episodes in the past is remembered as having been experienced prior to the other, so that arising out of the function of memory is the experience of a personal past time as an extended dimension in which past experiences bear a constant and linear relation to each other. Furthermore, these past experiences are all felt as being the experiences of the same person, hence it follows that memory is essential to the experience of personal identity.

There is also a function of memory which seems to be intermediate between the reproduction of a passage of jargon and the recollection of an isolated incident. This is the recall of an image built up as a result of repeated experiences as, for example, that of a house or a person with whom one is familiar. A similar function of remembering enters not only into the act of representing to oneself the familiar house or face in its absence, but also into the act of recognizing it when it is presented to one again.

Loss of memory is known as amnesia.

The Anatomical and Physiological Basis of Memory

This is discussed on page 1147.

Tests of Memory

It will be clear from what has been said that the function of remembering cannot be adequately tested by means of the ordinary simple tests which usually investigate the patient's power to retain and recall a series of digits or similar data. Inquiry must also be made into the patient's power to recall the events of his past life, both remote and recent, as well as his capacity for mechanical memory as illustrated by the recollection of digits or passages learnt by heart [see p. 1180]. Other tests designed to investigate other functions of memory described above will suggest themselves in particular cases.

Some Organic Causes of Amnesia

The importance of the temporal lobe in memory mechanisms has already been stressed [p. 1148] and it is well recognized that bilateral temporal lobe disease or resection may seriously impair memory. Among the conditions which may cause severe memory loss, characterized particularly by an inability to record, retain, and recall recent impressions with, as a rule, comparative sparing of the memory for remote events, are inflammatory and degenerative diseases of the brain which cause dementia (including general paresis, the presenile and senile dementias and diffuse cerebral atherosclerosis), temporal lobe tumours, herpes simplex encephalitis, severe anoxia, or hypoglycaemia, severe head injury with diffuse brain damage, chronic alcoholism and, in some cases, bilateral rostral leucotomy (Whitty and Lishman, 1966). Transient amnesia may occur as a result of various toxic confusional states, milder anoxic episodes, concussion, acute alcoholic or drug intoxication, encephalitis and meningitis, epilepsy (particularly of the temporal lobe type), migraine and other forms of cerebral ischaemia, and a variety of deficiency disorders (particularly of thiamine, giving the Korsakow syndrome—see below).

Transient Global Amnesia

This syndrome, believed to be due to transient ischaemia in one or both temporal lobes, as it usually occurs in middle-aged or elderly individuals with evidence of cerebral atherosclerosis, is a disorder of sudden onset (Fisher and Adams, 1958) It has already been mentioned on page 1148 that memory loss for recent events develops rapidly and in the attacks, despite their inability to register new impressions, the patients retain their personal identity, show no abnormality of behaviour apart from anxiety and no evidence of impaired perception. Recovery is usually complete within a few hours, and retrograde amnesia shrinks rapidly, leaving the patient with no disability other than amnesia for the events occurring in the attack itself (Fogelholm et al., 1975).

Hysterical Amnesia

This is considered on page 1190.

KORSAKOW'S SYNDROME

The characteristic feature of Korsakow's syndrome is a certain type of amnesia. The patient has a gross defect of memory for recent events so that he has no recollection of what has happened even half an hour previously. He is disorientated in space and time and he fills the gaps in his memory by confabulating, that is, by giving imaginary accounts of his activities. Thus a bedridden patient will describe a walk which he asserts he has just taken. The subject was reviewed by Lewis (1961).

The amnesia of Korsakow's syndrome appears to be due to a lesion in the same situation as that which causes amnesia for current events. Other psychological disorders include a reduced capacity for retention and a disturbance of perception except for the immediate apprehension of spatially and temporally unitary patterns (Talland, 1958, 1959; Talland and Ekdahl, 1959). Lidz (1942) stated that in this 'amnestic syndrome' the patient can neither evoke the past nor relate the current experience to it. However, Seltzer and Benson (1974), who compared by means of a multiple-choice questionnaire based upon well-known events of the past 50 years, the performance of 11 alcoholic subjects with Korsakow's syndrome with that of 50 control subjects, found in the patients a severe defect of recent memory but almost normal recall of events occurring in the remote past. The defect of appreciation of time is secondary to the amnesia.

Korsakow's psychosis is seen typically in chronic alcoholism, and Victor (1964) identified it with Wernicke's encephalopathy, speaking of the Korsakow-Wernicke syndrome. The lesions involve the medial parts of the medial, dorsal pulvinar and antero-ventral thalamic nuclei, the mammillary bodies, and the terminal portions of the fornices, and consist of loss of medullated fibres and nerve cells, large numbers of adventitial histiocytes and microglia, proliferation of capillaries, and in a few cases haemorrhages.

Korsakow's syndrome may result from other kinds of lesion involving the same structures, e.g. head injury, anoxia, carbon monoxide poisoning, epilepsy, electroconvulsive therapy, acute encephalitis, dementia paralytica, other forms of dementia, intracranial tumour, cerebral arteriosclerosis, subarachnoid haemorrhage and the operation of cingulectomy. It has also been described as a sequel of gastrectomy, malnutrition, malabsorption, and pancreatitis (Pallis and Lewis, 1974).

REFERENCES

FISHER, M., and ADAMS, R. D. (1958) Transient global amnesia, *Trans. Amer. neurol. Ass.*, **83**, 143.

FOGELHOLM, R., KIVALO, E., and BERGSTRÖM, L. (1975) The transient global amnesia syndrome, *Europ. Neurol.*, **13**, 72.

LEWIS, A. (1961) Amnesic syndromes: the psychopathological aspect, *Proc. roy. Soc. Med.*, **54**, 955.

LIDZ, T. (1942) The amnestic syndrome, *Arch. Neurol. Psychiat. (Chic.)*, **47**, 588.

PALLIS, C. A., and LEWIS, P. D. (1974) *The Neurology of Gastrointestinal Disease*, London.

ROSENBAUM, M., and MERRITT, H. H. (1939) Korsakoff's syndrome. Clinical study of the alcoholic form, with special regard to prognosis, *Arch. Neurol. Psychiat. (Chic.)*, **51**, 978.

SELTZER, B., and BENSON, D. F. (1974) The temporal pattern of retrograde amnesia in Korsakoff's disease, *Neurology (Minneap.)*, **24**, 527.

TALLAND, G. A. (1958) Psychological studies of Korsakow's psychosis. II. Perceptual functions, *J. nerv. ment. Dis.*, **127**, 197.

TALLAND, G. A. (1959) The interference theory of forgetting and the amnesic syndrome, *J. abnorm. soc. Psychol.*, **59,** 10.

TALLAND, G. A., and EKDAHL, M. (1959) Psychological studies of Korsakow's psychosis. IV. The note and mode of forgetting narrative material, *J. nerv. ment. Dis.*, **129,** 391.

VICTOR, M. (1964) RNA and brain function, memory and learning, in *Brain Function*, vol. ii, ed. Brazier, M. A. B., Berkeley, Calif.

WHITTY, C. W. M., and LISHMAN, W. A. (1966) Amnesia in cerebral disease, in *Amnesia*, ed. Whitty, C. W. M., and Zangwill, O. L., London.

DISORDERS OF MOOD

The neural basis of the registration of emotion and the integration of the accompanying bodily changes have been discussed on page 1146. It is to disorders of this mechanism and of its relationship with higher levels of the nervous system that we must look for the explanation of disorders of mood occurring as a result of organic nervous disease. For more detailed commentaries upon disorders of mood and emotion consequent upon affective and psychotic disorders the reader is referred to textbooks of psychiatry; such conditions will only be mentioned here in so far as they enter into the differential diagnosis of those mood changes which occur in organic nervous disease.

Emotional Instability

Emotional instability or lability is a very common symptom of nervous diseases, especially of those in which the lesions are diffuse. The patient is easily moved by almost any form of emotion. He is quickly irritated or angered, easily becomes apprehensive, is readily depressed or reduced to tears. Less often, he experiences pleasurable emotion with abnormal facility and is readily moved to laughter. Emotional instability of this kind is commonly encountered after head injury, after massive cerebral infarction, and in patients with diffuse cerebral arteriosclerosis. It is frequently present in the early stages of dementia, however produced, and is highly characteristic of the later stages of multiple sclerosis. The animal experiments already quoted suggest that this exaggerated emotional activity common to so many disorders is the result of an impairment of the control which higher levels of the nervous system normally exercise over the thalamus and hypothalamus.

Impulsive Disorders of Conduct

The emotional instability described in the previous paragraph does not usually lead to disorder of conduct, perhaps because conduct is normally more strongly inhibited than feeling. Exceptionally, however, impairment of higher control releases emotions which pass into action. This most often happens in children or adolescents in whom the control of impulsive action, which it is the object of education to impose, is as yet incomplete. The misdemeanours and acts of violence sometimes committed by children and adolescents who have had encephalitis lethargica or other disorders causing diffuse brain damage are examples of this, and similar acts may be committed by aggressive psychopaths, and rarely by epileptics, either before an epileptic attack or in the phase of post-epileptic automatism or in the intervals between attacks. Such acts of aggression seem most likely to occur in patients with temporal lobe lesions.

Emotional Apathy

A general loss of emotional responsiveness without a proportionate intellectual deterioration was once most characteristically seen in association with Parkinsonism due to encephalitis lethargica. In view of the known predilection of the virus of this disease for the diencephalic grey matter, it was reasonable to attribute the apathy to injury to the posterior hypothalamus. A similar picture is seen associated with mental deterioration in the later stages of dementia from any cause. Here it is probable that the apathy is in part, at least, secondary to the deterioration of thought and perception. However, apathy may also be observed as a consequence of many forms of organic encephalopathy, degenerative brain diseases and in some psychotic disorders, especially severe melancholia and schizophrenia. The apathetic patient loses all his former interests and affections and, lacking the drive of the instinctive life, becomes incapable of effort, and sinks into a vegetative existence.

Euphoria

Euphoria is the term used to indicate a mood characterized by feelings of cheerfulness and happiness, a sense of mental well-being. Transitory euphoria is induced in many people by the consumption of alcohol. As a prevailing mood, it is seen most characteristically in multiple sclerosis. Some sufferers from this disease remain persistently serene and happy in spite of their increasing physical disabilities. Euphoria is also encountered occasionally in patients with intracranial tumours, especially when the tumour is situated in the temporal lobe or, less frequently, in the frontal lobe or corpus callosum. Euphoria is common also in general paralysis and is the predominating emotional state in the milder degrees of maniacal excitement. The psychophysiological basis of euphoria is little understood.

Excitement

Excitement is a term somewhat loosely applied to several forms of mental over-activity, which may predominantly involve the intellectual, emotional, or psychomotor spheres. All three may be affected together, as in acute mania, characterized by flight of ideas, elation, and psychomotor restlessness. Disordered ideas may be linked with excitement in some delirious and confusional states, and in catatonic schizophrenia. Delirium has been defined as confusion with an overlay of excitement. It may occur as a result of head injury, diffuse inflammation of the brain or in a variety of toxic and metabolic confusional states including those resulting from drug withdrawal. Psychomotor restlessness is associated with anxiety in agitated depression; and the prevailing mood may be one of rage in the outbursts of aggressive psychopaths. Meyer (1944) discussed the evidence for the view that states of excitement may be caused by lesions of the anterior hypothalamus.

Depression

Depression may be regarded as the opposite of euphoria. It is a mood of dejection and gloom for which frequently the patient can offer no explanation. It is encountered in a variety of states. It is sometimes produced by infections, especially influenza, and certain drugs, especially the sulphonamides. It may be a reaction to an adequate external cause, such as failure or bereavement, or a neurotic reaction to personal difficulties (reactive depression). In sufferers from cyclothymia, depression is liable to occur as a recurrent disorder of mood, sometimes alternating with phases of excitement, though often these are no more than a mild general sense of elation. In cyclothymic individuals the depression is likely to be associated with psychomotor retardation, manifesting itself in a difficulty in concentrating, and with insomnia and loss of appetite. Such patients typically wake early and feel at their worst in the early part of the day. Depression also occurs as the predominant feature of endogenous depression or involutional melancholia, in which it may be associated with agitation. Patients suffering from psychotic depression in a severe form often have delusions of guilt or of a hypochondriacal nature. Individuals with such a so-called endogenous depression frequently have physical symptoms including headache, fatigue, and facial and/or limb or low back pain; often they, too, show a typical pattern of early-morning waking. Depression is also a mood which is common in patients suffering from organic disease of the brain. This may be in part a natural reaction to their disabilities and it is most likely to occur in individuals of a cyclothymic temperament in whom the nervous disease may be regarded as having released a pre-existing tendency to depression. Thus we sometimes encounter depression after head injury, in some patients suffering from multiple sclerosis, and sometimes in those with intracranial tumour, general paresis, Parkinsonism and a variety of other neurological disorders.

Anxiety

Fear is the emotional reaction to an imminent danger; anxiety is the reaction to a possible future danger—fear linked with anticipation. Anxiety may be produced in a variety of ways. It may, of course, be a normal emotional reaction. It may be the effect of certain toxins which appear to stimulate directly the nervous centres concerned. These are all toxins which have a stimulating effect upon the sympathetic nervous system, namely adrenaline, ephedrine, amphetamine, nicotine, and thyroxine. Anxiety may be the prevailing mood in patients suffering from organic disease of the brain, for example, following head injury, and it is then probably in part the outcome of diminished control of emotional reactions by higher centres, and in part a reaction to the disability produced by the injury or disease. Fear may be very evident in delirious states, when it appears as the reaction to terrifying hallucinations, and may be linked with depression in involutional melancholia. In very many cases, however, anxiety is neurotic—that is, it is the product of unconscious mental processes.

REFERENCES

AGRANOFF, B. W. (1975) Biochemical strategies in the study of memory formation, in *Nervous System*, ed. Tower, D. B., vol. 1, *The Basic Neurosciences*, ed. Brady, R. O., New York.
COTTRELL, S. S., and WILSON, S. A. K. (1926) The affective symptomatology of disseminated sclerosis, *J. Neurol. Psychopath.*, **7**, 1.
FULTON, J. F., and INGRAHAM, F. D. (1929) Emotional disturbances following experimental lesions of the base of the brain (pre-chiasmal), *J. Physiol. (Lond.)*, **67**, 27.
MEYER, A. (1944) The Wernicke syndrome, *J. Neurol. Neurosurg. Psychiat.*, **7**, 66.
REITAN, R. M., and DAVISON, L. A. (Eds.) (1974) *Clinical Neuropsychology: Current Status and Applications*, Washington, D.C.
SMYTHIES, J. R. (1966) *The Neurological Foundations of Psychiatry*, Oxford.

THE INVESTIGATION OF MENTAL CHANGES
AFTER CEREBRAL LESIONS

It is only comparatively recently that much attention has been devoted to the psychological investigation of patients with lesions of the brain, and the Second World War gave a great impetus to this study. The complexity of mental function makes progress slow, but certain facts of theoretical and practical importance have emerged already. Numerous tests and several batteries of tests have been employed (Babcock, 1930; Wechsler, 1941; Reynell, 1944; Klein and Mayer-Gross, 1957; Reitan and Davison, 1974). Though there is much of theoretical interest to be learned from patients in states of confusion, the chief practical importance of psychometric investigation is in the diagnosis of dementia, and the assessment of the nature of the residual psychological change after head injury or other cerebral lesions in relation to prognosis and rehabilitation.

Specific Defects of Speech and Perception

It is first necessary to recognize defects of a specific kind, such as aphasia, acalculia, and the various forms of apraxia and agnosia. Two types of defect are of special importance, as emphasized by Zangwill (1945). Minor degrees of aphasia, which are a substantial handicap to a patient in formulating and expressing his thoughts with fluency, may be shown only by special tests of high-grade comprehension and reasoning. And disorders of spatial judgement and manipulative skill—minor degrees of spatial agnosia or constructive apraxia—may interfere with the performance of skilled and semi-skilled manual occupations. These disorders are discussed elsewhere in this book [see pp. 102 and 115 and Geschwind, 1974]. The Wechsler intelligence scale for children (W.I.S.C.) is particularly useful in childhood, when a discrepancy between the results obtained on the verbal and performance scales may indicate a specific inability to carry out certain performance tasks (motor skills) thus indicating some degree of apraxia (Gubbay, 1975). The assessment of Schonell's 'reading age' is also valuable in the assessment of suspected dyslexia. Similar tests are available for adults; thus the Wechsler Adult Intelligence Scale (W.A.I.S.) is widely employed; Critchley (1972) describes current techniques for assessing disorders of communication.

Intellectual Defects

The study of intellectual defects by appropriate tests has brought to light the fact that after damage to the brain 'certain abilities or attainments, such as vocabulary, general information, and powers of comprehension suffer less in deterioration than do such capacities as reasoning ability, attention, recent memory, and "relational thinking"' (Reynell, 1944). Babcock's and Reynell's batteries were designed to detect this difference. It is clear that the functions which suffer are themselves complex. Trist and Trist (1942-3) found Weigl's 'form-colour sorting test' of special value as a test of conceptual thought: failure is interpreted as meaning that the patient cannot abstract from the perceptual fields. Piercy (1964) and Oldfield (1972) have given valuable reviews of current methods, and Allison (1962) described techniques of particular value in the elderly. A simple test commonly employed is to ask the patient to subtract serial sevens from 100 aloud (the 100—7 test); the patient's performance may be impaired as a consequence of dementia but also by acalculia. In this and other tests it is important as far as possible to ascertain and bear in mind the patient's premorbid intellectual and educational status. Many of the psychometric methods commonly employed (e.g. the W.A.I.S. and W.I.S.C.) are capable of demonstrating not only intellectual impairment but also give an assessment of the premorbid intelligence quotient. It is also useful on occasion to test the patient's powers of abstract thought by asking him to interpret proverbs such as 'People who live in glass houses should not throw stones'. A concrete interpretation ('They would break the glass') may occur in dementia but is more often a consequence of thought disorder such as schizophrenia.

Defects of Memory

Memory defects are common after cerebral lesions and are often, but not invariably associated with defects of intellect (Newcombe, 1972). Inquiry should first be made about everyday events in the patient's immediate past. His memory for remote events is also tested. He should be asked to name notable personalities (e.g. the last three Prime Ministers or American Presidents). Specific tests are also useful. Some form of digit test is simple to carry out. Zangwill (1942–3) first ascertains the normal span, i.e. the number of digits which the patient can repeat correctly after one hearing, and then the number of hearings necessary for correct repetition when one more digit is added. The deteriorated patient will be able to repeat fewer than normal (7) and may exhibit a sharp threshold, i.e. he may fail completely to remember one more. Reynell scores the total number of digits repeated forwards correctly added to the number repeated backwards, the average being $7+5$. It is also customary to use the name, address, and flower test, in which the patient is given a name, an address, and the name of a flower to recall several minutes later after other tests have been interposed. Zangwill also uses the Rey Davis performance test and one of the Babcock Sentences, No. 23, which runs as follows: 'One thing a nation must have to become rich and great is a large, secure supply of wood.' The observer ascertains the number of hearings necessary before the patient can repeat it correctly. More than four is abnormal.

Emotional Factors and Personality Changes

Psychometric tests have also proved of value in distinguishing between failures of performance due to intellectual defects and those resulting from emotional disturbances. Thus Zangwill (1942–3) found the 'organic' reaction-type characterized by impairment of learning capacity and the 'neurotic' reaction-type by exaggerated variability of response and a tendency to fail on easy tasks. Tests such as the Minnesota Personality Inventory (M.M.P.I.) and many others are useful in the assessment of personality traits and of alterations consequent upon disease (Humphrey, 1972). The importance of personality change needs no emphasis. It can be interpreted only in the light of the patient's previous personality, of which the new personality is often a 'caricature' as Patterson (1942) pointed out; i.e. the previous trends are exaggerated. In other cases the change is rather an inversion (Reynell), and the previously cheerful, sociable, alert person may become depressed, unsocial, and lacking in initiative. After brain damage the distinction made by Zangwill between 'organic' and 'neurotic' would perhaps be better described as between intellectual and emotional; for it is artificial to distinguish between organic and psychogenic symptoms in such patients: once again we are dealing with a brain-mind unity.

REFERENCES

ALLISON, R. S. (1962) *The Senile Brain*, London.

BABCOCK, H. (1930) An experiment in the measurement of mental deterioration, *Arch. Psych.*, **117**, 5, New York.

CRITCHLEY, M. (1972) Communication: recognition of its minimal impairment, in *Scientific Foundations of Neurology*, ed. Critchley, M., O'Leary, J. L., and Jennett, W. B., London.

GESCHWIND, N. (1974) *Selected Papers on Language and the Brain*, Dordrecht, Holland.

GUBBAY, S. S. (1975) *Clumsy Children*, London.

HUMPHREY, M. E. (1972) Intelligence, in *Scientific Foundations of Neurology*, ed. Critchley, M., O'Leary, J. L., and Jennett, W. B., London.

KLEIN, R., and MAYER-GROSS, W. (1957) *The Clinical Examination of Patients with Organic Cerebral Disease*, London.

NEWCOMBE, F. (1972) Memory, in *Scientific Foundations of Neurology*, ed. Critchley, M., O'Leary, J. L., and Jennett, W. B., London.

OLDFIELD, R. C. (1972) Intelligence, in *Scientific Foundations of Neurology*, ed. Critchley, M., O'Leary, J. L., and Jennett, W. B., London.

PATTERSON, A. (1942) Emotional and cognitive changes in the post-traumatic confusional state, *Lancet*, **ii**, 717.

PIERCY, M. (1964) The effects of cerebral lesions on intellectual function: a review of current research trends, *Brit. J. Psychiat.*, **110**, 310.

RAPAPORT, D. (1945) *Diagnostic Psychological Testing*, Chicago.

REITAN, R. M., and DAVISON, L. A. (Eds.) (1974) *Clinical Neuropsychology: Current Status and Applications*, Washington, D.C.

REYNELL, W. R. (1944) A psychometric method of determining intellectual loss following head injury, *J. ment. Sci.*, **90**, 710.

TRIST, E. L., and TRIST, V. (1942–3) Discussion on the quality of mental test performance in intellectual deterioration, *Proc. roy. Soc. Med.*, **36**, 243.

WECHSLER, D. (1941) *Measurement of Adult Intelligence*, Baltimore.

ZANGWILL, O. L. (1942–3) Clinical tests of memory impairment, *Proc. roy. Soc. Med.*, **36**, 576.

ZANGWILL, O. L. (1945) A review of psychological work at the brain injuries unit, Edinburgh, 1941–5, *Brit. med. J.*, **2**, 248.

DEMENTIA

Dementia is the term applied to a diffuse deterioration in the mental functions, resulting from organic disease of the brain and manifesting itself primarily in thought and memory and secondarily in feeling and conduct. It may be produced by a large number of pathological agencies and the clinical picture varies somewhat according to the previous temperament of the patient, the age of onset, the localization, rate of progress, and nature of the causal disorder.

SYMPTOMS

Judgement and Reasoning

The earliest disability is often an impairment of judgement and reasoning manifesting itself in a failure to grasp the meaning of a situation as a whole and hence to react to it appropriately. At this stage a man's business judgement begins to fail, though in the semi-automatic activities of life no defect may be noticed.

Memory

Memory becomes impaired, the recollection of recent events suffering more than that of early periods of life [see p. 1173]. Even when both are grossly defective, mechanical memory may remain for a time. In more severe stages of dementia, defect of memory linked with defective perception leads to disorientation in space and time.

The Emotional Life

Although in some patients the emotional life is little disturbed, in others impairment of higher control leads to emotional instability which finds expression in irritability and impulsive conduct. Acts of violence, alcoholic excess, and sexual aberrations are thus explained. The prevailing mood may be one of euphoria, with hilariousness and hyperactivity, or of depression, anxiety, or maniacal excitement, and will be influenced by the pre-existing psychological constitution. In the late stages the patient is apathetic.

Delusions

Delusions are comparatively uncommon in dementing disorders, but may be noted, for instance, in the fatuous euphoric state which sometimes results from general paresis and occasionally in other conditions; when they do occur they are usually associated with impairment of judgement and defective appreciation of reality. Delusions centred on the self are likely to be grandiose in a state of euphoria and self-condemnatory or hypochondriacal in a state of depression. Delusions regarding others are often hostile and express fear, suspicion, or jealousy.

Care of the Person

In the later stages of dementia the patient becomes careless in dress and in personal cleanliness, and finally incontinent. This may be attributed at first to a decay of the self-regarding sentiment and later also to the lack of perception and frontal lobe damage.

Speech

In the later stages also, speech sometimes undergoes a progressive disintegration. Though the forms of aphasia caused by focal lesions of the brain may be present in dementia, there may also be destruction of speech function as a whole, so that it becomes increasingly meaningless and ends in jargon or isolated words or phrases, 'logoclonia'. Agnosia and apraxia may also develop.

Physical Concomitants

The condition of the somatic nervous functions will depend upon the causal disorder, but, whatever the cause, there is usually a general physical deterioration with loss of weight, and depression of endocrine function.

AETIOLOGY

The more important causes of dementia, many of which have already been considered in detail, are:

1. Syphilis—general paresis, cerebral meningovascular syphilis, etc.
2. Cerebral arteriosclerosis and other vascular disorders.
3. The presenile dementias—a mixed group of degenerative diseases of unknown origin—Pick's disease, Alzheimer's disease, Huntington's

chorea and other degenerative diseases, including progressive multi-system degeneration (the Shy–Drager syndrome).
4. Intracranial tumour, carcinomatous meningitis, reticulosis and 'low-pressure' or communicating hydrocephalus.
5. Non-syphilitic inflammatory diseases—encephalitis (various forms), intracranial abscess, meningitis, sarcoidosis, granulomatous angiitis, and other collagen diseases, cryptococcosis and slow virus infections including Creutzfeld–Jakob disease, and progressive multifocal leuko-encephalopathy.
6. Intoxications and deficiency diseases—alcoholism, drug addiction, carbon monoxide poisoning, uraemia, vitamin B_{12} neuropathy, pellagra, Wernicke's encephalopathy, myxoedema, liver failure.
7. Dementia supervening in chronic psychotic states.
8. Miscellaneous demyelinating and metabolic disorders, including multiple sclerosis, the diffuse cerebral scleroses and leukodystrophies, the lipidoses, and tuberous sclerosis, many of which may cause dementia in childhood.
9. Injury to the brain.
10. Severe and diffuse brain damage due to anoxia (as in some cases of intractable epilepsy), hypoglycaemia or heat stroke.
11. Dementia in neurofibromatosis and the hereditary ataxias (some forms).

Since in most of these disorders the dementia is an inconstant and sometimes a rare symptom, an account of them must be sought in the appropriate sections of this book. The presenile dementias, however, which, with the exception of Huntington's chorea, normally present with disorders of memory, intellect, and personality, are most conveniently considered at this point, and will also provide an opportunity of considering the diagnosis of dementia.

THE PRESENILE DEMENTIAS

Alzheimer's Disease

Alzheimer's disease is a progressive cerebral degeneration with the pathological picture of senility occurring in middle life. It is not inherited and has been described in one monozygotic twin (Hunter et al., 1972). The essential lesion is a diffuse degeneration of the cerebral cortex involving all its layers and most marked in the frontal lobes. The basal ganglia and the cerebellum escape. The brain is atrophic. Histologically, besides degeneration of the ganglion cells of the cortex there is a profusion of senile plaques in the cortex. These are silver-staining masses, often ring- or star-shaped. In addition, there are intraneural fibrillary tangles. These changes are regarded as characteristic of senile degeneration of the cortex. Their occurrence in middle age is unexplained, but there seems no doubt that Alzheimer's disease is essentially a premature senile change. Neurofibrillary tangles are most numerous in various basal nuclei and the thalamus, and are less common in the lenticular nuclei and pontine reticular substance. Similar changes are seen in many other degenerative brain diseases but in a different distribution. Thus in progressive supranuclear palsy, these tangles, by contrast, are found especially in the subthalamic nuclei, globus pallidus, midbrain reticular formation, and pontine nuclei (Ishino and Otsuki, 1975). Ultrastructural studies have shown that senile plaques are composed of degenerating neuronal terminals with 'twisted tubules', amyloid, and reactive cells (microglia, macrophages, and astrocytes) and three varieties of plaque have been characterized (Wisniewski and Terry, 1973). Neurochemical studies have shown that the plaques consistently contain certain combinations of amino acids and that their cones also contain phosphorus and sulphur (Nikaido et al., 1971), while neurofibrillary tangles appear to show an increased content of silicon (Nikaido et al., 1972). Recently, an increased concentration of aluminium has been found in the brains of affected patients (Crapper et al., 1976). The activities of levodopa decarboxylase, glutamic-acid decarboxylase, and beta-galactosidase are substantially reduced in various parts of the brain (Bowen et al., 1974). However, no specific biochemical findings have yet been identified to indicate the primary cause of the degenerative process; analgesic abuse, postulated as one factor (Murray et al., 1971) is unlikely to play a major role. Woodard (1962) has shown that granulovacuolar degeneration in the nerve cells of the hippocampal pyramidal layer can be even more closely correlated with dementia than senile plaques in the cortex. Tomlinson et al. (1968) have shown that all of the changes described, with the possible exception of granulo-vacuolar degeneration, can be found in the brains of non-demented elderly people, but there is a quantitative relationship between the severity of dementia and the severity and ubiquity of the pathological changes described (Roth et al., 1966; Tomlinson et al., 1970).

Alzheimer's disease usually develops between the ages of 40 and 60. The symptoms are generally those of a progressive dementia with apraxia and speech disturbances. The onset is insidious. In the early stages the patient suffers from loss of memory and becomes careless in dress and conduct. Epileptiform attacks may occur. Speech becomes slurred, and there is difficulty in recalling words. As the disease progresses there is complete disorientation. The patient recognizes none of his friends, becomes restless, and may wander about. A progressive deterioration takes place in the faculty of speech, which, from paraphasic talkativeness, becomes reduced to isolated words and phrases, so-called 'logoclonia'. Movements become stereotyped and the snout and sucking reflexes are often elicitable in the late stages. Spastic contractures sometimes develop. The duration of the disease is from one and a half to 15 years.

Since the discovery that 'low-pressure hydrocephalus' [p. 225] may give rise to dementia and that the condition may be relieved by ventriculo-atrial shunting, there have been a number of reports suggesting that this operation may be beneficial in Alzheimer's disease (Appenzeller and Salmon, 1967) and that CSF hydrodynamics may be abnormal in this disease (Sohn et al., 1973). However, in a comprehensive study Coblentz et al. (1973) concluded that the abnormalities of CSF dynamics reported were due to misleading findings on pneumoencephalography and isotope cisternography and that shunting was of no benefit in true Alzheimer's disease. Indeed, there is no evidence that any form of treatment influences this progressive disorder.

Pick's Disease

Synonym. Circumscribed cortical atrophy.

This condition is characterized by circumscribed atrophy of the cerebral cortex, usually confined to the frontal and temporal regions. The upper three cortical layers are principally affected, exhibiting chromatolysis and disappearance of ganglion cells. There is some glial increase in the atrophic areas. On light microscopy, cortical neurones show typical amphophilic and argentophilic Pick bodies with ballooning and central chromatolysis; senile plaques are relatively infrequent and neurofibrillary tangles are absent. The senile plaques are typical save for the fact that the twisted tubules seen in Alzheimer's disease are absent (Wisniewski *et al.*, 1972). The Pick bodies are made up of filaments, ribosomes, vesicles, and lipochrome and occasional tubules; there is thus a clear difference between the histological changes observed in Alzheimer's disease and Pick's disease, in that in the former lesions of the so-called twisted tubule type predominate, while the latter shows predominantly neurofilamentary changes (Brion *et al.*, 1973). The cause of the disease is unknown. It appears to be a form of primary degeneration developing in middle life. Multiple cases have been described in one sibship. The age of onset is usually between 50 and 60, and the disease has a duration of from three to 12 years, always terminating fatally. Females are said to be affected more often than males. It is characterized by a progressive dementia and aphasia. Restlessness and loss of normal inhibitions are prominent in the early stages. The patient is often voluble and tends to make jokes and puns. At first the more abstract intellectual functions suffer, but the more concrete type of behaviour is well preserved and the patient emotionally accessible. Later, mental dullness becomes pronounced and epileptic attacks may occur. Speech is reduced to a few stereotyped phrases. In the terminal stages there is much loss of weight, and the patient becomes bed-ridden, and tends to develop contractures. It is uninfluenced by treatment.

SENILE DEMENTIA

Many of the causes of dementia listed on pages 1182–3 may operate in old age. Is there a distinctive senile dementia apart from them, and especially from cerebral atheromatosis? This has been much debated (see McMenemey, 1958), but current evidence indicates that 'idiopathic' senile dementia is Alzheimer's disease of late onset and that it simply represents an ageing process which is observed in lesser degree in elderly non-demented subjects (see Pearce and Miller, 1973). Pathological evidence indicates that except in the presence of a history of recurrent cerebral infarction, atherosclerotic dementia is uncommon, even in old age and cerebral softening must be severe and widespread for 'multi-infarct' dementia to occur (Tomlinson *et al.*, 1968; Hachinski *et al.*, 1974).

THE DIAGNOSIS OF THE CAUSE OF DEMENTIA

The cause of dementia is sometimes obvious, as when the condition follows head injury, acute encephalitis, severe epilepsy, or chronic alcoholism. Dementia of syphilitic origin, whether due to general paresis or meningovascular syphilis, is associated with characteristic serological reactions and usually with abnormal physical signs in the nervous system. In cases of intracranial tumour the history is usually short, and the course of the dementia steadily progressive. The diagnosis is easy if symptoms and signs of increased intracranial pressure are present. In their absence full investigation with electroencephalography, gamma-encephalography, computerized transaxial tomography, and other specialized neuroradiological studies is often necessary. Electroencephalography frequently shows marked slowing of the dominant rhythms in the presenile dementias but rarely gives specific or diagnostic findings except in Creutzfeld-Jakob disease or subacute sclerosing panencephalitis. Air encephalography is usually diagnostic in cases of low-pressure or communicating hydrocephalus which may present with fluctuating confusion, dementia, and ataxia. Air will outline dilated ventricles but in this condition none passes over the cortex and deterioration often follows the procedure. Isotope encephalography may confirm the diagnosis but false positive results are not uncommon and the findings must be interpreted with care (Coblentz *et al.*, 1973). Occasionally, brain biopsy may be justified to confirm the exact nature of the pathological change; the indications for this procedure are reviewed by Pearce and Miller (1973). Arteriosclerotic dementia is usually encountered after the age of 60. The onset is usually insidious, and there is almost always a history of focal cerebral vascular lesions, slight 'strokes'. Evidence of arteriosclerosis is to be found as a rule in the retinal and peripheral circulation, with or without high blood pressure. Psychometric testing with the Wechsler Adult Intelligence Scale (W.A.I.S.) has been shown to give a consistently poorer performance on tests of cognitive and intellectual ability in patients with Alzheimer's disease than in those with multi-infarct dementia (Perez *et al.*, 1975). Indeed, detailed psychometric testing is invariably indicated in cases of suspected dementia. Measurement of regional cerebral blood flow may also be helpful (Simard *et al.*, 1971) as this is usually normal in Alzheimer's disease but impaired in patients with cerebrovascular disease.

The differentiation of the presenile dementias may be difficult. These usually begin between 45 and 60. Other common causes of dementia can readily be excluded. Pneumoencephalography or the EMI scan usually demonstrate some general dilatation of the cerebral ventricles with an excess of air over the anterior part of the hemispheres in Pick's disease, but more diffuse in Alzheimer's disease. Early psychomotor restlessness and jocularity and a family history of presenile dementia would favour Pick's disease as against Alzheimer's disease.

The possibility of a metabolic or endocrine cause for dementia must always be borne in mind. In vitamin B_{12} deficiency, dementia may antedate symptoms and signs of anaemia and spinal cord involvement and estimation of the serum B_{12} or a Schilling test may be necessary for diagnosis. Myxoedema will usually be apparent clinically, if considered. The fluctuating confusion of subdural haematoma is sometimes mistaken for dementia, but there is usually associated drowsiness and headache and an angiogram will give diagnostic findings.

It must also be remembered that the retardation of severe endogenous depression may be misconstrued as being due to dementia, while many patients with receptive aphasia due to focal cerebral lesions are wrongly regarded as suffering from dementia in view of their failure to communicate and a similar error is not infrequently made in patients with delirium and/or toxic confusional states, or with specific disturbances of memory such as Korsakow's syndrome or transient global amnesia (Pearce and Miller, 1973). Impairment of memory without evidence of any change in personality or intellectual function, like psychomotor retardation alone, gives insufficient grounds for the diagnosis of dementia. Hysteria in young patients and hysterical 'pseudodementia' in adults, sometimes arising as a result of a desire for financial compensation after relatively minor head injury may also give rise to occasional difficulty. Marsden and Harrison (1972) found that in a series of 106 patients admitted to hospital with a presumptive diagnosis of dementia, 15 had some other condition, usually a depressive illness, and 15 a disorder which was amenable to treatment. Among the 84 patients shown to have impairment of intellect and/or learning capacity and memory, several proved to have intracranial mass lesions, diffuse arterial disease, or alcoholism as the presumptive cause.

REFERENCES

ALLISON, R. S. (1962) *The Senile Brain*, London.

APPENZELLER, O., and SALMON, J. H. (1967) Treatment of parenchymatous degeneration of the brain by ventriculo-atrial shunting of the cerebrospinal fluid, *J. Neurosurg.*, **26**, 478.

BENEDEK, L., and LEHOCZKY, T. (1939) The clinical recognition of Pick's disease. Report of three cases, *Brain*, **62**, 104.

BOWEN, D. M., WHITE, P., FLACK, R. H. A., SMITH, C. B., and DAVISON, A. N. (1974) Brain-decarboxylase activities as indices of pathological change in senile dementia, *Lancet*, **i**, 1247.

BRION, S., MIKOL, J., and PSIMARAS, A. (1973) Recent findings in Pick's disease, in *Progress in Neuropathology*, vol. II, ed. Zimmerman, H. M., New York.

COBLENTZ, J. M., MATTIS, S., ZINGESSER, L. H., KASOFF, S. S., WISNIEWSKI, H. M., and KATZMAN, R. (1973) Presenile dementia. Clinical aspects and evaluation of cerebrospinal fluid dynamics, *Arch. Neurol. (Chic.)*, **29**, 299.

CONSTANTINIDIS, J. (1971) Demence presenile d'Alzheimer et demence senile alzheimerisée. Étude statistique des correlations anatomocliniques, in *Psychiatry* (Excerpta Medica International Congress Series No. 274), Amsterdam.

CRAPPER, D. R., KRISHNAN, S. S., and QUITTKAT, S. (1976) Aluminium, neurofibrillary degeneration and Alzheimer's disease, *Brain*, **99**, 67.

DELAY, J., BRION, S., and BADARACIO, J. G. (1955) Le diagnostic différentiel des maladies de Pick et de Alzheimer, *Encéphale*, **44**, 454.

GRÜNTHAL, E. (1926) Ueber die Alzheimersche Krankheit, *Z. ges. Neurol. Psychiat.*, **101**, 128.

GRÜNTHAL, E. (1930) Über ein Brüderpaar mit Pickscher Krankheit, *Z. ges. Neurol. Psychiat.*, **129**, 350.

HACHINSKI, V. C., LASSEN, N. A., and MARSHALL, J. (1974) Multi-infarct dementia. A cause of mental deterioration in the elderly, *Lancet*, **ii**, 207.

HENDERSON, D. K., and MACLACHAN, S. H. (1930) Alzheimer's disease, *J. ment. Sci.*, **76**, 646.

HUNTER, R., DAYAN, A. D., and WILSON, J. (1972) Alzheimer's disease in one monozygotic twin, *J. Neurol. Neurosurg. Psychiat.*, **35**, 707.

ISHINO, H., and OTSUKI, S. (1975) Distribution of Alzheimer's neurofibrillary tangles in the basal ganglia and brain stem of progressive supranuclear palsy and Alzheimer's disease, *Folia Psychiat. Neurol. Japonica*, **29**, 179.

LARSSON, T., SJÖGREN, T., and JACOBSON, G. (1963) Senile dementia, *Acta psychiat. (Kbh.)*, **39**, Suppl. 167.

McMENEMEY, W. H. (1958) in *Neuropathology*, ed. Greenfield, J. G., Blackwood, W., McMenemey, W. H., Meyer, A., and Norman, R. M., p. 475, London.

MALAMUD, W., and LOWENBERG, K. (1929) Alzheimer's disease, *Arch. Neurol. Psychiat. (Chic.)*, **21**, 805.

MANSVELT, J. VAN (1954) *Pick's Disease*, Enschede.

MARSDEN, C. D., and HARRISON, M. J. G. (1972) Outcome of investigation of patients with presenile dementia, *Brit. med. J.*, **2**, 249.

MAYER-GROSS, W., CRITCHLEY, M., and MEYER, A. (1937–8) Discussion on the presenile dementias: symptomatology, pathology and differential diagnosis, *Proc. roy. Soc. Med.*, **31**, 1443.

MURRAY, R. M., GREENE, J. G., and ADAMS, J. H. (1971) Analgesic abuse and dementia, *Lancet*, **ii**, 242.

NICHOLS, I. C., and WEIGNER, W. C. (1938) Pick's disease—a specific type of dementia, *Brain*, **61**, 237.

NIKAIDO, T., AUSTIN, J., RINEHART, R., TRUEBB, L., HUTCHINSON, J., STUKENBROK, H., and MILES, B. (1971) Studies in ageing of the brain. I. Isolation and preliminary characterization of Alzheimer plaques and cores, *Arch. Neurol. (Chic.)*, **25**, 198.

NIKAIDO, T., AUSTIN, J., TRUEB, L., and RINEHART, R. (1972) Studies in ageing of the brain. II. Microchemical analyses of the nervous system in Alzheimer patients, *Arch. Neurol. (Chic.)*, **27**, 549.

PEARCE, J., and MILLER, E. (1973) *Clinical Aspects of Dementia*, London.

PEREZ, F. I., RIVERA, V. M., MEYER, J. S., GAY, J. R. A., TAYLOR, R. L., and MATHEW, N. T. (1975) Analysis of intellectual and cognitive performance in patients with multi-infarct dementia, vertebrobasilar insufficiency with dementia, and Alzheimer's disease, *J. Neurol. Neurosurg. Psychiat.*, **38**, 533.

ROTH, M., TOMLINSON, B. E., and BLESSED, G. (1966) Correlation between scores for dementia and counts of 'senile plaques' in cerebral grey matter of elderly subjects, *Nature (Lond.)*, **209**, 109.

SIMARD, D., OLESEN, J., PAULSON, O. B., LASSEN, N. A., and SKINHØJ, E. (1971) Regional cerebral blood flow and its regulation in dementia, *Brain*, **94**, 273.

SJÖGREN, T., SJÖGREN, H., and LINDGREN, A. G. H. (1952) Morbus Alzheimer and Morbus Pick, *Acta psychiat. scand.*, Suppl. 82.

SOHN, R. S., SIEGEL, B. A., GADO, M., and TORACK, R. M. (1973) Alzheimer's disease with abnormal cerebrospinal fluid flow, *Neurology (Minneap.)*, **23**, 1058.

THORPE, F. T. (1932) Pick's disease (circumscribed senile atrophy) and Alzheimer's disease, *J. ment. Sci.*, **78**, 303.

TOMLINSON, B. E., BLESSED, G., and ROTH, M. (1968) Observations on the brains of non-demented old people, *J. neurol. Sci.*, **7**, 331.

TOMLINSON, B. E., BLESSED, G., and ROTH, M. (1970) Observations on the brains of demented old people, *J. neurol. Sci.*, **11**, 205.

WISNIEWSKI, H. M., COBLENTZ, J. M., and TERRY, R. D. (1972) Pick's disease. A clinical and ultrastructural study, *Arch. Neurol. (Chic.)*, **26**, 97.

WISNIEWSKI, H. M., and TERRY, R. D. (1973) Re-examination of the pathogenesis of the senile plaque, in *Progress in Neuropathology*, vol. II, ed. Zimmerman, H. M., New York.

WOODARD, J. S. (1962) Clinico-pathological significance of granulo-vacuolar degeneration in Alzheimer's disease, *J. Neuropath. exp. Neurol.*, **21**, 85.

HYSTERIA

Definition. A disorder characterized by mental dissociation leading in severe cases to multiple personality and amnesia, but more often to somatic symptoms such as 'fits', paralysis, and sensory disturbances in the absence of organic disease of the nervous system.

AETIOLOGY

In hysteria the type of abnormal reaction exhibited by the patient is determined by the peculiar tendency of the hysterical personality to mental dissociation. In response to mental stress of a kind to be described later, the personality becomes split, certain psychophysiological elements becoming separated from the conscious life. In general, all hysterical syndromes may be regarded as representing the subconscious results of an attempt to escape from some stressful situation. In the most severe cases the dissociated part of the mental life is so extensive that the patient may be regarded as suffering from multiple personality, since his body is at different times under the control of different personalities, which exhibit differences in temperament and which may or may not have access to each other's memories. A similar profound mental dissociation is responsible for the state known as hysterical fugue, in which the patient disappears from home and wanders about, having lost his sense of identity. During the period of fugue he has no access to the memories of his normal personality, and on recovery he may have no recollection of the events of his fugue. Such profound degrees of dissociation are, however, uncommon, and usually the splitting of the personality finds expression at the physiological level, part of the body being functionally cut off from the rest of the mental life, so that the patient is unable to move it or to feel with it, hysterical paralysis or anaesthesia resulting.

The nature of the hysterical tendency to dissociation is little understood. It appears to be associated with a peculiarity of the emotional life of the hysterical patient. The poverty of the affective reactions of such individuals is well known—*la belle indifférence* of Janet—and Golla showed that in spite of the violence of their somatic reactions the psycho-galvanic response to nocuous stimuli is greatly depressed in hysterical patients. The underlying abnormality which finds expression in hysteria may well in many cases be inborn or at least may develop at an early age. But certain organic nervous diseases seem to predispose to hysteria, especially multiple sclerosis, and typically hysterical symptoms may occur in patients with a focal abnormality in the temporal lobe, which suggests that mental dissociation may sometimes have an organic basis. Women suffer from hysteria more frequently than men.

It is also important to recognize that hysterical manifestations occurring for the first time in adult life, unless there is some obvious motive (such as, for instance, escape from stress, or the desire for material gain such as compensation after injury) may be the result of either an underlying organic disorder (such as early dementia) or else of a more serious psychiatric illness (such as endogenous depression). Slater (1965) has drawn attention to the frequency with which symptoms regarded by experienced clinicians as being due to hysteria may conceal evidence of underlying organic disease of the nervous system. He suggests that all too often this diagnosis is 'a disguise for ignorance and a fertile source of clinical error'. His warning that such a diagnosis does not necessarily imply the absence of, as yet, unrecognized organic disease, was timely but Carter (1972) argues that hysteria, nevertheless, deserves continuing recognition as a disease entity in which patients respond to stress by converting their emotional problems into physical disabilities.

The Mode of Production of Hysterical Symptoms

The hysterical symptom is at the same time (1) a product of suggestion, (2) the expression of an idea in the patient's mind, and (3) a means to achieve a purpose.

1. The precise nature of a hysterical symptom in a given case is usually, probably always, determined by suggestion. The suggestion frequently emanates from an organic disorder from which the patient actually suffers. Thus laryngitis may lead to aphonia, which is perpetuated as a hysterical symptom. Accidents of all kinds, for reasons which are discussed elsewhere, are apt to cause hysterical symptoms which perpetuate or exaggerate the disabilities produced by an injury. A doctor, nurse, or friend of the patient may unwittingly evoke a hysterical symptom by seeming to imply that a disability is to be expected. There are fashions in hysterical symptoms which seem partly to be determined by the expectations of doctors interested in the subject at the time. Finally, the symptom may be an imitation of an organic disorder in a person whom the patient has seen and with whom for some reason he identifies himself.

2. Suggestion operates through the patient's acceptance on irrational grounds of the idea that he is suffering from a certain symptom. It follows that the hysterical symptom is always the expression of an idea in the patient's mind. Thus hysterical aphonia expresses the idea 'I have lost my voice', hysterical

paralysis the idea 'I cannot move my limb', and so on. This fact is of great diagnostic importance, for it is unlikely, except in doctors and nurses, where diagnosis may present exceptional difficulties, that the patient's idea of a symptom will correspond with a similar symptom produced by organic disease, and the resulting discrepancy renders possible the diagnosis of the one from the other.

3. The purposive character of the hysterical symptom is important in connection with treatment. The purpose served by the symptom can usually be expressed as the unconscious solution, however unsatisfactory, of a mental conflict. The patient finds himself in a situation in which a course of action which he desires to follow conflicts with his sense of duty or self-respect. The development of the hysterical symptom unconsciously solves this conflict, though at the price of a neurotic disability. For example, a girl was compelled to give up her work to look after her invalid mother. She developed a hysterical paralysis of her right hand which prevented her from doing housework, and assistance had to be obtained to look after both her mother and herself. Her hysterical illness saved her from her unpleasant duty and also preserved her self-respect, since she felt that no one could blame her for being ill. At the same time she ceased to do any work at all, unconsciously revenged herself on her exacting parent, and became an object of sympathy to those with whom she came in contact. It is important to recognize that hysteria may fulfil other purposes than the solution of such a conflict, and that one symptom may achieve more than one object. The symptom frequently expresses a demand for sympathy, especially when the patient feels that he is neglected or insufficiently appreciated. Tyrannical parents and unfaithful spouses excite such a demand directly, while invalid parents and delicate brothers and sisters evoke it competitively. The hysterical symptom frequently possesses the further significance of being a symbol which expresses the patient's feelings. An example is the adoption of a crucifixion attitude in a hysterical fit.

The patient suffering from hysteria is thus often an individual confronted with a mental difficulty, often a conflict between two opposing wishes. While in this situation he receives a suggestion of ill health emanating either from an actual organic disease or from some outside source. He accepts this suggestion and manifests hysterical symptoms which provide a solution, albeit a pathological and unsatisfactory one, of his difficulty, and may also express in symbolic form his emotional reaction to his problem.

SYMPTOMS

Amnesia and Multiple Personality

Loss of memory and multiple personality are among the most striking symptoms of hysteria, and in outspoken forms are rare. The commonest example is the hysterical fugue, in which the patient disappears from home and wanders about, having lost his sense of identity. This state may last for hours, days, or even months, and on recovery the patient usually has no recollection of the events of his period of fugue. During the fugue he may be dazed and confused or he may be apparently normal and live as a normal individual, carrying on an occupation and exhibiting a mode of life different from his usual one. Hysterical amnesias and fugues are usually reactions to difficulties which render normal life intolerable. A wife has been known to react in this way to the infidelity of her husband and to adopt during her fugue the name of his mistress. A patient already in financial difficulties had a quantity of uninsured stock stolen from his car. He drove for miles in a state of fugue, subsequently returning home exhausted and without any recollection of the events of the day, including the theft. In such a case the fugue and the amnesia constituted an escape from an unbearable situation which composed so large a part of the patient's life that he could only escape from it by suppression of a large field of consciousness. Amnesia may also occur in association with hysterical fits, the events of the attack being subsequently forgotten. Patients suffering from hysterical fugue may justly be regarded as examples of multiple or dissociated personality, since they exhibit alternating phases of consciousness with mutually isolated memories. More complicated cases of multiple personality have been described in which more than two sub-personalities alternated or coexisted, some having access to the memories of the others. It is interesting to note that it has sometimes been possible to produce these dissociations of personality by hypnotic suggestion, and that the subject-matter of a hysterical amnesia can often be restored to consciousness under hypnosis.

By no means all cases of 'loss of memory' are hysterical in origin [p. 1173]. Many other disorders lead to mental confusion or impairment of memory such that the patient may become lost and be unable to give an account of himself.

Pseudodementia

Hysterical pseudodementia, or the Ganser syndrome, is characterized by failure of memory, and the acting out of the patient's idea of a psychosis, i.e. bizarre behaviour, excitement, or stupor.

Hysterical 'Fits'

It is sometimes difficult to decide from the history whether attacks are hysterical or epileptic, but the question is usually easily settled if the doctor is fortunate enough to witness a fit himself. The hysterical fit is often a dramatic performance appropriately staged, hence it does not occur when the patient is alone or at least out of reach of an audience. Often the attack is directly precipitated by the emotional situation responsible for the neurosis. The onset is usually gradual and never of the fulminating suddenness of an epileptic fit. Whereas the epileptic falls to the ground with alarming violence and may injure himself, the hysteric subsides with some care, leaning, for example, against a wall or slipping slowly from a chair on to the ground. The epileptic fit follows a more or less stereotyped course, beginning sometimes with a cry and passing through a tonic phase, a phase of clonic, purposeless, jerking movements, and ending in post-convulsive coma of variable length, sometimes followed by automatism. In hysterical fits these phases do not occur. Crying-out often occurs during the attack, but unlike the convulsive cry of the epileptic, which is merely an inarticulate phonation, consists of emotional reactions, e.g. laughing and crying, or the articulate utterance of words or sentences. The movements of the hysterical fit are not of a low order like the clonic movements of epilepsy, but are co-ordinated and purposive. The hysteric clutches at surrounding objects, struggles, and may attempt to fall out of bed or to tear off his clothes. Opisthotonus is common, and bizarre attitudes may be adopted. The tongue is not bitten in a hysterical convulsion, and incontinence of urine does not usually occur, but if the patient becomes aware that micturition is a characteristic of epileptic attacks, this symptom may be reproduced. Some hysterical 'fits', particularly in adolescent girls, are not accompanied by movement, but the patient simply slumps to the floor and gets up again a few minutes later. These attacks may be difficult to distinguish from akinetic epilepsy but they usually occur at work or at school, do not cause injury, and usually fail to respond to anticonvulsant drugs. Similar attacks, occurring sometimes with great frequency, may occur in adults after trivial head injury in a compensation setting and resolve after financial settlement. In the convulsions of epilepsy consciousness is lost at the onset, so that the patient during and immediately after the fit makes no response to external simuli. The hysteric when in a 'fit', though in an abnormal state of consciousness, is not completely unconscious and can usually be roused by sufficiently firm handling, whence the time-honoured practice of administering a douche of cold water. The corneal reflex accordingly is absent in an epileptic during a fit and during the phase of post-convulsive coma. The corneal reflex is sometimes absent in hysteria, but an attempt to elicit it during a hysterical fit often evokes a violent contraction of the orbicularis oculi. The hysterical 'fit', unlike the epileptic, has no well-defined termination but tails away in sighs and groans and motor restlessness. After the attack the hysterical patient, though shaken and exhausted, does not usually exhibit the tendency to sleep which follows most epileptic fits. The plantar reflexes are for a time extensor after a proportion of epileptic fits. Flexor plantar responses after a fit do not exclude epilepsy, but extensor responses in similar circumstances exclude hysteria as the cause of the fit, provided there is no coexisting corticospinal tract lesion to which they are attributable and provided the patient has not learned, as in some cases of the 'von Munchausen syndrome' [p. 1197], to simulate the response.

Paralysis

Hysterical paralysis may affect any part of the body over which there is normally voluntary control. Most commonly it involves one limb or part of a limb, the movements at one joint being alone affected. Less frequently more than one limb is affected, as in hysterical hemiplegia, paraplegia, and diplegia. The paralysis may be associated with flaccidity or rigidity, or there may be no gross disturbance of muscle tone. Hysterical paralysis of the face and tongue is rare and is usually associated with spasm of the corresponding muscles on the opposite side. The diagnosis of hysterical paralysis rests upon the following points:

Anomalies of Distribution. Since the paralysis corresponds to the patient's idea, there are inevitably discrepancies between hysterical paralysis and that produced by organic lesions of the nervous system. The distribution of the weakness is often anomalous. Thus in hysterical hemiplegia there is no weakness of the face. Paralysis limited to the movements at one joint is almost unknown in organic disease.

Contraction of Antagonistic Muscles. It is very common in hysterical paralysis to find that when the patient attempts to move the limb he contracts the antagonistic muscles as well as the prime movers. Thus extension of the elbow is associated with active contraction of the biceps, flexion of the knee with contraction of the quadriceps. Such antagonistic contractions can easily be detected by the observer if he places a finger upon the biceps tendon and patella respectively. Electromyography can give useful confirmation. Such a disorder of movement expresses mental conflict at the physiological level in a simultaneous contraction of the muscles which would carry out a movement and of those which would prevent it. Antagonistic contraction is absent when the paresis is so great that the prime movers hardly contract at all. It is often characteristic that in hysterical weakness or paralysis the patient may demonstrate a massive expenditure of effort in his attempts to move the paralysed member, but to little effect.

Muscular Wasting and Contractures. These are absent except in cases of long standing, in which these phenomena may supervene upon the prolonged muscular inactivity. Thus when hysterical flexion of the fingers (which may literally dig into the palm) [FIG. 170] or hysterical inversion of the foot, say, has

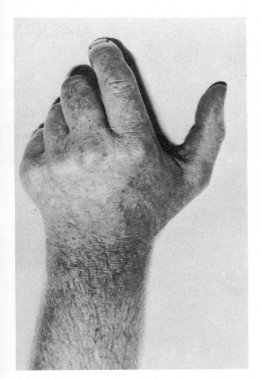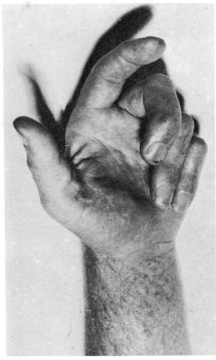

FIG. 170. Hysterical contracture of the middle, ring, and little fingers following upon a trivial industrial injury (photograph kindly supplied by Dr. J. D. Spillane)

been present for many months or years, shortening of tendons and muscles may eventually occur. Even so, considerable relaxation and an almost normal range of movement may still be achieved by electrical stimulation of antagonistic muscles or under anaesthesia.

The Reflexes. The tendon reflexes in hysteria depend upon a number of variable factors. There is often a symmetrical and moderate exaggeration. Extreme rigidity may make them difficult to elicit. Moderate unilateral rigidity may render them exaggerated on the affected side, but if adequate muscular relaxation can be obtained they are never asymmetrical, and never diminished. The same is true of the abdominal reflexes, and the plantar reflexes are flexor unless the patient has learned the pathological significance of an extensor plantar response. True ankle clonus does not occur, though a few clonic jerks may be evoked if the lower limb is incompletely relaxed.

Gait

Hysterical disorders of gait may be associated with hysterical paralysis of one or both lower limbs, and are sometimes a perpetuation of the normal instability which occurs on first getting out of bed after an illness. A hysterical gait is usually easily recognized on account of its bizarre character and its dissimilarity from any disorder of gait produced by organic disease. In hysterical hemiplegia the affected lower limb is ostentatiously dragged along the ground and not circumducted, as in hemiplegia due to a corticospinal lesion. When the disorder involves both lower limbs, stiffness and ataxia are present to a varying extent. Not infrequently a patient who, while lying in bed, exhibits normal power and co-ordination, walks with the greatest difficulty, clinging to the bed and the furniture. There is often a tendency to fall, especially when other patients are present, but the fall does not lead to injury. In severe cases there is a complete astasia-abasia, and two persons may have difficulty in supporting the patient, for whereas a patient with organic disease leading to difficulty in walking does his best to support himself, the unconscious efforts of the hysterical patient are directed to falling.

Rigidity

Hysterical rigidity may be localized to a paralysed limb, or generalized, as in hysterical trance. It is distinguished from all forms of rigidity due to organic disease by the fact that it increases in proportion to the effort made by the observer to move the rigid part, whereas in organic disease of the nervous system the rigidity is a definite quantum which can be overcome by the exercise of a slightly greater force. Moreover, in hysteria a successful attempt to break down the rigidity almost always leads to an intense emotional reaction in the patient.

Involuntary Movements

Tremor is a common hysterical involuntary movement. It may be fine or coarse, generalized or localized. A coarse tremor is often associated with hysterical paralysis, being intensified when the patient attempts to move the paralysed limb. It is increased when attention is directed to it, and may be absent in movements carried out when the attention is distracted. Hysterical involuntary movements may simulate chorea, though not with sufficient accuracy to deceive the skilled observer. In such cases movements do not usually involve the face.

Sensory Symptoms and Signs

Hysterical sensory impairment is common. It is most often confined to a limb which is the site of other hysterical symptoms, for example, paralysis. It may affect some forms of sensibility only, especially appreciation of light touch and cutaneous pain, or all forms may be lost. When cutaneous sensibility is lost over the peripheral segments of the limb, the anaesthetic area is demarcated from the area of normal sensibility by a sharp upper border which encircles the limb and usually coincides with a joint. Sensation may be lost over half of the body, and in such cases there may be loss of smell and taste on the same side as well as loss of vibration sense on the same side of the skull and half of the sternum. Anaesthesia of the whole body is less frequent. Anaesthesia of the cornea, palate, and pharynx, with loss of the corresponding reflexes, is an unexplained symptom of hysteria, which may be present without other sensory disturbances.

Hysterical sensory loss is distinguished from that due to organic disease of the nervous system by its failure to correspond with the distribution of the loss resulting from lesions of the sensory tracts, spinal segments, or peripheral nerves. Anaesthesia of the 'glove and stocking' distribution may simulate that found in polyneuritis and in subacute combined degeneration, but in these disorders the transition from impaired to normal sensibility is usually gradual. Hysterical patients often exhibit striking discrepancies in their sensory symptoms which are incompatible with an organic origin. Thus co-ordination may be perfect in spite of complete loss of postural sensibility and appreciation of passive movement in a limb. Or a patient with hysterical hemianaesthesia may state that he is unable to feel a vibrating tuning-fork placed over the affected half of the sternum or skull, although the bone conducts the stimulus perfectly to the opposite side. In hysterical persons sensory loss can readily be, and perhaps always is, produced by suggestion; it may be possible to 'find' islands of normal sensation within an anaesthetic area by suggesting to an observer, in the patient's hearing, that such findings are common.

Deafness. There is little difficulty in detecting hysterical deafness when examination reveals that the ears and vestibular reactions are normal, but the diagnosis is more difficult when hysterical deafness is superimposed upon a reduction of hearing due to organic disease of the ears. Hysterical deafness may disappear during sleep, so that the patient can be aroused by sounds, and the blinking reflex on auditory stimulation may be retained by the hysterically deaf. When Bárány's noise-box is used, a patient suffering from hysterical deafness will raise his voice, but this does not occur when deafness is due to disease of the ear. Hysterical vertigo is rare, but feelings of giddiness, instability and depersonalization are common.

Pain. There has been some discussion as to whether hysterical pain is qualitatively the same as the pain produced by organic disease, and this has been denied on the ground that the hysterical patient, though complaining of severe pain, usually exhibits none of the physical reactions which are associated with pain of organic origin and presents an appearance which belies his allegations of intense suffering. Nevertheless, since pain is essentially a psychical state, there seems no reason why it should not sometimes be psychogenic, and it does not follow that pain thus induced would necessarily be associated with the physiological concomitants of pain excited at lower levels of the nervous system. Hysterical pain is especially common in the head. The recognition of its nature depends upon the absence of symptoms of organic disease sufficient to explain it, its failure to respond to analgesic drugs, often including morphine, and to local anaesthetic block of the nerves innervating the affected region, and upon the mental state of the patient, who is usually distressed and agitated by the pain to an abnormal degree. Walters (1961) preferred the title 'psychogenic regional pain' to 'hysterical pain'. Among common syndromes of psychogenic pain, discussed elsewhere in this volume, are atypical facial neuralgia, chest pain in the effort syndrome, low back pain as a consequence of anxiety and depression, proctalgia fugax (attacks of anal pain often wakening the patient from sleep) and many more varieties. Methods of management of psychogenic pain are discussed in Bonica (1974).

Ocular Symptoms

Hysterical blindness may be unilateral or bilateral and may be complete or consist merely of a reduction of visual acuity. Bilateral blindness may be a perpetuation of the transitory visual impairment associated with syncope or with head injury. Unilateral blindness may be associated with hysterical hemianaesthesia on the same side. In hysterical blindness the optic discs and the pupillary reactions to light are normal, and it may be possible to evoke blinking by a sudden feint with the hand towards the eyes. Moreover, the blind hysteric may avoid obstacles in his path, but so, too, may the patient with visual agnosia due to organic brain disease. There are a number of tests for the detection of unilateral hysterical blindness. Diplopia may be produced by covering one eye with an appropriate prism, or one eye may be covered with a red, and the other with a green glass, the patient being then asked to read a word-test of alternate red and green letters. Since one colour is invisible to each eye, if all the letters are read the patient must be using both eyes. Visual field defects are common in hysteria and are usually the result of suggestion at the time of examination. The commonest type is a concentric defect of the field which takes the form of a spiral with the field progressively diminishing with each circuit of the test object but 'tubular vision' may also occur.

Disturbances of the ocular movements include spasm of convergence, which is almost always hysterical, and may be associated with spasm of accommodation. Defects and dissociation of conjugate ocular movements in the lateral and vertical planes may be produced by spasm of the ocular muscles, and a coarse nystagmus may occur. Hysterical ptosis is the result of spasm of the palpebral fibres of the orbicularis oculi, and when the lid is passively raised this spasm can be felt to increase. Blepharospasm is similarly produced.

Symptoms referred to the Alimentary Canal

Hysterical dysphagia may occur, but is rare. Air-swallowing is common and is usually begun by straining to bring up wind. It may lead to extreme gastric distension. Globus hystericus, described as a sensation of constriction or a lump in the throat, is sometimes but not always the result of air-swallowing and is a referred sensation produced by the presence of air in the lower part of the oesophagus. It must be distinguished from the similar sensation which can occur in some patients with hiatus hernia.

Hysterical vomiting when mild may lead to no loss of weight, when severe may cause marked acidosis and emaciation. Cyclical vomiting in childhood is often psychogenic. It is usually symbolic of an intense aversion from some task or situation, of which the patient is literally, as well as metaphorically, sick.

Hysterical anorexia—'anorexia nervosa'—may arise as a primary hysterical reaction to the patient's difficulties, or may be secondary to other hysterical symptoms referred to the alimentary canal, and which the patient believes are exacerbated by taking food. It occurs in adolescent girls and young women, and may lead to extreme emaciation, and to amenorrhoea. It may follow a period of dieting in order to lose weight, leading to an aversion to food, and the affected girls may go to remarkable lengths to avoid eating and often find many methods of disposing of the food they are given. Hirsutism is common and the tendon reflexes may be prolonged (Fowler et al., 1972). The many endocrine and metabolic abnormalities observed in such cases are secondary to caloric deficit and carbohydrate deprivation (Kanis et al., 1974).

Hysterical diarrhoea and constipation may occur, and it is probable that many of the abdominal and pelvic symptoms which used to be attributed to visceroptosis are in part or entirely hysterical.

Cardiac Symptoms

Tachycardia and palpitation play a prominent part in the symptoms of neurotic anxiety. In hysteria, however, such symptoms may occur in a patient who is outwardly placid. The recognition of their nature is of great importance, lest sufferers from these symptoms should be restricted in their activity for long periods with a mistaken diagnosis of organic heart disease or thyrotoxicosis.

Respiratory Symptoms

Respiratory tics have already been described. Hysterical hyperpnoea is sometimes seen and usually follows a fright. It also occurs in some panic attacks of the phobic anxiety-depersonalization syndrome. The excessive ventilation of the lungs may lead to tetany and even to syncope. The hysterical nature of the symptom can usually be detected by the fact that the hyperpnoea disappears or is much diminished when the patient is engaged in conversation, whereas talking increases the dyspnoea due to organic disease.

Urinary Symptoms

Nocturnal enuresis in childhood is the perpetuation of, or a reversion to, the infantile lack of control over the bladder. Its motive is frequently a desire to attract attention, and the symptom tends to be maintained by punishment and by suggestions emanating from a household in which the lapse comes to be expected. Pathological polyuria and organic causes of enuresis, especially spina bifida occulta, must be excluded, but psychogenic polydypsia (compulsive water-drinking) may be a contributory factor. Hysterical retention of urine occasionally occurs in young girls.

The Skin

'Dermatitis artefacta' is the term applied to cutaneous lesions voluntarily produced by a hysterical patient, either by scratching or rubbing, or by the use of external agents, including corrosives. These are usually easily recognized by their appearance and by the fact that they quickly heal when covered by an occlusive dressing. Pruritus is frequently a hysterical symptom. Cyanosis and oedema may occur in a limb which is the site of hysterical paralysis and has been described as a result of the purposive use of tight elastic bands applied to the limb by the hysterical patient.

The Spine

The spine may be the site of hysterical pain and tenderness, and occasionally remarkable deformities occur in hysteria, sometimes leading to a grossly flexed posture or an apparent shortening of several inches in the vertebral column.

Pyrexia

Probably in most cases of apparent pyrexia occurring in hysteria, the thermometer is manipulated by the patient. This source of error can readily be detected by adequate supervision when the temperature is taken. In certain cases, however, it appears that an actual rise of body temperature may occur as a hysterical symptom.

The 'von Munchausen Syndrome'

The 'desire to be ill' is classified by some authorities as a condition which shows some affinities with hysteria though it would appear that many of the affected individuals have psychopathic personalities. Not only may the patients feign illness by manipulation of clinical thermometers but some may actually produce illness in themselves by injecting themselves with insulin or with their own bath water. *E. coli* arthritis is invariably due to this cause. This type of phenomenon is almost always seen in nurses or doctors.

The 'von Munchausen syndrome' is a name given to a group of patients who move from hospital to hospital, cleverly feigning physical illness, including cardiac infarction, renal colic, perforated peptic ulcer or even cerebral vascular accidents. While some such individuals are addicted to morphine or pethidine and simply seek injections of the appropriate drugs and others seek nothing more than a bed for the night, others undertake these activities for complex psychological reasons related to the 'desire to be ill' (Mayer-Gross *et al.*, 1960).

Speech

Hysterical speech disturbances—mutism and aphonia—are described elsewhere [p. 102].

DIAGNOSIS

The diagnosis of individual hysterical symptoms has already been considered. In general it may be said that the diagnosis of hysteria depends upon the presence of positive signs of hysteria already described in connection with individual symptoms, and the absence of signs of organic disease. It is also essential, when possible, to identify a motive. It is essential in every case, therefore, that a thorough examination should be made both of the nervous system and of other systems to which symptoms may be referred. The organic nervous disease most likely to be confused with hysteria is multiple sclerosis, on account of the transitory occurrence in the early stages of this disorder of weakness and sensory disturbances. Careful examination of a patient with multiple sclerosis, however, will almost always reveal signs of organic disease of the nervous system, the commonest of which are pallor of the optic discs, nystagmus, diminution or absence of the abdominal reflexes, and extensor plantar responses. The possibility that overt hysterical manifestations may be superimposed upon the subclinical features of an underlying organic disease such as intracranial neoplasia or dementia or a psychotic depression must also be considered. Undoubtedly some such symptoms are in a sense iatrogenic in that symptoms may be exaggerated or distorted by emotional factors in patients who find themselves unable to persuade a doctor that they are genuinely ill.

The distinction between hysteria (subconscious motivation) and malingering (conscious motivation) may be a matter of considerable difficulty in individuals who are seeking compensation after injury or in others accused of criminal offences (who may feign amnesia) as the clinical manifestations of the two conditions are similar. Unfortunately we possess no definitive objective tests by means of which this distinction can be made (Miller, 1966).

PROGNOSIS

The prognosis as to recovery from an individual symptom of hysteria is good in most cases, though relapses are frequent unless the patient can be induced to carry out a considerable psychological readjustment or unless the causal stress can be abolished or modified substantially. Chronic cases are common in which a single symptom persists for years, often because it is the patient's reaction to

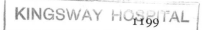

a domestic situation which also persists unchanged. Victims of chronic hysteria are often persons in whom the expectation of compensation for an injury or the receipt of a pension puts a premium upon the persistence of their disability.

TREATMENT

General Considerations

When a hysterical symptom is a neurotic solution of a mental conflict, symptomatic treatment alone is inadequate. It is essential that the cause of the conflict should be discovered and that the patient should be induced to deal with it in a manner which does not involve resort to a neurosis. Analytical psychological methods, however, are often rendered difficult by lack of intelligence or by resistance in the patient, and in severely dissociated individuals with amnesia, hypnosis or narco-analysis may be necessary to recover forgotten episodes. When the cause of the symptom has been discovered and dealt with, treatment may also be directed towards the relief of the symptom itself. A careful physical examination must be made in order that the patient may be assured that no organic cause for the disability exists. The patient must be convinced that he can overcome the disability, but care should be taken to avoid the suggestion that this requires a great effort of will, since this attitude implies that the achievement is difficult. In some cases recovery is best effected by a gradual process of persuasion and re-education extending over a considerable time. Some, however, prefer to attempt to remove the symptom at one sitting. This method requires great tact and patience on the part of the physician and is not without risk, since the failure of a protracted attempt to cure will only reinforce the patient's belief in the intractable nature of his disorder. The removal of a symptom by hypnotic suggestion is usually undesirable in adult patients, since it tends to strengthen the abnormal suggestibility which is an undesirable characteristic of the hysteric. This method, however, is admissible in dealing with children, in whose education suggestion plays a legitimate part.

The management of hysteria, especially if symptoms are intractable or recurrent, is often extremely difficult and some cases are in effect incurable. Psychotropic drugs play a useful part in some cases especially in dealing with associated symptoms of anxiety and/or depression. While the measures mentioned here and below are often effective in promoting the resolution of some hysterical phenomena, long-term psychiatric support and supervision is often needed in the more intractable cases.

Treatment of Individual Symptoms

Hysterical 'Fits'. A hysterical attack can usually be quickly terminated by firm handling, especially if the patient is isolated from a sympathetic audience.

Paralysis and Rigidity. These symptoms are commonly associated, and, since they depend in part upon involuntary muscular contraction, this should be explained to the patient, who should first be directed to relax the muscles of the affected region and should be told that when the muscles are relaxed movement will be easy. Electrical stimulation may be employed to demonstrate that the muscles are still capable of contraction, the patient then being made to imitate the movements excited electrically.

Hysterical gait. This is a symptom which sometimes lends itself to cure at a single treatment. The patient is first encouraged to walk with adequate support, the doctor or physiotherapist walking on one side. The support is gradually diminished until the patient can be told that he is now walking alone, and finally he should be induced to run.

Enuresis. Before regarding enuresis in childhood as a neurosis it is necessary to exclude irritative lesions of the urinary tract, polyuria, and organic lesions which impair sphincter control, especially spinal dysraphic syndromes associated with spina bifida occulta. An attempt should be made to ascertain the cause of the symptom, which may be the symbol of a wish to remain infantile or of a desire to attract attention. Both the parents and the patient should be encouraged to expect a cure, and neither blame nor punishment for lapses should be permitted. Propantheline or ephedrine in full doses given before retiring may be used to depress reflex evacuation of the bladder until the habit of continence is established. Alternatively, drugs such as imipramine given to lighten sleep are also helpful in some cases. Hypnotic suggestion or various deconditioning techniques will often bring about a cure in hitherto intractable cases (Kolvin *et al.*, 1973).

Vomiting. The psychological cause of the vomiting must first be ascertained and discussed with the patient, who must be reassured that no organic cause for it exists. Special diets, alkalies, and other drugs may often have been employed in treatment. These should be withdrawn. An ordinary light meal should then be obtained and the patient persuaded to consume it with the assurance that no vomiting will follow. An attempt can often be made to cure hysterical vomiting at one sitting, a cure once effected usually being permanent.

Anorexia Nervosa. The patient should be isolated from relatives and friends and the cause of the anorexia ascertained. It is often necessary to explain that the symptoms which the patient attributes to taking food are really the result of taking too little. A beginning should be made with frequent small feeds, and no effort should be spared to make the diet attractive. In severe cases admission to hospital is usually required. Chlorpromazine in increasing doses has been found to be helpful in some cases but for details the reader is referred to textbooks of psychiatry.

OCCUPATIONAL NEUROSIS

Synonyms. Craft palsy; occupational cramp.

Definition. A functional nervous disorder prone to afflict those whose occupation entails the persistent use of finely co-ordinated movements, especially of the hand, and characterized by a progressive occupational disability, due to spasm of the muscles employed, which are often the site of pain and sometimes of tremor.

AETIOLOGY

Occupational neurosis was once attributed to fatigue of cortical ganglion cells or to a disorder of the basal ganglia. It now seems evident, however, that it is primarily psychogenic. We know of no organic disorder in which the movements are impaired when they take part in one co-ordinated act but remain unaffected in others. The muscular spasm evoked by an attempt to carry out the act involves both prime movers and their antagonists, and thus resembles the disorder of function which occurs in hysterical paralysis. The disability in occupational neurosis may be influenced by external factors in a manner which would be inexplicable if it were due to an organic disorder. For example, a lawyer who suffered from severe writers' cramp was almost totally unable to write when sitting, but could write quite well when standing. Occupational neurosis, moreover, may be associated with typical hysterical symptoms, and investigation may elicit an adequate psychological cause. Thus a woman who developed writers' cramp after an unhappy marriage suffered also from vaginismus. Finally, in some cases, occupational neurosis is curable by psychotherapy. It thus presents many points of resemblance to stammering, another functional disorder of finely co-ordinated movements; indeed, occupational neurosis may be described as a manual stammer. It must be admitted, however, that sufferers from occupational neurosis may possess a physiological predisposition which determines the character of their neurosis, as, for example, left-handedness appears sometimes to predispose to stammering.

Fatigue and the effort to carry out accurate work against time are important precipitating factors, and since in most cases the sufferer's livelihood depends upon his speed and accuracy, an impairment of his efficiency evokes anxiety, which probably plays a part in the psychogenesis of the disorder. Numerous occupational neuroses have been described, writers', telegraphists', goldbeaters', violinists', and piano-players' cramps being the most familiar, but there is probably no occupation involving the repetition of fine movements which is immune. Both sexes are affected, but males more often than females.

SYMPTOMS

The symptoms of writers' cramp will alone be described, since the disorder is essentially the same in other occupations. The onset of symptoms is gradual, and the disorder shows itself at first only when the patient is fatigued, when a difficulty in controlling the pen leads to inaccurate writing. When the condition is well developed the attempt to write evokes a spasm of the muscles concerned in holding and moving the pen, and this may spread to the whole of the upper limb. The whole limb may thus become rigid, so that the act is brought to an abrupt stop. More usually the attempt to write leads to jerky and inco-ordinate movements of the fingers, so that the writing is completely illegible. The pen may be driven into the paper. In some cases a tremor of the hand develops. No two patients present precisely the same disorder of function. An attempt is often made to circumvent the disability by various tricks and unusual methods of holding the pen. Extension of the muscular spasm beyond the upper limb is rare. Sensory symptoms are common and are the result of the muscular spasm, the patient complaining of a sense of fatigue or an aching pain in the muscles, not only of the upper limb but sometimes also of the neck. Muscular wasting, sensory loss, and reflex changes are absent. In the early stages the disability is limited to the single act in which it originates. Later it may extend to other acts which are carried out by the same hand. Thus the woman already mentioned, after developing writers' cramp, learned to use a typewriter. Her disability then extended to typing and finally to the use of a paint-brush in water-colour sketching. The sufferer from writers' cramp who learns to write with the left hand may develop the same disorder in this.

Q q

DIAGNOSIS

Occupational neurosis must be distinguished from organic disorders of the nervous system which may lead to a difficulty in carrying out fine movements. A careful history and physical examination usually render the diagnosis easy, since in such cases signs of organic disease are always present and the disability usually involves all finely co-ordinated acts, and not writing alone, to an equal extent from the beginning.

PROGNOSIS

The prognosis of occupational neurosis is usually poor, since in many cases the disability is progressive, though recovery rarely occurs and some patients may be able to continue their occupation in spite of their disorder. Some find a change of occupation to one not involving writing beneficial, but this is rarely possible.

TREATMENT

Prolonged rest from the occupation is sometimes helpful but rarely practicable. The way in which muscular spasm interferes with the act should be explained to the patient, and he should be taught muscular relaxation under skilled supervision. This should later be combined with re-educational exercises for the affected limb, and return to work should be gradual, fatigue being avoided. Learning to write with the other hand, or using a typewriter may be helpful, but not infrequently the second hand, and even the movements involved in typewriting, may later be affected. Liversedge and Sylvester (1955) have devised a method of 'deconditioning' the patient. Some patients obtain benefit from the use of drugs such as chlordiazepoxide (*Librium*), 10 mg three or four times a day, or diazepam (*Valium*), 2–5 mg three or four times daily, but while these may partially relieve muscular spasms they are in no sense curative.

REFERENCES

BONICA, J. J. (Ed.) (1974) *Pain*, vol. 4 in Advances in Neurology, New York.

CARTER, A. B. (1972) A physician's view of hysteria, *Lancet*, **ii,** 1241.

EYSENCK, H. J. (1960) *Handbook of Abnormal Psychology*, London.

FOWLER, P. B. S., BANIM, S. O., and IKRAM, H. (1972) Prolonged ankle reflex in anorexia nervosa, *Lancet*, **ii,** 307.

KANIS, J. A., BROWN, P., FITZPATRICK, K., HIBBERT, D. J., HORN, D. B., NAIRN, I. M., SHIRLING, D., STRONG, J. A., and WALTON, H. J. (1974) Anorexia nervosa: a clinical, psychiatric, and laboratory study, *Quart. J. Med.*, **43,** 321.

KOLVIN, I., MACKEITH, R. C., and MEADOW, S. R. (Eds.) (1973) *Bladder Control and Enuresis*, Clinics in Developmental Medicine, Nos. 48/49, London.

KRETSCHMER, E. (1952) *A Textbook of Medical Psychology*, trans. STRAUSS, E. B., 2nd ed., London.

LIVERSEDGE, L. R., and SYLVESTER, J. D. (1955) Conditioning techniques in the treatment of writer's cramp, *Lancet*, **i,** 1147.

MAYER-GROSS, W., SLATER, E., and ROTH, M. (1960) *Clinical Psychiatry*, 2nd ed., London.

MILLER, H. (1966) Mental sequelae of head injury, *Proc. roy. Soc. Med.*, **59,** 257.

SIM, M. (1975) *Guide to Psychiatry*, 3rd ed., Edinburgh.

SLATER, E. (1965) Diagnosis of 'hysteria', *Brit. med. J.*, **1,** 1395.

WALTERS, A. (1961) Psychogenic regional pain alias hysterical pain, *Brain*, **84,** 1.

INDEX

A-alpha and beta-lipoproteinaemia, polyneuritis in, 941, 942
A-band, 989
abdominal
  pain in porphyria, 827
  reflexes, 55
abducens nerve palsy, 167
a-beta-lipoproteinaemia, 655
abortion, selective, in carriers of Duchenne dystrophy, 996
abreaction in torticollis, 610
abscess
  cerebellar, 431, 434–5
  cerebral, 431–7
    as a cause of coma, 1160
    EEG in, 147
    EMI scan in, 435
    papilloedema in, 158
  extradural, 407, 431, 434
  haematogenous, 431
  intracranial, 431–7
    aetiology, 432–3
    and meningitis, 412
    diagnosis, 435–6
      from tumour, 285
    due to typhoid, 442
    focal signs, 434–5
    investigation, 435
    pathology, 431
    prognosis, 436–7
    symptoms, 433–5
    treatment, 437
  intramedullary spinal, 738, 779
  otogenic, 431
  spinal extradural, 738
    surgery in, 758
  spinal subdural, 738
  subdural, 407, 431, 434
Abstem, 794
acalculia, 107, 119
acanthocytosis, 655, 863
accessory nerve, 214–16
  lesions of, 215
accommodation
  of nerve in tetany, 1140
  paralysis of, 91
    in botulism, 822
    in diphtheria, 976
  reflex, 92
acetazolamide
  in epilepsy, 1123
  in familial periodic paralysis, 1035, 1036
acetylcholine, 1068
  and botulinum toxin, 822
  and epilepsy, 1094–5
  at the myoneural junction, 988
  receptor, and myasthenia, 1023
achlorhydria in B$_{12}$ neuropathy, 858
achondroplasia
  and cord compression, 738, 1091
  surgery in, 757
acid maltase
  deficiency, 1033–4

in treatment of Pompe's disease, 1034
acidosis, metabolic, in subarachnoid haemorrhage, 360
acoustic neuroma
  and facial nerve, 181
  and neurofibromatosis, 666
  caloric tests in, 193
  deafness in, 193
  diagnosis, 289
  pathology, 241
  skull radiography in, 256
  symptomatology, 281
  vertigo in, 199
acousticomotor epilepsy, 1106
acrocephalosyndactyly, 1087
acrodermatitis chronica atrophicans, 984
acrodynia, 974–5
acrodystrophic neuropathy, 767
acromegaly, 246, 276, 837
  carpal tunnel syndrome in, 905
  muscular weakness in, 1032
  myopathy in, 1032
acroparaesthesiae, 898
acrosclerosis, 1014
acrylamide polyneuropathy, 961
ACTH
  in delirium tremens, 794
  in facial palsy, 184
  in infantile spasms, 1107
  in multiple sclerosis, 558
  in myasthenia, 1024
  in myelitis, 781
  in optic neuritis, 165
  in petit mal status, 1124
  in polymyositis, 1015
  in post-infective polyneuritis, 952
  myopathy, 1033
  secretion, by carcinomas, 873
actin, 989
action myoclonus, 1133, 1135
action potentials
  evoked, of muscle, in myasthenia, 1053
  motor unit, 988
    in myopathy, 1052
    in the EMG, 882–6
  of muscle, 12
  of nerve, 12
action tremor, 573, 585
acuity, visual, 65, 155
acute
  haemorrhagic conjunctivitis, 517
  haemorrhagic leucoencephalitis, 527, 541–2
  multiple sclerosis, 554
adamantinoma, 245
addiction
  to drugs, 796–804
    tremor in, 590
  to synthetic analgesics, 796–8
Addisonian crisis, coma in, 1165
Addison's disease, 837
  coma in, 1165
  myopathy in, 1032
Addison–Schilder's disease, 567

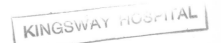